INHERITED EYE DISEASES

INHERITED EYE DISEASES

Diagnosis and Management

SECOND EDITION

Saul Merin
Hadassah-Hebrew University Medical Center
Jerusalem, Israel

The University of Illinois College of Medicine at Chicago
Chicago, Illinois, U.S.A.

With contributions by
Joel Zlotogora and Dror Sharon

Taylor & Francis
Taylor & Francis Group

Boca Raton London New York Singapore

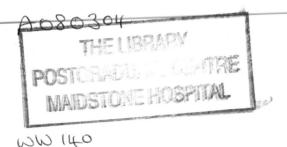

Published in 2005 by
Taylor & Francis Group
6000 Broken Sound Parkway NW, Suite 300
Boca Raton, FL 33487-2742

Printed in the United States of America on acid-free paper
10 9 8 7 6 5 4 3 2 1

International Standard Book Number-10: 1-57444-839-0 (Hardcover)
International Standard Book Number-13: 978-1-57444-839-9 (Hardcover)

Library of Congress Cataloging-in-Publication Data

Catalog record is available from the Library of Congress

T&F informa
Taylor & Francis Group
is the Academic Division of T&F Informa plc.

Visit the Taylor & Francis Web site at
http://www.taylorandfrancis.com

To three remarkable women:

Aniela Zawacka-Szwajcer,
who saved two small children from the Holocaust

Sara Feld-Splewinski,
who turned on the light in darkness

Rachela Siton-Merin,
who made it all worthwhile

Preface to Second Edition

Since the publication of the first edition of this book, genetics has remained in the forefront of human medical research. The Human Genome Project is, in fact, almost complete, with the entire human DNA sequence documented. A large number of human disease-bearing genes, were located, identified and even cloned. Many genes with thousands of mutations are now recognized. The old and accepted view that one gene causes one disease is no longer valid. The advent of molecular genetics has revolutionized all clinical subjects related to genetics including, of course, clinical ophthalmology, a discipline heavily dependent on genetics. Many human diseases have been found to be polygenic (caused by more than one gene), while in other cases, one gene may be responsible for several, sometimes very different, diseases. These were surprising and unexpected findings. As a result, we can not use the name of the gene in place of the name of the disease. They are, rather, supplementary terms. The name of a disease, which represents the clinical findings of this particular disease (or "phenotype"), will remain the nomenclature for the clinician. The name and chromosomal location of the disease-causative gene, as well as the involved mutation or mutations, will all become part of the accepted clinical terminology.

This book will continue to be based on tissues and diseases as in the first edition. However, it will be enormously expanded to include all the new developments in this field of genetics and ophthalmology. New chapters have been added, such as my introductory chapter on the changing face of genetics in ophthalmology, a chapter on molecular genetics written by Dror Sharon, a chapter on thrombophilia and genetically triggered retinal vascular diseases, and others. In addition, multiple new sub-chapters have been added to the first edition. Some are devoted to important genes, recently identified, and others to new diseases and their management. The rapid expansion of genetics research makes it extremely difficult to currently record all genes and mutations in a single book. I have decided to keep the book as a practical handbook for the clinician. It may be possible to find some of the rare genes and mutations online at the *National Center for Biotechnology Information's OMIM-Online Mendelian Inheritance in Man* website (http://www.ncbi.nlm.nih.gov/Omim/) and other related sites.

In the preparation of this second edition, I was assisted by several people. I would like to acknowledge the help of Jose Pulido, MD and Margaret Chervinko from the University of Illinois at Chicago College of Medicine; Dana Bigelow from Taylor & Francis in New York; Sandra Beberman and her colleagues from Taylor & Francis, the publisher of this edition; Sara Katineri, and Israel Barzel from Hadassah University Medical Center in Jerusalem. Financial support was given by a grant from the University of Illinois Nelson Sisters Fund.

Saul Merin

Foreword to First Edition

The ability to visualize and photographically document genetically determined cellular abnormalities has made the study of inherited human eye disease both fascinating and feasible. Indeed, genetic disorders of ocular tissues have intrigued physicians for hundreds of years. Garrod, for one, utilized ophthalmic observations in generating his pivotal ideas about inborn errors of metabolism. Other authors around the world have periodically summarized knowledge about many types of inherited eye disease, sometimes in huge compendia. Professor Merin's splendid and interesting book is now at the vanguard of this historical continuum of clinical and scientifiic ideas and observations.

This book has several appealing characteristics. It is almost completely written by one person. That person, Saul Merin, is more than a compiler or sifter of information. He is internationally admired for his personal and active contributions to the field of ophthalmic genetics. Moreover, he is not afraid to take a stand. The contents of this book are sprinkled with a therapeutic dose of personal pronouns; for example, "I believe that..." or "In my opinion..." Thus, this book differs from many literary efforts in the modern medical world, in which the author's identity, ideas, and opinions are deftly deleted by editors hoping to effect a certain impersonal style.

Moreover, unlike many edited works, this book has a uniform style and a standardized format for each chapter; both promote easy reading. Clinical and historical descriptions are followed by diagnostic procedures, histopathologic data, pathogenetic ideas, epidermiologic and genetic concepts, and, where applicable, principles and techniques of clinical management.

Finally, Professor Merin's book is current and comprehensive. The explosively expanding recent literature is nicely summarized and integrated with the author's personal clinical experience.

The appeal of this book to a great variety of readers and the present exponential growth of genetic knowledge virtually assure the book's success, but also places an added burden on Dr. Merin, who will almost certainly feel compelled to issue a second edition in only a few year's time.

Morton F. Goldberg, M.D.
The Wilmer Ophthalmologic Institute
Baltimore, Maryland

Preface to First Edition

The writing of *Inherited Eye Diseases* was inspired by my residents. Many years of teaching this subject to them resulted in an accumulation of lectures, which were finally turned into chapters of this book.

The purpose of this book is to provide a standard textbook of inherited eye diseases. I hope that it will provide the practicing general ophthalmologist and the resident-in-training with a text to consult when dealing with an inherited eye disease. My intent is to enable the reader to find the most likely diagnosis w[illegible] the context of the various types and subtypes of genetic diseases to obtain an in-depth understanding of the specific disease, the various available tests, and the management of patients with inherited eye diseases. Many of the genetic eye diseases are untreatable by medical means and inoperable by surgical methods, but in every case the patient is amenable to management. In some cases, this may mean visual rehabilitation with any of the many low-vision aids; in others, genetic counseling alone is necessary; in still others, prophylactic measures to prevent deterioration and future complications should be advised. All these measures are part of the standard medical practice. The recent increase in the number of legal suits against physicians for improper genetic counseling proves that the general public views genetic counseling as an indispensable and integral part of the medical management of inherited diseases.

The first chapters of this book were written about five years ago but have been updated. During this period, I witnessed an enormous expansion in the knowldege of inherited eye diseases. New techniques of molecular genetics enabled a totally new approach to genetic disease in general and to ocular disease in particular. These basic scientific methods turned into laboratory science and are in the process of incorporation into clinical practice. The process of a better understanding of genetic diseases becomes the process of better clinical management. The use of molecular probes turns into reality, the dream of every geneticist: to have a complete map of all human genetic diseases. I have little doubt that such a complete map will be available in the not too distant future. This will open new pathways for accurate diagnosis, prenatal determination of a genetic disease and accurate genetic counseling, and, most probably, for new methods of treatments directed at the cellular level.

In preparing this book, I found that the subject is much larger than I expected, for two reasons. First, genetic knowledge has expanded in new directions, molecular genetics being just one example. Second, the sheer number of genetic eye diseases is enormous. About 1% of all newborns suffer from a unifactorial genetic disease (7% autosomal dominant, 2.5% autosomal recessive, and 0.5% X-linked) (1). In about a quarter of all inherited diseases the eye is affected (2).

Genetic diseases in which the eye is involved in a minor way are not included in this book. Metabolic diseases, multisystem and systemic diseases, chromosomal anomalies, muscular dystrophics, and skin diseases are not discussed unless the ocular involvement is the principal or important part of the syndrome. Sometimes such diseases are mentioned for the sake of comparison and differential diagnosis.

The chapters in this book, with one exception, evolved from lectures given by one person. This means that the presentation is heavily dependent on the personal views of the author. It is possible that some experts may have different views on a certain point. I hope that such experts will excuse me for emphasizing my personal views and be compensated by the ability to compare different views.

Several people helped me by giving advice or supplying photographs. I would like to pay special acknowledgment to Norman Blair, MD, Marilyn Farber, PhD, Gerald Fishman, MD, Morton F. Goldberg, MD, David R. Pepperberg, PhD, John Read, MS, Robert Spector, MD, Joel Sugar, MD, Ramesh Tripathi, MD, Mark Tso, MD, Charles Vygantus, MD, Virgina Weiss, MD, and Fulton Wong, PhD, all from Chicago; and, for providing the necessary illustration, photographers Norbert Jednock from Chicago and Aric Zelichovsky, Ruth Wesis, and Israel Barzel from Jerusalem. Editorial assistance was provided by Maxine Gere for most of the chapters and by Kathleen Louden for the rest. Secretarial help was efficiently provided by Hilda Ortiz. I acknowledge with special affection the invaluable help in literature research provided by librarian Mary Winnike. The preparation of this book was supported (in part) by the Samuel and Abraham Goldstein Foundation and the Jeanne and Albert Micsri Fund.

REFERENCES

1. Emery AEH, Rimoin D: Nature and incidence of genetic disease. In Emery AEH, and Rimoin DL (ed): Principles and Practice of Medical Genetics. Churchill-Livingstone, Edinburgh, 1983:1–3.
2. Goldberg MF: An introduction to basic genetic principles applied to ophthalmology. Trans Am Acad Ophthalmol Otolaryngol 1972; 76:1137–1159.

Saul Merin

Contents

1

Introduction: The Changing Place of Genetics in Clinical Ophthalmology

For more than a hundred years since the first experiments of Gregor Mendel, whose work is considered to be the foundation of modern genetics, very little changed. Then an exponential increase in knowledge occurred. In 1970, the first report of the linkage of a human disease to a chromosome was published (1). The discovery related to ophthalmology and described the linkage of congenital cataract to the Duffy blood group on chromosome 1. The location of the gene was later identified as position 22–23 on the long arm of chromosome 1 (1q22–1q23) (2,3). The gene was cloned in 1945 and in 1998 a mutation was identified on the gene for gap-junction protein alpha-8 (GJA8) (3). This gene encodes a connexin protein, which is about 50 kDa (kilodalton) in size, and primarily and abundantly expressed in the crystalline lens (3). The mutation identified was the substitution of serine for proline at codon 88 (Pro88Ser).

In the last 30 years the chromosomal location of most ocular diseases has become known. For many ocular diseases the disease-bearing gene has been identified, its structure and its encoded protein described. In some cases, the function of the gene, in relation to the disease caused by it, has also been discovered. However, many unexpected problems have arisen. These will be discussed in greater detail.

MOLECULAR GENETICS

The development of polymerase chain reaction (PCR) in 1985 revolutionized DNA analysis. In vitro enzymatic amplification of a specific DNA segment, allowing for the synthesis of millions of copies of that segment, was now possible (4). Genes were localized and identified by one of three approaches (5–7). *Positional cloning* involved genetic linkage studies in families bearing a specific disease. *Candidate gene approach* involved the search for the function of the protein, the amino acid sequence, or underlying biochemical defect. In the *positional candidate approach*, after the locus was identified, attractive candidate genes were identified and surveyed (see Chapter 3).

THE HUMAN GENOME PROJECT

The sequence and organization of the human mitochondrial genome (HGM) was established in 1981 (8). The fully sequenced mitochondrial DNA (mtDNA) was found to be circular in form, containing 16,569 base pairs (8). The origin of mtDNA is almost exclusively maternal. The ocular effect of disease-bearing mutations will be discussed in various chapters of this book.

The sequencing of nuclear DNA was much more complicated. Human chromosomal DNA contains 3 billion base pairs. The enormous task of sequencing began in the 1990s, with the view of completing it by 2005 (9,10). By the year 2000, 97% of the human genome was mapped and 85% of the DNA was sequenced (11). The map of the human genome was almost complete (more than 99.9%) by 2001, using two different modes of approach (12–14). The number of genes defined as "distinct transcription units" (transcribed to produce mRNA and protein coding) was estimated as 52,000–64,000 (15). Previous estimates ranged from 20,000 to 300,000 (15). By 1996, more than 16,000 human genes had been mapped (16) and by 2000, 38,000 genes were identified (11). The published maps of DNA sequences indicate that any two individuals may differ by only 1 base for every 1000 bases. An average gene contains 12 variations that are common within the population studied and usually not disease-bearing (17).

The HGP accelerated the discovery of human disease-bearing genes (18) and changed our classical understanding of the genotype–phenotype relationship. Gene expression profile analysis allowed automatic, reliable screening of genes (19).

GENES, GENOTYPES AND PHENOTYPES

For most inherited human diseases, the causative gene and the disease-bearing mutations were identified. The number of different mutations of one gene varies greatly, from just one or two to, literally, hundreds of mutations. In autosomal recessive diseases the two abnormal alleles may be the same (homozygote) or different (compound heterozygote). Different mutations, responsible for the same disease, may produce phenotypes of differing severity and thus be of prognostic value. Retinitis pigmentosa due to rhodopsin gene mutations may be more or less severe according to the involved autosomal dominant mutation.

An unexpected result of the extensive studies on genotype–phenotype relationship was the discovery that one disease may be the result of mutations in a variety of genes and, conversely, different mutations in a single gene may cause a variety of diseases (phenotypes) (20). Different mutations of the peripherin/*RDS* gene may, for example, cause autosomal dominant retinitis pigmentosa (adRP), retinitis punctata albescens, butterfly pattern macular dystrophy, adult-onset vitelliform macular dystrophy, and others. In fact, the same mutation, consisting of a three-base deletion at codon 153 of the peripherin/*RDS* gene, has been shown to cause different phenotypes in different members of one family (21). The expressed diseases were adRP, pattern dystrophy, and fundus flavimaculatus. This may imply the importance of other genes, in addition to the disease-bearing mutation, in controlling its effect. Furthermore, the 60 known additional mutations of the peripherin/*RDS* gene may also cause different phenotypes, including isolated macular diseases and diffuse cone-rod dystrophy and adRP (22).

More mutations are found in males when compared to females. This may result from the higher rate of cell divisions during spermatogenesis (23).

A high proportion of mutations are not disease-causative variants and are termed polymorphisms. Their frequent occurrence complicates the research of disease-bearing genes. Not every amino acid sequence change is a cause of a disease and therefore any association studies must have a genetically matched control population for comparison (24).

OCULAR GENE THERAPY

Recent developments in ocular genetics enable us to help the patient with an ocular genetic disease in several ways. In some cases, such as in families with open angle glaucoma, an individual can be diagnosed as carrying the disease-causative mutation, before it becomes symptomatic, while in others, a better understanding of the pathogenetic mechanism may enable treatment by biochemical or other means to change the outcome. Gene-based therapies can be divided into two general groups (18): those that supply the missing or defective gene or other protein particle, and those that remove or replace the defective gene. Abetalipopreteinemia belongs to the first group. The supply of vitamins A and E at an early age prevents later retinal damage. Replacement of the gene or its product includes direct RNA antisense therapy, ribozyme therapy, and transfection with a modified gene (18). Genes can be introduced in order to replace the mutant gene by viral or nonviral methods. Virus infection carries the recombinant DNA into many cells of the body including the target cell. The virus, usually an adeno-associated virus or a retrovirus, is modified so that it carries the genetic information but is unable to replicate or cause disease (25). Nonviral vectors involve the transfection of target cells with recombinant DNA by intracellular microinjection, liposome-mediated methodology, electropolation (electrical transfer of DNA across membrane), or cell surface receptor-mediated endocytosis (inward folding of the cell membrane to introduce a substance) (25).

Gene therapy for inherited eye disease is currently not available, but may be in the not-too-distant future. Its first application will very likely be in the treatment of recessive diseases, in which we have to supply the missing or defective gene (26). In animal research, recombinant replication-defective adenovirus was injected into the subretinal space of mice affected by an autosomal recessive retinal degeneration. The adenovirus caused the rescue of photoreceptors and delayed photoreceptor death by six weeks (27). Many such rescue studies have been performed and are discussed in the appropriate chapters. Gene therapy may be more difficult for dominant diseases in which the mutated gene is functional. Possible applications of gene therapy may include the suppression of the gene at the DNA/RNA level, the suppression of the protein product, or the elimination of the whole cell altogether (25). Viral-mediated gene transfer may be a powerful technique for treatment of various ocular nongenetic diseases as well. An adeno-associated modified virus carrying the appropriate gene and injected into the vitreous has been successfully used in the treatment of optic neuritis in guinea pigs (28,29). Proliferative vitreoretinopathy was successfully treated in rabbits by retroviral vector-mediated transfer of suicide genes (30). Photoreceptor death in retinal dystrophies is related to apoptosis, a programmed cell death that starts in embryonic life or very early in life. Rescue genes carrying factors that prevent apoptosis such as fibroblast growth factors may be effective against photoreceptor cell death (31). Old and dying ocular cells may extend their life by inserting a gene for the protein component of telomerase enzyme. Such a gene may re-extend the chromosomal telomeres to the lengths found in young cells (32).

GENETIC COUNSELING AND PRENATAL DIAGNOSIS

Genetic counseling, in its classical sense, continues to be an essential part of the management of genetic diseases. Parents have the right to make the decision to start a pregnancy or terminate it when a very serious disease is likely to occur. Prenatal diagnosis is a suitable companion to counseling for many diseases. An excellent review article on this subject was written by Bruno Brambati (33). The widespread use of amniocentesis began in the 1960s. It involved the withdrawal of amniotic fluid surrounding the fetus and the examination of its cells. It was good for diagnosing chromosomal abnormalities, biochemical abnormalities, and structural changes in the fetus. Fetoscopy, developed in the 1970s, enables us to visualize the fetus, obtain blood, perform skin biopsy and in some cases, facilitates intrauterine treatment. In the 1980s, real-time ultrasound became essential for routine amniocentesis. In 1983, chorionic villus sampling (CVS), guided by advanced ultrasound, enabled prenatal diagnosis as early as the first trimester. Utilizing CVS, a placental biopsy enables a wide range of tests to be performed. Single-gene defects may, in some cases, be diagnosed by recombinant DNA technology or PCR technique. All of these examinations carry the risk of about 1% of fetal loss and parents should be made aware of this risk.

In high-risk genetic diseases, pre-implantation genetic diagnosis (PGD) can be performed. In embryos created by in vitro fertilization, single cells are removed and analyzed using FISH or PCR techniques (see Chapter 3) (33,34). Single-gene defects can also be diagnosed. The risks of PGD can be reduced by removing and testing only the polar body instead of a whole cell (35). Prenatal diagnosis can also be used in the detection of mitochondrial genetic diseases (36). In spite of the risks involved, a survey of affected families indicates that most approve of prenatal diagnosis (37). They use the information obtained in one of three ways: to terminate the pregnancy, prepare for life with a visually disabled child, or receive reassurance when the results are negative (37).

ETHICS OF GENETIC EYE DISEASES

The great advances in the knowledge and management of genetic eye diseases has, unfortunately, not been paralleled by similar advances in solutions to the serious ethical problems involved in genetic testing. What should we do with the brother of our patient who tests positively for the mutation of Leber's hereditary optic neuropathy or open angle glaucoma but is asymptomatic? Should we tell him? Should we do the test at all? I have no doubt that such an individual can benefit from this knowledge. He may even reduce the risk of the symptomatic disease by changing behavior such as the cessation of smoking. On the other hand, he may suffer from the knowledge of his genetic pre-disposition. Genetic testing may be used as a tool by insurance companies to increase the cost of or deny a patients' medical coverage. Hopefully, future legislation will prevent insurance companies from requiring or using this method of pre-screening to the detriment of the insured. Presently, no guidelines are available on these difficult issues, (38,39).

REFERENCES

1. Renwick JH. Eyes on chromosomes. Med Genet 1970; 7:239–243.
2. Church RL, Wang JH, Steele E. The human lens intrinsic membrane protein MP70 (CX50) gene: clonal analysis and chromosome mapping. Curr Eye Res 1995; 14: 215–221.
3. Shiels A, Mackay D, Ionides A, et al. A missense mutation in the human connexin50 gene (GJA8) underlies autosomal dominant "zonular pulverulent" cataract, on chromosome 1q. Am J Hum Genet 1998; 62:526–532.
4. Albert DM. Molecular genetics, an increasingly important tool for ophthalmology. Arch Ophthalmol 1995; 113:565.
5. Della NG. The revolution in molecular genetics and its impact on ophthalmology. Austr NZ J Ophthalmol 1996; 24:85–95.
6. Della NG. Molecular biology in ophthalmology. A review of principles and recent advances. Arch Ophthalmol 1996; 114:457–463.
7. Damji KF, Allingham RR. Molecular genetics is revolutionizing our understanding of ophthalmic disease. Am J Ophthalmol 1997; 124:530–543.
8. Anderson S, Bankier AT, Barrell BG, et al. Sequence and organization of the human mitochondrial genome. Nature 1981; 290:457–465.
9. Weber JL. Know thy genome. Nat Genet 1994; 7:343–344.
10. Dib C, Favre S, Fizames C, et al. A comprehensive genetic map of the human genome based on 5,264 microsatellites. Nature 1996; 380:152–154.
11. Butcher J. "Working draft" of human genome completed. The Lancet 2000; 356:47.
12. The International Human Genome Mapping Consortium. A physical map of the human genome. Nature 2001; 409:934–941.
13. Venter JC, Adams MD, Myers EW, et al. The sequence of the human genome. Science 2001; 291:1304–1351.
14. Bentley DR, Deloukaj P, Dunham A, et al. The physical maps for sequencing human chromosomes 1, 6, 9, 10, 13, 20, and X. Nature 2001; 409:942–943.
15. Fields C, Adams MD, White O, Venter JL. How many genes in the human genome? Nat Genet 1994; 7:345–346.
16. Schuler GD, Boguski MS, Stewart EA, et al. A gene map of the human genome. Science 1996; 274:540–546.
17. Little P. The end of all human DNA maps? Nature Genetics 2001; 27:229–230.
18. Wiggs JL. The human genome project and eye disease: clinical implications. Arch Ophthalmol 2001; 119:1710–1711.
19. King HD Sinha AA. Gene expressions profile analysis by DNA microarrays. Promise and pitfalls. J Am Med Assoc 2001; 286:2280–2288.
20. Bird AC. Retinal photoreceptor dystrophies (51st Edward Jackson Memorial Lecture). Am J Ophthalmol 1995; 119:543–562.
21. Weleber RG, Carr RE, Murphey WH, et al. Phenotypic variation including retinitis pigmentosa, pattern dystrophy, and fundus flavimaculatus in a single family with a deletion of codon 153 or 154 of the peripherin/RDS gene. Arch Ophthalmol 1993; 111: 1531–1542.
22. Grover S, Fishman GA, Stone EM. Atypical presentation of pattern dystrophy in two families with peripheral RDS mutations. Ophthalmology 2002; 109:1110–1117.
23. Lessells K. More mutations in males. Nature 1997; 390:236–237.
24. Gorin MB. The ABCA4 gene and eye-related macular degeneration Editorial. Arch Ophthalmol 2001; 119:752–753.
25. Stout T. Gene therapy in ocular disease. Ophthalmology 1995; 102:1415–1416.
26. Zack DJ. Ocular gene therapy, from fantasy to foreseeable reality. Arch Ophthalmol 1993; 111:1477–1478.
27. Bennett J, Tanabe T, Jun D, et al. Photoreceptor cell rescue in retinal degeneration- (rd) mice by in vivo gene therapy. Nat Med 1996; 2:649–654.

28. Guy J, Qi X, Muzyczka N, Hauswirth WW. Receptor expression persists 1 year after a gene-associated virus- mediated gene transfer to the optic nerve. Arch Ophthalmol 1999; 117:929–937.
29. Guy J, Qi X, Wang H, Hauswirth WW. Adenoviral gene therapy with catalase suppresses experimental optic neuritis. Arch Ophthalmol 1999; 117:1533–1539.
30. Sakamoto T, Kimura H, Scuric Z, et al. Inhibition of experimental proliferative vitreoretinopathy by retroviral vector- medicated transfer of suicide gene. Can proliferative vitreoretinopathy be a target of gene therapy? Ophthalmology 1995; 102:1417–1524.
31. Adler R. Mechanisms of photoreceptor death in retinal degenerations. Arch Ophthalmol 1996; 114:79–83.
32. Fossel M. Telomerase and the aging cell: implications for human health. J Am Med Assoc 1998; 279:1732–1735.
33. Brambati B. Prenatal diagnosis of genetic diseases. Eur J Obstet Gynecol Reprod Biol 2000; 90:165–169.
34. Findlay I. Pre-implantation genetic diagnosis. Br Med Bull 2000; 56:672–690.
35. Strom CM, Levin R, Strom S, et al. Neonatal outcome of preimplantation genetic diagnosis by polar body removal: The first 109 infants. Pediatrics 2000; 106:650–653.
36. Poulton J, Marchington DR. Progress in genetic counseling and prenatal diagnosis of maternally inherited mtDNA diseases. Neuromuscul Disord 2000; 10:484–487.
37. Evans K, Gregory CY, Fryer A, et al. The role of molecular genetics in the prenatal diagnosis of retinal dystrophies. Eye 1995; 9:24–28.
38. Gieser JP. Ethics and human fetal retinal pigment epithelium transplantation. Arch Ophthalmol 2001; 116:899–900.
39. Parker M, Lucassen A. Working towards ethical management of genetic testing. Lancet 2002; 360:1685–1688.

2
The Basics of Genetics

MONOGENIC INHERITANCE

Introduction

When a mutation of only one gene leads to an abnormal phenotype, the pattern of inheritance is said to be *monogenic*. All genes, except those on the X chromosome in the male, are found in two copies in every person; each copy is an allele of the gene. When an individual has one mutant allele and one normal *allele* the individual is referred to as a *heterozygote*. If both alleles are mutants then the individual is *homozygous* for the mutation. Because males have only one X chromosome, they are *hemizygotes* for each of the genes on this chromosome.

If the abnormal trait is clinically manifested in a heterozygote, then the mutant allele is *dominant* to the normal allele, whereas, if the heterozygote has a normal phenotype, and only the homozygote is affected, then the mutant allele is *recessive*. *Codominance* is a team used for both normal and mutant alleles that express themselves fully.

If the gene is located on one of the autosomes, then the inheritance is *autosomal* whereas if the gene is one one of the "sex" chromosomes, the inheritance is *sex-linked*.

Autosomal Dominant Inheritance

In autosomal dominant inheritance (Fig. 1), the affected individual is generally heterozygous for the abnormal allele: one of the alleles is abnormal and is dominant to the normal allele. In general, one of the parents of an affected individual is also affected. An affected individual has a risk of 50% to transmit the mutant allele to his or her offspring, males or females; normal individuals will not transmit the disease to their offspring.

New Mutations

New mutations are seen relatively often in dominant disorders. In a dominant disorder, a new mutation will express itself in the first individual in whom the mutation appeared. In diseases in which the fitness of the affected individual is reduced or null (the fitness measures the ability to reproduce), most or all cases of the disease must be new mutations. New mutations may arise in one of the gametes of one of the parents or in a cell that later produces a germinal line. Therefore, a disease may remain a unique event in the family if the mutation occurred in one of the gametes of one parent; but it may appear again in another child if the mutation

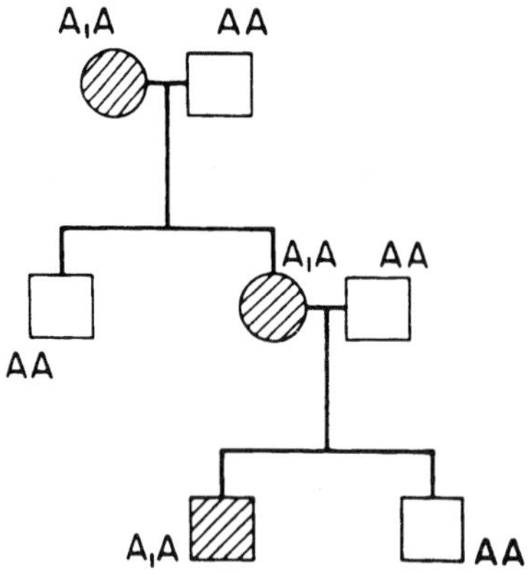

Figure 1 Autosomal dominant inheritance: A is the normal allele and A_1 is the mutant allele, which is dominant. Note that the transmission of the disease is from generation to generation; males and females are affected.

was in a germinal cell. An increased frequency of new mutations has been reported among older fathers in many dominant diseases.

Homozygosity

In autosomal dominant disorders the affected individual is usually heterozygous for the mutant allele. Homozygotes for autosomal dominant alleles are rare because practically always both parents must be affected. Homozygotes may be found in particular if the marriage of the parents is related to the abnormal trait. Assortative mating, as such marriages are termed, include, for instance, blindness, deafness, and short stature. Another possibility for the existence of homozygotes in autosomal dominant disorders is consanguineous marriages. In many autosomal dominant disorders the disease is more severe in the homozygote than in the heterozygote. All offspring of such a homozygote will be affected, except in reduced penetrance.

Autosomal Recessive Inheritance

In autosomal recessive inheritance (Fig. 2) the affected individual must be homozygous for the mutant allele. In general, both parents of an affected individual are healthy, carriers of the abnormal allele (heterozygotes), and have a 25% risk of their children, males or females, being affected (homozygotes).

The *carriers* of autosomal recessive traits are, by definition, healthy, without any clinical manifestation of the disease. However, in some inherited diseases, mild clinical symptoms may be found in the carriers. For instance, the carrier of sickle cell anemia may become symptomatic under conditions of low oxygen tension. In some autosomal recessive diseases, there are laboratory tests that allow one to differentiate the carrier from the normal homozygote: in some inborn errors of metabolism, such as TaySachs disease, the enzyme is absent in the affected homozygotes, whereas the heterozygote shows decreased activity. However, most heterozygotes for autosomal recessive disorders cannot be discovered until after the birth of an affected child because most cannot be distinguished from the normal homozygotes by clinical or by laboratory examinations.

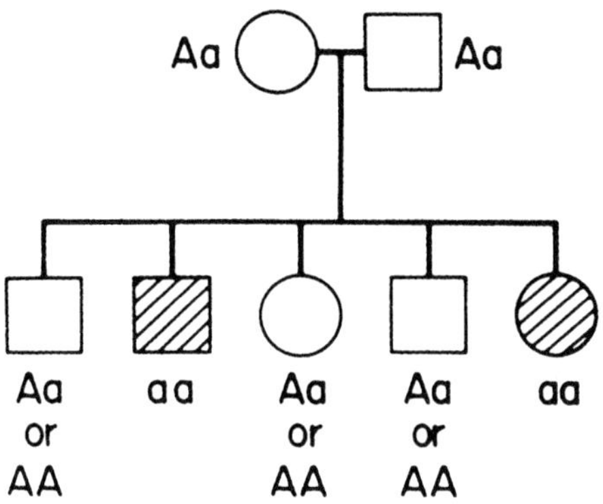

Figure 2 Autosomal recessive inheritance: A is the normal allele and a the mutant allele, which is recessive. The parents are healthy carriers, heterozygotes. Both males and females are affected, homozygotes.

The probability that two carriers of a mutant allele will marry is related to the frequency of the allele and mating habit of the population: therefore, when the allele is very rare, most of the affected children will be born to parents who are related to one another and in whom the mutant allele has a common origin (common ancestor). Conversely, when the allele is frequent in the population, usually the parents of affected children are not related. In endogamous communities, specific autosomal recessive disorders have been reported with a high frequency, because a common ancestor carried the mutant gene (founder effect).

When the allele is frequent and the fitness (ability to reproduce) of the homozygote is normal, a homozygote may marry a heterozygote for the same mutant gene. Here, there is a 50% risk that children of both sexes will be affected and, since the transmission is vertical, this type of inheritance is often referred to as *pseudodominance*. The marriage of two homozygotes for the same mutant allele is also possible, especially in assortative mating, and here, 100% of the children will be affected.

X-Linked Dominant Inheritance

X-linked dominant inheritance (Fig. 3) is relatively rare. Affected individuals are generally heterozygous for a mutant allele on the X chromosome. There is a 50% risk that the children of an affected individual will also be affected, as in autosomal dominant inheritance, but in X-linked dominant disorders, an affected male will never transmit the disease to his sons (since they receive the Y from their father), whereas his daughters will always be affected. Because females have two X chromosomes, there are statistically twice as many affected women as affected males, who have only one X chromosome.

X-Linked Recessive Inheritance

In X-linked recessive inheritance (Fig. 4), males are affected, whereas affected women are very rare. The affected male is hemizygous for the mutant allele. A woman with only one abnormal allele is a heterozygote and has a 50% risk that her children will receive the X chromosome with the abnormal allele; if the child is a male, he will then be a hemizygote and affected, and if the child is a female, she will be a heterozygote,

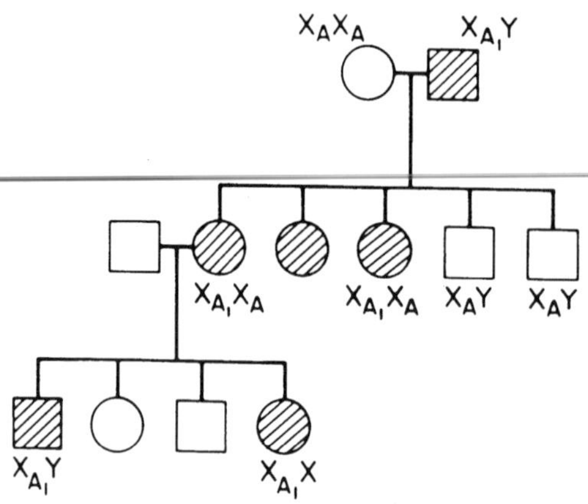

Figure 3 X-linked recessive inheritance: XA is the normal allele and XA_1 the mutant allele, which is dominant. Note that all the daughters of the affected man are affected, whereas his sons are always normal.

carrier of the mutant allele. All the daughters of an affected male are carriers, and all his sons are healthy.

In women, only one X chromosome is active (whereas the other is randomly inactivated (Lyon hypothesis). As a result, in an average half of the cells of a carrier for an X-linked recessive disorder, the X chromosome with the normal allele is active, and in the other half of the cells, the X chromosome with the mutant allele is active. Such women, having a normal allele in 50% of their cells should be healthy, as are women carriers of autosomal recessive disorders. Sometimes this is true, but in a large percentage of X-linked disorders the carriers are symptomatic and mildly affected. This permits the detection of carriers among women related to the affected patients: for instance, most carriers of Lowe disease or Fabry's disease may have the disease diagnosed by clinical ophthalmological examination. In some diseases, the carriers may even be as severely affected as affected males, for instance, in Fabry's disease.

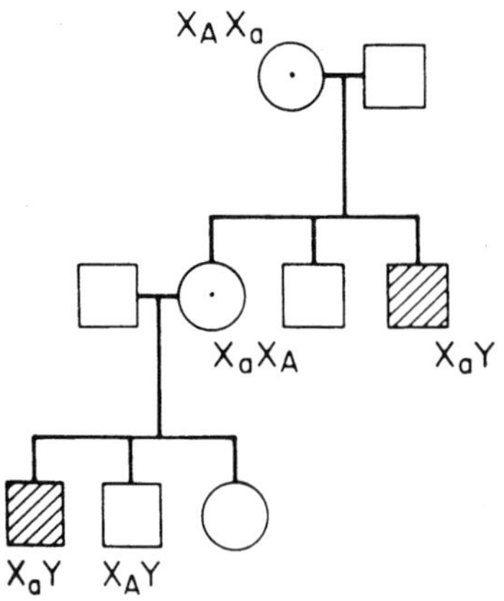

Figure 4 X-linked recessive inheritance: XA is the normal allele and Xa the mutant allele, which is recessive. Note that the disease is transmitted by healthy women, who are heterozygotes, to half their sons.

A woman may be affected with one of the X-linked recessive disorders for one of four reasons:

1. *Manifesting heterozygote*: A woman may be a heterozygote and present some or most symptoms of the disease as explained in the foregoing. She is then referred to as a manifesting heterozygote.
2. *Homozygote for the mutant allele*: In some cases, when the father is affected and the mother is a carrier, their daughter may be a homozygote for the mutant allele and affected. This may be seen, in particular, if the parents are related or if the mutant allele is frequent in the population.
3. *Hemizygote*: A woman with only one X chromosome and carrier of a mutant allele on this chromosome will be affected with the corresponding disease, exactly as the affected male; for instance, a woman with Turner's syndrome with only one sex chromosome (45,X0) or with testicular feminization in whom the phenotype is of a female and the genotype is of a male (46,XY).
4. *Nonrandom inactivation of the X chromosome*: In a woman with a structural aberration of the X chromosome the inactivation is not at random. Three different cases may be distinguished. First, if the X chromosome is abnormal, such as when a part of it is absent (deletion), the inactivation will be preferentially of the abnormal chromosome, most probably because of selection in favor of the cell with the normal chromosome. Second, if a translocation between an X chromosome and an autosome exists, the inactivation will be of the normal X chromosome to protect the autosome because, if the translocated X is inactivated, the process of inactivation may also involve a part of the autosome. If the woman had inherited the mutant allele on the structurally normal X chromosome, then the nonrandom inactivation would lead to the presence of the mutant allele in all cells, and the woman will be affected. In the second example, if the mutation is on the translocated X chromosome, then the woman will be affected. Third, if in this type of translocation, the break of the X chromosome causes a disruption of a gene and, as a result, the gene becomes abnormal, the X chromosome with the translocation is the only one active. Such a woman will be affected by the disease caused by the disrupted gene, even though she has not inherited this abnormal gene. Such cases of women affected with an X-linked disease, without a family history of the disease and in whom a translocation of the X chromosome is found in cytogenetic examination, always at the same break point, have enabled us to localize the gene of the disorder to this break point. This was particularly useful in location of the gene for Duchenne's muscular dystrophy.

Genetic Heterogeneity

Often two or more genotypes lead to the same abnormal phenotype. In isolated retinitis pigmentosa, many genes are known to be involved, and a mutation of any of them may cause the disease. Some of these genes are dominant, others recessive, autosomal, or X-linked, and often the clinical picture does not allow one to differentiate among these different genotypes. In some cases, only the family history gives the clue for the type of inheritance involved. Within each type of inheritance, different genes are known to be involved; therefore, heterogeneity exists (Fig. 5).

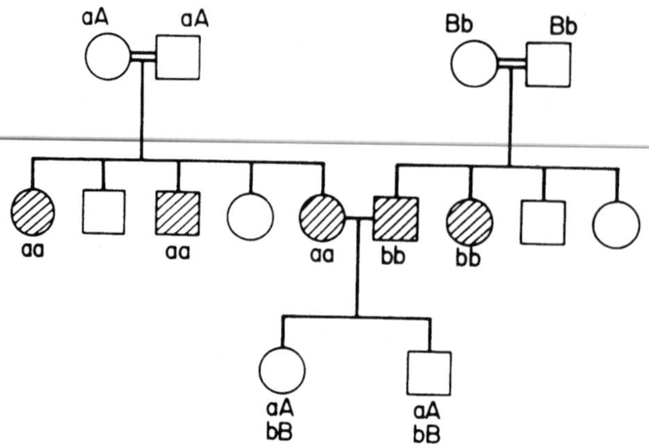

Figure 5 Genetic heterogeneity: Two individuals, affected with the same disease, married. In each of the families the disease is transmitted as an autosomal recessive disorder. Since the children of the couple are healthy, one may conclude that the mutation in each family is of a different gene. One parent is an affected homozygote aa and normal at locus BB and the other parent is homozygote bb and normal AA. The children are heterozygote at each loci: Aa and Bb are healthy.

DIGENIC INHERITANCE

When the existence of two different mutations each in a different gene is necessary for the abnormal phenotype to be present the inheritance is said to be digenic. In the case in which one allele of each gene is mutated, the digenic inheritance is biallelic. For instance, for some of the mutations in the photoreceptor-specific genes *ROM1* and peripherin/*RDS*, only double heterozygotes develop retinitis pigmentosa. The carriers of a single of these mutations either in peripherin/*RDS*, or in *ROM1* are healthy. (Fig. 6).

Another type of digenic inheritance is said to be triallelic, since the phenotype is present only when the two alleles of one of the genes are mutated and one allele in the other gene. This situation was reported in Bardet–Biedl syndrome, an autosomal recessive disorder including mental retardation, obesity, polydactyly, and retinal degeneration. Several patients were found to be carrier of two mutations at the *BBS2* locus and one mutation at the *BBS6* locus, while individuals that were carriers of two mutations at the *BBS2* locus were unaffected.

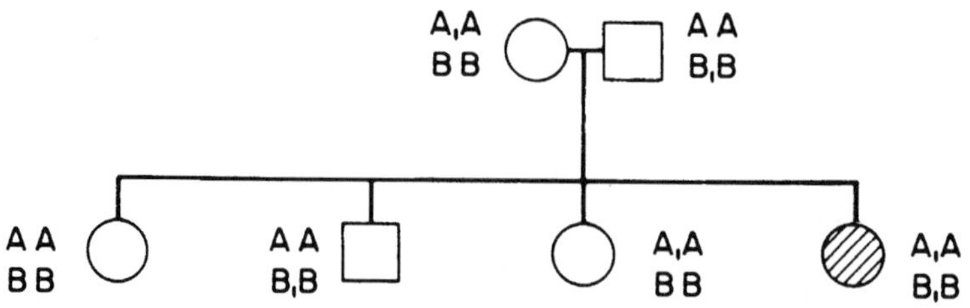

Figure 6 Digenic inheritance. A and B are the normal alleles at two different loci; A_1 and B_1 are mutated alleles. The double heterozygote A_1A, B_1B only is affected.

UNUSUAL PATTERNS OF INHERITANCE

Penetrance

A genotype that may or may not produce a clinical trait is said to be incompletely penetrant (Fig. 7). The penetrance of a genotype is defined by the probability that a person carrying it will present clinical manifestations. Only if after a complete examination there are no clinical signs of the syndrome in an obligate carrier, can it be concluded that the mutation is nonpenetrant in the individual. The degree of penetrance is specific for each mutant gene and this figure is important for genetic counseling.

Variable Expressivity

Mutations in the same gene may cause different clinical symptoms in affected individuals. This variation may range from very mild to severe in individuals carrying the same genotype, including members of the same family.

Sex Limitation

When the abnormal trait expresses itself only in one gender, but the mutant allele is transmitted in both genders, then the trait is sex limited (Fig. 8). The limitation to one gender may sometimes result because the organ affected exists only in one gender.

Imprinting

Both parental genomes are essential for normal growth and development. In mice, and later in humans, it was demonstrated that some of the genes are imprinted, expressed only from either the maternal or the paternal chromosome. A mutation in one of these imprinted genes will be expressed only if present on the chromosome of the parent who transmits the active copy of the gene. In the example of maternal imprinting (Fig. 9), only the allele originating from the father is active. Therefore,

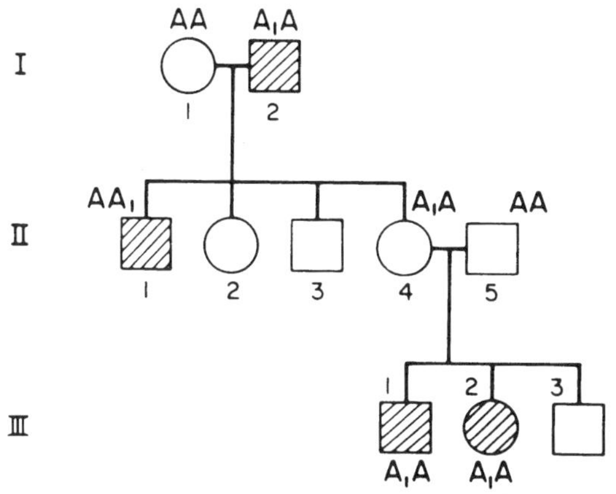

Figure 7 Autosomal dominant inheritance, incomplete penetrance: II_4 is healthy but transmits the allele to her children. The allele is nonpenetrant in this individual.

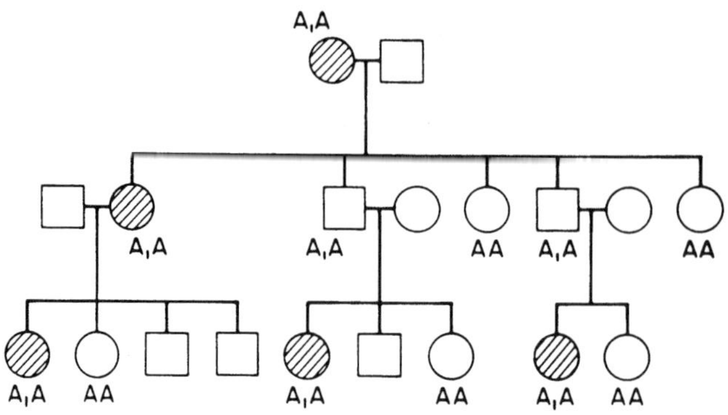

Figure 8 Sex limitation: The disease is transmitted as a dominant trait, but only women are affected; male carriers of the mutant allele are healthy and transmit the allele to half their children, whereas only the females are affected.

while half of the offspring of a male or a female carrier will also be carriers, only those born to a male carrier will be affected.

Anticipation

Anticipation is a term used to describe the transmission of a dominant disorder with more severe manifestations from one generation to the other. The classical example is myotonic dystrophy, in which late-onset cataracts are often the only symptom in the first generations. Later on more severe symptoms appear among the carriers of the mutation, often presenting at earlier ages.

MULTIFACTORIAL INHERITANCE

Most human traits and inherited diseases are controlled by more than one gene; this type of inheritance is called polygenic: each gene has an additive effect on the trait. The expression of the trait is continuous and, in the population, the distribution of a polygenic trait may be described by a "normal" (Gaussian) curve. In humans there

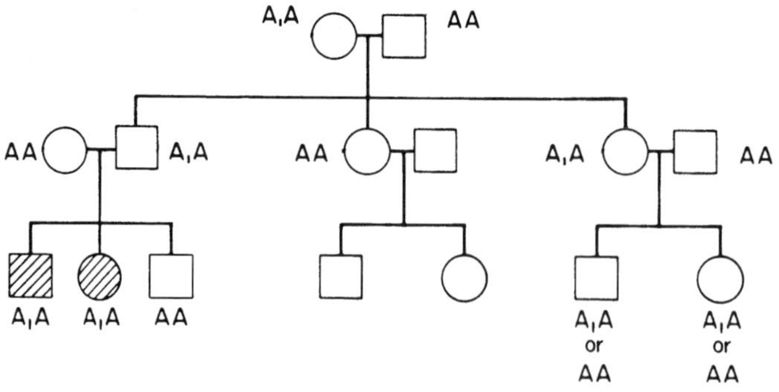

Figure 9 Maternal imprinting. A_1 is the mutated allele. Note that among the carriers of the mutation those who received it from their mother are healthy (only the allele received from the father is active) while those who received it from their father are affected (the normal allele is imprinted and inactive).

are very few examples of pure polygenic inheritance, and usually, the trait is also influenced by environmental factors. This type of inheritance, involving polygenic and environmental factors, is referred to multifactorial inheritance. The disorders that are multifactorial are relatively frequent and represent significant morbidity in the population. Generally, the genes involved are not known, and in only very few diseases have the environmental factors involved been delineated. There are many examples of this type of inheritance for normal traits, as well as for diseases: height, intelligence, blood pressure, coronary heart disease, hypertension, schizophrenia, and many birth anomalies such as neural tube defects, congenital heart defects, and others. In ophthalmology, primary glaucoma and strabismus are considered to be of multifactorial inheritance.

A theoretical model of multifactorial inheritance has been described from clinical observations. There are five important points in evaluating the risk for an individual to be affected:

1. The degree of relationship with the patient. The risk is highest for first-degree relatives, such as children or siblings; much lower for second-degree relatives, such as grandchildren, uncle, aunt; and almost the same as in the general population in third-degree relatives.
2. The number of affected patients in the family. In a family with two affected children, the risk for a third child to be affected will be higher than in a family in whom only one child is affected.
3. The severity of the disease in the patient. The risk is higher for relatives if the patient is more severely affected.
4. The sex of the affected patient. In disorders in which one sex is affected more than the other, the risk is higher in families in whom the affected child is from the less-affected sex.
5. The risks are empiric, calculated from families with patients affected with the disorder.

CHROMOSOMAL INHERITANCE

One refers to chromosomal inheritance when the disorder is due to a chromosomal aberration that is visible by the cytogenetic methods used in the laboratory. Chromosomal disorders may mimic simple Mendelian inheritance.

Chromosomal Inheritance Mimicking a Recessive Disorder

A carrier of a balanced translocation is an individual in whom all the genetic material is present but some has been translocated from one chromosome to another. After meiosis, half of the chromosomes are found in the gametes. In a carrier of a balanced translocation, the gamete will be normal if it contains a set of all normal chromosomes. The gamete will also be normal if it includes both chromosomes with the translocation, meaning that all the genetic material is present. The third possibility exists when within a set of chromosomes, where only one chromosome carries the translocation, the gamete becomes unbalanced. Some of the genetic material appears twice, whereas some material is not present at all. When one parent is a carrier of a balanced translocation, some children may receive an abnormal gamete and will be affected with a clinical disorder because of the unbalanced chromosomal aberration, whereas other children who received a normal gamete or a gamete with the translocation will be healthy. The family will present as healthy parents with some affected children, whereas others are normal, mimicking a recessive disorder. The diagnosis must be confirmed by chromosomal examination of one affected child.

Chromosomal Disorders Mimicking Autosomal Dominant Inheritance

An individual with a chromosomal aberration will transmit it to half of his or her offspring, if the aberration does not lead to infertility. The findings in this type of family will mimic a dominant disorder. For diseases that are transmitted vertically from generation to generation, but their exact inheritance is not known, chromosomal analysis of one of the affected patients is mandatory.

Chromosomal Disorders Mimicking X-Linked Inheritance

A female carrier of a discrete aberration of the X chromosome will generally not be affected because this chromosome will be preferentially inactivated. Half her sons will receive this chromosome and will be affected, whereas the daughters who received it will be carriers. Again, in these disorders of unknown X-linked inheritance, chromosomal studies should be performed.

MITOCHONDRIAL INHERITANCE

The mitochondrial DNA (mtDNA) of an individual is derived exclusively from the mother, because the mtDNA from the father's sperm degenerates after the fertilization of the egg. Therefore, the mtDNA is inherited from mothers through the generations. If a mutation has occurred in the mtDNA and causes an abnormal trait or disease, this trait or disease will be transmitted by the mother to both daughters and sons. An affected male forms the end of the vertical line of transmission, but women will continue to transmit it to their offspring. The genes coded by mtDNA are not well known, but some diseases have been suspected to be of mitochondrial inheritance, in particular, some muscular dystrophies. It has been proposed that Leber's hereditary optic neuroretinopathy is a maternally inherited disease of mitochondrial inheritance, with sex limitation; accordingly, only males are affected.

DIAGNOSTIC TESTS IN GENETIC DISEASES OF THE EYES

Family History

Information concerning the family, including origin, consanguinity, and age of the parents at the time of conception, must be collected.

Origin: Some of the rare genetic disorders have been reported in small ethnic groups, and the origin of the family may be a clue for the diagnosis.

Consanguinity: In rare genetic disorders, consanguinity may suggest that the disease is inherited as an autosomal recessive disorder.

Age of the parents: In an isolated patient, an older father may suggest that the disease is due to a new dominant mutation.

Details concerning the relatives of the patients, including siblings, parents, and close relatives, are recorded and, in particular, all diseases and malformations in the family members are noted. *Since variability of genetic disorders may be wide, a search should be made for even discrete signs of the disorder*. The best way for such information to be recorded is by drawing a family tree and asking specifically about every member of the family.

Clinical Examination

A complete clinical examination is performed in an attempt to identify all the abnormalities, to establish whether the disease is confined to the eyes, or is part of a more complex syndrome. In many cases, examination of close relatives for discrete signs of the disease is worthwhile because it may identify mildly affected relatives or symptomatic carriers. Additional investigations must be performed including radiography, biochemical tests, biopsy, or other diagnostic procedures according to the findings and suspected diagnosis.

Chromosomal Studies

Chromosomal morphology usually may be studied in cells during mitosis in metaphase. The analysis is made in peripheral blood after the growth of leukocytes, for 72 hr in suitable medium and in the presence of a mitotic agent. The mitoses are arrested at metaphase by adding colchicine. After appropriate treatment, including staining, the chromosomes are microscopically analysed and photographed.

Each human cell contains 46 chromosomes; of these, 44 are autosomes (22 pairs of chromosomes), and the other two are the sex chromosomes X or Y. The *karyotype* is the analysis of the chromosomes of the individual. The autosomes are classified according to their length and the position of the centromere, and are assigned a number: the largest chromosome is number 1, and the smallest is chromosome 22. In addition to their size and morphologic structure, various staining techniques (banding) permit to differentiate each chromosome and to make a precise analysis of the karyotype. The centromere divides the chromosome into two unequal parts: the small arm, p, and the long arm, q.

Two basic processes are responsible for most of the aberrations in chromosomes: a deviation of the normal number: aneuploidy and structural alterations. Among the aneuploidies the most common are the trisomies (three times the same chromosome instead of twice), with trisomy 21 Down syndrome being the most frequent. The monosomies are another type of aneuploidy (only one chromosome, instead of a pair) the most frequent is Turner syndrome in which only one X is present, without another sex chromosome. Among the structural alternations, one must distinguish between balanced alterations, in which all the genetic material is present, from those in which a part is additional or absent, leading to a partial trisomy or partial monosomy, respectively. Among the balanced alterations, translocations are the most frequent and are the result of a process by which there is a transfer of chromosomal material from one chromosome to another. The unbalanced alterations may be secondary to translocation deletion or duplication of a part of a chromosome.

Fluorescent in situ hybridization (FISH) is a molecular technique that has been introduced in recent years for chromosome analysis. On a microscope slide (in situ) the chromosomal DNA is denatured (single strained) and then renatured in the presence of a fluorescent DNA probe. The probe may be chosen as the complementary sequence of a chromosomal region or a single gene. Therefore, it is expected that the probe will hybridize with the complementary DNA if present in the patient. FISH allows for diagnosis of situations that often cannot be seen under a light microscope, in particular subtle translocations or deletions and single gene disorders.

Chromosomal disorders are diagnosed at the light microscopic level, and when one sees an aberration at this level, many genes must be involved. Therefore, as a rule, in most chromosomal syndromes many malformations are found, often with mental retardation. Ocular defects are frequently found in chromosomal disorders, but rarely as an isolated malformation.

Gene Mapping and Linkage

Human gene mapping is concerned with the assignement of individual genes to specific parts of the chromosomes. Many clinical applications are of importance, in particular prenatal diagnosis of genetic disorders. With the application of molecular genetics in recent years, the progress of gene mapping has been rapid, and the location of many genes responsible for monogenic disorders is now known.

Methods used for gene mapping include mainly inheritance pattern (for X-linked genes), gene dosage, somatic and in situ hybridization, and linkage analysis, the latter being the most important for its clinical applications. Genes on the same chromosome are not necessarily passed on together to an offspring. A physical exchange of material occurs between pairs of homologous chromosomes during meiosis; crossovers lead to recombination. Two genes on the same chromosome that are close to each other are rarely separated by a crossover. They will remain together in the children, as they were in the parents, with very few recombinations. If the two genes are on the same chromosome, but are far apart, they will act as if completely independent. In the children, they will appear as they were in the parents or as recombinants, each with a same frequency (50%). The number of recombinants in the offspring measures the degree of linkage between the two loci, from 0 (very tightly linked) to 50 units [no linkage; 1 unit = 1 centimorgan (cM) = 1% recombination]. This distance is not physical, but it represents the number of crossovers between the two loci. It may be that two loci, physically very close, are not linked, because the area represents a high spot for recombination, at which crossovers are frequent.

In humans, two difficulties arise in the calculation of linkage. First, matings are observed, but not constructed, such as in experimental animals, and, second, the size of the families is small. To circumvent these difficulties a mathematical method was developed: the lod score analysis. The *lod score* is the lod (logarithm of the odds) of a probability ratio that divides two numbers: first, that the segregation among offspring in a family is observed, since the two genes are linked at a distance θ, and, second, the probability that this same segregation is observed without any linkage between the two genes. The linkage between two loci must be evaluated for different possible distances (θ) between 0 and 50 cM and the lod score, therefore, is a calculated program. Statistical evidence for linkage exists when the lod score is over 3 (a probability of >0.999 that there is linkage) at a specific value of θ. When the lod score is -2 or less, the linkage is rejected. Intermediate results are due to too little information and more data are needed.

When linkage is known between two genes, it may be used for diagnosis only in informative families. For instance, in an autosomal dominant disease, the patient is heterozygous for the mutant gene. A family is informative if the analysis of the gene that is linked to the gene of the disease enables us to distinguish between the allele of the disease and the normal allele in the patients of this family. In an autosomal recessive disease, the affected patient is homozygous for the mutant allele, and each of his or her parents is heterozygous. Here, an informative family will be a family for whom one will be able to distinguish between the normal and mutant allele in the parents by examination of the gene that is linked to the gene of the disease, in other words, if the parents are heterozygous for both loci.

Historically, linkage was first established between diseases and blood groups; thereafter, many other biochemical markers were used for delineation of linkage groups, sometimes even without precise knowledge of the location on the chromosome. The problem with this type of markers is that there are relatively few genes for which allelism frequently occurs in the normal population (polymorphism). Therefore, informative families were rarely found.

In recent years together with the near completion of the Human Genome Project many DNA polymorphic sites were characterized and mapped (often repeated sequences, or single-base polymorphisms). In parallel, detailed maps of these markers on each chromosome have been produced. With the increase in technological abilities, methods were developed to perform "whole-genome studies" for linkage analysis. These type of studies are performed using markers dispersed in the whole genome at relatively small distances from each other. After obtaining the first hint for a region, further detailed analysis is performed for more precise gene localization.

The mapping of genes involved in complex disorders is much more difficult and other types of analysis and methods are necessary such as association analysis, sib-pair analysis, transmission disequilibrium test.

Gene Amplification

When the sequence of the gene responsible for the disease is known, it is possible to amplify this gene, or a part of it, by a relatively simple method. The polymerase chain reaction (PCR) uses a pair of short oligonucleotide primers, each complementary to one end of the sequence of interest: one to the (+) strand and the other to the (−) strand. Repeated cycles of DNA denaturation, reannealing, and synthesis, in the presence of DNA polymerase, are used for the amplification of the sequence. The DNA may be amplified hundreds of times and, therefore, even a very small initial DNA sample may be used, such as the amount of one single cell. The DNA obtained is a perfect copy of the gene or of the part amplified and may then be used for diagnosis.

REFERENCES

1. De Grouchy J, Truleau C. Clinical Atlas of Human Chromosomes. 2nd ed. New York: John Wiley & Sons, 1984.
2. Emery AE, Rimoin DL. Principles and Practice of Medical Genetics. Edinburgh: 4th edition Churchil-livingston, 2002.
3. Nussbaum RL, McInnes RR, Willard HF. Thompson and Thompson Genetics in Medicine. 6th ed. Philadelphia: WB Saunders, 2004.
4. Vogel F, Motulsky AG. Human Genetics Problems and Approach. 2nd ed. New York: Springer-Verlag, 1986.

3
Introduction to Human Molecular Genetics

INTRODUCTION TO MOLECULAR BIOLOGY

Deoxyribonucleic acid (DNA) is the genetic molecule of all cellular organisms and DNA viruses. DNA exists in every cell in the human body; it is localized predominantly to the nucleus, and contains all the molecular information needed for replication, transcription, and translation. The DNA molecule consists of two strands of nucleotides which form the double-helix structure. The two strands are composed of four DNA nucleotides and complement each other: adenine (A) forms two hydrogen bonds with thymine (T) and cytosine (C) forms three hydrogen bonds with guanine (G). The human genome contains ~3.2 billion nucleotides arranged in 22 pairs of autosomal chromosomes (chromosomes 1–22), and two sex chromosomes (X and Y). Both female and male genomes contain the 22 pairs of autosomal chromosomes, but the female genome contains a pair of X chromosomes, and the male genome contains one copy of the X chromosome and one copy of the Y chromosome. The chromosomes differ in sequence, gene content, size, and structure.

Each chromosome contains functional units, the genes, and each of the two copies of a gene is called an allele. Each gene usually harbors the information for the production of one protein in the right cell(s), at the right timing, and in the right amount. A typical gene contains coding and noncoding regions: the coding region contains the information needed to produce the protein in the right order of amino acids, and is divided into exons (Fig. 1), and the noncoding region contains the promoter region, transcription initiation and termination signals, intronic sequences (in between the exons), splicing sequences, and others (Fig. 1). Most of the DNA, however, is not arranged in functional units, and only 3% of the human genome encodes proteins. Noncoding DNA has been considered as "junk" DNA in the past, but there is accumulative evidence indicating that it has many important functions including various regulatory roles.

The DNA molecule is a template for two main kinds of machinery in molecular biology: replication and transcription. The DNA molecule can replicate itself based on the sequence information of one of the strands and base pairing of A–T and G–C. The new strand is then a template for synthesizing the complementary strand. This machinery ensures that the DNA is kept in its original sequence for many generations. The process, however, is not 100% accurate, allowing changes to occur at a low rate. These changes are subjected to evolutionary forces and establish the

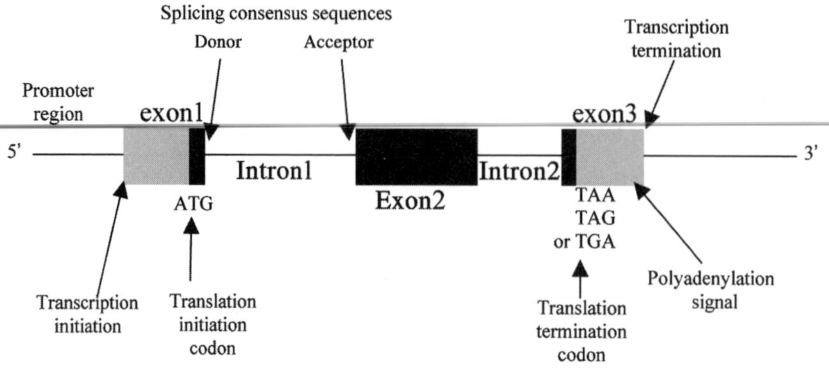

Figure 1 Schematic structure of a typical human gene.

fundamental step of molecular evolution as well as inherited diseases, as will be discussed further in this chapter. The second machinery, transcription, is the first step toward the production of proteins (Fig. 2). This step includes the synthesis of many single-stranded ribonucleic acid (RNA) molecules based on the DNA template. A newly synthesized RNA molecule is complementary to the original DNA strand except for one difference: the RNA molecule contains a uracil (U) base instead of thymidine. The freshly transcribed RNA molecule contains the original entire sequence presented in the gene starting with the initiation of transcription signal and ending with the termination of transcription signal. The RNA molecule includes

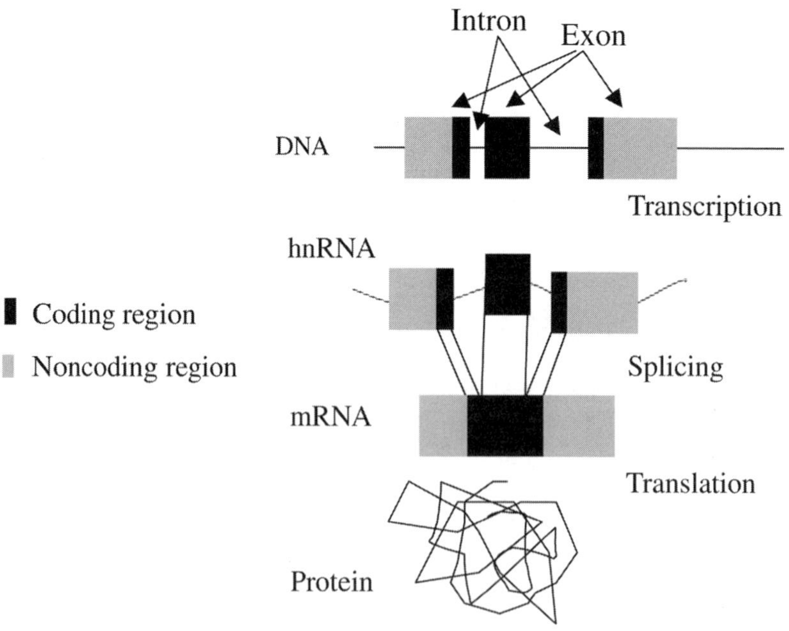

Figure 2 From DNA to protein: human genes consist of exons (which include the coding sequence) and introns. The gene is transcribed and the initial RNA (heteronuclear RNA or hnRNA) is produced. The hnRNA is processed and the introns are removed. The resulting mRNA molecule serves as a template for protein translation. Only the coding regions (black) code for amino acids.

coding exonic sequences as well as noncoding exonic and intronic sequences and thus has to be edited before producing the protein. The editing step is called RNA splicing and occurs in the spliceosome. The introns are being removed (spliced-out) and the messenger RNA (mRNA) molecule is ready for the next step, the translation (Fig. 2). Protein translation occurs in the ribosomes, which are molecular factories for protein synthesis, based on the mRNA template. The basic units of proteins are amino acids which are carried by transfer RNA (tRNA) that recognizes a codon (a sequence of three bases) in the mRNA molecule. Each tRNA contains a sequence complementary to the mRNA codon and carries the corresponding amino acid. The process of protein synthesis is highly accurate and the correct amino acid sequence is important for the function of the protein.

DNA MUTATIONS

Inherited human diseases are caused by mutations in the DNA molecule. A mutation is a mistake that occurs during DNA replication resulting in a difference between the newly synthesized DNA molecule and its template. Mutations can occur in any base or region in the genome, but particular DNA sequences (such as repetitive regions) are more prone to mutations. Because only a small fraction of the human genome encodes proteins, most of the mutations do not have any effect on the phenotype and are designated as neutral mutations (or polymorphisms). Moreover, the vast majority of germ line mutations disappear from the population within a few generations, and the likelihood that a mutation will both survive and have an effect on the protein function is slim. For the study of inherited human diseases we are usually interested in disease-causing mutations that occur within coding regions of genes. There is substantial evidence that many disease-causing mutations occur in noncoding regions within genes, as well as in intergenic regions. A sequence change can affect one specific base, a sequence of a few bases, a whole gene, and even whole chromosomes. It can also cause substitution, deletion, or insertion. The most common mutations implicated in inherited diseases are missense, nonsense, frameshift, and splice-site mutations which will be discussed below. Other types of pathogenic mutations will be mentioned briefly.

Point mutations or single-base substitutions result in the change of one base with another. The most common point mutation is the change of cytosine to thymine within C_pG dinucleotides which are frequently methylated in genomic DNA. Methylated cytosine can undergo spontaneous deamination and be converted to thymine. Based on the effect of the mutations on the codon sequence, point mutations are classified into three groups: isocoding (or silent), missense, and nonsense. Isocoding mutations will result in a codon that codes for the same amino acid (i.e., an A to G mutation that changes the TGA codon to TGG: both code for the same amino acid, glycine). Most of the isocoding mutations occur in the third base of a codon. Missense mutations will result in a codon that codes for a different amino acid, and thus affects the protein sequence. Most of the missense mutations occur in the second or first base of a codon. If the original and newly coded amino acids have a similar chemistry, the mutation is conservative; otherwise it is nonconservative and is more likely to affect the protein function. An excellent example of a nonconservative missense mutation in an ocular disease is the Pro23His mutation in the rhodopsin gene (1). The original amino acid in position 23 in rhodopsin is proline (Pro), which is nonpolar. About 8% of patients with autosomal dominant retinitis pigmentosa in North America have a mutation in which codon 23 codes for histidine (His), which is polar. This was the first mutation to be associated with retinitis pigmentosa, and was found only in North America and probably arose in a single ancestor. Another type of point mutation is nonsense mutation that causes a premature stop codon and thus a premature termination of the protein sequence.

Splice-site mutations result in an aberrant splicing of the mRNA molecule. They can affect a single base or a large number of bases. They usually change the sequence of a conserved donor or acceptor splice-site located at the beginning or at the end of an intron (Fig. 1). Interestingly, point mutations in the coding region can also cause splice-site mutations. They can create a novel splice-site, destroy a nearby splice-site, or affect exonic sequences that are necessary for efficient and accurate splicing (2). Splice-site mutations might lead to the deletion of a whole exon or part of it, or even to the inclusion of intronic sequences. Such mutations are likely to create a premature stop codon, the mRNA molecule will be usually destroyed by the nonsense-mediated mRNA decay (NMD) pathway (3), and will not be translated.

Small deletions or insertions can result in either the insertion or the deletion of at least one amino acid (inframe mutations) or in the shift of the reading frame (frameshift mutations). Inframe mutations might be pathogenic or not, depending on the mutation location and the type of inserted or deleted amino acid(s). Frameshift mutations, on the other hand, are likely to be pathogenic because they usually cause a premature stop codon prior to the terminal exon and will be thus destroyed by the NMD pathway. Frameshift mutations in the terminal exon are likely to be pathogenic as well because they will change the amino terminus of the encoded protein. For example, frameshift mutations in any exon of the most common X-linked retinitis pigmentosa gene, *RPGR*, including the terminal *ORF15* exon, are all pathogenic. Many nonpathogenic inframe mutations have been identified in *ORF15*, some are frequent in the normal population, and are assumed not to affect the protein function (4).

An unusual type of mutation, expanding repeats, has been reported in many genes associated with autosomal dominant neurodegenerative disorders (5). Expansion mutations occur in trinucleotide repeats within coding regions (usually CAG, coding for glutamine) or in the introns. These sequences are unstable due to slippage of the replicating enzyme and are thus more prone to mutations than nonrepetitive sequences. This results in a high mutation rate and a variable number of repeat units. Many of the neurodegenerative disorders contain an ocular phenotype: for example, expansion of CAG repeats in the *SCA7* gene is a cause of dominant spino-cerebellar ataxia with macular or retinal degeneration (6).

IDENTIFICATION OF DISEASE-CAUSING GENES

The "almost finished" human genome sequence, which is freely available to the public, changed dramatically the efficiency of identifying genes that cause genetic diseases. The concept of gene identification, however, has not been dramatically shifted. Current human genetic studies have the advantage of using better DNA markers, resulting in more accurate genome maps, improved technologies, and enriched gene expression and sequence databases. I will discuss here two approaches for gene identification, the "candidate gene approach" and "positional cloning," and will mention some tools that can be used to make these methods more efficient.

Many recent studies used a combination of the two methods, which has been shown to be highly efficient and crucial for gene identification.

The Candidate Gene Approach

The use of the candidate gene approach for identifying retinal degeneration genes was first introduced in 1990 (1,7,8). The main advantage of this approach is that no preliminary mapping information is needed. A gene is considered a candidate if it is expressed in the affected tissue, and there is previous information pointing to its importance for that tissue. This information might be based on the protein sequence alone, which might point to a specific biochemical pathway on the known protein function, or on a knock-out animal showing a retinal phenotype. In many cases, however, preliminary mapping information helped to zoom in on a specific gene. In the pure sense of this approach, a large collection of DNA samples is gathered from patients with a genetically heterogenous disease. The DNA is screened for mutations in candidate genes which are predicted to cause the disease, when mutated. The candidate gene approach, with or without previous mapping information, was proved to be useful in identifying genes causing retinitis pigmentosa (1,9).

Positional Cloning

The first step of the positional cloning approach is to identify a link between the phenotype and a genomic region harboring the causative gene. This is usually done by analyzing the genotype of individuals in a specific pedigree using highly polymorphic markers. These markers, usually microsatellites, are evenly spaced along the human genome. Once the gene has been assigned to a particular chromosomal region, it is highly important to reduce the suspected linked region by using fine mapping tools. This reduces the number of candidate genes that must be screened for mutations. After reducing the linked interval, the physical map of the genomic region needs to be built using either molecular genetic techniques or bioinformatics. Because of the success of the human genome project, physical maps are already available for most of the human genome, and can be used to assemble and build the actual sequence of the linked region. Alternatively, large DNA segments covering the linked region can be cloned into yeast artificial chromosomes and studied. Once a full or partial sequence is available, one will focus on the transcribed genes in the region. This can be done by studying the gene expression data available in public databases as will be discussed later. Otherwise, the content of genes expressed in the region can be studied using in vitro transcription techniques. These methods are likely to result in a number of genes expressed in the region. An educational effort should then be applied to sort the genes based on the potential importance to the affected tissue(s). The candidate genes should then be subjected to mutational analysis tools, preferably sequence analysis of one affected and one unaffected individual. In the first step, coding regions and splice-sites are being screened for mutations, and only if no potential mutation is detected, other regions, such as 5′ and 3′ untranslated regions, promoter region, and intronic sequences should also be screened. Potential pathogenic mutations are those detected in affected individuals in the pedigree and are likely to affect the protein production, transport, or function.

Using Gene Expression Data

The recent revolution in developing methods that enable the simultaneous detection of expression pattern of thousands of genes has had a major impact on the identification of disease-causing genes. These comprehensive gene expression methods allow us to theoretically study the expression of all the genes in the human genome in a single experiment in a reasonable time frame and at a reasonable cost. The information being generated using these methods is routinely incorporated into the genomic databases and thus can be used by the whole scientific community. Detailed below are the most useful comprehensive gene expression methods.

Expressed Sequence Tags

Aiming to identify all the major genes expressed in the human genome, a large sequencing project was initiated in 1991 (10). The idea was to clone mRNAs from a variety of human tissues and perform large-scale sequencing of thousands of clones from each library. Although the quality of the sequencing reaction is relatively low, the sequence information obtained is enough to link it to the correct gene or genomic region. Expressed sequence tags (ESTs) were found to be highly useful in gene identification, and over 5 million ESTs have been sequenced so far from many different human tissues (data are updated frequently and can be found at http://www.ncbi.nlm.nih.gov/dbEST/). The human EST project was followed by similar projects in other organisms and over 15 million ESTs have been generated so far. One should always keep in mind, however, that the poor sequence quality and other sequencing and assignment errors might lead to wrong conclusions, and thus it is essential to verify the EST data.

Gene Expression Microarrays

Gene expression microarrays are the most common tools for studying comprehensive gene expression in a tissue. The detection of gene expression is done by hybridizing the mRNA isolated from the studied tissue to probes (either oligonucleotides or cDNAs) which are attached to a solid surface on the array. Microarrays usually have a high density and include all known and predicted genes in the genome (oligonucleotide array) or in a specific tissue (cDNA-based array). Gene expression microarrays have been successfully used to study cancer and mainly to distinguish between different malignancies (11). A few studies have been published recently with initial gene expression data in different ocular tissues using microarrays (12–18). One should keep in mind, however, that accurate information on the level of expression of each gene is limited due to hybridization differences between such a diverse population of sequences.

Serial Analysis of Gene Expression

Serial analysis of gene expression (SAGE) is an elegant way to count the number of transcripts generated by each gene in a specific tissue. The technique is highly useful in species with completed or nearly completed sequence information, e.g., humans and mice. The simple idea of SAGE is to sequence a tag, which is a short fragment ($\sim$14 bases) from each mRNA molecule in the tissue, to identify the corresponding gene, and to calculate the expression frequency of each gene. The output is thus a digital one, and can be easily compared to results obtained in different experiments, different tissues, and even different laboratories. The initial purpose of SAGE was to accurately compare the expression level of genes in different malignant tissues, but later on it was used to profile gene expression in specific tissues including the human retina, macula and retinal pigment epithelium (19), and the mouse retina (20). A large set of expression data has been presented in these studies including the identification of a large number of candidates for retinal diseases, and many novel photoreceptor-specific genes. The advantages of SAGE are the high number of mRNAs that can be counted (usually 50,000–100,000, but is unlimited), and the digital output which permits straightforward downstream analyses. The disadvantages are the cost of sequencing thousands of clones, and the inability to correspond some tags to the correct gene.

Using Genomic Databases

The public human genome database is very active, and is frequently being updated. The starting point for collecting information on a gene or sequence of interest is the National Center for Biological Information at www.ncbi.nlm.gov. This front page will lead you to many useful databases including the heavily used Pubmed, where you can search for relevant publications, as well as many genomic databases. The most useful ones will be mentioned here:

1. *UniGene* is a database designed to gather mapping and expression information into a unique, nonredundant set of clusters, many of which correspond to unique genes.
2. *LocusLink* provides sequence and descriptive information about genetic loci. This includes information about the presumed or known protein function, official nomenclature, sequence accessions for Complementary DNA (cDNA) and genomic clones, links to genomic organization of the gene, mapping information and more.
3. *MapView* provides a very useful sequence or gene content view at the whole-genome level, the chromosome level, or the specific interval you are interested in. The MapView can be retrieved by text queries or sequence alignment. In one MapView you can obtain information on the order of genetic markers, order and content of genes, ESTs' location along the chromosome, and more. The view can be controlled by the user who can display the desired multiple information on one map.
4. *BLAST (Basic Local Alignment Search Tool)* is a set of similar search programs designed to find DNA or protein sequences that are identical or similar to your query sequence. The BLAST programs search among all the publicly available sequences and rank the match based on the length of the matched sequence, and the degree of similarity.

REFERENCES

1. Dryja TP, McGee TL, Reichel E, Hahn LB, Cowley GS, Yandell DW, Sandberg MA, Berson EL. A point mutation of the rhodopsin gene in one form of retinitis pigmentosa. Nature 1990; 343:364–366.
2. Liu HX, Cartegni L, Zhang MQ, Krainer AR. A mechanism for exon skipping caused by nonsense or missense mutations in BRCA1 and other genes. Nat Genet 2001; 27:55–58.
3. Hentze MW, Kulozik AE. A perfect message: RNA surveillance and nonsense-mediated decay. Cell 1999; 96:307–310.

4. Vervoort R, Wright AF. Mutations of RPGR in X-linked retinitis pigmentosa (RP3). Hum Mutat 2002; 19:486–500.
5. Fischbeck KH. Polyglutamine expansion neurodegenerative disease. Brain Res Bull 2001; 56:161–163.
6. David G, Abbas N, Stevanin G, Durr A, Yvert G, Cancel G, Weber C, Imbert G, Saudou F, Antoniou E, Drabkin H, Gemmill R, Giunti P, Benomar A, Wood N, Ruberg M, Agid Y, Mandel JL, Brice A. Cloning of the SCA7 gene reveals a highly unstable CAG repeat expansion. Nat Genet 1997; 17:65–70.
7. Dryja TP. Human genetics. Deficiencies in sight with the candidate gene approach. Nature 1990; 347:614.
8. Pittler SJ, Baehr W, Wasmuth JJ, McConnell DG, Champagne MS, vanTuinen P, Ledbetter D, Davis RL. Molecular characterization of human and bovine rod photoreceptor cGMP phosphodiesterase alpha-subunit and chromosomal localization of the human gene. Genomics 1990; 6:272–283.
9. Morimura H, Saindelle-Ribeaudeau F, Berson EL, Dryja TP. Mutations in RGR, encoding a light-sensitive opsin homologue, in patients with retinitis pigmentosa. Nat Genet 1999; 23:393–394.
10. Adams MD, Kelley JM, Gocayne JD, Dubnick M, Polymeropoulos MH, Xiao H, Merril CR, Wu A, Olde B, Moreno RF, et al. Complementary DNA sequencing: expressed sequence tags and human genome project. Science 1991; 252:1651–1656.
11. Clarke PA, te Poele R, Wooster R, Workman P. Gene expression microarray analysis in cancer biology, pharmacology, and drug development: progress and potential. Biochem Pharmacol 2001; 62:1311–1336.
12. Jun AS, Liu SH, Koo EH, Do DV, Stark WJ, Gottsch JD. Microarray analysis of gene expression in human donor corneas. Arch Ophthalmol 2001; 119:1629–1634.
13. Kennan A, Aherne A, Palfi A, Humphries M, McKee A, Stitt A, Simpson DA, Demtroder K, Orntoft T, Ayuso C, Kenna PF, Farrar GJ, Humphries P. Identification of an IMPDH1 mutation in autosomal dominant retinitis pigmentosa (RP10) revealed following comparative microarray analysis of transcripts derived from retinas of wild-type and Rho(−/−) mice. Hum Mol Genet 2002; 11:547–557.
14. Livesey FJ, Furukawa T, Steffen MA, Church GM, Cepko CL. Microarray analysis of the transcriptional network controlled by the photoreceptor homeobox gene Crx. Curr Biol 2000; 10:301–310.
15. Mu X, Zhao S, Pershad R, Hsieh TF, Scarpa A, Wang SW, White RA, Beremand PD, Thomas TL, Gan L, Klein WH. Gene expression in the developing mouse retina by EST sequencing and microarray analysis. Nucleic Acids Res 2001; 29:4983–4993.
16. Seftor EA, Meltzer PS, Kirschmann DA, Pe'er J, Maniotis AJ, Trent JM, Folberg R, Hendrix MJ. Molecular determinants of human uveal melanoma invasion and metastasis. Clin Exp Metastasis 2002; 19:233–246.
17. Swaroop A, Zack DJ. Transcriptome analysis of the retina. Genome Biol 3:reviews1022.1–1022.4.
18. Yoshida S, Yashar BM, Hiriyanna S, Swaroop A. Microarray analysis of gene expression in the aging human retina. Invest Ophthalmol Vis Sci 2002; 43:2554–2560.
19. Sharon D, Blackshaw S, Cepko CL, Dryja TP. Profile of the genes expressed in the human peripheral retina, macula, and retinal pigment epithelium determined through serial analysis of gene expression (SAGE). Proc Natl Acad Sci USA 2002; 99:315–320.
20. Blackshaw S, Fraioli RE, Furukawa T, Cepko CL. Comprehensive analysis of photoreceptor gene expression and the identification of candidate retinal disease genes. Cell 2001; 107:579–589.

4
Cornea

INTRODUCTION

Inherited corneal disorders were first reported in 1890 by Groenouw, who described two patients with bilateral corneal opacifications in a nodular form (1). About half a century later, Bücklers stated that at least three different types of such corneal disorders exist and stressed their familial nature and their different modes of inheritance (2). In the next 50 years, thousands of articles were published on the subject of inherited corneal diseases, resulting in frequent confusion in the clinical understanding of these diseases. Most of these publications described the clinical appearance of various corneal dystrophies.

A corneal dystrophy is defined as an inherited, bilateral, noninflammatory corneal opacification. It may take different shape and forms, affect mainly certain layers of the cornea, be stationary or progressive, cause mild or severe visual deterioration, or not affect visual acuity at all. A corneal dystrophy often causes secondary corneal erosions, with photophobia and pain. It may cause secondary inflammation, as was the presenting symptom Groenouw's first patient (1), and it may even cause secondary neovascularization.

The subject of corneal dystrophies is difficult to describe and difficult to learn. It cannot be properly presented by photographs. For best clinical evaluation of a dystropic cornea, slit-lamp biomicroscopy, with its direct, indirect, and specular modes should be used. In addition, a great variability of the clinical appearance exists among different patients with the same dystrophy, and in the same patient in different stages of development of the disease. Drawings may be more suitable in presenting the basic changes of each dystrophy.

Most corneal dystrophies can be accurately diagnosed by their clinical appearance (3). However, for some, the clinical picture may be completely misleading. The individual diagnosis of such unusual cases and our understanding of corneal dystrophies, in general, were greatly enhanced by the increasing use of corneal transplantation in the 1960s and 1970s. This surgery enabled the extensive study of corneal dystrophies by light and electron microscopy. Later, tissue culture of skin and corneal fibroblasts (4), and newer biochemical, histochemical, immunohistochemical, and cell culture techniques (5), greatly enhanced our knowledge of the corneal dystrophies.

The breakthrough in our understanding of corneal dystrophies came in the 1990s with the advent of molecular genetics and the surprising discovery that the main group of corneal dystrophies is caused by different mutations of one single gene mapped to chromosome 5q31. The gene initially named BIGH3, was later renamed TGFBI. This finding led to a reclassification of the corneal dystrophies which have been clinically determined to be one disease, but genetically heterogenous.

The management of corneal dystrophies, which was based mainly on corneal transplantation, changed in the last decade with the use of the excimer laser, superficial keratectomies, and limbal stem cell transplants. We are probably on the eve of using genetic therapy for corneal dystrophies.

The inherited disorders of the cornea will be discussed in this chapter under separate headings. Traditionally, corneal dystrophies were categorized as those affecting the anterior limiting membranes, those affecting the stroma, and those affecting the posterior limiting membranes. For the benefit of the clinician I will hold on to this tradition, but additional subchapters will group together same-gene-associated dystrophies and discuss separately heterogenous disorders. Other subchapters will be devoted to changes in corneal thickness and size, to corneal disorders resulting from multisystem syndromes, and to some rare disorders.

CORNEAL DYSTROPHIES AFFECTING THE ANTERIOR LIMITING MEMBRANES

Description

The epithelium and Bowman's membrane are primarily affected in two corneal dystrophies, the epithelial basement membrane dystrophy and Meesman's dystrophy. The first is quite common and often not diagnosed properly. The second is subtle and rather uncommon (Fig. 1; Table 1).

One type of Reis–Bücklers corneal dystrophy, renamed Thiel–Behnke type II corneal dystrophy, is a disorder that affects primarily Bowman's membrane and the epithelium. This type was mapped to locus CDTB (corneal dystrophy of Thiel–Behnke) on chromosome 10q23–q24 (Fig. 1).

The Clinical and Genetic Types

Epithelial Basement Membrane Dystrophy

Several synonyms are used in conjunction with this disorder. The most commonly used are map–dot–fingerprint dystrophy and Cogan's microcystic dystrophy. It was first described by Cogan and colleagues (7) in five patients, all women. Few symptoms were present. Slit-lamp examination revealed grayish-white, usually discrete spheres (or cysts), measuring 0.1–0.5 mm in diameter within the superficial cornea, together with larger, irregular, or comma-shaped opacities (7). Family members were not examined. Later, its familial nature was clarified (8), and its autosomal dominant transmission was confirmed by the existence of three generations of affected members (8).

The disease is asymptomatic in the first decades of life, but after the age of 30 it may become symptomatic. Usually, the earliest symptom is mild blurring of vision, which is caused by an irregular astigmatism resulting from the irregular epithelium (3). At this stage, careful slit-lamp examination will reveal the characteristic changes

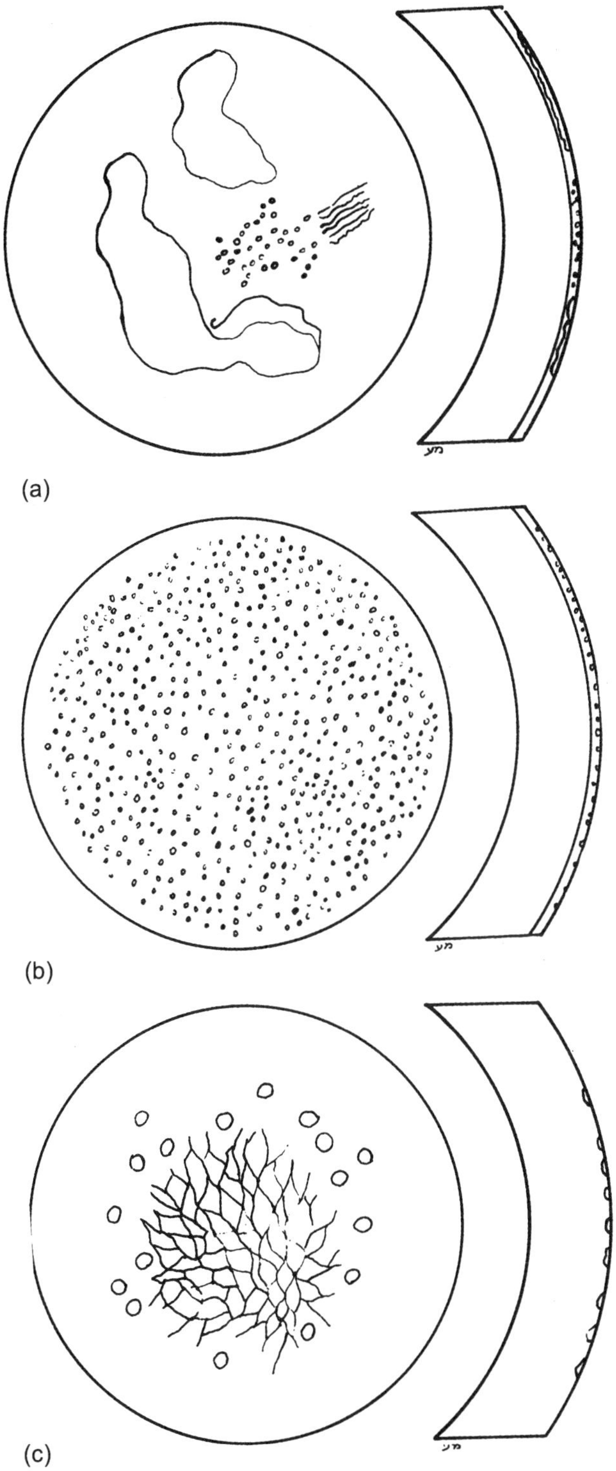

Figure 1 The corneal dystrophies affecting mainly the anterior limiting membranes: (a) epithelial basement membrane, (b) Meesman's, and (c) Thiel–Behnke type II (formerly Reis–Bücklers). (Drawings by M. Ivry.)

Table 1 Corneal Dystrophies Affecting the Anterior Limiting Membranes

Name	Synonyms	OMIM (6)	Inheritance	Gene and chromosomal location	Clinical findings			Main pathological findings
					Early	Periphery of cornea	Late	
Epithelial basement membrane dystrophy	Map–dot–fingerprint; Cogan's microcystic	121820	AD[a]	Unknown	Superficial maps, dots, fingerprints	Clear	Irregular astigmatism; recurrent cornea	Multilaminar basement membrane; subepithelial deposit of fibrogranular protein; abnormal epithelial cells
Meesman's dystrophy	Juvenile hereditary epithelial	122100	AD	KRT12 at 17ql2 KRT3 at 12ql3	Small vacuoles in epithelium	Affected	Remains asymptomatic, or irregular astigmatism, or corneal erosion	Epithelial, intracellular deposit; thickened epithelial basement membrane; cysts
Thiel–Behnke dystrophy	Vogt's anterior crocodile-shagreen; corneal dystrophy of Bowman layer, type II	602082	AD	CDB2 at 10q24	Ring form of sub-epithelial opacities in different forms; recurrent erosions	Clear	Superficial corneal scarring; reduced vision	Missing basement membrane and parts of Bowman's membrane; "curly" filaments deposits

[a]AD, autosomal dominant.

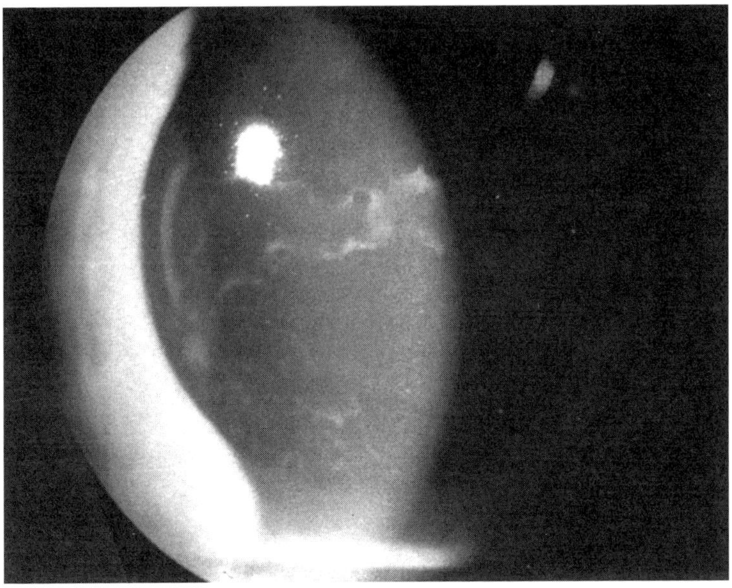

Figure 2 Epithelial basement membrane dystrophy. The maplike configuration is the most clearly seen sign. (Courtesy of J. Sugar, MD, Chicago.)

at the level of the corneal epithelium and Bowman's membrane. Dots representing the microcysts in the epithelium, maplike configuration, and fingerprint pattern may be found in any combination (Fig. 2). In a study of 78 patients who were followed up for eight years, Laibson (9) found that 48 had familial cases, 71 had bilateral involvement, and 7 had unilateral involvement. About one-third of the affected eyes showed symptoms. Maplike changes, with or without microcysts, were the most common, followed by fingerprintlike changes. Dots as the only sign of the disease are probably extremely rare (9,10). Maps are seen as large areas of haziness in the depth of the epithelium, circumscribed by scalloped borders; dots are seen as small round-, oval-, or comma-shaped opacities; and the fingerprintlike pattern represents deep epithelial curvilinear and parallel lines. The periphery of the cornea is unaffected.

The most common symptom of epithelial basement membrane dystrophy is pain associated with recurrent corneal erosion. This is usually the presenting symptom. Recurrent corneal erosion may occur as a sporadic phenomenon caused by trauma (11), but in about 50% of the patients with recurrent corneal erosion, signs of epithelial basement membrane dystrophy are found (3).

A condition termed "hereditary recurrent corneal erosion" was described in several families (12). It is possible that many of these suffer from an undetected epithelial basement membrane dystrophy. Recurrent attacks of erosions, after several years, may stop (3,13), possibly because of scarring at the level of the epithelial basement membrane.

Epithelial basement membrane corneal dystrophy is a distinct entity, given the OMIM number 121820. The causative gene and its chromosomal mapping are still unknown.

Meesman's Dystrophy

Meesman's corneal dystrophy, also known as juvenile hereditary epithelial dystrophy or juvenile epithelial dystrophy of Meesman, was first described in 1935 in an 8-year-old boy (14). Later, Meesman studied three families and described the characteristic clinical findings along with their histologic background (15). The autosomal dominant inheritance of this dystrophy is well established (16,17).

Small vacuoles are seen in the epithelium and are best seen by retroillumination. Some may reach the epithelial surface, rupture, and stain by fluorescein (18). The disease may be noticed in early childhood or remain asymptomatic and unnoticed until late in life. When symptomatic, recurrent corneal erosion with pain, tearing, and photophobia are the most common symtpoms, followed by mild reduction of visual acuity from epithelial irregularity.

The vacuoles are seen in their myriads (Fig. 3). Unlike most dystrophies, they extend over the whole cornea, from limbus to limbus, a fact noticed early by Pameijer (14).

Irvine and associates investigated families with Meesman corneal dystrophy for mutations in those known genes encoding cornea-specific cytokeratins (18,19): the type I keratin cluster on the long arm of chromosome 17 (cytokeratin K12, KRT12), and the type II keratin cluster on the long arm of chromosome 12 (cytokeratin K3, KRT3). Mutations were identified in one of the two genes in all the families studied. KRT12 cornea-specific keratin has been mapped to chromosome 12q13 and KRT3 to chromosome 17q12.

Thiel–Behnke Corneal Dystrophy, Type II

There has been some confusion on the proper nomenclature for the third corneal dystrophy affecting Bowman's membrane and the corneal epithelium, in particular that between Thiel–Behnke corneal dystrophy and Reis–Bücklers corneal dystrophy.

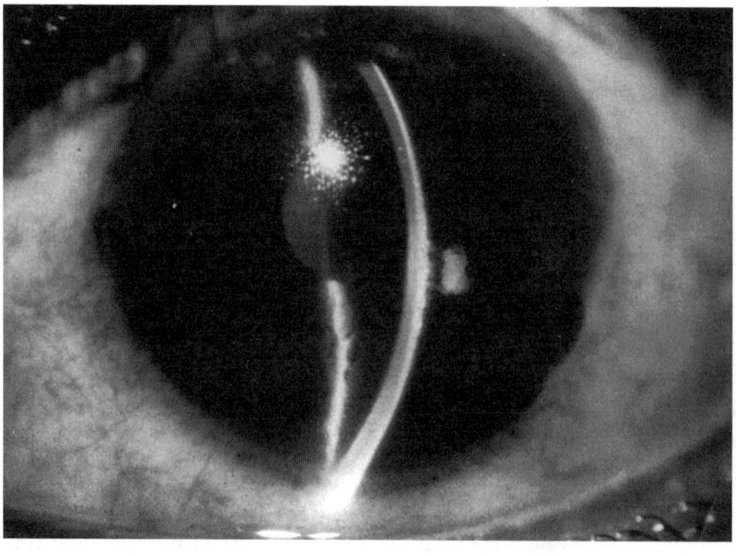

Figure 3 Meesman's corneal dystrophy. Irregular epithelium and multiple dots are seen. By retroillumination these dots are seen as fine vesicles. (Courtesy of J. Sugar, MD, Chicago.)

The disorder was named "familial corneal dystrophy of Reis" in 1949 by Bücklers (20), and later it became known as Reis–Bücklers ring-shaped dystrophy, anterior crocodile-shagreen (3), or Vogt's crocodile-shagreen (21). In 1965, Thiel and Behnke described a honeycomb dystrophy (22), which was similar to many cases described as Reis–Bücklers dystrophy. In 1995, after studying corneal specimens of both Reis–Bücklers and Thiel–Behnke dystrophy, Küchle and colleagues (23) concluded that two distinct clinical and histological phenotypes exist, both at the level of Bowman's layer. Corneal dystrophy at Bowman's membrane (CDB) type I is deeper in the cornea, clinically more severe, with vision more affected; CDB type II, a milder disease with less visual loss and recurrent corneal erosions. Kuckle and colleagues proposed the term Thiel–Behnke for type II and Reis–Bücklers for type I. Later, the distinction between these two entities was confirmed by the identification of two different loci: CDB2 on chromosome 10q24 for Thiel-Behnke (24) and 5q31 for Reis–Bücklers. Thiel–Behnke corneal dystrophy is a rather rare disease, occurring early in life in the form of recurrent corneal erosions. A slit-lamp examination will reveal irregular opacities and thickening of Bowman's membrane. These subepithelial opacities may take on different forms, including linear, fishnet, or mottled (Fig. 4), and their increased number in the midperiphery gives a ring appearance to the opacity (18). Perry and coworkers (25) found, in eight patients, a visual acuity ranging from 20/30 to finger counting, a decreased corneal sensation in most of the patients, prominent corneal nerves in two, and recurrent corneal erosion in all.

Episodes of recurrent corneal erosions typically occur in the first two decades of life (3,13,25), although they may start even in the fifth decade (25). The attacks tend to continue for 10–20 years and then stop, together with cessation of the periodic pain, tearing, photophobia, and inflammation. Usually, these symptoms will then be replaced by reduced visual acuity, resulting from scarring of Bowman's membrane.

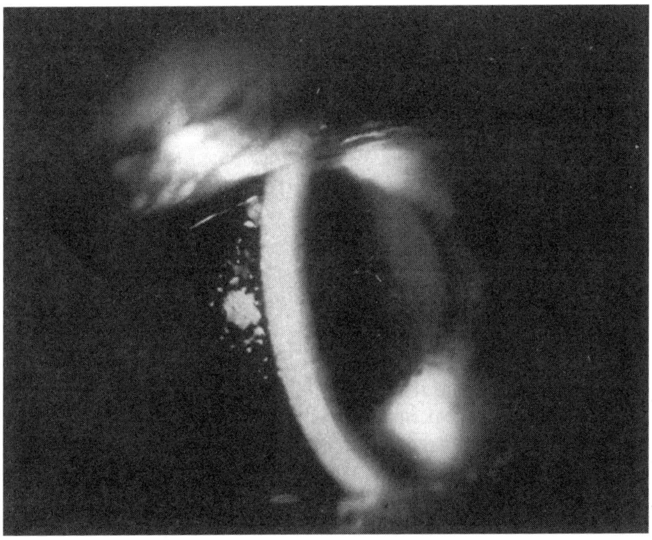

Figure 4 Reis–Bücklers corneal dystrophy. Diffuse cloudiness with multiple dense opacities at the level of Bowman's membrane can be seen. (Courtesy of J. Sugar, MD, Chicago.)

Reis–Bücklers dystrophy is transmitted by an autosomal dominant gene. It is more severe than either epithelial basement membrane dystrophy or Meesman's dystrophy, both in intensity and frequency of the recurrent corneal erosions and in the final reduction of visual acuity.

The disorder was described to recur in the corneal graft tissue of a patient with Reis–Bücklers dystrophy, 15 years after the keratoplasty (26).

The honeycomb dystrophy of Thiel and Behnke (22) and the anterior membrane dystrophy of Grayson and Wilbrandt (27) seem to be the same disease.

Diagnosis

The diagnosis of the dystrophies of the anterior limiting membrane is based on clinical manifestation including the family history of autosomal dominant transmission, the symptoms of variably blurred vision and recurrent episodes of pain, photophobia, tearing, and inflammation. The corneal abnormalities are found in the epithelium and in the region of Bowman's membrane.

The differences among the three disorders are listed in Table 1 and are drawn in Figure 1.

Pathology and Pathogenesis

Light and electron microscopic studies have been performed in all three disorders of the anterior limiting membrane.

In epithelial basement membrane dystrophy, three pathologic changes seem to represent the three basic clinical findings (28). A multilaminar basement membrane in abnormal quantities represents the fingerprintlike changes. Collagenous tissue in placoid or mushroom form is found in the space between the basal epithelial cells and Bowman's membrane. Inverted basal cells were found to desquamate into intra-epithelial pockets, representing the microcysts (28). The material between Bowman's and basement membranes is a fibrogranular protein (29). Production of a faulty multilaminar basement membrane may be the primary change of the disease (9). As a result, poor adherence to Bowman's membrane occurs, thereby causing recurrent erosions (3,13).

In Meesman's dystrophy, three pathologic changes have been described, and when present together, are specific for the disease (30). They are (1) cysts filled by a homogenous substance found near the epithelial surface; (2) scattered epithelial cells filled by an intracytoplasmic peculiar substance, which ultrastructurally is a fibrillo-granular material; and (3) a variably thickened epithelial basement membrane. The chemical substance of the intracytoplasmic substance in the epithelial cells is not known, but it has been suggested that the chemical composition is that of glycogen (3). These intracellular accumulations are probably the primary pathology of the disease, the rest being secondary changes (18).

The pathologic changes of Reis–Bücklers dystrophy are also characteristic. They occur more posteriorly than in the other two diseases; the subepithelial space, Bowman's membrane, and the anterior stroma are involved. Basal cell membrane, hemidesmosomes, and basement membranes of the epithelial cells seem largely absent (31). Dense collagen fibrils in conglomerates displace Bowman's membrane, which is absent in several areas. Characteristically, these deposits are composed of masses of "curly" filaments with a diameter of about 100 nm (25). The anterior stroma manifests degenerative keratocytes (31). The exact pathogenesis and the primary abnormality of the disease is yet to be discovered, but Perry and associates suggested that the primary disorder lies within the epithelial basal cell, which causes a secondary disintegration of Bowman's membrane. Then, as a response, curly filaments are produced by basal cells.

Using electron microscopy, Küchle and colleagues (23) found subepithelial fibrocellular tissue with an undulant configuration, absence of epithelial basement membrane, and "curly" collagen fibers.

Epidemiology and Genetics

Epithelial basement membrane dystrophy is a common disorder. It is estimated to affect almost 2% of the population (3). Its prevalence may be even much higher; if subclinical, asymptomatic cases are also accounted for, it may be quite frequent (32). Meesman's dystrophy and Reis–Bücklers dystrophy seem to be rare diseases; they are infrequently, if at all, diagnosed in the average ophthalmic practice.

All three diseases are transmitted by single autosomal dominant genes. Meesman's dystrophy shows complete penetrance in family studies (16,17) Behnke and Thiel (17) showed that the 120 patients with the disorder, living in Schleswig-Holstein, are descendants of a person living in 1620. Reis–Bücklers dystrophy is an autosomal dominant disorder, with complete or incomplete penetration autosomal (24). The variable expression and the occurrence of asymptomatic carriers of the gene make an accurate genetic study difficult.

Most reported families with Meesman's dystrophy are of German origin, but the disease was also described in a Saudi tribe (33). It is not clear whether Lisch corneal dystrophy (34) is the same entity as Meesman's dystrophy. The clinical appearance and mild symptomatology are similar, but this may be a genetically distinct entity transmitted by an X-linked gene (35).

Genetic counseling may be assisted by gene studies for K3 and K12 keratins (19,36) in cases of Meesman's dystrophy and of locus CDB2 on chromosome 10q23 for Thiel–Behnke dystrophy (24). A preliminary, comprehensive database of corneal gene expression was produced after microarray analysis (37). This should facilitate gene identification.

Management

Medical and Surgical

Medical treatment of the three aforementioned corneal dystrophies should be initiated in symptomatic cases. Usually this includes the use of lubricating agents, tear substitutes, and hyperosmotic agents. Both drops (more often used during the day) and ointments (more often used at night) can be applied. A multitude of commercial preparations are available. I usually find that the best preparation must be specifically selected for each patient, and that the response of individual patients varies for each preparation.

During the acute attack of a corneal erosion, patching along with cycloplegic and antibiotic preparations may be used. Soft contact lenses used as therapeutic bandage lenses were successful for more difficult cases (13). Corneal abrasion of the recurrent eroding area, together with lactic acid-induced, circumscribed inflammation, was also suggested (13). In cases of recurrent erosions not healed by all these conventional methods, a total superficial keratectomy and soft lens bandage has been successful in relieving symptoms in 85% of treated patients with epithelial basement membrane dystrophy (38).

In patients with Reis–Bücklers dystrophy, reduction of visual acuity with the progression of the disease is common and necessitates surgical treatment. In the past, lamellar or penetrating keratoplasty was performed. In some cases, a recurrence of the disease in the graft has been reported (26). Wood and associates (39) advised a simple surgical approach of removing the subepithelial fibrous tissue by scraping off the epithelium after using a cyclodialysis spatula to form a space and accomplish blunt dissection. This method seems to be effective for most patients with Reis–Bücklers dystrophy.

In the last decade, the excimer laser, in a procedure called phototherapeutic keratectomy (PTK), has been used use for the treatment of anterior corneal dystrophies. The objectives are to ablate corneal opacities, smooth out surface irregularities, heal corneal wounds, and improve visual acuity (40). Results seem effective, stable, and safe (41). The most common indication for this treatment is recurrent corneal erosion, mainly that of the epithelial basement membrane corneal dystrophy (40,42). However, one study indicated that in a substantial percentage, the disease recurs after laser (43). Of the treated patients 42% suffered recurrence in less than nine months (43). Other surgical methods were also suggested and are sometimes used. For prevention of recurrent corneal erosion, these other methods include stromal micropuncture of the Nd-YAG laser and a diamond burr superficial keratectomy (44).

Genetic Counseling

Counseling is based on the assumption of autosomal dominant inheritance meaning 50% chance of an affected child of either sex. The variable degree of expression of these disorders should be stressed. Gene studies can be performed.

CHROMOSOME 5q31 ASSOCIATED CORNEAL DYSTROPHIES

Description

Studies performed in recent years acknowledged the surprising fact that most of the classic autosomal dominant corneal dystrophies affecting the stroma result from mutations of a single locus mapped to chromosome 5q31. They include several types of granular corneal dystrophy, several types of lattice corneal dystrophy, and one variant of Thiel–Behnke corneal dystrophy. Figure 5 presents drawings of the main corneal dystrophies primarily affecting the stroma and Table 2 describes chromosome 5q31 associated dystrophies. At least nine different genes have been found to be responsible for corneal dystrophies (45). In addition, six other dystrophies have been located to specific chromosomal locations (45).

The Locus at Chromosome 5q31

Corneal dystrophies of this group were considered distinct clinical and genetic entities for many years. In 1994, Folberg and associates, after examining histopathologically 23 corneal buttons from two families with lattice corneal dystrophy and 13 corneal buttons from two families with granular corneal dystrophy, concluded that these two distinct entities are probably caused by mutations within one gene (46). The pathologic diagnosis in corneas clinically diagnosed as lattice corneal dystrophy, was lattice in six corneas, granular in six, and lattice/granular in nine. In the same year, Stone and associates (47) concluded that it is likely that lattice dystrophy type I, granular dystrophy, and Avellino corneal dystrophy, three phenetypically distinct entities, are caused by mutations in the same gene. Linkage analysis mapped the locus to chromosome 5q28.6. Later, Munier, Korvatska, and associates recovered the gene using a yeast artificial chromosome, named it BIGH3, mapped it to chromosome 5q31, and identified several mutations in families with four distinct clinical entities (48,49). The term stemming from human transforming growth factor beta-induced gene was therefore changed to TGFBI. The gene consists of 17 exons, coding for a unique protein of 683 aminoacids produced by both mesenchymal stromal keratocytes and corneal epithelial cells (50). The protein keratoepithelin can be found in numerous tissues. In the eye, the gene is expressed almost exclusively in the corneal epithelium and stromal keratocytes (50).

The Clinical and Genetic Types of TGFBI/BIGH3 Gene Associated Corneal Dystrophies

Granular corneal dystrophy (GCD) was described by Groenouw (1) and named the nodular dystrophy of Groenouw by Bücklers (2). It was also called Groenouw's type I corneal dystrophy. It is now often named Groenouw granular corneal dystrophy

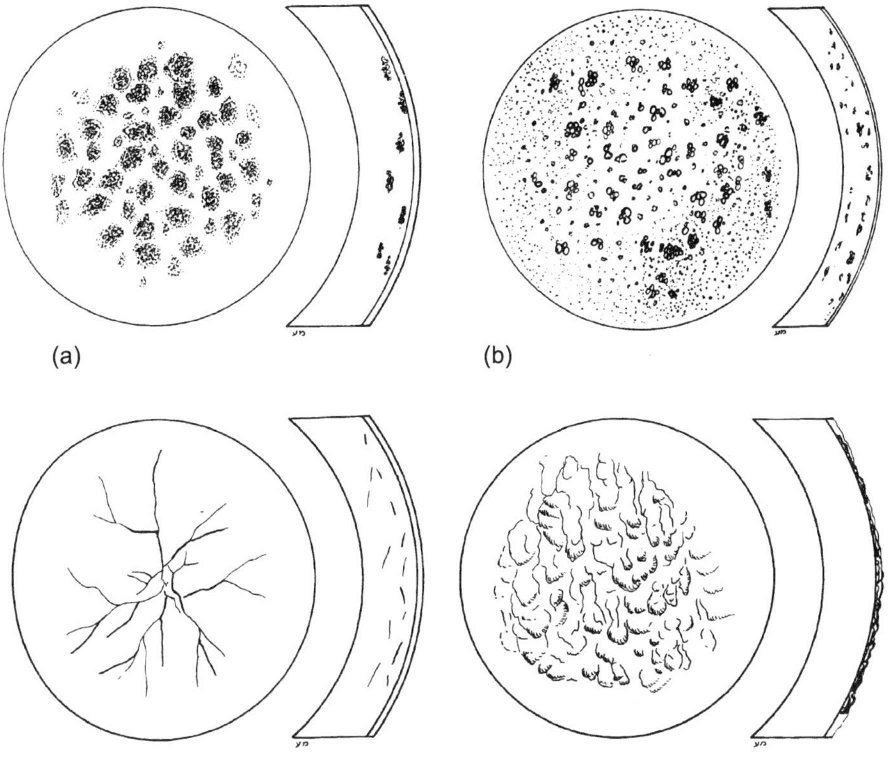

(a) (b) (c) (d)

Figure 5 The corneal dystrophies affecting mainly the stroma: (a) granular, (b) macular, (c) lattice; (d) gelatinous droplike, (e) central crystalline of Schnyder, (f) fleck, (g) central cloudy, (h) congenital hereditary stromal, (i) posterior amorphous, and (j) pre-Descemet membrane. (Drawings by M. Ivry.) Note that (e, see p. 40) may have a noncrystalline form manifested by hazy stroma and that (f) and (g) seem to be one disorder with variable manifestation.

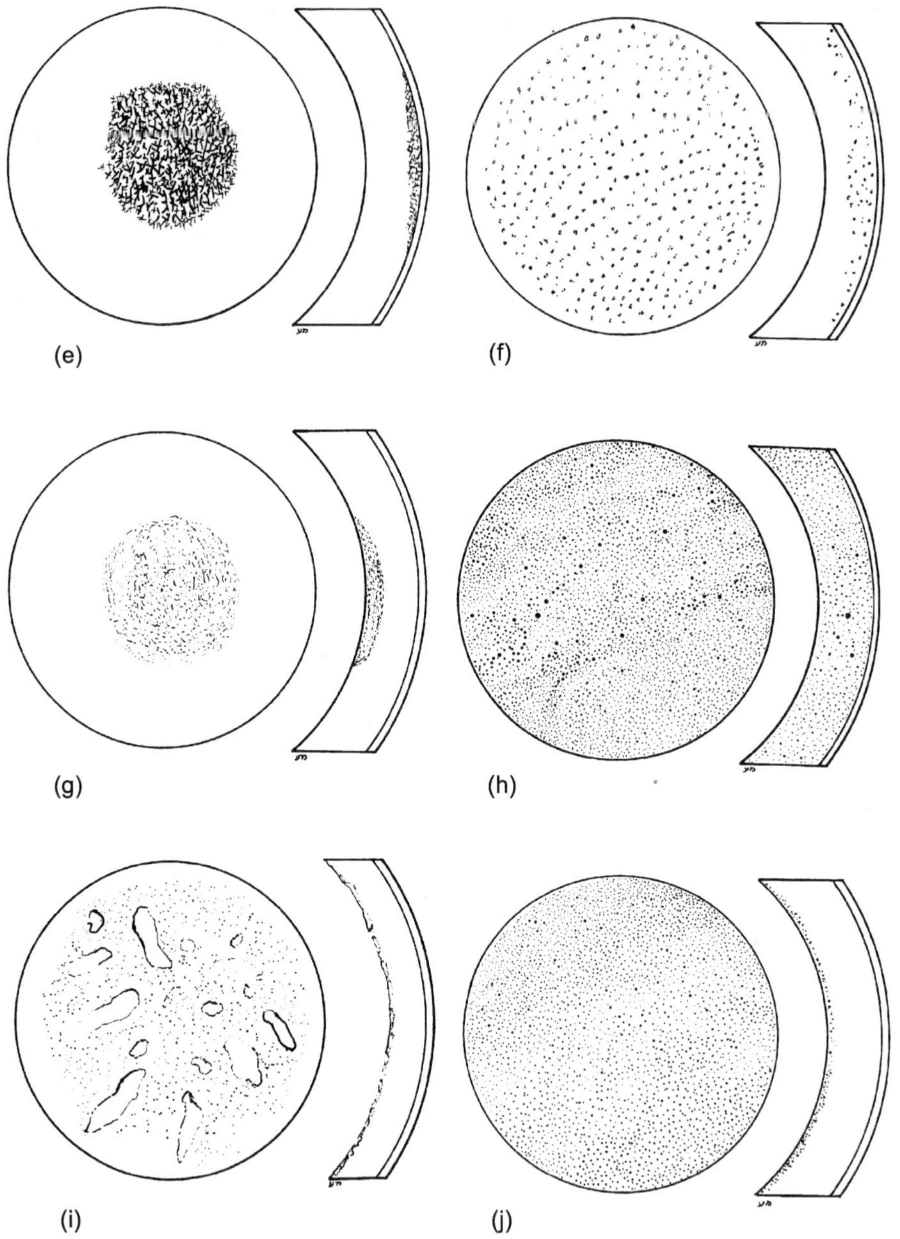

Figure 5 (*Continued*)

type I and marked CDGG1. It is transmitted by an autosomal dominant gene. It can be clinically detected by slit-lamp examination in the first decade of life, by the presence of large (0.1–0.4 mm), discrete, prominent opacities seen mainly in the superficial stroma. The stroma between the spots and in the corneal periphery is normal.

As the disease progresses, opacities increase in size and density and involve the deeper stroma, and the clear stroma between the spots becomes cloudy (51). At this stage, visual acuity is reduced and keratoplasty may be necessary when useful vision decreases.

Table 2 Comeal Dystrophies Associated with TGFBI Gene Mutations

Name/ symbol	Synonyms	OMIM (6)	Inheritance	Clinical findings: Early	Clinical findings: Late	Main pathological findings	Mutations
Granular corneal dystro-phy, CDGG1	Groenouw's type l	121900	AD	Large discrete opaque nodules	Stroma between nodules turns cloudy	Hyaline substance (noncollagenous protein) in extracellular pockets in stroma; rod- shaped structures	Arg555Trp
Lattice corneal dystrophy (LCD), type I CDL1	Biber–Haab–Dimmer	122200	AD	Short rodlike white or gray lines; recurrent erosion	Lines become thicker; opacification; scarring	Accumulation of amyloid in anterior stroma and subepithelial space, curly structures	Argl24Cys
Avellino corneal dystrophy (ACD)		601692	AD	Discrete opaque nodules and rod-like lines	Corneal erosion; haze of stroma	Granular-proteinaceous and amyloid	Argl24His
Superficial granular corneal dystrophy (SGCD)	Bowman type 1 corneal dystrophy CDB1 Reis–Bücklers	121900	AD	Large discrete nodules	Rapid coalescence of nodules	Absent Bowman; rod-shaped structures	Argl24Leu Arg555Gln 540 3bpdel Gly623Asp

(*Continued*)

Table 2 Comeal Dystrophies Associated with TGFBI Gene Mutations (*Continued*)

Name/symbol	Synonyms	OMIM (6)	Inheritance	Clinical findings: Early	Clinical findings: Late	Main pathological findings	Mutations
	CDRB						
Lattice corneal dystrophy type III A	LCD3A	—	AD	Thick lines of late onset	Corneal erosions	Amyloid deposits in stroma	Pro501Thr
Lattice corneal dystrophy type III B (French type)	LCD3B	—	AD	Thick lines of late onset	Corneal erosions	Amyloid deposits	Ala546Thr
Assymetric lattice corneal dystrophy	ALCD	—	AD	Lines, late onset	Corneal erosions	Amyloid deposits	His626Arg Asn622His
Lattice corneal dystrophy variant	CDL1 variant	—	AD	As in LCD type I	As in LCD type I	—	Leu518Pro Leu527Arg
Granular corneal dystrophy variant	CDGG1 variant	—	AD	As in LCD type I	As in LCD type I	—	Compound heterozygosity

Note: In all disorders: anterior stroma is mainly affected and in all the corneal periphery remains clear.

Variable expressivity occurs in GCD. Different affected members of the same family may show, to a certain extent, a variable course and severity of the corneal opacification. The interfamilial differences may be even greater. Forsius and associates (52) described five families with GCD in Finland. Four of these had mild disease, and their visual acuity never fell below reading ability. The cornea of the affected members showed opacities in the form of spots, bows, or lines. In the fifth family, the corneal flecks were smaller, but much denser, and some family members needed keratoplasty for reduced vision.

There is little doubt that the variable expressivity is related to different mutations in the TGFBI gene. Figure 6 is a photograph of a typical case of CDGG1 and

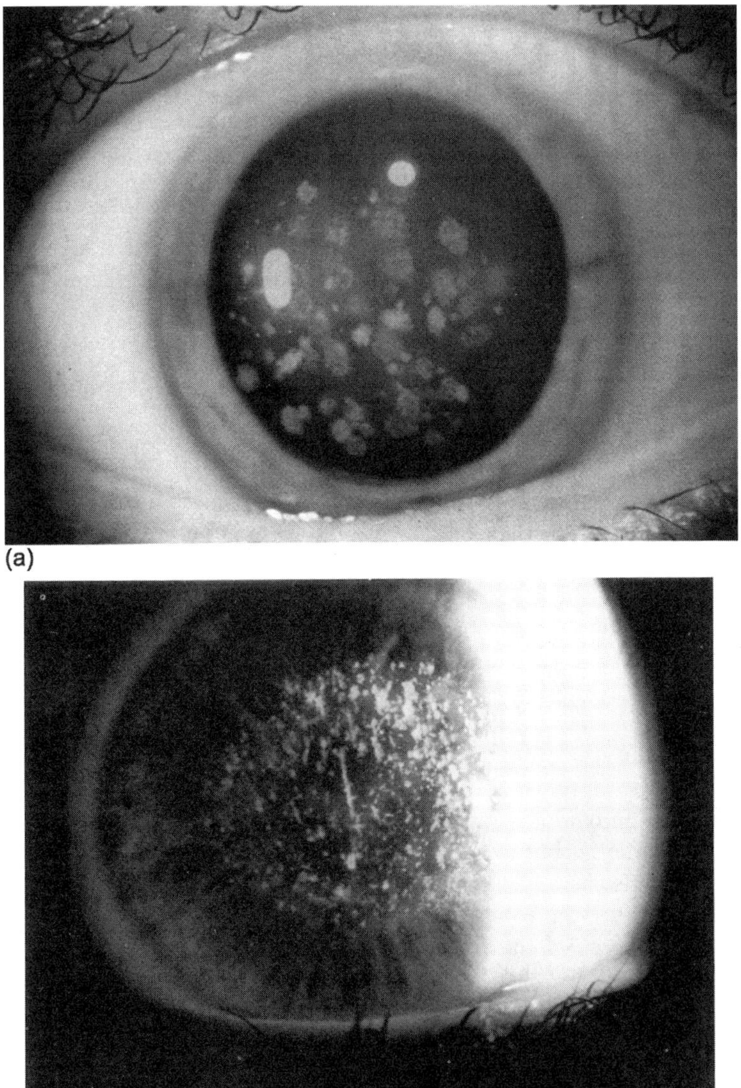

(a)

(b)

Figure 6 Granular corneal dystrophy. The nodules of opacification in the anterior stroma vary from (a) large to (b) small. (Courtesy of J. Sugar, MD, Chicago.)

Table 2 shows the clinical and pathologic findings of the stromal corneal dystrophies associated with mutations of the TGFBI gene.

The mutation of CDGG1 is Arg555Trp (the replacement of arginine by tryptophane at codon 555) (48,49,53–56). It is one of the more common macular dystrophies in Europeans, but is uncommon in Japanese (54).

Lattice Corneal Dystrophy

Lattice corneal dystrophy (LCD) was termed by Bücklers the lattice-like dystrophy of Haab (2) and, later, especially in Europe, lattice dystrophy of Biber–Haab–Dimmer, named after the authors who first described the condition (57). In 1967, Klintworth (58) identified the corneal deposits in LCD as amyloid substance and, thus, its nature as an inherited localized amyloidosis was clarified. More recently, the occurrence of other inherited varieties of corneal amyloidosis became known; therefore, classic LCD should best be termed lattice corneal dystrophy type I, as, in fact, it was called in several articles (59,60).

Corneal dystrophy lattice type I marked as CDL1 is caused by replacement of arginine by cysteine at codon 124 (Arg124Cys)(48,49,53,61). As it is an autosomal dominant disorder, heterozygotes show the classic appearance of the disorder. However, homozygotic occurrence was reported and its phenotypical expression is different (see later). Assymetric involvement is also known and even pure unilateral involvement of CDL1 was reported in several cases (62,63).

Characteristically, the corneal opacities occur in the form of thickened radiating lines resembling thick corneal nerves (Fig. 7). In the first and second decades of life, short, rodlike, white or gray lines can be seen in the anterior stroma. The stroma between the lines and the corneal periphery is clear. Later, the lines become progressively thicker, the epithelium becomes irregular, and there is some reduction in vision; then recurrent corneal erosions, with attacks of pain, frequently occur. White spots and stromal haze can then be seen between the radiating lattice lines, and the opacification of the cornea continues to involve the deeper stroma. When the central opacities become thick, corneal erosions stop recurring (13). At that stage, reduction in visual acuity usually necessitates keratoplasty.

Intrafamilial variability occurs. In one study of primary keratoplasties of 34 patients with LCD, the average age at surgery was 47 years, with a wide range of ages from 20 to 76 (64).

Interfamilial variability is even greater. Families were described with mild disease, very late onset of symptoms, and retention of useful vision into the seventh decade of life, with many individuals remaining asymptomatic (65). The disease is usually bilateral and symmetric, but unilateral cases have been described.

It is likely, that in some cases, the diagnosis of lattice corneal dystrophy or even LCD type I was erroneously given to a patient whose mutation in the TGFBI gene was not Argl24Cys and therefore the phenotypical appearance should be termed differently.

Keratoplasty usually has a favorable outcome, with good final visual acuity (64). In one study, 30 patients who were followed for up to 11 years after keratoplasty did not show any recurrence (57). In another study of 61 penetrating keratoplasties, 29 transplants (57) (48%) showed clinical signs of recurrent LCD after periods ranging from 3 to 26 years (66). Recurrence usually took the form of subepithelial opacities or anterior stromal haze, or both, with lattice figures rarely seen (66).

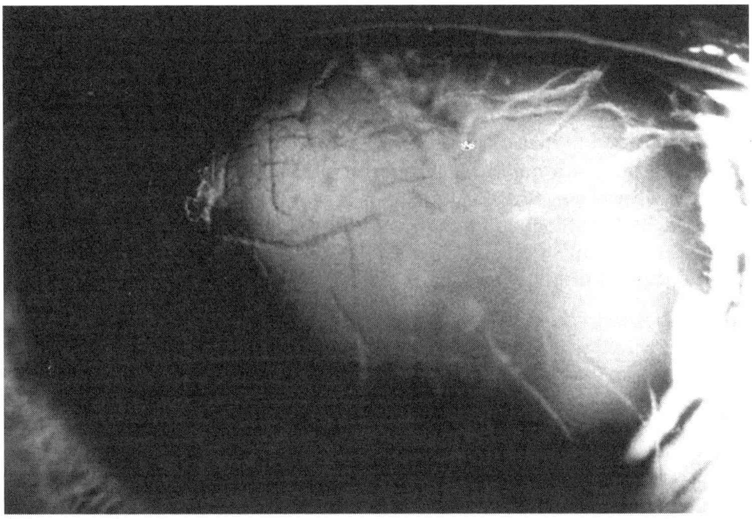

(a)

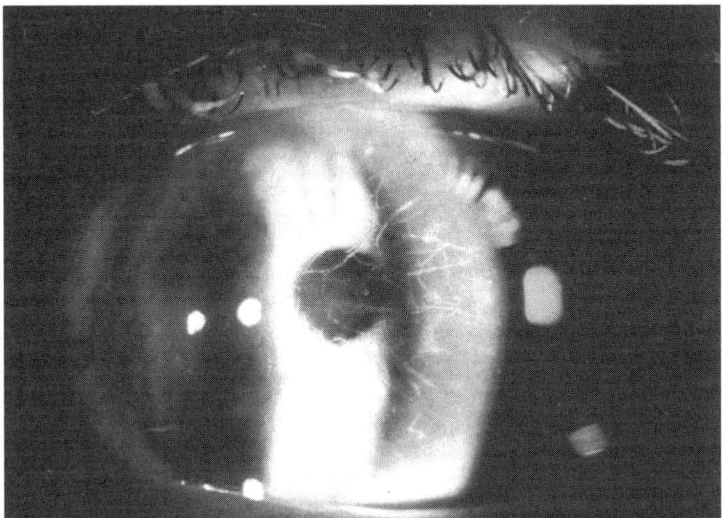

(b)

Figure 7 Lattice corneal dystrophy, type I. Note (a) the typical lattice-like configuration in high magnification and (b) the opacities between the lattice lines. (Courtesy of J. Sugar, MD, Chicago.)

Avellino Corneal Dystrophy

Avellino corneal dystrophy (ACD) (Fig. 8) presents the combined deposits of both granular and lattice forms. This was already shown in the pathologic studies of corneal buttons by Folberg and colleagues (46) with the finding of granular-proteinaceous and amyloid deposits in the cornea. The mutation identified in the TGFBI/BIGH3 gene was a replacement of arginine by histidine at codon 124 (Argl24His). It was suggested by Korvatska and associates (49) that amyloid-related phenotypes carry a codon 124 mutation while nonamyloid (granular) phenotypes carry a codon 555 mutation (49).

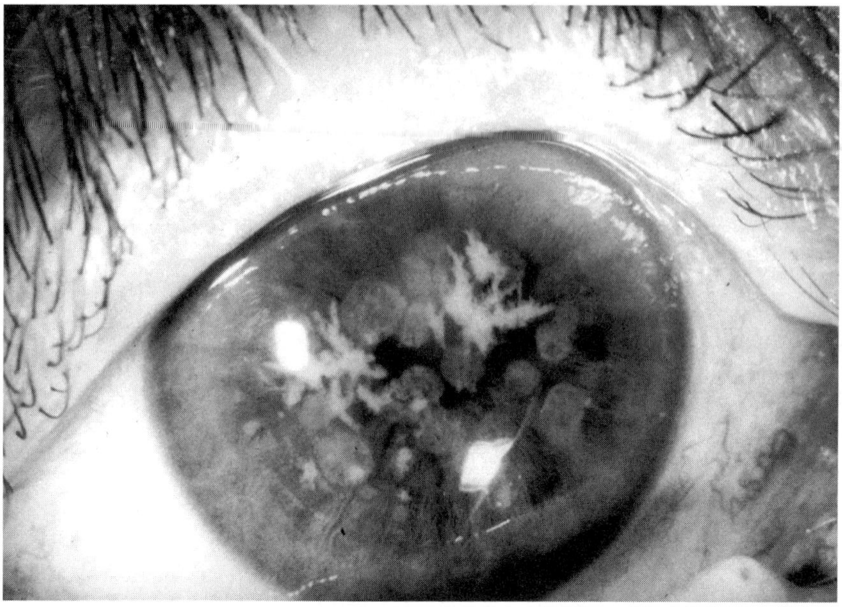

Figure 8 Avellino corneal dystrophy. Both granular and lattice-like deposits can be seen, (Courtesy of J. Sugar, MD, Chicago.)

Avellino CD (ACD) shows pathologically both rod-shaped bodies and amyloid deposits (50).

Avellino corneal dystrophy was first described in members of families who originated from Avellino in Italy (67). Later it was shown that the disorder ACD with the same Argl24His mutation is not uncommon among corneal dystrophies in Japan (54,68,69). In one study, it was responsible for 72% of Japanese patients with corneal dystrophies (70).

In another study (71), 91% of Japanese patients clinically diagnosed as granular corneal dystrophy turned out to carry the Argl24His mutation of ACD. Today, therefore, two clusters of families are known: those who originate from Italy, Avellino and other places in Campania (72), a family from Germany, and the second cluster from Japan.

Phenotypically, ACD shows findings of both granular type I and lattice type I. In younger patients, granular deposits are manifested in the cornea. Later in life, anterior stromal haze appears between deposits and affects vision (67). Also, the lattice component appears later in life (72). At that time glare and disturbed night vision may be marked, and visual acuity may become reduced up to 20/200 (72). Recurrent corneal erosions are infrequent and PKP is the exception (71). The periphery of the cornea is relatively free from deposits (73).

Noninherited Corneal Amyloidoses

Clinical and histopathologic studies showed that corneal amyloidosis may occur as a nonhereditary degeneration of the cornea of unknown etiology (74,75) or as a secondary amyloid degeneration after injury or another ocular disease (76). Glasslike deposits in the deeper layers of the cornea, with surrounding normal stroma, without visual dysfunction, can be found by clinical examination (74). Various terms were used for such amyloid degeneration, including posterior crocodile shagreen and polymorphic amyloid degeneration. This condition can be confused with LCD and other corneal dystrophies. It is probably age-related.

Superficial Granular Corneal Dystrophy

This rather rare condition is caused by Argl24Leu mutations in the TGFBI/BIGH3 gene. Granular deposits in the superficial layers of the cornea are detected by histopathology (77). Superficial granular corneal dystrophy (SGCD) is probably the same condition named as corneal dystrophy of Bowman's layer type I (CDB1), also referred to as Reis-Bücklers corneal dystrophy (original form) (78) and as the superficial variant of granular corneal dystrophy type 1 (CDB1) (79). Histopathology reveals deposits in the anterior layers of stroma with the often absent Bowman's layer. By electron microscopy, irregular electron-dense, rod-shaped structures are seen in the extracellular space (78).

Onset is early, often in the first decade of life. Perforating keratoplasty may be needed by the early 20s (56). The phenotype of Japanese patients with the same mutation of Argl24Leu was reported to be similar, with early onset of recurrent corneal erosions, rod-shaped deposits near Bowman's membrane, and early severe deterioration (80). This mutation has been shown to be similar or identical to the original Reis-Bücklers geographic corneal dystrophy (81). It is now commonly referred to as Thiel–Behnke corneal dystrophy In this disease, severe rapid progression of corneal opacities occurs along with severe impairment of vision in the teens (81) (Fig. 9).

A different mutation at codon 555, (in which arginine is replaced by glutamine (Arg555Gln)), is traditionally considered to be the cause of Reis-Bücklers corneal dystrophy with milder severity (48,49,54). Okada and associates (81) and Mashima and associates (70) considered the Arg555Gln mutation to cause Reis-Bücklers

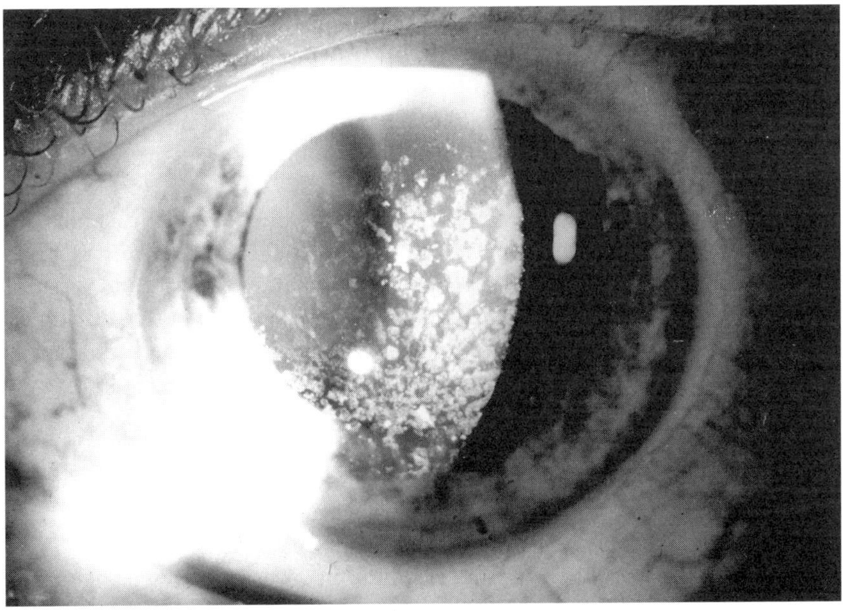

Figure 9 Superficial granular corneal dystrophy, Reis–Bücklers corneal dystrophy. Note the large coalescing opaque nodules in the superficial stroma. (Courtesy, of J. Sugar, MD, Chicago.)

corneal dystrophy (CDRB), also named CDB2. The Argl24Leu mutation caused the original German form of CDRB, or the "geographic form." Two additional mutations caused a similar disease, which Afshari and colleagues also considered CDRB (55). These had a three-pair deletion at codon 540 (82) and a Gly623Asp missense mutation (55). Clearly, allelic heterogeneity exists, and since 1996 (83) it has been debated whether each of these diseases is a separate entity or one disease. In some articles, CDB1 is referred to as CDRB and CDB2 is referred to as Thiel–Behnke corneal dystrophy.

Other Lattice and Granular Corneal Dystrophies

LCD type II or lattice corneal dystrophy of Meretoja will be described separately as it is caused by mutations in another gene. Several mutations in the TGFBI/BIGH3 gene are associated with a lattice-like corneal dystrophy and manifest deposits of amyloid material in the stroma. Lattice corneal dystrophy type III is another term used for gelatinous droplike corneal dystrophy, a recessive disease which will be discussed later. Lattice corneal dystrophy (LCD) type IIIA (LCD3A) was first described in two families in Sicily and given this name because it resembled the phenotypic appearance of LCD type III (84). Yamamoto and colleagues described it in Japanese families and identified a Pro501Thr mutation in the TGFBI gene in all affected family members (85). The disorder is of late onset, sometimes in the eighth, ninth, or tenth decade of life. Characteristically, thick ropy lattice lines are seen in the stroma and corneal erosions are common (85).

LCD3A-like disorder was clinically diagnosed in a large French family and found to have an Ala546Thr mutation in the TGFBI gene (86). This French lattice CDIIIA is clinically similar to LCD3A of the Japanese families. Onset is late with deposits seen beneath Bowman's membrane and stroma. Klintworth refers to this disorder as LCD type IIIB (45).

Assymetric lattice corneal dystrophy was the name given to a corneal dystrophy in three families. The affected members had disease onset in middle life. The cornea manifested recurrent erosions, progressive deepening of stromal involvement, and asymmetry of progression. In two families a His626Arg mutation was identified. In the third family, a Asn622His was identified. Both mutations were missense mutations in exon 14 of the TGFBI gene (87).

Endo and colleagues (88) described a condition phenotypically similar to LCD1 and identified a novel mutation Leu518Pro in exon 12 of the TGFBI gene. Onset of the disorders is early, and it becomes symptomatic in the second or third decade in life. Initially, only the central cornea is affected. Later the periphery becomes cloudy and corneal transplants may be needed. The condition should more accurately be termed LCD type I variant. A similar phenotypic condition was described with a nearby mutation of Leu527Arg (88).

Dighiero and colleagues (89) described an atypical variant of granular corneal dystrophy caused by association of two mutations in the TGFBI gene. The first was Argl24Leu, the mutation of classic granular corneal dystrophy and the second a novel mutation causing deletion of threonine and glutamic acid of codons 125 and 126. Phenotypically, the condition was intermediate in severity between the classic (milder) and superficial (severe) variant. Round or snowflake-like deposits can be seen in the anterior layer of the cornea (89). This condition was described in a large French family and was termed French granular corneal dystrophy variant (79).

Homozygotic Patients with TGFBI Mutations

A mutation of the kerato-epithelin gene is clinically expressed only in the cornea. Therefore, even in the homozygous state of this autosomal dominant disorder the expression remains local and, of course, is not lethal. Several cases of such homozygous condition were reported and their phenotypes seemed similar. The condition is much more severe than in the heterozygous state. It was described with the Argl24-His mutation (90–93) and the Arg555Trp mutation (94). The homozygous state, typically has a very early onset with severe symptoms and visual reduction requiring keratoplasty in the first decade of life (90,91). The corneal cloudiness involved a spot-like opacity or a reticular opacity with round translucent spaces in the anterior stroma (93). Early disease involvement of the corneal transplant seems the rule in homozygous cases (92,94), thus causing an extremely difficult clinical problem.

Diagnosis and Laboratory Tests

Most patients with a dystrophy affecting the stroma can be diagnosed by clinical evaluation, which will include history-taking of the dystrophic progression, a careful biomicroscopic examination, the family history, and examination of first-grade relatives. In other cases, the diagnosis, based on clinical grounds only, may be erroneous, and a number of such cases were reported. The correct diagnosis was made by histopathologic studies of the removed corneal button.

Granular corneal dystrophy had the clinical appearance of Reis-Bücklers dystrophy in two young patients without a positive family history (95). The rapid progression of the lesions, early loss of vision, and the anteriorly located deposits at Bowman's membrane, misled the ophthalmologist to diagnose Reis-Bücklers dystrophy. The opposite diagnostic error may also occur. Figure 4 presents a patient with Reis–Bücklers dystrophy in whom a clinical diagnosis of granular corneal dystrophy was made (96). Four patients, stemming from four Italian families, had the clinical appearance of granular corneal dystrophy, but histopathologic analysis showed the deposits to be of the amyloid nature of lattice corneal dystrophy (97).

Lattice corneal dystrophy (LCD) is easy to diagnose when the typical lattice-like changes are seen. However, these signs are not seen in young children and in the late stages of involution when scarring of the cornea masks the lines. The early signs found in seven children, ranging in age from 3 to 13 years were as follows: (1) subepithelial round or oval whitish opacities, (2) diffuse axial anterior stromal haze, and (3) anterior stromal dots and fine filamentary lines (98). Any of these signs may indicate the presence of LCD. The absence or disappearance of lines in the late stages may cause the erroneous diagnosis of GCD (99).

On the other hand, the mild variant of LCD can also be misdiagnosed. In one family, no fewer than five affected members were diagnosed as suffering from herpes simplex virus (65)!

Molecular genetics may soon play a major role in accurately diagnosing the different entities of corneal dystrophies. The identification of the involved mutation enables the determination of the progress and a better management.

Pathology and Pathogenesis

The availability of tissue of dystrophic corneas, mainly through keratoplasties, has enabled extensive pathologic studies. These included light microscopy, electron microscopy, histochemistry, immunohistology, and tissue cultures. These will be presented briefly.

In granular corneal dystrophy, a hyaline substance and an eosinophihc granular material, can be found in extracellular pockets, mainly in the anterior stroma and in the subepithelial space in front of Bowman's membrane (Fig. 10). The deposits consist principally of noncollagenous protein, containing tyrosine, tryptophan, arginine, and sulfur-containing amino acids (100).

The epithelium has variable thickness and the basement membrane is missing in many places. Electron microscopy shows deposits of small rods of electron-dense material (101). The origin of the abnormal protein is unknown. Garner suggested in 1969 that the protein could originate in the corneal epithelium, in the keratocytes, or from an extracorneal source (100). Some evidence supports the stromal keratocyte origin, as the electron-dense material was found near these cells (101). Other studies support the epithelial origin of the abnormal deposits. In one study, the rod-shaped electron-dense structures were found within the cytoplasm of epithelial cells, mostly within the basal epithelial cells, but also within the wing cells (102). In addition, extracellular deposits were conspicuous within the epithelial basement membrane (102). In another study, similar involvement of the epithelium, subepithelial tissue, and anterior stroma was found (103). The granular deposits are electron-dense material surrounded by microfibrils of 8–10 nm (51). The stored material seemed to be a microfibrillar protein, and increased amounts of 65 and 110 kDa proteins and of phospholipids were found (51).

LCD type 1 was shown to be localized amyloidosis by Seitelberger and Nemetz in 1961 (104).

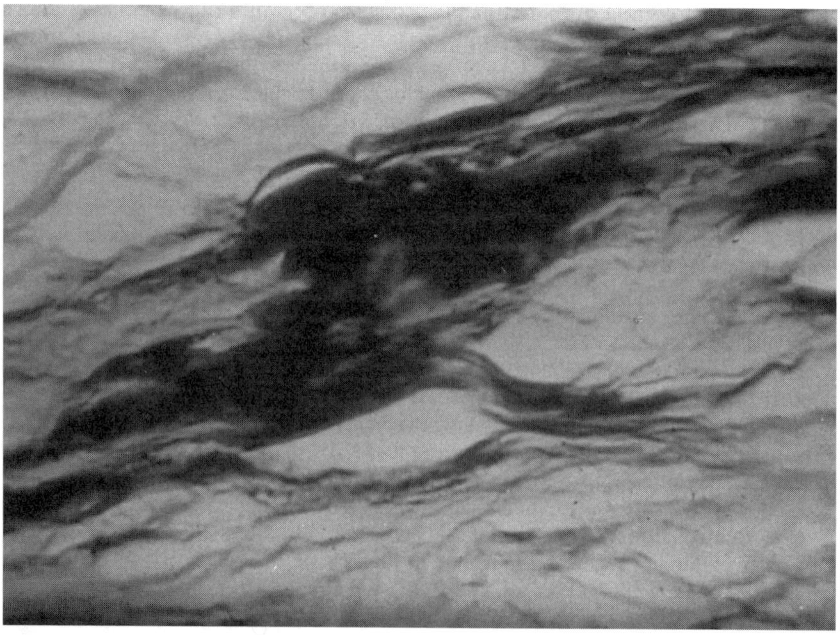

Figure 10 Histopathologic appearance of a cornea with granular corneal dystrophy, displaying the typical hyaline deposits between stromal lamellae. These were stained red with Masson trichromatic stain.

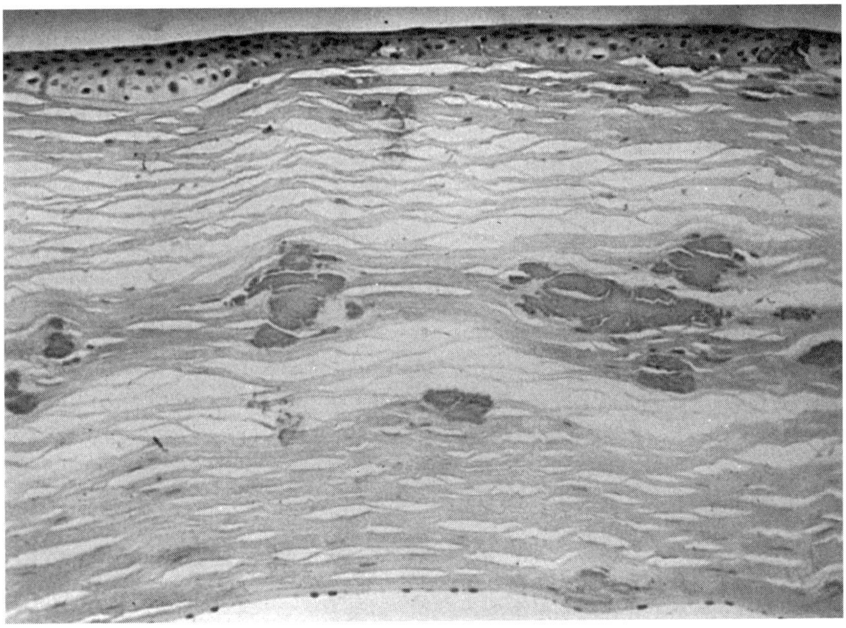

Figure 11 Histopathologic appearance of a cornea with LCD. Note the large deposits of the abnormal amyloid material in the midstroma and multiple small deposits elsewhere.

By light microscopy, the corneal stroma shows multiple deposits of a eosinophilic substance, especially in the anterior stroma. A similar substance is found in the subepithelial space anterior to Bowman's membrane (Fig. 11). Special stains show it to be amyloid (58). Electron microscopy shows the presence of electron-dense, nonbranching fibrils 8–10 nm in diameter, without periodicity in the extracellular spaces (58,105). These were assumed to be produced by the keratocytes in addition to normal collagen fibers (58) or, possibly, instead of normal collagen (105). Francois and Victoria-Troncoso suggested (105) that LCD is a primary disease of the lysosomes of the keratocytes, which then, by autolysis, destroy the keratocytes and the extracellular collagen, which is, in turn, replaced by amyloid. In such a case, the production of amyloid could be related to activation of mononuclear cells (107). On the other hand, some evidence indicates that the stromal extracellular deposits might be the product of keratocytic synthetic activity and that the filamentous material in the basement membrane is a product of epithelial cells (99). By electron microscopy, LCD can be readily distinguished from granular dystrophy, by the presence of distinct filaments in the former and a homogenous hyaline mass in the latter (99).

The histologic and electron microscopic findings in all types of amyloidosis are uniform (108). Light microscopy shows a homogneous, eosinophlic, extracellular substance, and electron microscopy displays intertwined, randomly arrayed, nonbranching fibrils 7.5–10 nm in diameter (108). However, amyloid is chemically heterogenous and probably has a different chemical composition for each type of amyloidosis.

Several studies attempted to elucidate the chemical composition of amyloid in LCD. In one study (109), both AA protein and AP protein were found in the amyloid deposits. AA protein is unrelated to immunoglobulins and is associated with secondary amyloidosis, especially with familial Mediterranean fever, whereas AP protein is related to the light chain of immunoglobulins and is a structural protein found in the plasma and tissues in both primary and secondary amyloidosis (109). Another study could not confirm the presence of AA protein in eight LCD corneas studied (110). The abnormal deposits were found to consist, in part, of glycoconjugates containing oligosaccharides (111). The deposits have a significant linkage with haptoglobulin (5).

The determination that GCDs and LCDs are related disorders and caused by mutations of the same gene enabled a better understanding of all corneal dystrophies and a better classification. The pathologic hallmark of rod-shaped bodies is found in granular dystrophy, in the superficial variant of granular corneal dystrophy, and in the French variant of granular corneal dystrophy. Curly fibers are found in Thiel–Behnke corneal dystrophy (CDB2, CDRB); amyloid deposits in LCD1, in assymetric LCD, and in French LCDIIIA; rod-shaped bodies with amyloid deposits are found in Avellino corneal dystrophy (79) and in the superficial variant of granular corneal dystrophy (112). Immunolocalization of keratoepithelin, the protein product of TGFBI/BIGH3 gene, showed strongest response in the Bowman layer and less at stromal interlamellar junctions (113). In all TGFBI-associated dystrophies the pathological deposits are found in the area of the Bowman membrane and anterior stroma associated with keratocytes (53,78,114). The function of keratoepithelin in the normal cornea is unknown, but it is assumed to be important in cell adhesion (50). Confocal microscopy provides better resolution than biomicroscopy and allows, in vivo, a better localization of the deposits (115).

Management

Patients with symptoms stemming from epithelial desquamation should be treated as was outlined for the dystrophies of the anterior limiting membranes. Treatments include tear substitutes, lubricants, hyperosmotic topical agents, and, occasionally, soft contact lenses.

For progressive stromal dystrophies of this group, keratoplasty may be necessary. The entities may be classified into early-onset, rapidly progressing, severe types such as the superficial variant of granular dystrophy or homozygotic patients, and mild types such as the classic granular, classic lattice, asymmetric type, and others. An intermediate type also exists that includes the French variant of granular dystrophy and others. Keratoplasty is usually needed in the first group.

The results of keratoplasty are usually good, with a high percentage of successful results and good visual acuity (64). Recurrence of the disorder in the graft may be a problem, but it usually takes many years before the patient again becomes handicapped. In such cases, repeated grafting may be necessary (64,66). A simple technique for removal of the recurring deposits of GCD in grafts was advised by Lempert and coauthors (116). These authors used forceps and an interposed cyclodialysis spatula in front of Bowman's membrane to incise and lift the opaque epithelium and deposits (116). Re-epithelialization occurred in 5 days.

Genetic counseling should be given according to the genetic transmission as outlined in the foregoing discussion. The diagnosis must be properly made and the patient's family examined. The different subtypes and the variability in expressivity of these diseases should be taken into consideration. Prenatal diagnosis is not yet possible.

A multicenter study of 164 pediatric keratoplasties of all etiologies indicated a relatively high initial success rate with a subsequent increasing failure rate (117).

Graft survival after 1 year was 80% and reduced to 67% at two years (117). Similarly, long-term results in adult keratoplasties are far below the usual results for this successful operation. Recurrence rate for granular corneal dystrophy was reported as 43–94% after three to five years and for LCDs 38% after nine years (118).

Donor-derived limbal stem cells may remain as donor-derived epithelial cells on the surface of the host cornea for several or many years in some cases. These stem cells may be obtained from a donor transplant or from a layer of cultivated cells and transplanted in the denuded limbal area (119,120). In successful cases, the donor-origin epithelium will contain the wild-type gene. This may be a long-term solution for prevention of recurrency after transplants in cases of corneal dystrophies (119).

Another approach to corneal surgery is limbokeratoplasty. In this procedure, eccentric trephination of the donor graft is performed, so as to include about 40% of the limbus of the donor transplant. This eccentric donor graft is fitted into a central trephination of the recipient (121). Sundmacher and colleagues (121) performed nine operations, five on GCDs and four on LCD (121). Immunosuppression by administration of systemic cyclosporine for six months was given and topical corticosteroids were administered indefinitely. Successful results were reported (121). Another possible approach, not yet performed in humans, could be a virally transduced keratolimbal autograft containing the wild-type gene transplanted into the limbal area of the diseased cornea (122). We may well be at the beginning of an era of the therapeutic use of limbal stem cell transplantation for severe corneal dystrophies (118).

The results of treatment by Excimer laser of corneal dystrophies primarily affecting the stroma seem much worse than the results of this treatment in dystrophies of the anterior limiting membranes. Most researchers consider this treatment contraindicated.

In one study, PTK gave good results in a mild heterozygous case. A severe, homozygous case of Argl24His mutations in the TGFBI gene had poor results with rapid and severe recurrence (123). In all patients operated by LASIK (124,125), Avellino corneal dystrophy increased in severity with recurrence.

Genetic counseling is based on the assumption that all TGFBI/BIGH3 associated dystrophies are transmitted by the autosomal dominant mode with practically full penetrance. Great interfamilial variability (52) indicates that different mutations of the same gene, allelic heterogeneity, are now known to exist. Prognosis is different in mutations causing a mild variant, such as the classic type of granular dystrophy, or a severe variant, such as the superficial variant of granular dystrophy.

The identification of the exact mutation in the TGFBI gene, is now an essential step in properly diagnosing and advising the patient. Prenatal diagnosis may be used in severe cases.

AUTOSOMAL RECESSIVE CORNEAL DYSTROPHIES PRIMARILY AFFECTING THE STROMA

Description

Two major corneal dystrophies transmitted by the autosomal recessive mode primarily affect the stroma. These are macular corneal dystrophy and gelatinous drop-like corneal dystrophy. Both are relatively severe and often require corneal transplants. The third LCD type III is a milder disorder (Fig. 2; Table 3).

Table 3 Autosomal Recessive Corneal Dystrophies

Name	Synonyms	OMIM (6)	Inheritance	Clinical findings: Early	Clinical findings: Late	Part of stroma mainly affected	Periphery of cornea	Main pathological Findings	Chromosomal location	Gene	Mutations
Macular corneal dystrophy MCDC1[a]	Groenouw's type 2	217800	AR	Small white-gray spots, photophobia, corneal thinning	Spots coalesce into large nodules with intense stromal cloudiness	Anterior	Affected	Accumulation of a glycosaminoglycanlike substance in keratocytes, stroma and histiocytes	16q22	CHST6 (sulphonyl-transferase)	Many, missense, deletions, insertions
Gelatinous droplike[b] dystrophy CDGDL GDLD	Primary familial amyioidosis	204870	AR	Photophobia, pain, superficial opacities	Gelatinous subepithelial mulberrylike masses	Anterior	Clear	Massive accumulation of amyloid in subepithelial space	1p32	M1S1	GLU118Stop (78%) and others
LCD type 3	—	—	AR	Thick short radiating lines	Mild gradual progression	Anterior	Clear (narrow rim)	As in type 1, but epithelium and Bowman's membrane better preserved	?	?	?

[a]Three varieties exist: type1: keratan sulfate-negative; type 2: keratan sulfate-positive; type1A: KS-negative but positive in keratocytes.
[b]Common in Japan.

The Clinical and Genetic Types

Macular Corneal Dystrophy and the Sulphotransferase (CHST6) Gene

Macular corneal dystrophy (MCD), also called Groenouw's type II corneal dystrophy or corneal dystrophy of Fehr, is the only autosomal recessive disorder of this group. It is usually much more severe than granular corneal dystrophy. The patient, although asymptomatic, shows by slit-lamp multiple small white-gray nodules or spots in the superficial stroma in the first decade of life (Fig. 12).

Gradually, the disease progresses by coalescence of the multiple spots into larger nodules, with intense cloudiness between the nodules, and by involvement of all layers of the stroma and of the corneal periphery. Most patients lose useful vision and need keratoplasty in about the third decade of life (17). Photophobia is a common and peculiar feature of MCD, despite uncommon recurrent corneal erosions (17). Corneal sensitivity is reduced, and corneal thinning seems to be a constant feature. Donnenfeld and associates found (126), by pachymetry, a central corneal thickness ranging from 0.36 to 0.45 mm, with a mean of 0.45 mm (normal 0.51 mm) in six patients with MCD.

MCD is one of the more common corneal dystrophies. The incidence varies, depending on the population gene frequency and rate of consanguinity. MCD comprises between 10% and 75% of all corneal dystrophies (127), with the highest known rate occurring in Iceland (128).

Vance and colleagues (129) mapped the locus of MCD in American and Icelandic families by linkage analysis to chromosome 16q22. Based on immunohistochemical studies two subgroups of MCD were diagnosed, which later were divided into three subgroups (127–134). MCD was found to be caused by a defect in the biosynthesis of a keratan sulfate-containing proteoglycan (129). In MCD type I there is typically a virtual absence of keratan sulfate in the serum or in the cornea. In MCD type II serum, keratan sulfate responds normally, while in the cornea, the corneal accumulates demonstrate antigenic reaction to keratan sulfate (127–129). A subtype of

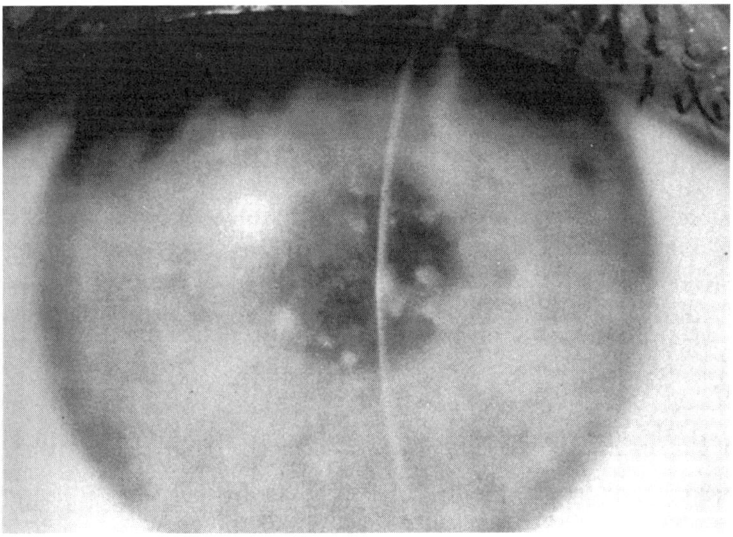

Figure 12 MCD. Note the nodules of opacification (best seen opposite the black pupil) and the diffuse cloudiness of the whole cornea. (Courtesy of J. Sugar, MD, Chicago.)

MCD type I, named MCDIA, demonstrates a strong positive reaction to keratan sulfate antibodies only at the stromal keratocytes (132). Otherwise its immunological responses are similar to those in MCD I. Linkage analysis showed that all types of MCD are linked to the locus at chromosome 16q22 (129). It is likely that the three types are caused by different allelic mutations on the same gene. Klintworth and associates (132) studied MCD in Saudi Arabia and demonstrated that the majority, 56%, were MCD type I, 30% type Ia, and 12% type II. A somewhat similar distribution was found in Germany (134). The subtypes were determined to be allelic, as demonstrated by the fact that families reported with some siblings with MCD I and others with MCD II (127). A genealogical study in Iceland demonstrated that all subtypes stem from the same family with a common ancestor in the 15th century (128). In 1997, Hassell and Klintworth (131) suspected that the enzyme sulfotransferase for *N*-acetylglucosamine is deficient and causes the disease. In 2000, Akama and associates identified the gene for carbohydrate sulphotransferase 6 CHST6 (135). The gene encodes the enzyme *N*-acetylglucosamine-6-sulfotransferase. Several missense mutations that inactivate the gene in the gene were identified in MCD type I. Large deletions or insertions upstream of CHST6 were identified in MCD type II. Studies performed in Iceland and in the United Kingdom identified several different missense mutations and insertions. Patients were homozygotic or compound heterozygotic, and the mutations were likely to cause loss of function of the sulfotransferase enzyme (136,137).

No correlation exists between the phenotypic appearance of the cornea and the specific subtype of MCD.

The results of keratoplasty for corneas with MCD are better than in other corneal dystrophies. Recurrence of the disease after keratoplasty is rare but has been reported, usually many years after the original operation (138,139). In one patient with MCD type II, the cornea became opaque 49 years after the original penetrating keratoplasty (140).

Gelatinous Droplike Corneal Dystrophy and the M1S1 Gene

This dystrophy is a localized corneal amyloidosis, which is clinically and genetically distinct from LCD. It is rather rare, except in Japan, where it was extensively studied. Gelatinous droplike dystrophy of the cornea is probably the most used term, but other names were also used, including primary familial amyloidosis of the cornea (76,141), familial subepithelial amyloidosis (141), and amyloid corneal dystrophy, Japanese type (6).

Gelatinous droplike dystrophy is transmitted as an autosomal recessive disorder. It starts in the first or second decade of life with severe symptoms of photophobia, lacrimation, and pain. Epithelial erosions may be present. Characteristically, central, raised, subepithelial gelatinous masses resembling a mulberry are seen (Fig. 13). These changes are progressive; visual acuity is reduced early in the course of the disease, and the patient often needs keratoplasty in the third decade of life.

Gelatinous droplike corneal dystrophy (GDLCD) is a severe disease leading to visual reduction early in life. Shimazaki and associates studied seven GDLCD patients, followed up for a mean period of 21 years. A total of 35 keratoplasties were performed, each after a severe recurrence of the disease (142). In each case, subepithelial haze was the first sign of recurrence; amyloid deposition was seen after a few years. There was a high incidence of postoperative complications, such as wound dehiscence, glaucoma, and cataract (142). GDLCD is transmitted by an autosomal

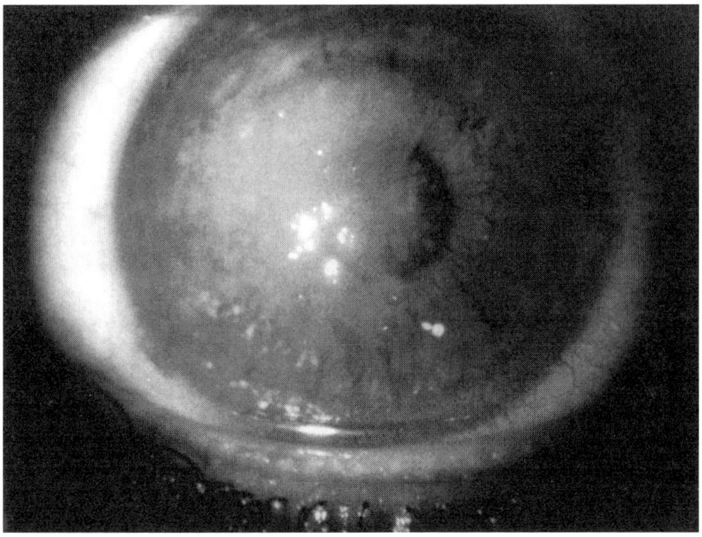

Figure 13 Gelatinous drop-like corneal dystrophy. Note the typical mulberry-like opacity. (Courtesy of J. Sugar, MD, Chicago.)

recessive gene (76,143). The search for the causative gene led to the negation of the 5q31 locus for this dystrophy (144) and to identification of the responsible gene mapped to chromosome 1p32 (145). The disease-associated gene is M1S1, considered a carcinoma-associated antigen. Four different nonsense mutations in this gene were identified in Japan, where there is a high predilection to GDLCD (145). The most common mutation was Gl118Stop found in 82.5% of Japanese GDLCD patients. A similar high percentage of this mutation is found in GDLCD patients in other populations (146), with 6 other mutations accounting for 20% of all patients (145–147).

The gene M1S1 is expressed in many tissues in the body, such as the comea, kidneys, lungs, pancreas, prostate, and placenta. Its function is not well understood (145). It has a single exon and encodes a 35.7 kD protein predicted to contain 323 amino acids. In disease, the mutated, truncated protein aggregates in the perinuclear region (145).

The name M1S1 stands for membrane component, chromosome 1, surface marker 1. The former name TACSTD2 referred to "tumor-associated calcium signal transducer 2." However, no excessive incidence of tumors was reported in patients with GDLCD. Gelatinous drop-like corneal dystrophy may have variable expressivity. For unknown reasons, the disease may have a different expressivity in two members of a single family, in spite of both having the same mutation in the M1S1 gene. Two brothers with the same M1S1 gene mutation Gln1118Stop suffered, one from a severe corneal opacity with classic GDLCD and the other from band keratopathy (148). Possibly other modulating genes are important for the phenotype. However, in one study the presence of a Pro501Thr mutation in the BIGH3 gene in addition to the mutation in the M1S1 gene did not influence the phenotypic appearance (149).

LCD type III

LCD type III (LCD 3) was described as a separate clinical entity, by Hida and associates in 1987 (60). In contrast to LCD types I and II, the hereditary mode of transmission in LCD3 was autosomal recessive (60). The onset was very late, in the seventh or eighth decade of life. The lattice lines in the cornea were much thicker than in the other types.

No extraocular involvement was noted. The corneal disease was mild, no recurrent corneal erosions were experienced, and no corneal transplants were needed (60). In two other patients, LCD3 appeared as a unilateral disorder which necessitated a corneal transplant (150). The authors stressed the typical clinical phenotype of LCD3, which included strikingly thickened lattice lines, radially oriented and located in the anterior cornea and midstroma (150). The gene was not identified and its location is unknown.

Diagnosis, Pathology, and Pathogenesis

MCD, since the 1960s, is known to be a disease of abnormal mucopolysaccharide metabolism. Intially, it was assumed that the acid mucopolysaccharides, or glycosaminoglycans, as they later became known, are stored intracellularly, whereas the extracellular deposits, are of a different nature (151,152). However, it is now clear that a glycosaminoglycanlike substance is accumulated, both intracellularly and extracellularly, surrounding the keratocytes.

Light microscopy shows deposits within the superficial stroma and extended keratocytes, and degeneration of basal epithelial cells, with partial absence of Bowman's membrane (Fig. 14). Special stains show accumulation of a glycosaminoglycanlike substance within keratocytes and within histiocytes in the subepithelial region and, later, in stroma, Descemet's membrane, and endothelium (17,154). A local deficiency of the hydrolytic enzyme α-galactosidase in the keratocytes was assumed to be the cause (153,154), but this has not yet been confirmed.

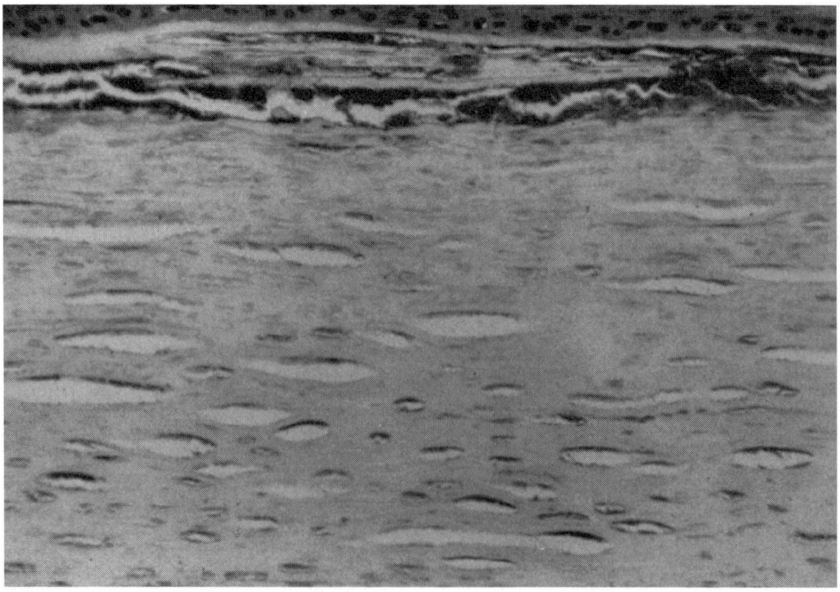

Figure 14 Histopathologic appearance of a cornea with MCD showing the accumulation of an abnormal (glycosaminoglycan-like) substance in the subepithelial space, Bowman's membrane, and within stromal keratocytes.

Electron microscopy demonstrates intracytoplasmic vacuoles distending the keratocytes and containing a clear or a granular–fibrillar material or lamellar bodies. A fibrillogranular substance can also be found within vesicles extracellularly (155).

Organ culture techniques enabled Klintworth and Smith to demonstrate that in MCD the normal synthesis of keratan sulfate proteoglycans is diminished and replaced by production of an abnormal glycoprotein of lower molecular weight (156). It was therefore suggested that an error in the synthesis of keratan sulfate, possibly involving a specific sulfotransferase, causes the disease (157). Stromal keratocytes have a reduction or absence of sulfation of keratan chains (158).

A low level or absence of keratan sulfate was found in both the cornea and the serum of patients with MCD, indicating that it is a systemic disease (159,160). Serum keratan sulfate is derived mostly from the body cartilage, and its absence from serum indicated that the enzymatic defect is not confined to the cornea, as previously considered. A recent study, using five different monoclonal anti-keratan sulfate antibodies on 88 corneas from 67 patients with MCD, indicated that keratan sulfate is present in the accumulations in some cases, whereas it is absent in others (161). These investigators concluded that MCD has at least two distinct varieties: keratan sulfate-negative (type 1) and keratan sulfate-positive (type 2).

A type 3 MCD, another allelic type of MCD, was later reported and is described in this chapter.

A laboratory test may now be available for diagnosing MCD. An enzyme-linked immunosorbent assay (ELISA) performed on sera from 16 patients with histologically confirmed MCD, showed sulfated keratan sulfate levels that were absent or extremely diminished in the serum (159,160). The serum keratan sulfate level was determined to be less than 2 ng/mL. In normal patients and in other corneal diseases and dystrophies, the level is more than 100 times this amount. The ELISA should be useful for making the diagnosis of MCD in young individuals before clinical changes become conspicuous (160).

Pathologic studies of corneal grafts, in which there had been a recurrence of macular dystrophy, demonstrated that host keratocytes did not invade the graft and that graft stromal keratocytes synthesized normal proteoglycans (138). However, endothelial cells of the graft and keratocytes in the periphery of the graft were affected by the process (139).

This may well be the reason for the relative by successful corneal implantations in MCD, and the rarity of a recurrence (140). If recurrence occurs and another corneal graft is needed, pathological studies demonstrated a wide involvement of the host cornea by the disease process. Deposits of glycosaminoglycans were manifested beneath Bowman's layer, throughout the stroma and even in the Descemet and endothelium (140). The deposits were noticed, both intracellularly and extracellularly (140) by transmission electron microscopy.

In gelatinous droplike dystrophy, massive subepithelial deposits of amyloid were found in the space between epithelial cells and Bowman's membrane, with a total absence of the epithelial basal membrane (143).

In the stroma, fusiform deposits of amyloid were found, mainly in the anterior two-thirds of the stroma. The amyloid deposits were found in cytoplasmic inclusions of stromal macrophages by Takahashi and coworkers (162). These authors suggested that in gelatinous drop-like dystrophy, amyloid fibrils are produced by epithelial cells and that stromal macrophages participate in collecting the abnormal material as phagocytic scavengers. The deposits of gelatinous drop-like corneal dystrophy contain AP protein, but not AA protein.

In GDLCD, corneal transplantation is frequent. A study of the removed corneal buttons, demonstrated subepithelial haziness, subepithelial nodular lesions, and amyloid deposits between basal cells and Bowman's layer (142).

In LCD type III, amyloid deposits were seen scattered throughout the stroma much larger than in LCD types I and II (108).

Management

Management of the autosomal recessive corneal dystrophies should be as described above for autosomal dominant disorders. When visual acuity becomes severely reduced, a corneal transplant is the treatment of choice. In macular the results seem better than in other corneal dystrophies, but even here recurrence is not unusual. In GDLCD, which may be manifested as a severe disorder with a drop in vision, a new approach of transplantation of limbal stem cells may be considered. Limbal stem cells, if taken from an unaffected close relative, may be a source of supply of the normal wild-type gene. Postoperative immunosuppressive therapy should be administered and, if necessary at a later stage, a corneal transplant performed.

MERETOJA-TYPE AMYLOIDOSIS AND THE GELSOLIN GENE

The Clinical and Genetic Entity

LCD type II: LCD type II, LCD of Meretoja, familial amyloidosis with corneal lattice dystrophy cranial neuropathy, LCD with generalized amyloidosis, amyloidosis type V, Finland type amyloidosis, Meretoja-type amyloidosis, amyloid cranial neuropathy with LCD, and Meretoja's syndrome, all are synonyms used for the same disease. Meretoja first described this corneal dystrophy with generalized amyloidosis in 1972 (59). The corneal disease is milder in type II than in LCD type I. The visual acuity is usually good until the seventh decade of life. The radiating lattice lines in the cornea are longer, thinner, and fewer than in type I, but the corneal periphery is also affected. The stroma is clear between the lines. Open-angle glaucoma seems to be much more common than in the general population (59). The onset of symptoms of the generalized disease is usually between the ages of 20 and 35 years. Its signs are sagging facial skin, with drooping eyelids and blepharochalasis (59). Facial nerve palsy may occur, with occasional exposure keratitis (163). Other cranial nerves may be affected. It is transmitted by an autosomal dominant gene.

Meretoja syndrome was initially reported in 207 Finnish individuals (163) and was believed to be a disorder associated only with Finns and especially with two regions of Finland (59,163). Later, the syndrome was reported in Japan (164) and other places, including Denmark, Netherlands, and the United States (165).

The ocular disease, initially asymptomatic, may become symptomatic after the age of 40 or later. Corneal erosions may also occur. Generally, the ocular disease is mild and rarely necessitates additional surgical treatment. However, an unusually severe phenotype occurs in individuals homozygous for the mutation, resulting in a serious ocular and systemic disease (166).

Meretoja syndrome is a systemic amyloidosis resulting in amyloid deposits along the nerves, skin, heart and kidneys. Slowly progressing cranial and peripheral nerve palsies are common (165). The skin becomes dry, itchy, and loose (cutis laxa), including blepharochalasis. Polycythemia, ventricular hypertrophy and renal failure all have been described (165). In one study of Finnish patients, all 30 patients examined showed some cranial neuropathy, especially facial nerve palsy, while peripheral neuropathy including sensory nerves was detected in 26 of the 30 patients (167).

The disorder is transmitted by an autosomal dominant gene. In 1991 a mutation in the gelsolin (GSN) gene was identified in one American family and three Finnish families with Meretoja syndrome (168,169). The authors demonstrated that a variant gelsolin protein molecule is deposited in the cornea and other tissues of patients (169). The mutation was an adenine for guanine substitution at nucleotide 654 of the GSN gene, (168,169). This results in replacement of aspartic acid by asparagine at codon 187 (Aspl87Asn mutation).

Gelsolin is a protein found in leukocytes, platelets, and other cells. It is known to be involved in the clearance of actin, a common protein found in most tissues, but its exact effect in the normal eye is unknown.

The identified mutation, Aspl87Asn, is the only disease-bearing mutation identified in the GSN gene. It was found in 100% of Finnish patients with Meretoja syndrome (170) and in all the patients examined.

Diagnosis and Pathology

The diagnosis of Meretoja syndrome is based on the characteristic ocular findings, especially the typical lattice lines in the cornea, the autosomal recessive transmission, and the characteristic systemic findings such as cranial neuropathy. The diagnosis can be confirmed by finding the characteristic mutation in the GSN gene.

In LCD type II (Meretoja's syndrome), amyloid deposits are found along the lattice lines in the stroma and in a thick layer along Bowman's membrane (105). Amyloid accumulation was found in the cornea, conjunctiva, and skin of the lower eyelid (171). No AA or AP amyloid protein or prealbumin was found in the deposits (171).

CENTRAL CRYSTALLINE DYSTROPHY

The Clinical and Genetic Entity

Central Crystalline Dystrophy

Variably named as Schnyder's crystalline dystrophy, crystalline stromal dystrophy, or hereditary crystalline stromal dystrophy of Schnyder, central crystalline dystrophy is an autosomal dominant, relatively rare disorder. Delleman and Winkelman proved that it is a cholesterol storage disorder (107). The disease begins in early childhood as a bilateral, usually symmetric disease. Subepithelial opacities can be seen by slit-lamp in the form of multiple, small, needlelike crystals limited to the central portion of the cornea and to the anterior one-third of the stroma (107). The clear peripheral cornea is initially wide and becomes, with time, narrower. A white peripheral girdle is a frequent finding (107).

Lisch and coworkers followed up patients with central crystalline dystrophy (172). In addition to the crystalline opacities, small punctate opacities caused a corneal haze. Stromal opacities never regressed, whereas progression, when it occurred, was more frequent in the diffuse opacities type than in the crystalline type.

In some families, the coexistence with abnormally elevated plasma lipoproteins has been reported (173). Increased frequency of xanthelasmas and corneal arcus may be seen in these families, without any other obvious systemic abnormality. As such patients have a high predisposition for cardiovascular disease, all patients with central crystalline dystrophy should be evaluated for hyperlipidemia. No correlation was found between the severity of the corneal changes and systemic lipid metabolism abnormalities (172).

At least four reports indicated the coexistence in families of central crystalline dystrophy with genu valgum (174).

While Schnyder central crystalline dystrophy is frequently nonprogressive after childhood, significant progression of the disease may occur (175). Weiss studied several families with Schnyder dystrophy who lived in Massachusetts but were of Swedish–Finnish origin. Bilateral, central disklike corneal opacifications were the most prominent clinical finding up to the age of 23 years (176). After 23 years, a lipoidal arcus became more and more prominent, and after the age of 40 years, all had diffuse stromal haze (176). Weiss considered the characteristic corneal crystals not to be an essential part of the entity. In fact, in the Massachusetts cohort, she found only about 50% manifesting those crystals (176,177). In the noncrystalline cases, the stroma becomes progressively more opaque with age. Shearman and colleagues, studying the same families in Massachusetts, located the gene causative of Schnyder dystrophy to chromosome 1p34.1–p36 (178). The authors and others suggested some candidate genes, such as the gene encoding fatty acid-binding protein 3 (FABP3), methylene tetrahydrofolate reductase gene (MTHFR), and B120, a gene associated with lipid transport (178,179). As of 2005, none have been confirmed.

Diagnosis

The characteristic clinical picture, the family history, and the progression of the disease are the basis for diagnosing Schnyder corneal dystrophy. Arcus lipoides, xanthelasmas and hyperlipidemia may be found (172–174). The possibility of Schnyder corneal dystrophy "sine crystals" should be considered. The use of the confocal microscope may be helpful. Highly reflective deposits can be seen accumulating in the anterior stroma and along subepithelial nerves (180). Both normal and elevated serum levels of cholesterol/lipids can be found in patients with Schnyder corneal dystrophy (178). Therefore, blood tests should be taken for each patient.

Differential diagnosis is with other corneal dystrophies and with cystinosis, a systemic disease of abnormal amino acid metabolism.

Pathology and Pathogenesis

Several studies were performed on corneas of patients with central crystalline dystrophy (Schnyder's). The crystals in the stroma were shown by histology, special stains, polarized light, and electron microscopy, to consist of cholesterol (107,181–183). Cholesterol esters were also found, but no triglyceride or free fatty acids were present (182). The superficial stroma, Bowman's membrane, and basal epithelial cells were affected with many disruptions of Bowman's membrane (181–183). Extracellular lipid droplets (not in crystal form) can also be found.

Corneal deposits are rich in unesterified cholesterol, but also contain cholesterol esters and phospholipids (184,185). Electromicroscopy manifested abnormal accumulation of phospholipids and dissolved cholesterol in the epithelium, Bowman layer, and stroma, with sparing of the Descemet layer and endothelium (184). The distribution of the deposits fits three zones: a central zone of cloudiness, a ring of the most translucent cornea, and peripheral arcus lipoides (184).

Quantitative biochemical analysis of a corneal button demonstrated the deposit of 23.6 mg/g of phospholipids (about five times normal), 6.99 mg/g of free cholesterol (about 13 times normal) and 3.16 mg/g of cholesterol ester (about 12 times normal) (184). Sphingomyelin is the main phospholipid deposited (186).

Management

Visual acuity is rarely reduced in Schnyder corneal dystrophy to the degree that a corneal graft is necessary, however, it does occur. Patients with recurrent corneal erosions and photophobia should be treated by lubricating agents. A case report described the spontaneous disappearance of corneal crystals in the corresponding area of a recurrent corneal erosion, and suggested the consideration of superficial debridement for treatment in some cases of Schnyder corneal dystrophy (185). Genetic counseling is based on the fact that central crystalline dystrophy (of Schnyder) is an autosomal dominant disease. It is not clear whether or not more than one genetic type actually exists. Possibly, three types exist: (1) type 1—disease limited to the cornea (107); (2) type 2—corneal disease associated with hyperlipidemia (173); and (3) type 3—corneal disease associated with genu valgum (174). Families tend to show the same pattern of disease according to these types.

OTHER CORNEAL DYSTROPHIES PRIMARILY AFFECTING THE STROMA

Several corneal dystrophies mainly affecting the stroma must be considered separately. They are rare or very rare and their disease causative genes have not been identified. In most, the gene location is also unknown (Table 4).

Francois Corneal Dystrophy

Fleck corneal dystrophy, also called speckled corneal dystrophy of Francois and Neetens, and central cloudy dystrophy of Francois, are according to Klintworth (45) one and the same genetic entity. He argues that both clinical phenotypes can be found in the same family and even in the same affected individual (45). These two terms will be named here "Francois corneal dystrophy" as both bear his name.

Francois and Neetens, in their first report of fleck corneal dystrophy, called it *héredo-dystrophie mouchetée* (fleck dystrophy) (187), which became widely known as the speckled corneal dystrophy of Francois and Neetens. It is a rare autosomal dominant disorder. Fleck dystrophy is usually asymptomatic and can be found in early childhood as an accidental finding. Multiple, small, gray-white, irregularly shaped opacities (discrete flecks, dots, commas, or wreathlike forms) can be seen throughout all layers of the stroma and up to the periphery, but the central cornea is affected more than the periphery, and midstromal and deep stromal levels are affected more than the superficial layers (188). In one family, the number of opacities number ranged from 6 to more than 20 (188). Although the opacities remain unchanged in size, they may increase in number with time (189). Some members of an affected family may have a partial distribution or a unilateral distribution of the flecks (189,190). The corneal sensitivity is usually normal, but sometimes is reduced (190).

Table 4 Other Corneal Dystrophies, Primarily Affecting the Stroma

Name	Synonyms	OMM (6)	Inheritance	Clinical findings: Early	Clinical findings: Late	Part of stroma mainly affected	Periphery of cornea	Main pathological findings	Remarks	Chromosomal location	Gene	Mutations
LCD type2	Meretoja's	105120	AD[a]	Longer, thinner, fewer lattice lines	Less severe than type 1	Anterior	Affected	Accumulation of amyloid in cornea, conjunctiva, and eyelids	Generalized amyloidosis; cranial nerve palsies and facial skin involvement	9p34	GSN (gelsoline)	Asp 187Asn
Central crystalline dystrophy	Schnyder's	121800	AD	Multiple small needlelike crystals	Tiny opaci-ties increase to form stromal haze	Anterior	Clear	Cholesterol and cholesterol-esters accumulate in anterior stroma and basal epithelial cells	May have three clinicogenetic entities: (1) corneal involvement only, (2) with hyperlipidemia, and (3) with genu valgum	lp34.1	?	?
Fleck corneal dystrophy	Francois and Neetens; speckled	121850	AD	Small gray-white flecks in multiple forms	Number of flecks may increase	Midstroma or all of stroma	Affected	Keratocytes filled with two types of vacuoles containing muco-polysaccharide and lipid material	Fleck and central cloudy corneal dystrophies are likely one disease: Francois corneal dystrophy	2q35	?	?

Central cloudy	Francois; posterior crocodile-shagreen	—	AD	Small cloudy gray spots with cracklike polygonal structure	Unchanged	Posterior	Clear	—	Rare; not confirmed as a separate entity	2q35	?	?
Congenital hereditary stromal dystrophy	Familial corneal parenchymatous	—	AD	Diffuse cloudiness since birth; normal corneal thickness	Unchanged	All of stroma	Affected	Stromal collagen filaments about half of their normal thickness	Rare			
Posterior amorphous corneal dystrophy	—	—	AD	Large thin sheets of opacification; thin cornea; congenital	Unchanged	In front of Descemet's membrane	Affected	Keratocytes in front of Descemet's membrane filled by vacuoles containing lipofuscin-like lipoprotein	Could be an age-related degenerative disease and not an inherited dystrophy			

[a]AD, antosonal dominant.

Central cloudy corneal dystrophy is a very rare autosomal dominant disease described first by Francois in 1956 (191). It is often referred to as the central cloudy corneal dystrophy of Francois. The central one-third of the cornea is affected by small, cloudy, gray spots within a disk area of indistinct borders (192). The posterior stroma is most affected. The epithelium and endothelium are unaffected. Visual acuity is good, and the condition is not progressive (192). The lesions were described as polygonal or rounded gray opacities surrounded by normal stroma (193).

Posterior crocodile shagreen dystrophy, in which a mosaic of opacities is surrounded by a cracklike polygonal structure of clear stroma, may be the same condition (13,18).

Francois corneal dystrophy is inherited by an autosomal dominant gene, with high penetrance and variable expressivity (188–192). Nonpenetrant carriers were reported (194). Mode of transmission is autosomal dominant (184), with somewhat reduced penetrance. Variable expressivity and assymetric involvement of the two eyes were all reported (194).

Recently, Jiao and colleagues (194) mapped the causative gene to chromosome 2q35. Several candidate genes exist in this area but none was confirmed as the associated gene.

The visual acuity is usually good to very good, with some patients diagnosed in the course of a routine eye examination. The flecks, which vary in the number of tiny small opacities scattered throughout the entire corneal stroma (with an increase in the central area) are not related to cloudiness of the cornea between them.

Pathologic examination of a rare corneal button after corneal transplant showed stromal staining for acid mucopolysaccharidoses (195). Transmission electron microscopy manifested extracellular vacuoles, some filled by a fibrillogranular material. The primary defect appears to be in the keratocyte. The keratocytes displayed accumulation of two types of vacuoles: single-membrane-limited vacuoles, filled with acid mucopolysaccharidelike substance, and smaller vacuoles containing apparently a lipid material (188). This would place the corneal findings within the pathologic group of metabolic diseases termed mucolipidoses.

Congenital Hereditary Stromal Dystrophy

This rare congenital autosomal dominant condition was first described by Desvignes and Vigo, in 1955, and termed familial corneal parenchymatous dystrophy (196). It is present at birth, mostly nonprogressive, and shows a diffuse corneal cloudiness affecting the stroma (197,198). Although nonprogressive, the reduction in vision is severe and keratoplasty may be necessary (197,198). The cornea has a normal thickness.

Congenital hereditary stromal dystrophy displays characteristic, abnormal corneal lamellae composed of collagen filaments of abnormally small diameter (196). Loose lamellae of such filaments are related to keratocytes (198).

Posterior Amorphous Corneal Dystrophy

This autosomal dominant disorder, reported for the first time by Carpel and colleagues in 1977 (199), is extremely rare. A second family was reported by Dunn and associates (200). It has the characteristic appearance of diffuse, irregular, large sheets of opacifications in the posterior stroma, just in front of Descemet's membrane

(199,200). The cornea appears to be thinner than usual, and other abnormalities include hyperopia, flat cornea, iris abnormalities, and extensive fine iridocorneal processes (200). Autosomal dominant inheritance was found. The disorder is probably congenital, is nonprogressive, and the visual acuity remains good.

The entity is very rare. Only a few families are known and in two cases the corneal button after corneal transplant was studied (201,202). Dense opacification, sheet-like in the posterior stroma was found (201,202). Two forms prevail in the affected families. In one, high hypermetropia, flat cornea (less than 41.0 D), and low central thickness are seen. In the second, the central cornea is also thinner than 500 μm but less hyperopia or even myopia is seen, as the cornea is not as flat. Ultrasound biomicroscopy may be helpful in the clinical assessment and diagnosis of posterior amorphous corneal dystrophy (203). In two cases, a gray-white, sheetlike posterior stromal opacity with superior corneal thinning was noted. Stromal opacification was deep, just anterior to Descemet's membrane. Corneal thickness was measured as less than 450 μm (203).

A light microscopic, study of a corneal button of a 5-year-old boy with posterior amorphous corneal dystrophy (204) revealed fracturing of the most posterior stromal layer of collagen and loss of endothelial cells. Electron microscopy revealed disorganized collagen fibers and Descemet membrane interrupted by collagen fibers. The authors conclude that posterior amorphous corneal dystrophy is a developmental abnormality in the formation of posterior stroma and Descemet membrane (204).

Posterior amorphous corneal dystrophy is transmitted by the autosomal dominant mode (199,200), but the causative gene has not yet been identified or located.

Pre-Descemet's Membrane Corneal Dystrophy

Opacities of the stroma, just in front of Descemet's membrane, are usually caused by an aging, noninherited, degenerative process and should be distinguished from the corneal dystrophies. They include the not infrequently found cornea farinata, in which a multitude of fine, dustlike or flourlike opacities are found in the deep stroma (17). Filiform dystrophy, described by Maeder and Danis in 1947 (205), is probably a similarly degenerative condition.

In 1967, Grayson and Wilbrandt described a clinically similar condition occurring in families and transmitted through two generations (206). It is not yet clear whether it is a separate clinical and genetic entity.

Confocal microscopy was used to diagnose this rare condition (207,208). Small irregular particles, all extracellular deposits, were found just in front of the Descemet membrane (207,208). It also allowed the comparison to Francois fleck corneal dystrophy, in which both tiny intracellular deposits (less than 1 mm in size) and large extracellular deposits (50–70 μm in size) were scattered throughout the whole cornea (207,208).

In pre-Descement's membrane corneal dystrophy, the anterior part of the stroma, Bowman's membrane and epithelium are normal. Deep keratocytes were filled with vacuoles having clear or fibrillogranular material (209). The surrounding stromal collagen seemed normal. The authors concluded (209) that the accumulation is probably a lipofuscin-like lipoprotein. This would indicate the degenerative nature of the disorder as part of an aging process.

Stromal dystrophies affecting mainly the posterior stroma must be differentiated from dystrophies of the posterior limiting membranes. In congenital hereditary stromal dystrophy, the cornea has normal thickness and no edema, in contrast to congenital hereditary endothelial dystrophy, which manifests a thickened cornea with epithelial and stromal edema.

CORNEAL DYSTROPHIES PRIMARILY AFFECTING THE POSTERIOR LIMITING MEMBRANE

Description

This group of corneal dystrophies affects principally the endothelium and Descemet's membrane. They include three well-defined diseases: Fuchs' endothelial dystrophy, posterior polymorphous dystrophy, and congenital hereditary endothelial dystrophy (Fig. 15 and Table 5).

The term "primary corneal endotheliopathies" was used to describe this group of diseases (210), in addition to other forms not discussed here, such as iridocorneal endothelial syndrome, which is not an inherited condition, and some intermediate forms, not yet defined.

The Clinical and Genetic Types

Congenital Hereditary Endothelial Dystrophy

Congenital hereditary endothelial dystrophy (CHED) was first described by Maumenee, in 1960, in eight patients (211). All patients had a cloudy edematous cornea, with the edema extending up to the periphery and into the epithelium (211). The condition is now known to occur in two genetic forms, an autosomal recessive and an autosomal dominant form. The cornea is affected at birth. It is variably cloudy and thickened, and the epithelium is irregular.

In autosomal recessive CHED, photophobia, epiphora, and inflammation are absent; often a pendular nystagmus is seen; and the condition tends to be stationary (212). The entire cornea is uniformly cloudy. The epithelium and the endothelium show irregular surfaces. In some cases of autosomal recessive CHED, the condition becomes worse with time.

In autosomal dominant CHED, a similar milky opacification of the whole cornea, detected at birth or early in life, has been reported (213,214). Photophobia and epiphora may precede the corneal cloudiness and may be severe. Toward the end of the first year of life, the initially mild edema turns into cloudiness, with reduction in the photophobia (213). The severity varies, with visual acuities ranging from finger counting to useful vision (213).

Nystagmus occurs rarely; secondary changes may occur later in life, including corneal scarring and neovascularization (213).

Both autosomal dominant and autosomal recessive CHED may occasionally be progressive (215), especially in early childhood. Figure 16 shows the corneas of two brothers affected by autosomal recessive CHED. The younger brother had a mild edema and a corneal thickness of 1.0 mm. The older brother had a severe edema and a corneal thickness of 1.2 mm. The recessive form has an earlier onset and is usually more severe than the dominant form.

The autosomal dominant form was named type 1 (CHEDl) and the autosomal recessive form type 2 (CHED2). The disease-causative genes were localized for both forms. In 1995, Toma and associates mapped CHEDl to the centromeric region of

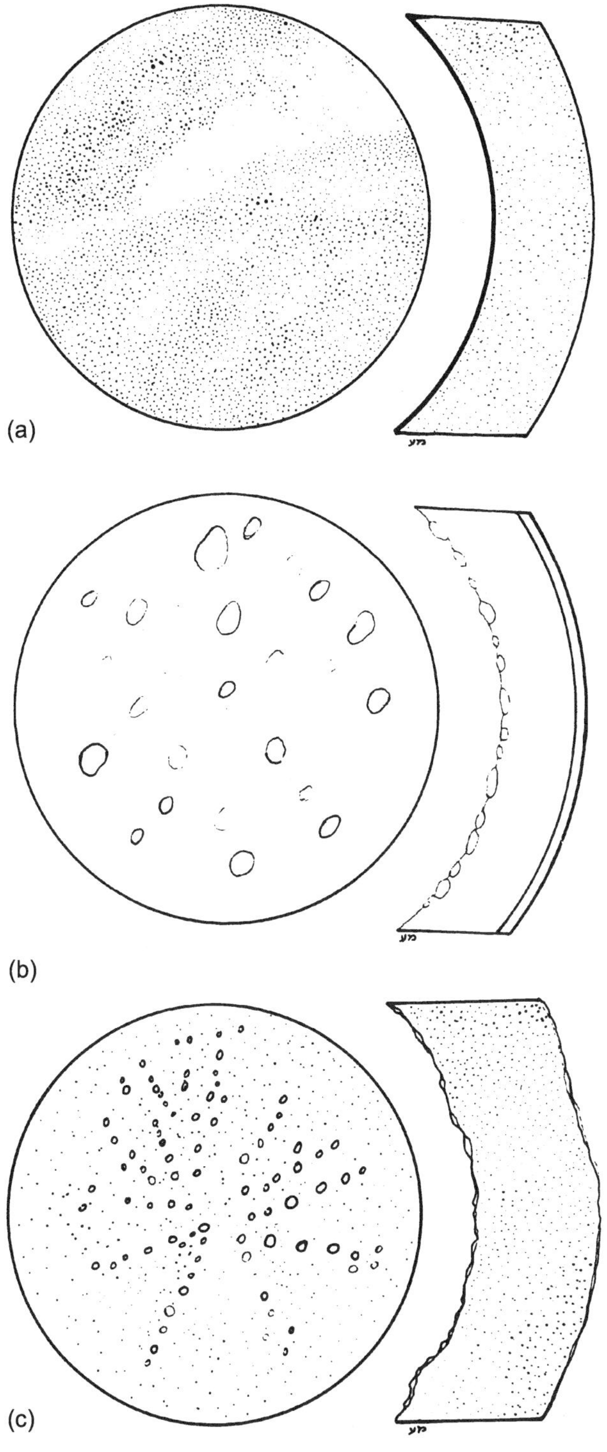

Figure 15 The corneal dystrophies affecting mainly the posterior limiting membranes: (a) congenital hereditary endothelial, (b) posterior polymorphous, and (c) Fuchs' endothelial. (Drawings by M. Ivry.)

Table 5 Corneal Dystrophies Affecting the Posterior Limiting Membranes

Name	Synonyms	MIM	Inheritance[a]	Clinical findings: Early	Clinical findings: Late	Pathological findings	Chromosomal Location	Gene
Congenital hereditary endothelial dystrophy (CHED), type 1, AD	Congenital hereditary corneal edema of Pearce CHED1	121700	AD	Milky cloudiness of whole cornea since birth; thickened cornea	Unchanged or slowly progressive (infrequently)	Disorganization of corneal lamellae; endothelium denuded areas covered by connective tissue	20p12–q13.1	
CHED, AR type 2	Congenital hereditary corneal edema of Maumenee	217700	AR	Photophobia, epiphora; corneal cloudiness since birth or early childhood	Unchanged or slowly progressive (frequently)	Similar to AD form	20pl3	
Posterior poly-morphous corneal dystrophy (PPCD)	Polymorphous deep corneal dystrophy of Schlichting	122000	AD	Cysts and vesicles at Descemet's level without or with corneal edema (marked variability)	Unchanged or slowly progressive (infrequently)	Epithelial-like cells replace a portion of endothelial cells; abnormal posterior layer of Descemet's membrane	20p11.2 1p34.3–p32	VSX1 COL8A2
Fuchs' endothelial dystrophy	Fuchs' epithelial endothelial corneal dystrophy	136800	AD	Guttate excrescences, opacification of Descemet's membrane	Stromal and epithelial edema and scarring	Posterior layer of Descemet's membrane multilayered and markedly thickened	1p34.3–p32	COL8A2

[a]AD, autosomal dominant; AR, autosomal recessive.

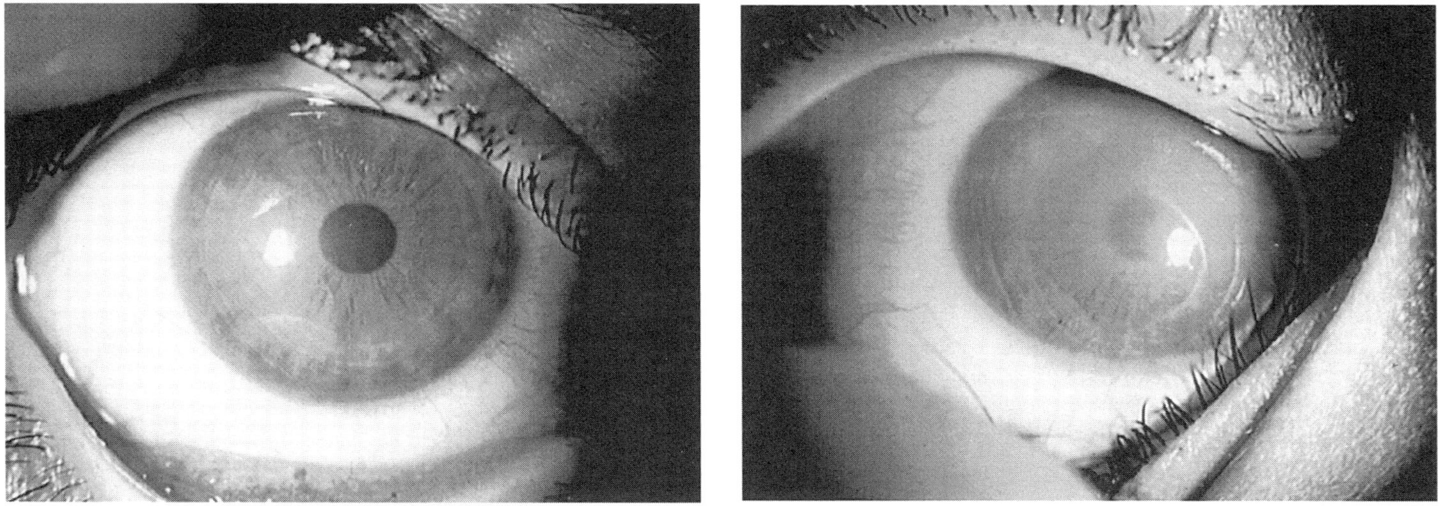

Figure 16 Two brothers with autosomal recessive CHED. Note the milder disease in one brother (left) and the more severe affliction of the brother on right. (Courtesy of U. Rehani, MD Nahariya.)

chromosome 20 (20p12–q13.1) In 1999, Hand and associates mapped CHED2 to chromosome 20pl3 and stressed that it is a separate locus (217).

Posterior Polymorphous Corneal Dystrophy

Posterior polymorphous corneal dystrophy (PPCD) was described by Schlichting in 1941 as an endothelial dystrophy, with cysts and vesicles in the posterior layers (218), and is thus often termed "PPCD of Schlichting" (219). Characteristically, great intrafamilial variability occurs, with a clinical picture ranging from a few isolated endothelial vesicles to severe stromal and epithelial edema (220). Onset of the disorder may be at birth, early childhood, or later in life (220). It is bilateral, usually nonprogressive and often asymptomatic. Good vision is usually present (220–223). Its inheritance is usually autosomal dominant (220–223), but an autosomal recessive variety (220) and sporadic cases have been described. Open-angle glaucoma is common (219,223) and may substantially reduce the chance for favorable results of keratoplasty if needed (223).

At the level of Descemet's membrane, blisters and vesicles, can be found in linear form or in groups. White patches of a thickened Descemet's membrane projecting into the anterior chamber or having bandlike lesions are less frequently found (220,223). Gonioscopy can reveal occasional iridocorneal adhesions. In severe cases, the cornea is cloudy from edema with bullous keratopathy and even calcific and lipoid degenerative changes (223).

A specular microscopic study of 48 patients with PPCD manifested vesicles in 42%, bands in 48%, and diffuse abnormality of Descemet in 10% (229).

After performing a genome-wide study, Heon and colleagues (225) determined linkage of the PPCD-associated gene to chromosome 20p11, in the same region as the CHED1-associated gene. This raises the possibility of an allelic heterogeneity of the two conditions.

In some cases of PPCD, a mutation in the COL8A2 gene was identified (226). This gene, mapped to chromosome 1p34.3–p32 is associated with Fuchs' endothelial corneal dystrophy (FECD) (225).

Fuchs' Endothelial Dystrophy

In 1910, Fuchs first described a corneal endothelial dystrophy that affected the aged, more women than men, that reduced the sensitivity of the cornea, that began inferiorly and that led to opacification and inflammation (227).

All these remain the primary clinical findings of the disease. Fuchs suspected that the endothelium might be affected and might be the origin of the disease, despite not using a slit-lamp in his time, and despite the obvious clinical involvement of the epithelium (227).

The first clinical evidence of possible Fuchs' dystrophy is cornea guttata. In this stage, multiple spots or guttae can be seen projecting as excrescences at the level of the endothelium (Fig. 17). Later mild hazy opacification of Descemet's membrane takes place. Some patients will be asymptomatic and will not progress beyond this stage. Other cases will progress to Fuchs' dystrophy, in which the stroma and, later, the epithelium will become edematous.

The disease is bilateral, but often asymmetric. Early symptoms include fluctuating vision, especially blurred vision in the mornings; this results from increased tear osmolarity in the morning caused by a decreased tear evaporation at night (228). Visual acuity will gradually be reduced with the onset of the edema. Later, frank

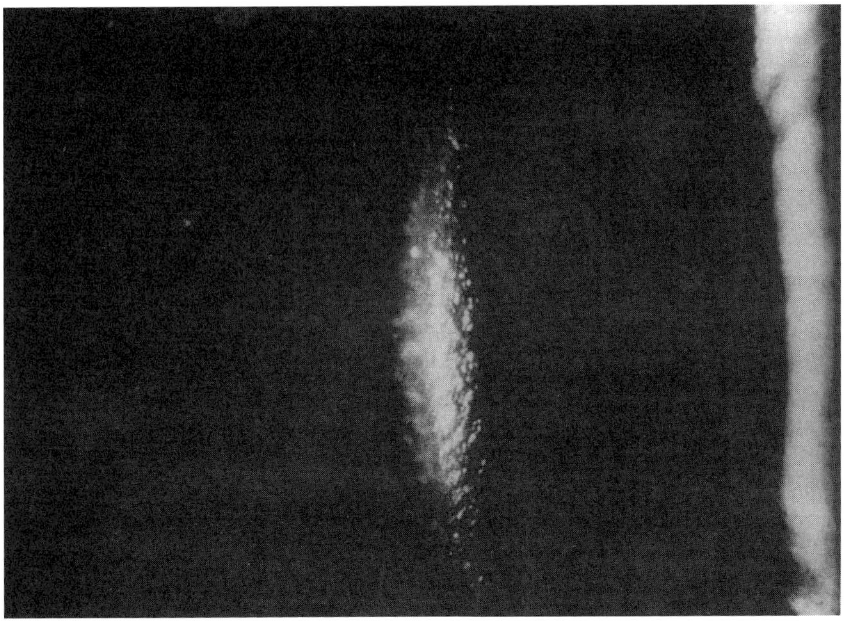

Figure 17 Cornea guttata. Note the myriad of excrescences.

bullous keratopathy, with secondary inflammation is seen. Open-angle glaucoma may be associated.

Fuchs' dystrophy was considered a nongenetic disease because of the inability to conduct a proper familial investigation of a disease affecting the elderly. Also, the high female preponderance could not be easily explained. However, more recent evidence points to a disease of autosomal dominant inheritance (see later discussion).

Biswas and associates examined several families with Fuchs' endothelial corneal dystrophy (FECD) and identified two missense mutations in the COL8A2 gene, a Glu455Lys mutation in several families, and a Argl55Glu mutation in another family (226). The gene COL8A2 encodes a short 703 amino acid, alpha-2 chain of type VIII collagen. This collagen is a component of endothelial basement membranes. The gene was mapped to chromosome 1p34.3–p32 (226). However, in other cases of FECD, no mutation was identified.

Other Endothelial Dystrophies

Other dystrophies affecting the endothelium have been reported, but their existence as distinct clinicogenetic entities is yet to be confirmed.

Harboyan and coworkers described a corneal disorder similar to CHED, with progressive sensorineural deafness in one family (229). Behrens-Baumann and colleagues reported a "hereditary ocular dysproteinhydria" in which multiple-colored crystalline deposits were seen on the corneal endothelium in members of one family (230).

Meretoja described, in Finland, an autosomal dominant disorder in which myriads of small, round, oval, or corkscrew opacities on the endothelium and

Descemet's membrane were associated with later increasing endothelial pigmentation (231). Cutaneous disturbance in pigmentation was also common.

EDICT syndrome was the name given to a disorder that included corneal thinning and steeping, microcornea, endothelial abnormalities resembling PPCD or Fuchs' dystrophy, iris hypoplasia, and congenital anterior polar cataracts (232). It is transmitted as an autosomal dominant trait and mapped to chromosome 15q22.1–q25.3 (232).

Diagnosis

The differential diagnosis between CHED and PPCD is based on the following: (1) the different clinical picture: (2) the fact that most cases of CHED are autosomal recessive, whereas most cases of PPCD are autosomal dominant; and (3) the extremely variable expression of PPCD in members of the same family. Other possible causes of congenital or early childhood cloudiness of the cornea must be considered. These include sporadic cases of bilateral congenitally opaque corneas of unknown etiology (233), the mucopolysaccharidoses, and some mucolipidoses. However, the most important differential diagnosis is with primary infantile glaucoma. In one study, five patients had glaucoma surgery (215). I have seen two patients with CHED who had previous unnecessary glaucoma surgery. Findings that may help in the differential diagnosis are the size of the cornea, which is usually enlarged in congenital glaucoma and normal in CHED; the presence of breaks in Descemet's membrane in glaucoma; and, of course, if visible, the appearance of the disk.

Pathology and Pathogenesis

A large number of pathologic studies, both by light microscopy and by electron microscopy, enhance our understanding of the dystrophies of the posterior limiting membranes.

In CHED, the entire cornea is affected, mostly by nonspecific changes in the form of disorganization of stromal lamellae by the edema and variations in the thickness of Bowman's membrane, epithelial basement membrane, and Descemet's membrane (234). Pearce and his colleagues (213) noted a thickening of the nonbanded portion of Descemet's membrane and a marked reduction in the number of endothelial cells. An absence of endothelial cells in the central portion of the posterior cornea, without an associated defect in Descemet's membrane, was detected in a 36-hour-old neonate with corneal edema resulting from CHED, who died of respiratory distress (235). Kanai and Kaufman (214) reported the finding of fibroblastlike cells, which replaced most of the absent endothelial cells. Descemet's membrane had an anterior normal portion and a posterior thickened one, consisting of an acellular, basement membranelike material (236). Kirkness and coworkers (215) reported only subtle histologic differences between autosomal dominant and autosomal recessive CHED. Endothelial cells were in some areas normal, whereas in others, they were absent or showed vacuolation.

In endothelium-denuded areas, a thick retrocorneal membrane of fine fibrils can be seen (237).

It seems, therefore, that in CHED the primary disease is of the endothelium, which for an unknown reason is lost or undergoes degenerative changes in utero. Later, secondary changes occur in Descemet's membrane and nonspecific changes of edema occur in the stroma and epithelium. The timing of these events has been suggested as after the fifth month of gestation (237) and after the eighth month of gestation (215).

The hallmark of the pathologic findings in PPCD is the finding of epithelial cells partially lining the posterior cornea. This was first reported in 1971 (238) and has been confirmed in many studies.

There is a loss and degeneration of endothelial cells, which show, in addition to reduced numbers, variability in cellular size and guttatelike excrescences. These cells are partially replaced by epithelial-like cells containing desmosomes, microvilli, and intracellular keratofibrils (222,238–240). Descemet's membrane is composed of a normal anterior banded layer and an abnormal, irregular, posterior homogenous collagenous layer (241).

Cell cultures of endothelial cells from four corneas of patients with PPCD showed that two different populations of cells can be found: normal endothelial and epithelial-like cells displaying microvilli, stratifications, desmosomes, and 8 nm cytoplasmic filaments (242).

McCartney and Kirkness (243) compared the histology of 20 corneal buttons taken in transplants of CHED to that of 10 corneal buttons taken from PPCD cases. The typical findings were different for each distinct disorder. In CHED1, spheroidal degeneration of the stroma was characteristic. In CHED2, Descemet's membrane was completely abnormal, and in PPCD a calcific band was found. A fibrillary posterior collagen layer was manifested in both CHED1 and PPCD (243).

Several theories were proposed on the pathogenesis of PPCD. A basic mesothelial cell has the potential to develop into (1) normal endothelium, (2) an epithelium-like cell, or (3) a fibroblast-like cell (244). One possibility is that the mesothelial cell in PPCD most often turns into the epithelium-like cell, and in CHED it most often turns into the fibroblast-like cell. A second possibility is that abnormal endothelial cells will transform into epitheliallike cells (241). Henriquez and coworkers suggested (222) that the disorder starts with focal degeneration of endothelial ceils. This causes abnormal secretion of a basement membrane and of an abnormal posterior collagen layer, with the formation of guttate excrescences. Endothelial defects are repaired by abnormal neighboring endothelium that undergoes fibroblastic or epithelial-like transformation. Stromal edema depends on the number of functioning endothelial cells.

The results of immunohistochemical analysis of corneas of PPCD support the hypothesis that epitheliallike cells arise from the endothelium by a metaplastic process in which they become progressively abnormal (245).

In Fuchs' dystrophy, the anterior prenatal portion of Descemet's membrane is normal. The posterior collagenous portion is markedly thickened by the presence of several additional layers (246). This thickening was reported to appear much earlier than any clinical signs of the disease, as it was seen even in the first two decades of life (246). The structure of the guttate excrescences is similar to that of Descemet's membrane (247). They may be hidden within the abnormal new layers of Descemet's or may project into the anterior chamber, just covered by thin, attenuated endothelium (247). The presence of stromal and epithelial edema is related to the thickening of Descemet's membrane (246). Nonspecific findings of edema in the stroma and basal epithelial cells, together with later fibrous proliferation, can be found.

Excessive apoptosis may be an important mechanism in the pathogenesis of Fuchs' dystrophy (248).

Epidemiology and Genetics

Congenital hereditary endothelial dystrophy is an uncommon disease. It is most frequently reported in its autosomal recessive variant (212).

The loci of both forms were mapped, CHED1 to chromosome 20pl2–ql3.1 and CHED2 to chromosome 20pl3. Neither gene has yet been identified.

In contrast, PPCD is usually reported as an autosomal dominant disorder. It may not be uncommon, as many asymptomtic cases may go unnoticed and undiagnosed. Its penetrance is not complete. Skipped generations have been reported (219). Its expressivity is extremely variable.

PPCD seems to be a heterogeneic disorder. One PPCD-associated gene was mapped to chromosome 20q11 and could be allelic with the gene associated with CHED1. Mutations of another gene, COL8A2, mapped to chromosome 1p34.3–p32 were identified as causative of PPCD in several families (see earlier).

Segregation analysis of patients with Fuchs' dystrophy suggests an autosomal dominant mutation as the most likely cause (249). The female preponderance could not be explained by greater female longevity. The authors also considered the possibility of a heterogenous disorder, with autosomal dominant transmission being responsible for a portion of the cases (249). A prospective study of 69 families showed that 38% of patients' relatives aged over 40 were affected (250). This observation considerably strengthens the possibility of autosomal dominant transmission. Some family pedigrees indicate autosomal dominant transmission with full penetrance (251).

As mentioned above, the COL8A2 gene was identified and at least two mutations were found to be causative of FECD. The same mutation was found in all affected members of the same family.

Management

Fuchs' dystrophy, CHED, and PPCD all should be treated when symptomatic.

In Fuchs' dystrophy, the earliest symptoms of "morning blur" can be treated by hyperosmotic drops or by a current of hot air (228). Later, as edema increases, hypertonic solutions and soft contact lenses may be considered. With the reduction in visual acuity, keratoplasty may be necessary.

In both CHED and PPCD, keratoplasty may be necessary when vision is seriously reduced. It is better not to perform surgery on very young children, as their visual acuity is usually difficult to ascertain. The visible amount of edema may not well represent the reduction in visual acuity. Pearce and coworkers (213) warned of the poor results of keratoplasty in autosomal dominant CHED.

Of 40 patients with CHED, who were operated mostly in childhood, graft survival was only 56.5% at five years of age (252). Almost all surgically treated cases in this report were type 2 autosomal recessive (252). In another study of 21 transplants of children with CHED, the 2-year graft survival was almost identical at 71% (253). It is not clear whether earlier or delayed surgery is preferable. This important decision should be probably decided on a case-by-case basis (254).

High intraocular pressure should be controlled before keratoplasty is undertaken.

Genetic counseling is based on the known hereditary transmission in each family. Variable expressivity, should be considered, especially in the autosomal dominant diseases.

DISORDERS INVOLVING CORNEAL THINNING AND SIZE

Description

A series of disorders with hereditary background cause diminution of the thickness of the cornea or changes in its size. In some of these disorders, the genetic, Mendelian transmission is clear and in others it may be non-mendelian. The most common of these is keratoconus. This and the other disorders will be discussed under the different types.

The Clinical and Genetic Types

Keratoconus

In keratoconus (KC), the cornea assumes a conical shape because of thinning and protrusion (254). At the apex, the cornea is half to one-fifth of its normal thickness. Hemosiderin pigment at the base of the cone, situated in the deep epithelial layers, produces the Fleischer ring. Bowman's membrane may show lines of rupture and scarring. Striae may be seen anteriorly to Descemet's membrane (255).

The diagnosis is based on the history of decrease in vision, usually in a young adult, and on the clinical findings. Munson's sign is usually positive; on downgaze, the lower eyelid becomes angulated instead of rounded. Placido disk shows irregular rings and usually inferior steepening. Retinoscopy displays myopia, astigmatism, and a "scissors effect." Keratometry shows a steep and irregular corneal surface, usually above the 50 D point.

Increased serum immunoglobulin E, both total and specific (to house dust mites), was found in a study of one family with keratoconus (256), but this study was not confirmed. Linkage to any HLA antigens is also not yet confirmed. One group of investigators claimed an increased frequency of HLA-B5 and a decreased frequency of HLA-B7 in patients with keratoconus (257,258).

In another study, 90 consecutive Japanese keratoconus patients were studied. A significant association was found between KC patients diagnosed before age 20, and three HLA antigens: A26, B40, and DR90 (259).

Histopathology usually reveals a cornea of conical shape, with focal thinning at the cone, a thickened epithelial basement membrane, disruption of Bowman's membrane, and fibrous tissue between the two (260). Iron pigment may be deposited in the deep epithelial layers. Quantities of lysinonorleucine far exceeding the normal were demonstrated in corneal buttons of keratoconus removed at surgery, possibly indicating that the synthesis of an abnormal collagen takes place in keratoconus (261).

Keratoconus is neither rare nor common. In a 48-year follow-up of a specific population in Minnesota, Kennedy and associates (262) found a generally stable incidence rate of 2.0:100,000 new cases per year. The overall prevalence was 54.5:100,000 population. Of the cases, 59% were bilateral and the rest unilateral. An overview from many studies points to a prevalence of between 50:100,000 and 230:100,000 population, with large variability in different populations (255), but found in individuals of all races.

The literature is controversial concerning the etiology of keratoconus. Studies in some families indicated direct genetic transmission (263), but such observations are rare. Most studies indicate an increased frequency of keratoconus in relatives of patients, variously reported as 6% in Minnesota (262), 10% in Germany (264),

9% in southern Finland, and 19% in northern Finland (264). These studies suggested an irregular dominant transmission or an autosomal dominant transmission, with incomplete penetrance and variable expressivity (264,265).

The genetic background of KC became more evident with the introduction of computerized topography which could identify cases of "forme fruste," unusually high astigmatism, and more peripheral keratoconus. Using such methods, an incidence of keratoconus was detected which was 15–67 times higher in first-degree relatives of patients than in the general population (266). Significant topographic abnormalities were detected in asymptomatic relatives of KC patients (267,268). Positive family history was found in 6–19% of all keratoconus patients (269). Twin studies comparing monozygotic to dizygotic twins led to the conclusion that KC is primarily an inherited condition (270,271).

On the other hand, many studies demonstrate environmental factors associated with keratoconus. The foremost of these is eye rubbing. Eye rubbing was reported in 25–60% of patients in various studies (262), but in one study, 73% of patients with keratoconus had a history of eye rubbing (272). Leber's congenital amaurosis, in which fist pressure on the ocular globes commonly occurs in childhood (Franceschetti's oculodigital sign) (273), has the most frequent later association with adolescent KC of any disease. Other ocular conditions associated with eye rubbing are vernal catarrh, allergic blepharoconjunctivitis, and chronic blepharoconjunctivitis of Down's syndrome. Psychogenic factors may play a role. A higher frequency of KC is also found in generalized abnormalities of the connective tissue, such as Ehlers–Danlos syndrome, osteogenesis imperfecta, and pseudoxanthoma elasticum (255,272). Acute KC, a condition in which a sudden rupture of Descemet's membrane and endothelium causes corneal edema, is not uncommon in Down syndrome, possibly due to eye rubbing (275).

In summary, it seems that both hereditary and nonhereditary factors are associated with the occurrence of KC. The most likely explanation for such findings is that KC is a multifactorial disorder (275), having a genetic background, with environmental factors modifying it. The most important of these factors are eye rubbing and generalized connective tissue disorders; possibly both play a role by weakening the corneal collagen fibers. Less common environmental factors may be pregnancy and heavy reading (265).

In some families, KC is transmitted by an autosomal dominant gene. Clusters of families with an increased frequency of KC were described in populations manifesting a "founder effect," such as the populations in Northern Finland (276) or in northwest Tasmania (277). It is possible that the same gene with a different mutation may need varying degrees of modifying factors (including other genes or environmental influence), to manifest the phenotype of KC.

Recently, two different loci for KC were mapped. The "Finnish locus" was mapped to chromosome 16q22.3–q23.1 (276) and the "Tasmania locus" was mapped to chromosome 20ql2 (277). At the same time, mutations in the VSX1 gene were identified in Toronto, Canada in families with KC or posterior polymorphous corneal dystrophy (278). In humans the VSXl gene was detected in the retina, embryonic craniofacial tissue and adult cornea, It also plays a role in the development of retinal bipolar cells (278). VSX1 was mapped to the centromer region of chromosome 20 (20p11–q11) (278), but it is not clear whether it is the same locus as the "Tasmanian gene." Different mutations cause PPCD and KC. This may explain the existence of both KC and PPCD in the same individual (279).

Management of KC involves the prescription of glasses; fitting of hard, soft, or "piggyback" contact lenses; and surgery. Surgery is usually performed when other methods fail or the visual acuity is reduced by corneal opacities. Perforating keratoplasty is probably most often done, but other methods, such as epikeratophakia, thermokeratoplasty, lamellar keratoplasty, and even radial keratotomy, were also suggested.

Genetic counseling should be based on the contributory factors known for the specific family. In unknown cases, it is probably safest to assume a 10% chance for occurrence of KC in each child.

Posterior Keratoconus

Posterior KC is a very rare condition, in which a sharp change in the curvature of the posterior corneal surface occurs.

It may be unilateral, as a secondary phenomenon after trauma or disease. However, bilateral inherited cases have been reported (280,281). Associated systemic abnormalities in these families included growth retardation, clefting syndrome, hypertelorism with displacement of lateral canthi, and stiff gait. The inheritance seems to be autosomal recessive (281).

Histologic studies in one case (281) indicated a mesenchymal dysgenesis.

Brittle Cornea with Keratoglobus

Keratoglobus is a generalized thinning of the cornea that assumes a globular condition. The cornea may have only 20% of its normal thickness (255). It may occur as a rare, bilateral condition of unknown cause. However, it is reported with growing frequency in association with the brittle cornea syndrome, as an inherited condition. The brittle cornea syndrome consists of a triad of findings: (1) keratoglobus, a thin cornea of about one-fifth of its normal thickness; (2) brittle cornea, frequent corneal ruptures, occurring spontaneously or after minor trauma; and (3) blue sclera. A fourth finding of red hair was reported in three unrelated Jewish families of Tunisian origin in Israel (282–284) and in one Syrian family (285). Other reports did not mention hair color (280–288).

All studies of the brittle cornea syndrome report similar ocular findings of corneal perforations, which have often a disastrous effect on the eye, as the very thin cornea is not amenable for proper suturing.

In most reports, the inheritance seems to be autosomal recessive, but an X-linked recessive inheritance was suggested in some cases (287). Hyperextensibility of joints and hearing defects were also reported in some families (284,285).

In my opinion, the brittle cornea syndrome is a distinct entity, not to be confused with Ehlers–Danlos type VI ("ocular type of Ehlers–Danlos"). It was termed Stein Syndrome as Stein and colleagues first described it as a distinct entity.

Management of perforations may be very difficult. Patching or the use of glue may occasionally be effective treatments.

Blue sclerae with keratoconus, hearing loss owing to a middle ear conduction defect, and spondylolisthesis were described in one family (289).

Megalocornea

Megalocornea is a bilateral condition, in which the corneal diameter is enlarged beyond 13 mm without the presence of infantile glaucoma. It has been described as a not infrequent inherited disorder transmitted by the X-linked recessive mode and, sometimes, by the autosomal dominant or recessive mode (290). Clinically, these patients show, in addition to the increased corneal diameter, a deep anterior chamber, often atrophy of iris stroma with miosis, often iridodonesis with lens subluxation, and frequent cataracts (290). Megalocornea is found with high frequency in association with Marfan syndrome (291) and with mosaic dystrophy of the cornea, a mosaic pattern at the level of Bowman's membrane (292).

In a study of a family with megalocornea, by specular microscopy, Skuta and coworkers (290) found a normal endothelial cell density and structure, and they concluded that the number of these cells must be almost double the normal number.

Microcornea

Microcornea is a condition in which the cornea is smaller than normal, less than 11 mm in diameter. It was reported to occur sporadically or as an inherited condition, usually autosomal dominant. Autosomal dominant microcornea with cataract was reported in several large families (293,294). It was sometimes associated with myopia (293) and sometimes with sclerocornea or Peter's anomaly (293). The cataract is congenital, but at first, may be only partial in density. Sometimes, aniridia may also occur (295). Microcornea with macrophthalmia (increased axial length), posterior staphyloma, high myopia, and uveal coloboma were reported in another autosomal dominant family (296). Autosomal recessive microcornea with myopia also has been reported (297).

OTHER INHERITED CORNEAL ABNORMALITIES

Band-shaped opacities of the superficial cornea are not uncommon as secondary phenomena in eyes with chronic diseases such as uveitis, glaucoma, or phthisis bulbi. They were described as inherited disorders in several families. Bilateral, symmetric, small, yellowish to amber, oily lobules form the band keratopathy in the superficial interpalpebral cornea (298,299). The onset is early in life. Photophobia is a common symptom (300). Visual acuity slowly and progressively decreases.

Most reports demonstrate an autosomal recessive inheritance (298–301), but autosomal dominant inheritance has also been reported (302).

In patients with band-shaped keratoplathy light microscopy and electron microscopy revealed thickened epithelium and Bowman's membrane, and deposits composed of a protein and acid-fast lipoid material mainly in the anterior stroma and subepithelial space (298–301).

Sclerocornea is usually a sporadic, rare, congenital occurrence, which can be unilateral or bilateral. One family, with nine affected members, displayed sclerocornea with cornea plana (303). The transmission was autosomal dominant.

Autosomal dominant corneal hypesthesia was described in three families. In one family, the sharply decreased corneal sensation was associated with severe, diffuse, but asymptomatic, punctate corneal erosions (304). In another family, it was associated with congenital distichiasis (305). In the third family, nodular corneal opacities were also present (306).

An autosomal recessive condition, termed *congenital insensitivity to pain with anhidrosis*, was reported (307). Corneal sensation is absent in both eyes, a neurotrophic keratitis develops, and corneal ulcers with corneal leucomas are common.

In Peter's anomaly, unilateral or bilateral congenital corneal opacities linked to various signs of anterior chamber and angle dysgenesis are not common. It may occur as a sporadic, nongenetic congenital disorder, or as a genetically induced disease. Associated chromosomal anomalies have been described (308–310). Families may manifest an autosomal dominant or autosomal recessive mode of transmission. A missense mutation (Arg266Gly) in the PAX6 gene was identified in affected members of one family (311). The PAX6 gene, located at chromosome 11 p13 is the causative gene for aniridia and its protein product is a transcriptional regulator. In children with poor visual acuity, a corneal transplant may be the only therapeutic approach. Reports on such surgery presented controversial results, from a reasonable success of 62% graft survival at three years (312) to poorer results of 44% graft survival at three years and 35% at ten years (313).

CORNEAL DISORDERS ASSOCIATED WITH SYSTEMIC DISEASES OR SYNDROMES

This book does not deal with inherited systemic disorders, unless the major affected organ is the ocular globe. However, for the sake of completeness and to aid in the differential diagnosis, corneal disorders that are associated with, or that result from, systemic inherited diseases or that are part of a syndrome will be briefly mentioned. Rare or minor corneal abnormalities will be omitted.

Disorders of Carbohydrate Metabolism

In all mucopolysaccharidoses (MPSs), the cornea may become cloudy, and the clinical manifestations may appear so early in life that a differential diagnosis with congenital hereditary endothelial dystrophy should be taken into account. In all MPSs, however, the corneal clouding is a result of accumulation of a mucopolysaccharide in the cornea, and this usually takes time; consequently, the cloudiness becomes visible not at birth, but later. The cloudiness is most severe and early in MPS I-H (Hurler syndrome) and MPS I-S (Scheie's syndrome) and is least noticed in MPS III (San-filippo's syndrome). Retinitis pigmentosa or optic atrophy may be the main cause of visual deterioration in some MPSs.

An ophthalmologist can diagnose MPS given the combined findings of corneal cloudiness, systemic changes seen in the body and the face, and conjunctival biopsy. Electron microscopic evaluation of the conjunctiva always shows characteristic findings. All MPSs are transmitted by the autosomal recessive mode, except MPS II (Hunter syndrome), transmitted by a sex-linked recessive gene.

The enzymatic abnormality and chromosomal localization have been identified for most genes and their mutations (314). The corneal cloudiness may be successfully repaired by corneal transplantation (315), but this does not repair other ocular abnormalities such as retinitis pigmentosa or optic atrophy. Successful results were obtained with intravitreal gene replacement animal experiments (316). Beta-galactosidase gene was successfully transduced into human keratocytes (317), thus opening a possible future venue of genetic therapy.

Disorders of Lipid Metabolism

In Fabry's disease, an X-linked recessive lysosomal storage disorder, whorl-like opacities can be seen in the subepithelial layers within or near Bowman's membrane. Typically, they are cream-colored to golden brown and found more in the lower parts of the cornea (318). The opacities are seen in both heterozygotes and homozygotes, even at a very young age (319). The whorls are more pronounced in heterozygotes, in whom they may assume a more pronounced picture of cornea verticillata, previously assumed to be a dystrophy.

Gaucher disease, another disorder of lipid metabolism, caused by glucocerebrosidase deficiency, has three subtypes. Hepatosplenomegaly is marked. Corneal opacities in the form of small, linear, and dotlike corneal opacities in the posterior stroma were described (320). All three types of Gaucher disease are associated with mutations in the gene encoding acid-base glucosidase (GBA), mapped to chromosome Iq21 (314).

In Tangier disease, an autosomal recessive disease, in which generalized accumulation of cholesterol esters is found, diffuse fine opacities were reported scattered in the corneal stroma, especially later in life (321).

Familial lecithin-cholesterol acyltransferase (LCAT) deficiency is a rare autosomal recessive disorder. Central corneal haze caused by deposition of myriads of minute gray dots in the stroma and an arcus corneae is found in all patients (322). Heterozygotes may have a higher incidence of arcus-like corneal changes (321). The corneal deposits consist of multilaminar figures, which contain phospholipids and cholesterol, with reduced cholesteryl esters (323).

In fish-eye disease, a rare autosomal dominant disease described in Sweden (324), massive corneal opacities are associated with a generalized dyslipoproteinemia. Corneal opacities cause slight visual impairment in childhood, but increase gradually (324). Normal LCAT levels differentiate this disease from LCAT deficiency (325).

Fish-eye disease and LCAT deficiency are caused by mutations in the same gene (326), but the first disease occurs in the heterozygotic state (autosomal dominant transmission), while familial LCAT deficiency occurs in the homozygotic state (autosomal recessive transmission).

Arcus corneae is frequently found in familial hyperlipoproteinemia types II and III. The arcus occurs in the first decades of life in patients with hyperlipoproteinemia type II (327,328), a rather common autosomal dominant disease. Corneal arcus seems to be correlated with plasma low-density lipoproteins, and recognition of the disease and appropriate treatment may reduce the risk of ischemic heart disease (329).

The Mucolipidoses

The mucolipidoses are a group of metabolic disorders, in which both mucopolysaccharides (glycosaminoglycans) and lipids are accumulated in the tissues. In mucolipidoses I, II, III, and IV, corneal cloudiness may occur. However, in mucolipidosis IV, it is severe and early and may necessitate corneal transplantation (330). All mucolipidoses are autosomal recessive disorders.

Corneal clouding is also a prominent feature in Goldberg's syndrome (331), in which there is accumulation of lipids and glycosaminoglycans.

Disorders of Protein Metabolism

Cystinosis is an autosomal recessive disorder of amino acid metabolism, with accumulation of cystine in various tissues of the body. The cornea is always affected. Fine crystals can be seen in the superficial stroma (332) and can resemble central crystalline dystrophy of Schnyder.

The nephropathic form of cystinosis is the more common form. It has the highest incidence in French Canada (333). The nonnephropathic form is also named ocular cystinosis, as the main manifestation of the disorder is ocular. All forms of cystinosis are caused by mutations in the same gene, CTNS (334). In patients with ocular cystinosis a compound heterozygosity was detected, with one mild and one severe mutation in each patient. This combination may be the basis for the mild systemic disease. In the severe disease of nephropathic cystinosis, two severe mutations with loss of protein function occur.

The gene was mapped to chromosome 17pl3 (335) and identified and named CTNS (336). CTNS encodes an integral membrane protein, cystinosin. Mutations causing loss of function were identified in the nephropathic form (336,337).

Blindness in both infantile cystinosis and ocular cystinosis may result from the corneal cloudiness, retinopathy, or glaucoma. Crystals of cystine were detected, by UBM, in the trabecular meshwork (338).

Oral cysteamine, a cystine-depleting agent, is the therapy of choice, but does not affect the eye (339). The ocular condition manifests itself in reduction of vision due to increasing amounts of cystine crystals in the cornea, in photophobia, and in recurrent erosions. This can be efficiently treated by cysteamine 0.5% eye drops administered 6–12 times a day (339–341). In severe cases, a corneal transplant can be performed with good chances of graft survival (342), or both surgery and topical cysteamine are administered (343).

In tyrosinemia type II (Richner–Hanhart syndrome), a rare autosomal recessive error of metabolism of amino acids, the cornea is affected by subepithelial dendritic lines resembling herpes simplex lesions (344). They may look like snowflakes (345) and later be associated with secondary corneal neovascularization (346). Photophobia and tearing may be early findings (346).

Patients with tyrosinemia type II suffer, in addition to the herpetiform ocular condition, from a characteristic palmar and plantar hyperkeratosis, elevated serum tyrosine and phenylalanine, and sometimes mental retardation, usually mild. The disorder is caused by point mutations in the TAT gene, which encodes tyrosine transaminase and is mapped to chromosome 16q22 (347) Tyrosine- and phenylalanine-restricted diet, for life, is the treatment of choice. The corneal lesions have been resolved with the diet therapy that was continued for nine months (348).

Miscellaneous Disorders

In X-linked recessive ichthyosis, a thin, irregular layer of confluent gray-white opacities (349), or small punctate, filiform opacities resembling pre-Descemet's dystrophy can be seen (350). Corneal opacities were found in 14 of 28 patients with X-linked ichthyosis and steroid sulfatase deficiency (351).

Clinically, the cornea may manifest a punctate keratopathy, nodular swellings of the corneal nerves, filiform to punctate opacities in the deep stroma and a posterior embryotoxon. Pathologic studies showed a thick amorphous, subepithelial proteinaceous material, disorganized collagen fibers, and round, elongated spaces anterior to the Descemet layer (352). Electron-dense granular material accumulates in the stroma (352).

In Wilson's disease the corneal Kayser–Fleischer ring is seen as a characteristic ring of different colors, according to the concentration of copper. It can be easily seen by slit-lamp, situated in front of Descemet layer near the corneal limbus. Mutations in the Wilson disease gene, ATP78, were identified (359). The gene encodes a copper transporting ATP-ase and was mapped to chromosome 13ql4.3–q21.1

Corneal abnormalities were described in Bietti crystallin corneoretinal dystrophy and they will be discussed in the chapter on retinitis pigmentosa. Hereditary endotheliopathy with retinopathy, nephropathy, and stroke will be discussed along with other retinal diseases. Corneal changes in Marfan disease will be discussed in the chapter on lens disorders.

Corneal opacities with vascularization are seen in the autosomal dominant KID syndrome, with the triad of *k*eratitis, *i*chthyosis, and *d*eafness (353). Another disease affecting the skin and cornea is the ACL syndrome (*a*cromegaloid features, *c*utis verticis gyrata, and *l*eukoma corneae) (354). Pathologic study showed accumulation of granular material in the stroma and abnormal collagen fibers (354).

Severe corneal scarring, neovascularization, and photophobia were described in the EEC syndrome (*e*ctrodactylia, *e*ctodermal dysplasia, *c*left lip and palate) (355). In this autosomal dominant disorder, lobster-claw deformities of hands and feet, abnormal hair, abnormal teeth, and a cleft lip and palate are found.

Familial spinocerebellar degeneration with corneal dystrophy is an autosomal recessive disorder (356). Bilateral corneal opacification starts in the second year of life and progresses to severe visual impairment (356).

A severely cloudy cornea has been described in cases of severe congenital malformations associated with chromosomal anomalies (357,358).

REFERENCES

1. Groenouw A. Knotchenformige Hornhauttriibungen (noduii corneae). Arch Augenheilkd 1890; 21:281–289.
2. Bücklers M. The three forms of familial corneal degeneration and their hereditary transmission. Arch Ophthalmol 1937; 18:331–332.
3. Waring GO, Rodrigues MM, Laibson PR. Corneal dystrophies: I Dystrophies of the epithelium, Bowman's layer and stroma. Surv Ophthalmol 1978; 23:71–122.
4. Klintworth GK. Tissue culture in the inherited corneal dystrophies: possible applications and problems. Birth Defects 1976; 12:115–132.
5. Rodrigues MM, Krachmer JH. Recent advances in corneal stromal dystrophies. Cornea 1988; 7:19–29.
6. OMTM at: http://www.ncbi.nlm.nih.gov/omim/
7. Cogan DG, Donaldson DD, Kuwabara T, Marshall D. Microcystic dystrophy of the corneal epithelium. Trans Am Ophthalmol Soc 1964; 62:213–235.
8. Laibson PR, Krachmer JH. Familial occurrence of dot (microcystic), map, fingerprint dystrophy of the cornea. Invest Ophthalmol 1975; 14:397–399.
9. Laibson PR. Microcystic corneal dystrophy. Trans Am Ophthalmol Soc 1976; 74: 488–531.
10. Lisch W, Lisch C. Die epitheliale Hornhautbasalmembran dystrophie. Klin Monatsbl Augenheilkd 1983; 183:251–255.
11. Pau H. Pathogenese und Therapie der primaren und secondaren rezidevierenden ergion. Klin Monatsbl Augenheilkd 1982; 180:259–263.

12. Remler O. Beitrag zur hereditaren rezidivierenden Hornhaut erosion. Klin Monatsbl Augenheilkd 1983; 183:59.
13. Sugar J. Defects of the cornea. In: Emery AEH, Remoin DL, eds. Principles and Practice of Medical Genetics. Edinburgh: Churchill-Livingstone, 1983:497–508.
14. Pameijer JK. Ueber eine fremdartige familiäre oberflachliche Hornhautveranderung. Klin Monatsbl Augenheilkd 1935; 95:516–517.
15. Meesmann A, Wilke F. Klinische und anatomische Untersuchungen ueber eine bisher unbekannte, dominant vererbte Epitheldystrophie der Hornhaut. Klin Monatsbl Augen-heilkd 1939; 103:361–391.
16. Stocker FW, Holt LB. A rare form of hereditary epithelial dystrophy of the cornea: a genetic clinical and pathologic study. Trans Am Ophthalmol Soc 1954; 52: 133–144.
17. Behnke H, Thiel HJ. Ueber die hereditare Epitheldystrophie der Hornhaut (Typ Mees-man-Wilke) in Schleswjg-Holstein. Klin Monatsbl Augenheilkd 1965; 147: 662–672.
18. Miller CA, Krachmer JH. Corneal diseases. In: Reinie WA, ed. Goldberg's Genetic and Metabolic Eye Disease. 2nd ed. Boston: Little, Brown & Co., 1986:297–367.
19. Irvine AD, Corden LD, Swensson O, et al. Mutations in cornea-specific keratin K3 or K12 genes cause Meesmann's corneal dystrophy. Nat Genet 1997; 16:184–187.
20. Bücklers M. Ueber eine weitere familiare Hornhautdystrophie (Reis). Klin Monatsbl Augenheilkd 1949; 114:386–397.
21. Pouliquen Y, Dhermy P, Presles D, Tollard MF. Dégénérescence en Chagrin de crocodile de Vogt on dégénérescence en mosaique de Valerio. Arch Ophthalmol (Paris) 1976; 36:395–417.
22. Thiel HJ, Behnke H. Eine bisher unbekannte subepitheliale hereditare Hornhautdystrophie. Klin Monatsbl Augenheilkd 1967; 150:862–874.
23. Kuchle M, Green WR, Volcker HE, Barraquer J. Reevaluation of corneal dystrophies of Bowman's layer and the anterior stroma (Reis-Bücklers and Thiel-Behnke types): a light and electron microscopic study of eight corneas and a review of the literature. Cornea 1995; 14:333–354.
24. Yee RW, Sullivan LS, Montiero MP, Daiger SP. Refined linkage mapping and candidate screening for Thiel–Behnke corneal dystrophy (CDB2) on 10q23–q24 (abstract). Invest Ophthalmol Vis Sci , 1998; 39(suppl):739.
25. Perry HD, Fine BS, Caldwell DR. Reis-Bücklers dystrophy. Arch Ophthalmol 1979; 97:664–670.
26. Caldwell DR. Postoperative recurrence of Reis-Bücklers corneal dystrophy. Am J Ophthalmol 1978; 85:567–568.
27. Grayson M, Wilbrandt H. Dystrophy of the anterior limiting membrane of the cornea (Reis-Bücklers type). Am J Ophthalmol 1966; 61:345–349.
28. Rodrigues MM, Fine BS, Laibson PR, Zimmerman LE. Disorders of the corneal epithelium: a clinicopathologic study of dot, geographic and fingerprint patterns. Am J Ophthalmol 1974; 92:475–482.
29. Brodrick JD, Dark AJ, Peace GW. Fingerprint dystrophy of the cornea. A histologic study. Am J Ophthalmol 1974; 92:483–489.
30. Fine BS, Yanoff M, Pitts E, Slaughter FD. Meesman's epithelial dystrophy of the cornea. Am J Ophthamol 1977; 83:633–642.
31. Kanai A, Kaufman HE, Polack FM. Electron microscopic study of Reis-Bücklers dystrophy. Ann Ophthalmol 1973; 5:953–962.
32. Werblin TP, Hirst LW, Stark WJ, Maumenee IH. Prevalence of map-dot-fingerprint changes in the cornea. Br J Ophthalmol 1981; 65:401–409.
33. Badr IA, Basaffar S, Jabak M, Wagoner MD. Meesmann corneal epithelial dystrophy in a Saudi Arabian family. Am J Ophthalmol 1998; 125:182–186.
34. Lisch W, Steuhl KP, Lisch C, et al. A new, band-shaped and whorled microcystic dystrophy of the corneal epithelium. Am J Ophthalmol 1992; 114:35–44.

35. Lisch W, Büttner A, Oeffner F, et al. Lisch corneal dystrophy is genetically distinct from Meesmann corneal dystrophy and maps to xp22.3. Am J Ophthalmol 2000; 130: 461–468.
36. Nishida K, Adachi W, Shimizu-Matsumoto A, et al. A gene expression profile of human corneal epithelium and the isolation of human keratin 12 cDNA. Invest Ophthalmol Vis Sci 1996; 37:1800–1809.
37. Jun AS, Liu SH, Koo EH, et al. Microarray analysis of gene expression in human donor corneas. Arch Ophthalmol 2001; 119:1629–1634.
38. Buxton JN, Fox ML. Superficial epithelial keratectomy in the treatment of epithelial basement membrane dystrophy. A preliminary report. Arch Opthalmol 1983; 101: 392–395.
39. Wood TO, Fleming JC, Dotson RS, Cotten MS. Treatment of Reis-Bücklers corneal dystrophy by removal of sub-epithelial fibrous tissue. Am J Ophthaimol 1978; 85:360–362.
40. Orndahl M, Fagerholm P, Fitzsimmons T, Tengroth B. Treatment of corneal dystrophies with excimer laser. Acta Ophthalmol 1994; 72:235–240.
41. Orndahl MJ, Fagerholm PP. Phototherapeutic keratectomy for map-dot-fingerprint corneal dystrophy. Cornea 1998; 17:595–599.
42. Fagerholm P. Phototherapeutic keratectomy: 12 years of experience. Acta Ophthalmol Scand 2003; 81:19–32.
43. Dinh R, Rapuano CJ, Cohen EJ, Laibson PR. Recurrence of corneal dystrophy after excimer laser phototherapeutic keratectomy. Ophthalmology 1999; 106:1490–1497.
44. Soong HK, Farjo Q, Meyer RF, Sugar A. Diamond burr superficial keratectomy for recurrent corneal erosions. Br J Ophthalmol 2002; 86:296–298.
45. Klintworth G. The molecular genetics of the corneal dystrophies—current status. Front Biosci 2003; 8:2687–713.
46. Folberg R, Stone EM, Sheffield VC, Mathers WD. The relationship between granular, lattice type 1, and Avellino corneal dystrophies A histopathologic study. Arch Ophthalmol 1994; 112:1080–1085.
47. Stone EM, Mathers WD, Rosenwasser GO, et al. Three autosomal dominant corneal dystrophies map to chromosome 5q. Nat Genet 1994; 6:47–51.
48. Munier FL, Korvatska E, Djemai A, et al. Kerato-epithelin mutations in four 5q31-linked corneal dystrophies. Nat Genet 1997; 15:247–251.
49. Korvatska E, Munier FL, Djemai A, et al. Mutation hot spots in 5q31-linked corneal dystrophies. Am J Hum Genet 1998; 62:320–324.
50. Dighiero P, Niel F, Ellies P, et al. Histologic phenotype-genotype correlation of corneal dystrophies associated with eight distinct mutations in the TGFBI gene. Ophthalmology 2001; 108:818–823.
51. Rodrigues MM, Streeten BW, Krachmer JH, et al. Microfibrillar protein and phospholipid in granular corneal dystrophy. Arch Ophthalmol 1983; 101:802–810.
52. Forsius H, Eriksson AW, Kama J, et al. Granular corneal dystrophy with late manifestation. Acta Ophthalmol 1983; 61:514–528.
53. Klintworth GK. Advances in the molecular genetics of corneal dystrophies. Am J Ophthalmol 1999; 128:747–754.
54. Konishi M, Mashima Y, Yamada M, et al. The classic form of granular corneal dystrophy associated with R555W mutation in the BIGH3 gene is rare in Japanese patients. Am J Ophthalmol 1998; 126:450–452.
55. Afshari NA, Mullally JE, Afshari MA, et al. Survey of patients with granular, lattice, avellino, and Reis-Bücklers corneal dystrophies for mutations in the BIGH3 and gelsolin genes. Arch Ophthalmol 2001; 119:16–22.
56. Ellies P, Renard G, Valleix S, et al. Clinical outcome of eight BIGH3-linked corneal dystrophies. Ophthalmology 2002; 109:793–797.
57. Durand L, Resal R, Burillon C. Mise au point sur une entite anatomoclinique la dystrophie grillagee de Biber-Haab-Dimmer. J Fr Ophtalmol 1985; 8:729–734.

58. Klintworth GK. Lattice corneal dystrophy. An inherited variety of amyloidosis restricted to the cornea. Am J Pathol 1967; 50:371–400.
59. Meretoja J. Comparative histopathological and clinical findings in eyes with lattice corneal dystrophy of two different types. Ophthalmologica 1972; 165:15–37.
60. Hida T, Tsubota K, Kigasawa K, et al. Clinical features of a newly recognized type of lattice corneal dystrophy. Am J Ophthalmol 1987; 104:241–248.
61. Gupta SK, Hodge WG, Damji KF, et al. Lattice corneal dystrophy type 1 in a Canadian kindred is associated with the Arg124 → Cys mutation in the kerato-epithelin gene. Am J Ophthalmol 1998; 125:547–549.
62. Rabb MF, Blodi F, Boniuk M. Unilateral lattice dystrophy of the cornea. Trans Am Acad Ophthalmol Otolaryngol 1974; 78:440–444.
63. Sridhar MS, Laibson PR, Eagle RC, et al. Unilateral corneal lattice dystrophy. Cornea 2001; 20:850–852.
64. Lanier JD, Fine M, Togni B. Lattice corneal dystrophy. Arch Ophthalmol 1976; 94:921–924.
65. Sturrock AD. Lattice corneal dystrophy: a source of confusion. Br J Ophthalmol 1983; 67:629–634.
66. Meisler DM, Fine M. Recurrence of the clinical signs of lattice corneal dystrophy (type I) in corneal transplants. Am J Ophthalmol 1984; 97:210–214.
67. Holland EJ, Daya SM, Stone EM, et al. Avellino corneal dystrophy. Clinical manifestations and natural history. Ophthalmology 1992; 99:1564–1568.
68. Santo RM, Yamaguchi T, Kanai A, et al. Clinical and histopathologic features of corneal dystrophies in Japan. Ophthalmology 1995; 102:557–567.
69. Nakamura T, Nishida K, Dota A, et al. Gelatino-lattice corneal dystrophy: clinical features and mutational analysis. Am J Ophthalmol 2000; 129:665–666.
70. Mashima Y, Yamamoto S, Inoue Y, et al. Association of autosomal dominantly inherited corneal dystrophies with BIGH3 gene mutations in Japan. Am J Ophthalmol 2000; 130:516–517.
71. Yamamoto S, Okada M, Tsujikawa M, et al. The spectrum of beta ig-h3 gene mutations in Japanese patients with corneal dystrophy. Cornea 2000; 19(suppl) 3:S21–S23.
72. Rosenwasser GO, Sucheski BM, Rosa N, et al. Phenotypic variation in combined granular-lattice (Avellino) corneal dystrophy. Arch Ophthalmol 1993; 111:1546–1552.
73. Lucarelli MJ, Adamis AP. Avellino corneal dystrophy. Arch Ophthalmol 1994; 112:418–419.
74. Mannis MJ, Krachmer JH, Rodrigues MM, Pardos GJ. Polymorphic amyloid degeneration of the cornea: a clinical and histopathologic study. Am J Ophthalmol 1981; 99:1217–1223.
75. Krachmer JH, Dubord PJ, Rodrigues MM, Mannis MJ. Corneal posterior crocodile shagreen and polymorphic amyloid degeneration. A histopathologic study. Arch Ophthal mol 1983; 101:54–59.
76. Kirk HQ, Rabb M, Hattenhauer J, Smith R. Primary familial amyloidosis of the cornea. Trans Am Acad Ophthalmol Otolaryngol 1973; 77:411–417.
77. Konishi M, Yamada M, Nakamura Y, Mashima Y. Immunohistology of kerato-epithelin in corneal stromal dystrophies associated with R124 mutations of the BIGH3 gene. Curr Eye Res 2001; 21:891–896.
78. Dighiero P, Valleix S, D'Hermies F, et al. Clinical, histologic, and ultrastructural features of the corneal dystrophy caused by the R124L mutation of the BIGH3 gene. Ophthalmology 2000; 107:1353–1357.
79. Dighiero P, Niel F, Ellies P. Histologic phenotype-genotype correlation of corneal dystrophies associated with eight distinct mutations in the TGFBI gene. Ophthalmology 2001; 108:818–823.
80. Mashima Y, Nakamura Y, Noda K. A novel mutation at codon 124 (R124L) in the BIGH3 gene is associated with a superficial variant of granular corneal dystrophy. Arch Ophthalmol 1999; 117:90–93.

81. Okada M, Yamamoto S, Tsujikawa M, et al. Two distinct kerato-epithelin mutations in Reis–Bücklers corneal dystrophy. Am J Ophthalmol 1998; 126:535–542.
82. Rozzo C, Fossarello M, Galleri G. A common beta ig-h3 gene mutation (delta f540) in a large cohort of Sardinian Reis–Bücklers corneal dystrophy patients. Hum Mutat 1998; 12:215–216.
83. Small KW, Mullen L, Barletta J, et al. Mapping of Reis–Bücklers' corneal dystrophy to chromosome 5q. Am J Ophthalmol 1996; 121:384–390.
84. Stock EL, Feder RS, O'Grady RB, et al. Lattice corneal dystrophy type IIIA. Clinical and histopathologic correlations. Arch Ophthalmol 1991; 109:354–358.
85. Yamamoto S, Okada M, Tsujikawa M, et al. A kerato-epithelin (betaig-h3) mutation in lattice corneal dystrophy type IIIA. Am J Hum Genet 1998; 62:719–722.
86. Dighiero P, Drunat S, Ellies P, et al. A new mutation (A546T) of the betaig-h3 gene responsible for a French lattice corneal dystrophy type IIIA. Am J Ophthalmol 2000; 129:248–251.
87. Stewart H, Black GC, Donnai D, et al. A mutation within exon 14 of the TGFBI (BIGH3) gene on chromosome 5q31 causes an asymmetric, late-onset form of lattice corneal dystrophy. Ophthalmology 1999; 106:964–970.
88. Endo S, Nguyen TH, Fujiki K, et al. Leu518Pro mutation of the beta ig-h3 gene causes lattice corneal dystrophy type I. Am J Ophthalmol 1999; 128:104–106.
89. Dighiero P, Drunat S, D'Hermies F, et al. A novel variant of granular corneal dystrophy caused by association of 2 mutations in the TGFBI gene-R124L and DeltaT125-DeltaE126. Arch Ophthalmol 2000; 118:814–818.
90. Mashima Y, Imamura Y, Konishi M, et al. Homogeneity of kerato-epithelin codon 124 mutations in Japanese patients with either of two types of corneal stromal dystrophy. Am J Hum Genet 1997; 61:1448–1450.
91. Fujiki K, Hotta Y, Nakayasu K, Kanai A. Homozygotic patient with beta ig-h3 gene mutation in granular dystrophy. Cornea 1998; 17:288–292.
92. Kaji Y, Amano S, Oshika T, et al. Chronic clinical course of two patients with severe corneal dystrophy caused by homozygous R124H mutations in the beta ig-h3 gene. Am J Ophthalmol 2000; 129:663–665.
93. Watanabe H, Hashida Y, Tsujikawa K, et al. Two patterns of opacity in corneal dystrophy caused by the homozygous BIG-H3 R124H mutation. Am J Ophthalmol 2001; 132:211–216.
94. Okada M, Yamamoto S, Watanabe H, et al. Granular corneal dystrophy with homozygous mutations in the kerato-epithelin gene. Am J Ophthalmol 1998; 126:169–176.
95. Haddad R, Font RL, Fine BS. Unusual superficial variant of granular dystrophy of the cornea. Am J Ophthalmol 1977; 83:213–218.
96. Sugar J. Personal communication.
97. Folberg R, Alfonso E, Croxatto JO, et al. Clinically atypical granular corneal dystrophy with pathologic features of lattice-like amyloid deposits. A study of three families. Ophthalmology 1988; 95:46–51.
98. Dubord PJ, Krachmer JH. Diagnosis of early lattice corneal dystrophy. Arch Ophthalmol 1982; 100:788–790.
99. Yanoff M, Fine BS, Colosi NJ, Katowitz JA. Lattice corneal dystrophy: report of an unusual case. Arch Ophthalmol 1977; 95:651–655.
100. Garner A. Histochemistry of corneal granular dystrophy. Br J Ophthalmol 1969; 53:799–807.
101. Akiya S, Brown SI. Granular dystrophy of the cornea. Characteristic electron microscopic lesions. Arch Ophthalmol 1970; 84:179–192.
102. Johnson BL, Brown Si, Zaidman GW. A light and electron microscopic study of recurrent granular dystrophy of the cornea. Am J Ophthalmol 1981; 92:49–58.
103. Rodrigues MM, Gaster RN, Pratt MV. Unusual superficial confluent form of granular corneal dystrophy. Ophthalmology 1983; 90:1507–1511.

104. Seitelberger F, Nemetz UR. Beitrag zur Frage der gittrigen Hornhautdystrophie. Graefes Arch Clin Exp Ophthalmol 1961; 169:102–111.
105. Francois J, Feher J. Light microscopical and polarisation optical study of the lattice dystrophy of the cornea. Ophthalmologies 1972; 164:1–18.
106. Francois J, Victoria-Troncoso V. Histopathogemic study of the lattice dystrophy of the cornea. Ophthalmic Res 1975; 7:420–431.
107. Delleman JW, Winkelman JE. Degeneratio corneae cristallinea hereditaria. A clinical, genetical and histological study. Ophthalmologica 1968; 155:409–426.
108. Hida T, Prioa AD, Kigasawa K, et al. Histopathologic and immunochemical features of lattice corneal dystrophy type III. Am J Ophthalmol 1987; 104:249–254.
109. Mondino BJ, Raj CVS, Skinner M, et al. Protein AA and lattice corneal dystrophy. Am J Ophthalmol 1980; 89:377–380.
110. Gorevic PD, Rodrigues MM,, Krachmer JH, et al. Lack of evidence for protein AA reactivity in amyloid deposits of lattice corneal dystrophy and amyloid corneal degeneration. Am J Ophthalmol 1984; 98:216–224.
111. Panjwani N, Rodrigues M, Free K, et al. Lectin receptors of amyloid in corneas with lattice dystrophy. Arch Ophthalmol 1987; 105:688–691.
112. Owens SL, Sugar J, Edward DP. Superficial granular corneal dystrophy with amyloid deposits. Arch Ophthalmol 1992; 110:175–176.
113. Streeten BW, Qi Y, Klintworth GK, et al. Immunolocalization of beta ig-h3 protein in 5q31-linked corneal dystrophies and normal corneas. Arch Ophthalmol 1999; 117: 67–75.
114. Akhtar S, Meek KM, Ridgway AE, et al. Deposits and proteoglycan changes in primary and recurrent granular dystrophy of the cornea. Arch Ophthalmol 1999; 117:310–321.
115. Werner LP, Werner L, Dighiero P. Confocal microscopy in Bowman and stromal corneal dystrophies. Ophthalmology 1999; 106:1697–1704.
116. Lempert SL, Jenkins MS, Johnson BL, Brown SI. A simple technique for removal of recurring granular dystrophy in corneal grafts. Am J Ophthalmol 1978; 86:89–91.
117. Dana MR, Moyes AL, Gomes JA, et al. The indications for and outcome in pediatric keratoplasty. A multicenter study. Ophthalmology 1995; 102:1129–1139.
118. Dunaief JL, Ng EW, Goldberg MF. Corneal dystrophies of epithelial genesis: the possible therapeutic use of limbal stem cell transplantation. Arch Ophthalmol 2001; 119:120–122.
119. Tsubota K, Satake Y, Kaido M, et al. Treatment of severe ocular-surface disorders with corneal epithelial stem-cell transplantation. N Engl J Med 1999; 340:1697–1703.
120. Koizumi N, Inatomi T, Suzuki T, et al. Cultivated corneal epithelial stem cell transplantation in ocular surface disorders. Ophthalmology 2001; 108:1569–1574.
121. Sundmacher R, Spelsberg H, Reinhard T. Homologous penetrating central limbokeratoplasty in granular and lattice corneal dystrophy. Cornea 1999; 18:664–670.
122. Bradshaw JJ, Obritsch WF, Cho BJ, et al. Ex vivo transduction of corneal epithelial progenitor cells using a retroviral vector. Invest Ophthalmol Vis Sci 1999; 40:230–235.
123. Inoue T, Watanabe H, Yamamoto S, et al. Different recurrence patterns after phototherapeutic keratectomy in the corneal dystrophy resulting from homozygous and heterozygous R124H BIG-H3 mutation. Am J Ophthalmol 2001; 132:255–257.
124. Dogru M, Katakami C, Nishida T, Yamanaka A. Alteration of the ocular surface with recurrence of granular/avellino corneal dystrophy after phototherapeutic keratectomy: report of five cases and literature review. Ophthalmology 2001; 108:810–817.
125. Wan XH, Lee HC, Stulting RD. Exacerbation of Avellino corneal dystrophy after laser in situ keratomileusis. Cornea 2002; 21:223–226.
126. Donnenfeld ED, Cohen EJ, Ingraham JH, et al. Corneal thinning in macular corneal dystrophy. Am J Ophthalmol 1986; 101:112–113.
127. Liu NP, Baldwin J, Lennon F. Coexistence of macular corneal dystrophy types I and II in a single sibship. Br J Ophthalmol 1998; 82:241–244.

128. Jonasson F, Oshima E, Thonar EJ, et al. Macular corneal dystrophy in Iceland. A clinical, genealogic, and immunohistochemical study of 28 patients. Ophthalmology 1996; 103:1111–1117.
129. Vance JM, Jonasson F, Lennon F, et al. Linkage of a gene for macular corneal dystrophy to chromosome 16. Am J Hum Genet 1996; 58:757–762.
130. Edward DP, Yue BY, Sugar J, et al. Heterogeneity in macular corneal dystrophy. Arch Ophthalmol 1988; 106:1579–1583.
131. Hassell JR, Klintworth GK. Serum sulfotransferase levels in patients with macular corneal dystrophy type I. Arch Ophthalmol 1997; 115:1419–1421.
132. Klintworth GK, Oshima E, al-Rajhi A, et al. Macular corneal dystrophy in Saudi Arabia: a study of 56 cases and recognition of a new immunophenotype. Am J Ophthalmol 1997; 124:9–18.
133. Edward DP, Thonar EJ, Srinivasan M, et al. Macular dystrophy of the cornea. A systemic disorder of keratan sulfate metabolism. Ophthalmology 1990; 97:1194–1200.
134. Cursiefen C, Hofmann-Rummelt C, Schlotzer-Schrehardt U, et al. Immunohistochemical classification of primary and recurrent macular corneal dystrophy in Germany: subclassification of immunophenotype I A using a novel keratan sulfate antibody. Exp Eye Res 2001; 73:593–600.
135. Akama TO, Nishida K, Nakayama J. Macular corneal dystrophy type I and type II are caused by distinct mutations in a new sulphotransferase gene. Nat Genet 2000; 26:237–241.
136. Liu NP, Dew-Knight S, Rayner M. Mutations in corneal carbohydrate sulfotransferase 6 gene (CHST6) cause macular corneal dystrophy in Iceland. Mol Vis 2000; 6:261–264.
137. El-Ashry MF, El-Aziz MM, Wilkins S, et al. Identification of novel mutations in the carbohydrate sulfotransferase gene (CHST6) causing macular corneal dystrophy. Invest Ophthalmol Vis Sci 2002; 43:377–382.
138. Newsome DA, Hassall JR, Rodrigues MM, et al. Biochemical and histological analysis of "recurrent" macular corneal dystrophy. Am J Ophthalmol 1982; 100:1125–1131.
139. Klintworth GK, Reed J, Stainer GA, Binder PS. Recurrence of macular corneal dystrophy within grafts. Am J Ophthalmol 1983; 95:60–72.
140. Küchle M, Cursiefen C, Fischer DC, et al. Recurrent macular corneal dystrophy type II 49 years after penetrating keratoplasty. Arch Ophthalmol 1999; 117:528–531.
141. Mondino BJ, Rabb MF, Sugar J, et al. I. Primary familial amyloidosis of the cornea. Am J Ophthalmol 1981; 92:732–736.
142. Shimazaki J, Hida T, Inoue M, et al. Long-term follow-up of patients with familial subepithelial amyloidosis of the cornea. Ophthalmology 1995; 102:139–144.
143. Weber FL, Babel J. Gelatinous drop-like dystrophy. A form of primary corneal amyloidosis. Arch Ophthalmol 1980; 98:144–148.
144. Dota A, Nishida K, Honma Y, et al. Gelatinous drop-like corneal dystrophy is not one of the beta ig-h3-mutated corneal amyloidoses. Am J Ophthalmol 1998; 126:832–833.
145. Tsujikawa M, Kurahashi H, Tanaka T, et al. Identification of the gene responsible for gelatinous drop-like corneal dystrophy. Nat Genet 1999; 21:420–423.
146. Ren Z, Lin PY, Klintworth GK, et al. Allelic and locus heterogeneity in autosomal recessive gelatinous drop-like corneal dystrophy. Hum Genet 2002; 110:568–577.
147. Ha NT, Chau HM, Cung LX, et al. A novel mutation of M1S1 gene found in a Vietnamese patient with gelatinous droplike corneal dystrophy. Am J Ophthalmol 2003; 135:390–393.
148. Yoshida S, Kumano Y, Yoshida A, et al. Two brothers with gelatinous drop-like dystrophy at different stages of the disease: role of mutational analysis. Am J Ophthalmol 2002; 133:830–832.
149. Ha NT, Fujiki K, Hotta Y, et al. Q118X mutation of M1S1 gene caused gelatinous drop-like corneal dystrophy: the P501T of BIGH3 gene found in a family with gelatinous drop-like corneal dystrophy. Am J Ophthalmol 2000; 130:119–120.
150. Seitz B, Weidle E, Naumann GO. Unilateral type III (Hida) lattice stromal corneal dystrophy (German). Klin Monatsbl Augenteilkd 1993; 203:279–285.

151. Teng CC. Macular dystrophy of the cornea, a histochemical and electro-microscopic study. Am J Ophthalmol 1966; 62:436–454.
152. Francois J, Feher J. Light microscopical and polarisation optical study of the macular dystrophy of the cornea. Ophthalmologica 1972; 164:19–34.
153. Livni N, Abraham FA, Zauberman H. Groenouw's macular dystrophy: histochemistry and ultrastructure of the cornea. Doc Ophthalmol 1979; 37:327–345.
154. Bruner WE, Dejak TR, Grossniklaus HE, et al. Corneal alpha-galactosidase deficiency in macular corneal dystrophy. Ophthalmic Paediatr Genet 1985; 5:179–183.
155. Francois J, Hanssens M, Tenchi H, Subruijns M. Ultrastructural findings in corneal macular dystrophy (Groenouw type II). Ophthalmic Res 1975; 7:80–89.
156. Klintworth GK, Smith CF. Abnormalities of proteoglycans synthesized by corneal organ cultures derived from patients with macular corneal dystrophy. Lab Invest 1983; 48:603–612.
157. Nakazawa K, Hassell JR, Hascall VC, et al. Defective processing of keratan sulfate in macular corneal dystrophy. J Biol Chem 1984; 259:13751–13757.
158. Sundar-Raj N, Barbacci-Tobin E, Howe WE, et al. Macular corneal dystrophy: immuno-chemical characterization using monoclonal antibodies. Invest Ophthalmol Vis Sci 1987; 28:1678–1686.
159. Klintworth GK, Meyer R, Dennis R, et al. Macular corneal dystrophy. Lack of keratan sulfate in serum and cornea. Ophthalmic Paediatr Genet 1986; 7:139–143.
160. Thonar EJ, Meyer RF, Dennis RF, et al. Absence of normal keratan sulfate in the blood of patients with macular corneal dystrophy. Am J Ophthalmol 1986; 102:561–569.
161. Yang CJ, Sundar-Raj N, Thonar EJ, Klintworth GK. Immunohistochemical evidence of heterogeneity in macular corneal dystrophy. Am J Ophthalmol 1988; 106:65–71.
162. Takahashi M, Yokota T, Yamashita Y, et al. Unusual inclusions in stromal macrophages in a case of gelatinous drop-like corneal dystrophy. Am J Ophthalmol 1985; 99:312–316.
163. Meretoja J. Genetic aspects of familial amyloidosis with corneal lattice dystrophy and cranial neuropathy. Clin Genet 1973; 4:173–185.
164. Akiya S, Nishio Y, Ibi K, et al. Lattice corneal dystrophy type II associated with familial amyloid polyneuropathy type IV. Ophthalmology 1996; 103:1106–1110.
165. Rothstein A, Auran JD, Wittpenn JR, et al. Confocal microscopy in Meretoja syndrome. Cornea 2002; 21:364–367.
166. Maury CP. Homozygous familial amyloidosis, Finnish type: demonstration of glomerular gelsolin-derived amyloid and non-amyloid tubular gelsolin. Clin Nephrol 1993; 40:53–56.
167. Kiuru S. Familial amyloidosis of the Finnish type (FAF). A clinical study of 30 patients. Acta Neurol Scand 1992; 86:346–353.
168. Hiltunen T, Kiuru S, Hongell V, et al. Finnish type of familial amyloidosis: cosegregation of Asp187—Asn mutation of gelsolin with the disease in three large families. Am J Hum Genet 1991; 49:522–528.
169. Gorevic PD, Munoz PC, Gorgone G, et al. Amyloidosis due to a mutation of the gelsolin gene in an American family with lattice corneal dystrophy type II. N Engl J Med 1991; 325:1780–1785.
170. Sipila K, Aula P. Database for the mutations of the Finnish disease heritage. Hum Mutat 2002; 19:16–22.
171. Purcell JJ Jr, Rodrigues M, Chishti MI, et al. Lattice corneal dystrophy associated with familial systemic amyloidosis (Meretoja's syndrome). Ophthalmology 1983; 90: 1512–1517.
172. Lisch W, Weidle EG, Lisch C, et al. Schnyder's dystrophy. Progression and metabolism. Ophthalmic Paediatr Genet 1986; 7:45–56.
173. Bron AJ, Williams HP, Carruthers ME. Hereditary crystalline stromal dystrophy of Schnyder I. Clinical features of a family with hyperlipoproteinemia. Br J Ophthalmol 1972; 56:383–399.

174. Hoang-Xuan T, Pouliquen Y, Gasteau J. Dystrophie cristalline de Schnyder. II. Association a un genu valgum. J Fr Ophtalmol 1985; 8:743–747.
175. Ingraham HJ, Perry HD, Donnenfeld ED, Donaldson DD. Progressive Schnyder's corneal dystrophy. Ophthalmology 1993; 100:1824–1827.
176. Weiss JS. Schnyder's dystrophy of the cornea. A Swede-Finn connection. Cornea 1992; 11:93–101.
177. Weiss JS. Schnyder crystalline dystrophy sine crystals. Recommendation for a revision of nomenclature. Ophthalmology 1996; 103:465–473.
178. Shearman AM, Hudson TJ, Andresen JM, et al. The gene for Schnyder's crystalline corneal dystrophy maps to human chromosome 1p34.1-p36. Hum Mol Genet 1996; 5: 1667–1672.
179. Takeuchi T, Furihata M, Heng HH, et al. Chromosomal mapping and expression of the human B120 gene. Gene 1998; 213:189–193.
180. Vesaluoma MH, Linna TU, Sankila EM, et al. In vivo confocal microscopy of a family with Schnyder crystalline corneal dystrophy. Ophthalmology 1999; 106:944–951.
181. Garner A, Tripathi RC. Hereditary crystalline stromal dystrophy of Schnyder: II histopathology and ultrastructure. Br J Ophthalmol 1972; 56:400–408.
182. Weller RL, Rodger FC. Crystalline stromal dystrophy, histochemistry and ultrastructure of the cornea. Br J Ophthalmol 1980; 64:46–52.
183. Hoang-Xuan T, Pouliquen Y, Savoldelli M, Gasteau J. Dystrophie cristalline de Schnyder. 1. Etude d'un cas en microscopie optique et en ultrastructure. J Fr Ophtalmol 1985; 8:735–742.
184. Weiss JS, Rodrigues MM, Kruth HS, et al. Panstromal Schnyder's corneal dystrophy. Ultrastructural and histochemical studies. Ophthalmology 1992; 99:1072–1081.
185. Chern KC, Meisler DM. Disappearance of crystals in Schnyder's crystalline corneal dystrophy after epithelial erosion. Am J Ophthalmol 1995; 120:802–803.
186. Yamada M, Mochizuki H, Kamata Y, et al. Quantitative analysis of lipid deposits from Schnyder's corneal dystrophy. Br J Ophthalmol 1998; 82:444–447.
187. Francois J, Neetens A. Nouvelle dystrophie heredofamiliale du parenchyme corneen (heredo-dystrophie mouchetee). Bull Soc Beige Ophthalmol 1957:114–641.
188. Nicholson DH, Green WR, Cross HE, et al. A clinical and histopathological study of Francois-Neetens speckled corneal dystrophy. Am J Ophthalmol 1977; 83:554–560.
189. Aracena T. Hereditary fleck dystrophy of the cornea: Report of a family. J Pediatr Ophthalmol 1975; 12:223–227.
190. Goldberg MF, Krimmer B, Sugar J, et al. Variable expression in flecked (speckled) dystrophy of the cornea. Ann Ophthalmol 1977; 9:889–896.
191. Francois J. Une nouvelle dystrophie heredofamiliale de la cornee. J Genet Hum 1956; 5:189–196.
192. Strachan IM. Cloudy central corneal dystrophy of Francois. Br J Ophthalmol 1969; 53:192–194.
193. Bramsen T, Ehlers N, Baggesen LH. Central cloudy corneal dystrophy of Francois. Acta Ophthalmol 1976; 54:221–226.
194. Jiao X, Munier FL, Schorderet DF, et al. Genetic linkage of Francois-Neetens fleck (mouchetee) corneal dystrophy to chromosome 2q35. Hum Genet 2003; 112:593–599.
195. Karp CL, Scott IU, Green WR, et al. Central cloudy corneal dystrophy of Francois. A clinicopathologic study. Arch Ophthalmol 1997; 115:1058–1062.
196. Desvignes P, Vigo A. A propos d'un cas de dystrophie corneenne parenchymateuse familiale a heredite dominante. Bull Soc Ophthalmol Fr 1955; 55:220–225.
197. Odnald M. Dystrophia corneae parenchymatosa congenita. A clinical, morphological and histochemical examination. Acta Ophthalmol 1968; 46:477–485.
198. Witschel H, Fine BS, Grutzner P, McTigue JW. Congenital hereditary stromal dystrophy of the cornea. Arch Ophthalmol 1978; 96:1043–1051.
199. Carpel EF, Sigelman RJ, Doughman DJ. Posterior amorphous corneal dystrophy. Am J Ophthalmol 1977; 83:629–632.

200. Dunn SP, Krachmer JH, Ching SS. New findings in posterior amorphous corneal dystrophy. Arch Ophthalmol 1984; 102:236–239.
201. Moshegov CN, Hoe WK, Wiffen SJ, Daya SM. Posterior amorphous corneal dystrophy. A new pedigree with phenotypic variation. Ophthalmology 1996; 103:474–478.
202. Roth SI, Mittelman D, Stock EL. Posterior amorphous corneal dystrophy. An ultrastructural study of a variant with histopathological features of an endothelial dystrophy. Cornea 1992; 11:165–172.
203. Castelo Branco B, Chalita MR, Casanova FH, et al. Posterior amorphous corneal dystrophy: ultrasound biomicroscopy findings in two cases. Cornea 2002; 21:220–222.
204. Johnson AT, Folberg R, Vrabec MP, et al. The pathology of posterior amorphous corneal dystrophy. Ophthalmology 1990; 97:104–109.
205. Maeder G, Danis P. Sur une nouvelle forme de dystrophie corneenne (dystrophia fili-formis profunda corneae) associee a un keratocone. Ophthalmologica 1947; 114:2467–248.
206. Grayson M, Wilbrandt H. Pre-Descemet dystrophy. Am J Ophthalmol 1967; 64:276–282.
207. Holopainen JM, Moilanen JA, Tervo TM. In vivo confocal microscopy of Fleck dystrophy and pre-Descemet's membrane corneal dystrophy. Cornea 2003; 22:160–163.
208. Grupcheva CN, Malik TY, Craig JP, et al. Microstructural assessment of rare corneal dystrophies using real-time in vivo confocal microscopy. Clin Experiment Ophthalmol 2001; 29:281–285.
209. Curran RE, Kenyon KR, Green WR. Pre-Descemet's membrane corneal dystrophy. Am J Ophthalmol 1974; 77:711–716.
210. Bourne WM. Primary corneal endotheliopathies. Am J Ophthalmol 1983; 95:852–853.
211. Maumenee AE. Congenital hereditary corneal dystrophy. Am J Ophthalmol 1960; 50:1114–1124.
212. Judisch FG, Maumenee IH. Clinical differentiation of recessive congenital hereditary endothelial dystrophy and dominant hereditary endothelial dystrophy. Am J Ophthal mol 1978; 85:606–612.
213. Pearce WC, Tripathi RC, Morgan G. Congenital endothelial corneal dystrophy. Clinical, pathological, and genetic study. Br J Ophthalmol 1969; 53:577–591.
214. Kanai A, Kaufman HE. Further electron microscopic study of hereditary corneal edema. Invest Ophthalmol 1971; 10:545–554.
215. Kirkness CM, McCartney A, Rice NSC, et al. Congenital hereditary corneal oedema of Maumenee: its clinical features, management and pathology. Br J Ophthalmol 1987; 71:130–144.
216. Toma NM, Ebenezer ND, Inglehearn CF, et al. Linkage of congenital hereditary endothelial dystrophy to chromosome 20. Hum Mol Genet 1995; 4:2395–2398.
217. Hand CK, Harmon DL, Kennedy SM, et al. Localization of the gene for autosomal recessive congenital hereditary endothelial dystrophy (CHED2) to chromosome 20 by homozygosity mapping. Genomics 1999; 61:1–4.
218. Schlichting H. Blasen und dellenformige Endotheldystrophie der Hornhaut. Klin Monatsbl Augenheilkd 1941; 107:425–435.
219. Hansen TE. Posterior polymorphous corneal dystrophy of Schlichting. A clinical study on four families. Acta Ophthalmol 1983; 61:454–460.
220. Cibis GW, Krachmer JH, Phelps CD, Weingeist TA. The clinical spectrum of posterior polymorphous dystrophy. Arch Ophthalmol 1977; 95:1529–1537.
221. Hirst LW, Waring GO. Clinical specular microscopy of posterior polymorphous endothelial dystrophy. Am J Ophthalmol 1983; 95:143–155.
222. Henriquez AS, Kenyon KR, Dohlman CH, et al. Morphologic characteristics of poste rior polymorphous dystrophy. A study of nine corneas and review of the literature. Surv Ophthalmol 1984; 29:139–147.
223. Krachmer JH. Posterior polymorphous corneal dystrophy: a disease characterized by epithelial-like endothelial cells which influence management and prognosis. Trans Am Ophthalmol Soc 1985; 83:413–475.

224. Laganowski HC, Sherrard ES, Muir MG. The posterior corneal surface in posterior polymorphous dystrophy: a specular microscopical study. Cornea 1991; 10:224–232.
225. Heon E, Mathers WD, Alward WL, et al. Linkage of posterior polymorphous corneal dystrophy to 20q11. Hum Mol Genet 1995; 4:485–488.
226. Biswas S, Munier FL, Yardley J, et al. Missense mutations in COL8A2, the gene encoding the alpha2 chain of type VIII collagen, cause two forms of corneal endothelial dystrophy. Hum Mol Genet 2001; 10:2415–2423.
227. Fuchs E. Dystrophia epithelialis corneae. Graefes Arch Clin Exp Ophthalmol 1910; 76:478–508.
228. Waring GO, Rodrigues MM, Laibson PR. Corneal dystrophies: II Endothelial dystrophies. Surv Ophthalmol 1978; 23:147–168.
229. Harboyan G, Mamo J, Der Kaloustian V, Karam F. Congenital corneal dystrophy and progressive sensorineural deafness in a family. Arch Ophthalmol 1971; 85:27–32.
230. Behrens-Baumann W, Schott K, Vogel M, et al. Hereditary ocular dysproteinhydria of the aqueous humour with crystalline deposits. Graefes Arch Clin Exp Ophthalmol 1984; 221:187–191.
231. Meretoja J. Inherited corneal snowflake dystrophy with oculocutaneous pigmentation disturbances and other symptoms. Ophthalmologica 1985; 191:197–205.
232. Jun AS, Broman KW, Do DV, et al. Endothelial dystrophy, iris hypoplasia, congenital cataract, and stromal thinning (edict) syndrome maps to chromosome 15q22.1-q25.3. Am J Ophthalmol 2002; 134:172–176.
233. Speakman JS, Crawford JS. Congenital opacities of the cornea. Br J Ophthalmol 1966; 50:68–78.
234. Kenyon KR, Maumenee AE. The histological and ultrastructural pathology of congenital hereditary corneal dystrophy. A case report. Invest Ophthalmol 1968; 7:475–500.
235. Antine B. Histology of congenital corneal dystrophy. Am J Ophthalmol 1970; 69: 964–969.
236. Kenyon KR, Maumenee AE. Further studies of congenital hereditary endothelial dystrophy of the cornea. Am J Ophthalmol 1973; 76:419–439.
237. Kenyon KR, Antine B. The pathogenesis of congenital hereditary endothelial dystrophy of the cornea. Am J Ophthalmol 1971; 72:787–795.
238. Boruchoff SA, Kuwabara T. Electron microscopy of posterior polymorphous degeneration. Am J Ophthalmol 1971; 72:879–887.
239. Weber U, Bernsmeier H. Endothelial changes in posterior polymorphous corneal dystrophy. Klin Monatsbl Augenheilkd 1983; 182:328–330.
240. Paolo de Felice G, Braidotti P, Viale G, et al. Posterior polymorphous dystrophy of the cornea. An ultrastructural study. Graefes Arch Clin Exp Ophthalmol 1985; 223:265–271.
241. Matsumoto K, Weber PA, Makley TA. Posterior polymorphous dystrophy—a histopathologic presentation. Ann Ophthalmol 1988; 20:388–390.
242. Rodrigues MM, Newsome DA, Krachmer JH, Sun TT. Posterior polymorphous dystrophy of the cornea. Cell culture studies. Exp Eye Res 1981; 33:535–544.
243. McCartney AC, Kirkness CM. Comparison between posterior polymorphous dystrophy and congenital hereditary endothelial dystrophy of the cornea. Eye 1988; 2:63–70.
244. Rodrigues MM, Waring GO, Laibson PR, Weinreb S. Endothelial alterations in congenital corneal dystrophies. Am J Ophthalmol 1975; 80:678–689.
245. Ross JR, Foulks GN, Sanfilippo FP, Howell DN. Immunohistochemical analysis of the pathogenesis of posterior polymorphous dystrophy. Arch Ophthalmol 1995; 113: 340–345.
246. Rodrigues MM, Krachmer JH, Hackett J, et al. Fuchs' corneal dystrophy. A clinicopathologic study of the variation in corneal edema. Ophthalmology 1986; 93:789–796.
247. Hogan MJ, Wood I, Fine M. Fuchs' endothelial dystrophy of the cornea. Am J Ophthalmol 1974; 78:363–383.
248. Li QJ, Ashraf MF, Shen DF, et al. The role of apoptosis in the pathogenesis of Fuchs endothelial dystrophy of the cornea. Arch Ophthalmol 2001; 119:1597–1604.

249. Cross HE, Maumenee AE, Caontolino SJ. Inheritance of Fuchs' endothelial dystrophy. Arch Ophthalmol 1971; 85:268–272.
250. Krachmer JH, Purcell JJ, Young CW, Bucher KD. Corneal endothelial dystrophy: a study of 64 families. Arch Ophthalmol 1978; 96:2036–2039.
251. Magovern M, Beauchamp GR, McTigue JW, et al. Inheritance of Fuchs' combined dystrophy. Ophthalmology 1979; 86:1897–1920.
252. al-Rajhi AA, Wagoner MD. Penetrating keratoplasty in congenital hereditary endothelial dystrophy. Ophthalmology 1997; 104:956–961.
253. Schaumberg DA, Moyes AL, Gomes JA, Dana MR. Corneal transplantation in young children with congenital hereditary endothelial dystrophy. Multicenter Pediatric Keratoplasty Study. Am J Ophthalmol 1999; 127:373–378.
254. Adachi W, Mitsuishi Y, Terai K, Nakayama C, et al. The association of HLA with young-onset keratoconus in Japan. Am J Ophthalmol 2002; 133:557–559.
255. Krachmer JH, Feder RS, Belin MW. Keratoconus and related noninflammatory corneal thinning disorders. Surv Ophthalmol 1984; 28:292–322.
256. Kemp EG, Lewis CJ. Measurement of total and specific IgE levels in the management of a family exhibiting a high incidence of keratoconus. Acta Ophthalmol 1984; 62: 524–529.
257. Klouda PT, Syrbopoulos EK, Entwistle CC, et al. HLA and keratoconus. Tissue Antigens 1983; 21:397:399.
258. Klouda PT, Harrison R, Corbin SA, et al. HLA-A, B and DR antigens in patients with keratoconus. Tissue Antigens 1986; 27:114–115.
259. Wang Y, Rabinowitz YS, Rotter JI, Yang H. Genetic epidemiological study of keratoconus: evidence for major gene determination. Am J Med Genet 2000; 93:403–409.
260. Flanders M, Lapointe ML, Brownstein S, Little JM. Keratoconus and Leber's congenital amaurosis: a clinicopathological correlation. Can J Ophthalmol 1984; 19:310–314.
261. Cannon DJ, Forster CS. Collagen crosslinking in keratoconus. Invest Ophthalmol Vis Sci 1978; 117:63–65.
262. Kennedy RH, Bourne WM, Dyer JA. A 48-year clinical and epidemiologic study of keratoconus. Am J Ophthalmol 1986; 101:267–273.
263. Forstot SL, Goldstein JH, Damiano RE, Dukes DK. Familial keratoconus. Am J Ophthalmol 1988; 105:92–93.
264. Hammerstein W. Zur Genetik des Keratoconus. Graefes Arch Clin Exp Ophthalmol 1974; 190:293–308.
265. Ihalainen A. Clinical and epidemiological features of keratoconus Genetic and external factors in the pathogenesis of the disease. Acta Ophthalmol Suppl 1986; 178:5–64.
266. Morrow GL, Stein RM, Racine JS. Computerized videokeratography of keratoconus kindreds. Can J Ophthalmol 1997; 32:233–243.
267. McMahon TT, Shin JA, Newlin A, et al. Discordance for keratoconus in two pairs of monozygotic twins. Cornea 1999; 18:444–451.
268. Rabinowitz YS. Major review: keratoconus. Surv Ophthalmol 1998; 42:297–319.
269. Valluri S, Minkovitz JB, Budak K, et al. Comparative corneal topography and refractive variables in monozygotic and dizygotic twins. Am J Ophthalmol 1999; 127:158–163.
270. Edwards M, McGhee CN, Dean S. The genetics of keratoconus. Clin Experiment Ophthalmol 2001; 29:345–351.
271. Tyynismaa H, Sistonen P, Tuupanen S, et al. A locus for autosomal dominant keratoconus: linkage to 16p22.3-p23.1 in Finnish families. Invest Ophthalmol Vis Sci 2002; 43:3160–3164.
272. Karseras AG, Ruben M. Aetiology of keratoconus. Br J Ophthalmol 1976; 60:522–525.
273. Merin S, Auerbach E. Retinitis pigmentosa. Surv Ophthalmol 1976; 20:303–346.
274. Pierse D, Eustace P. Acute keratoconus in Mongols. Br J Ophthalmol 1971; 55:50–54.
275. Hallermann W, Wilson EJ. Genetische Betrachtungen ueber den Keratokonus. Klin Monatsbl Augenheilkd 1977; 170:906–908.

276. Fullerton J, Paprocki P, Foote S, et al. Identity-by-descent approach to gene localisation in eight individuals affected by keratoconus from north-west Tasmania, Australia. Hum Genet 2002; 110:462–470.
277. Heon E, Greenberg A, Kopp KK, et al. VSX1: a gene for posterior polymorphous dystrophy and keratoconus. Hum Mol Genet 2002; 11:1029–1036.
278. Blair SD, Seabrooks D, Shields WJ, et al. Bilateral progressive essential iris atrophy and keratoconus with coincident features of posterior polymorphous dystrophy: a case report and proposed pathogenesis. Cornea 1992; 11:255–261.
279. Yagev R, Levy J, Shorer Z, Lifshitz T. Congenital insensitivity to pain with anhidrosis: ocular and systemic manifestations. Am J Ophthalmol 1999; 127:322–326.
280. Haney WP, Falls HF. The occurrence of congenital keratoconus posticus circumstriptus. In two siblings presenting a previously unrecognized syndrome. Am J Ophthalmol 1961; 52:53–57.
281. Streeten BW, Karpik AG, Spitzer KH. Posterior keratoconus associated with systemic abnormalities. Arch Ophthalmol 1983; 101:616–622.
282. Stein R, Lazar M, Adam A. Brittle cornea. A familial trait associated with blue sclera. Am J Ophthalmol 1968; 66:67–69.
283. Ticho U, Ivry M, Merin S. Brittle cornea blue sclera and red hair syndrome (the brittle cornea syndrome). Br J Ophthalmol 1980; 64:175–177.
284. Hyams SW, Dar H, Neumann E. Blue sclerae und keratoglobus. Ocular signs of a systemic connective tissue disorder. Br J Ophthalmol 1969; 53:53–58.
285. Steinhorst U, Kohlschutter A, Steinmann B, von Domarus D. "Brittle cornea syndrome": Eine hereditäre Erkrankung des Bindegewebes mit spontaner Hornhautperforation. Fortschr Ophthalmol 1988; 85:659–661.
286. Bertelsen TI. Dysgenesis mesodermalis corneae et sclerae. Rupture of both corneae in a patient with blue sclerae. Acta Ophthalmol 1968; 46:486–491.
287. Gregoratos N, Bartosocas C, Papas K. Blue sclerae with keratoglobus and brittle cornea. Br J Ophthalmol 1971; 55:424–426.
288. Behrens-Baumann W, Gebauer H, Langenbeck U. Blaue-sklera-syndrom und Keratoglobus. Graefes Arch Clin Exp Ophthalmol 1977; 204:235–246.
289. Greenfield G, Romano A, Stein R, Goodman RM. Blue sclerae and keratoconus. Key features of a distinct heritable disorder of connective tissue. Clin Genet 1973; 4:8–16.
290. Skuta GL, Sugar J, Ericson ES. Corneal endothelial cell measurements in megalocornea. Arch Ophthalmol 1983; 101:51–53.
291. Maumenee IH. The cornea in connective tissue disease. Ophthalmology 1978; 85:1014–1017.
292. Young AI. Megalocornea and mosaic dystrophy in identical twins. Am J Ophthalmol 1968; 66:734–735.
293. Mollica F, Li Volti S, Tomarchio S, et al. Autosomal dominant cataract and microcornea associated with myopia in a Sicilian family. Clin Genet 1985; 28:42–46.
294. Salmon JF, Wallis CE, Murray ADN. Variable expressivity of autosomal dominant microcornea with cataract. Arch Ophthalmol 1988; 106:505–510.
295. Yamamoto Y, Hayasaka S, Setogawa T. Family with aniridia, microcornea and spontaneously reabsorbed cataract. Arch Ophthalmol 1988; 106:502–504.
296. Bateman JB, Maumenee IH. Colobomatous macrophthalmia with microcornea. Ophthalmic Paediatr Genet 1984; 4:59–66.
297. Batra DV, Paul SD. Microcornea with myopia. Br J Ophthalmol 1967; 51:57–60.
298. Meisler DM, Tabbara KF, Wood IS, et al. Familial band-shaped nodular keratopathy. Ophthalmology 1985; 92:217–222.
299. Hida T, Akiya S, Kigasawa K, Hosoda Y. Familial band-shaped spheroid degeneration of the cornea. Am J Ophthalmol 1984; 97:651–652.
300. Hida T, Kigasawa K, Tanaka E, et al. Primary band-shaped spheroidal degeneration of the cornea: Three cases from two consanguineous families. Br J Ophthalmol 1986; 70:347–353.

301. Ticho U, Lahav M, Ivry M. Familial band-shaped keratopathy. J Pediatr Ophthalmol Strabismus 1979; 16:183–185.
302. Kloucek F. Familial band-shaped keratopathy and spheroidal degeneration. Clinical and electromicroscopic study. Graefes Arch Clin Exp Ophthalmol 1977; 205:47–59.
303. Elliott JH, Feman SS, O'Day DM, Garber M. Hereditary sclerocornea. Arch Ophthalmol 1985; 103:676–679.
304. Purcell JJ, Krachmer JH. Familial corneal hypesthesia. Arch Ophthalmol 1979; 97: 872–874.
305. Kremer I, Weinberger D, Cohen S, Ben Sira I. Corneal hypoaesthesia in asymptomatic familial distichiasis. Br J Ophthalmol 1986; 70:132–134.
306. Hirst LW, Farmer ER, Green WR, et al. Familial corneal scarring: a new dystrophy? Ophthalmology 1984; 91:174–178.
307. Dichtl A, Jonas JB, Naumann GO. Atypical Peters' anomaly associated with partial trisomy 5p. Am J Ophthalmol 1995; 120:541–542.
308. Bateman JB, Maumenee IH, Sparkes RS. Peters' anomaly associated with partial deletion of the long arm of chromosome 11. Am J Ophthalmol 1984; 97:11–15.
309. Wertelecki W, Dev VG, Superneau DW. Abnormal centromere-chromatid apposition (ACCA) and Peters' anomaly. Ophthalmic Paediatr Genet 1985; 6:247–255.
310. Hanson IM, Fletcher JM, Jordan T, et al. Mutations at the PAX6 locus are found in heterogeneous anterior segment malformations including Peters' anomaly. Nat Genet 1994; 6:168–173.
311. Dana MR, Schaumberg DA, Moyes AL, Gomes JA. Corneal transplantation in children with Peters anomaly and mesenchymal dysgenesis. Multicenter Pediatric Keratoplasty Study. Ophthalmology 1997; 104:1580–1586.
312. Yang LL, Lambert SR, Lynn MJ, Stulting RD. Long-term results of corneal graft survival in infants and children with Peters anomaly. Ophthalmology 1999; 106:833–848.
313. OMIM Online Mendelian Inheritance in Man at http://www.ncbi.nlm.nih.gov/Omim.
314. Varssano D, Cohen EJ, Nelson LB, Eagle RC Jr. Corneal transplantation in Maroteaux-Lamy syndrome. Arch Ophthalmol 1997; 115:428–429.
315. Hennig AK, Levy B, Ogilvie JM, et al. Intravitreal gene therapy reduces lysosomal storage in specific areas of the CNS in mucopolysaccharidosis VII mice. J Neurosci 2003; 23:3302–3307.
316. Seitz B, Moreira L, Baktanian E, et al. Retroviral vector-mediated gene transfer into keratocytes in vitro and in vivo. Am J Ophthalmol 1998; 126:630–639.
317. Guemes A, Kosmorsky GS, Moodie DS, et al. Corneal opacities in Gaucher disease. Am J Ophthalmol 1998; 126:833–835.
318. Sher NA, Letson RD, Desnick RJ. The ocular manifestations in Fabry's disease. Arch Ophthalmol 1979; 97:671–676.
319. MacRae WG, Ghosh M, McCulloch C. Corneal changes in Fabry's disease: a clinicopathologic case report of a heterozygote. Ophthalmic Paediatr Genet 1985; 5:185–190.
320. Skretting G, Prydz H. An amino acid exchange in exon I of the human lecithin: cholesterol acyltransferase (LCAT) gene is associated with fish eye disease. Biochem Biophys Res Commun 1992; 182:583–587.
321. Chu FC, Kuwabara T, Cogan DG, et al. Ocular manifestations of familial high-density lipoprotein deficiency (Tangier disease). Arch Ophthalmol 1979; 97:1926–1928.
322. Vrabec MP, Shapiro MB, Koller E, et al. Ophthalmic observations in lecithin-cholesterol acyltransferase deficiency. Arch Ophthalmol 1988; 106:225–229.
323. Winder AF, Garner A, Sheraidah GA, Barry P. Familial lecithin:cholesterol acyltransferase deficiency. J Lipid Res 1985; 26:283–287.
324. Carlson LA, Philipson B. Fish eye disease. A new familial condition with massive corneal opacities and dyslipoproteinemia. Lancet 1979; 2:921–923.
325. Carlson LA, Holmquist L. Evidence for deficiency of high density lipoprotein lecithin: cholesterol acyltransferase activity (alpha-LCAT) in fish eye disease. Acta Med Scand 1985; 218:189–196.

326. Richler M, Milot J, Quigley M, O'Regan S. Ocular manifestations of nephropathic cystinosis. The French-Canadian experience in a genetically homogeneous population. Arch Ophthalmol 1991; 109:359–362.
327. Jaeger W, Eisenhauer GG. Der diagnostische Wert des arcus corneae als Hinweis auf Lipoidstoffwechselstörungen. Klin Monatsbl Augenheilkd 1977; 171:321–330.
328. Hayasaka S, Honda M, Kitaoka M, Chiba R. Corneal arcus in Japanese family with type IIa hyperlipoproteinemia. Jpn J Ophthalmol 1984; 28:254–258.
329. Editorial: Corneal arcus. Lancet 376, 1984.
330. Merin S, Nemet P, Livni N, Lazar M. The cornea in mucolipidosis IV. J Pediatr Ophthalmol 1976; 13:289–295.
331. Goldberg MF, Cotlier E, Fichenscher LG, et al. Macular cherry red spot, corneal clouding, and galactosidase deficiency. Clinical, biochemical and electron microscopic study of a new autosomal recessive storage disease. Arch Intern Med 1971; 128:387–398.
332. Kenyon KR, Sensenbrenner JA. Electron microscopy of cornea and conjunctiva in childhood cystinosis. Am J Ophthalmol 1974; 78:68–76.
333. McDowell G, Isogai T, Tanigami A, et al. Five mapping of the cystinosis gene using an integrated genetic and physical map of a region within human chromosome band 17p13. Biochem Mol Med 1996; 58:135–141.
334. Anikster Y, Lucero C, Guo J, et al. Ocular nonnephropathic cystinosis: clinical, biochemical, and molecular correlations. Pediatr Res 2000; 47:17–23.
335. Town M, Jean G, Cherqui S, et al. A novel gene encoding an integral membrane protein is mutated in nephropathic cystinosis. Nat Genet 1998; 18:319–324.
336. Attard M, Jean G, Forestier L, et al. Severity of phenotype in cystinosis varies with mutations in the CTNS gene: predicted effect on the model of cystinosin. Hum Mol Genet 1999; 8:2507–2514.
337. Mungan N, Nischal KK, Heon E, et al. Ultrasound biomicroscopy of the eye in cystinosis. Arch Ophthalmol 2000; 118:1329–1333.
338. Iwata F, Kuehl EM, Reed GF, et al. A randomized clinical trial of topical cysteamine disulfide (cystamine) versus free thiol (cysteamine) in the treatment of corneal cystine crystals in cystinosis. Mol Genet Metab 1998; 64:237–242.
339. Kaiser-Kupfer MI, Fujikawa L, Kuwabara T, et al. Removal of corneal crystals by topical cysteamine in nephropathic cystinosis. N Engl J Med 1987; 316:775–779.
340. Gahl WA, Kuehl EM, Iwata F, et al. Corneal crystals in nephropathic cystinosis: natural history and treatment with cysteamine eyedrops. Mol Genet Metab 2000; 71: 100–120.
341. Kaiser-Kupfer MI, Datiles MB, Gahl WA. Clear graft two years after keratoplasty in nephropathic cystinosis. Am J Ophthalmol 1988; 105:318–319.
342. Katz B, Melles RB, Schneider JA. Crystal deposition following keratoplasty in nephropathic cystinosis. Arch Ophthalmol 1989; 107:1727–1728.
343. Natt E, Kida K, Odievre M, et al. Point mutations in the tyrosine aminotransferase gene in tyrosinemia type III. Proc Nat Acad Sci USA 1992; 89:9297–9301.
344. Margules LJ, Mannis MJ. Dendritic corneal lesions associated with soft contact lens wear. Arch Ophthalmol 1983; 101:1551–1553.
345. Burns RP, Gipson IK, Murray MJ. Keratopathy in tyrosinemia. Birth Defects 1976; 12:169–180.
346. Sammartino A, De Crecchio G, Balato N, et al. Familial Richner-Hanhart syndrome: genetic, clinical, and metabolic studies. Ann Ophthalmol 1984; 16:1069–1074.
347. Macsai MS, Schwartz TL, Hinkle D, et al. Tyrosinemia type II. nine cases of ocular signs and symptoms. Am J Ophthalmol 2001; 132:522–527.
348. Kempster RC, Hirst LW, de la Cruz Z, Green WR. Clinicopathologic study of the cornea in X-linked ichthyosis. Arch Ophthalmol 1997; 115:409–415.
349. Grala PE. Cornea changes in X-linked ichthyosis. J Am Optom Assoc 1985; 56:315–317.
350. Sever RJ, Frost P, Weinstein G. Eye changes in ichthyosis. J Am Med Assoc 1968; 206:2283–2286.

351. Lykkesfeldt G, Hyer H, Ibsen HH, Brandrup F. Steroid sulphatase deficiency disease. Clin Genet 1985; 28:231–237.
352. Shah AB, Chernov I, Zhang HT. Identification and analysis of mutations in the Wilson disease gene (ATP7B): population frequencies, genotype-phenotype correlation, and functional analyses. Am J Hum Genet 1997; 61:317–328.
353. Tuppurainen K, Fraki J, Karjalainen S, et al. The KID-syndrome in Finland. A report of four cases. Acta Ophthalmol 1988; 66:692–698.
354. Azar P Jr, Rothschild H, Rosenthal JW, Ichinose H. Histopathology of corneal leukoma and fibroma in the ACL syndrome. Hum Pathol 1983; 14:188–190.
355. Mawhorter LG, Ruttum MS, Koenig SB. Keratopathy in a family with the ectrodactyly-ectodermal dysplasia-clefting syndrome. Ophthalmology 1985; 92:1427–1431.
356. der Kaloustian VM, Jarudi NI, Khoury MJ, et al. Familial spinocerebellar degeneration with corneal dystrophy. Am J Med Genet 1985; 20:325–339.
357. MacDonald IM, Clarke WN, Clifford BG, et al. Corneal pathology and aniridia associated with partial trisomy 2q, due to a maternal (2;6) translocation. Ophthalmic Paediatr Genet 1984; 4:75–80.
358. Kivlin JD, Fineman RM, Williams MS. Phenotypic variation in the del (12p) syndrome. Am J Med Genet 1985; 22:769–779.
359. Petrukhin K, Lutsenko S, Chemov I, et al. Characterization of the Wilson disease gene encoding a p-type copper transporting ATPate: genomic organization, alternative splicing, and structure/function predictions Hum Mol Genet 1994; 3:1647–1656.

5
The Iris

INTRODUCTION

The iris may be involved in a series of inherited anomalies and diseases and plays a role in disorders of the filtering angle or pupil. This chapter includes a discussion of aniridia, Waardenburg's syndrome, anterior chamber angle, and congenital iris anomalies, and the possible relationship between iritis and other inherited forms of uveitis.

ANIRIDIA AND PAX6 GENE MUTATIONS

Although uncommon, aniridia is usually a familial disease and, thus, is important to the ophthalmologist for its genetic implications, its association with a slowly progressive form of glaucoma, and its relationship with extraocular abnormalities.

Description and Clinical Findings

The most obvious clinical manifestation of aniridia is the absence of the iris. However, in most cases, gonioscopy shows the presence of a rudimentary stump. Some patients may have quite a large portion of peripheral iris. Iris abnormalities tend to be bilaterally symmetric in each patient, but vary considerably among the affected members of the same family. It is not rare to find in one family some members with a totally absent iris, others with a large stump, and still others with an iris coloboma (1,2) (Fig. 1).

Gonioscopy commonly reveals peripheral iridocorneal processes and an anteriorly inserted iris. Grant and Walton have documented (3,4), with repeated gonioscopic evaluations, a gradually increasing obstruction of the filtering angle in the first two decades of life in 60 children with aniridia. This initially represented an increase in the number of iridocorneal processes, which was later followed by an enlarging anterior extension of the anterior stromal layer of the iris stump. The cause was suggested to be an invisible contractile membrane covering the angle and extending between the iris and the cornea.

Gradual changes in the anatomy of the angle increasingly impair the function of the filtering angle. In advanced cases, the iris stump may be totally adherent to the

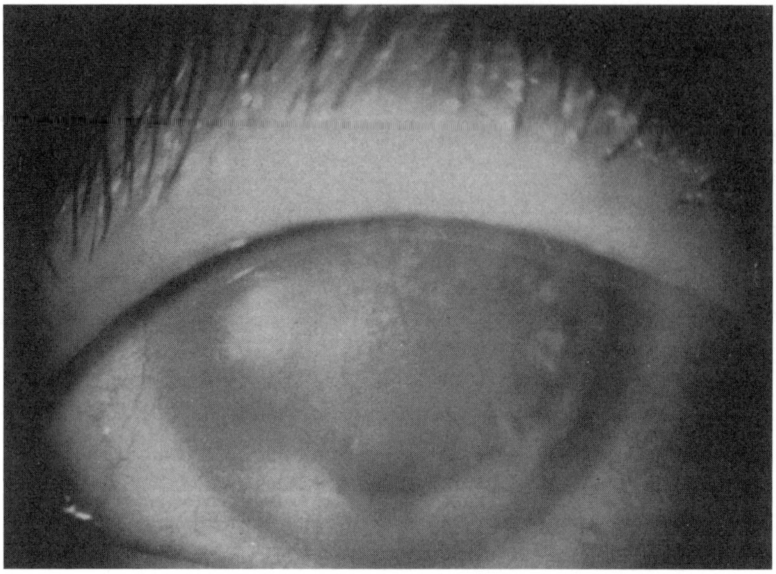

(a)

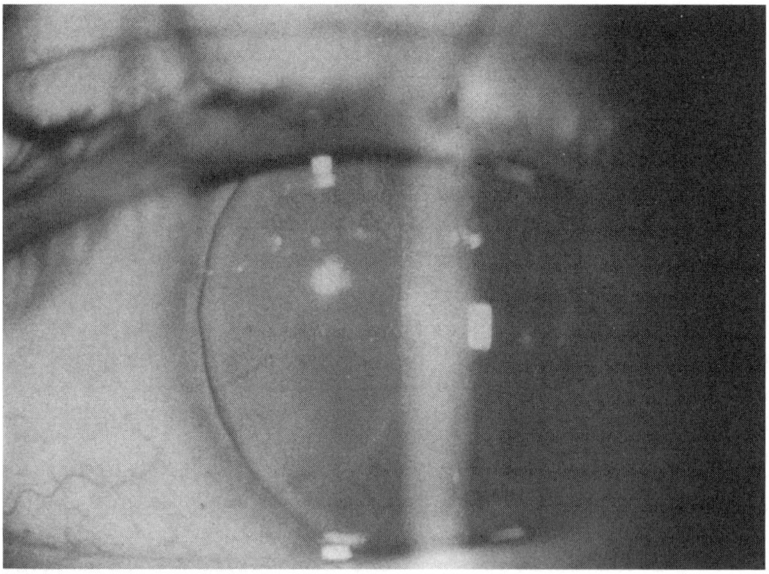

(b)

Figure 1 A mother (a) and her son (b) have aniridia. The mother, aged 45, also has severe keratopathy and advanced nuclear cataracts. Her iris stump was 1 mm in diameter. The son, aged 8, had no visible iris stump and only slight lens opacities. (Courtesy of M.F. Goldberg, MD.)

posterior corneal surface. In the review of reported series, 6–75% of all patients with aniridia had glaucoma (5).

Foveal hypoplasia or aplasia (a partial or total absence of the foveal pit) commonly occurs in aniridia, although its cause is not clear. It may result from an abnormally developed retina, visual deprivation because of poor vision in early life, the phototoxic effect of light reaching the fovea, or a combination of a three (6). The frequent association of optic nerve hypoplasia [(75% in one series) (7)] may support the theory of an abnormally developed retina in which fewer nerve axons are formed. An abnormally formed fetal neuroectoderm may result in anomaheso or absent iris pigment epithelium, iris musculature, and retina, all derived from this structure (7).

Secondary changes occur frequently in any of the different genetic and clinical types of aniridia. In addition to glaucoma, these include corneal and lens changes. The corneal changes are progressive. They start with epithelial disease in the corneal periphery and progress to stromal scarring (Fig. 1) and central corneal involvement (8) with severe reduction in vision. Lens changes begin with fine opacities, which may gradually progress to vision-reducing cataracts (1,2,5). The lens may subluxate (ectopia lentis).

Corneal changes now seem to be an intrinsic part of the aniridia syndrome. Tseng (9) proposed a model of limbal stem cell deficiency as causing the corneal abnormalities in aniridia. This model was later elaborated by Nishida and colleagues (10) who showed that limbal stem cell deficiency results in the invasion of the cornea by conjunctival epithelium.

Visual acuity is low in most patients with aniridia, and is seldom greater than 20/200 in the better eye (5,6), except in families with a clinically milder disease (aniridia type II). When present, this amblyopia is usually accompanied by horizontal, pendular nystagmus, and often by strabismus.

In summary, a young patient with aniridia may have poor visual acuity caused by primary abnormalities, such as lack of iris tissue, macular hypoplasia or aplasia, and optic nerve hypoplasia. Later in life, secondary changes such as glaucoma, cataract, and corneal opacification may affect vision.

The Clinical and Genetic Types of Aniridia

Several clinical and genetic types of aniridia are well-defined entities; others are still being debated.

Aniridia (Hereditary Aniridia; Congenital Aniridia; Autosomal Dominant Aniridia; Aniridia Type I)

The most common clinicogenetic type of aniridia was described in an early 1960s report of two large families (11,12). The clinical findings included poor vision in the majority of affected members, a typical feature of this disease (5,6,11,12). This form of aniridia is transmitted by a single autosomal dominant gene, with almost complete penetrance.

Another clinical entity was identified, in which autosomal dominant aniridia is associated with preserved visual acuity, no nystagmus, no optic nerve hypoplasia, minimal abnormalities in the fovea in some affected patients, and glaucoma in a few (2). Whether "familial aniridia with preserved ocular function," or aniridia type II, exists as a separate entity is still uncertain because of the highly variable iris and other ocular abnormalities found among the affected members within the same family (1). Nevertheless, the conspicuous discrepancy between families with definite type I (11,12) and those with preserved visual functions in almost all, referred to as type II (1,2), indicates a different clinical manifestation. It now seems (13) that the same gene is involved in both types, possibly with a different mutation The locus for aniridia was mapped to chromosome 11p13.

Gillespie's Syndrome

Incomplete aniridia, cerebellar ataxia, and mental retardation compose Gillespie's syndrome. Transmitted by autosomal recessive inheritance, it is a rare, but definite, separate entity. A similar clinical picture is reported in all affected families. The central part of the iris is absent; this is described as bilateral circumpupillary aplasia of the iris. The ataxia is nonprogressive, and the mental retardation varies from mild to profound (14–17).

The 11p-/Aniridia Syndromes

The association of nonfamilial aniridia with Wilms' tumor and with hemihypertrophy and other congenital malformations was reported by Miller and colleagues in 1964 (18). The 35 cases that were described by 1971 (19) almost doubled by 1982 to 60 (20). In 1977 and 1978 (21,22), it was noted that these abnormalities occurred in patients with a deletion of a part of the short arm of chromosome 11:del (11p), which was later confirmed to be on band 13 (Fig. 2). Clinically, the following types of 11pl3 deletion can be recognized.

Aniridia–Wilms' Tumor Association: The syndrome of aniridia associated with Wilms' tumor includes congenital aniridia, Wilms' tumor, mental retardation in 75%, craniofacial abnormalities in 75%, and growth retardation. Among the

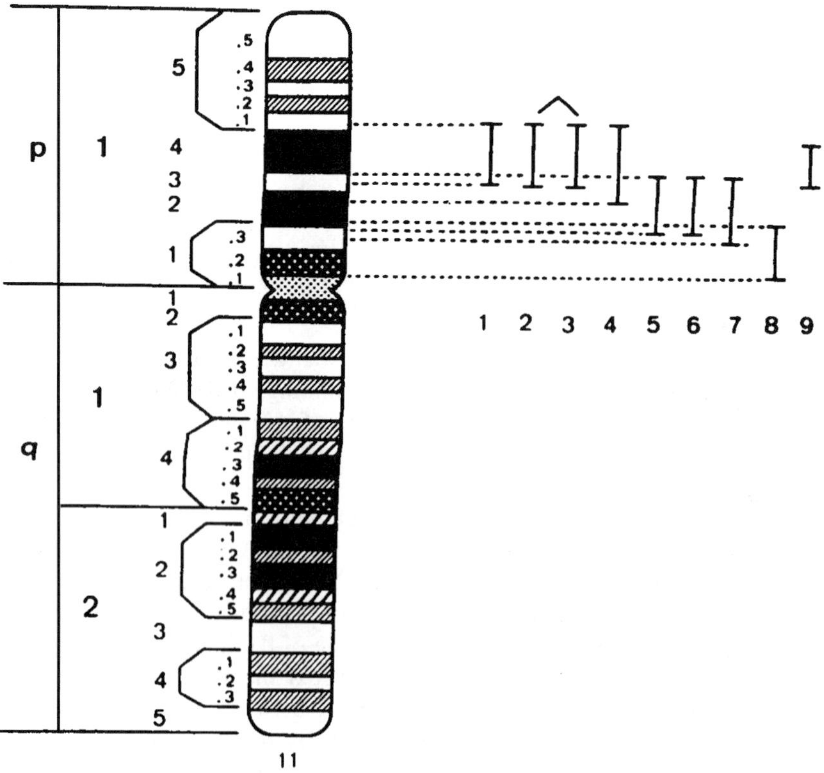

Figure 2 Chromosome 11 in nine reported cases of interstitial deletion of the short arm. All except case 8 had aniridia. All cases are missing the distal part of band 13 (from Ref. 23).

associated facial abnormalities are long face, high and prominent root of nose, low-set ears, ptosis, small palpebral fissures, and, sometimes, microcephaly. The full-blown syndrome is termed WAGR for *W*ilms' tumor, *a*niridia, *g*enitourinary anomalies, and mental *r*etardation.

About one-fifth of the nonfamilial cases of aniridia also have Wilms' tumor (5,20). Approximately 20% of these cases have bilateral tumors, an extremely rare occurrence for nonfamilial Wilms' tumor (24). The facial hemihypertrophy described in this syndrome (18) has been found in a few cases.

AGR-1: *A*niridia, ambiguous *g*enitalia (or genitourinary malformations), and mental *r*etardation have been described in several patients with deletion of 11p13 (25).

AGR-2: Aniridia, bilateral gonadoblastoma, and mental retardation, with deletion of 11p13 and no Wilms' tumor, has been reported (30).

Aniridia with other congenital malformations and no Wilms' tumor: Mild craniofacial dysmorphism or mild mental retardation may be the only signs of an aniridia associated chromosomal abnormality.

It appears likely that all four clinical syndromes associated with a deletion of band 11pl3 are one entity. The deletion practically always leads to congenital aniridia and predisposes to Wilms' tumor in many, but not all cases (23). The two-event model, as suggested by Knudson for retinoblastoma (26), could also fit hereditary Wilms' tumor and the aniridia–Wilms' tumor association (AWTA).

In most cases, Wilms' tumor is sporadic, although as many as 38% of cases are inherited. According to the two-event model, affected persons have had one mutation in the germinal line of one parent and are highly predisposed to a second event in one of the millions of kidney cells. This second event, being a somatic mutation, affects a cell that has had a germinal mutation by turning it into a malignant Wilms' tumor cell (24). According to statistical analysis, 48% of individuals with an inherited germinal mutation will have a second somatic mutation (or more than one in one kidney) and develop a unilateral malignant tumor; 37% have no additional mutation and no tumor; and 15% will have two or more additional somatic mutations, with at least one in each kidney, and exhibit bilateral tumors (24). In patients with sporadic tumors, both events are somatic, which explains the two characteristics of inherited Wilms' tumor: early occurrence and high rate of bilaterality (24).

A similar sequence of events can be theorized for AWTA. The chromosomal abnormality of 11p13 replaces the first event of germinal mutation and causes the first clinical event, which is aniridia, and some of the other congenital anomalies. Wilms' tumors develop in those who also demonstrate the second event, the somatic mutation. Germinal mutation alone explains the cases of 11p13 deletion without Wilms' tumor (27). It also accounts for the cases of monozygotic twins concordant for aniridia, but not for Wilms' tumor, which occurred in only one of genetically identical twins (28,29). One of the identical twins had only one mutation (the germinal), the other had both (the germinal and the sporadic).

Knudson's theory that the mutational events at 11pl3 caused Wilms' tumor was confirmed by molecular genetics methods. Lewis and colleagues (30) used probe p2.3 (locus D11S87) to show a homozygous deletion at 11p13 in both a patient with a constitutional deletion of 11p and a patient with sporadic Wilms' tumor.

Molecular genetics methods also indicated that the Wilms' tumor and aniridia are separate loci within band 11p13 (31,32). The area can be subdivided into 16 subregions, and this fact can explain the variable phenotypic appearance of 11pl3 deletions. In patients with a complete deletion, the full-blown WAGR syndrome will occur; with partial deletions the different subtypes, as described, will be manifest.

Recent evidence indicates an etiologic heterogeneity for Wilms' tumor. By using polymorphic DNA markers and multipoint linkage analysis, the 11p13 band was excluded as the locus for the Wilms' tumor predisposing mutation in two separate families with hereditary Wilms' tumor (33,34).

Other Associations of Aniridia. One reported family with aniridia also had no patella, as transmitted by an autosomal dominant trait (35). Another family with partial trisomy of the long arm of chromosome 2 (2q+) had aniridia, marked corneal disease, and extraocular changes, including microcephaly, a prominent forehead, hypertelorism, a broad nose with a flat nasal bridge, a long philtrum, micrognathia, and low-set ears (36).

Another possible aniridic variant appears primarily as a corneal disease and was termed autosomal dominant keratitis (37). A band of corneal opacification and vascularization is prominent at the level of Bowman's membrane (37). The true nature of aniridia is manifested by iris abnormality, ectropion uveae, and macular hypoplasia.

Diagnosis and Laboratory Tests

The diagnosis of aniridia is based on the total or partial lack of clinically evident iris. Gonioscopy appears the most important single examination to follow up the patient and monitor secondary glaucoma (3). Intraocular pressures should be measured early in life and observed thereafter. The macula and optic dist should be examined for characteristic findings. The corneal changes should be closely watched.

Supernormal electro–oculograms (EOG) were demonstrated in this disease, as in albinism (38). The significance of this finding is as of yet unclear, but may indicate light-induced retinal damage.

Retinal dysfunction can be confirmed electrophysiologicaily. The ERG b-wave is reduced to various extents (39,40).

In patients with nonfamilial aniridia, the karyotype should always be examined by the new banding techniques (41). I recommend that such studies be performed even in familial cases, if the family is small (only one or two generations affected) and extraocular abnormalities are present. Several cases of 11p deletion in association with chromosomal translocation have been described (23,27,42), and, hence, familial cases may occur.

It is not currently clear if studies to measure the activity of enzymes, the genes for which are on a locus near or on band 13 of 1lp, will become a useful clinical test. Loci for two enzymes were detected: red blood cell catalase, presumably assigned to 11pl3 (43), and lactate dehydrogenase A, assigned to 11p13 (23). The assignment of the gene for catalase to 11pl3 was recently confirmed by molecular genetic analysis (44).

Pathology

Margo performed a histologic study on seven eyes with aniridia from children six days to 14 years of age (45). He found iris hypoplasia, ciliary body hypoplasia, incomplete cleavage of the anterior chamber, attenuation of Bowman's membrane, and secondary changes in the form of corneal pannus, peripheral iridocorneal synechiae, and

lenticular degeneration. In the two oldest children, the angle was completely closed. In two other eyes with a chromosomal abnormality, the anterior chamber angle was abnormally developed.

Epidemiology and Molecular Genetics

Aniridia was studied in the southern part of the Michigan peninsula. The incidence was 1.8×10^{-5} (1:56,000), and the calculated mutation rate was 4.0×10^{-6} per locus per generation (11). Aniridia type I is transmitted by the autosomal dominant mode, with complete penetrance (Fig. 3) and variable expressivity. In the homozygote state the condition is probably lethal. Two pairs of parents with aniridia had no children, a stillbirth, or children with aniridia who died on the first day of life (12). Another couple of first-degree cousins with aniridia also had a stillbirth (2). Aniridia type II is also transmitted by an autosomal dominant gene (1,2) (Fig. 4), that is not different from the gene inherited in type 1 (13).

Linkage assignment of aniridia to chromosome 1 (46) or to chromosome 2 (47) has been suggested, but not yet confirmed. In one family, pericentric inversion of chromosome 9 was detected in all three affected individuals (48). This could have been a coincidence, and it has not been confirmed in any other family.

It is now clear that the gene for aniridia on 11p13 in AWTA is not identical with, but is very close to, the gene for Wilms' tumor. Theoretically, however, both possibilities exist: it could be one or two separate, close, genes (19).

Since the early 1990s, the localization of the causative gene of autosomal dominant aniridia to chromosome 11p13 was confirmed. The causative gene was confirmed as *PAX6,* a gene with high sequence conservation throughout evolution. The term *PAX6* was given because of the homology to mouse *Pax-6.* The human gene *PAX6* spans 22 kb and is divided into 14 exons. Various intragenic mutations were identified (40,49–52). All mutations were found between exon 5 and exon 12 (52). The mutations were identified as single–base substitutions (50%), splicing errors, and deletion or insertion events (51). They mostly were nonsense mutations and a truncated protein with loss of function (51,53).

The *PAX6* gene appears to be the only gene causing aniridia transmitted by the autosomal dominant route (51). However, the *PAX6* gene may also be responsible for additional clinical entities including some cases of Peters anomaly with cataract, congenital cataract, autosomal dominant congenital keratitis, isolated foveal hypoplasia, ectopia pupillae, and ocular coloboma. These reported isolated cases may all be variants of aniridia. The Wilms tumor gene, WT1, is also mapped to chromosome 11p13. Its genomic organization and the sequence of all 10 exons and their flanking introns was established in 1992 (54). Deletion of the whole seament of chromosome 11p13 may cause WAGR, including Wilms tumor, aniridia, genitourinary anomalies, mental retardation, or any part or combination of the syndrome. Additional abnormalities such as limbal cysts or microphthalmus may also occur, (55). Sporadic cases of aniridia carry a substantial risk of the development of a Wilms tumor and patients may undergo DNA tests in order to establish their risk of developing this tumor (142,143). Gillespie's syndrome, in which foveal hypoplasia, hypoplasia of the iris and superior colobomas, together with brain anomalies occur, is transmitted by an autosomal recessive gene. It is located nearto, but is not associated with the *PAX6* gene (56).

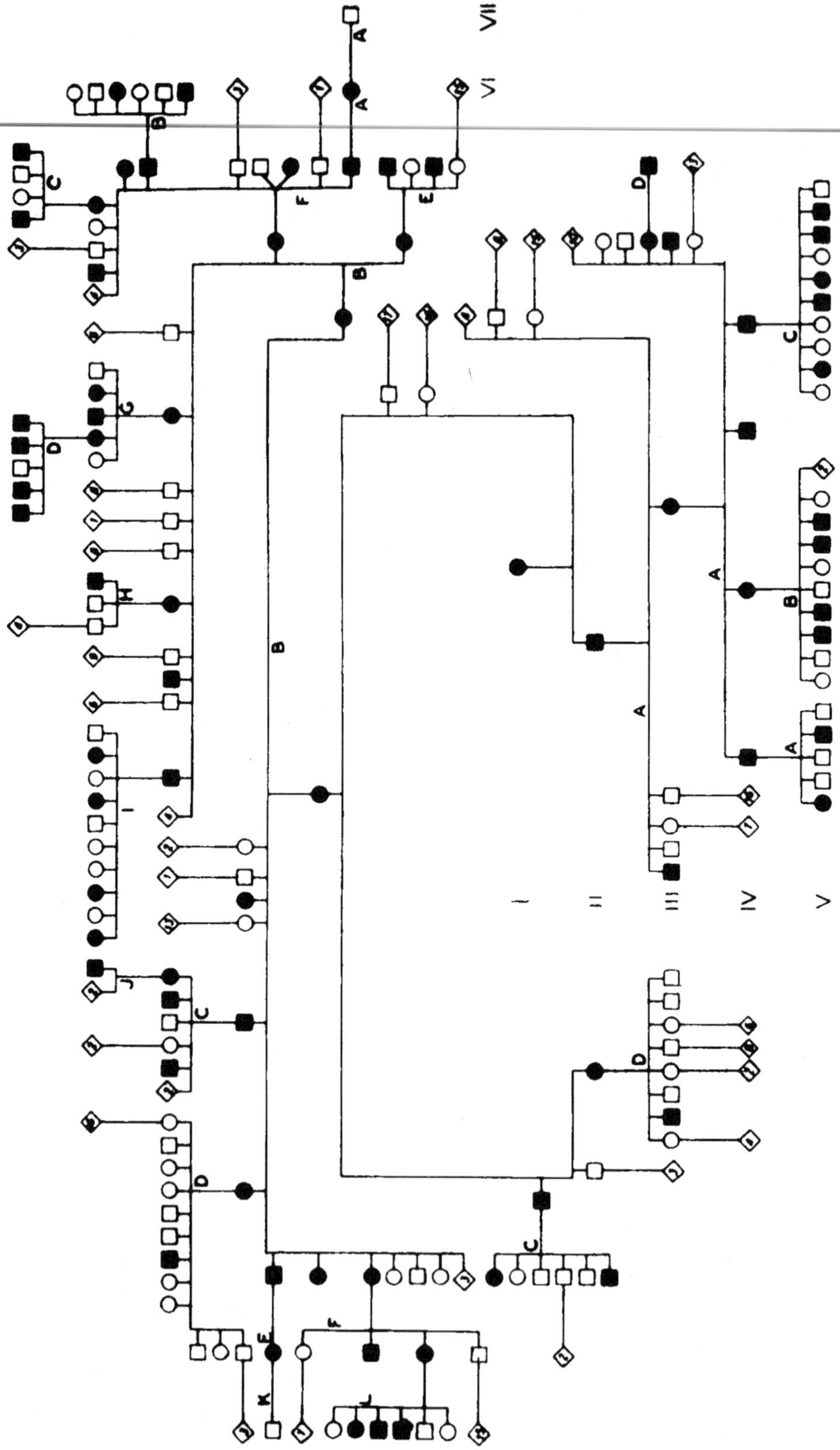

Figure 3 Pedigree of large Canadian family with aniridia: note typical autosomal dominant transmission with complete penetrance. The dark symbols indicate those with aniridia (from Ref. 12).

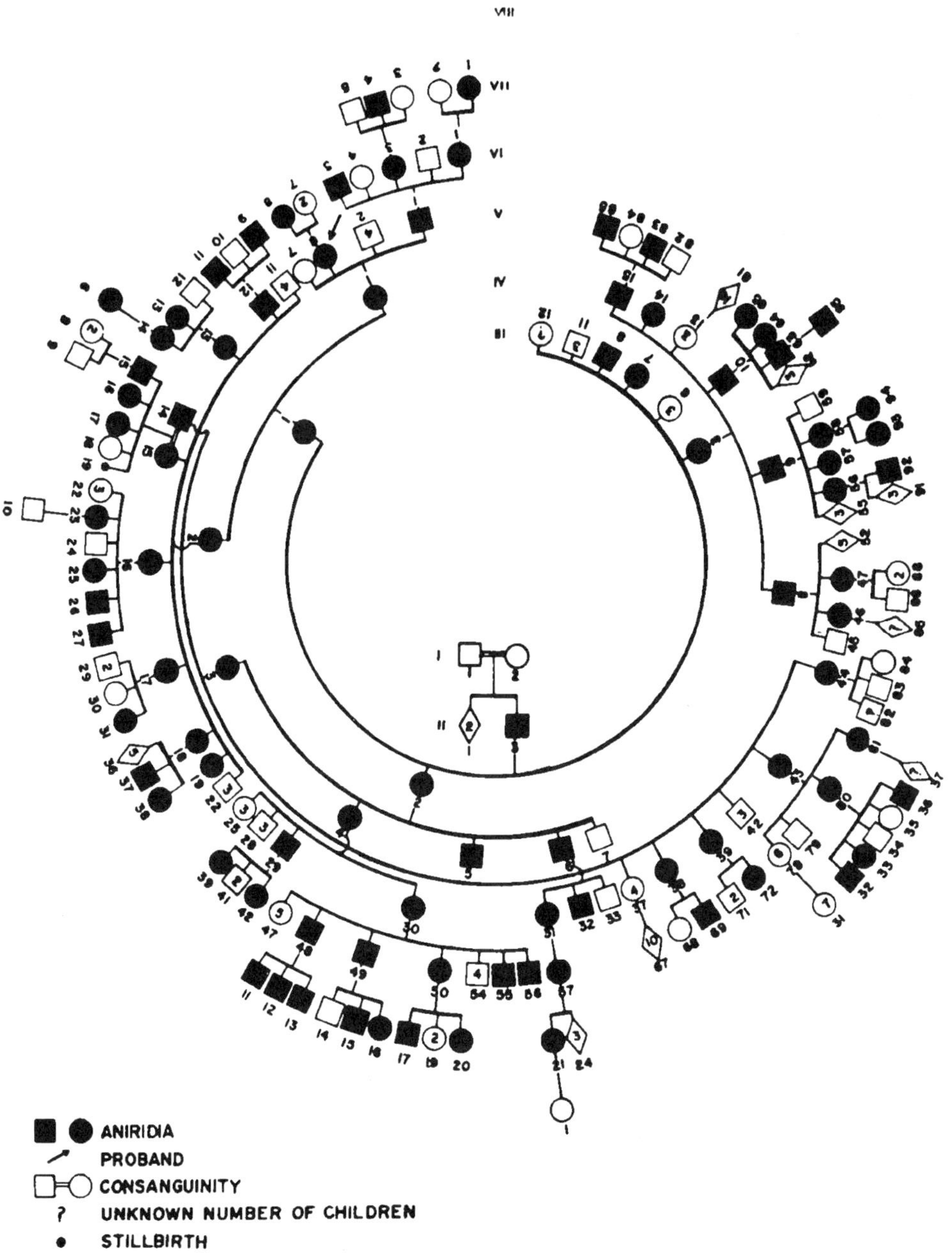

Figure 4 Pedigree of a family with aniridia and preserved ocular function (aniridia type II). Transmission is autosomal dominant with complete penetrance (from Ref. 2).

Management

Surgical and Medical Treatment

Glaucoma in the patient with aniridia is very difficult to treat. Both medical and surgical methods carry poorer results than in other types of glaucoma. Preventive treatment by goniotomy has been suggested if the intraocular pressure is not too high (3), and this approach has been confirmed in an additional 28 eyes of 16 aniridia patients (4). Usually, two procedures were required for each eye, but good results were claimed. Medical treatment should be attempted. If it fails, trabeculectomy or cyclocryopexy may succeed, whereas goniotomy, trabeculotomy, or full-thickness filtering procedures commonly fail (5).

In a more recent study, aniridic glaucoma was successfully treated in 83% of the patients with one or two surgeries (57). The operation of choice was trabulectomy. If the first operation fails to control the intraocular pressure, Molteno valve was suggested as the second procedure (58). The average follow-up of 55 eyes (operated by 200° of goniosurgery as a preventive measure) approximately ten years after the procedures, demonstrated that prophylactic goniotomy may be effective in selected cases (59). Reinhard and associates (60) designed a black diaphragm intraocular lens and implanted it into the sulcus of 19 aniridic eyes. They claimed good results but warned of deterioration of the glaucoma after cataract surgery. Holland and colleagues (61) claimed the successful treatment of the corneal abnormalities of aniridia by a keratolimbal allograft (KLAL) in 31 eyes of 32 patients. In early cases, this operation was sufficient to overcome the stem cell deficiency of aniridic eyes. In advanced cases with stromal scarring, perforating keratoplasty is needed as a second procedure. In all cases, immunosuppression given orally for a prolonged period of time was essential to success (61).

Genetic Counseling

In the cases of autosomal dominant or autosomal recessive (Gillespie's syndrome) aniridia, genetic counseling should be given accordingly. In the autosomal dominant cases, penetrance is practically complete, but expressivity varies. Boys and girls are affected equally.

In sporadic cases, of which some must be new mutations of the autosomal dominant gene, the disease may be transmitted to 50% of their offspring, but the risk to subsequent children is very small.

In other sporadic cases, a chromosomal anomaly may be found. If this is not a translocation-associated anomaly, the risk to siblings is low. The theoretical risk to offspring, if a patient survives and has children, is 50%, as with any autosomal dominant gene.

Prenatal diagnosis cannot be performed for autosomal dominant aniridia. Amniocentesis may, however, confirm a suspected 11p deletion, and abortion may be chosen (62). Preimplantation genetic diagnosis may be considered in severe cases.

AXENFELD–RIEGER SYNDROMES

The anterior chamber cleavage syndromes, or mesodermal dysgenesis, are a group of congenital diseases that result from defectively developed structures lining the anterior chamber. The anterior chamber angle and iris are mainly affected, although other structures, such as the cornea and the lens, are implicated in the process. Glaucoma is the most common secondary ocular complication. Patients with Rieger syndrome demonstrate systemic abnormalities as well.

Clincally, several different phenotypes are known and traditionally they are termed as separate diseases. Genetically, they are a heterogenous group, caused by mutations in at least three causative genes. However, the clinical entities cannot be distinguished by the specific causative gene.

The Clinical and Genetic Types

Several types of anterior chamber cleavage syndromes are recognized; some are well delineated, and others are still questionable.

Rieger's Anomaly and Rieger Syndrome

Since Rieger's original description in 1935 (63) many cases and families have been reported. In most patients, both ocular and systemic abnormalities can be detected, and the term Rieger syndrome is used. Rieger's anomaly implies that the ocular findings are present, without extraocular involvement. The ocular findings include a partial loss of iris stroma (hypoplasia or dysplasia), often causing an irregular pupil updrawn in one direction and not central. Iris atrophy may lead to iris holes and polycoria. Angle changes are conspicuous; multiple iridocorneal processes traverse the angle. Schwalbe's line is prominent and anteriorly set. These iris and angle changes are progressive, even without glaucoma or miotic treatment (64). The cornea may be smaller than usual.

A 15-year follow-up of a patient with Rieger syndrome disclosed a changing pupil (by traction), additional loss of anterior iris stroma, accumulated pigment, a broader synechial band in the periphery, and the appearance of an iris hole (64).

Among the several extraocular findings described, a characteristic facies is the most obvious; because of maxillary hypoplasia, the face is mostly flat, except for a bulging chin (prognathism) and protruding lower lip. The characteristic face imparts a similarity to affected family members. Dental anomalies are common (63,64), and several recent reports have described protuberant periumbilical skin (65) or an umbilical hernia. Hypospadias may be present.

Glaucoma may be a common sequela to Rieger syndrome. Its frequency increases with time; it has been reported as 8% at birth, 50% by the second decade, and 60% thereafter (66). In one series of 136 cases of infantile glaucoma, 7 were a result of Rieger's anomaly, all bilateral (67). In another series, 6 of 133 cases of infantile glaucoma had Rieger's anomaly (68).

Both Rieger's anomaly and Rieger syndrome are transmitted by the autosomal dominant mode (69), with incomplete penetrance and variable expressivity. Most probably, it is one and the same gene, a statement confirmed by recent genetic studies.

Axenfeld Syndrome

Axenfeld syndrome is described as an ocular condition in which an abnormally thickened and anteriorly placed Schwalbe's line occurs congenitally, with multiple iridocorneal processes in the angle. No extraocular findings are associated with it. Glaucoma may be found, as in Rieger's anomaly, and may exist as a congenital condition (66–68). Transmission is autosomal dominant.

Axenfeld's syndrome is not a separate entity but a milder expression of Rieger's anomaly (70). Waring and colleagues (71) have suggested that the entire group of mesodermal dysgeneses be divided into three groups of anomalies. The first of these are the peripheral anomalies, including Rieger's and Axenfeld's, with frequently associated glaucoma.

Posterior embryotoxon describes a congenitally thickened, prominent, and anteriorly placed Schwalbe line. It is transmitted as an autosomal dominant trait, and probably represents the mildest form of Rieger's anomaly.

Axenfeld-Rieger Syndrome

It is probably best to use the term Axenfeld–Rieger syndrome for all diseases earlier called various terms, syndromes, and anomalies (72). Molecular genetics studies, performed in the last decade indicate the grouping together of these various entities, although they may be caused by mutations in different genes.

Autosomal Dominant Iris Hypoplasia

In this condition, the iris is atrophic and has a slate gray to chocolate brown color with a pronounced tan coloring at sphincter (73). Glaucoma occurs early and is very difficult to treat. Molecular genetic studies confirmed the linkage to the RIEG1/PITX2 gene responsible for Axenfeld–Rieger syndrome (73,74).

Peters Anomaly

Peters anomaly is a rather rare condition in which the iris is hypoplastic, as in Rieger's anomaly, but the angle may or may not demonstrate the typical forms of mesodermal dysgenesis. In addition, a defect in Descemet's membrane causes a central corneal leukoma adherent to the iris near the pupil, and sometimes, to the lens. Infantile glaucoma is not infrequent (66–68) and is usually bilateral. In Waring's "step-ladder classification" of mesodermal dysgenesis, Peters' anomaly would be classified with the group of central or combined (peripheral and central) anomalies (71).

Peters anomaly is reportedly transmitted by the autosomal recessive mode.

Autosomal Dominant Iridogoniodysgenesis

Autosomal dominant iridogoniodysgenesis is distinctly separate from Rieger's anomaly. Glaucoma develops in almost all affected family members in the first and second decade of life, Hypoplasia of iris stroma and mesodermal remnants in the angle may be associated with an abnormal vasculature that covers the angle structures (75). This condition is probably the same as reported by Berg in 1932 (76), and later referred to as juvenile glaucoma, hereditary juvenile glaucoma, or dysgenic glaucoma (77–79). In one family, associated somatic anomalies were described (80).

The disease is transmitted by a single autosomal dominant gene, with complete penetrance, some variation in expressivity, and a remarkably symmetric involvement of the two eyes (75) (Fig. 5). The family described by Weatherill and Hart (81) probably had this genetic entity.

It is controversial whether autosomal dominant iridogoniodysgenesis is generally separate from Axenfeld–Rieger syndrome (72,82). It is likely that autosomal dominant iridogoniodysgenesis is a heterogenous entity with some families suffering from juvenile glaucoma with iris anomalies without the typical angle cleavage anomalies found in Axenfeld–Rieger syndrome. In other families, they represent variants of Axenfeld–Rieger and are caused by mutations of the same genes (72,82,83). Autosomal dominant iridogoniodysgenesis will also be discussed in the chapter on glaucoma.

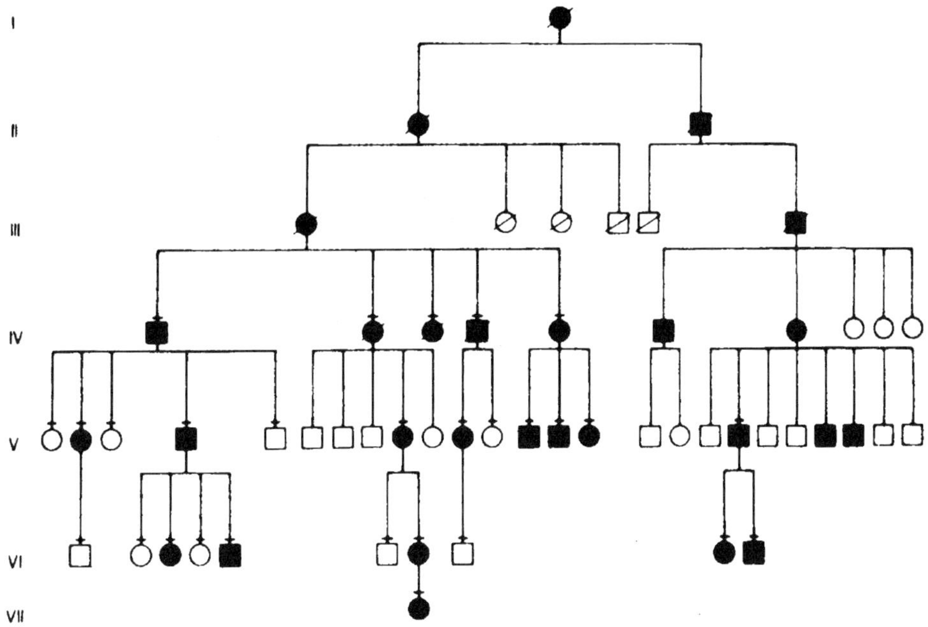

Figure 5 Pedigree of a family with autosomal dominant iridogoniodysgenesis: note the regular transmission of an autosomal dominant trait (from Ref. 75).

Other Associations of Mesodermal Dysgenesis

A dominantly inherited syndrome of iris hypoplasia, with Rieger's-type angle and pupillary anomalies, hypertelorism, strabismus, and systemic abnormalities, including mental retardation, short stature, lax joints, hypotonia, and deafness, was described in one family (84). It may represent a different expression of Rieger syndrome.

Another syndrome related to Axenfeld–Rieger included atrial septal defect and sensorineural hearing defect transmitted as an autosomal dominant trait (85).

The familial occurrence of a unilateral or bilateral coloboma with pannuslike corneal changes, transmitted by an autosomal dominant mode (86), may also belong to this group.

Wolf–Hirschhorn syndrome is associated with a deletion of a part of the short arm of chromosome 4 (4p−). Multiple ocular anomalies have been described. All three patients reported by Wilcox and coworkers (87) had anterior segment anomalies, including one with Rieger's anomaly.

Anterior chamber cleavage syndrome is associated with both oculocutaneous (autosomal recessive) and ocular (X-linked recessive) albinism (88–91). It is speculated that the mesodermal dysgenesis is a developmental anomaly related to the lack of pigmentation in the tissues.

Molecular Genetics

Several genes and loci were found to be associated with Axenfeld–Rieger syndromes.

The RIEG1 Locus

The first significant linkage of Rieger syndrome to chromosome 4q25–q26 was reported in 1992 at the same locus of EGF, the epidermal growth factor (EGF) (92). This linkage was confirmed in a patient with a balanced translocation (93). The locus RIEG1 was identified as homologus to murine Rieg-1. It is a small gene containing four exons and predicted to encode a protein of 271 amino acids; several missense and splicing mutations were identified (94). The gene was named PITX2 for paired-like homeo-domain transcription factor-2 as it represents a paired homeobox gene (72). It is causative of Rieger syndrome and anomaly, and Axenfeld syndrome and anomaly It is associated with the clinical entity of autosomal dominant iris hypoplasia (73,74), and some cases of autosomal dominant iridodysgenesis (82), sometimes referred to as iridodysgenesis syndrome type 2 and autosomal recessive syndromic goniodysgenesis (82).

The RIEG2 Locus

A second locus for Rieger syndrome has been mapped to chromosome 13q14 (95). In this family, the ocular findings were indistinguishable from Rieger syndrome including posterior embryotoxon, iris hypoplasia, peripheral synechiae, high incidence of glaucoma, and premature loss of teeth with hearing loss (95). Additional families were identified later.

The FOXC1/FKHL7 Gene

A third locus associated with the development of the anterior segment of the eye IRID1 has been mapped to chromosome 6p25 (96). Several families with Axenfeld–Rieger syndrome manifested mutations in the FKHL7 (forkhead drosophila homolog transcription factor 7) gene at this location (72,96–98). The gene is now named FOXC1 (forkhead box C1). Various mutations in the FOXC1 gene were identified as associated with Axenfeld–Rieger anomaly and syndrome, Peters anomaly, some with cardiac abnormalities (98), iridogoniodysgenesis (83), and familial glaucoma iridogoniodysgenesis (99).

Diagnosis

A mesodermal dysgenesis is diagnosed by clinical findings. No laboratory test is available to support or confirm the diagnosis. Suggested linkage to chromosome 4q (100,101) has been confirmed. It is now possible, therefore, to confirm the diagnosis by demonstration of the mutation of one of the genes associated with Axenfeld–Rieger syndrome. However, all three genes mentioned here are causative of only about one-third of all Rieger–type families.

If the diagnosis of one of these mesodermal dysgenesis syndromes is determined or suspected, the intraocular pressure must be checked and followed up. Congenital or infantile glaucoma is not rare. In the two series mentioned, 28 of 269 children with infantile glaucoma (or about 10%) had Rieger's, Axenfeld's, or Peters anomaly (62,68). The frequency of glaucoma increases rapidly in the second decade of life, with the progressive changes occurring in the iris and in the angle (64).

One problem facing the ophthalmologist is the differential diagnosis of nonhereditary diseases that constitute the iridocorneal endothelial (ICE) syndromes (144), and the unilateral situation in the noninherited condition. Schwalbe's line, which is always prominent in the inherited condition, is usually normal in the ICE syndrome.

Management

The main problem in the anterior chamber cleavage is to manage the glaucoma. The findings in autosomal dominant iridogoniodysgenesis are probably typical of the entire group of disorders. The intraocular pressure responds poorly to medical treatment, but the optic nerve seems more resistant to pressure damage than in the primary glaucomas (102). Surgery is often unsuccessful, but filtering operations are preferred over goniotomy (91).

Genetic counseling should be handled according to the following information:

1. In the Rieger's-type disorder (Rieger's anomaly, Rieger's syndrome, posterior embryotoxon, Axenfeld's syndrome), the transmission is autosomal dominant, with incomplete penetrance and highly variable expressivity. Most likely, the same gene is involved in this whole group and in the differences of expressivity.
2. Peters anomaly is transmitted by an autosomal recessive trait.
3. Autosomal dominant iridogoniodysgenesis (hereditary juvenile glaucoma) is transmitted by an autosomal dominant gene, with complete penetrance and fairly regular expressivity. Some cases are just a variant of Rieger's anomaly.

IRIS CYSTS

Although rare, cysts of the iris or of the iris and ciliary body may be hereditary. In a study of 62 patients, Shields found that most had cysts of the iridociliary pigment epithelium, with 42 so affected (103). Familial cases also were described (104,105). In one family, the transmission was not clear, although three generations were affected in six other families; an autosomal dominant transmission was suggested (87,148). The condition was usually bilateral in hereditary cases. Angle closure glaucoma could develop from the pressure of the large cysts on the iris (87). Therapy may be palliative, with the use of pilocarpine, or curative, with laser treatment or surgery. The argon or krypton laser can be used for pigmented cysts, and the Nd:YAG laser for nonpigmented cysts.

CONGENITAL MIOSIS (MICROCORIA)

A congenitally narrow pupil may be associated with other anomalies of the anterior segment, such as microcornea, megalocornea, mesodermal dysgenesis, and hypoplasia of the iris. It may also be an isolated finding. The narrow pupil ranges from 0.5 mm to a maximum of 3.5 mm in diameter, usually around 1.5 mm. Little or no response is obtained with mydriatics. The disorder is probably caused by a congenital absence of hypoplasia of the dilator muscle of the pupil.

This disorder was reported to be familial. It was described as an autosomal dominant trait in one family, as an autosomal recessive trait in a second (107), as an autosomal dominant trait linked with goniodysgenesis in a third family (108), and as autosomal dominant microcoria with hereditary, nonprogressive spastic ataxia in a fourth family (109).

In one large family with autosomal dominant microcoria, a strong association between the small pupil (2 mm or less) and myopia, astigmatism, or glaucoma due to angle structure abnormalities was detected (110). The condition is rare and may be unilateral, bilateral, or asymmetric (anisocoria). A molecular genetics study mapped the congenital microcoria of one large French family to chromosome 13q31–q32 (111). One pathological study of congenital microcoria (112) demonstrated a defect of the intermediate filaments in the anterior pigmented cells of the iris, with the absence of myofilaments and failure of development of the dilator pupillae muscle.

IRIS COLOR

It is not known by what mode the color of the iris is inherited. Since the beginning of the century, the theory of Davenport and Davenport has served as the basis for genetic counseling. According to these authors (113), dark colors are dominant and light colors are recessive, with blue being recessive to gray, and gray being recessive to brown. Therefore, blue-eyed parents will always have blue-eyed offspring, gray-eyed parents may have blue- or gray-eyed children, whereas the children of brown-eyed parents may have any eye color. Even using the 16 colors of the Martin–Schultz scale, Rufer and associates (114) found the Davenport theory to be basically true.

Stable eye color is achieved in humans by six years of age except in a subgroup of 10–15%, in which it continues to change (115).

However, there are serious doubts that iris color is transmitted by a single gene. The heritability of eye color is extremely high. Jensen (116) found a concordance of 100% in 50 pairs of monozygotic twins, but only 52% in 50 pairs of dizygotic twins. Therefore, although the genetic factors are extremely powerful, the mode of inheritance is not simple. In a more recent study, dominance played no role in determining eye color, and the additive action of three (117) or four genes (118) was suggested.

Iris color, therefore, seems to be inherited by the multifactorial mode. The additive action of a few genes, without any environmental influence, appears the most likely mode of transmission.

VARIOUS IRIS ANOMALIES

The hallmark of ocular manifestations of Smith–Magenis syndrome are iris anomalies. Patients suffer from psychomotor retardation, brachycephaly, midface hypoplasia, delayed speech, and other signs. Iris anomalies were found in 68%, consisting of lack of iris colarette, nasal corectopia, stromal dysplasia, and white-elevated nodules in the peripheral iris (119). Microcornea, myopia, and strabismus are quite frequent (119). The locus for the syndrome was mapped in several families to a deletion of chromosome 17p11.2. In several families, a deletion of this chromosomal region was identified (119). EDICT syndrome was the name given by the authors to an autosomal dominant entity combining endothelial dystrophy resembling posterior polymorphous corneal dystrophy, iris hypoplasia, stromal thinning leading to corneal thinning and congenital anterior polar cataract (120). EDICT syndrome has been mapped to chromosome 15q22.1–q25.3 (120).

Waardenburg's syndrome in which iris heterochromia is a frequent finding, will be discussed in Chapter 22.

IRITIS AND OTHER UVEITIS

In spite of the fact that iritis, cyclitis, and choroiditis are inflammatory diseases, reports of familial cases of pars planitis (121–123) and iritis have led to the speculation of a genetic influence. This hypothesis has been supported by studies of the human leucocyte antigen (HLA) system, which correlated uveitis in specific diseases with inborn and inherited predisposition. The mode of action of these genes is not yet known. An explanation for this inflammatory disease has been interaction between HLA-linked genes and environmental factors or a triple interaction between HLA-linked genes, non-HLA-linked genes, and environmental factors (124). Such HLA-linked activity could be responsible, for example, for the antiviral activity of individual cells (124). The HLA-linked genes are located on the short arm of chromosome 6 (70).

Behçet's Disease and Posterior Uveitis

The well-known triad of iritis, aphthous stomatitis, and ulcerations on the genitalia laid down by Behcet is still the basis for the clinical diagnosis of Behcet's disease. Other ocular associations are usually retinal vasculitis and occlusion of retinal vessels, posterior uveitis, neuritis, and neuroretinitis, and later cataract. Familial cases are frequently described, as is the association with HLA-B5. Siblings were affected in addition to the proband in seven reported families, including a father and son in one (125). In another family, four generations were affected (126). The association of HLA-B5 antigen, especially its B51 split, with Behcet's disease was reported from Japan and Turkey, where this disease is common, and from Britain, where it is uncommon (127). Behcet's disease was also reported in two Swedish brothers who were raised in separate homes and lived apart, which eliminated the possibility of one infecting the other (128).

It has been suggested that the disease is more severe in familial cases and that the HLA-B5-Behcet's association is stronger in males than in females (128).

Over 100 HLA-associated diseases were identified. The HLA complex is spread over approximately 4000 kb of DNA on the short arm of chromosome 6 (129). About half of it is comprised of genes associated with class I HLA molecules: HLA-A, B, and C. The rest are associated with class II, HLA-DR, DQ and DP, or class III. About 100 genes are encoded in this area (129).

Birdshot retinochoroidopathy has a strong association with HLA A29.2 (2902) and can be found also with HLA A29.1 (2901). It is not associated with other subtypes of HLA-A 29 (145). Other posterior pole inflammatory diseases are associated with class II HLA antigens and their association is less prominent. Acute retinal necrosis was reported to be associated with HLA DR9 or HLA DQW7, presumed ocular histoplasmosis with HLA-DR2 (129) and intermediate uveitis with HLA-DR15 (130), a subtype of HLA-DR2 (131). The same antigen was also associated with multiple sclerosis and/or optic neuritis (130). A high association was also detected between APMPPE and HLA-B7 and HLA-DR2 (146).

Anterior Uveitis

Acute anterior uveitis has been found in association with antigen HLA-B27. The presence of this antigen increases the risk of acute anterior uveitis 20-fold (132). This is particularly true in recurrent anterior uveitis associated with ankylosing spondylitis in males (133). It has been proposed that an association with additional antigens, such as A2 with B27 in American whites and blacks or A9 (w24) with B27 in Asian Indians, also occurs (134). Other investigators have found the association of acute anterior uveitis with the monozygotic α_1-antitrypsin phenotype (135). Also, HLA-DR5 has been associated with chronic iridocyclitis and juvenile rheumatoid arthritis with onset in early childhood (136). However, except for HLA-B27, all other associations are unconfirmed (124).

Juvenile rheumatoid arthritis (JRA), which is sometimes associated with anterior uveitis and the presence of HLA-B27, can be classified into one of three subtypes (132): (1) In polyarthritis with severe systemic symptoms (Still's disease), no uveitis occurs. (2) In polyarthritis without severe systemic symptoms, a disease that occurs mostly in females, no uveitis occurs. (3) In monoarthritis or pauciarthritis (few joints affected) in males, 10–20% are affected by acute anterior uveitis, 75% of whom have positive HLA-B27 and negative antinuclear and rheumatic factors. In females, 50% develop a chronic anterior uveitis, HLA-B27 is mostly negative, and antinuclear factors are positive in 60–90%.

The highest frequency of HLA-B27 association is found in males, with acute anterior uveitis and ankylosing spondylitis or Reiter's disease (138). It is not clear whether the outcome of HLA-B27 associated uveitis is worse than in HLA-B27 negative cases. Controversial results of follow-up have been reported (139,140).

A significantly high incidence of acute anterior uveitis was found in first-degree relatives of patients with HLA-B27-positive anterior uveitis (141). Thirteen percent of such relatives were positive for HLA-B27 and had acute anterior uveitis. In the general Dutch population, 1% are positive for HLA-B27 and about 1% of these have anterior uveitis, whereas approximately 50% of all patients with acute anterior uveitis are also HLA-B27-positive (141).

REFERENCES

1. Hittner HM, Riccardi VM, Ferrell RE, et al. Variable expressivity in autosomal dominant aniridia by clinical, electrophysiologic and angiographic criteria. Am J Ophthalmol 1980; 89:531–539.
2. Esas FJ, Maumenee IH, Kenyon KR, Yoder F. Familial aniridia with preserved ocular function. Am J Ophthalmol 1977; 83:718–724.
3. Grant WM, Walton DS. Progressive changes in the angle in congenital aniridia, with development of glaucoma. Am J Ophthalmol 1974; 78:842–847.
4. Walton DS. Aniridic glaucoma: the results of goniosurgery to prevent and treat this problem. Trans Am Ophthaimol Soc 1986; 84:59–70.
5. Nelson LB, Spaeth GL, Nowrnski TS, et al. Aniridia. A review. Surv Ophthalmol 1984; 28:621–642.
6. Shaffer RN, Cohen JS. Visual reduction in aniridia. J Pediatr Ophthalmol 1975; 12: 220–222.
7. Layman PR, Anderson DR, Flynn JT. Frequent occurrence of hypoplastic optic disks in patients with aniridia. Am J Ophthalmol 1974; 77:513–516.

8. Mackman G, Brightbell FS, Opitz JM. Corneal changes in aniridia. Am J Ophthalmol 1979; 87:497–502.
9. Tseng SCG. Concept and application of limbal stem cells. Eye 1989; 3:141–157.
10. Nismida K, Kinoshita S, Ohashi Y, et al. Ocular surface abnormalities in aniridia. Am J Ophthalmol 1995; 120:368–375.
11. Shaw MW, Falls HF, Neel JV. Congenital aniridia. Am J Hum Genet 1960; 12:389–415.
12. Grove JH, Shaw MW, Bourque G. A family study of aniridia. Arch Opthalmol 1961; 65:81–94.
13. Lyons LA, Martha A, Mintz-Hittner HA, et al. Resolution of the two loci for autosomal dominant aniridia AN1 and AN2, to a single locus on chromosome 11p13. Genomics 13:925–930.
14. Gillespie FD. Aniridia, cerebellar ataxia and oligophrenia in siblings. Arch Ophthalmol 1965; 73:338–341.
15. Sarsfield JK. The syndrome of congenital cerebellar ataxia, aniridia and mental retardation. Dev Med Child Neurol 1971; 13:508–511.
16. Francois J, Lentini F, de Rouck F. Gillespie's syndrome (incomplete aniridia, cerebellar atxia and oligophrenia). Ophthalmic Paediatr Genet 1984; 4:29–32.
17. Witting EO, Moreira CA, Freire–Maia N, Vianna-Morgante AM. Partial aniridia, cerebellar ataxia, and mental deficiency (Gillespie syndrome) in two brothers. Am J Med Genet 1988; 30:703–708.
18. Miller RW, Fraumeni JF, Manning MD. Association of Wilms' tumor with aniridia, hemihypertrophy and other congenital malformations. N Engl J Med 1964; 270:922–927.
19. Haicken BN, Miller DR. Simultaneous occurrence of congenital aniridia, hamartoma and Wilms' tumor. J Pediatr 1971; 78:497–502.
20. Francois J, Verschraegen-Spae MR, DeSutter E. The aniridia-Wilms' tumor syndrome and other associations of aniridia. Ophthalmic Paediatr Genet 1982; 1:125–138.
21. Smith AC, Sujansky E, Riccardi VM. Aniridia, mental retardation and genital abnormality in 2 patients with 46,XY,11p. Birth Defects 1977; 13:257.
22. Francke U. Interstitial del(11p) as a cause of the aniridia Wilms' tumor association. Band localization and a heritable basis. Am J Hum Genet 1978; 30:81A.
23. Francke U, Holmes LB, Atkins L, Riccardi VM. Aniridia-Wilms' tumor association: evidence for specific deletion of 11p13. Cytogenet Cell Genet 1979; 24:185–192.
24. Knudson AG, Strong LC. Mutation and cancer. A model for Wilms' tumor of the kidney. J Natl Cancer Inst 1972; 48:313–324.
25. Riccardi VM, Sujansky E, Smith AC, Francke U. Chromosomal imbalance in the aniridia-Wilms' tumor association, 11p interstitial deletion. Pediatrics 1978; 61:604–610.
26. Knudson AG. Mutation and cancer: Statistical study of retinoblastoma. Proc Natl Acad Sci USA 1971; 68:820–823.
27. Hittner HM, Riccardi VM, Franke U. Aniridia due to a heritable chromosome 11 deletion. Ophthalmology 1979; 86:1173–1183.
28. Cotlier E, Rose M, Moel SA. Aniridia, cataracts and Wilms' tumor in monozygous twins. Am J Ophthalmol 1978; 86:129–132.
29. Maurer HS, Pendergrass TW, Borges W, Honig GR. The role of genetic factors in the etiology of Wilms' tumor. Two pairs of monozygous twins with congenital abnormalities (aniridia, hemihypertrophy) and discordance for Wilms' tumor. Cancer 1979; 43:205–208.
30. Lewis WH, Yegev H, Bonetta L, et al. Homozygous deletion of a DNA marker from chromosome 11p13 in sporadic Wilms' tumor. Genomics 1988; 3:25–31.
31. Davis LM, Stallard R, Thomas GH, et al. Two anonymous DNA segments distinguish the Wilms' tumor and aniridia loci. Science 1988; 241:840–842.
32. Gessler M, Thomas GH, Couillin P, et al. A deletion map of the WAGR region on chromosome 11. Am J Hum Genet 1989; 44:486–495.
33. Grundy P, Koufos A, Morgan K, et al. Familial predisposition to Wilms' tumor does not map to the short arm of chromosome 11. Nature 1988; 336:374–376.

34. Huff V, Compton DA, Chao LY, et al. Lack of linkage of familial Wilms' tumour to chromosomal band 11p13. Nature 1988; 336:377–378.
35. Mirkinson AE, Mirkinson NK. A familial syndrome of aniridia and absence of patella. Birth Defects 1975; 11:129–131.
36. MacDonald IM, Clarke WN, Clifford BG, et al. Corneal pathology and aniridia associated with partial trisomy 2q, due to a maternal (2;6) translocation. Ophthalmic Paediatr Genet 1984; 4:75–80.
37. Pearce WG, Mielke BW, Hassard DTR, et al. Autosomal dominant keratitis: a possible aniridia variant. Can J Opthalmol 1995; 30:131–137.
38. Reeser F, Weinstein GW, Feiock BK, Oser RS. Electro-oculography as a test of retinal function. The normal and supernormal EOG. Am J Ophthalmol 1970; 70:505–514.
39. Tremblay F, Gupta SK, DeBecker I, et al. Effects of PAX6 mutations on retinal function: an electroretinographic study. Am J Ophthalmol 1998; 126:211–218.
40. Gupta SK, DeBecker I, Tremblay F, et al. Genotype/phenotype correlations in aniridia. Am J Ophthalmol 1998; 126:203–210.
41. Riccardi VM, Borges W. Aniridia, cataracts and Wilms' tumor. Am J Ophthalmol 1978; 86:577–578.
42. Yunis JJ, Ramsay NKC. Familial occurrence of the aniridia-Wilms' tumor syndrome with deletion 11p13-14.1. J Pediatr 1980; 96:1027–1030.
43. Barletta C, Castello MA, Ferrante E, et al. 11p13 deletion and reduced RBC catalase in a patient with aniridia, glaucoma and bilateral Wilms' tumor. Tumori 1985; 71: 119–121.
44. Couillin P, Azoulay M, Metezeau P, et al. The gene for catalase is assigned between the antigen loci *MIC4* and *MIC11* Genomics 1989; 4:7–11.
45. Margo CE. Congenital aniridia: a histopathologic study of the anterior segment in children. J Pediatr Ophthalmol Strabismus 1983; 20:192–198.
46. Sloderbeck JD, Maumenee IH, Elsas FE, et al. Linkage assignment of aniridia to chromosome 1 (Abstract). Am J Hum Genet 1975; 27:83A.
47. Ferrel RE, Chakrovarte A, Hittner HM, Ricardi VM. Autosomal dominant aniridia—probable linkage to acid phosphatase-1 locus on chromosome 2. Proc Natl Acad Sci USA 1982; 77:1580–1582.
48. Karmon G, Savir H, Shabtai F. Chromosome 9 pericentric inversion in familial aniridia. Metab Ophthalmol 1978; 2:213–214.
49. Jordan T, Hanson I, Zaletyev D, et al. The human PAX6 gene is mutated in two patients with aniridia. Nat Genet 1992; 1:328–332.
50. Glaser T, Walton DS, Maas RL. Genomic structure, evolutionary conservation and aniridia mutations in the human PAX6 gene. Nat Genet 1992; 2:232–239.
51. Prosser J, Van Heyningen V. PAX6 mutations reviewed. Hum Mutat 1998; 11:93–108.
52. Chao LYM, Huff V, Strong LC, Saunders GF. Mutation in the PAX6 gene in twenty patients with aniridia. Hum Mutat 2000; 15:332–339.
53. Martha AD, Strong LC, Ferrell RE, Saunders GF. Three novel aniridia mutations in the human PAX6 gene. Hum Mutat 1995; 6:44–49.
54. Gessler M, Konig A, Bruns GA. The genomic organization and expression of the WT1 gene. Genomics 1992; 12:807–813.
55. Kawase E, Tanaka K, Honna T, Azuma N. A case of atypical WAGR syndrome with anterior segment anomaly and microphthalmus. Arch Ophthalmol 2001; 119:1855–1856.
56. Dollfus H, Joanny-Flinois O, Doco-Fenzy M, et al. Gillespie syndrome phenotype with a t(X;11)(p22.32;pl2) de novo translocation. Am J Ophthalmol 1998; 125:397–399.
57. Adachi M, Dickens CJ, Hetherington J, et al. Clinical experience of trabeculotomy for the surgical treatment of aniridic glaucoma. Ophthalmology 1997; 104:2121–2125.
58. Wiggins RE, Tomey KF. The results of glaucoma surgery in aniridia. Arch Ophthalmol 1992; 110:503–505.
59. Chen TC, Walton DS. Goniosurgery for prevention of aniridic glaucoma. Arch Ophthalmol 1999; 117:1144–1148.

60. Reinhard T, Engelhardt S, Sundmacher R. Black diaphragm aniridia intraocular lens for congenital aniridia: long-term follow up. J Cataract Refract Surg 2000; 26:375–381.
61. Holland EJ, Djililian AR, Schwartz GS. Management of aniridic keratopathy with keratolimbal allograft: a limbal stem cell transplantation technique. Ophthalmology 2003; 110:125–130.
62. Stern RJ, Hunter WS, Moross T, Gardner HA. Prenatal diagnosis of del(11)(pl3pl5). Prenat Diagn 1988; 8:1–6.
63. Rieger H. Beitraege zur Kenntnis seltener Missbildungen der Iris: Ueber Hypoplasia des Irisvorderblattes mit Verlagerung und Entrundung der Pupille. Graefes Arch Ktin Exp Ophthalmol 1935; 133:602–635.
64. Judisch GF, Phelps CD, Hanson J. Rieger's syndrome: a case report with a 15 year follow-up. Arch Ophthalmol 1979; 97:2120–2122.
65. Jorgenson RJ, Levin LS, Cross HE, et al. The Rieger syndrome. J Med Genet 1978; 15:30–34.
66. Heckenlively J, Isenberg S. Glaucoma and buphthalmus. In: Emery AEH, Rimoin DL (eds). Principles and Practice of Medical Genetics. Edinburgh: Churchill-Livingstone 1983:488–496.
67. Azuma I. Ein Bericht zum Kongenitalen Glaukom. Klin Monatsbl Augenheiikd 1984; 184:287–289.
68. Bardelli AM, Hadjistilianou T, Frezzotti R. Etiology of congenital glaucoma. Genetic and extragenetic factors. Ophthalmic Paediatr Genet 1985; 6:265–270.
69. Alkemade PPH. Dysgenesis Mesodermalis of the Iris and the Cornea. A Study of Rieger's Syndrome and Peters' Anomaly. Assen: Van Gorcum, 1969.
70. McKussick VA. Mendelian Inheritance in Man. 6th ed. Baltimore: Johns Hopkins University Press, 1983.
71. Waring GO, Rodrigues MM, Laibson PR. Anterior chamber cleavage syndrome: a step-ladder classification. Surv Ophthalmol 1975; 20:3–27.
72. Alward WLM. Axenfeld-Rieger syndrome in the age of molecular genetics. Am J Ophthalmol 2000; 130:107–115.
73. Alward WLM, Semina EV, Kalenak JW, et al. Autosomal dominant iris hypoplasia is caused by a mutation in the Rieger syndrome (RIEG/PITX2) gene. Am J Ophthalmol 1998; 125:98–100.
74. Heon E, Sheth BP, Kalenak JW, et al. Linkage of autosomal dominant iris hypoplasia to the region of the Rieger syndrome locus (4q 25). Hum Mol Genet 1995; 4:1435–1439.
75. Pearce WG, Wyatt HT, Boyd TA, et al. Autosomal dominant iridogoniodysgenesis: genetic features. Can J Ophthalmol 1983; 18:7–10.
76. Berg F. Erbliches jugendliches Glaukom. Acta Ophthalmol 1932; 10:568–587.
77. Jerndal T. Goniodysgenesis and hereditary juvenile glaucoma. A clinical study of a Swedish pedigree. Acta Ophthalmol Suppl 1970; 107.
78. Martin JP, Zorab EC. Familial glaucoma in nine generations of a South Hampshire family. Br J Ophthalmol 1974; 58:536–542.
79. Jerndal T. Congenital glaucoma due to dominant goniodysgenesis. A new concept of the heredity of glaucoma. Am J Hum Genet 1983; 35:645–651.
80. Chisholm 1A, Chudley AE. Autosomal dominant iridogoniodysgenesis with associated somatic anomalies: four generation family with Rieger's syndrome. Br J Ophthalmol 1983; 67:529–534.
81. Weatherill JR, Hart CT. Familial hypoplasia of the iris stroma associated with glaucoma. Br J Ophthalmol 1969; 53:433–438.
82. Walter MA, Mirzayans F, Mears AJ, et al. Autosomal-dominant iridogoniodysgenesis and Axenfeld-Rieger syndrome are genetically distinct. Ophthalmology 1996; 103:1907–1915.
83. Mears AJ, Mirzayans F, Gould DB, et al. Autosomal dominant iridogoniodysgenesis anomaly maps to 6p25. Hum Genet 1996; 59:1321–1327.

84. De Hauwere RC, Leroy JG, Adiaenssens K, van Heule R. Iris hypoplasia, orbital hyper telorism and psychomotor retardation: a dominantly inherited developmental syndrome. J Pediatr 1973; 82:679–681.
85. Cunningham ET, Eliott D, Miller NR, et al. Familial Axenfeld-Rieger anomaly, atrial septal defect, and sensorineural hearing loss: a possible new genetic syndrome. Arch Ophthalmol 1998; 116:78–82.
86. Soong HK, Raizman MB. Corneal changes in familial iris coloboma. Ophthalmology 1986; 93:335–339.
87. Wilcox LM, Bercovitch L, Howard RO. Ophthalmic features of chromosome deletion 4p- (Wolf-Hirschhorn syndrome). Am J Ophthalmol 1974; 86:834–839.
88. Lubin JR. Oculocutaneous albinism associated with corneal mesodermal dysgenesis. Am J Ophthalmol 1981; 91:347–350.
89. Benson W. Oculocutaneous albinism with Axenfeld's anomaly. Am J Ophthalmol 1981; 92:133–134.
90. Ricci B, Lacerra F. Oculocutaneous albinism and corneal mesodermal dysgenesis. Am J Ophthalmol 1981; 92:587.
91. van Dorp BD, Delleman JW, Loewer-Sieger DH. Oculocutaneous albinism and anterior chamber cleavage malformations. Not a coincidence. Clin Genet 1984; 26:440–444.
92. Murray JC, Bennett SR, Kwitek AE, et al. Linkage of Rieger syndrome to the region of the epidermal growth factor gene of chromosome 4. Nat Genet 1992; 2:46–49.
93. Makita T, Masuno M, Imaizumi K, et al. Rieger syndrome with de novo reciprocal translocation t (1;4) (q 23.1 ;q 25). Am J Med Genet 1995; 57:19–21.
94. Semina E, Reiter R, Leysens N, et al. Cloning and characterization of a novel bicoid-related homeobox transcription factor gene, RIEG, involved in Rieger syndrome. Nat Genet 1996; 14:392–399.
95. Phillips JC, del Bono EA, Haines JL, et al. A second locus for Rieger syndrome maps to chromosome 13q14. Am J Hum Genet 1996; 59:613–619.
96. Mears AJ, Jordan T, Mirzayans F, et al. Mutations of the forkhead/winged-helix gene, FKHL7, in patients with Axenfeld-Rieger anomaly. Am J Hum Genet 1998; 63:1316–1328.
97. Mirzayans F, Gould DB, Heon E, et al. Axenfeld-Rieger syndrome resulting from mutation of the FKHL7 gene on chromosome 6p25. Eur J Hum Genet 2000; 8:71–74.
98. Honkanen RA, Nishimura DY, Swiderski RE, et al. A family with Axenfeld-Rieger syndrome and Peters anomaly caused by a point mutation (Phel 12Ser) in the FOXC1 gene. Am J Ophthalrnol 2003; 135:368–375.
99. Jordan T, Ebenezer N, Manners R, et al. Familial glaucoma iridogoniodysplasia maps to a 6p25 region implicated in primary congenital glaucoma and iridogoniodysgenesis anomaly. Am J Hum Genet 1997; 61:882–888.
100. Hittner HM, Ferrell RE, Antoszyk JH, Kretzer FL. Autosomal dominant anterior segment dysgenesis with variable expressivity—probable linkage to MNS blood group on chromosome 4 (abstract). Pediatr Res 1981; 15:563.
101. Ligutic I, Brecevic L, Petkovic I, et al. Interstitial deletion of 4q and Rieger syndrome. Clin Genet 1981; 20:323–327.
102. Wyatt HT, Pearce WG, Boyd TA, et al. Autosomal dominant iridogoniodysgenesis: glaucoma management. Can J Ophthalmol 1983; 18:11–14.
103. Shields JA. Primary cysts of the iris. Trans Am Ophthalmol Soc 1981; 79:771–809.
104. Vela A, Rieser JC, Campbell DG. The heredity and treatment of angle-closure glaucoma secondary to iris and ciliary body cysts. Ophthalmology 1984; 91:332–337.
105. Balacco-Gabrieli C, Castellano L, Palmisano C, et al. Iris cysts in three generations conveyed by means of a genetic process connected with sex. Ophthalmic Paediatr Genet 1985; 6:319–324.
106. Lee BL, Lanier AB, Bateman JB. Autosomal-dominant anomalies of the iris pigment epithelium. Ophthalmology 1996; 103:1696–1699.
107. Polomeno RC, Milot J. Congenital miosis. Can J Ophthalmol 1979; 14:43–46.

108. Tawara A, Inomata H. Familial cases of congenital microcoria associated with late onset congenital glaucoma and goniodysgenesis. Jpn J Ophthalmol 1983; 27:63–72.
109. Dick DJ, Newman PK, Cleland PG. Hereditary spastic ataxia with congenital miosis: Four cases in one family. Br J Ophthalmol 1983; 67:97–101.
110. Toulemont PJ, Urvoy M, Coscas G, et al. Association of congenital microcoria with myopia and glaucoma. A study of 23 patients with congenital microcoria. Ophthalmology 1995; 102:193–198.
111. Rouillac C, Roche O, Marchant D, et al. Mapping of a congenital microcoria locus to 13q31-q32. Am J Hum Genet 1998; 62:1117–1122.
112. Simpson WAC, Parsons MA. The ultrastructural pathological features of congenital microcoria. A case report. Arch Ophthalmol 1989; 107:99–102.
113. Davenport CG, Davenport CB. Heredity of eye colour in man. Science 1907; 26:589–592.
114. Rufer V, Bauer J, Soukup F. On the hereditary of eye colour. Acta Univ Carol 1971; 16:429–434.
115. Bito LZ, Matheny A, Cruickshanks KJ, et al. Eye color changes past early childhood. The Louisville Twin Study. Arch Ophthalmol 1997; 115:659–63.
116. Jensen AR. Estimation of the limits of heritability of traits by comparison of monozygotic and dizygotic twins. Proc Natl Acad Sci 1967; 58:148–156.
117. Bräuer G, Chopra VP. Schätzungen der Heritabilitat van Haar-und Augenfarbe. Anthropol Anz 1978; 36:109–120.
118. Francois J. Multifactorial or polygenic inheritance in ophthalmology. Dev Ophthalmol 1985; 10:1–39.
119. Chen RM, Lupski JR, Greenberg F, Lewis RA. Ophthalmic manifestations of Smith-Magenis syndrome. Ophthalmology 1996; 103:1084–1091.
120. Jun AS, Broman KW, Do DV, et al. Endothelial dystrophy, iris hypoplasia, congenital cataract, and stromal thinning (EDICT) syndrome maps to chromosome 15q22.1-q25,3. Am J Ophthalmol 2002; 134:172–176.
121. Giles CL, Tanton JH. Peripheral uveitis in three children of one family. J Pediatr Ophthalmol Strabismus 1980; 17:297–299.
122. Augsburger JJ, Annesley WH, Sergott RC, et al. Familial pars planitis. Ann Ophthalmol 1981; 13:553–557.
123. Doft BH. Pars planitis in identical twins. Retina 1983; 3:32–33.
124. Woodrow JC. Genetic aspects of the spondyloarthropathies. Clin Rheum Dis 1985; 11:1–24.
125. Dündar SV, Gencalp U, Simsek H. Familial cases of Behcet's disease. Br J Dermatol 1985; 113:319–321.
126. Berman L, Trappler B, Jenkins T. Behcet's syndrome: a family study and the elucidation of a genetic role. Ann Rheum Dis 1979; 38:118–121.
127. Yazici H, Chamberlain MA, Schreuder GM, et al. HLA B5 and Behcet's disease. Ann Rheum Dis 1983; 42:602–603.
128. Aronsson A, Tegner E. Behcet's syndrome in two brothers. Acta Dermatol Venereol 1983; 63:73–74.
129. Davey MP, Rosenbaum JT. The human leukocyte antigen complex and chronic ocular inflammatory disorders. Am J Ophthalmol 2000; 129:235–243.
130. Tang WM, Pulido JS, Eckels DD, et al. The association of HLA-DR15 and intermediate uveitis. Am J Ophthalmol 1997; 123:70–75.
131. Raja SC, Jabs DA, Dunn JP, et al. Pars planitis: clinical features and class II HLA associations. Ophthalmology 1999; 106:594–599.
132. Brewerton DA. The genetics of acute anterior uveitis. Trans Ophthalmol Soc UK 1985; 104:248–249.
133. Wakefield S, Wright J, Penny R. HLA antigens in uveitis. Hum Immunol 1983; 7:89–93.
134. Mehra NK, Khan MA, Vaidya MC, et al. HLA antigens in acute anterior uveitis and spondyloarthropathies in Asian Indians and their comparison with American whites and blacks. J Rheumatol 1983; 10:981–984.

135. Leclercq SA, Percy JS, Russel AS. Genetic markers for acute anterior uveitis. J Rheumatol 1983; 10:998–1000.
136. Miller ML, Fraser PA, Jackson JM, et al. Inherited predisposition to iridocyclitis with juvenile rheumatoid arthritis: selectivity among HLA-DR5 haplotypes. Proc Natl Acad Sci U S A 1984; 81:3539–3542.
137. Lisch K. Genetische Aspekte bei Morbus Behcet und juveniler rheumatoider Arthritis. Klin Monatsbl Augenheilkd 1985; 187:460–463.
138. Brewerton DA. The genetics of acute antereior uveitis. Trans Ophthalmol Soc UK 1985; 104:248–249.
139. Linssen A, Meenken C. Outcomes of HLA-B27-positive and HLA-B27-negative acute anterior uveitis. Am J Ophthalmol 1995; 120:351–361.
140. Power WJ, Rodriguez A, Pedroza-Seres M, Foster CS. Outcomes in anterior uveitis associated with the HLA-B27 haplotype. Ophthalmology 1998; 105:1646–1651.
141. Derhaag PJFM, Linssen A, Broekema N, et al. A familial study of the inheritance of HLA-B27-positive acute anterior uveitis. Am J Ophthalmol 1988; 105:603–606.
142. Crolla JA, Cawdry JE, Oley CA, et al. A FISH approach to defining the extent and possible clinical significance of deletions at the WAGR locus. J Med Genet 1997; 34:207–212.
143. Gupta SK, DeBecker I, Guernsey DL, Neumann PE. PCR-based risk assessment for Wilms tumor in sporadic aniridia. Am J Ophthalmol 1998; 125:687–692.
144. Eagle RC, Font RL, Yanoff M, Fine BS. Proliferative endotheliopathy with iris abnormalities: the iridocorneal endothelial syndrome. Arch Ophthalmol 1979; 97:2104–2111.
145. Levinson RD, Rajalingam R, Park MS et al. Human leukocyte antigen A29 subtypes associated with birdshot netinochoroidopathy. Am J Ophthalmol 2004; 128:631–635.
146. Wolf MD, Folk JC, Panknen CA, Goeken NE. HLA-B7 and HLA-DR2 antigens and acute posterior multifocal placoid pigment epitheliopathy. Arch Ophthalmol 1990; 108:698–700.

6
Inherited Cataracts

INTRODUCTION

Cataract is a common denominator of many hereditary diseases, especially congenital and infantile cataracts. In fact, it may be the most common single sign of a large group of heterogenous hereditary diseases, which primarily affect such diverse organs as the central nervous system (CNS), genitourinary tract, gastrointestinal tract, the skeletal system, and others.

Cataracts may be classified according to age of appearance (congenital, infantile, juvenile, presenile, and senile), etiology (hereditary-isolated, hereditary-associated, nonhereditary known causes, and idiopathic), and morphologic appearance. It is often not possible to distinguish between a cataract present at birth (congenital) and one that develops in the first few weeks or months of life (infantile cataract), so these terms will be used here synonymously. Most hereditary cataracts occur in the congenital-infantile group, but isolated hereditary cataracts do not exceed 25% of all cases of congenital cataracts (1). Judging from other studies on the etiology of congenital cataract (2,3), 25% may be an exaggerated figure. However in one study the assumption was that one-third of all congenital cataracts are of hereditary origin (4). The various etiologies of congenital cataract should, therefore, be considered in each case individually. Tables 1 and 2 list the results of two large studies on the etiology of congenital cataracts (1,2). These may be helpful for etiologic considerations when there is no obvious family history. Congenital rubella, which was an important cause of congenital cataracts only two decades ago, has declined in frequency and importance owing to large-scale immunizations, but other congenital viral diseases may be factors (5).

Several attempts to classify human cataracts morphologically have been made (6–8). These use a photographic technique for the recognition of lens changes, especially the color of the lens nucleus, for nuclear sclerosis and nuclear cataract. However, these classifications are not suitable for congenital and hereditary cataracts. The simplified morphologic classification, as previously suggested by Merin (9), is probably more appropriate for this type of cataract. According to this scheme, the cataract is classified as total (mature), polar (anterior or posterior), zonular (nuclear, lamellar, or sutural), or membranous.

Table 1 Etiology of Infantile Cataract in 386 Cases

Etiology	%
Hereditary isolated	8.3
Congenital rubella	19.1
Hereditary and nonhereditary associated	11.9
Other ocular disease	6.0
Convulsive disorder or CNS disease	22.8
Unknown	31.9

Source: From Merin and Crawford

Table 2 Etiology of Congenital Cataract in 300 Cases

Etiology	%
Hereditary	25
Embryopathy	10
Genetic systemic	6
Idiopathic	59

Source: From Francois (1).

Other hereditary lens anomalies are relatively rare, and they will be discussed separately in Chapter 7.

ISOLATED CONGENITAL CATARACTS

Introduction

The term isolated nonsyndromic congenital cataract is used when the sole manifestation of the gene or the disease is congenital cataract. In some of these cases, nystagmus, microphthalmos, and deprivation amblyopia are related secondarily to the cataract. An isolated congenital cataract may be familial owing to hereditary causes or sporadic owing to hereditary or nonhereditary causes. Hereditary cases may be transmitted as an autosomal dominant, autosomal recessive, or X-linked trait. It is now well known that many different genes cause isolated cataract. In 1974 Merin estimated (9) that at least 8–12 autosomal dominant genes, at least two to three autosomal recessive genes, and at least one X-linked recessive gene may cause isolated hereditary congenital cataract.

We now know that these figures are an underestimation, as I suggested in the previous edition. The number of known distinct loci for congenital cataract is more than double these figures.

Genetic and Clinical Types

It is logical to classify cataracts according to their genetic trait, a consistent and stable factor. Morphologic similarities in individual families usually exist, but not always. However, the morphologic structure of the cataract (Table 3) may serve to subclassify individual genetic entities.

Table 3 Morphologic Types of Isolated Hereditary Congenital Cataracts

Type		Heredity[a]
A	Anterior polar cataracts	
	With zonular lens opacities	AD
	With microphthalmia	AD
	With persistent hyperplastic pupillary membrane	AD
B	Posterior polar cataracts	
	Autosomal dominant type	AD
	Autosomal recessive type	AR
C	Zonular cataracts	
	Nuclear	AD, AR, XL
	Lamellar	AD
	Sutural	XL
D	Total cataracts	
	Autosomal dominant type	AD
	Autosomal recessive type	AR
E	Membranous cataracts	

[a]AD, autosomal dominant; AR, autosomal recessive; XL, X-linked.

Autosomal Dominant Cataract

The most common form of transmission of isolated hereditary congenital cataract is the autosomal dominant mode (Fig. 1). Many family pedigrees of this transmission have been reported, indicating the full penetrance of the gene. As the gene is not lethal and does not reduce the normal life span or fertility, very large pedigrees have been published.

Earlier studies have assigned the genes causing congenital cataract to specific chromosomes and loci. Three methods of assignments have been used (10): the classic pedigree analysis, the somatic cell hybridization technique, and the recombinant DNA technique. Most studies used the first method. At present, the assignment of two human autosomal dominant congenital cataracts has been successful. Renwick and Lawler (11) showed, by complicated statistical evaluation of linkage, that the locus for a congenital cataract is closely linked to the locus for Duffy (Fy) blood group on chromosome 1. The same cataract, which was originally described by Nettleship and Ogilvie, in 1906 (12), consists of multiple spots of opacity in the nucleus. It was named "Coppock cataract," after John Coppock, who described the original large family. The assignment of this cataract to chromosome 1 has been confirmed by Conneally et al. (13) through linkage studies of another family with a similar nuclear cataract with scattered spots and riders.

The cataract, as seen in the Coppock family, was zonular pulverulent but also polymorphic, as variable phenotypes could be seen in one family. In 1997, the locus of the Coppock-type cataract, cataract zonular pulverulent (CZP1), was mapped to chromosome 1q21.1 (14). The gene GJA8 gap junction alpha protein 8 (GJA8) encodes the lens intrinsic protein MP70, also named CX50, one of the gap junction proteins (14,15). A morphologically similar cataract, CZP3 locus, was mapped to chromosome 13q11–q12, near the centromere of chromosome 13. The gene GJA3 encodes CX46. Both proteins belong to the gap junction proteins. Mutations in these genes cause the Coppock-type congenital cataracts (14–17) and a variety of

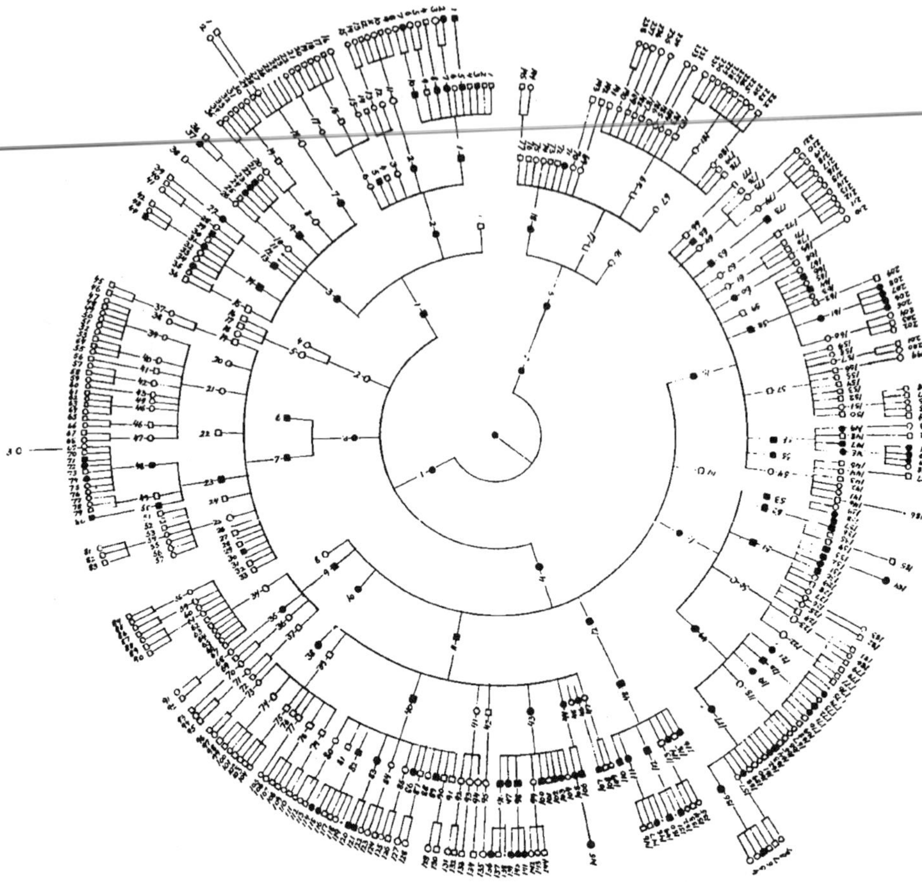

Figure 1 Autosomal dominant inheritance of congenital cataract in eight generations. Note the regular transmission with full penetrance of the gene: no affected child was born to an unaffected parent. However, the fertility of nonaffected members of the family is higher than that of the affected, resulting in a much higher number of nonaffected than affected in the seventh and eighth generations. The cataract was lamellar in this family (''zonular and central'') [from Marner (35)].

other disorders such as deafness, neuropathy, skin disorders, heart defects (16). These proteins, of which there are at least 10, mediate the intercellular transport of small biomolecules (16).

Using complex techniques of molecular genetics, Lubsen and associates (18) showed that the locus for a Coppock-like cataract is closely linked to the γ-crystallin gene cluster, with a very high lod (log of the odds) score of 7.58 at recombination rate zero. The genes for the human γ-crystallins are located in the 2q33–2q36 region of chromosome 2 and are a family of seven closely homologous genes (18).

In the first half of the 1990s several other congenital cataract loci had been mapped. Later, more and more genes and their disease-causing mutations were identified. Table 4 lists the phenotypically and genetically different types of autosomal dominant congenital cataracts.

The human lens has the highest cellular density of any tissue. Ninety-five percent of its proteins are crystallins. They are the alpha, beta, and gamma crystallins.

Table 4 Autosomal Dominant Nonsyndromic (Isolated) Congenital Cataracts in Humans

Cataract description	Symbol	MIM	Chromosomal location	Gene	References
Early total	CC	116700	?	?	(50)
Total with anterior dysgenesis		602669	10q25	PITX3	(4)
Zonular–lamellar Marner	CAM	116800	16q21–q22.1	HSF4	(35–38)
Lamellar, Coppock-like	CCL1	604307	2q33–q35	CRYGC	(28,29)
Lamellar, Coppock-like	CCL2	607133	22q11.2	CRYBB2	(16,17)
Lamellar, Coppock-like	CCL3	123660	2q33–q35	CRYGE	(31,51)
Zonular, aculeiform/ polymorphic	ADPCC	601286	2q33–q35	CRYGB	(30,52)
Zonular, polymorphic		154050	12q14	MIP	(42)
Zonular, nuclear, pulverulent Coppock-type	CZP1	116200	Iq21.1	GJA8	(11–15)
Zonular, nuclear, pulverulent Coppock-type	CZP3	601885	13q11–q12	GJA3	(15,30)
Cerulean/ pulverulent	CCA1	115660	17q24	?	(40)
Cerulean/ pulverulent		600929	22q11.2	CRYBB1	(20,24)
Zonular, central nuclear	ADCC2	123580	21q22.3	CRYAA	(19)
Zonular, nuclear progressive		607304	2p12	?	(41)
Zonular, Volkman type	CCV	115665	1pter–p36.13	?	(39)
Zonular and sutural progressive	CCZS	600881	17q11.1–q12	CRYBA1	(21–23)
Anterior polar	CTAA1	115650	14q24–qter	?	(53,54)
Anterior polar	CTAA2	601202	17p13	?	(43,53,54)
Posterior polar	CPP1	116600	1pter–p36.1	?	(33,43,46,55)
Posterior polar	CPP2	123590	11q22.3–q23.1	CRYAB	(20)
Posterior polar	CPP3	605387	20p12–q12	?	(46)
Cataract with microphthal-mus	CATM	156850	16p13.3	?	(56–58)

The genes are mapped to separate locations. Alpha-crystallins and beta-crystallins appear each in two forms, A for acidic and B for basic. Gamma-crystallins genes are lumped together as a cluster of seven genes.

A central nuclear cataract is caused by a missense mutation (Arg116Cys) of the alpha crystalline A (CRYAA) gene, mapped to chromosome 21q22.3 (19). A mutation (450delA) in the CRYAB gene located on chromosome 11q22–q22.3 was identified in patients with congenital autosomal dominant posterior polar cataracts (20).

Beta-crystallin genes are located in at least two locations. Crystalline beta A1 (CRYBA1) is located at chromosome 17q11–q12. A mutation was identified resulting in a protein with a single globular domain and causing zonular–sutural cataract (21–23). Beta-crystallin genes were mapped to chromosome 22q11.2. Cataract-causing mutations were identified in crystalline-beta-basic-1 (CRYBB1) (Gly220Stop) (24) and in CRYBB2 (chain termination mutation) (17) and in a mutation in exon 6 (25). The phenotype of the congenital cataract caused by mutations in the beta-crystallin genes was variable but zonular in all. They included lamellar–nuclear Coppock-like cataract, polymorphic, being of variable appearance in the same family, pulverulent lamellar–zonular (Coppock-like), and cerulean (multiple blue flecks) (17,24–26). All of these were usually mild with visual acuity only minimally affected in early childhood.

The cluster of gamma-crystallin genes was mapped to chromosomes 2q33–q35. Polymorphic, aculeiform, Coppock-like, lamellar, and nuclear were the terms used to describe the cataract by the researchers. The descriptions fit a congenital mild cataract, in some cases visual acuity is not reduced with a cataractous cloudiness in the form of multiple dots, lamellar around or in the nucleus. Sometimes other parts, such as the lens sutures or posterior pole, are also affected. It is usually not progressive. Cataract-causing mutations were identified in the crystalline gamma B (CRYGB) gene (27), CRYGC (28,29), CRYGD (29,30), and CRYGE (31,32).

An assignment of a locus for posterior polar cataract to chromosome 16 has been reported by Maumenee (33), and by Richard and associates (34). Also, strong evidence was provided that the gene for Marner's cataract, a lamellar congenital cataract involving nine generations of one family, is linked to haptoglobin on chromosome 16 (36).

The disease-causing gene for the Mamer family lamellar cataract was identified in both Danish and Chinese families as HSF4, a gene which regulates the expression of heat-shock proteins, in the eye which are components of lens development (37). A missense Leu115Pro mutation was identified in all affected (37). The gene maps to chromosome 16q21–q22.1.

Some rare zonular cataracts of the lamellar–nuclear type are caused by mutations in other genes. The Volkman–type cataract, a mild cataract in which opacities in the nucleus and sutures can be seen, was mapped to chromosome 1pter–p36.13 (38,39). Unlike the Marner cataract, congenital cataract Volkman (CCV) is progressive and may require surgery in the second decade of life (38). A cerulean mild cataract, in which blue dots surround the nucleus, is slowly progressive. It has been mapped to chromosome 17q24 (40). A nuclear cataract was recently mapped to chromosome 2p12 (41).

PITX3, the homeobox gene associated with cataract and anterior segment dysgenesis was mapped to chromosome 10q25 (4). Mutations that cause mainly congenital cataracts with mild dysgenesis were identified (4).

A polymorphic lamellar cataract was associated in two families with mutations in the MTP gene, the gene encoding the major (42) intrinsic protein of the lens fiber membrane.

Anterior polar cataracts were mapped to chromosomes 17p13 (43) and 14q24 (44). Posterior polar congenital cataracts were reported as at least three distinct loci mapped to chromosomes 1pter–p36.1 (45), 11q22–q22.3 associated with mutations in the CRYAB gene (20), and 20p12–q12 (46), indicating heterogeneity of posterior polar cataract.

Other families with autosomal dominant cataract do not show linkage (11,13), including in large studies using multiple phenotypic gene markers (47) or DNA restriction fragment length polymorphisms, detected by lens-specific DNA probes (48). Many linkage studies were inconclusive (47). Table 4 is an attempt to list all phenotypically different types of autosomal dominant congenital cataracts. It seems that 12 different genetic and clinical entities can now firmly be identified. Some of these entities display heterogeneity, in that several separate autosomal dominant genes are expressed in the same phenotype. Lamellar cataracts are usually expressed somewhat differently in individual family members, and it is often difficult to compare different families. The same may be said about nuclear cataracts. Anterior polar cataracts are usually sporadic and nonhereditary, but a familial occurrence in association with other anterior segment anomalies, such as microcornea, microphthalmos, and persistent hyperplastic pupillary membrane, have been well established by family studies as separate clinical and genetic entities.

The largest group (about 40%) of these autosomal dominant diseases is manifested by a lamellar cataract, followed (in 30%) by nuclear cataract (9) (Fig. 2). Sutural (stellate) cataracts have been reported to regress over the course of some 20 years in one patient, whereas nuclear opacities increased enormously at the same time (49). Also, stellate cataracts have been described in some members of one family, whereas other members had nuclear cataracts (9). This may indicate a relationship between these two morphologic types.

About 25% of all sporadic bilateral cataracts have been estimated to be new mutations (2).

Autosomal Recessive Cataract

Isolated congenital cataract transmitted as an autosomal recessive disease is relatively uncommon. However, in populations with endogamous marriages (59,60), or with a high percentage of consanguineous marriages, autosomal recessive isolated congenital cataract composes about 25% of all hereditary isolated cataracts (9). In fact, it may be the most common form of hereditary cataract in some populations (Fig. 3). In Egypt, the average consanguinity rate is 33%, whereas in a group of patients with congenital cataract, the rate of parental consanguinity has reached 56.5% (61).

In a study of congenital cataract in 13 states of India, Vanita and coauthors (62) found that autosomal recessive inheritance is more common than dominant (21% vs. 15%). Fifty percent of autosomal recessive patients originated from a consanguineous marriage (62). In contrast, in southeast Wales, in 36 families with known type of hereditary transmission of congenital cataract, 30 were dominant, 4 X-linked, and only 2 autosomal recessive (63).

The list of autosomal recessive congenital cataracts (ARCC) is, in fact, very short. It is possible that the majority are not yet known. It should be remembered

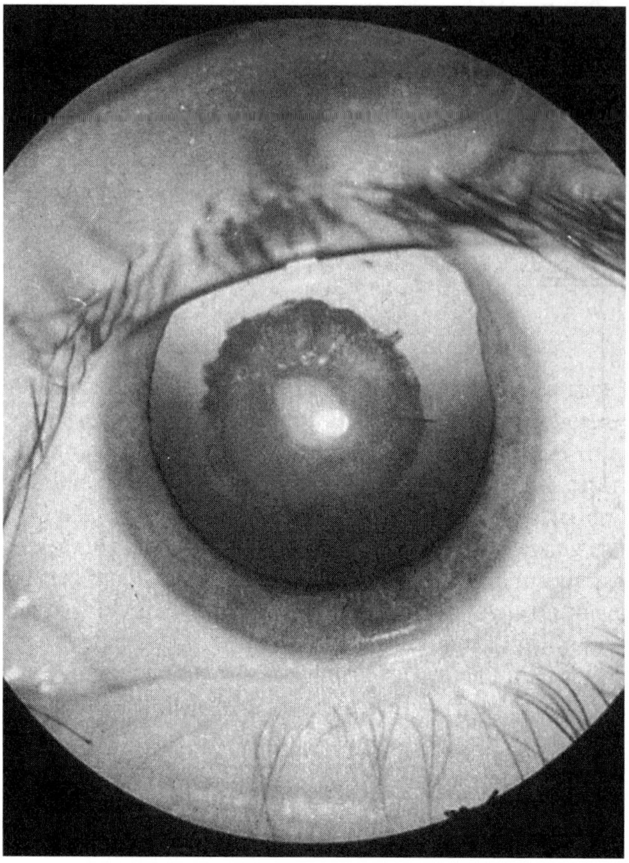

Figure 2 The most common appearance of a hereditary congenital cataract—the lamellar type. In this patient it is combined with a nuclear cataract.

that most genes for ARCC are associated with manifestation of a systemic disease (discussed later) and are not the cause of isolated congenital cataract. Also, the classification into the different entities is much less reliable than for autosomal dominant diseases.

Figure 3 demonstrates the typical pedigrees of families with ARCC and with autosomal dominant congenital cataract. Table 5 describes some possible isolated congenital cataracts of autosomal recessive and X-linked recessive inheritance.

Only one disease-causative gene was identified. Pras and coauthors (64) identified a homozygous mutation, Trp9Stop, in CRYAA, the gene encoding alpha-crystallin A and mapped to chromosome 21q22.3, in all affected members of a Jewish family of Persian origin. The cataract was dense and all affected required surgery in the first three months of life (64). Another ARCC was described among the Hutterites, a group of people living in Saskatechewan and Alberta in Canada and in Montana in the United States (60,65) and in the Aland Islands (66). The cataract may be congenital or may appear as juvenile cataract. Nuclear ARCC were also described (67,68) and there is no doubt that some other families with ARCC suffer from different genetic entities (64,69). Cataract marked as 212550 in OMIM (70) consists of a congenital cataract with microphthalmia and nystagmus (71). The location of the gene is unknown. Its phenotype is polymorphic.

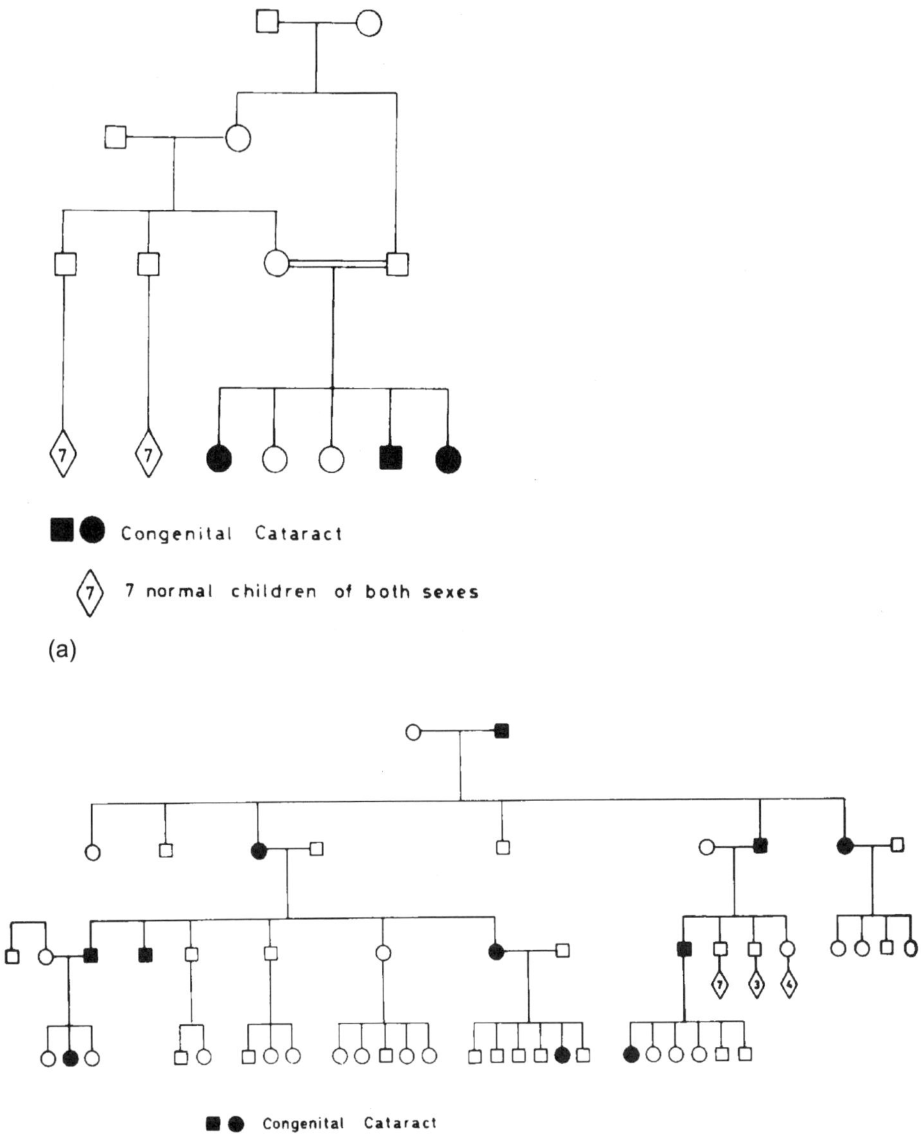

Figure 3 (a) Autosomal recessive cataract. Rate of consanguinity of parents is high in this mode of inheritance. (b) Autosomal dominant cataract in a family from Jerusalem.

X-Linked Cataract

X-linked isolated congenital cataract is a rare finding. At least one clinical and genetic entity exists for an X-linked recessive cataract. In the affected male, the cataract starts at the posterior Y-suture, continues to a lamellar–perinuclear opacification, and later progresses through total nuclear cataract to total lens opacification (72,78). Female carriers display characteristic posterior Y-sutural opacities (72–75). In some cases, females are affected by a progressing cataract and poor vision, as predieted by the Lyon theory on X-chromosomal inactivation (79). This X-linked cataract is possibly linked to the Xg blood group locus on the chromosome

Table 5 Autosomal Recessive and X-Linked Recessive Congenital Cataract

Cataract description	Heredity	MIM	Chromosomal location	Gene	References
Hutterite type[a]	AR	212500	?	?	(65,66,69)
Nuclear	AR	—	?	?	(67,68)
Persian Jewish[a]	AR	—	21q22.3	CRYAA	(64)
Other congenital	AR	—	?	?	(64,69)
With microphthalmus and nystagmus	AR	212550	?	?	(71)
Total	X-L	302200	?	?	(72–75)
With microcornea	X-L	302300		?	(70,74,75)
Total with or without heart defect	X-L	—	Xp22.2	?	(77)

[a]See text.

(72–75) and is numbered 302200 in OMIM (70). The cataract in the affected boys is total, while both hemizygotes and heterozygotes manifest posterior sutural opacities, as explained earlier.

It is not clear whether microcomea and microphthalmos are part of this genetic disease, or if they are a separate entity. These two findings are common in some members of families affected by X-Iinked congenital cataracts (74–76), but not in others (72,73,78). The microphthalmos may be a secondary phenomenon to the cataract, but it is also possible that we are dealing with two separate genetic and clinical entities. Congenital cataract with microcomea's is OMIM number 302300 (70).

Another X-linked congenital cataract was mapped to chromosome Xp22.2 (77). The cataract was dense and all affected members of the family were operated in the first months of life. Some had also a congenital heart disease (77).

The existence of a Y-chromosome-linked cataract has been suggested (47), but not yet confirmed.

Pathology and Pathogenesis

Very little is known about the pathogenesis of human isolated congenital cataract. Even its pathology can hardly be studied, as the cataract is not removed intracapsularly. Attempts to study cells from human lenses that display hereditary congenital cataracts by tissue culture (81) have not revealed its true pathology and pathogenesis. We rely, therefore, on studies from animal experiments. Mice most studied species in hereditary cataracts. Table 6 lists hereditary cataracts in varieties of mice that have been widely investigated and that have potential value for extrapolation to the human condition. In the Nakano mouse (82), hereditary cataract is transmitted by an autosomal recessive gene: Cat^{Nakano}. The homozygotic mouse has an inherited deficiency of the sodium–potassium (Na–K) ATPase, which leads to a subnormality of the cation pump mechanism (83). This deficiency has been found in 13-day-old mice before any structural lens abnormality could be detected. An increase in the sodium and water content of the lens on day 20 was followed by a nuclear opacity on days 23 through 25, and later by a mature cataract (83). Scanning electron microscopy has shown that the opacity starts at the posterior pole, that the lens cells are

Table 6 Hereditary Cataract in Experimental Strains of Mice

Strain	Heredity[a]	Reference
Nakano	AR	82
Fraser ("Shrivelled")	AD	88
Philly	AD	90
Lop	AD	95
Deer	AR	96
Emory	AD	97

[a]AD, autosomal dominant; AR, autosomal recessive.

irregular in size, and that there are numerous intercellular cysts, all probably due to increased accumulation of water (84). The deficiency in Na–K ATPase is probably caused by excess of an inhibitor, a polypeptide, as its activity can be abolished by peptidases (85). Once the cataractogenic process starts, these lenses show an abnormal synthesis, degradation, and leakage of protein (86). It is interesting that there is variable expressivity of the disease in the Nakano mouse, similar to most human hereditary cataracts, Four types of expression occur (87): (1) a cataract is manifest in both eyes within 35 days (89% of about 300 homozygotic mice); (2) asymmetric cataract occurs in the two eyes within 35 days (8%); (3) cataracts present after 50 days (0.9%); and (4) no cataract is apparent, but lens fiber changes are detected histologically (1.5%).

Another well-studied mouse cataract, "shrivelled," is found in the house mouse and is caused by an autosomal dominant gene, Cat^{fraser} (*Svl*). The heterozygote manifests the disease, but it is slow in developing; the homozygote develops the cataract rapidly (50,58). The opacification starts in the anterior (apical) end of the lens and is related to water accumulation intra- and intercellularly (84). Biochemically, some normal lens proteins, such as gamma-crystallins and beta-crystallins are absent or decreased, others such as alpha-crystallins are increased, and several abnormal soluble proteins, which are never observed in a normal lens, are detectable in the cataractous lens (89).

Recently, a widely investigated hereditary cataract was found in a strain called the Philly mouse, a mutant of Swiss-Webster mice. The cataract develops progressively. Faint anterior opacities seen at 15 days are followed by sutural cataracts at 25 days, nuclear cataracts at 30 days, lamellar–perinuclear opacities at 35 days, and total nuclear with anterior and posterior polar cataracts at 45 days (90). As in the autosomal recessive Nakano cataract, cataractogenesis parallels an intralenticular increase in water, sodium, and calcium, and a decrease in potassium, glutathione, and ATP. However, unlike the recessive cataract, no enzyme abnormality is detected. Instead, a defect in membrane permeability is the cause of an increased outward leak, with a similar net result of increased osmotic pressure and osmotic cataract (90). Morphologic changes are seen earlier than clinical changes. One cytologic study revealed the presence of intracellular, membrane-bound, amorphous dense particles from the eighth day (91). This was followed by a loss of the normal lens denucleation process and swelling of the lens fibers. The characteristic bow configuration of the nuclei in the lens cortex was replaced by a fan-shaped configuration (91).

The Philly mouse cataract is inherited as an autosomal dominant trait, but, like the Fraser mouse, the cataract develops much faster in homozygotes than in heterozygotes (92). It was found that the Philly lens fails to synthesize a beta-crystallin polypeptide of 27 kDa and that it lacks a functional messenger RNA (mRNA) responsible for this polypeptide (92,93). This is consistent with a transcriptional or posttranscriptional deficiency in expression of the appropriate gene. Homozygotes are completely deficient in the 27kDa beta-crystallin polypeptide, whereas heterozygotes have a reduced amount (92).

A recent study indicated that in the Philly mouse lens, the normal beta-crystallin basic principal polypeptide is absent, an mRNA encoding for this polypeptide is present, and that, an abnormal protein that is not heat-stable is present (94).

The *Lop* (lens opacities) gene that causes autosomal dominant cataract in mice has been assigned to chromosome 10 by Lyon et al. (95).

Two additional strains, the deer mouse cataract (96) and the Emory mouse cataract (97), are examples of a late-developing hereditary cataract and serve as models for human senile or metabolic cataract. The Emory mouse also has a hereditary retinal degeneration.

About 30 mutations of lens anomalies have been described in the mouse (98). Many of these are hereditary cataracts. However, only some have been investigated in depth.

Hereditary cataracts also have been described in many other species, such as fish, fowl (98), several breeds of cattle, rats (99), and dogs (100). One strain of an autosomal recessive cataract in rats may serve as a model for developmental or juvenile hereditary cataract, as diffuse opacities start in the posterior subcapsular area at about two four months of age and mature later (101).

Many breeds of dog suffer from hereditary cataracts (100). These may be congenital, usually in a syndrome with microphthalmos or developmental abnormalities occurring during the first year of life. Autosomal recessive cataracts have been described in the Boston terrier, Staffordshire, bull terrier, miniature schnauzer, Afghan hound, Welsh springer spaniel, German shepherd, and American cocker spaniel. In all breeds, the cataract starts at several weeks or months of age and progresses to blindness (100). An autosomal dominant, nonprogressive cataract has been found in the golden retriever and Labrador retriever (100). All of these, and hereditary cataracts in other breeds of dogs, have not been investigated as thoroughly as those in mice.

In addition to the continuing identification of novel mutations in laboratory animals, two main lines of research continued in the last decade: one, the use of the high degree of genetic homology between human and mouse genome, which enables the study of the homologous gene in inbred strains of mice (102), and two, the study of transgenic models for cataracts and other ocular congenital anomalies in a large series of existing mouse models (103).

Management

Surgical and Medical Treatment

The treatment of an isolated congenital cataract, whether unilateral or bilateral, remains basically surgical. Developments in instrumentation and techniques, the routine use of the surgical microscope, and a better understanding of the process of deprivation amblyopia have revolutionized the results of such treatment in the last two decades. However, controversy still exists over the best surgical approach, the indications and timing of surgery, the preferred method of optical correction, and the prevention of amblyopia.

Surgical approach: Older methods of cataract surgery produced discouraging results (104). Enormous improvements have been noted with the irrigation–aspiration method (105). Any one of the available mechanized methods is probably preferable to the 25-year-old single-syringe-needle irrigation–aspiration technique. The main problem with the current method is the high incidence of postoperative opacification of the posterior capsule, which occurs in the majority of patients. In one study, 19 of 28 patients had repeated operations for pupillary opacity (106). To prevent this complication, a routine posterior capsulectomy (107) or capsulotomy (108) is suggested, even though such patients will have an open vitreous face, in contrast to a clear posterior capsule, if capsulotomy and capsulectomy are not performed.

Since the early 1990s, posterior capsulotomy and anterior vitrectomy in every case of congenital cataract surgery in early childhood have increased in popularity. Buckley et al. (109) advised that the postcapsule be opened and vitrectomy performed through the pars plana. Basti and associates (110) advised that anterior capsulorhexis of 6 mm and posterior capsulorhexis of 4 mm be performed. BenEzra and Cohen (111) considered anterior vitrectomy necessary in cataract surgery in younger children.

Some surgeons prefer a planned anterior vitrectomy with cataract removal, using a vitreous suction-cutter for both cataract irrigation–aspiration and vitrectomy. A limbal (112,118) pars plana or pars plicata approach (114–117) may be used.

Complications include a high percentage of posterior capsule opacification or secondary membrane formation, and secondary glaucoma. In one study (117), these were found in 10% and 11%, respectively.

Glaucoma continues to be a serious problem, appearing in the late postoperative period. In one study glaucoma was diagnosed in 24% of operated eyes in a period of 60–105 months after the operation (118). Asrani and Wilensky found open angle glaucoma in 80% (!) of 64 operated eyes (119). In the majority, topical medications were sufficient to control the glaucoma, but usually the diagnosis was made late after onset, with a mean of 12 years postoperatively (119), often already with serious damage to the optic nerve. High prevalence of ocular hypertension was also found in a prospective study of 107 subjects who were followed for five years (120).

Indications and timing of surgery: A patient with congenital cataract should be operated if the visual acuity is expected to be low. Although there is no doubt about the poor outcome of an unexcised complete congenital cataract, the prediction of future visual acuity in an eye with incomplete cataract may be difficult. Except in cases of very small cataract (less than 2 mm) and of other concurrent ocular anomalies, the visual outcome seems to be determined by the density of the opacity (121). Surgery should be performed before eight weeks of age (122). Prolonging the surgery results in the appearance of pendular nystagmus in patients with dense cataracts. Good visual results may be obtained with surgery as late as 1 year (122), if the cataracts are incomplete.

In bilateral cataracts, the interval between operations on the two eyes must be short, not exceeding five days, to prevent deep amblyopia in one eye (123).

Optical correction of aphakia: The treatment of congenital cataract includes the correction of surgical aphakia. Glasses or contact lenses for bilateral cases and contact lenses for monocular cases are usual used (123–125). Most patients are fitted with extended-wear contact lenses (126). Although contact lenses are a good optical solution, they also have many disadvantages, such as the need for close cooperation of the parents, their relatively high cost, and frequent need for replacement (sometimes 10 or more in the first year alone). In addition, a high frequency of complications has been reported in children (125).

The vastly expanded use of intraocular implants for the correction of aphakia (127,128) has focused attention on the possibility of their use in children. Intraocular lens implantation (IOL) for congenital cataract has been advocated by Binkhorst and Gobin since 1970 (129), but only in children 12 months of age or older (130). Results with intraocular implants have been conflicting. The prognosis is good in older children and in those with traumatic cataracts (130,131), and it has been reported as good, safe, and effective by Hiles (132) and as poor by others (133,134) in unilateral cases. Good visual acuities have been reported in 59% of bilateral congenital cataracts (133) and in one report on lens implantation in monocular congenital cataract (135). One technique used was different. The implantation of a posterior chamber IOL into the epilenticular space as the initial step was followed by a pars plana endo-capsular lensectomy (136).

My own approach is to implant intraocular lenses in selected patients with bilateral congenital cataract, such as those with mental retardation or severe nystagmus, and in patients with monocular cataracts when it is obvious that the child will not use a contact lens. Most patients will have IOL implants, anyhow. Epikeratophakia, has become a competitive method for the optical correction of pediatric aphakia (137). In relatively large series, the reported rates of successful grafts were 89% (138) and 95% with repeated surgery (139). In some cases, lensectomy and epikeratophakia were performed as one primary procedure (136).

Treatment of amblyopia: Essential parts in the treatment of congenital cataract are the management of deprivation amblyopia resulting from the opaque lens and the prevention of ametropic amblyopia (in bilateral cases) and anisometropicametropia (in unilateral cases) resulting from the aphakic state. Those with monocular congenital cataract have the poorest results, both because of amblyopia and because of a high incidence of associated ocular anomalies (140). In the last few years, the visual outcome for monocular congenital cataract has improved dramatically (124) as a result of early successful surgery, better fitting of contact lenses in difficult situations, such as high hypermetropia, small corneal diameter, and steep corneal curvature, and early and vigorous postoperative treatment. Contact lenses should be fitted and patching therapy started within four days of surgery (123,141). The extended-wear contact lenses should be periodically exchanged and readjusted for better fit and for changing ocular refraction. Patching of the good eye must be done carefully, adjusted individually, and monitored by visual acuity (as measured by visual-evoked potentials (VEP) (141) or by the preferential looking technique) (122,142).

Undoubtedly, the successful management of unilateral congenital cataract necessitates all of the following: early recognition of the problem, early surgery, early contact lens fitting, and aggressive amblyopia therapy with compliance (143–145). Early surgery means by two months of age in some studies (144) and by 17 weeks, at the latest, in others (145), contact lens fitting may be replaced by other means of optical correction, such as intraocular lens implantation.

Since the beginning of the 1990s, the approach of correction by IOL implantation into the posterior chamber has become the treatment of choice (146–149). Extended–wear contact lenses or daily wear contact lens continued to be used by others (150).

Controversy continues in reported results. Some report the results as poor (151,152), others report more favorable results (153,154). Undoubtedly, visual results are poorest in monocular cataracts, followed by bilateral total cataracts, and best in partial and mild cataracts, such as lamellar cataracts.

Genetic Counseling

In familial cases of autosomal dominant isolated congenital cataract, gene penetrance is practically complete. A study of the family pedigree, including as many affected members as possible, will reveal phenotypic variance in expressivity of the gene and intrafamilial differences. Expectation of a possible advanced or total cataract will help with arrangements for early postnatal surgery.

As listed, families with autosomal recessive and X-linked cataracts are less common. From the structure of the cataract and pedigree, the diagnosis should be properly made and the family counseled accordingly. In most cases, female carriers of X-linked recessive cataract can be recognized by the posterior Y-suture opacification.

The ability to make a molecular diagnosis revolutionizes our approach to genetic counseling. The identification of the gene and of the mutation enables the physician to estimate the prognosis, assists him with management decisions, and can sometimes enable prenatal diagnosis by amniocentesis. In severe cases with a known and identified mutation, preimplantation genetic diagnosis may be considered.

CONGENITAL CATARACTS ASSOCIATED WITH MULTISYSTEM DISEASES

Introduction

Congenital cataracts are not uncommon in a large number of congenital anomalies and diseases. Some are now well-recognized syndromes; others are multiple congenital malformations with questionable hereditary transmission. Table 7 lists most recognized associations of congenital cataracts. Because many organs and tissues may be affected, the classification is somewhat arbitrary according to the extraocular finding that is most likely to draw the physician's attention.

Genetic and Clinical Types

Microcephaly, Mental Retardation, or Neurologic Abnormalities

The syndromes of Torsten Sjögren, Marinesco–Sjögren, Crome, and Martsolf involve congenital cataract, with mental retardation and other abnormalities. The hereditary transmission is autosomal recessive. Each is caused by a different gene and has a somewhat different phenotype. The association of congenital cataract and mental retardation is termed Sjögren syndrome (155), whereas that with the additional finding of cerebellar ataxia is termed Marinesco–Sjögren syndrome (156,157). It should not be confused with Sjögren–Larsson syndrome of mental retardation with congenital ichthyosis and spastic disorder (158). In this syndrome, retinal changes occur. The locus of Marinesco–Sjögren syndrome has been mapped to chromosome 18qter (159). Merlini and associates considered three phenotypes, the Marinesco–Sjögren, the CCFDN (congenital cataract, facial dysmorphism,

Table 7 Congenital Cataracts Associated with Hereditary Multisystem Disease

Group	Syndrome	MIM	Heredity
Microcephaly, mental retardation and/or neurologic abnormalities	T. Sjögren	NM	AR
	Marinesco–Sjögren	248800	AR
	Crome	218900	AR
	Martsolf	212720	AR
	Lenz dysmorphogenetic	309800	XR
	CAMFAK	212540	AR
	Smith-Lemli-Opitz	270400	AR
	Menkes	309400	XR
	Optic atrophy and neurologic disorder	165300	AD
Skeletal abnormalities	Conradi–Hühnerman	215100	AR
	Marfan	154700	AD
	Albright hereditary osteodystrophy	300800	XL
	Majewski	263520	AR
Renal abnormalities	Lowe oculocerebrorenal	309000	XR
	Alport	203780, 104200, 301050	AD or AR or XR
	Zellweger	214100	AR
	Fabry	301500	XR
Mandibulofacial dysostoses	Francois dyscephalic (Hallerman–Streiff)	234100	AR
	Pierre Robin	261800	AD
	Treacher Collins (Franceschetti–Klein)	154500	AD
Other associations	Nance–Horan	302350	XL
	Cerebrotendinous xanthomatosis	213700	AR
	Cataract and cochleosaccular degeneration	120040	AD
Chromosomal aberrations	Trisomy 13		
	Trisomy 18		
	Trisomy 21		
Inborn errors of metabolism	Galactosemia	230400	AR
	Galactosemia deficiency	230200	AR
	Mannosidosis	248500	AR

Note: See text for description of syndromes. AD, autosomal dominant; AR, autosomal recessive; XR, X-chromosome-linked recessive; XD, NE, exact mode of hereditary transmission not established; NM, not mentioned in OMIM.

neuropathy), and peripheral neuropathy with nyoglobinuria as one genetic entity with a single-founder mutation (159). In Crome's syndrome, congenital cataract is associated with mental retardation, small stature, and epileptic seizures (160). Small stature, psychomotor retardation, abnormal physiognomy, minor digital abnormalities, primary hypogonadism, and congenital cataract, without ataxia, originally had been described by Martsolf et al. in two brothers (161). It was earlier suggested that the findings of the Marinesco–Sjögren syndrome may be linked to another genetic condition: hypergonadotropic hypogonadism (162).

Microcephaly occurs in several of these syndromes. Lenz dysmorphogenetic syndrome, sometimes called "Maine microphthalmos" after a large family investigated in Maine, consists of cataract, colobomatous microphthalmos, nystagmus, esotropia, ptosis, microcephaly, mental retardation, short stature, kyphoscoliosis, anteverted simple pinnae, and dental anomalies (163). Not all affected members have cataracts. The CAMAK syndrome (cataract, microcephaly, arthrogryposis, and kyphosis) (164) and the CAMFAK syndrome (cataract, microcephaly, *failure* to thrive, and kyphosis) (113), are autosomal recessive traits and may be the same genetic entity.

In the Smith–Lemli–Opitz syndrome, multiple ocular and systemic anomalies are found. Congenital cataracts (in 15% of all patients), corneal endothelial microvesicles, choroidal hemangiomas, optic atrophy, and palpebral and other ocular anomalies have been described clinically and histopathologically (166). Most lens fibers are found to be abnormal, vesiculated, and laced (166). Systemically, affected children have microcephaly, mental retardation, hypotonia, failure to thrive, and gastrointestinal, urogenital, and other anomalies. Life expectancy is short.

In some cases of Menkes syndrome (severe mental retardation, coarse unpigmented hair, demineralization of bones, and frequent fractures related to low serum iron and copper levels), cataracts have been described (167). Congenital cataract with optic atrophy and neurologic disorder, reported by Garcin et al. in 1961 (168), has not yet been confirmed as a clinical entity.

The locus for Lenz microphthalmia was mapped to chromosome Xq27–q28 (169). Its gene is not yet known. The disease-causative gene for Smith–Lemli–Opitz syndrome is DHCR7 located on chromosome 11q12–q13. DHCR7 encodes the protein enzyme dehydrocholesterol reductase. Its deficiency causes an enormous increase in blood levels of 7-dehydrocholesterol, up to 2000-fold the normal (170).

Skeletal Abnormalities

The syndrome of congenital stippled epiphyses (Conradi's syndrome, Conradi–Hühnerman syndrome, chondrodysplasia punctata, chondrodysplasia calcificans congenita) has several features including short stature, short neck, frontal bossing, saddle nose, high arched palate and hypertelorism, hip dislocation, flexion contracture, short upper limbs-rhizomelia (sometimes), and stippled epiphyses. Congenital cataracts are usually found (2,171) together with other ocular anomalies such as hetero-chromia iridis and optic atrophy.

The locus for Conradi–Hühnerman, rhizomelic chondrodysplasia punctata was mapped to chromosome 6q22–q24. The responsible gene, PEX7, encodes the receptor for peroxisomal matrix proteins, and disease-causing mutations were identified (70).

In some cases of Marfan syndrome, infantile cataract is found instead of, or in addition to, the much more common subluxation of lens related to this disease. In Albright's hereditary osteodystrophy type I, short stature, subcutaneous calcification's, brachydactyly, and sometimes cataract are related to hypocalcemia, with an elevated serum parathyroid hormone level (172). The disease is genetic, although the mode of transmission is not clear.

The association of neonatal dwarfism with polydactyly, narrow thorax ("short rib"), cleft lip and palate, and visceral and ocular abnormalities is known as Majewski's syndrome. Ocular abnormalities include cataract, papilledema, optic atrophy, hypertelorism, absent lashes and brows, and persistent pupillary membrane (173).

Renal Disease

The most common and best known in this group of renal diseases is the oculocerebrorenal syndrome of Lowe, an X-linked recessive disease (Fig. 4). The affected hemizygous male has mental retardation, renal aminoaciduria, and ocular anomalies. Congenital cataract occurs in every case (175). Other ocular anomalies found are glaucoma, caused by an abnormal "embryonic-type" angle; miosis, resulting from segmental hypoplasia of the dilator pupillae; and corneal keloids (174). In one study, the cataractous lens was found to be small and discoid, with retained nuclei in the lens cells and posterior lenticonus (174).

It is now clear that female carriers of Lowe's disease may be recognized by characteristic lens opacities (174–177). These are spokelike opacities in the posterior cortex or diffuse punctate or flakelike opacities. At least 82% (177), and possibly every obligate carrier of the disease (178), show these lens opacities.

By examining obligatory carriers, Fagerholm and colleagues (179) found that all women with more than 100 lenticular opacities were carriers of the mutant gene, whereas those with fewer than 100 were not.

Tripathi and associates (180) suggested that the pathogenesis of the cataract in Lowes' syndrome is based on a genetic defect causing defective formation and subsequent degeneration of the primary posterior lens fibers. In affected hemizygotes all fibers are thus affected; in female carriers, a proportion of fibers are affected, according to Lyon's theory. The gene for Lowe's syndrome was found to be closely linked to the locus *DXS42* and to markers in the Xq24–q26 region. This can be used to detect carriers by molecular genetics methods (179).

Later, the gene responsible for Lowe syndrome was cloned and more accurately mapped, initially to chromosome Xq25–q26 (181) and then to Xq26.1 (182).

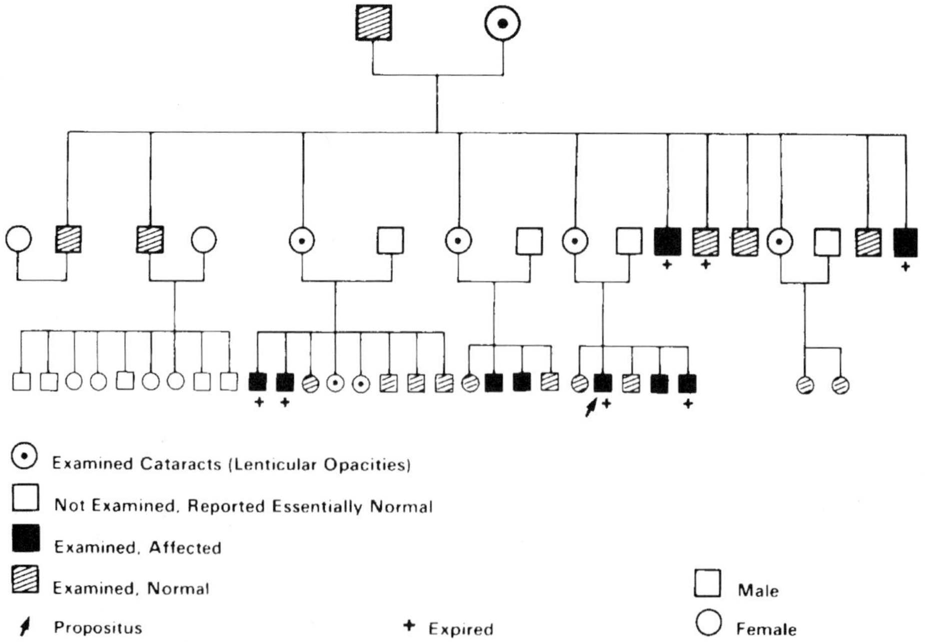

Figure 4 Pedigree of a family with Lowe syndrome, transmitted by the characteristic X-linked mode. The female carriers had lenticular opacities (from Ref. 174).

Mutations in the oculocerebrorenal syndrome of Lowe (OCRLl) gene were identified. They included nonsense mutations or deletion of a whole exon, or frameshifts and premature termination (182–185). Few missense mutations were also identified. The heterogeneity in phenotype is most likely due to the different mutations. Each of the usual clinical manifestations, such as congenital cataract, buphthalmus, renal disease, aminoaciduria, reduced ammonia production in kidney, and mental retardation, may be more or less prominent.

Lenticonus is the usual manifestation of Alport's syndrome. Rarely are infantile cataracts found (see Chapter 7).

In the cerebrohepatorenal syndrome of Zellweger, abnormal development of the skull, face, ear, hands, and feet, some mental retardation, hepatic interstitial fibro- sis, renal cortical cysts, and ocular abnormalities are seen. Zonular cataracts have been noted in all four cases studied by Hittner et al. (186). Cloudy cornea, retinal dystrophy with an extinct electroretinogram (ERG), and optic atrophy are also observed. The serum iron and iron-binding capacities are high. Ultrastructurally, the lens fibers are abnormal, with a high density of mitochondria and inclusion bodies. Obligatory heterozygotes may have lens opacities in the form of curvilinear lens condensations (186).

Mutations were identified in all of the five PEX genes, involved in peroxisome biogenesis (70). These are PEX1 located on chromosome 7q21, PEX2 on 8q, PEX3 on 6q, PEX5 on chromosome 12, and PEX6 on 6p (70).

In Fabry's disease, cataract appears later in life, and the female carrier can be recognized by lens opacities. The cataractous changes characteristically are spokelike opacities.

Mandibulofacial Dysostoses

Of this group, only in Francois dyscephalic syndrome is congenital or infantile cataract common. Cataract is found in 81–90% of all patients. It is always bilateral, usually complete, and has a milky liquid consistency (187,188). Spontaneous resorption is not rare and may produce uveitis (187). The mode of hereditary transmission is unclear. In most cases, occurrence is sporadic and nonfamilial. In others, autosomal dominant, autosomal recessive, or multifactorial inheritance has been suggested.

Congenital cataract is sometimes found in the two other diseases in this group.

TCS, the locus for Treacher Collins syndrome, was mapped to chromosome 5q31.3–q32 (189). At least 35 different mutations were identified, almost all inducing a premature termination. They represent a 60% detection rate of Treacher Collins syndrome (189).

Other Associations

Congenital X-linked cataracts with dental anomalies (supernumerary incisors, wide spanning of teeth), short metacarpals, and anteverted pinnae were reported in one family by Nance et al. (190). Female carriers have posterior sutural opacities. Five generations of a second family with the same disease (191) have confirmed the existence of this separate genetic entity.

NHS, the locus symbol for Nance–Horan syndrome was mapped to chromosome Xp22.13 (192). Several candidate genes exist at this location but none has been proven.

Another systemic disease, in which congenital or juvenile cataract very frequently occurs, is cerebrotendinous xanthomatosis (CTX). Mental deterioration, neurologic abnormalities, tendon xanthomas, cataracts and premature atheromatosis are the main manifestations of this inherited disorder (193,194). According to some studies, cataracts were found in all affected. Pale optic disks are the second most common ocular finding, in a quarter to half of patients (194,195). The disease-causing mutations were identified on CYP27A1 (cytochrome P450 subfamily 27A), mapped to chromosome 2q33-qter. The gene has nine exons, eight introns and spans 18.6 kb of DNA (193). There are an unusually high frequency of disease-bearing mutations in Moroccan Jews (193).

Progressive sensorineural hearing loss caused by cochleosaccular degeneration with congenital cataract that later progresses to maturation, was described by Nadol and Burgess (196). It is transmitted by an autosomal dominant gene.

Ectodermal dysplasia, with deafness and ocular anomalies, including cataract, has been described by Marshall as being transmitted by an autosomal dominant gene (197, see section V.B).

Congenital cataract may be associated with chromosomal aberrations. In trisomy 13 and 18 it may be secondary to other intraocular abnormalities, and in Down syndrome (trisomy 21) the etiology is unknown. Thirteen percent of infants and children with Down syndrome have cataracts (198).

Established inborn errors of metabolism are discussed in the next section.

Management

Surgical and Medical

The management of an associated congenital cataract is similar to that of an isolated congenital cataract. However, there may be more reasons to implant an intraocular lens in debilitated patients if they are over one year old at the time of surgery. These children may never be able to use any other optical correction, as the daily insertion of contact lenses may not be possible, the use of extended-wear contact lenses bears a higher risk than in normal children, and the patients may not be willing to use glasses. In such cases, even the use of binocular implants may be justified.

Genetic Counseling

Genetic counseling is rather simple, once the proper diagnosis is established, as most associated hereditary cataracts are transmitted by a single autosomal dominant, autosomal recessive, or X-linked gene.

INFANTILE CATARACTS WITH INBORN ERRORS OF METABOLISM

Introduction

The biochemical background of some systemic diseases associated with cataracts is now well defined and will be described here. It is possible that some of the multisystem diseases previously described, especially the autosomal recessive ones, also result from an enzymatic deficiency, which is still unknown.

The association of an abnormal galactose metabolism with cataract has been known since the 1950s, when infantile cataracts occurring in galactosemia were described (199). Later, when cataracts were found in all patients homozygous for galactokinase deficiency, it became clear that a whole group of diseases induce the occurrence of infantile cataract through the accumulation of a sugar polyol in the lens. These opacities are now known as "sugar cataracts," and their study in experimental animals has enhanced our knowledge of the pathogenesis, prevention, and treatment of infantile cataracts. The term "infantile cataract" is probably better than "congenital" in this case because a cataract resulting from a biochemical abnormality takes some time to form.

In addition to sugar cataracts, other infantile cataracts related to abnormal metabolism are also known.

Genetic and Clinical Types

Galactosemia and Galactokinase Deficiency

The metabolism of galactose into glucose involves three steps, each assisted by an enzyme (Fig. 5). Deficiency in the enzyme galactokinase (GALK), causes an autosomal recessive inherited disease, galactokinase deficiency (200). Deficiency in galactose-1-phosphate uridyltransferase (GALT) causes classic galactosemia in homozygotes. In both diseases the accumulation of dulcitol, a metabolite of galactose (Fig. 6), causes the development of infantile cataracts in most untreated patients. Deficiency of the third enzyme, uridine diphosphogalactose-4-epimerase, is not known to cause cataracts.

In galactosemia (GALT deficiency), cataracts are part of multiple abnormalities including nutritional failure, mental and motor retardation, hepatosplenomegaly, and cirrhosis. The disease is caused by a single autosomal recessive gene, with a locus on chromosome 9 (201). After screening some six million newborns, the rate of homozygosity to this gene was estimated to be 1:40,000, with a heterozygous rate of about 1:100 (202).

In GALK deficiency, cataracts are the sole or main manifestation in homozygotes. Homozygotes have abnormal galactose tolerance curves, elevated fasting blood galactose levels, and sometimes hepatosplenomegaly. The locus for the gene of GALK deficiency has been assigned to the long arm of chromosome 17 in the

1. GALACTOSE + ATP $\xrightarrow{\text{GALACTOKINASE}}$ GALACTOSE-1-P + ADP
2. GALACTOSE-1-P + UDP GLUCOSE $\rightleftarrows$ GLUCOSE-1-P + UDP GALACTOSE (GAL-1-P URIDYL TRANSFERASE)
3. UDP GALACTOSE $\rightleftarrows$ UDP GLUCOSE (UDP GAL-4- -EPIMERASE)

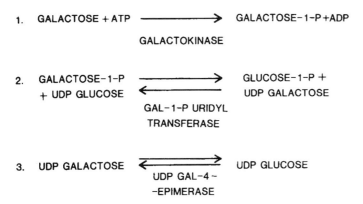

Figure 5 The three steps of galactose–glucose metabolism. Deficiency in the enzymes regulating the first or second steps (galactokinase or transferase) frequently causes cataract. Deficiency of epimerase, the enzyme regulating the third step, was not reported to cause cataracts. ATP, adenosine triphosphate; ADP, adenosine diphosphate; P, phosphate; UDP, uridine diphosphate; GAL, galactose.

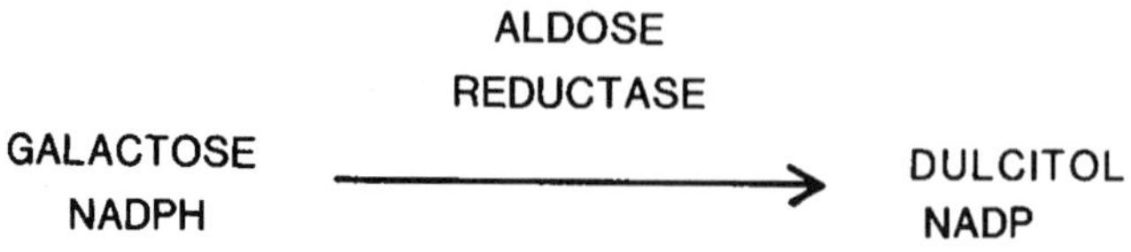

Figure 6 Galactose–dulcitol metabolism is regulated by aldose reductase. It represents similar reactions for all sugar-polyol reductions. NADP, nicotinamide adenine dinucleotide phosphate.

region of bands 21–22 (203). The description of a simplified method for the assay of GALK activity in erythrocytes (204) has enabled wide-scale population surveys (202,205,206), which have established the frequency of the heterozygote state to be about 1:310. Therefore, homozygosity is rare.

The morphologic structure of the cataract in both diseases, if untreated, is similar. Initially, a zone of the lens becomes opacified. This can be nuclear (involving the embryonal nucleus), sutural, lamellar, posterior cortical, or any combination of these (207).

The opacification progresses to total mature cataract. The cataract is usually diagnosed in the first year of life; the earliest has been described on the 24th day of life (207), but an incomplete cataract may go unnoticed until the second or third decade of life.

Does reduced GALK or reduced GALT activity, as found in heterozygotes, predispose to infantile cataract? The answer seems to be affirmative for two groups of patients: some of the heterozygous infants and infants whose mothers have reduced enzyme activity.

Analysis of family pedigrees indicates that most heterozygotes show no abnormal lens opacities. However, infantile cataracts are found in some heterozygotes. The risk for the development of cataracts in heterozygotes is high for GALK deficiency and very low for GALT deficiency (208). It has been suggested that a combined heterozygosity to two enzymes increases the risk of developing a cataract (209).

In 1974, Harley and co-workers described infantile cataracts in a child whose mother had low activity of GALK because of heterozygosity (210). This etiology of infantile cataract seems to have been confirmed, and preventive measures have been suggested (208,209); however, such indirect maternal effects seem to be variable, modest, and not obviously causal (211,212).

Classic type galactosemia is caused by mutations in the GALT gene, mapped to chromosome 9p13 (70). More than 35 mutations are known and different mutations cause different variants of the disease (213).

The GALK gene was cloned and mapped to chromosome 17q24 (214). Disease-bearing mutations were identified and several alleles were recognized (215). Cataracts are the hallmark of the disease with only the rather uncommon manifestation of pseudotumor cerebri occurring in this disease (215).

Other Metabolic Cataracts

The association of infantile cataracts with other inborn errors of metabolism is far less certain than the association with abnormal galactose metabolism. Infantile cataract may be associated with mannosidosis type I (216) and type II (217), both autosomal recessive, rare, and fatal infantile diseases. They are caused by mutations in the MANB gene encoding lysosomal alpha B mannosidase and mapped to chromosome 19cen–ql2. (70). Many disease-bearing mutations have been described.

In one family with infantile cataract, an abnormally low activity of sorbitol dehydrogenase in the red blood cells (218) could be related to cataract formation.

Infantile cataracts have been described in all three types of hypoglycemia: neonatal, idiopathic, and ketotic (219). Summarizing the literature, Wets et al. found that 37.5% of all reported cases of infantile hypoglycemia developed cataract (220). However, the condition is not hereditary.

Pathology and Pathogenesis

Results of investigations on experimental animals form the basis for our present understanding of the pathology and pathogenesis of sugar cataracts.

In galactose-fed rats, a mature cataract occurs after 20 days, but ultrastructural changes are apparent after three days (221). These early changes consist of maligned fibers, with single, membrane-bound vesicles, and small electron-dense aggregates in the fiberplasm. At seven days the aggregates enlarge and the intercellular spaces increase. At nine days, the fibers swell because of disruption and folding of the fiber membrane. At 12–15 days the damage is much more extensive and the boundaries between fibers are ill-defined (221).

The cataract in galactosemia is produced through accumulation of dulcitol (galactitol) in the lens (222). Galactose, with the aid of the enzyme aldose reductase, is metabolized into dulcitol, its sugar alcohol. Dulcitol, in turn, accumulates in the lens and causes an osmotic cataract (222). In rats, a similar mechanism causes a hyperglycemic (diabetic) and hyperxylotic cataract. However, in mice that have a very low activity of aldose reductose (about 1/10 of the activity of this enzyme in rats), a hyperglycemic cataract does not develop (223). The smaller amount of sorbitol produced in these mice is metabolized, by polyol dehydrogenase in the sorbitol pathway, into fructose (Fig. 7). The high levels of polyol dehydrogenase combined with the limited levels of aldose reductase in the normal and diabetic human lens (224) are probably responsible for the infrequency and delay in manifestation of the human hyperglycemic lens, when compared with the frequent and early occurrence of the galactosemic cataract. Nuclear magnetic resonance studies may enable a better understanding of the metabolic processes in the clear human lens and in human cataract (225).

Hypoglycemic cataract seems to result from deactivation of lens hexokinase following the depletion of its substrates, ATP and glucose (226). In the rat, younger lenses are more susceptible. The initial loss of lenticular ATP can be reversed by restoring normal glucose levels, but after 8 hours, hexokinase activity becomes irreversibly subnormal (227).

Clinical Management

Strict restriction of dietary intake of galactose, which means the limitation of milk ingestion in infants, is the accepted treatment of galactosemia. Such treatment prevents the severe systemic abnormalities of this disease and associated cataracts. It may, in fact, reverse early opacifications of the lens in galactosemic patients.

Withdrawal of galactose from the diet yields dramatic results in affected infants. Lifelong galactose restriction remains the basis for treatment of both galactosemia and galactokinase deficiency (228).

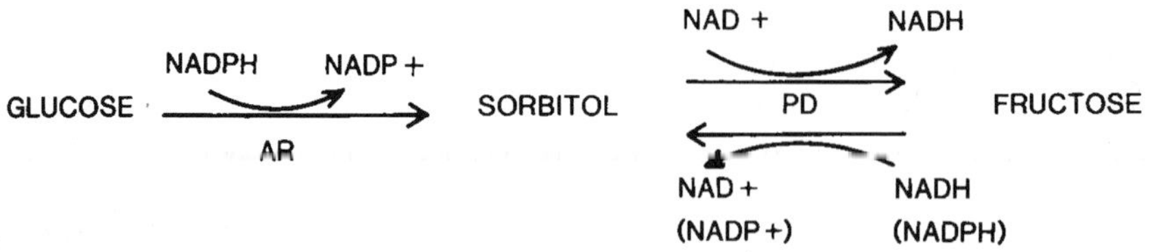

Figure 7 The two steps of the sorbitol pathway by which glucose is converted into fructose. NADP, nicotinamide adenine dinucleotide phosphate; AR, aldose reductase; PD, polyol dehydrogenase.

Dietary galactose control may similarly prevent the cataract associated with galactokinase deficiency (207). Heterozygotic women who are known to have low levels of galactokinase activity may have a child affected by infantile cataracts, and should restrict galactose in their diet during pregnancy (208,209).

The prevention of sugar cataracts by oral drugs is still in an experimental stage. Since it has been proved that sugar cataracts in animals can be prevented by the inhibition of aldose reductase (229), several of these inhibitors have been developed. The best known include AY 22,284 (alrestatin) (230,231) and the newer, potent sorbinil (*d*-6-fluorospiro[chroman-4,4′-imidazolidinel]-2′,5′-dione) (232). In rats, sorbinil, in a dose of 60 mg/kg/day, prevented the sugar cataract of diabetes (233) and that from galactose feeding (234,235). Sorbinil was as effective as removing galactose from the diet in preventing cataracts, but did not do so after the changes became irreversible (after five days of galactose feeding) (236). It is probably the one drug of the current long list that may be useful in the future in humans (237). It is interesting that corneal re-epithelialization, which is abnormal in galactosemic rats, becomes normal when these rats are given sorbinil medication (238,239).

JUVENILE, PRESENILE, AND SENILE CATARACTS

Introduction

Most cataracts that occur later in life are not known to be hereditary, but they may be caused by a genetic disease, and this factor should be considered in every case of unexplained cataract (Table 8). A genetic background for postinfantile cataract is known in five groups of diseases: metabolic diseases, syndromes and multisystem diseases, skin diseases, diseases secondary to another hereditary eye disease, and hereditary juvenile cataract.

Genetic and Clinical Types

Metabolic Diseases

The cataract related to GALK deficiency or to galactosemia (GALT deficiency) may be manifested not only in infancy, but later in life. The cataract of GALK deficiency was diagnosed in a patient aged nine years (207), and I have diagnosed it in a 16-year-old girl.

Reduced activity of GALK or GALT, as found in the heterozygous state as the cause of juvenile and presenile cataract is still controversial. In some studies, one-third to almost one-half of patients with presenile cataract had a red blood cell GALK or GALT activity reduced more than 2 SD from normal (240,241). In other studies,

Table 8 Postinfantile Hereditary Cataracts: Childhood, Juvenile, and Presenile

Group	Disease	Mode of transmission	Frequency of cataract
Metabolic	GALK deficiency, homozygote	AR	Common
	GALK deficiency, heterozygote	AR	Uncommon
	Galactosemia (GALT deficiency), homozygote	AR	Common
	Galactosemia (GALT deficiency), heterozygote	AR	Rare
	Double heterozygote for galactose enzymes	2 × AR	Uncommon
	Diabetes mellitus	MF	Uncommon
	Glucose-6-phosphate dehydrogenase deficiency	XR	Rare
	Wilson's disease	AR	Uncommon
	Fabry's disease	XR	Common
Multisystem disease	Myotonic dystrophy	AD	Common
	Late distal hereditary myopathy	AD	Rare
	Myotubular myopathy	AD	Rare
	Mitochondria-lipid-glycogen myopathy	AR	Rare
	Myopathy with cataract and hypogonadism	AR	Common
	Kearns–Sayre syndrome	AD	Common
	Cerebrotendinous xanthomatosis	AR	Common
	Osteogenesis imperfecta and cataract	AR	
	Congenital nystagmus, foveal hypoplasia, and presenile cataract	AD	
	Trichomegaly and hereditary spherocytosis	AD	
Skin diseases	Rothmund–Thomson syndrome	AR	Common
	Werner syndrome	AR	Common
	Marshall syndrome	AD	Common
	Bloch–Sulzberger syndrome	NE	Uncommon
	Ichthyosis	AD, XR	Rare
With ocular diseases	Microphthalmos	AD, AR, XR	Uncommon
	Microcornea	AD	Uncommon
	Aniridia	AD	Uncommon
	Rieger's anomaly	AD	Uncommon
	Persistent hyperplastic pupillary membrane		
	PHPV	AD	Common
	Norrie's disease	XR	Common
	Bloch–Sulzberger syndrome	NE	Uncommon
	Retinitis pigmentosa	AD, AR, XR	Intermediate
	Cone-rod degeneration	AD, AR	Intermediate
	Usher syndrome	AR	Intermediate
	Refsum disease	AR	Intermediate
	Kearns–Sayre syndrome	AD	Uncommon

(Continued)

Table 8 Postinfantile Hereditary Cataracts: Childhood, Juvenile, and Presenile (*Continued*)

Group	Disease	Mode of transmission	Frequency of cataract
	Gyrate atrophy	AR	Common
	Choroideremia	XR	Intermediate
	Bardet–Biedl syndrome	AR	Intermediate
	Cockayne's syndrome	AR	Common

Note: AR, autosomal recessive; AD, autosomal dominant; XR, X-linked recessive; MF, multifactorial; PHPV, persistent hyperplastic primary vitreous; NE, not finally established—indicates a rare syndrome that includes cataracts. In the retinal dystrophies frequency of cataracts depends on age. In most it is common after the third decade of life.

such an association has not been found (242–244). In still other studies, a small percentage, but much higher than expected in the general population, showed the combination of presenile cataract and abnormal GALK or GALT activity (245–247). It is difficult to explain these controversial results, but it seems safe to say that most heterozygotes do not manifest cataracts, but that some heterozygotes, especially those for GALK deficiency, do. It may be that an additional unknown factor is needed to cause the cataract, or that red cell enzyme activity does not reflect lens activity (244). It is also possible that different forms or variants of the GALK enzyme predispose the patient to cataract formation, or that a combination of two heterozygous states increases galactose intolerance (248), Interestingly, one patient heterozygous for GALT deficiency developed cataracts during the lactating period (249).

It is probable that other postinfantile sugar cataracts may also occur in humans. This is seen in some patients with diabetes.

An increased incidence of presenile cataract has been reported in males hemizygous for X-linked glucose-6-phosphate dehydrogenase (G6PD) deficiency (250). Such patients have no activity of G6PD in their lenses (251). However, among the 100 million people worldwide who suffer from G6PD deficiency (250), only a few are afflicted by cataract caused by this deficiency. In Wilson's disease (hepatolenticular degeneration), a typical "sunflower cataract" occasionally develops (252). In Fabry's disease, a characteristic cataract develops with time.

Syndromes and Multisystem Diseases

Myotonic dystrophy is an autosomal dominant disease affecting primarily the neuromuscular system. Typical lens changes occur in most patients. Usually, these appear in the second decade of life as multiple spots of opacity, with colored crystals localized in the anterior and posterior subcapsular layers in the form of a thin band. Later, the cataract progresses to maturity. Additional ocular findings include ptosis, subnormal dark adaptation, subnormal ERG findings in most or all patients, and dry eyes, blepharitis, and retinal lesions in others (253). The characteristic colored crystals are caused by myelin-like figures of intracellular multilaminated whorls in vacuoles (254,255).

Myotonic dystrophy of adult onset occurs in two forms. In type I, the locus symbol is DM1 (for dystrophia myotonica), and has been mapped to chromosome 19q13.2-q13.3 (256). The disease-associated gene is dystrophia myotonica protein kinase (DMPK) and the disease is caused by an enormous amplification of a trinucleotide repeat. In type 2, the second locus, DM2, was mapped to chromosome 3q13.3–q24 (257) and the disease is caused by a mutation in the Z9F9 gene (257). Cataracts, developmental and typical, as outlined above, are found in both types. In several other myopathies a developmental cataract is rare (258). These are listed in Table 8. In Kearns-Sayre syndrome (external ophthalmoplegia, retinal degeneration, and cardiomyopathy), cataract is common and develops secondary to the retinal degeneration.

CTX (cerebrotendinous xanthomathosis), a rare autosomal recessive trait, is definitely associated with cataract. Large deposits of cholesterol and cholestanol in most tissues cause the typical tendon xanthomata, particularly in the Achilles tendon, and xanthelasmata. Cataracts are an early finding and may help to diagnose the condition. Later, cholesterol deposits in the brain may produce neurologic abnormalities and mental debility. The gene has a high frequency in one community of Israel (259). Other families have been described with presenile cataracts, but the association has not been confirmed. This includes the association of foveal hypoplasia, congenital nystagmus, corneal pannus, and subalbinotic fundus with presenile cataracts, that is transmitted as an autosomal dominant trait in four generations of one family (260). Another possible autosomal dominant syndrome is the association of trichomegaly (long lashes), spoke-like lens opacities, and hereditary spherocytosis (261). One family with autosomal recessive osteogenesis imperfecta (similar to type II of this disease) and cataracts also has been described (262).

Skin Diseases

In several hereditary skin diseases, cataract is a common phenomenon. It manifests at birth as congenital cataract (8), but more frequently it occurs as a childhood, juvenile, or presenile finding.

In the Rothmund-Thomson syndrome (poikiloderma atrophicans and cataract), a hereditary dermatosis (plaques of erythema, teleangiectases, skin atrophy and pigmentation, and edema) is frequently associated with a saddle nose and hypogonadism. About half of all patients manifest developmental cataract; the usual onset is at three to six years of age (263). The disease is transmitted as an autosomal recessive trait.

Werner syndrome, another autosomal recessive disease, has more pronounced skin changes in the form of atrophy of skin and muscles, facial abnormality, early graying of hair, and short stature, all giving the appearance of premature senility. Juvenile and presenile cataracts are common (263).

A family with anhidrotic or hypohidrotic ectodermal dysplasia, associated with partial deafness, various facial anomalies (depressed nasal bridge, hypoplastic maxilla, and thick lips), and ocular anomalies has been described by Marshall (197). Patients have congenital or juvenile cataracts and glaucoma or lens dislocation. The trait is autosomal dominant.

In the Bloch-Sulzberger syndrome (incontinentia pigmenti) eye defects are rather common, with retinal dysplasia being the most important congenital malformation. Other ocular defects are juvenile cataracts (most common), strabismus, optic atrophy, uveitis, chorioretinitis, microphthalmos, and nystagmus (264). The hereditary transmission is not yet established. Of 361 cases reported until 1975, only 6 were males (160). It was, therefore, suggested that the disease is X-linked dominant, with lethality in the hemizygous male. However, cytoplasmic inheritance also may be a factor.

Juvenile cataracts also have been described in both forms of the common hereditary ichthyosis, the autosomal dominant form (OMIM No. 146700), and the X-linked form (OMIM No. 308100) (265,266).

Other Hereditary Eye Diseases

Cataracts, which may be congenital but usually are developmental, may be a major manifestation of other hereditary eye diseases. These diseases may involve the whole eye, result in abnormalities in the anterior segment or the vitreous structure, or occur as hereditary retinal degenerations.

Microphthalmos and microcornea: Microphthalmos is the most frequent ocular abnormality associated with infantile cataract. Microcornea, with or without Peters anomaly, and infantile cataract is transmitted by the autosomal dominant mode and shows extremely variable expressivity (267,268). Microphthalmos and microcornea with cataract may be transmitted as an autosomal recessive trait (71); microcornea with iris coloboma and nystagmus may be an autosomal dominant (56) or an X-linked recessive disease (75,76).

Abnormalities of anterior segment: Aniridia and Rieger's anomaly may be associated with early cataracts (2). Several families with a persistent hyperplastic pupillary membrane and cataract transmitted by an autosomal dominant gene have been described (269). The cataract is anterior, polar, and mild. The visual reduction is not severe.

Abnormalities of vitreous structure: The most common association of early cataract in this group is with persistent hyperplastic primary vitreous (PHPV), which is usually nonhereditary (2). Retinal dysplasia with PHPV, as found in Norrie's disease (270) or in the Bloch-Sulzberger syndrome, also causes early cataracts as a secondary phenomenon.

Hereditary retinal degeneration: Cataracts are found in at least one-third of all patients with hereditary retinal degenerations (271,272). They occur in retinitis pigmentosa, cone-rod degenerations, Usher syndrome, and other syndromes with retinitis pigmentosa, choroideremia (271), the Kearns-Sayre syndrome (273) and other myopathies (258), and gyrate atrophy of the retina and choroid (274).

Typically, the cataract develops in the third or fourth decade of life; the youngest patient to manifest this cataract was seven years old (272). It seems to occur earlier in patients with gyrate atrophy (274). The cataract has a characteristic appearance: it is posterior and subcapsular, with or without stellate projections, and with or without a nuclear opacity.

The cause of cataract in hereditary retinal degenerations is uncertain. It has been suggested that the cataract is a result of vitreal degeneration or that the retina ceases to produce a substance necessary for lens clarity (271). My own study has suggested that, like uveitis in which morphologically similar lens opacities are found, the pseudoinflammatory vitreous response seen in all hereditary retinal degeneration causes the cataract (272).

Hereditary Juvenile Cataract

Several pedigrees of families with a hereditary cataract occurring in young adolescents were reported (Fig. 8). The hereditary trait is autosomal dominant, and the condition is uncommon. It may be a late manifestation of a congenital cataract in some cases.

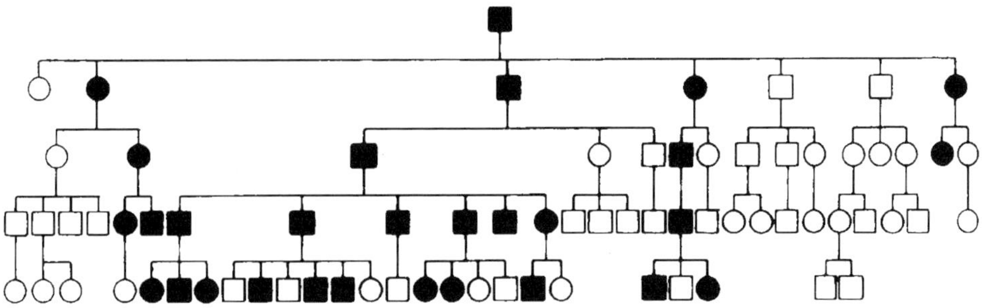

Figure 8 Typical autosomal dominant inheritance in a family with juvenile cataract (from Ref. 1).

Adult-Onset Cataracts

Some kind of heritability exists regarding the onset of age-related cataract. Hammond and colleagues compared the formation of cataract and its severity in the worse eye of 226 monozygotic twins to that of 280 dizygotic twins (275). All were females. They concluded that the transmission is multifactorial, and that an additive genetic and environmental influence exists. They calculated that the influencing factors were 48% genetic, 38% due to age, and 14% environmental (275). The mean age of twins in the groups was 62 years, and about 20% had significant cataracts (276).

Three genes are known to be associated with hereditary transmission of presenile cataracts. All three are considered to have autosomal recessive transmission. Heon and colleagues (277) described a large family with adult-onset pulverulent cataract, mostly cortical opacities in the form of dots and spots, progressing so that surgery was required at a mean age of 44. The locus mapped to chromosome 9q13-q22 (277). Pras and associates examined two different families and were the first to show that an autosomal recessive adult-onset cataract is transmitted on the short arm of chromosome 3 (278). In another identified family, a presenile cataract consisted of bluish and white opacifications in concentric layers with prominent sutures. Pras identified a homozygous mutation, Phe105Val, in the LIM2 gene on chromosome 19. This gene encodes MP20, a protein likely to have a transport or enzymatic function (279).

Pathology and Pathogenesis

Studies on the ultrastructure of the cataract in myotonic dystrophy revealed two kinds of changes (254,255). The first are similar to those found in other cataracts, such as enlarged intercellular spaces or watery vacuoles, loss of plasma membranes, abnormal cell organelles, compression in cytoplasmic density, and occasional pyknotic cells. The second kind of changes are specific for this cataract and are the typical clinical finding of multicolored spots or crystals. These include intracellular vacuoles containing whorls of multilaminated membranes. It has been suggested that these large myelinlike figures produce an interference phenomenon that results in the multicolored dots (254), and that the primary defect in the lens of myotonic dystrophy lies in a defect in the plasma membranes of the lens fibers (255).

The cataract of retinitis pigmentosa shows disruption of fibers in the posterior lens, a finding described in all reported posterior subcapsular cataracts (280). The same authors also found an additional posterior lens capsule that resulted from posterior migration of lens epithelial cells. These ultrastructural abnormalities are remarkably similar to those found in cataracts of gyrate atrophy, which show a backward extension of the lens epithelium and a two-layered thickened posterior lens capsule (274). The inner layer composed of multiple basal laminae and fine filaments, and the outer layer of homogenous granular substance. Pigment deposits occur on the vitreal side.

It is interesting that a defect in the lens membrane, in the form of an increase in permeability, without a defect in the cation pump mechanism has been suggested as the cause of the osmotic imbalance in human senile cataract (281).

A hereditary cataract found in the deer mouse could serve as a model for presenile and senile human cataracts (96). Inherited as an autosomal recessive trait, the cataract develops after two months to three years; the normal life span is eight years. An associated syndactyly of two toes identifies the homozygous animals. Vacuolation of equatorial lens fibers marks the beginning of the intralenticular changes.

Clinical Management

The management of developmental cataracts is similar to that of cataracts in general. Surgery is performed when vision is impaired enough to justify this approach. The presence of a metabolic or multisystem disease is not a contraindication to cataract extraction. Patients with retinal degeneration and progressive cataract benefit from the removal of the cataract, as long as they have, to a certain extent, a functional retina and macula. The question of an intraocular implant must be decided individually, taking into account the age of the patient, the general medical condition, other ocular problems, and the etiology of the cataract. Usually, I find that patients with multisystem diseases need intraocular implants, as they have difficulty in handling contact lenses. On the other hand, patients with other ocular diseases may do poorly with implants.

In many cases of developmental cataracts in this group, the cataract is an early sign of a metabolic, systemic, or multisystem disease. It is the duty of the ophthalmologist, who may be the first physician to see the patient, to raise the possibility of a hereditary progressive systemic disease before irreversible changes occur.

Preventive measures should be taken to stop the progress of the cataract whenever feasible. These include dietary restrictions for patients with abnormal galactose metabolism. It is possible that even the juvenile cataract of GALK deficiency is influenced by a specially constructed diet (S. Merin and S. Yatziv, in preparation). Patients with CTX should be treated both by diet and by cholesterol-lowering drugs. In experimental diabetic rats the diabetic cataract has been prevented by daily injections of vitamin E, but the mechanism of action is not clear (206).

Genetic counseling is usually simple once the etiologic background of the cataract is diagnosed.

REFERENCES

1. Francois J. Genetics of cataract. Ophthalmologica 1982; 184:61–71.
2. Merin S, Crawford JS. The etiology of congenital cataracts: a survey of 386 cases. Can J Ophthalmol 1971; 6:178–182.

3. Fraser GR, Friedman AI. The Causes of Blindness in Childhood: A Study of 776 Children with Severe Visual Handicaps. Baltimore: Johns Hopkins University Press, 1967.
4. Semina EV, Ferrell RE, Mintz-Hittner HA, et al. A novel homeobox gene PITX3 is mutated in families with autosomal-dominant cataracts and ASMD. Nat Genet 1998; 19:167–170.
5. Hertzberg R. Rubella and virus induced cataracts. Trans Ophthalmol Soc UK 1982; 102:355–358.
6. Chylack LT. Classification of human cataracts. Arch Opthalmol 1978; 96:888–892.
7. Chylack LT, Lee MR, Tung WH, Cheng HM. Classification of human senile cataractous change by the American Cooperative Cataract Research Group (CCRG) Method I. Instrumentation and technique. Invest Opthalmol Vis Sci 1983; 24:424–431.
8. Marcantonio JM, Duncan G, Davies PD, Bushell AR. Classification of human senile cataracts by nuclear colour and sodium content. Exp Eye Res 1980; 31:227–237.
9. Merin S. Congenital cataracts. In: Goldberg MF, ed. Genetic and Metabolic Eye Disease. Boston: Little, Brown & Co., 1974:337–355.
10. Jay M. Linkage and chromosomal studies in congenital cataract. Trans Ophthalmol Soc UK 1982; 102:350–354.
11. Renwick JH, Lawler SD. Probable linkage between a congenital cataract locus and the Duffy blood group locus. Ann Hum Genet 1963; 27:67–76.
12. Nettleship E, Ogilvie FM. A peculiar form of hereditary congenital cataract. Trans Ophthalmol Soc UK 1906; 26:191–206.
13. Conneally PM, Wilson AF, Merritt AD, Helveston EM, Palmer CG, Wang LY. Conformation of genetic heterogeneity in autosomal dominant forms of congenital cataract from linkage studies. Cytogenet Cell Genet 1978; 22:295–297.
14. Geyer DD, Church RL, Steele EC, et al. Regional mapping of the human MP70 (Cx50; connexin 50) gene by fluorescence in situ hybridization to 1q21.1. Mol Vis 1997; 3:13.
15. Mackay D, Ionides A, Kibar Z, et al. Connexin46 mutations in autosomal dominant congenital cataract. Am J Hum Genet 1999; 64:1357–1364.
16. Mackay D, Ionides A, Berry V, et al. A new locus for dominant "zonular pulverulent" cataract, on chromosome 13. Am J Hum Genet 1998; 60:1474–1478.
17. Litt M, Carrero-Valenzuela R, LaMorticella DM, et al. Autosomal dominant cerulean cataract is associated with a chain termination mutation in the human beta-crystallin gene CRYBB2. Hum Mol Genet 1997; 6:665–668.
18. Lubsen NM, Renwick JH, Tsui LC, et al. A locus for a human hereditary cataract is closely linked to the gamma-crystallin gene family, Proc Natl Acad Sci USA 1987; 84:489–492.
19. Litt M, Kramer P, LaMorticella DM, et al. Autosomal dominant congenital cataract associated with a missense mutation in the human alpha crystallin gene CRYAA. Hum Mol Genet 1998; 7: 471–474.
20. Berry V, Francis P, Reddy MA, et al. Alpha-B crystallin gene (CRYAB) mutation causes dominant congenital posterior polar cataract in humans. Am J Hum Genet 2001; 69:1141–1145.
21. Basti S, Hejtmancik JF, Padma T, et al. Autosomal dominant zonular cataract with sutural opacities in a four-generation family. Am J Ophthalmol 1996; 121:162–168.
22. Padma T, Ayyagari R, Murty JS, et al. Autosomal dominant zonular cataract with sutural opacities localized to chromosome 17q11–12. Am J Hum Genet 1995; 57: 840–845.
23. Kannabiran C, Wawrovsek E, Sergeev Y, et al. Mutation of beta A3/A1 crystallin gene in autosomal dominant zonular cataract with sutural opacities results in a protein with single globular domain. Invest Ophthalmol Vis Sci 1999; 40:5786.
24. Mackay DS, Boskovska OB, Knopf HL, et al. A nonsense mutation in CRYBB1 associated with autosomal dominant cataract linked to human chromosome 22q. Am J Hum Genet 2002; 71:1216–1221.

25. Gill D, Klose R, Munier FL, et al. Genetic heterogeneity of the Coppock-like cataract: a mutation in CRYBB2 on chromosome 22q11.2. Invest Ophthalmol Vis Sci 2000; 41:159–165.
26. Kramer P, Yount J, Mitchell T, et al. A second gene for cerulean cataracts maps to the beta crystallin region on chromosome 22. Genomics 1996; 35:539–542.
27. Rogaev EI, Rogaeva EA, Korovaitseva GI, et al. Linkage of polymorphic congenital cataract to the gamma-crystallin gene locus on human chromosome 2q33–35. Hum Mol Genet 1996; 5:699–703.
28. Santhiya ST, Shyam Manohar M, Rawlley D, et al. Novel mutations in the gamma-crystallin genes cause autosomal dominant congenital cataracts. J Med Genet 2002; 39:352–358.
29. Heon E, Priston M, Schorderet DF, et al. The gamma-crystallins and human cataracts: a puzzle made clearer. Am J Hum Genet 1999; 65:1261–1267.
30. Stephan DA, Gillanders E, Vanderveen D, et al. Progressive juvenile-onset punctate cataracts caused by mutation of the gamma D-crystallin gene. Proc Natl Acad Sci 1999; 96:1008–1012.
31. Brakenhoff RH, Henskens HA, van Rossum MW, et al. Activation of the gamma E-crystallin pseudogene in the human hereditary Coppock-like cataract. Hum Mol Genet 1999; 3:279–283.
32. Pande A, Pande J, Asherie N, et al. Crystal cataract: human genetic cataract caused by protein crystallization. Proc Natl Acad Sci 2001; 98:6116–6120.
33. Maumenee IH. Classification of hereditary cataracts in children by linkage analysis. Ophthalmology 1979; 86:1554–1558.
34. Richard J, Maumenee IH, Rowe S, Lourien EW. Congenital cataract possibly linked to haptoglobin. Cytogenet Cell Genet 1984; 37:570.
35. Marner E. A family with eight generations of hereditary cataract. Acta Ophthalmol 1949; 27:537–551.
36. Eiberg H, Marner E, Rosenberg T, Mohr J. Marner's cataract (CAM) assigned to chromosome 16: linkage to haptoglobin. Clin Genet 1988; 34:272–275.
37. Bu L, Jin Y, Shi Y, et al. Mutant DNA-binding domain of HSF4 is associated with autosomal dominant lamellar and Marner cataract. Nat Genet 2002; 31:276–278.
38. Lund AM, Eiberg H, Rosenberg T, Warburg M, et al. Autosomal dominant congenital cataract, linkage relations, clinical and genetic heterogeneity. Clin Genet 1992; 41:65–69.
39. Eiberg H, Lund AM, Warburg M, Rosenberg T. Assignment of congenital cataract Volkmann type (CCV) to chromosome 1p36. Hum Genet 1995; 96:33–38.
40. Armitage MM, Kivlin JD, Ferrell RE. A progressive early onset cataract gene maps to human chromosome 17q24. Nat Genet 1995; 9:37–40.
41. Khaliq S, Hameed A, Ismail M, et al. A novel locus for autosomal dominant nuclear cataract mapped to chromosome 2p12 in a Pakistani family. Invest Ophthalmol Vis Sci 2002; 43:2083–2087.
42. Berry V, Francis P, Kaushal S. Missense mutations in MIP underlie autosomal dominant 'polymorphic' and lamellar cataracts linked to 12q. Nat Genet 2000; 25:15–17.
43. Berry V, Ionides AC, Moore AT, et al. A locus for autosomal dominant anterior polar cataract on chromosome 17p. Hum Mol Genet 1996; 5:415–419.
44. Francis PJ, Berry V, Bhattacharya SS, Moore AT. The genetics of childhood cataract. J Med Genet 2000; 37:481–488.
45. Ionides AC, Berry V, Mackay DS, et al. A locus for autosomal dominant posterior polar cataract on chromosome 1p. Hum Mol Genet 1997; 6:47–51.
46. Yamada K, Tomita HA, Kanazawa S, et al. Genetically distinct autosomal dominant posterior polar cataract in a four-generation Japanese family. Am J Ophthalmol 2000; 129:159–165.
47. Bateman JB, Spence MAA, Marazita ML, Sparkes RS. Genetic linkage analysis of autosomal dominant congenital cataracts. Am J Ophthalmol 1986; 101:218–225.

48. Barrett DJM, Sparkes RS, Gorin MB, et al. Genetic linkage analysis of autosomal dominant congenital cataracts with lens specific DNA probes and polymorphic phenotypic markers. Ophthalmology 1988; 95:538–544.
49. Bercovitch L, Donaldson DD. The natural history of congenital sutural cataracts: case report with long-term follow up. J Pediatr Ophthalmol Strabismus 1982; 19:108–110.
50. Meissner M. Augenarztliches aus dem Blindinstitut. Z Augenheilkd 1933; 80:48–58.
51. Hejtmancik JF. The genetics of cataract: our vision becomes clearer. Am J Hum Genet 1998; 62:520–525.
52. Heon E, Liu S, Billingsley G, et al. Gene localization for aculeiform cataract, on chromosome 2q33–35. Am J Hum Genet 1998; 63:921–926.
53. Harman NB. Congenital cataract, a pedigree of five generations. Trans Ophthalmol Soc UK 1909; 29:101–108.
54. Harman NB. New pedigrees of cataract, posterior polar, anterior polar and microphthalmia and lamellar. Trans Ophthalmol Soc UK 1909; 29:296–306.
55. Tulloh CG. Heredity of posterior polar cataracts with report of a pedigree. Br J Ophthalmol 1955; 39:374–379.
56. Polomeno RC, Cummings C. Autosomal dominant cataracts and microcornea. Can J Ophthalmol 1979; 14:227–229.
57. Stefaniak E, Zaremba J, Cieslinska I, Kropinska E. An unusual pedigree with microcornea-cataract syndrome. J Med Genet 1995; 32:813–815.
58. Yokoyama Y, Narahara K, Tsuji K, et al. Autosomal dominant congenital cataract and microphthalmia associated with a familial (2;16) translocation. Hum Genet 1992; 90:177–178.
59. Merin S, Lapithis AG, Horovitz D, Michaelson IC. Childhood blindness in Cyprus. Am J Ophthalmol 1972; 74:538–542.
60. Pearce WG, MacKay JA, Holmes TM, et al. Autosomal recessive juvenile cataract in Hutterites. Ophthalmic Paediatr Genet 1987; 8:119–124.
61. Mostafa MSB, Temtamy S, El-Gammal MY, Abdel-Sayed SI, Abdel-Salam M, El-Baroudy R. Genetic studies of congenital cataract. Metab Pediatr Ophthalmol 1981; 5:233–242.
62. Vanita, Singh JR, Singh D. Genetic and segregation analysis of congenital cataract in the Indian population. Clin Genet 1999; 56:389–393.
63. Wirth MG, Russell-Eggitt IM, Craig JE, et al. Aetiology of congenital and paediatric cataract in an Australian population. Br J Ophthalmol 2002; 86:782–786.
64. Pras E, Frydman M, Levy-Nissenbaum E. A nonsense mutation (W9X) in CRYAA causes autosomal recessive cataract in an inbred Jewish Persian family. Invest Ophthalmol Vis Sci 2000; 41:3511–3515.
65. Shokeir MH, Lowry RB. Juvenile cataract in Hutterites. Am J Med Genet 1985; 22:495–500.
66. Forsius H, Arentz-Grastvedt B, Eriksson AW. Juvenile cataract with autosomal recessive inheritance. A study from the Aland Islands, Finland. Acta Ophthalmol 1992; 70:26–32.
67. Rados A. Central pulverulent (discoid) cataract and its hereditary transmission. Arch Ophthalmol 1947; 38:57–77.
68. Wagner H. Recessive vererbter angeborener Star. Klin Monatsbl Augenheilkd 1940; 104:337–338.
69. Saebo J. An investigation into the mode of hereditary of congenital and juvenile cataracts. Br J Ophthalmol 1949; 33:601–629.
70. OMIM at http://www.ncbi.nlm.nih.gov/omim/.
71. Temtamy SA, Shalash BA. Genetic heterogeneity of the syndrome: microphthalmos with congenital cataract. Birth Defects 1974; 10:292–293.
72. Krill AE, Woodbury G, Bowman JE. X-chromosomal-linked sutural cataracts. Am J Ophthalmol 1969; 68:867–872.
73. Fraccardo M, Morone G, Manfredini U, Sanger R. X-linked cataract. Ann Hum Genet 1967; 31:45–50.

74. Walsh EB, Wegman ME. Pedigree of hereditary cataract, illustrating sex-limited type. Bull Johns Hopkins Hosp 1937; 61:125–135.
75. Pavone L, Larosa M, Sorge G, Scaletta S, Li Volti S, Mollica F. Ocular manifestations in a family with probably X-linked cataracts. Clin Genet 1981; 20:243–246.
76. Capella JA, Kaufman HE, Lill FJ, Cooper G. Hereditary cataracts and microphthalmia. Am J Ophthalmol 1963; 56:454–458.
77. Francis PJ, Berry V, Hardcastle AJ, et al. A locus for isolated cataract on human Xp. J Med Genet 2002; 39:105–109.
78. Falls HF. The role of the sex chromosome in hereditary ocular pathology. Trans Am Ophthalmol Soc 1952; 50:421–467.
79. Lyon MF. Sex chromatin and gene action in the mammalian X-chromosome. Am J Hum Genet 1962; 14:135–148.
80. Feingold J, Raoul O, See G, Delthil S, Crovzet J, Demailly ML, Morel J. Existence possible d'une forme de cataracte congenitale liee au chromosome Y. J Genet Hum 1979; 27:67–69.
81. Russell P, Uga S, Zigler JS, Kaiser-Kupfer M, Kuwabara T. Studies using human lenses from a family displaying hereditary congenital cataracts. Vision Res 1981; 21:169–172.
82. Nakano T, Yamamoto S, Kutsukake G, Ogawa H, Nakajima A, Takano E. Hereditary cataract in mice. Jpn J Clin Ophthalmol 1960; 14:196–200.
83. Iwata S, Kinoshita JH. Mechanism of development of hereditary cataract in mice. Invest Ophthalmol 1971; 10:504–512.
84. Sakuragawa M, Kuwabara T, Kinoshita JH, Fukui HN. Swelling of the lens fibers. Exp Eye Res 1975; 21:381–394.
85. Fukui HN, Merola LO, Kinoshita JH. A possible cataractogenic factor in the Nakano mouse lens. Exp Eye Res 1978; 26:477–485.
86. Piatigorsky J, Fukui HN, Kinoshita JH. Differential metabolism and leakage of protein in an inherited cataract and in normal lens cultured with ouabain. Nature 1978; 274:558–562.
87. Lipman RD, Muggleton-Harris AL, Aroian MA. Phenotypic variation of cataractogenesis in the Nakano mouse. Exp Eye Res 1981; 32:255–256.
88. Fraser FC, Schabtach A. "Shrivelled" a hereditary degeneration of the lens in the house mouse. Genet Res 1962; 3:383–387.
89. Garber AT, Stirk L, Gold RJM. Abnormalities of crystallins in the lens of the Cat Fraser mouse. Exp Eye Res 1983; 36:165–169.
90. Kador PF, Fukui HN, Fukushi S, Jernigan HM, Kinoshita JH. Philly mouse: a new model of hereditary cataract. Exp Eye Res 1980; 30:59–68.
91. Uga S, Kador PF, Kuwabara T. Cytological study of Philly mouse cataract. Exp Eye Res 1980; 30:79–92.
92. Carper D, Shinohara T, Piatigorsky J, Kinoshita JH. Deficiency of functional messenger RNA for a development ally regulated β-crystallin polypeptide in a hereditary cataract. Science 1982; 217:463–464.
93. Piatigorsky J, Treton JA, King CR, Nickerson JM, Carper D, Shinohara T, Inana G, Hejtmancik JF, Norman B. A molecular genetic approach to vision research crystallin gene expression in the lens. Ophthalmic Pediatr Genet 1983; 3:61–72.
94. Nakamura M, Russell P, Carper DA, et al. Alteration of a developmentally regulated, heat-stable polypeptide in the lens of the Philly mouse. Implications for cataract formation. J Biol Chem 1988; 263:19218–19221.
95. Lyon MF, Jarvis SE, Sayers I, Holmes RS. Lens opacity: a new gene for congenital cataract on chromosome 10 of the mouse. Genet Res 1981; 38:337–341.
96. Burns RP, Feeney L. Hereditary cataract in deer mice (*Peromycuns inaniculatus*). Am J Ophthalmol 1975; 80:370–378.
97. Kuck JF, Kuwabara J, Kuck KO. The Emory mouse cataract: an animal model for human senile cataract. Curr Eye Res 1981–1982; 1:643–649.

98. Zwaan J. Genetically determined lens abnormalities. In: Stivastava SK, ed. Red Blood Cell and Lens Metabolism. Amsterdam: Elsevier, 1980:415–422.
99. Vainisi SJ, Goldberg MF. Animal models of inherited human eye disease. In: Goldberg MF, ed. Genetic and Metabolic Eye Disease. Boston: Little Brown & Co., 1974: 215–231.
100. Barnett KC. Lens opacities in the dog as models for human eye disease. Trans Ophthalmol Soc UK 1982; 102:346–349.
101. Ihara N. A new strain of rat with an inherited cataract. Experientia 1983; 39:909–911.
102. Smith RS, Sundberg JP, Linder CC. Mouse mutations as models for studying cataracts. Pathobiology 1997; 65:146–154.
103. Gotz W. Transgenic models for eye malformations. Ophthalmic Genet 1995; 16:85–104.
104. Francois J. Late results of congenital cataract surgery. Ophthalmology 1979; 86: 1586–1598.
105. Stark WJ, Taylor HR, Michels RG, Maumenee AE. Management of congenital cataracts. Ophthalmology 1979; 86:1575–1578.
106. Taylor DSI. Choice of surgical technique in the management of congenital cataracts. Trans Ophthal Soc UK 1981; 101:114–117.
107. Parks MM. Posterior lens capsulectomy during primary cataract surgery in children. Ophthalmology 1983; 90:344–345.
108. Gelbart SS, Hoyt CS, Jastrebski G, Marg E. Long-term visual results in bilateral congenital cataract. Am J Ophthalmol 1982; 93:615–621.
109. Buckley EG, Klombers LA, Seaber JH, et al. Management of the posterior capsule during pediatric intraocular lens implantation. Am J Ophthalmol 1993; 115:722–728.
110. Basti S, Ravishankar U, Gupta S. Results of a prospective evaluation of three methods of management of pediatric cataracts. Ophthalmology 1996; 103:713–720.
111. BenEzra D, Cohen E. Posterior capsulectomy in pediatric cataract surgery: the necessity of a choice. Ophthalmology 1997; 104:2168–2174.
112. Douvas NG. Phakectomy with shallow anterior vitrectomy in congenital and juvenile cataracts. Dev Ophthalmol 1981; 2:163–174.
113. Parks MM. Visual results in aphakic children. Am J Ophthalmol 1982; 94:441–449.
114. Girard LJ. Lensectomy through the pars plana by ultrasonic fragmentation (USF). Ophthalmology 1979; 86:1985–1993.
115. Peyman GA, Raichand M, Oesterle C, Goldberg MF. Pars plicata lensectomy and vitrectomy in the management of congenital cataracts. Ophthalmology 1981; 88:437–439.
116. Grossman SA, Peyman GA. Long-term visual results after pars plicata lensectomy-vitrectomy for congenital cataracts. Br J Ophthalmol 1988; 72:601–606.
117. Keech RV, Tongue AC, Scott WE. Complications after surgery for congenital and infantile cataracts. Am J Ophthalmol 1989; 108:136–141.
118. Simon JW. Mehta N. Simmons ST, et al. Glaucoma after pediatric lensectomy/vitrectomy. Ophthalmology 1991; 98:670–674.
119. Asrani SG, Wilensky JT. Glaucoma after congenital cataract surgery. Ophthalmology 1995; 102:863–867.
120. Egbert JE, Wright MM, Dahlhauser KF, et al. A prospective study of ocular hypertension and glaucoma after pediatric cataract surgery. Ophthalmology 1995; 102:1098–1101.
121. Merin S, Crawford JS. Assessment of incomplete congenital cataract. Can J Ophthalmol 1972; 7:56.
122. Rogers GL, Tishler CL, Tsou BH, Hertle RW, Fellows RR. Visual acuities in infants with congenital cataracts operated on prior to six months of age. Arch Ophthalmol 1981; 99:999–1003.
123. Pratt-Johnson JA, Tillson G. Visual results after removal of congenital cataracts before the age of one year. Can J Ophthalmol 1981; 16:19–21.
124. Hoyt CS. Monocular congenital cataract. J Pediatr Ophthalmol Strabismus 1982; 19:127–128.

125. Taylor DSI. Risks and difficulties of the treatment of aphakia in infancy. Trans Ophthalmol Soc UK 1982; 102:403–406.
126. Levin AV, Edmonds SA, Nelson LB, et al. Extended-wear contact lenses for the treatment of pediatric aphakia. Ophthalmology 1988; 95;1107–1113.
127. Stark WJ, Leske MC, Worthen DM, Murray GC. Trends in cataract surgery and intraocular lenses in the United States. Am J Ophthalmol 1983; 96:304–310.
128. Stark WJ, Worthen DM, Holladay JT, et al. The FDA report on intraocular lenses. Ophthalmology 1983; 90:311–317.
129. Binkhorst CD, Gobin MH. Treatment of congenital and juvenile cataract with intraocular lens implants (pseudophakoi). Br J Ophthalmol 1970; 54:759–765.
130. Binkhorst CD. The iridocapsular (two loop) lens and the iris clip (four loop) lens in pseudophakia. Trans Am Acad Ophthalmol Otolaryngol 1973; 77:589–617.
131. Hiles DA. The need for intraocular Iens implantation in children. Ophthalmic Surg 1977; 8(3):162–169.
132. Hiles DA. Intraocular lens implantation in children with monocular cataracts: 1974–1983. Ophthalmology 1984; 91:1231–1237.
133. Maida JW, Sheets JH. Pseudophakia in children: a review of results of eighteen implant surgeons. Ophthalmic Surg 1979; 10(12):61–66.
134. Menezo JL, Taboada J. Assessment of intraocular lens implantation in children. J Am Intraocul Implant Soc 1982; 8:131–135.
135. Ben-Ezra D, Paez JH. Congenital cataract and intraocular lenses. Am J Ophthalmol 1983; 96:311–314.
136. Tablante RT, Lapus JV, Cruz ED, Santos AM. A new technique of congenital cataract surgery with primary posterior chamber intraocular lens implantation. J Cataract Refract Surg 1988; 14:149–157.
137. Morgan KS, Arffa RC, Marbefli TL, Verity JM. Five year follow-up of epikeratophakia in children. Ophthalmology 1986; 93:423–432.
138. Morgan KS, McDonald MB, Hiles DA, et al. The nationwide study of epikeratophakia for aphakia in children. Am J Ophtalmol 1987; 103:366–374.
139. Uusitalo RJ, Lehtosalo J. Visual refractive and keratometric results of epikeratophakia in children. A two year follow-up. Arch Ophthalmol 1989; 107:358–363.
140. Helveston EM, Saunders RA, Ellis FD. Unilateral cataract in children. Ophthalmic Surg 1980; 11:102–108.
141. Beller R, Hoyt CS, Marg E, Odom JV. Good visual function after neonatal surgery for congenital monocular cataracts. Am J Ophthalmol 1981; 91:559–565.
142. Jacobson SG, Mohinora I, Held R. Development of visual acuity in infants with congenital cataracts. Br J Ophthalmol 1981; 65:727–735.
143. Nelson LB. Diagnosis and management of cataracts in infancy and childhood. Ophthalmic Surg 1984; 15:688–697.
144. Birch EE, Stager DR. Prevalence of good visual acuity following surgery for congenital unilateral cataract. Arch Ophthalmol 1988; 106:40–43.
145. Drummond GT, Scott WE, Keech RV. Management of monocular congenital cataracts. Arch Ophthalmol 1989; 107:45–51.
146. Wilson ME, Apple DJ, Bluestein EC, Wang XH. Intraocular lenses for pediatric implantation: biomaterials, designs, and sizing. J Cataract Refract Surg 1991; 20: 584–591.
147. Crouch ER Jr, Pressman SH, Crouch ER. Posterior chamber intraocular lenses: long-term results in pediatric cataract patients. J Pediatr Ophthalmol Strabismus 1995; 32:210–218.
148. Brady KM, Atkinson CS, Kilty LA, Hiles DA. Cataract surgery and intraocular lens implantation in children. Am J Ophthalmol 1995; 120:1–9.
149. BenEzra D. Cataract surgery and intraocular lens implantation in children, and intraocular lens implantation in children. Am J Ophthalmol 1996; 121:224–225.

150. Neumann D, Weissman BA, Isenberg SJ, et al. The effectiveness of daily wear contact lenses for the correction of infantile aphakia. Arch Ophthalmol 1993; 11:927–930.
151. Robb RM, Petersen RA. Outcome of treatment for bilateral congenital cataracts. Ophthalmic Surg 1992; 23:650–656.
152. Menezo JL, Esteve JT, Perez-Torregrosa VT. IOL implantation in children—17 years experience. Eur J Implant Refract Surg 1994; 6:251–256.
153. Parks MM, Johnson DA, Reed GW. Long-term visual results and complications in children with aphakia. A function of cataract type. Ophthalmology 1993; 100:826–841.
154. Zwaan J, Mullaney PB, Awad A, et al. Pediatric intraocular lens implantation. Surgical results and complications in more than 300 patients. Ophthalmology 1998; 105:112–119.
155. Sjögren T. Klinische und vererbungsmedizinische Untersuchungen über Oligophrenia mit kongenitaler Katarackt. Z Ges Neurol Psychiatr 1935; 152:263–292.
156. Marinesco G, Draganesco ST, Vasiliu D. Nouvelle maladie familiale caractérisee parune catracte congenitale et un arret du developement somato-neuro-psychique. Encephale 1931; 26:97–109.
157. Sjögren T. Hereditary congenital spinocerebellar ataxia accompanied by congenital cataract and oligophrenia: a genetic and clinical investigation. Confin Neurol 1950; 10: 293–308.
158. Sjögren T, Larsson T. Oligophrenia in combination with congenital ichthyosis and spastic disorders: a clinical and genetic study. Acta Psychiat Neurol Scand 1957; 32(suppl 113):1–112.
159. Merlini L, Gooding R, Lochmuller H, et al. Genetic identity of Marinesco-Sjogren/ myoglobinuria and CCFDN syndromes. Neurology 2002; 58:231–236.
160. Crome L, Duckett S, Franklin AW. Congenital cataracts, renal tubular necrosis and encephalopathy in two sisters. Arch Dis Child 1963; 38:505–515.
161. Martsolf JT, Hunter AGW, Haworth JC. Severe mental retardation, cataracts, short stature and primary hypogonadism in two brothers. Am J Med Genet 1978; 1:291–299.
162. Skre H, Berg K. Linkage studies on the Marinesco-Sjögren syndrome and hypergonadotropic hypogonadism. Clin Genet 1977; 11:57–66.
163. Goldberg MF, McKusick VA. X-linked colobomatous microphthalmos and other congenital anomalies. A disorder resembling Lenz's dysmorphogenetic syndrome. Am J Ophthalmol 1971; 71:1128–1133.
164. Lowry RB, MacLean R, McLean DM, Tischler B. Cataracts, microcephaly, kyphosis and limited joint movement in two siblings: a new syndrome. J Pediatr 1978; 79: 282–284.
165. Scott-Emaukpor AB, Heffelfinger J, Higgins IV. A syndrome of microcephaly and cataracts in four siblings: a new genetic syndrome. Am J Dis Child 1977; 131:167–169.
166. Kretzer FL, Hittner HM, Mehta RS. Ocular manifestations of the Smith-Lemli-Opitz syndrome. Arch Ophthalmol 1981; 99:2000–2006.
167. Sakano T, Okuda N, Yoshimitsu K, Hatano S, Nishi Y, Tanaka T, Usui T. A case of Menkes syndrome with cataracts. Eur J Pediatr 1982; 138:357–358.
168. Garcin R, Raverdy P, Delthil S, Man HX, Chimenes H. Sur une affection heredo-familiale associant cataract, atrophie optique, signes extra-pyramidaux et certains stigmates de la maladie de Friedrich. Rev Neurol 1961; 104:373–379.
169. Forrester S, Kovach MJ, Reynolds NM, et al. Manifestations in four males with and an obligate carrier of the Lenz microphthalmia syndrome. Am J Med Genet 2001; 98: 92–100.
170. Kelley RI. RSH/Smith-Lemli-Opitz syndrome: mutations and metabolic morphogenesis. Am J Hum Genet 1998; 63:322–326.
171. Abedi S. Syndromes with congenital cataract (Conradi Hunerman syndrome), a case report. Ann Ophthalmol 1982; 14:595–597.
172. McKusick VA. Mendelian Inheritance in Man. 6th ed. Baltimore: Johns Hopkins University Press, 1983:988–989.

173. Chess J, Albert DM. Ocular pathology of the Majewski syndrome. Br J Ophthalmol 1982; 66:736–741.
174. Tripathi RC, Cibis GW, Harris DJ, Tripathi B. Lowe's syndrome. Birth Defects 1982; 18:629–644.
175. Johnston SS, Nevin NC. Ocular manifestations in patients and female relatives of families with oculocerebrorenal syndrome of Lowe. Birth Defects 1976; 12:569–577.
176. Delleman JW, Bleekers-Wagemakers EM, Van Veelen AWC. Opacities of the lens indicating carrier status of the oculo-cerebro-renal (Lowe) syndrome. J Pediatr Ophthalmol 1977; 14:205–212.
177. Brown N, Gardner RJM. Lowe syndrome: identification of the carrier state. Birth Defects 1976; 12:579–591.
178. Cibis GW, Waeltermann JM, Whitcraft CT, et al. Lenticular opacities in carriers of Lowe's syndrome. Ophthalmology 1986; 93:1041–1045.
179. Fagerholm P, Pettersson U, Anneren G. Lowe oculocerebrorenal syndrome. DNA-based linkage of the gene to Xq24-q26, using tightly linked flanking markers and the correlation to lens examination in carrier diagnosis. Am J Hum Genet 1989; 44:241–247.
180. Tripathi RL, Cibis GW, Tripathi BJ. Pathogenesis of cataracts in patients with Lowe's syndrome. Ophthalmology 1986; 93:1046–1051.
181. Attree O, Olivos IM, Okabe I, et al. The Lowe's oculocerebrorenal syndrome gene encodes a protein highly homologous to inositol polyphosphate-5-phosphatase. Nature 1992; 358:239–242.
182. Leahey AM, Charnas LR, Nussbaum RL. Nonsense mutations in the OCRL-1 gene in patients with the oculocerebrorenal syndrome of Lowe. Hum Mol Genet 1993; 2: 461–463.
183. Lin T. Orrison BM. Leahey AM, et al. Spectrum of mutations in the OCRL1 gene in the Lowe oculocerebrorenal syndrome. Am J Hum Genet 1997; 60:1384–1388.
184. Kawano T, Indo Y, Nakazato H, et al. Oculocerebrorenal syndrome of Lowe: three mutations in the OCRL1 gene derived from three patients with different phenotypes. Am J Med Genet 1998; 77:348–355.
185. Lin T, Lewis RA, Nussbaum RL. Molecular confirmation of carriers for Lowe syndrome. Ophthalmology 1999; 106:119–122.
186. Hittner HM, Kretzer FL, Mehta RS. Zellweger syndrome. Lenticular opacities indicating carrier status and lens abnormalities characteristic of homozygotes. Arch Ophthalmol 1981; 99:1972–1982.
187. Francois J. Francois dyscephalic syndrome. Birth Defects 1982; 18:595–619.
188. Francois J. Francois' dyscephalic syndrome. Dev Ophthalmol 1983; 7:13–35.
189. Edwards SJ, Gladwin AJ, Dixon MJ. The mutational spectrum in Treacher Collins syndrome reveals a predominance of mutations that create a premature-termination codon. Am J Hum Genet 1997; 60:515–524.
190. Nance WE, Warburg M, Bixler D, Helveston EM. Congenital X-linked cataract, dental anomalies and brachymeta carpalia. Birth Defects 1974; 10:285–291.
191. Van Dorp DP, Delleman JW. A family with X-chromosomal recessive congenital cataract, microphthalmia, a peculiar form of the ear and dental anomalies. J Pediatr Ophthalmol Strabismus 1979; 16:166–171.
192. Toutain A, Dessay B, Ronce N, et al. Refinement of the NHS locus on chromosome Xp22.13 and analysis of five candidate genes. Eur J Hum Genet 2002; 10:516–520.
193. Leitersdorf E, Reshef A, Meiner V, et al. Frameshift and splice-junction mutations in the sterol 27-hydroxylase gene cause cerebrotendinous xanthomatosis in Jews or Moroccan origin. J Clin Invest 1993; 91:2488–2496.
194. Cruysberg JR, Wevers RA, van Engelen BG, et al. Ocular and systemic manifestations of cerebrotendinous xanthomatosis. Am J Ophthalmol 1995; 120:597–604.
195. Dotti MT, Rufa A, Federico A. Cerebrotendinous xanthomatosis: heterogeneity of clinical phenotype with evidence of previously undescribed ophthalmological findings. J Inherit Metab Dis 2001; 24:696–706.

196. Nadol JB, Burgess B. Cochleosaccular degeneration of the inner ear and progressive cataracts inherited as an autosomal dominant trait. Larynogoscope 1982; 92:1028–1037.
197. Marshall D. Ectodermal dysplasia. Report of kindred with ocular abnormalities and hearing defect. Am J Ophthalmol 1958; 45:143–156.
198. da Cunha RP, Moreira JB. Ocular findings in Down's syndrome. Am J Ophthalmol 1996; 122:236–244.
199. Patz A. Cataracts in galactosemia: observations in three cases. Am J Ophthalmol 1953; 36:453–462.
200. Gitzelman R. Hereditary galactokinase deficiency, a newly recognized cause of juvenile cataracts. Pediatr Res 1967; 1:14–23.
201. Benn PA, D'Ancona CG, Croce CM, Shows TB, Mellman WJ. Confirmation of the assignment of the gene for galactose-1-phosphate uridyltransferase (E.C. 2.7.7.12) to human chromosome 9. Cytogenet Cell Genet 1979; 24:37–41.
202. Levy HL, Hammersen G. Newborn screening for galactosemia and other galactose metabolic defects. J Pediatr 1978; 92:871–877.
203. Elsevier SM, Kucherlapati RS, Nichols EA, Creagan RP, Giles RE, Ruddle FH. Assignment of the gene for galactokinase to human chromosome 17 and its regional localization to band q21-22. Nature 1974; 251:633–636.
204. Beutler E, Matsumoto F. A rapid simplified assay for galactokinase activity in whole blood. J Lab Clin Med 1973; 82:818–821.
205. Tedesco TA, Miller KL, Rawnsley BE, Mennuti MT, Spielman RS, Mellman WJ. Human erythrocytic galactokinase and galactose-1-phosphate uridyltransferase: a population survey. Am J Hum Genet 1975; 27:737–747.
206. Magnani M, Cucchiarini L, Stocchi V, Stocchi D, Carnevali G, Dacha M, Fornaini G. Human erythrocyte galactokinase: a population survey. Hum Hered 1982; 32:274–279.
207. Levy NS, Krill AE, Beutler E. Galactokinase deficiency and cataracts. Am J Ophthalmol 1972; 74:41–48.
208. Winder AF. Laboratory screening in the assessment of human cataract. Trans Ophthalmol Soc UK 1981; 101:127–130.
209. Winder AF, Claringbold LJ, Jones RB, Jay BS, Rice NSC, Kissun RD, Menzies IS, Mount JN. Partial galactose disorders in families with premature cataracts. Arch Dis Child 1983; 58:362–366.
210. Harley JD, Irvine S, Mutton P, Gupta J. Maternal enzymes of galactose metabolism and the inexplicable infantile cataract. Lancet 1974; 2:259–261.
211. Winder AF, Fielder AR, Mount JN, Menzies IS. Direct and maternal aspects of the risk of cataract with partial disorders of galactose metabolism. Clin Genet 1985; 28:199–206.
212. Brivet M, Abadie V, Soni T, et al. Inexplicable infantile cataracts and partial maternal galactose disorder. Arch Dis Child 1986; 61:445–448.
213. Elsas LJ, Dembure PP, Langley S, et al. A common mutation associated with the Duarte galactosemia allele. Am J Hum Genet 1994; 54:1030–1036.
214. Stambolian D, Ai Y, Sidjanin D, et al. Cloning of the galactokinase cDNA and identification of mutations in two families with cataracts. Nat Genet 1995; 10:307–312.
215. Bosch AM, Bakker HD, van Gennip AM, et al. Clinical features of galactokinase deficiency: a review of the literature. J Inherit Metab Dis 2002; 25:629–634.
216. Murphree AL, Beaudet AL, Palmer EA, Nichols BL. Cataract in mannosidosis. Birth Defects 1976; 12:347–354.
217. Letson RD, Desnick RJ. Punctate lenticular opacities in type II mannosidosis. Am J Ophthalmol 1978; 85:218–224.
218. Vaca G, Ibarra B, Bracamontes M, Garcia-Cruz D, Sanchez-Corona J, Medina C, Wunsch C, Gonzales-Quiroga G, Cantu JM. Red blood cell sorbitol dehydrogenase deficiency in a family with cataracts. Hum Genet 1982; 61:338.
219. Merin S, Crawford JS. Hypoglycemia and infantile cataract. Arch Ophthalmol 1971; 86:495–498.

220. Wets B, Milot JA, Polomeno RC, Letarte J. Cataracts and ketotic hypoglycemia. Ophthalmology 1982; 89:999–1002.
221. Unakar NJ, Genyea C, Reddan JR, Reddy VN. Ultrastructural changes during the development and reversal of galactose cataracts. Exp Eye Res 1978; 26:123–133.
222. Kinoshita JH. Cataracts in galactosemia. Invest Ophthalmol Vis Sci 1965; 4:786–799.
223. Varma SD, Kinoshita JH. The absence of cataracts in mice with congenital hyperglycemia. Exp Eye Res 1974; 19:577–582.
224. Jedziniak JA, Chylack LT, Cheng HM, Gillis MK, Kalustian AA, Tung WH. The sorbitol pathway in the human lens: aldose reductase and polyol dehydrogenase. Invest Ophthalmol Vis Sci 1981; 20:314–326.
225. Gonzalez RG, Willis J, Aguayo J, Campbell P, Chylack LT, Schleich T. ^{13}C-Nuclear magnetic resonance studies of sugar cataractogenesis in the single intact rabbit lens. Invest Ophthalmol Vis Sci 1982; 22:808–811.
226. Chylack LT. Mechanism of "hypoglycemic" cataract formation in the rat lens. I. The role of hexokinase instability. Invest Ophthalmol 1975; 14:746–755.
227. Chylack LT, Schaefer FL. Mechanism of "hypoglycemic" cataract formation in the rat lens: II. Further studies on the role of hexokinase instability. Invest Ophthalmol 1976; 15:519–528.
228. Arn PH. Galactosemia. Curr Treat Options Neurol 2003; 5:343–345.
229. Chylack LT, Cheng HM. Sugar metabolism in the crystalline lens. Surv Ophthalmol 1978; 23:26–34.
230. Chylack LT, Henriques HF, Tung WH. Inhibition of sorbitol production in human lenses by aldose reductase inhibitor. Doc Ophthalmol 1979; 18:65–75.
231. Chylack LT, Henriques HF, Cheng HM, Tung, WH. Efficacy of alrestatin, an aldose reductase inhibitor, in human diabetic and nondiabetic lenses. Ophthalmology 1979; 86:1579–1585.
232. Peterson MJ, Sarges R, Aldinger CE, McDonald DP. CP -45, 634: a novel aldose reductase inhibitor that inhibits polyol pathway activity in diabetic and galactosemic rats. Metabolism 1979; 28(suppl 1):456–461.
233. Fukushi S, Merola LO, Kinoshita JH. Altering the course of cataracts in diabetic rats. Invest Ophthalmol Vis Sci 1980; 19:313–315.
234. Datiles M, Fukui H, Kinoshita JH. Galactose cataract prevention with sorbinil, an aldose reductase inhibitor: a light microscopic study. Invest Ophthalmol Vis Sci 1982; 22:174–179.
235. Unakar NJ, Tsui JY. Inhibition of galactose-induced alterations in ocular lens with sorbinil. Exp Eye Res 1983; 36:685–694.
236. Hu TS, Datiles M, Kinoshita JH. Reversal of galactose cataracts with sorbinil in rats. Invest Ophthalmol Vis Sci 1983; 24:640–644.
237. Kador PF. Overview of the current attempts toward the medical treatment of cataract. Ophthalmology 1983; 90:352–364.
238. Datiles MB, Kador PF, Fukus HN, Hu TS, Kinoshita JH. Corneal re-epithelialization in galactosemic rats. Invest Ophthalmol Vis Sci 1983; 24:563–569.
239. Unakar N, Tsui J, Johnson M. Aldose reductase inhibitors and prevention of galactose cataracts in rats. Invest Ophthalmol Vis Sci 1989; 30:1623–1632.
240. Prchal JT, Conrad ME, Skalka HW. Association of presenile cataracts with heterozygosity for galactosaemic states and with riboflavin deficiency. Lancet 1978; 1:12–13.
241. Skalka HW, Prchal JT. Presenile cataract formation and decreased activity of galactosemic enzymes. Arch Ophthalmol 1980; 98:269–273.
242. Beutler E, Matsumuto F. Galactokinase deficiency and cataracts. Lancet 1978; 1:1161.
243. Maraini G, Leardi E, Nuzzi G. Galactosemic enzyme levels in presenile cataracts. Graefes Arch Klin Exp Ophthalmol 1982; 219:100–101.
244. Magnani M, Cucchiarini L, Stocchi V, Dacha M. Red blood cell galactokinase activity and presenile cataracts. Enzyme 1983; 29:58–60.

245. Elman MJ, Miller MT, Matalon R. Galactokinase activity in patients with idiopathic cataracts. Ophthalmology 1986; 93:210–215.
246. Stambolian D, Scarpino-Myers V, Eagle RC, et al. Cataracts in patients heterozygous for galactokinase deficiency. Invest Ophthalmol Vis Sci 1986; 27:429–433.
247. Stevens RE, Datiles MB, Srivastava SK, et al. Idiopathic presenile cataract formation and galactosaemia. Br J Ophthalmol 1989; 73:48–51.
248. Winder AF, Fells P, Jones RB, Kissun RD, Menzies IS, Mount JN. Galactose intolerance and the risk of cataract. Br J Ophthalmol 1982; 66:438–441.
249. Avisar RA, Schwartzman S, Levinsky H, Allalouf D, Goldman J, Ninio A, Savir H. A case of cataract formation during the lactating period associated with galactose-1-phosphate uridyl transferase deficiency. Metab Pediatr Syst Ophthalmol 1982; 6:45–48.
250. Orzalesi N, Sorcinelli R, Guiso G. Increased incidence of cataracts in male subjects deficient in glucose-6-phosphate dehydrogenase. Arch Ophthalmol 1981; 99:69–70.
251. Orzalesi N, Sorcinelli R, Binaghi F. Glucose-6-phosphate dehydrogenase in cataracts of subjects suffering from favism. Ophthalmic Res 1976; 8:192–194.
252. Wiebers DO, Hollenhorst RW, Goldstein NP. The ophthalmologic manifestation of Wilson's disease. Mayo Clin Proc 1977; 52:409–416.
253. Burian HM, Burns CA. Ocular changes in myotonic dystrophy. Am J Ophthalmol 1967; 63:22–34.
254. Dark AJ, Streeten BW. Ultrastructural study of cataract in myotonia dystrophica. Am J Ophthalmol 1977; 84:665–674.
255. Eshaghian J, March WF, Goossens W, Rafferty NS. Infrastructure of cataract in myotonic dystrophy. Invest Ophthalmol Vis Sci 1978; 19:289–293.
256. Harley HG, Walsh KV, Rundle S, et al. Localisation of the myotonic dystrophy locus to 19q13.2–19q13.3 and its relationship to twelve polymorphic loci on 19q. Hum Genet 1991; 87:73–80.
257. Ranum LP, Rasmussen PF, Benzow KA, et al. Genetic mapping of a second myotonic dystrophy locus. Nat Genet 1998; 19:196–198.
258. Pepin B, Mikol J, Goldstein B, Aron JJ, Lebuisson DA. Familial mitochondrial myopathy with cataract. J Neurol Sci 1980; 45:191–203.
259. Berginer VM, Abeliovich D. Genetics of cerebrotendinous xanthomatosis (CTX): an autosomal recessive trait with high gene frequency in Sephardim of Morrocan origin. Am J Med Genet 1981; 10:151–157.
260. O'Donnell FE, Pappas HR. Autosomal dominant foveal hyperplasia and presenile cataracts. A new syndrome. Arch Ophthalmol 1982; 100:279–281.
261. Goldstein JH, Hutt AE. Trichomegaly cataract and hereditary spherocytosis in two siblings. Am J Ophthalmol 1972; 73:333–335.
262. Buyse M, Bull M. A syndrome of osteogenesis imperfecta and cataracts. Birth Defects 1978; 14:95–98.
263. Solomon LM, Esterly NB. The skin and the eye. In: Goldberg MF, ed. Genetic and Metabolic Eye Disease. Boston: Little, Brown & Co., 1974:504–505.
264. Scott JG, Friedmann AI, Chitters M, Pepler WJ. Ocular changes in the Bloch-Sulzberger syndrome (incontinentia pigmenti). Br J Ophthalmol 1955; 39:276–282.
265. Pinkerton OD. Cataract associated with congenital ichthyosis. Arch Ophthalmol 1958; 60:393–396.
266. Jay B, Blach RK, Wells RS. Ocular manifestations of ichthyosis. Br J Ophthalmol 1968; 52:217–226.
267. Green JS, Johnson GJ. Congenital cataract with microcornea and Peters' anomaly as expressions of one autosomal dominant gene. Ophthalmic Paediatr Genet 1986; 7:187–194.
268. Salmon JF, Wallis CE, Murray AD. Variable expressivity of autosomal dominant microcornea with cataract. Arch Ophthalmol 1988; 106:505–510.
269. Merin S, Crawford JS, Cardarelli J. Hyperplastic persistent pupillary membrane. Am J Ophthalmol 1971; 72:717–719.

270. Johnston SS, Hanna JE, Nevin NC, Bryars JH. Norrie's disease. Birth Defects 1982; 18:729–738.
271. Heckenlively J. The frequency of posterior subcapsular cataract in the hereditary retinal degeneration. Am J Ophthalmol 1982; 93:733–738.
272. Merin S. Cataract formation in retinitis pigmentosa. Birth Defects 1982; 18:187–191.
273. Nemet P, Godel V, Lazar M. Kearns-Sayre syndrome. Birth Defects 1982; 18:263–268.
274. Kaiser-Kupfer M, Kuwabara T, Uga S, Takki K, Valle D. Cataract in gyrate atrophy: Clinical and morphologic studies. Invest Ophthalmol Vis Sci 1983; 24:432–436.
275. Hammond CJ, Snieder H, Spector TD, Gilbert CE. Genetic and environmental factors in age-related nuclear cataracts in monozygotic and dizygotic twins. N Engl J Med 2000; 342:1786–1790.
276. Hammond CJ, Duncan DD, Snieder H, et al. The heritability of age-related cortical cataract: the twin eye study. Invest Ophthalmol Vis Sci 2001;42:601–605.
277. Heon E, Paterson AD, Fraser M, et al. A progressive autosomal recessive cataract locus maps to chromosome 9q13-q22. Am J Hum Genet 2001; 68:772–778.
278. Pras E, Pras E, Bakhan T, et al. A gene causing autosomal recessive cataract maps to the short arm of chromosome 3. Isr Med Assoc J 2001; 3:559–562.
279. Pras E, Levy-Nissenbaum E, Bakhan T, et al. A missense mutation in the LIM2 gene is associated with autosomal recessive presenile cataract in an inbred Iraqi Jewish family. Am J Hum Genet 2002; 70:1363–1367.
280. Eshaghian J, Rafferty NS. Ultrastructure of human cataract in retinitis pigmentosa. Invest Ophthalmol Vis Sci 1978; 17:289–293.
281. Pasino M, Maraini G. Cation pump activity and membrane permeability in human senile cataractous lenses. Exp Eye Res 1982; 34:887–893.

7
Inherited Anomalies of the Crystalline Lens

INTRODUCTION

The most cellular structure of the human body, the crystalline lens, is affected by a limited number of diseases. Apart from opacification of the lens (cataract formation), any other disease is relatively uncommon. The comparative rarity of abnormalities in the lens, for both acquired and inherited diseases, is mainly a result of its avascularity. Anomalies of the transparent crystalline lens include changes in its position *(ectopia lentis)*, shape *(lenticonus)*, size *(microspherophakia)*, and absence of the lens *(aphakia)*. These features will be discussed in this order.

ECTOPIA LENTIS IN SYSTEMIC AND MULTISYSTEM DISEASES

Introduction

Ectopia lentis, a condition in which the crystalline lens is abnormally positioned, has been known as a human familial disease since the 19th century. Clinically, this displacement is manifested as a "subluxation of the lens," whereby the lens remains attached to the ciliary body through abnormally elongated zonules. Such subluxation may be (1) minimal, recognizable only by a slight backward displacement of the lens and by iridodonesis; (2) intermediate, when the lens is displaced in any direction in the same plane or slightly more posteriorly, such that its equator can be seen through the dilated pupil; or (3) maximal, when the optical axis is aphakic and the free edge of the lens is barely seen at the pupillary edge. With more displacement the zonules are torn and the lens may float freely into the anterior chamber or vitreous, a condition termed dislocation of the lens.

Ectopia lentis is more often than not associated with a multisystem disease or an inborn error of metabolism (associated ectopia lentis). Although trauma is a common cause of ectopia lentis, it will not be discussed here. It seems that the common denominator of associated ectopia lentis is a weakness of zonules caused by an inherited disorder of connective tissue or an enzymatic deficiency. The list of known genetic diseases associated with ectopia lentis (Table 1) seems to grow from year to year. Several reviews summarize the subject, especially its ophthalmic

Table 1 Multisystem and Systemic Diseases Associated with Ectopia Lentis

Disease	MIM	Symbol/ locus	Mode of inheritance[a]	Chromosome location	Gene	Refe- rences
Marfan syndrome	154700	MFS	AD	15q21	FBN1	5,6,7
Homocystinuria	236200	—	AR	21q22.3	CBS	8,9,10
Weill–Marchesani I	277600	ARWMS	AR	19ql3.3–13.2	?	11
Weill–Marchesani II	—	ADWMS	AD	15q21.1	FBN1	12,13
Hyperlysinemia	238700		AR	7q31.3	AASS	14
Sulfite oxidase deficiency	606887	—	AR	12ql3.2–ql3.3	SUOX	15,16,17
Molybdenum Cofactor deficiency I	252150	MCD	AR	6p21.3	MOCS1	18
Molybdenum Cofactor deficiency II	252150	MCD	AR	5qll	MOCS2	18
Ehlers–Danlos I	130000	EDS1, EDS2	AD	9q34.2–q34.3	COL5A1	19,20
Ehlers–Danlos I	130000	EDS1	AD	2q31	COL5A2	19,20
Ehlers–Danlos I	130000	EDS1, EDS7	AD	17q21.3–q22	COL1A1	19

[a]AD—autosomal dominant; AR—autosomal recessive.

importance (1–4). Even though the different diseases have a single clinical manifestation in the form of lens displacement, their pathogenesis, clinical manifestations, diagnostic approach, genetic background, pathology, and management are not the same. Therefore, these will be discussed separately for each disease.

Clinical and Genetic Types of Associated Ectopia Lentis

Table 1 lists the different disorders of the group. Marfan syndrome is the most common, whereas in others, such as sulfite oxidase deficiency, only few cases have been reported.

Marfan Syndrome

Marfan syndrome (MFS) is an autosomal dominant multisystem disease with manifestations mainly in the form of skeletal, cardiovascular, and ocular abnormalities. As in many other autosomal dominant diseases, its severity varies considerably. In the same family mild cases can be seen, along with severely affected ones.

Extraocular manifestations: Characteristic of the disorder are the skeletal abnormalities, resulting in an apparent elongated figure with exceptionally long limbs. Marfan termed these changes dolichostenomelia (21). The fingers and toes are elongated (arachnodactyly); the face, chin, and nose may be longer than normal; the chest often has a sunken sternum, pectus excavatum, or pectus carinatum. Kypho-scoliosis may be prominent, giving the patient a somewhat bent figure.

Joint laxity is expressed in an abnormally large movement of the joints. Heart disease is common. About 60% of MFS patients have mitral or aortic regurgitation or other auscultary evidence of heart disease. Dilation of the ascending aorta is a major sign, dilation of the descending aorta is a minor sign, as is mitral valve prolapse with or without regurgitation or dilatation of the pulmonary artery (3).

An inherited weakness of other organs is also seen. Inguinal hernia is common. In addition, weak facial muscles and loss of subcutaneous fat give the patient's face a characteristic thin appearance. The life expectancy of patients with Marfan syndrome is about half that of normal persons (22).

Ocular manifestations: Several studies have been made on large groups of patients with Marfan syndrome, including 142 patients by Cross and Jensen in 1973 (23), 50 patients by Pyeritz and McKusick in 1979 (22), and 160 patients by Maumenee in 1982 (24). Results of these investigations give a well-defined picture of the multiple and variable ocular manifestations of Marfan syndrome.

Ectopia lentis is common, reportedly affecting 50–80% of all patients, with a mean of about 70%. The lens may be displaced in any direction (Fig. 1), but usually occurs upward, somewhat more superotemporally than superonasally (Fig. 2a).

Relatively uncommon is a backward displacement or dislocation of the lens into the vitreous. The zonules are elongated, but are usually normal in number and density (23). Because the zonules are tight, accommodation is present and seems to be normal in Marfan patients, in spite of the subluxated lens (22,24).

Myopia is another frequent ocular finding, caused by the increased axial length of the eye in about one-third of affected patients. Axial myopia is more prominent in patients with subluxated lenses. In one study (24), patients had an axial length of 25.96 mm, compared with 23.39 mm in patients without subluxated lenses.

The cornea in patients with Marfan syndrome is reported to be flatter than normal by about 2 D, as measured by keratometry, and its diameter is usually larger than normal.

Using orbscan, pachymetry and confocal microscopy, Sultan et al. (25) examined 60 eyes with MFS and frequently found a flat and thin cornea. The K-reading was 40.8 ± 1.4 (controls: 42.9 ± 1.1) and the corneal thickness was $50.2 \pm 41.9\,\mu m$ (controls: $55.2 \pm 23.6\,\mu m$). An opaque stromal matrix was also detected (25).

Other ocular abnormalities may be present. Enophthalmos is a result of reduced intraorbital fat. The iris may show decreased furrows (1), probably another

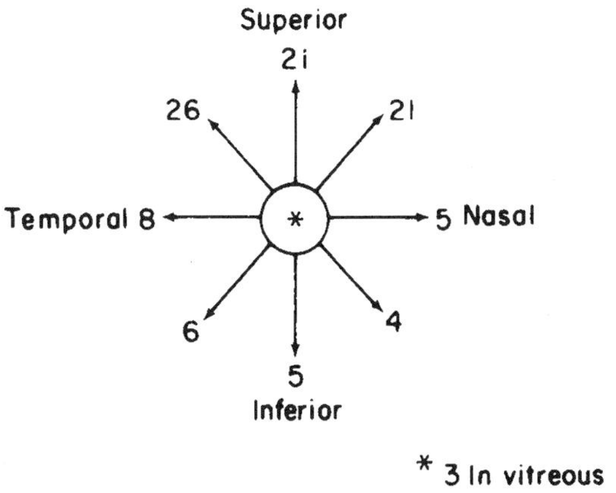

Figure 1 Direction of lens displacement in 159 eyes of patients with Marfan syndrome: the arrows point to the direction of displacement and the percentage of dislocations in each direction; 3% were displaced into the vitreous (from Ref. 23).

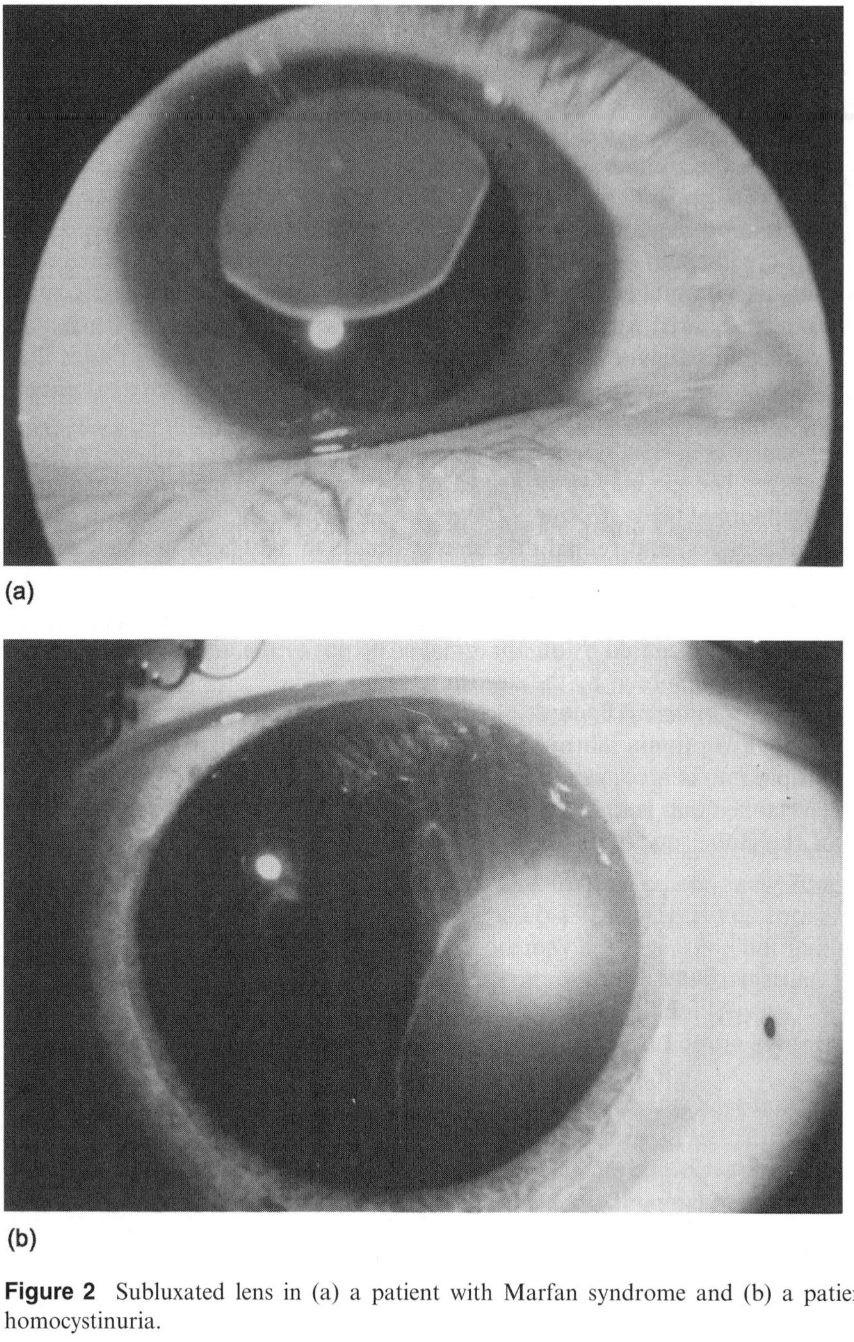

Figure 2 Subluxated lens in (a) a patient with Marfan syndrome and (b) a patient with homocystinuria.

manifestation of abnormal tissue structure. The retina frequently exhibits peripheral myopic degenerative changes, and retinal detachment occurs in 5–10% of phakic patients, and even more in aphakic patients. This incidence seems to be much higher than in comparably myopic patients and may be related to increased traction by the zonules on the retinal periphery. Glaucoma is not uncommon; about 8% has been reported in one study (23). It is caused by an abnormal structure of the angle, similar to congenital glaucoma, or rarely, by the dislocated lens.

Rare ocular abnormalities are spherophakia and lens colobomas.

With few exceptions, the ocular manifestations are bilateral and symmetric. The lens displacement can be congenital, or it may occur later in life, even in adulthood. It has been claimed that lens displacement may progress during one of two periods of growth of the globe: up to the age of five years and from 10 to 19 years (24).

Diagnosis: The diagnosis of Marfan's syndrome should be ruled out or confirmed in every patient with displaced lenses. It may be confirmed by the combination of the cardiovascular and skeletal abnormalities, the characteristic displacement of the lens, and a family history. If any of these findings is not present, the diagnosis may be more difficult to establish.

Echocardiography will confirm the characteristic prolapse of the posterior mitral leaflets in 80% of all patients (22). This is, therefore, a simple and very useful test. A chest x-ray film may also show the presence of cardiovascular abnormalities. A general physical examination should be performed, with measurements taken of body proportions, including a ratio of lower segment (from pubis to toes) to upper segment (from pubis to head) and a ratio of arm span to height (22). Both are markedly increased in Marfan syndrome. Two other simple tests can be performed in the clinician's office. The "thumb sign" is positive when the patient's thumb extends well beyond the ulner surface of the hand (26), with the thumb turned straight inward. The "wrist sign" is positive when the thumb and fifth finger on one hand overlap when embracing the opposite wrist (27).

The Ghent diagnostic criteria for MFS were established and revised (3). The necessary findings for diagnosis are two major criteria in two organ systems with a minor finding in a third organ. Alternatively, one of the major criteria and one other organ affected, plus a mutated disease-causative gene identified are sufficient for diagnosis. Major criteria include such findings as ectopia lentis, the wrist and thumb sign, or dilation of the ascending aorta (3). Another major criterion is the finding of four out of eight typical skeletal manifestations (3). Other classification systems of diagnostic criteria require fewer diagnostic findings (28). Dural ectasia was added as a major diagnostic criterion (28).

Pathology and pathogenesis: Several eyes of patients with Marfan syndrome have been studied by light and electron microscopy. Light microscopy shows that both zonular fibers and lens fibers are essentially normal (29), but electron microscopy demonstrates that the zonular fibers are randomly arranged instead of regularly, and that the lens fibers have poorly defined cellular borders and interdigitating processes (30). The most remarkable abnormality is the anterior zonular–capsular relationship. The zonules do not "fan-out" toward the attachment to the capsule (29), and the capsular fibers are abnormally large and contain gross granules (30). The iris does not show the usual circumferential ridges and furrows, is abnormally transparent, and has an underdeveloped dilator muscle, even in patients without lens displacement (29).

Marfan syndrome is the classic example of a "heritable disorder of connective tissue" (31). It was assumed that the collagen structure is basically abnormal, and that a defective organization of collagen results in reduced tensile strength of tissues, such as the zolunes, cardiac valves, and aorta (32).

In 1981, Boucek et al. (32) found reduced amounts of intermolecular cross-links in the collagen in both skin and aorta. The amount of total collagen and the ratio of type I to type III collagen fibers are normal. The authors have postulated that in Marfan syndrome abnormal nonenzymatic steps in maturation of collagen exist.

The 1991 discovery of mutations in the fibrillin gene being responsible for MFS, emphasized the important role of the fibrillins (FBNs) in the cornea. Fibrillin is a large glycoprotein, 350 kD in size and is a structural component of elastin-associated microfibrils (33). Extracellular microfibrils are 10–14 nm in diameter. One of their functions is to serve as a scaffold for the deposition of tropoelastin to form elastic fibers (34). A variety of proteins compose the structure of microfibrils, with FBN1 associated with MFS and FBN2 associated mainly with contractural arachnodactyly, a nonocular disorder. (34). The whole class of connective tissue microfibrils plays a key role in elastic fibrillogenesis and has an anchoring role in nonelastic tissues (35). Fibrillin is widely distributed in ocular tissues. It is found in the lens capsule and zonules, in the iris, ciliary body, and processes, in the conjunctiva, in the corneal basement membrane and endothelium, in Bruch's membrane, choroid, sclera, and lamina cribrosa (36).

Epidemiology, Genetics, and the MFS Genes

Marfan syndrome is an autosomal dominant disease, with almost full penetrance and variable expressivity. Its prevalence has been estimated as 4–5:100,000 of the population (22), but it is probably much more common. The prevalence is probably 1:5000 people (34) or even higher (37). About two-thirds of all patients have a positive family history, and the new mutation rate was estimated as 7.4×10^{-6} (24). The great variability in the manifestation of the disease raised the possibility of heterogeneity, however, it has never been proved.

The MFS locus was mapped to chromosome 15 in 1990, (5) and a year later both Lee and associates (6) and Dietz and associates (7) reported the cloning of the fibrillin gene and its mapping to chromosome 15ql5–q21. The mapping was refined to location 15q21, and a second fibrillin gene was cloned and mapped to chromosome 5q23 (6,33). Mutations in fibrillin-1 (FBN1) gene are associated with classic Marfan syndrome (7), while mutations in FBN2 gene are associated with another disorder, termed contractural arachnodactyly. (34) FBN1 is a large gene, containing 65 exons and spanning 110 kb (35). It encodes fibrillin-1, a large glycoprotein of 350 kD.

The number of mutations of the gene is very large. More than 50 mutations were reported by 1995 (34) and until now many or even most mutations identified seem to be novel, not previously reported. In 2002, in a study of 126 individuals Katzke and colleagues (38) identified 53 mutations, of which 33 were novel. The authors also reported that in patients diagnosed with MFS who did not fulfill the diagnostic criteria, the detection rate of abnormal mutations was 12% as compared with 42% for the whole group. Different mutations may result in strikingly different phenotypes of MFS and also in an isolated finding of ectopia lentis (39). The genetic mutations were missense, nonsense, splicing errors, and others. The missense mutations usually result in the milder forms of ectopia lentis or, less frequently, no ocular symptoms at all (39). In other cases, a mutation may cause only isolated skeletal features or familial ectopia lentis or full-blown MFS (35,40,41). Liu and associates (42) estimated that 10% of all MFS cases are caused by a silent mutation associated with skipping of an FBN1 exon (42). A splicing error in intron 63 was associated with classic MFS findings, microcomea and ectopia lentis (43).

A locus for another fibrillin gene MFS2 was assigned to chromosome 3p24.2–p25 (44). Mutations in the MFS2 gene cause a Marfan-like connective tissue disorder with the typical skeletal and cardiovascular features, but without the ocular involvement. It was marked in OMIM as No. 154705 (19).

Homocystinuria

In the 1970s, the first patients with increased homocystine in the urine, mental retardation, and ectopia lentis were described. Homocystinuria has since been defined as a separate entity from Marfan syndrome. The ophthalmologist who sees a patient with ectopia lentis must differentiate between homocystinuria and Marfan syndrome: the patient's life may be at risk.

Extraocular manifestations: A patient with homocystinuria has an external resemblance to one with Marfan syndrome, including the tall stature with an abnormal limb/body ratio, kyphoscoliosis, laxity of joints, and other skeletal abnormalities. However, these abnormalities are less frequent and are usually more subtle in homocystinuria. Osteoporosis is a common addition to the skeletal findings. Mental retardation is detected in at least 50% of all patients with homocystinuria, and it may become progressively worse (1).

Cardiovascular disorders in homocystinuria are related to hematologic abnormalities, such as the extraordinary tendency for intravascular thrombosis. The risk of thrombosis is greatly increased during general anesthesia and should be taken into consideration in these patients.

Increased risk of thromboembolic events and hypoglycemia applies also to children under anesthesia. Preoperative measures for prevention should be administered (see Management). The platelets have an abnormal tendency for increased adhesiveness, which may be related to the thrombotic phenomena. There is an increased prevalence of both cardiovascular and cerebrovascular diseases, even without anesthesia, and a reduced life expectancy in patients with homocystinuria. A malar flush and dilatation of vessels is frequent.

Ocular manifestations: Ectopia lentis occurs in about 90% of patients with homocystinuria (23). Subluxation can be in any direction, but most lenses are displaced in the inferior, inferonasal, and nasal directions (Figs. 2b and 3) (23,45). Contrary to Marfan syndrome, the zonules seem abnormally weak and tear easily, and the lens dislocates into the anterior chamber or into the vitreous. Accommodation is weak or totally absent. The lens displacement is not congenital in homocystinuria, but usually occurs during childhood or adulthood and may be progressive. Glaucoma is common (almost one-fourth of all patients), usually caused by pupillary block mechanism secondary to lens dislocation. Unlike patients with Marfan syndrome, the homocystinuric patient has no abnormal angle structure. Other complications, such as retinal detachment and spherophakia, also may be observed.

Other complications, reported in a series of 45 patients with homocystinuria were optic atrophy in 23%, iris atrophy in 21%, anterior staphyloma in 13%, lenticular opacities in 9%, and corneal opacities in 9% (8). Myopia was the most consistent initial finding. Seventy-one percent of a group of 34 patients had myopia of over −5.0 D and 47% had over −10.0 D. Ectopia lentis was found in 85% of patients (46).

Metabolic abnormalities and diagnosis: The detectable levels of homocysteine and homocystine in the urine are the hallmark of homocystinuria. In addition, increased levels of blood homocysteine, blood methionine, and urine methionine are found; blood cystathionine and cysteine concentrations are reduced (42).

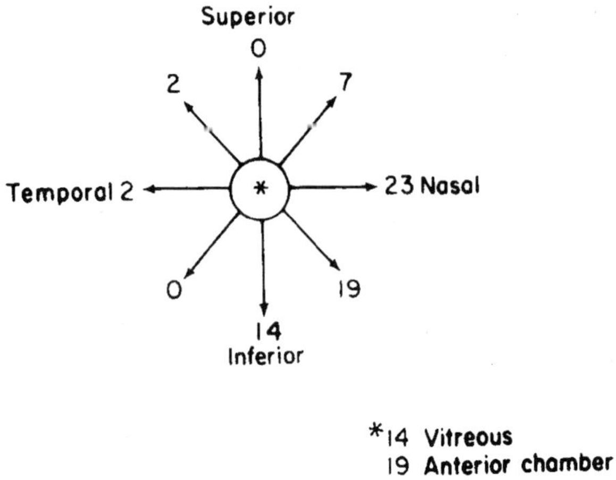

Figure 3 Direction of lens displacement in 57 eyes of patients with homocystinuria: arrows point to the direction of displacement and the percentage of dislocations in each direction; 14% were displaced into the vitreous, 19% into the anterior chamber (from Ref. 6).

The disease is commonly caused by an enzymatic deficiency of cystathionine β-synthetase. However, it is possible that other enzymatic defects involving methionine–homocysteine metabolism may have the same effect and may be responsible for some cases of homocystinuria.

The sodium nitroprusside test or the silver nitroprusside test are good screening methods for sulfur-containing amino acids in the urine. More detailed biochemical tests to confirm the diagnosis are necessary if these test results are positive.

Pyridoxine (vitamin B_6) may improve the biochemical abnormalities. It is tempting to postulate that "pyridoxine-positive" cases which respond to treatment by pyridoxine are genetically different from "pyridoxine-negative" cases which do not respond to pyridoxine. However, it seems that both types of pyridoxine response are found within the same family and that the pyridoxine-negative cases do respond to larger amounts of pyridoxine (47). These facts seem to negate the possibility of different genes.

Any abnormal platelet adhesiveness can be easily tested and, if positive, treated with dipyridamole therapy.

The delay in the correct diagnosis of homocystinuria is great. In one study, the mean age of diagnosis in a group of 34 patients was 24 years, with a range of 1–61 years (46). The authors found a mean delay in diagnosis of 11 years after the first manifestation of a major clinical sign (46). In suspicious cases or when a family history of homocystinuria is known, examinations should be performed immediately after birth (4) in order to confirm homocystinuria or rule it out.

Pathology and pathogenesis: Experimental homocystinemia has been achievedin baboon monkeys with loading doses of homocysteine (48). In these monkeys and in patients with homocystinuria, Harker et al. (48) has found that arterial thrombus formation results from sustained, homocystine-induced endothelial injury. Treatment with pyridoxine results in both reduced plasma homocystine and decreased platelet consumption (observed to be three times that of normal in the disorder). The risk of thrombotic phenomena increases when a patient with homocystinuria also has a hereditary deficiency in factor V Leiden (MTHFR) (49). While homocystinuria is rare, the heterozygotic and homozygotic state of MTHFR deficiency is common.

Epidemiology, Genetics, and the Cystathionine Beta-Synthase Gene

Homocystinuria is a rare autosomal recessive disease. Once considered to have an incidence of 1 in 350,000, it is undoubtedly more common, especially in some populations. Petterschmitt and associates (50) studied the results of the routine neonatal screening practiced in New England for several decades. The methionine cutoff value was reduced in 1990 from the initial 2 mg% to 1 mg% because of many false-negative results. The incidence is now established at 1 in 157,000 births (50). It is higher in populations with a high rate of consanguinity and in specific countries such as Ireland.

Homocystinuria is an inborn error of metabolism caused by one or more autosomal recessive genes. Although heterogeneity is suspected, it has never been confirmed. If more than one gene causes the disease, it is not known if it is allellic or not. Cystathionine β-synthetase deficiency, which could be pyridoxine-responsive or pyridoxine-unresponsive, is undoubtedly one of the most common genetic defects. Two other enzymes related to homocysteine metabolism may cause the same high levels of homocysteine in the blood (47). The deficient conditions are *N*-5,10-methylenetotrahydrofolate reductase (MTHFR) deficiency and *N*-5-methyltertrahydrofolate-homocysteine methyltransferase deficiency (47). Both have mild phenotypes, with increased thrombotic tendency as the main manifestation.

Spaeth (47) has suggested that an activator RNA is responsible for the coordinated activity of two (or more) genes, one associated with the production of cystathionine β-synthetase, the other with the autoregulation of homocysteine synthesis. A defect in the single "generator gene" responsible for the activity of the activator RNA could cause the phenotype of homocystinuria.

Obligatory heterozygotes of homocystinuria have been studied by Mudd et al. (51). They could not confirm an increased incidence of cardiovascular disease, but there was a mild degree of cystathionine synthetase deficiency.

The gene assignment to chromosome 21q22.3 is now known (8). The first description of the cystathionine beta-synthase (CBS) gene mapped it to this location (9). Many mutations were identified. By 1999, 92 different disease-associated mutations had been identified in the CBS gene in 310 homocystinuria patients examined worldwide (10). Most mutations were identified as missense mutations and the vast majority were private mutations. Kraus and colleagues (10) pointed out that two mutations were especially frequent: the pyridoxine-responsive Ile278Thr mutation and the pyridoxme-nonresponsive mutation, Gly307Ser (10).

Weill–Marchesani Syndrome

Weill–Marchesani syndrome, the third most frequent systemic disease associated with ectopia lentis, is often described as the "antithesis" of Marfan syndrome because patients manifest the "opposite" skeletal abnormalities. It is a hereditary disease, without known metabolic malfunction. Only a limited number of patients with this disorder have been reported, but probably it has not been properly diagnosed in many others. The disease is named after Weill and Marchesani, who separated it from the group of Marfan's syndrome and defined its clinical manifestations in the 1930s (52,53). Synonyms for this syndrome, such as spherophakia-brachymorphia syndrome and congenital mesodermal dysmorphodystrophy (19), stress the two major abnormalities found.

Extraocular manifestations: Patients with Weill–Marchesani syndrome have a prominent short stature, a short and large chest, and short and wide fingers. They have joint stiffness and limitation of mobility. Feet and hands are stubby and spade-like. The head is brachycephalic. However, the skeletal abnormalities may be mild (54), which makes diagnosis difficult.

Ocular manifestations: The ocular manifestations have been studied by Jensen et al. (54) in 10 patients from the Wilmer Eye Institute. Microspherophakia was found in almost all the patients (Fig. 4), with ectopia lentis occurring in about two-thirds of all eyes. The subluxation was usually downward, but sometimes it was backward. Two lenses had dislocated into the anterior chamber, when the pupils were dilated. Glaucoma was present in most of the patients, and usually of the angle closure type, owing to peripheral anterior synechiae or to pupillary block from lens dislocation (45). The visual outcome for these patients is often poor. Significant myopia frequently exists because of the small round lens.

Diagnosis: No single test is available to confirm the diagnosis of Weill–Marchesani syndrome. The diagnosis must be suspected in every patient with ectopia lentis or microspherophakia and the appropriate systemic manifestations. Mental development is normal. Examination of family members may be helpful in establishing the diagnosis.

Pathology and pathogenesis: Little is known about the pathology and pathogenesis of Weill–Marchesani syndrome. Like Marfan syndrome, it is assumed to be a generalized disorder of connective tissue. Both the lens and the zonular suspensory apparatus are abnormal. The overall lenticular mass is reduced by about 25%, the equatorial diameter is reduced to about 7 mm (normal: 9 mm), the sagittal diameter is increased, and the zonules are elongated, irregular, and broken (54).

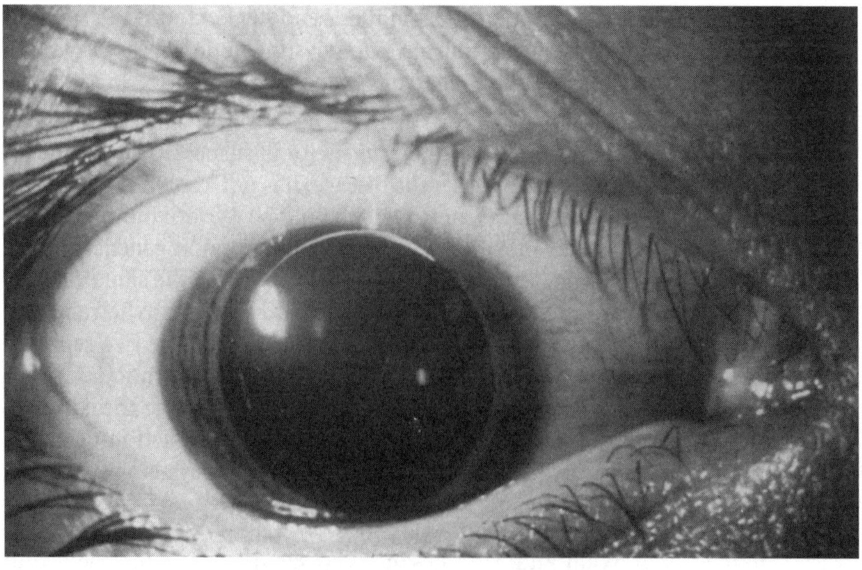

Figure 4 Microspherophakia in a patient with Weill–Marchesani syndrome. Note the edges of the small and round lens.

Genetics

The syndrome is transmitted as an autosomal recessive trait in most cases. Large families with consanguineous marriages were reported. It was suggested that an autosomal dominant form of a similar disease also occurred (19) and was debated for years. Recently, it was confirmed as a separate genetic entity.

A genome-wide study of two families with autosomal recessive Weill–Marchesani syndrome (ARWMS) mapped the Weill–Marchesani syndrome locus to chromosome 19pl3.3-pl3.2, near the COL5A3 gene (11). Faivre and colleagues (12) confirmed a previous suggestion (13) that the autosomal dominant form (ADWMS) mapped to chromosome 15q21.1. They identified a mutation (24nt inframe deletion) in exon 41 of the fibrillin 1 gene, the gene associated with MFS. In summary, the autosomal dominant and the autosomal recessive forms of Weill–Marchesani are genetically distinct but phenotypically similar (12). In contrast, ADWMS and Marfan are phenotypically different, but allelic in the fibrillin1 gene.

Familial Hyperlysinemia

A rare autosomal recessive metabolic disease was described in 1971 as being associated with ectopia lentis and spherophakia (55). The disease is caused by an inborn error of metabolism: deficiency of lysine ketoglutarate reductase results in increased blood levels of lysine. Smith et al. (55) have described four of the seven known cases. Extraocular manifestations include mental retardation, lax and weak ligaments, convulsions, and anemia.

Not enough patients have been identified to analyze how frequently these various abnormalities are found. Some patients with hyperlysinemia do not manifest the ocular changes or any of the extraocular abnormalities.

The gene associated with hyperlysinemia is AASS, the gene encoding alpha aminoadipic semialdehyde synthase. (14) The sequenced gene contains 24 exons, spanning 68 kb and maps to chromosome 7q31.3. A hyperlysinemia-causative mutation was identified in this gene. It is an out-of-frame 9 bp deletion in exon 15, resulting in a premature stop codon at position 534 (14).

Sulfite Oxidase Deficiency

A very rare hereditary disorder of sulfur metabolism is manifested by infantile hemiplegia, other neurologic disorders, and ectopia lentis (19,56). Increased urinary secretion of sulfite, thiosulfate, and *S*-sulfocysteine is found. Parallel findings are elevated blood levels of sulfite and *S*-sulfocysteine. The diagnosis can be confirmed by the absence of sulfite oxidase activity in skin fibroblasts. In one affected child (56), the lens was displaced superotemporally in one eye and inferiorly in the other eye. His parents (obligatory heterozygotes) both had markedly reduced activity of sulfite oxidase. The disorder is transmitted as an autosomal recessive trait.

The majority of the patients will have ectopia lentis. Severe and progressive neurologic disease is common, starting in infancy. Sequencing of the gene led to the identification of disease-causing mutations in the SUOX, the gene that encodes molybdohemoprotein sulfite oxidase (15–17). The gene was mapped to chromosome 12ql3.2–ql3.3 and produces a 466-amino acid molybdohemoprotein (17). The reported mutations include 11 disease-causative mutations, 2 frameshifts, 2 nonsense and 7 missense mutations.

Molybdenum Cofactor Deficiency

Another very rare autosomal recessive metabolic disorder includes deficiency of both sulfite oxidase and xanthine dehydrogenase. These two enzymes have a common cofactor, molybdenum, which is missing in this disorder. Two families have been described (19). Molybdenum is a trace element needed for the function of the cofactor. Most probably, the manifestations of the disorder result from sulfite oxidase deficiency and are in some aspects similar to the previously described disorder. Clinical findings include psychomotor retardation, dysmorphic features, seizures, and ectopia lentis in nearly all patients (57,58). Early death occurs. Spherophakia is the rule and the dislocation of the lens may occur during the second half of the first decade of life (58).

Two types of molybdenum cofactor deficiency are known and are separate genetic entities. Clinically the phenotype is similar. The two involved genes are molybdenum cofactor synthesis (MOCS1) the gene found in most European patients and mapped to chromosome 6p21.3, and MOCS2 mapped to chromosome 5q11 (18).

Other Systemic or Multisystem Diseases

Ectopia lentis is uncommonly found in three other inherited disorders related to abnormal connective tissue (39–61). Ehlers–Danlos' syndrome is an autosomal dominant disease of the mesenchymal tissues characterized by overelasticity of the skin and excessive extensibility of joints. Rupture of large vessels and hernias may occur. It is a heterogenous group with 11 recognized types. In some types an autosomal recessive transmission occurs, but the usual mode of inheritance is autosomal dominant. The common classic or type I Ehlers-Danlos syndrome has at least three different causative genes. These are COL5A1, the gene that encodes collagen alpha-1 V, COL5A2 gene, and COL1A1 gene (19,20). One of the types, EDS VI, is also named the ocular type due to frequent abnormalities in the cornea, sclera, and high myopia (62). Ectopia lentis does not occur in this type.

Kniest disease (metatropic dwarfism type II) is probably an autosomal dominant disease, with abnormally soft cartilage ("swiss–cheese type"), abnormally thin joint spaces, which prevent bending of fingers and fist formation, and a flat face. Wildervanck's syndrome, or cervico-oculo-acoustic syndrome, consists of congenital deafness, fused cervical vertebrae, and Duane-like syndrome. It is limited to females, and its mode of hereditary transmission is uncertain. It is not clear how frequently lens displacement occurs in these and other mesenchymal disorders.

Management

Medical and Surgical Treatment

Removal of displaced lens: There are no firm indications for removal of the displaced lens. The most common indication is displacement of the lens into the anterior chamber (129). The exact time to advise surgery varies among ophthalmologists. Generally, one of three factors may indicate the need for surgery: a lens-induced secondary ocular complication, poor visual acuity such as 20/80 or less (61), or annoying diplopia (63). Various surgical approaches have been advocated. The most popular is irrigation–aspiration (61), or phacoemulsification which leaves the posterior capsule intact. An alternative is pars plana lensectomy with shallow anterior vitrectomy (63).

Pars plana lensectomy with anterior vitrectomy gave good results (64–66). In cases of anterior dislocation of the lens a limbal approach was used (64). In one study, about half of all operations for displaced lenses was due to anterior dislocation into the anterior chamber (67). Another surgical approach was reported by Gerding (68). After a small capsulorhexis, manual endocapsular aspiration of the lens material was done. Then the 10L was fixed by sutures to the sulcus.

Specific treatment: Special attention should be given to the systemic or multisystem disease associated with ectopia lentis, as some patients require specific treatment. Patients with Marfan syndrome and homocystinuria may need preventive treatment for retinal holes, to reduce the risk of retinal detachment. The risk of thromboembolic phenomena and anesthesia should be considered for each homocystinuric patient before a decision for surgery is made. Pyridoxine and anti-sludging agents may be given to reduce the tendency to thrombotic phenomena (47,48).

Preparation of patients with homocystinuria for surgery includes preoperative, intraoperative, and postoperative measures (44). Preoperatively, strict dietary measures should be taken in order to lower serum methionine and homocysteine. During anesthesia, adequate hydration is important and stockings should be used to prevent embolization (44). High doses of vitamin B6 (pyridoxine), the cofactor of the deficient enzyme, should be given in pyridoxine-positive responders. In nonresponders, diet, folic acid, and betaine were given (46).

Miotics should not be given to patients with Weill–Marchesani syndrome, as they increase the pupillary block and may induce an acute-angle closure attack; mydriatics should not be given because the small round lens tends to move forward through the dilated pupil (45). Peripheral iridectomy has been used to treat the acute attack (54). More recently, Ritch and Wand have suggested the following therapy for an acute attack: put the patient in a supine position, give systemic glycerin, topical moxi-sylyte (thymoxamine), and perform a laser iridectomy (69).

In metabolic disorders, a proper diet may sometimes be helpful. A low-sulfur amino acid diet may be used in patients with a sulfite oxidase deficiency (56).

Dietary therapy was suggested for the mild form of sulphite oxidase deficiency and resulted in clinical improvement (70). The diet was low in protein from natural foods and restricted in protein and sulfur amino acids. A synthetic amino acid mixture without methionine and cysteine was administered (70).

Genetic Counseling

MFS is an autosomal dominant disorder, with probably full penetrance and very variable expressivity. Although 50% of the offspring of a patient will be affected, the severity of the disorder cannot reliably be predicted. About 15% of all Marfan syndrome patients result from a new mutation. All other disorders in this group result from autosomal recessive inheritance. Parental consaguinity is common, and 25% of siblings will be affected. The risk for offspring is low in the recessive diseases if the patient does not marry within the same family.

Identification of the mutated gene is extremely important in cases of doubtful diagnosis, especially when metabolic tests are useless, as in MFS. A somewhat simpler method for molecular diagnosis of MFS was used by Judge and associates (71).

Prenatal diagnosis is especially important in the serious disorders. Blaszczyk and colleagues (72) performed preimplantation genetic diagnosis (PGD) for suspected MFS. Nine of 13 oocytes, taken from IVF embryos on day 3, were fertilized. Four were found negative for the mutation and pregnancy was continued. All were born without signs of MFS (72). Prenatal diagnosis by chorionic villus sampling successfully predicted the outcome in one family with molybdenum cofactor deficiency (73). Both metabolic tests for sulfite oxidase activity and a search for MOCS1 mutations were performed.

ECTOPIA LENTIS AS AN ISOLATED OCULAR DISORDER

Introduction

Ectopia lentis in the form of a subluxated lens may occur as an isolated manifestation of a hereditary disease unassociated with any extraocular manifestations. In such cases, it may be congenital, or of late onset, or associated with another ocular anomaly such as displacement of the pupil.

It is difficult to know what the true incidence is of associated vs. isolated ectopia lentis. A study of 148 patients with ectopia lentis, published in 1950, has claimed that 6% were "associated with arachnodactyly," whereas 94% had systemic abnormalities (74). However, these figures only stress that an inadequate investigation of a patient with ectopia lentis may not reveal the systemic nature of the disorder. There is little doubt that the true figures for associated ectopia lentis are far higher than 6% of all subluxated lenses.

In Denmark a national register of all cases of congenital ectopia lentis documented 396 patients or 0.83 cases per 10,000 newborns (75). 68% had MFS, 21% had ectopia lentis of pupillae, 8% had autosomal dominant ectopia lentis, and about 1% each had homocystinuria, sulfide oxidase deficiency, and Weill–Marchesani syndrome (75).

As an isolated condition, ectopia lentis in its inheritedbilateral form should be distinguished from secondary lens subluxation caused by an enlarged eye (buphthalmos) or enlarged anterior segment (megalocornca) and from unilateral trauma.

Clinical and Genetic Types of Isolated Ectopia Lentis

Congenital Dominant Subluxaton of Lenses

This condition is transmitted by an autosomal dominant gene, usually with full penetrance and expressivity. The lenses are mostly displaced upward (76). The condition is not rare, and several families have been reported. The subluxation is bilateral, symmetric, and congenital.

Congenital dominant ectopia lentis is probably a heterogenous condition. In some families, linkage to the gene encoding fibrillin-1 (FBN1) associated with MFS, was found (33,77). These may, therefore, be allelic mutations on the FBN1 gene associated with a mild variant of MFS, which has no systemic or extraocular typical manifestations. Its sole expression in the family is ectopia lentis.

Congenital Recessive Subluxation of Lenses

Clinically similar to the dominant form, this condition is reportedly transmitted by an autosomal recessive gene (78), but its existence has yet to be confirmed (19).

Late-Onset Dominant Subluxation of Lenses

In this rare autosomal dominant disorder, subluxation occurs as a late phenomenon, with an onset between 20 and 65 years of age. The subluxation of the lenses is inferior (1), probably indicating a late degeneration of the zonules.

Ectopia Lentis et Pupillae

Ectopia lentis et pupillae (ELP) is a rare autosomal recessive disorder. Subluxation of the lenses is associated with displacement of the pupil (corectopia) and has been reported in several families (79,80).

Consanguinity of parents is frequently found. The condition seems to be congenital, nonprogressive, bilateral, and symmetric. In addition, patients have microspherophakia, miosis, and poor pupillary dilation with mydriatics (79). Some family members may have only lens subluxation without the pupillary displacement (79). The displacement of the lens may be in any direction, and the edge of the lens often bisects the pupil, causing diplopia. There is an increased transillumination of the iris periphery, possibly indicating a defect in the posterior pigmented layer of iris (79). This layer is of neuroectodermal origin, as are the zonule and the dilator iridis muscle, the three structures involved in this disorder.

The largest series of 16 patients with ELP was evaluated by Goldberg (81). He found variability of phenotypic expression between the eyes of the same patient and among different affected members of the same family. The clinical findings included displacement of the lens and pupil, severe axial myopia, abnormal iris transillumination, poor pupillary dilatation, persistent pupillary membranes, iridohyaloid adhesions, and prominent iris processes. Occasionally, enlarged corneal diameters, cataract, or retinal detachment were found. Poor vision was caused by a combination of various possible factors: ectopic and misshapen crystalline lenses, axial myopia, corneal astigmatism, and irreversible amblyopia (82).

Cataracts were seen before the age of 40 in all affected members of a three-generation family, probably manifesting pseudodominance (83). Lack of definition of the ciliary processes and a membrane-like structure attached anteriorly to the proximal pupillary margin may be related to the displacement of the lens and the pupil (84).

Other Conditions

One report of a family with congenital ectopia lentis, high myopia, and blepharoptosis, transmitted by an autosomal dominant gene, may indicate a separate disorder from congenital dominant subluxation of lenses (85).

Pathology and Pathogenesis

It is possible that the morphologic and the pathogenetic changes of different genetic types of ectopia lentis are not the same. The primary abnormality leading to the lens subluxation seems to lie with the zonules. Some insight into the early zonular changes, preceding the actual subluxation of the lens, can be obtained from animal investigations. A hereditary luxation of the lens occurs not infrequently in dogs, especially terriers that develop a spontaneous bilateral dislocation of the lens in early to late middle age (86). In a study of Tibetan terriers, which have such an autosomal recessive spontaneous dislocation of the lens in their adult life, Curtis found zonular abnormalities that preceded lens subluxation (87). Scanning and electron microscopy have shown abnormal fibrillar material and reticulate and cobweblike formations bridging the gap between the ciliary processes and lens equator. This abnormality seems to reduce the tensile strength of the zonules, preceding an increased mobility of the lens, and later an actual subluxation.

Management

The surgical management, decisions, and methods for isolated ectopia lentis are similar to the aforementioned approaches for associated ectopia lentis.

Vitrectomy was successfully used to treat a phacolytic glaucoma in a patient with ELP when the cataracts were very dense (88).

Genetic counseling should be given according to the mode of transmission of the disorder in any particular family. Autosomal dominant traits in this group are usually with full penetrance and so, on the average, 50% of the children will be affected. Patients and their families should be warned about the possible complications of a subluxated lens and about the possible danger of even mild trauma. Affected patients should probably not wear contact lenses because of the risks of ocular manipulations.

ANTERIOR LENTICONUS AND ALPORT SYNDROME

Anterior lenticonus, consisting of a bulge in the front part of the lens, is so intimately associated with Alport syndrome that the two will be discussed together. Alport syndrome is a multisystem disorder, with three major findings: chronic nephritis, nerve deafness, and specific ocular abnormalities.

Hereditary nephritis with hematuria and proteinuria is common in patients with Alport syndrome, but its severity varies. In families with Alport syndrome, males are affected more than females, and renal failure is much more common in affected males than in affected females. In one study 18 of 42 boys and only 2 of 16 girls had renal failure (89). Ultrastructurally, a kidney biopsy specimen shows abnormalities of glomerular basement membrane in the form of thickening, splitting, or thinning (89).

The hearing defect, a congenital disorder of the inner ear, is found in about half of all cases of Alport syndrome. As in the case of nephritis, males are affected with the hearing defect more than females, at a ratio of 3:2, respectively (90).

Anterior lenticonus seems to be exclusive to Alport syndrome (91), but other ocular abnormalities are also common. In the posterior pole, whitish gray dots in the superficial layers of the retina have been described (92,93). These small (20–100 μm) flecks are commonly found in the macular area and are nondetectable by fluorescein angiography. In addition, retinal flecks in the deeper layers are observed in the midperiphery (94). These deeper-lying flecks are larger and can be confluent. They often look like drusen or may be present along with drusen. Fluorescein angiography shows spots of "window defects."

The retinopathy may consist of a maculopathy and midperipheral retinopathy. In the macula, typical flecks similar to those seen in cone dystrophies, are manifested by fluorescein angiography as "bull's eye" maculopathy (95). In the periphery, yellow dots, or larger flecks, can often be seen in the nasal periphery (96–98). Usually, the EOG findings are normal, whereas the reported ERG studies were normal or somewhat impaired (99). The cornea may show variable signs of involvement of the posterior limiting membranes, similar to posterior polymorphous corneal dystrophy (100).

Sporadic, nonspecific ocular abnormalities in the form of cataract (posterior subcapsular), arcus cornealis (bilateral and symmetric), and myopia have been also described as frequent manifestations of Alport syndrome (94). All are age-dependent. Only 17% of patients in the first two decades of life have a corneal arc, whereas 100% of patients in the fourth decade of life manifest it (94).

The common denominator for the variety of findings in the eye and in other organs is an involvement of membranes. It is conceivable that Alport syndrome is a widespread disease of the basement membranes (94,100–102) in the intraocular abnormalities, in the middle ear, and in the kidney.

Spontaneous ruptures of the anterior capsule may occur due to the abnormal basement membranes (103).

Alport syndrome may well be underdiagnosed, as its incidence is 1:5000 (100,102).

The diagnosis is made when three criteria out of the following five are present: progressive intra-auricular deafness with high tones involved, the previously described eye anomalies, family history, glomerular abnormalities, and hematuria or microhematuria (104–106). Ocular signs occur in a proportion of cases; 24% according to one study (105).

Alport syndrome has been described in the literature as autosomal dominant, X-linked dominant, heterogenous (in some cases dominant: X-linked or autosomal, in others recessive), partially X-Iinked, or X-influenced (89). Father-to-son transmission has been described, but the risk to sons is lower when the father is affected and not the mother (13 vs. 42%), whereas the risk to daughters is not very different when the father is affected (53%) than when the mother is affected (45%) (90). Anterior lenticonus has been described in a female patient with a 45,XO karyotype (107).

It is now accepted that Alport syndrome may be transmitted by any one of three modes of transmission, indicating genetic heterogeneity, but phenotypically the disorder seems homogenous (100). X-linked transmission is the commonest, with 85% of all cases, autosomal recessive with 10%, and autosomal dominant with 5% (100). The gene associated with X-linked AS has been mapped to chromosome Xq22 (108,109,111,119–122). An intragenic deletion in the COL4A5 gene in the Xq22 region was identified in three patients with AS (109). The gene product is collagen alpha 5(IV), which is a specific component of the glomelular basement membrane within the kidney (109). A large number of mutations in patients with XLAS was described. These included deletions, rearrangement, frameshift mutations (110), missense mutations (111), splice-site mutations (112), and others. A wide variability of phenotypes is the result (110). Comparing missense mutations, Barker and colleagues (111) concluded that with the Cysl564Ser mutation, renal disease occurs earlier and is more severe than with the Lenl649Arg mutation (111). Jais et al. (112) showed that the risk for renal failure was much higher (90%) with large deletions or nonsense mutations or frameshifts when compared to missense mutations (112).

A nationwide search for AS in Finland detected 34 patients from 14 different families (113). 57% had COL4A5 mutations. Ocular abnormalities were rare in childhood, but increased with age. Terminal renal failure occurred in four of five males and in one of five females (113).

In autosomal recessive Alport syndrome (ARAS), mutations in the COL4A3 and in the COL4A4 were detected (114–116). The two genes have a head to head position with a common bidirectional promoter in the center (114,116). The genes were mapped to chromosomes 2q35–q37 (117). The disease occurs with nonsense mutation and it appears that most missense mutations are not pathogenic (115).

Disease-causing mutations transmitted as an autosomal dominant trait were also identified in the same gene as in ARAS (117). The COL4A4 gene was coded and characterized. It has 48 exons and spans 113 kb or more (118).

POSTERIOR LENTICONUS

Posterior lenticonus is a rare disorder, usually sporadic, unilateral, and of unknown etiology or pathogenesis. About 100 cases had been reported between 1888 and 1968 (46). Clinically it is observed as the "oil-drop" phenomenon, but posterior cortical cataract is found in front of the posterior lenticonus in about 80%, reducing vision even further.

In familial cases, the mode of transmission is autosomal dominant (46,47). In one family, two siblings were affected, whereas both parents were normal (47). This could indicate an autosomal recessive transmission or, more likely, incomplete penetrance. In hereditary cases the condition is always bilateral (120).

On the other hand, a recent study indicated that in Britain, the disease is usually transmitted by the X-linked recessive mode. Eleven out of 13 families with posterior lenticonus showed this mode of transmission (130).

Visual acuity is usually decreased early in life, and amblyopia and strabismus are common. In a report on the surgery of 19 eyes with posterior lenticonus, Crouch and Parks reported good results using the aspiration technique, occlusion therapy, and contact lens in unilateral cases (121).

MICROSPHEROPHAKIA

A small lens of abnormal shape is the typical manifestation of Weill–Marchesani syndrome. However, microspherophakia may be found in isolated form or in association with another syndrome. The lens may be subluxated or dislocated.

In one family, five of eight siblings were affected (122). In addition to the microspherophakia, clinical problems included lenticular myopia, poor accommodative reserves, and glaucoma of the acute-angle closure type. The mode of transmission was autosomal recessive, similar to that in another family displaying microspherophakia with arachnodactyly, dwarfism, beaked nose, micrognathia and microstomia, mental retardation, and tapetoretinal degeneration (123). It is possible that for all of these families the manifestation is a variant of Weill–Marchesani syndrome, transmitted by the same autosomal recessive gene or by another gene.

A study of the anatomy and ultrastructure of microspherophakia does not show the lens to be small and round but wider posteriorly and narrower in front, the exact opposite of normal (124). Both lens fibers and zonular fibers are abnormal. Lens fibers are abnormal in distribution, size (about one-fifth of normal in cross diameter), and structure, whereas zonular fibers are normal or abnormally large and attached only to the lens (124).

APHAKIA

Congenital aphakia is not known as an inherited disorder in humans. However, it has been well described in the mouse. In a strain of mutant mice, AK, aphakia is transmitted by an autosomal recessive gene (125). In spite of a normal developing retina, the whole eye remains microphthalmic because of lack of growth stimulation from the lens (126). In humans, spontaneous absorption of the lens in early childhood has been described in congenital rubella syndrome (127,128), but not in hereditary conditions.

REFERENCES

1. Nelson LB, Maumenee IH. Ectopia lentis. Surv Ophthalmol 1982; 27:143–160.
2. Koch HR, Wegener A. Anomalies of the lens. In: Emery AEH, Rimoin DL, eds. Principlesand Practice of Medical Genetics. Edinburgh: Churchill-Livingston, 1983: 509–521.
3. De Paepe A, Devereux RB, Dietz HC, et al. Revised diagnostic criteria for the Marfan syndrome. Am J Med Genet 1996; 62:417–426.
4. Taylor RH, Burke J, O'Keefe M, et al. Ophthalmic abnormalities in homocystinuria: the value of screening. Eye 1998; 12:427–430.
5. Kainulainen K, Pulkkinen L, Savolainen A, et al. Location on chromosome 15 of the gene defect causing Marfan syndrome. N Engl J Med 1990; 323:935–939.
6. Lee B, Godfrey M, Vitale E, et al. Linkage of Marfan syndrome and a phenotypically related disorder to two different fibrillin genes. Nature 1991; 352:330–334.
7. Dietz HC, Cutting GR, Pyeritz RE, et al. Marfan syndrome caused by a recurrent de novo missense mutation in the fibrillin gene. Nature 1991; 352:337–339.
8. Munke M, Kraus JP, Ohura T, Francke U. The gene for cystathionine beta-synthase (CBS) maps to the subtelomeric region on human chromosome 21q and to proximal mouse chromosome 17. Am J Hum Genet 1988; 42:550–559.
9. Chasse JF, Paul V, Escanez R, et al. Human cystathionine beta-synthase: gene organization and expression of different 5′ alternative splicing. Mamm Genome 1997; 8:917–921.
10. Kraus JP, Janosik M, Kozich V, et al. Cystathionine beta-synthase mutations in homocystinuria. Hum Mutat 1999; 13:362–375.
11. Faivre L, Megarbane A, Alswaid A, et al. Homozygosity mapping of a Weill-Marchesani syndrome locus chromosome 19pl3.3-pl3.2. Hum Genet 2002; 110:366–370.
12. Faivre L, Gorlin RJ, Wirtz MK, et al. In frame fibrillin-1 gene deletion in autosomal dominant Weill-Marchesani syndrome. J Med Genet 2003; 40:34–36.
13. Wirtz MK, Samples JR, Kramer PL, et al. Weill-Marchesani syndrome—possible linkage of the autosomal dominant form to 15q21.1. Am J Med Genet 1996; 65:68–75.
14. Sacksteder KA, Biery BJ, Morrell JC, et al. Identification of the alpha-aminoadipic semi-aldehyde synthase gene, which is defective in familial hyperlysinemia. Am J Hum Genet 2000; 66:1736–1743.
15. Garrett RM, Johnson JL, Graf TN, et al. Human sulfite oxidase R160Q: identification of the mutation in a sulfite oxidase-deficient patient and expression and characterization of the mutant enzyme. Proc Natl Acad Sci USA 1998; 95:6394–6398.
16. Edwards MC, Johnson JL, Marriage B, et al. Isolated sulfite oxidase deficiency: review of two cases in one family. Ophthalmology 1999; 106:1957–1961.
17. Johnson JL, Coyne KE, Garrett RM, et al. Isolated sulfite oxidase deficiency: identification of 12 novel SUOX mutations in 10 patients. Hum Mutat 2002; 20:74.
18. Reiss J. Genetics of molybdenum cofactor deficiency. Hum Genet 2000; 106:157–163.
19. http://www.ncbi.nlm.nih.gov/omim.

20. Loughlin J, Irven C, Hardwick LJ, et al. Linkage of the gene that encodes the alpha 1 chain of type V collagen (COL5A1) to type II Ehlers-Danlos syndrome (EDS II). Hum-Mol Genet 1995; 4:1649–1651.
21. Marfan AB. Un cas de déformation congénitale des quatre membres plus prononcée aux extrémitiés charactérisés par l'allongement dcs os avec un certain degré d'amincissement. Bull Mem Soc Med Hop Paris 1896; 13:220.
22. Pyeritz RE, McKusick VA. The Marfan syndrome. N Engl J Med 1979; 300:772–777.
23. Cross HE, Jensen AD. Ocular manifestations in the Marfan syndrome and homocystinuria. Am J Ophthalmol 1973; 75:405–420.
24. Maumenee IH. The eye in the Marfan syndrome. Birth Defects 1982; 18:515–524.
25. Sultan G, Baudouin C, Auzerie O, et al. Cornea in Marfan disease: orbscan and in vivo confocal microscopy analysis. Invest Ophthalmol Vis Sci 2002; 43:1757–1764.
26. Steinberg I. A simple screening test for the Marfan syndrome. Am J Roentgenol 1966; 97:118–124.
27. Walker BA, Murdoch JL. The wrist sign: a useful physical finding in the Marfan syndrome. Arch Intern Med 1970; 126:276–277.
28. Rose PS, Levy HP, Ahn NU, et al. A comparison of the Berlin and Ghent nosologies and the influence of dural ectasia in the diagnosis of Marfan syndrome. Genet Med 2000; 2:278–282.
29. Ramsey MS, Fine BS, Shields JA, Yanoff M. The Marfan syndrome: a histopathologic study of ocular findings. Am J Ophthalmol 1973; 76:102–116.
30. Farnsworth PN, Burke P, Dotto ME, Cinotti AA. Ultrastructural abnormalities in a Marfan's syndrome lens. Arch Ophthalmol 1977; 95:1601–1606.
31. Pyeritz RE, McKusick VA. Basic defects in the Marfan syndrome. N Engl J Med 1981; 305:1011–1012.
32. Boucek RJ, Noble NL, Gunja-Smith Z, Butler WT. The Marfan syndrome: a deficiency in chemically stable collagen cross-links. N Engl J Med 1981; 305:988–991.
33. Tsipouras P, Del Mastro R, Sarfarazi M, et al. Genetic linkage of the Marfan syndrome, ectopia lentis, and congenital contractural arachnodactyly to the fibrillin genes on chromosomes 15 and 5. The International Marfan Syndrome Collaborative Study. N Engl J Med 1992; 326:905–909.
34. Dietz HC, Pyeritz RE. Mutations in the human gene for fibrillin-l (FBN1) in the Marfan syndrome and related disorders. Hum Mol Genet 1995; 4:1799–1809.
35. Collod-Beroud G, Beroud C, Ades L, et al. Marfan Database (third edition): new mutations and new routines for the software. Nucleic Acids Res 1998; 26:229–233.
36. Wheatley HM, Traboulsi El, Flowers BE, et al. Immunohistochemical localization of fibrillin in human ocular tissues. Relevance to the Marfan syndrome. Arch Ophthalmol 1995; 113:103–109.
37. Loeys BL, Matthys DM, de Paepe AM. Genetic fibrillinopathies: new insights in molecular diagnosis and clinical management. Acta Clin Belg 2003; 58:3–11.
38. Katzke S, Booms P, Tiecke F, et al. TGGE screening of the entire FBN1 coding sequence in 126 individuals with Marfan syndrome and related fibrillinopathies. Hum Mutat 2002; 20:197–208.
39. Kainulainen K, Karttunen L, Puhakka L, et al. Mutations in the fibrillin gene responsible for dominant ectopia lentis and neonatal Marfan syndrome. Nat Genet 1994; 6:64–69.
40. Lonnqvist L, Child A, Kainulainen K, et al. A novel mutation of the fibrillin gene causing ectopia lentis. Genomics 1994; 19:573–576.
41. Montgomery RA, Geraghty MT, Bull E, et al. Multiple molecular mechanisms underlying subdiagnostic variants of Marfan syndrome. Am J Hum Genet 1998; 63: 1703–1711.
42. Liu W, Qian C, Francke U. Silent mutation induces exon skipping of fibrillin-1 gene in Marfan syndrome. Nat Genet 1997; 16:328–329.

43. Vital MC, Mintz-Hittner HA, Milewicz DM. Microcornea and subluxated lenses due to a splicing error in the fibrillin-1 gene in a patient with Marfan syndrome. Arch Ophthalmol 2003; 121:579–581.
44. Collod G, Babron MC, Jondeau G, et al. A second locus for Marfan syndrome maps to chromosome 3p24.2-p25. Nat Genet 1994; 8:264–268.
45. Cross HE. Differential diagnosis and treatment of dislocated lenses. Birth Defects 1976; 7:335.
46. Cruysberg JR, Boers GH, Trijbels JM, Deutman AF. Delay in diagnosis of homocystinuria: retrospective study of consecutive patients. Br Med J 1996; 313:1037–1040.
47. Spaeth GL. The usefulness of pyridoxine in the treatment of homocystinuria: A review of postulated mechanisms of action and a new hypothesis. Birth Defects 1976; 12: 347–354.
48. Harker LA, Slichter SJ, Scott CR, Ross R. Homocystinemia: Vascular injury and arterial thrombosis. N Engl J Med 1974; 291:537–543.
49. Mandel H, Brenner B, Berant M, et al. Coexistence of hereditary homocystinuria and factor V Leiden—effect on thrombosis. N Engl J Med 1996; 334:763–768.
50. Peterschmitt MJ, Simmons JR, Levy HL. Reduction of false negative results in screening of newborns for homocystinuria. N Engl J Med 1999; 341:1572–1574.
51. Mudd SH, Havlik R, Levy HL, McKusick VA, Feinleib M. A study of cardiovascular risk in heterozygotes for homocystinuria. Am J Hum Genet 1981; 33:883–893.
52. Weill G. Ectopie des cristallins et malformations generales. Ann Oculist 1932; 169: 21–44.
53. Marchesani O. Brachydaktylie und angeborene Kugellinse als Systemerkrankung. KlinMonatsbl Augenheilkd 1939; 103:392–406.
54. Jensen AD, Cross HE, Paton D. Ocular complications in the Weill-Marchesani syndrome. Am J Ophthalmol 1974; 77:261–269.
55. Smith TH, Holland MG, Woody NG. Ocular manifestations of familial hyperlysinemia. Trans Am Acad Ophthalmol Otolaryngol 1971; 75:355–360.
56. Shih VE, Abroms IF, Johnson JL, Carney M, Mandell BA, Robb RM, Cloherty JP, Rajagopalan KV. Sulfite oxidase deficiency: biochemical and clinical investigations of a hereditary metabolic disorder in sulfur metabolism. N Engl J Med 1977; 297:1022–1028.
57. Beemer FA, Deeleman JW. Combined deficiency of xanthine oxidase and sulfite oxidase; ophthalmological findings in a 3-week-old girl. Metab Pediatr Ophthalmol 1980; 4:49–52.
58. Parini R, Briscioli V, Caruso U, et al. Spherophakia associated with molybdenum cofactor deficiency. Am J Med Genet 1997; 73:272–275.
59. Thomas C, Cordier J, Algan B. Les alterations oculaires de la maladie d'Ehlers-Danlos. Arch Ophthalmol (Paris) 1954; 14:691–697.
60. Strisciuglio P. Vildervanck's syndrome with bilateral subluxation of lens and facial paralysis. J Med Genet 1983; 20:72–73.
61. Seetner AA, Crawford JS. Surgical correction of lens dislocation in children. Am J Ophthalmol 1981; 91:106–110.
62. Pollack JS, Custer PL, Hart WM, et al. Ocular complications in Ehlers-Danlos syndrome type IV. Arch Ophthalmol 1997; 115:416–419.
63. Peyman GA, Raichand M, Goldberg MF, Ritacca D. Management of subluxated and dislocated lenses with the vitrophage. Br J Ophthalmol 1979; 63:771–778.
64. Halpert M, BenEzra D. Surgery of the hereditary subluxated lens in children. Ophthalmology 1996; 103:681–686.
65. Koenig SB, Mieler WF. Management of ectopia lentis in a family with Marfan syndrome. Arch Ophthalmol 1996; 114:1058–1061.
66. Plager DA, Parks MM, Helveston EM, Ellis FD. Surgical treatment of subluxated lenses in children. Ophthalmology 1992; 99:1018–1023.

67. Harrison DA, Mullaney PB, Mesfer SA, et al. Management of ophthalmic complications of homocystinuria. Ophthalmology 1998; 105:1886–1890.
68. Gerding H. Ocular complications and a new surgical approach to lens dislocation in homocystinuria due to cystathionine-beta-synthetase deficiency. Eur J Pediatr 1998; 157(suppl 2):S94–S101.
69. Ritch R, Wand M. Treatment of the Weill-Marchesani syndrome. Ann Ophthalmol 1981; 13:665–667.
70. Touati G, Rusthoven E, Depondt E, et al. Dietary therapy in two patients with a mild form of sulphite oxidase deficiency. Evidence for clinical and biological improvement. J Inherit Metab Dis 2000; 23:45–53.
71. Judge DP, Biery NJ, Dietz HC. Characterization of microsatellite markers flanking FBNl: utility in the diagnostic evaluation for Marfan syndrome. Am J Med Genet 2001; 99:39–47.
72. Blaszczyk A, Tang YX, Dietz HC, et al. Preimplantation genetic diagnosis of human embryos for Marfan's syndrome. J Assist Reprod Genet 1998; 15:281–284.
73. Reiss J, Christensen E, Dorche C. Molybdenum cofactor deficiency: first prenatal genetic analysis. Prenatal Diag 1999; 19:386–388.
74. Lund A, Sjontoft F. Congenital ectopia lentis. Acta Ophthalmol 1950; 28:33–48.
75. Fuchs J, Rosenberg T. Congenital ectopia lentis. A Danish national survey. Acta Ophthalmol Scand 1998; 76:20–26.
76. Saureguy BM, Hall JG. Isolated congenital ectopia lentis with autosomal dominant inheritance. Clin Genet 1979; 15:97–109.
77. Edwards MJ, Challinor CJ, Colley PW, et al. Clinical and linkage study of a large family with simple ectopia lentis linked to FBNl. Am J Med Genet 1994; 53:65–71.
78. Ruiz C, Rivas F, Villar-Calvo VM, et al. Familial simple ectopia lentis. A probable autosomal recessive form. Ophthalmic Paediatr Genet 1986; 7:81–85.
79. Luebbers JA, Goldberg MF, Herbst R, Hattenhauer J, Maumenee AE. Iris transillumination and variable expression in ectopia lentis et pupllae. Am J Ophthalmol 1977; 83:647–656.
80. Cross HE. Ectopia lentis et pupiliae. Am J Ophthalmol 1979; 88:381–384.
81. Goldberg MF. Clinical manifestations of ectopia lentis et pupiliae in 16 patients. Ophthalmology 1988; 95:1080–1087.
82. Goldberg MF. Clinical manifestations of ectopia lentis et pupillae in 16 patients. Trans Am Ophthalmol Soc 1988; 86:158–177.
83. Cruysberg JR, Pinckers A. Ectopia lentis et pupillae syndrome in three generations. Br J Ophthalmol 1995; 79:135–138.
84. Byles DB, Nischal KK, Cheng H. Ectopia lentis et pupillae. A hypothesis revisited. Ophthalmology 1998; 105:1331–1336.
85. Gillum WN, Anderson RL. Dominantly inherited blepharoptosis, high myopia and ectopia lentis. Arch Ophthalmol 1982; 100:282–284.
86. Curtis R. Hereditary luxation of the canine lens. Trans Ophthalmol Soc UK 1982; 102:398–402.
87. Curtis R. Aetiopathological aspects of inherited lens dislocation in the Tibetan terrier. J Comp Pathol 1983; 93:151–163.
88. Rossiter JD, Morris AH, Etchells DE, Crick MP. Vitrectomy for phacolytic glaucoma in a patient with ectopia lentis et pupillae. Eye 2003; 17:243–244.
89. Gubler M, Levy M, Broyer M, Naizot C, Gonzales G, Perrin D, Habib R. Alport's syndrome: a report of 58 cases and a review of the literature. Am J Med 1981; 70:493–505.
90. Dahm K, Koch HR, Sieder M, Lerche W, Neumann OG, Passarge E. Familiares Alport syndrom mit vorderem Lenticonus. Dtsch Med Wachenschr 1974; 99:1252–1255.
91. Nielsen CE. Lenticonus anterior and Alport's syndrome. Acta Ophthalmol 1978; 56:518–530.
92. Polak BCP, Hogewind BL. Macular lesions in Alport's syndrome. Am J Ophthalmol 1977; 84:532–535.

93. Zylberman R, Silverstone B-Z, Brandes E, Drukker A. Retinal lesions in Alport's syndrome. J Pediatr Ophthalmol 1980; 17:255–260.
94. Govan JAA. Ocular manifestations of Alport's syndrome: a hereditary disorder of basement membranes. Br J Ophthalmol 1983; 67:493–503.
95. Setala K, Ruusuvaara P. Alport syndrome with hereditary macular degeneration. Acta Ophthalmol 1989; 67:409–414.
96. Gelisken O, Hendrikse F, Schroder CH, Berden JH. Retinal abnormalities in Alport's syndrome. Acta Ophthalmol 1988; 66:713–717.
97. Blasi MA, Rinaldi R, Renieri A, et al. Dot-and-fleck retinopathy in Alport syndrome caused by a novel mutation in the COL4A5 gene. Am J Ophthalmol 2000; 130:130–131.
98. Polak BC, Hogewind BL. Macular lesions in Alport's disease. Am J Ophthalmol 1977; 84:532–535.
99. Bhatnagar R, Kumar A, Pakrasi S. Alport's syndrome: ocular manifestations and unusual features. Acta Ophthalmol 1990; 68:347–349.
100. Colville DJ, Savige J. Alport syndrome: a review of ocular manifestations. Ophthalmic Genet 1997; 18:161–173.
101. Colville D, Savige J, Branley P, Wilson D. Ocular abnormalities in thin basement membrane disease. Br J Ophthalmol 1997; 81:373–377.
102. Colville D, Savige J, Morfis M, et al. Ocular manifestations of autosomal recessive Alport syndrome. Ophthalmic Genet 1997; 18:119–128.
103. Satish KR, Chandrashekar N, Pai V, et al. Spontaneous capsular ruptures in Alport syndrome. Ann Ophthalmol 2001; 33:131–135.
104. Junk AK, Stefani FH, Ludwig K. Bilateral anterior lenticonus: Scheimpflug imaging system documentation and ultrastructural confirmation of Alport syndrome in the lens capsule. Arch Ophthalmol 2000; 118:895–897.
105. Thompson SM, Deady JP, Willshaw HE, White RH. Ocular signs in Alport's syndrome. Eye 1987; 1:146–153.
106. Sabates R, Krachmer JH, Weingeist TA. Ocular findings in Alport's syndrome. Ophthalmologica 1983; 186:204–210.
107. Kapoor S, Dasgupta J. Chromosomal anomaly in a female patient with anterior lenticonus. Ophthalmologica 1979; 179:271–275.
108. Atkin CL, Hasstedt SJ, Menlove L, et al. Mapping of Alport syndrome to the long arm of the X chromosome. Am J Hum Genet 1988; 42:249–255.
109. Barker DF, Hostikka SL, Zhou J, et al. Identification of mutations in the COL4A5 collagen gene in Alport syndrome. Science 1990; 248:1224–1227.
110. Renieri A, Galli L, De Marchi M, et al. Single base pair deletions in exons 39 and 42 of the COL4A5 gene in Alport syndrome. Hum Mol Genet 1994; 3:201–202.
111. Barker DF, Pruchno CJ, Jiang X, et al. A mutation causing Alport syndrome with tardive hearing loss is common in the western United States. Am J Hum Genet 1996; 58:1157–1165.
112. Jais JP, Knebelmann B, Giatras I, et al. X-linked Alport syndrome: natural history in 195 families and genotype-phenotype correlations in males. J Am Soc Nephrol 2000; 11:649–657.
113. Pajari H, Setala K, Heiskari N, et al. Ocular findings in 34 patients with Alport syndrome: correlation of the findings to mutations in COL4A5 gene. Acta Ophthalmol Scand 1999; 77:214–217.
114. Mariyama M, Zheng K, Yang-Feng TL, Reeders ST. Colocalization of the genes for the alpha 3(IV) and alpha 4(IV) chains of type IV collagen to chromosome 2 bands q35-q37. Genomics 1992; 13:809–813.
115. Lemmink HH, Mochizuki T, van den Heuvel LP, et al. Mutations in the type IV collagen alpha 3 (COL4A3) gene in autosomal recessive Alport syndrome. Hum Mol Genet 1994; 3:1269–1273.

116. Mochizuki T, Lemmink HH, Mariyama M, et al. Identification of mutations in the alpha 3(1 V) and alpha 4(IV) collagen genes in autosomal recessive Alport syndrome. Nat Genet 1994; 8:77–81.
117. Jefferson JA, Lemmink HH, Hughes AE, et al. Autosomal dominant Alport syndrome linked to the type IV collagen alpha 3 and alpha 4 genes (COL4A3 and COL4A4). Nephrol Dial Transpl 1997; 12:1595–1599.
118. Boye E, Mollet G, Forestier L, et al. Determination of the genomic structure of the COL4A4 gene and of novel mutations causing autosomal recessive Alport syndrome. Am J Hum Genet 1998; 63:1329–1340.
119. Howitt D, Hornblass A. Posterior lenticonus. Am J Ophthalmol 1968; 66:1133–1136.
120. Pollard ZF. Familial bilateral posterior lenticonus. Arch Ophthalmol 1983; 101: 1238–1240.
121. Crouch ER, Parks MM. Management of posterior lenticonus complicated by unilateral cataract. Am J Ophthalmol 1978; 85:503–508.
122. Johnson GJ, Bosanquet RC. Spherophakia in a Newfoundland family: eight years' experience. Can J Ophthalmol 1983; 18:159–164.
123. Sierpinski-Bart J, Neumann E, Tirosh E, Atias D. Tapetoretinal degeneration and mental retardation associated with microspherophakia and mesodermal abnormalities: a new syndrome. Metab Pediatr Ophthalmol 1981; 5:225–231.
124. Farnsworth PN, Burke PA, Blanco J, Maltzman B. Ultrastructural abnormalities in a microspherical ectopic lens. Exp Eye Res 1978; 27:399–408.
125. Varnum DS, Stevens LC. Aphakia, a new mutation in the mouse. J Hereditary 1968; 59:147–150.
126. Zwaan J. Role of the lens in growth of the eye. Ophthalmic Res 1979; 12:145–146.
127. Boger WP, Peterson RA, Robb RM. Spontaneous absorption of the lens in the congenital rubella syndrome. Arch Ophthalmol 1981; 99:433–434.
128. Ehrlich LH. Congenital rubella syndrome. Arch Ophthalmol 1981; 99:1867–1868.
129. Harrison DA, Mullaney PB, Mesfer SA, et al. Management of ophthalmic complications of homocystinuria. Ophthalmology 1998; 105:1886–1890.
130. Russell-Eggitt IM. Non-syndromic posterior lenticonus a cause of childhood cataract: evidence for X-linked inheritance. Eye 2000; 14:861–863.

8
Inherited Macular Diseases

INTRODUCTION

The term *heredomacular dystrophies,* or inherited macular dystrophies, is usually applied to a group of inherited macular afflictions that cause visible macular changes.The best known are Stargardt disease and Best disease, or vitelliform macular dystrophy. However, the macula responds to various insults in a stereotypical way. The same morphologic changes can be seen in Stargardt disease, in some cases of retinitis pigmentosa, and in an acquired iatrogenic disease: chloroquine retinopathy. A diffuse disease of the neural retina or of the retinal pigment epithelium may manifest itself as a maculopathy, sometimes with few or no foveal changes. In this chapter, I shall classify as inherited macular diseases such genetically determined retinal or retinal pigment epithelial (RPE) disorders that affect predominantly the macular area, either morphologically (by visible macular abnormalities) or functionally (by decreased visual acuity), or both. Widespread functional disorders of the cones, which affect the cone-rich macula, will be discussed in another chapter. Similarly, widespread abnormalities of the rods or of the choriocapillaris will be dealt with separately, except as mentioned for purposes of differential diagnosis in this chapter.

In the last decade, the most important genes and their macular disease-causative mutations were identified. The surprising discovery was that the same disease may result from mutations on a variety of genes and, conversely, that different mutations on a single gene may cause a variety of phenotypes (1). In an article named "ABCR Unites What Ophthalmologists Divide," Van Driel and colleagues stated that different combinations of ABCR (ABCA4) mutations give rise to very different phenotypes (2) ranging from typical Stargardt disease to retinitis pigmentosa. In other words, a gene associated with macular disease may cause a generalized retinal disorder when specifically mutated, while another gene associated with a generalized retinal disease, such as RDS/peripherin, may cause only maculopathy in specific mutations (3).

In order to avoid confusion in such circumstances, we will classify all disorders and subdivide this chapter according to the clinical entities, as they are well-known to the practicing ophthalmologist. The genes and disease-causative mutations will be discussed under their relative clinical headings.

STARGARDT DISEASE AND FUNDUS FLAVIMACULATUS

Description and Clinical Findings

Stargardt disease, as originally described by Stargardt in the beginning of the century (4–6), affects predominantly the macula by pigmentary changes in a ring form, associated with depigmentation and atrophy of the RPE and often accompanied by whitish yellow extramacular spots. The whitish yellow spots and lines were "rediscovered" and termed fundus flavimaculatus by Franceschetti (7,8). It is probably a heterogenous group of diseases, most inherited. The classification is not final, but an attempt at classification may be carried out as follows.

For many years, Stargardt disease was thought to be transmitted as an autosomal recessive trait. However, within the last two decades it became clear that additional modes of genetic transmission existed. These included the rare autosomal dominant mode involving several genes, which will be discussed in this subchapter. Mitochondrial DNA inheritance associated with a Stargardt-like disorder will be discussed separately.

The Clinical and Genetic Types

Stargardt Disease Type I

This term corresponds to Stargardt original clinical description of, although similar cases were described earlier (9). This disease is often referred to as juvenile hereditary macular degeneration or juvenile hereditary macular dystrophy. The onset of symptoms usually occurs at age 6–12 years, and it usually parallels the appearance of macular pigmentation. It affects both sexes equally and is transmitted by the autosomal recessive mode.

The disease is bilateral and symmetric. In its typical full-blown form, the foveal reflex is not seen and abnormalities at the level of the RPE can be noticed. This usually takes the form of a brownish center ("beaten bronze appearance") with spots of hyperpigmentation and depigmentation around it (Fig. 1a). Sometimes, the brownish center is missing, and pigmentary mottling or multiple depigmented spots are seen (see Fig. 1b). The funduscopic appearance is of atrophic changes at the level of the pigment epithelium.

A high percentage of patients with Stargardt disease type I have extramacular changes in the form of flavimaculatus flecks. This led to confusion and controversy over whether fundus flavimaculatus and Stargardt disease are the same disease. The flecks are similar in appearance to those described in pure fundus flavimaculatus, but their distribution in the fundus is not always completely over the posterior pole as described for fundus flavimaculatus. In fact, three forms of distribution of flecks have been described: one row of flecks around the central lesion (10), several rows of perimacular flecks, and diffusely scattered flecks up to the equator (11) (Fig. 2). The single row of flecks is often indistinguishable from the macular atrophic lesion alone. The two other types were found in about one-third of 42 patients in one study (12). This figure may increase with time, because new appearance and increase in the number of flecks have been described in other reports (13,14).

Fluorescein angiography typically shows the "bull's-eye phenomenon" (Fig. 3). A dark hypofluorescent center is surrounded by a wide ring of hypofluorescent spots ("window effect") and often by another ring of hyperpigmentation. The significant hypofluorescence in the macular area by fluorescein angiography, named the "silent

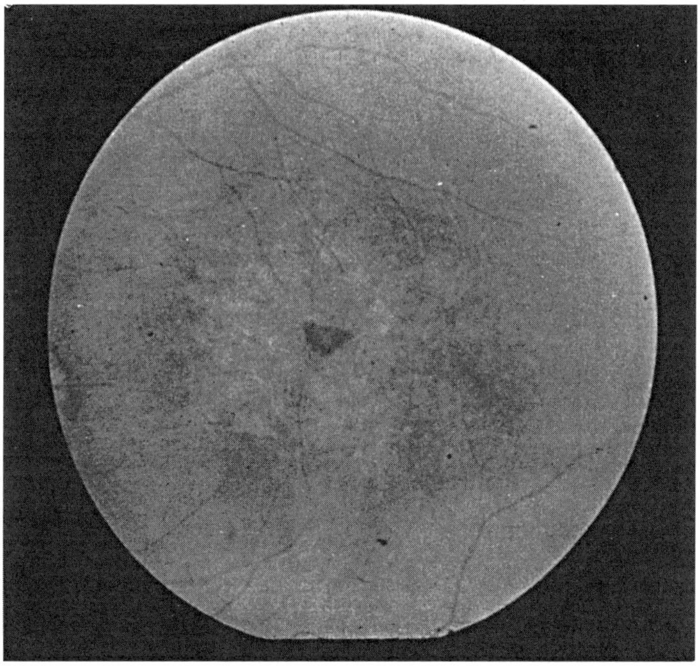

(a)

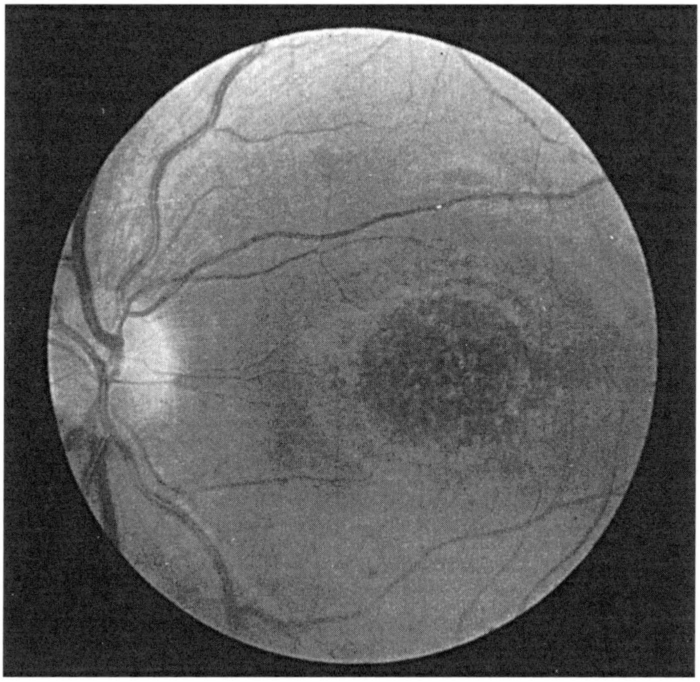

(b)

Figure 1 Two forms of macular dystrophy typical of Stargardt disease; (a)"beaten bronze" center with spots of depigmentation and hyperpigmentation around it and (b) spots of depigmentation and pigmentary mottling.

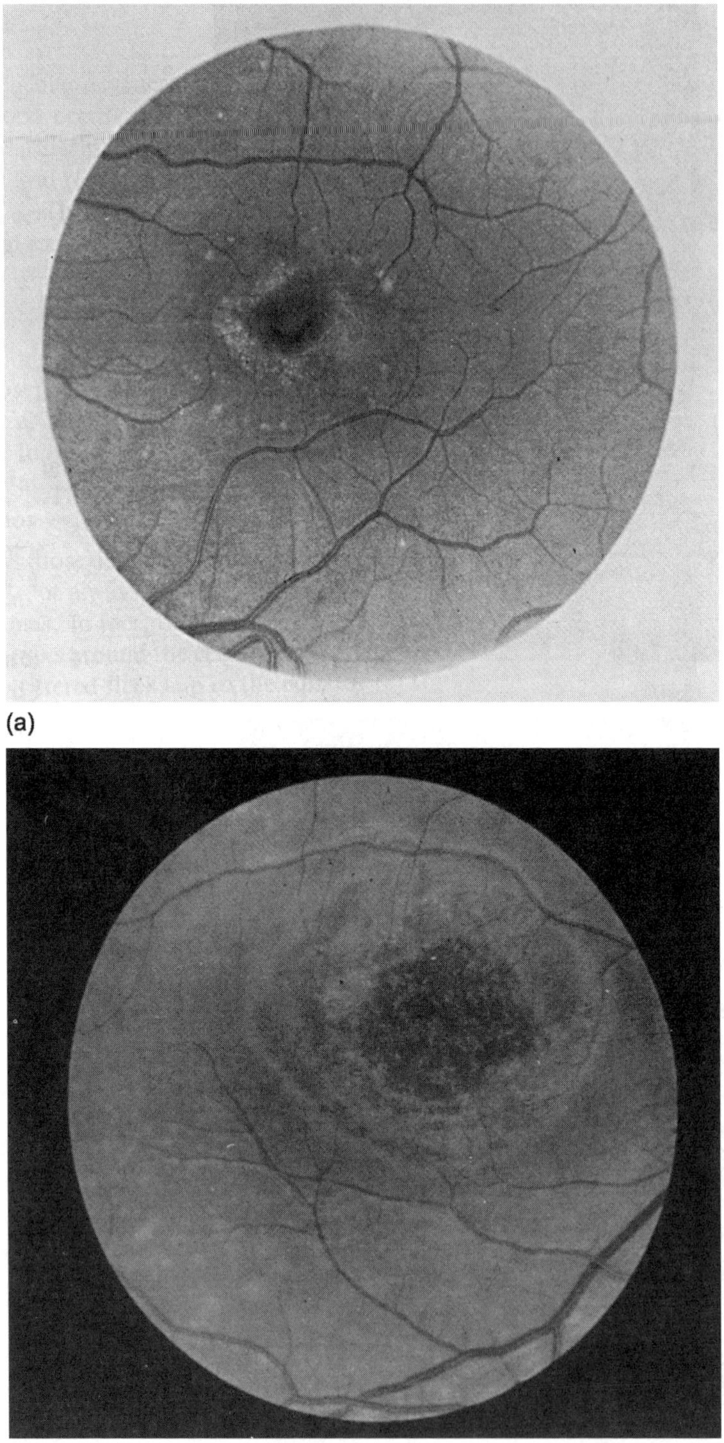

(a)

(b)

Figure 2 The relation of flavimaculatus flecks to the central lesion in three patients with Stargardt disease: (a) one row of flecks; (b) several circles of flecks in posterior pole; and (c) multiple flecks up to periphery.

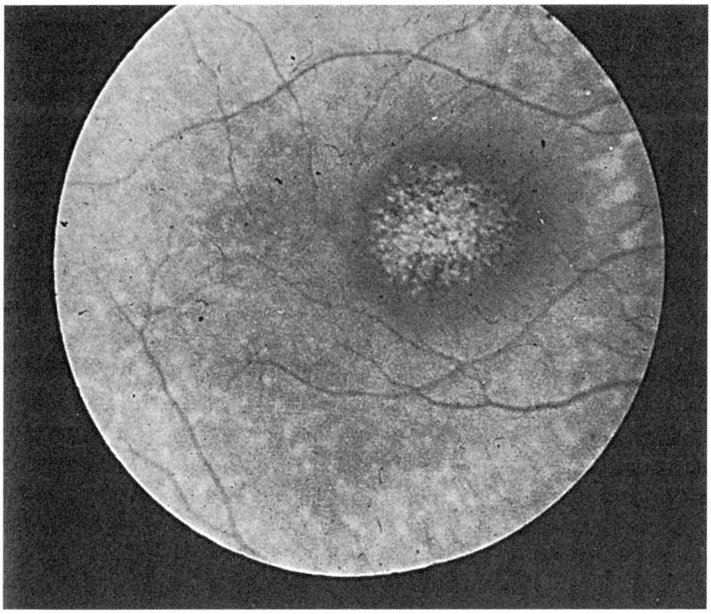

(c)

Figure 2 *(Continued)*

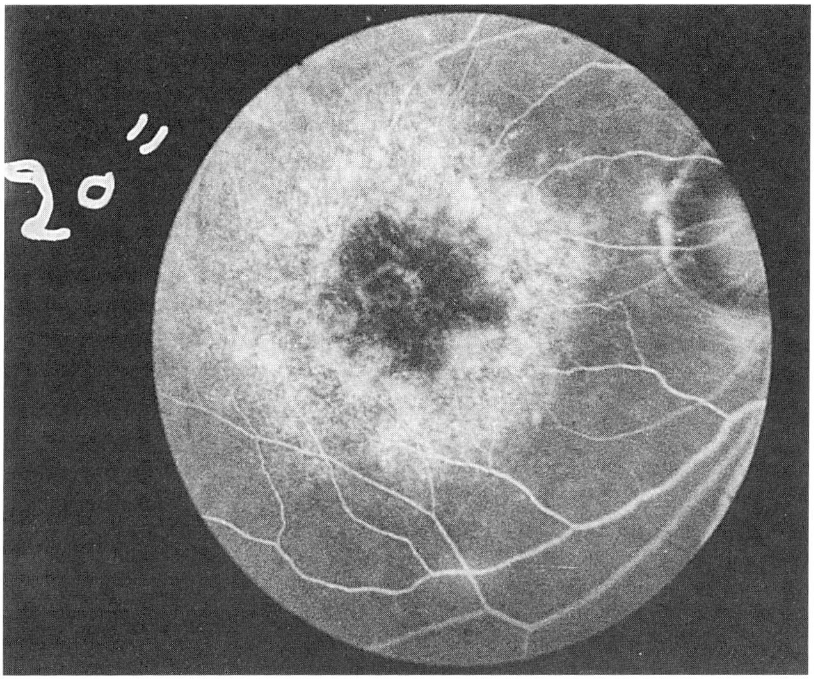

Figure 3 Fluorescein angiography of the fundus of Stargardt disease showing bull's-eye phenomenon 20 sec after injection.

AGE IN YEARS	NO.
6	4
7	4
8	9
9	2
10	5
12	4
13	1
15	1

Figure 4 Onset of visual symptoms in 30 patients with Stargardt diseases type I.

choroid" by Bonnin (15) and "dark choroid" by Fish et al. (16) is a peculiar finding of several heredomacular degenerations including Stargardt disease, and clinically suggests the deposition of an abnormal material in the RPE. Generally, the dark choroid phenomenon is family-specific. In one study of 14 families with heredomacular dystrophies, all but one had either a dark or a light choroid in all affected members (17). Fishman et al. (18) found that most of their 64 patients families with Stargardt disease showed the dark choroid sign by fluorescein angiography.

Stargardt disease type I is the term I use to describe a single clinical and genetic entity. It is an autosomal recessive disease with onset of symptoms most often in childhood (Fig. 4), although later occurrence has been described. The typical ("Stargardt-type") macular dystrophic changes occur in all affected individuals, and flavimaculatus flecks are apparent in some. The most important symptom is decrease in visual acuity, which usually begins at the same time as the abnormal macular changes, but sometimes may precede them (19). The deterioration in visual acuity is quite rapid (12,20) (Fig. 5), and the final visual outcome is poor. The distinction from other types of flavimaculatus or Stargardt disease is based on the symptomatology and its progression, the clinical examination, and fluorescein angiographic, psychophysical, and electrophysiologic evaluation (Table 1).

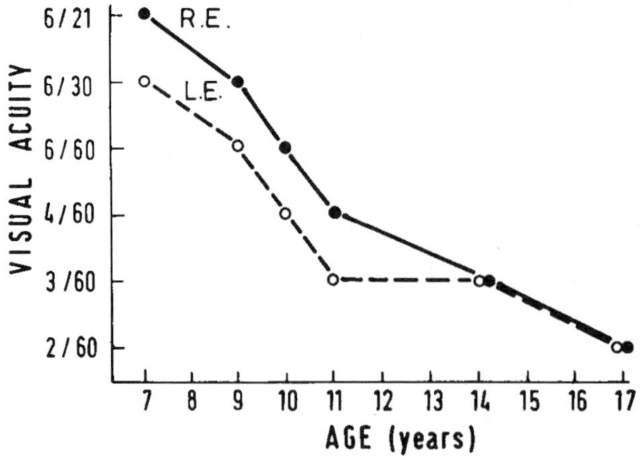

Figure 5 Stargardt disease type I: decrease of visual acuity in one patient over 10 years.

Table 1 Differential Diagnosis of Stargardt Disease and Fundus Flavimaculatus

	Stargardt disease type I	Stargardt disease type II	Fundus flavimaculatus	Atrophic maculopathy in cone and rod dystrophies
Usual age at onset of Symptoms (year)	6–10	18–35	Any age	10–40
Fundus: Macula	Atrophic maculopathy Stargardt-like	Similar to I	Normal	Similar to 1
Flavimaculatus flecks	In about one-third Usually not many	In all, many up to equator	In all, many up to equator	None or few
Other fundus changes	Mottling or RPE atrophy	Similar to I	None	None or bone corpuscular pigment
Visual acuity in final stages	1/60–6/60	1/60–6/60	Practically normal	1/60–6/30, sometimes lower
ERG, early	Normal	Normal	Normal	According to diagnosis
ERG, in late stages	Cones affected more than rods	Rods affected more than cones	Normal	According to diagnosis
Color vision	Predominant: deuteranopia	Predominant: unclassifiable	Normal	Various
EOG, early	Normal	Normal	Normal	Subnormal
EOG, in late stages	Slightly sub normal	Moderately sub normal	Normal	Moderately to severely sub-normal
Hereditary	Autosomal recessive	Nongenetic?	Autosomal recessive or nongenetic	Autosomal dominant or autosomal recessive

Visual acuity decreases gradually up to a point of stable, but low, visual acuity. A long-term follow-up of up to 22 years of 52 patients with Stargardt disease and 44 patients with fundus flavimaculatus indicated a reduction of visual acuity to a point usually about 20/200 and little change thereafter (21). Visual acuity was found to be related to the amount of macular pigment present. With normal pigment it was at least 20/40, with no pigment it was 20/200 or less, while with intermediate amounts, visual acuity ranged from 20/40 to 20/200 (22).

In 1993, Kaplan and associates (23) assigned the disease locus to chromosome 1p21–p13. About the same time, two autosomal dominant loci for Stargardt disease, another possible autosomal recessive locus, and the mitochondrial trait were recognized (24,25).

In 1997, Allikmets and colleagues (26), identified 19 different mutations in the gene ABCR after examining 48 families with Stargardt disease/fundus flavimaculatus. The locus STGD1 (for Stargardt disease) and the gene were mapped to chromosome 1p13–p21. The ABCR (R for retinal) gene was one of at least 21 human genes in the ATP-binding cassette transporter (ABC) superfamily of genes (26). The product of the gene, the ABCR protein, was localized within the photoreceptor cells. It was detected only in the disk membrane location of the rod outer segment and not in cones or any other retinal location (27). Gerber and associates (28) reported the structure of the gene. It is large, encompassing 50 exons. Immunofluorescence studies showed that ABCR protein is present in foveal and peripheral cones, as well as in rods (29). Later, the "official" name of the gene was changed to ABCA4, for ABC cassette, subfamily A, member 4. The early studies pointed to a large variety of disease-bearing mutations, with affected family members carrying homozygous or compound heterozygous alleles (26). By far, the most affected were compound heterozygotes, with both missense mutations or combined missense and nonsense mutations (26,28,30,31). Most mutations were in one of two ABC cassettes (see Fig. 6). The most frequently identified missense mutation in Caucasians was Gly863Ala (31).

Stargardt disease has a high allelic heterogeneity (32). Based on their studies of 40 patients with STGD1, Maugeri et al. hypothesized that there are mild mutations (usually missense) and severe mutations (usually nonsense or null mutations) (32). A mild mutation will be expressed phenotypically as severe disease only in conjunction with a severe allele. Webster and associates (33) also suggested that the phenotypic severity depends on the location of the mutation on the ABCA4 gene (33).

It became clear that a mutated ABCA4 gene may cause STGD1 or fundus flavimaculatus (FFM), as well as autosomal recessive retinitis pigmentosa (ARRP) or

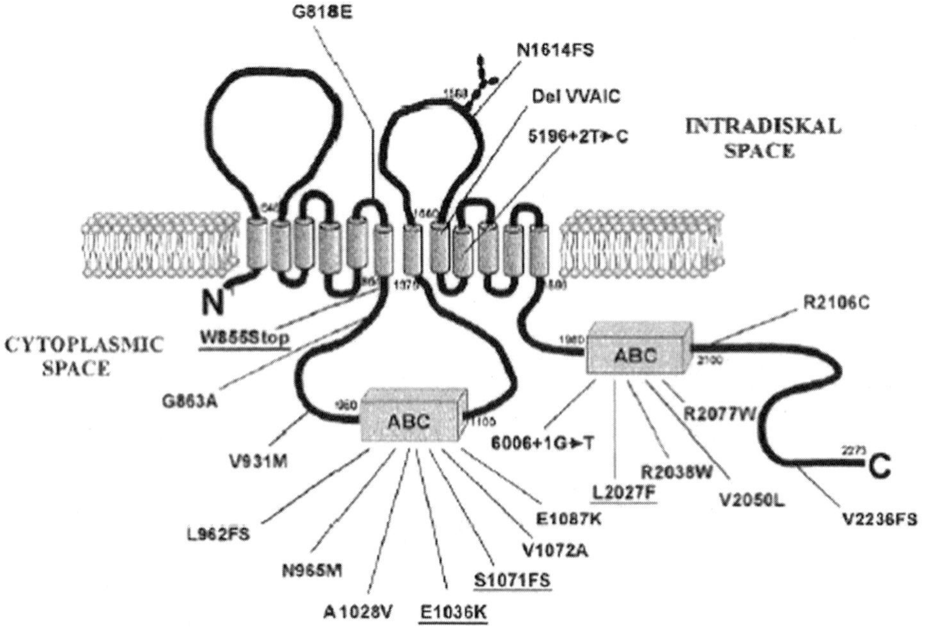

Figure 6 Model for the topological organization of the human ABCA4 gene. Disease bearing mutations are marked. Note the higher concentration of mutations in the ATP-binding cassettes (ABC) (from Ref. 30).

cone-rod dystrophy (34). Patients with two homozygous copies of a severe mutation manifested ARRP, while patients with two different severe mutations (compound heterozygosity) manifested cone-rod dystrophy (35,36). One of the ARRP loci colocalizes with STGD1 and FFM loci. The causative gene was identified as ABCA4 (37). The authors speculated that a homozygous severe mutation in exon 13, leading to a frameshift early in the coding region, results in the lack of both ATP-binding domains and nonfunctioning of the rod (37). This mutation results in RP19, a severe retinal disease. In patients clinically diagnosed with cone-rod dystrophy caused by mutations in the ABCA4 gene, the majority have cone ERG more affected than rod ERG. However, two of 12 patients had a non-recordable ERG (38).

Stargardt Disease of Late Onset

Different names have been attributed to this clinical entity, including Stargardt disease type II, Stargardt disease of late onset (12,39), fundus flavimaculatus with macular dystrophy (20), late-onset fundus flavimaculatus with macular dystrophy (40), and late-onset Stargardt disease (41). In the meantime, the term type II is used for another genetic entity of Stargardt disease, STGD2, an autosomal dominant entity of Stargardt.

In this disease, the typical atrophic macular changes of Stargardt disease occur together with widespread flavi maculatus flecks up to the equator (Fig. 7). The flavimaculatus flecks probably precede the macular changes, although this is difficult to verify, as it is the macular changes and the visual decrease that bring the patient to the ophthalmologist. In my patients (12,39), the age of onset was later than in Stargardt type I (Fig. 8), but it was younger in the patients of Moloney et al. (20). The decrease of vision was gradual and slow extending over many years (Fig. 9), with a final visual acuity stable at between 1/60 and 6/60. The rod system seemed more affected than the cone system, in contrast to Stargardt type I. None of my patients had a family history of a similar disease or was a descendant of a consanguineous marriage.

In summary, Stargardt disease type I predominantly has macular changes and, in some cases, flavimaculatus flecks, which are small in number and extent. Stargardt disease of late onset predominantly has multiple and widespread flavimaculatus flecks, with slowly developing atrophic macular changes indistinguishable from the morphologic macular abnormalities of Stargardt disease. The two diseases differ in age of onset, heredity, progression, and pathophysiologic and electrophysiologic changes as outlined in Table 1.

The locus for Stargardt disease of late onset was mapped to chromosome 1p13–p21 and was considered by Gerber and associates (40) as allelic to STGD1. In all their cases of late onset Stargardt, Yatsenko et al. (41) identified mild missense mutations in at least one of the two alleles in cases of compound heterozygosity. They speculated that the age of onset is correlated to the amount of residual ABCR activity left in cases of mild mutations. However, Stargardt disease of late onset may occur in cases of one heterozygous truncating (nonsense) mutation if the other allele is the mild type or mild mutation (42).

Fundus Flavimaculatus

Fundus flavimaculatus, a term introduced by Franceschetti, (7) Franceschetti and Francois (8), relates to the findings of multiple flecks in the posterior pole of the

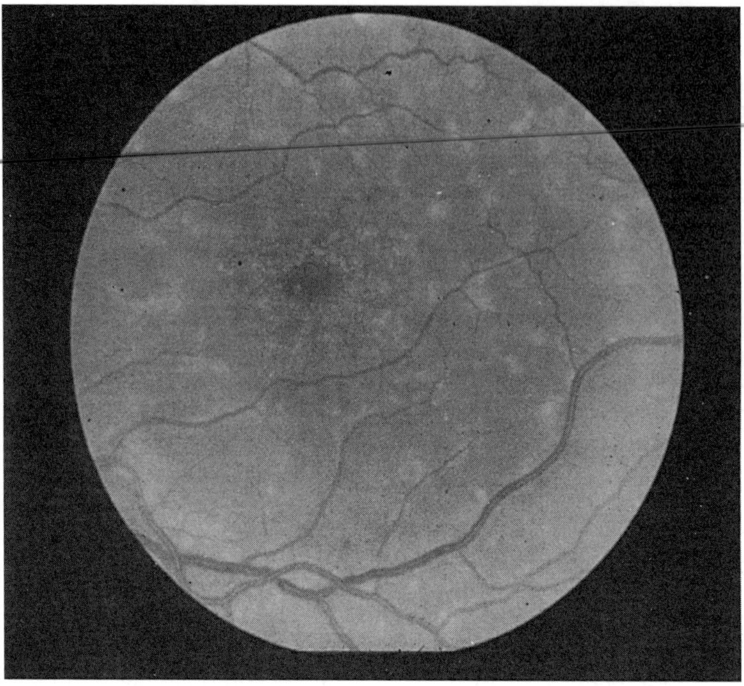

(a)

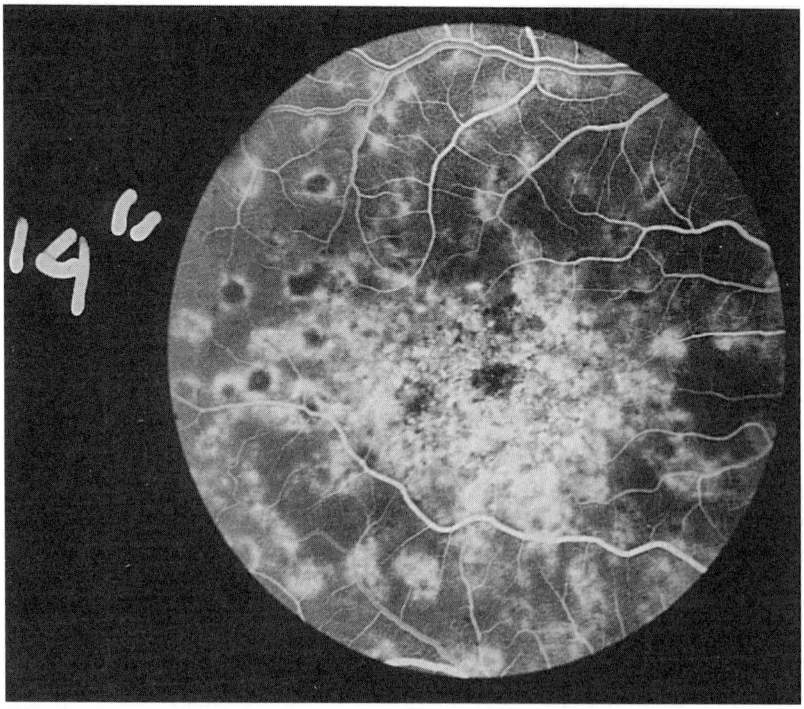

(b)

Figure 7 Stargardt disease of late onset: (a) clinical photograph and (b) fluorescein angiography. Note the characteristic beaten bronze center and bull's-eye phenomenon, (a) and (b) are eyes of the same patient.

AGE IN YEARS	NO.
18	1
22	3
23	1
25	1
33	1
35	1
40	1
49	1

Figure 8 Onset of visual symptoms in 10 patients with Stargardt disease of late onset.

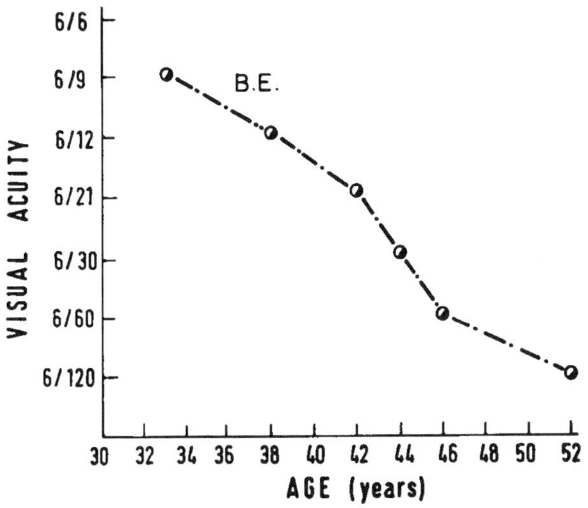

Figure 9 Stargardt disease of late onset: decrease of visual acuity over 20 years.

fundus. After their two articles were published in 1963 and 1965, many investigators noted the coexistence of such flecks with a Stargardt type macular dystrophy.

This finding led to the conclusion, accepted by many authors, that Stargardt disease (7) and fundus flavimaculatus are one and the same disease (9–11,13,19) (43–45). It seems to me, however, that classification of Stargardt disease into separate clinical and genetic entities is possible and feasible. In such classification, Stargardt disease type 1 sometimes (probably less than half of all cases) has flecks in the posterior pole, few in number, that develop after the macular dystrophy. Stargardt disease of late onset has macular dystrophy developing in a patient who has multiple flavimaculatus flecks up to the equator. Fundus flavimaculatus is the term I prefer to use for a condition of flavimaculatus flecks, without a macular dystrophy. It is sometimes called "pure fundus flavimaculatus" in the literature. The condition of pure fundus flavimaculatus is rather infrequently found. Noble and Carr (14) found only four such cases among 67 patients with Stargardt disease and/or flavimaculatus. Franceschetti and Francois (8) found 13 among 30, and Klein and Krill (46) found 9 among 27 patients. In the unusual family described by Merin and Landau (47), two boys had Stargardt disease type I, whereas their mother and one maternal aunt had fundus flavimacuiatus. It is possible that some patients with fundus flavimaculatus will display the macular atrophic changes and develop Stargardt disease of late onset later in their lives. On the other hand, it is also possible that many cases of fundus flavimaculatus, especially if nonfamilial, go unnoticed.

The typical patient with fundus flavimaculatus has no symptoms of the disease. The visual acuity, color vision, and visual fields are normal. Dark adaptation may be normal or slightly subnormal. The fundus shows a symmetric bilateral involvement. The macula and the retinal periphery are normal. Between the fovea and the equator, multiple gray-white to yellowish flecks are seen. These take up different forms: round, oval, elongated, commalike, split as in fishtail, or crescent. They may be confluent or separate, 200–300 μm in width and three to five times as much in length (Fig. 10). Several authors noticed the development of changes in the ophthalmoscopic appearance of the flecks (10,13,19,48). In addition to the eruption of new flecks, a certain chain of "evolutionary" changes occur. The flecks, initially yellowish and sharply outlined, become, over the course of years, gray and less defined and finally disintegrate, leaving an atrophic-looking RPE. Parallel to this, fluorescein angiographic findings become different with hypofluorescence turning into hyper-fluorescence. These changes in the flavimaculatus flecks are typically seen in all types of Stargardt disease, but they are less obvious in patients with pure fundus flavimaculatus.

It seems that both pure fundus flavimaculatus and late onset Stargardt disease are caused by mild mutations in the ABCA4 gene. All mutations identified in fundus flavimaculatus were missense mutations (49).

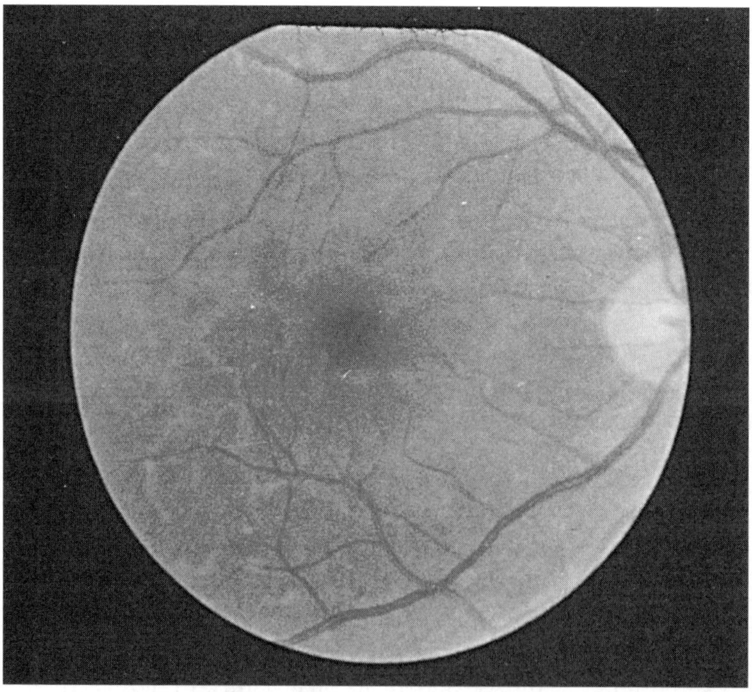

Figure 10 Fundus flavimaculatus in a 48-year-old patient: visual acuity was 6/9 in each eye. Both eyes were similarly affected.

Autosomal Dominant Stargardt Disease

For many years, controversy surrounded the existence of an autosomal dominant form of Stargardt disease. Isolated reports were published (50,51). Deutman (9) described such cases under the name of dominant progressive foveal dystrophy and cited a list of articles describing this condition. In the literature, however, this term has been used for a variety of different diagnoses, including dominant drusen and Best vitelliform dystrophy (BVMD).

Autosomal dominant Stargardt disease is rare, but is transmitted by at least four different genes.

- STGD1, the locus of the ABCA4 gene, may harbor mutations causing diseases in the heterozygous state and may be transmitted as an autosomal dominant trait (52). In one family, the mutation was Arg152Stop, a severe nonsense mutation. Phenotypically, the retina was Stargardt-like picture.
- STGD2 was located in chromosome 13q34, but the gene is yet unidentified (53). In one family with autosomal dominant disease, 29 members were affected, with a mean visual acuity of 20/160. The fundus manifested atrophic, Stargardt-like maculopathy and flavimaculatus flecks in all affected individuals (53).
- The locus STGD3 was located in chromosome 6q14 (54–57). The phenotype matched that of Stargardt type I. Normal vision exists in early childhood. Gradual reduction in vision started between 5 and 25 years of age. Flecks were seen around atrophic maculopathy. The flavimaculatus flecks preceded the maculopathy (54). Final visual acuity was between 20/300 and 20/800 (55). In one large North American family the mutation could be traced to a "founder" in the 18th century (58). The gene, at the STGD3 locus was identified in 2001 as ELOVL4 (for elongation of very long fatty acids-like 4) (59). The gene was found to be expressed exclusively in photoreceptor cells, both cones and rods. The mutation identified was a 5 bp deletion in exon 6 of ELOVL4 resulting in a frameshift (59). This was the first time that the biosynthesis of fatty acids was implicated in the pathogenesis of an inherited macular dystrophy. A second mutation of two 1 bp deletions was later identified (60). This results in a frameshift and a similar truncated protein as in the former mutation.
- STGD4 is the locus associated with Stargardt-like disease located at chromosome 4p (61,62).

Other Stargardt-Type Maculopathies

Several other diseases, some inherited and others not, may mimic the clinical appearance of Stargardt-type atrophic maculopathy (63). These diseases should be considered when a dark center in the fovea is surrounded by a ring of spots of hypopigmentation and hyperpigmentation, or any other atrophic type dystrophy of the macula.

RDS/peripherin gene mutations are frequent causes of maculopathies, including Stargardt-like disease (64). Remarkable variations in phenotype and disease expression were noted. Specific mutations in the RDS/peripherin gene were identified in eight families, and included five missense mutations, two nonsense mutations, and one single base insertion, all heterozygous (64).

A bull's-eye maculopathy was detected in a patient with a mitochondrial DNA mutation at position 11778 (65). Similarly, a Stargardt-like disease was described with mutations at position 15257. Both mutations lead to Leber's hereditary optic neuropathy (65).

Stargardt type atrophic macular degeneration was described in conjunction with olivopontocerebellar atrophy (66,67) and with other spinocerebellar and cerebellar spastic disorders (9). Other associated conditions were suggested, but not clearly defined.

A morphologic picture mimicking Stargardt type macular dystrophy may be seen not infrequently in two other groups of inherited diseases: the cone–rod dystrophies and the rod–cone dystrophies (retinitis pigmentosa). It may also be seen in nonhereditary diseases, such as the well-known bull's-eye phenomenon of chloroquine retinopathy or the rare late ocular effect of toxemia of pregnancy (68).

Diagnosis and Laboratory Tests

Table 1 outlines the clinical and laboratory findings in the various forms of Stargardt disease and fundus flavimaculatus. The four main clinical and genetic entities can be readily distinguished.

Fluorescein angiography in the typical form of Stargardt type macular dystrophy shows the bull's-eye phenomenon of a hypofluorescenfcenter [dark choroid of Fish (15)], a ring of hyperfluorescent spots around it, and a ring of hypofluorescence more peripherally. This picture is most probably a result of the combination of deposition of an abnormal storage material in RPE cells in the center, atrophy of other RPE cells, and the combination of surrounding atrophy and hypertrophy. In some cases, multiple spots of hypofluorescence, hyperfluorescence, or both, without formation of rings and without the dark choroid, can be seen. The flavimaculatus flecks are seen initially as spots of hypofluorescence; later spots of hyperfluorescence appear between these flecks. Finally, atrophy of RPE is indicated by disappearance of individual flecks and their replacement by irregular areas of hypofluorescence.

Background autofluorescence, as measured in vivo by confocal laser scanning, was found to be elevated in all forms of macular dystrophies, including Stargardt disease (69). It can be used for diagnosis when needed. Indocyanine green (ICG) angiography showed varying degrees of choroidal vascular closure in the macula and flecks blocking ICG fluorescence (70). In one asymptomatic, mutation-carrying individual, flecks were seen only by ICG (70).

Visual fields are normal in patients with fundus flavimaculatus and show a central scotoma in all patients with Stargardt disease.

The reports on the electroretinogram (ERG) in Stargardt disease are conflicting, ranging from a normal ERG in most cases to an abnormal ERG in other cases. The photopic function was selectively affected in a few cases in one study (14) and in most cases in another study (71). Fishman (10,13) considers that the ERG varies in different stages of Stargardt disease, starting with normal ERG responses, progressing into subnormal cone function, and then into subnormal rod and cone function in the final stages of the disease, when the RPE is widely affected. In my opinion, the ERG response depends on the type of the disease (12,39) and the extent of RPE involvement. In Stargardt disease type I, the ERG response initially may be normal, later cone function is predominantly affected, and finally both cone and rod functions are affected. In Stargardt disease of late onset, rod function is affected more than cone function. In fundus flavimaculatus, the ERG is normal or the rod function is somewhat subnormal.

The electro-oculogram (EOG) has also been reported to vary between normal and abnormal. It was reported to be normal in about three of every four patients (14,19). Fishman believes that the EOG becomes abnormal in the later stages of the disease (10,13). He suggested the use of an illuminated sphere, instead of a flat screen, for testing patients with Stargardt disease (72). With such a sphere most of the retina can be tested, not only the central part. Moloney et al. (20) found an EOG of 175 $\pm$ 6.6 in Stargardt disease type I and an EOG of 151 $\pm$ 4.6 in fundus flavimaculatus with macular dystrophy (Stargardt disease of late onset). Armstrong et al. (21) found abnormally low EOG in about half of all individuals with fundus flavimaculatus.

Color vision is normal in fundus flavimaculatus and abnormal in many or most patients with Stargardt disease type I and of late onset. The most common color vision defect in Stargardt disease type I was a tendency to deuteranopia, whereas in Stargardt disease of late onset, usually the defect was more severe and unclassifiable (12). The particular color vision defect probably relates to the extent and type of cones involved in the disease process. Figure 11 lists the color vision tests in the two types of Stargardt disease.

The c-wave of the human direct-current ERG reflects the dysfunction of the pigment epithelium. It was more reduced than the b-wave in Stargardt disease and in other heredomacular dystrophies (73).

Foveal densitometry revealed abnormally low two-way densities of visual pigment in all eight patients with Stargardt disease (74), indicating a subnormal concentration of visual pigments.

Vitreous fluorophotometry was tested in eight patients with Stargardt diseases who had normal results of electrophysiologic tests (75). A normal blood-retinal barrier was found.

Pathology

Klein and Krill, in 1967, published the first histologic report of fundus flavimaculatus in Stargardt disease (46). They claimed that acid mucopolysaccharides accumulate within the RPE cells. However, later these findings were disputed and were not supported by any of the following studies.

Several studies were performed on eyes with advanced Stargardt disease. The study of Maumenee and Maumenee (76) and other reports indicate that, in the late phase of Stargardt disease, a fairly similar histopathologic picture exists. In the center of the macula, most of the photoreceptors and pigment epithelial cells are lost.

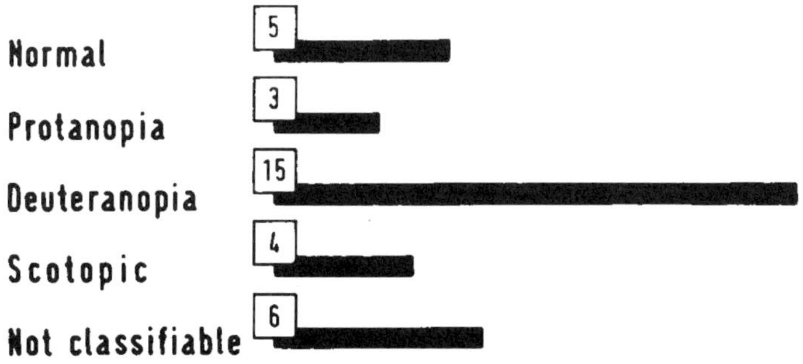

Figure 11 Color vision defects in 33 patients with Stargardt disease type I.

Other RPE cells are degenerated, with accumulation of lipofuscin. At the margin of the atrophic area, hyperplastic RPE cells can be seen.

Eagle et al. (77) examined the two eyes of a patient with typical and familial Stargardt disease type I, who died at age 24 in a road accident. They found a great variability in the size of RPE cells, which ranged from 14 μm in the periphery to 83 μm in the largest cells in the center. The larger RPE cells were packed with a granular substance, which had the ultrastructural, autofluorescent, and histochemical properties of an abnormal lipofuscin. There was a decrease in the amount of melanin, and melanin granules were displayed toward the inner part of the cell (Fig. 12). The flavimaculatus flecks seemed to be caused by the aggregation—in a commalike or fish-tail fashion—of large, hypopigmented RPE cells with large amounts of lipofuscin in their outer parts (Fig. 13). They concluded that the lack of melanin causes the pale appearance of the flecks and that the accumulation of lipofuscin causes the dark choroid effect by absorbing the blue light. Later, atrophy of the choroid causes the window effect seen by fluorescein.

McDonnel et al. (78) studied the eyes of a patient with fundus flavimaculatus, who at the age of 51 when he died, had no macular involvement. As in the previous study, the RPE cells showed great variability in size and shape. Some cells showed a domed configuration, with extended apices. In contrast, no abnormal accumulation of lipofuscin was found. The amounts of melanin, lipofuscin, and melanofuscin were normal. An abnormal tubulo-vesicular membraneous material was found accumulated within the extended apices of the abnormal RPE cells.

Birnbach and colleagues examined, by histopathology and immunocytochemistry, the retina of a patient with fundus flavimaculatus (79). They found accumulation of

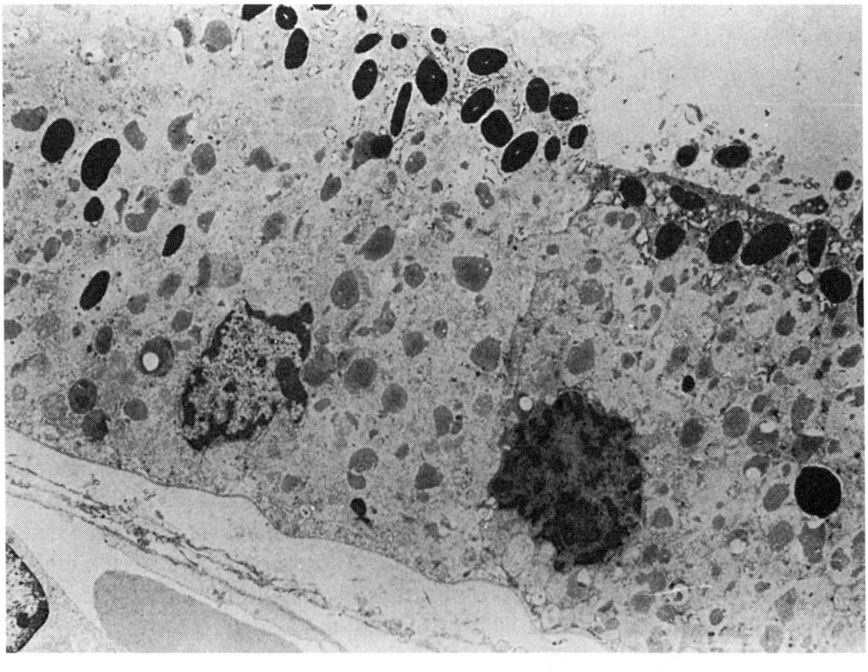

Figure 12 Massive accumulation of abnormal lipofuscin and apical displacement of melanin granules in peripheral RPE cells (from Ref. 37).

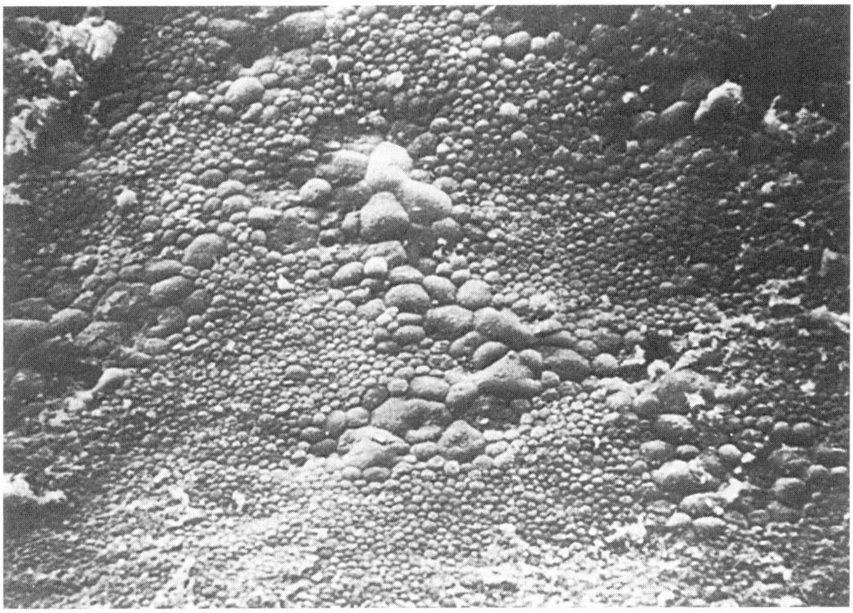

Figure 13 Scanning electron micrograph shows aggregations of large RPE cells, probably reflecting flavimaculatus flecks (from Ref. 77).

lipofuscin in photoreceptor inner segments, increased lipofuscin content in the RPE layer, and loss of RPE cells toward the macula.

It seems likely that both Stargardt disease and fundus flavimaculatus result from abnormal lipopigment metabolism, primarily affecting the photoreceptors, where the mutated disease-causative genes are expressed. The retinal transport mechanisms are affected and the RPE is secondarily affected.

The accumulated material may be different in the two conditions, and it seems that the loss of melanin granules and the degeneration of the RPE cells, with secondary atrophy of the adjacent photoreceptors, are typical of Stargardt disease. In fundus flavimaculatus, this degeneration and atrophy are not marked or are never seen.

Epidemiology and Genetics

The prevalence of Stargardt disease is not well known. It probably varies in different populations and is higher in populations with a high prevalence of consanguinity.

Management

Low-vision aids appear to be more useful in Stargardt disease than in other maculopathies (81,82). In fact, about 80% in our series of patients used low-vision aids successfully during a follow-up of two to three years. The low-vision aids seem especially useful for near vision. They should be prescribed for every patient with Stargardt disease. No other medical or surgical treatment is available.

Genetic counseling should be provided according to the type of the disease and the family history. Prenatal diagnosis is not possible.

Stargardt disease type I is the most common inherited macular disease. It comprises 7% all retinal dystrophies and is second in incidence only to retinitis pigmentosa.

Stargardt disease is usually transmitted by an autosomal recessive gene. The risk to siblings of an affected child is 25%, as expected. The gene ABCA4 (see Table 2) at the STGD1 locus may be associated with Stargardt disease type I, when one or both allelic mutations are of the severe type; with late-onset Stargardt when one or both mutations are of the mild type; with fundus flavimaculatus when both mutations are mild; and with autosomal dominant disease when the mutation is very severe. An overlap between mutations is seen. In very mild mutation, a homozygote may be asymptomatic. Different mutations may thus be associated with different phenotypes of Stargardt dystrophy (83). In the same family with severe ABCA4 mutations, affected members may phenotypically exhibit various manifestations, ranging from maculopathy to autosomal recessive cone–rod dystrophy or retinitis pigmentosa (36). This will be similar to mutated RDS/peripherin phenotypes, which may range from retinitis pigmentosa to pattern dystrophy, fundus flavimaculatus, and cone dystrophy (84,34). Autosomal dominant Stargardt disease definitely exists. It is transmitted by STGD1 or any one of the other three genes for Stargardt disease.

BVMD AND THE VMD2 GENE

Best described the first family with this condition in 1905 (85), but it is possible that a similar condition was described in an isolated case more than 20 years earlier by Adams [cited by Deutman (9)]. Since Best's report, a plethora of articles describing this condition, with different ophthalmoscopic manifestations, resulted in numerous names being given to it. Congenital macular dystrophy, congenital vitelliform cysts of the macula, vitelliform macular degeneration, vitelliform macular dystrophy, Best disease, Best's familial macular degeneration, and hereditary vitellieruptive macular degeneration are just some names given to the disease. I will use the term BVMD, for Best Vitelliform Macular Dystroply, which probably is now the most accepted term.

Description and Clinical Findings

BVMD refers to an autosomal dominant, congenital bilateral disorder, typically affecting the macula by displaying yellow cysts, good visual acuity, and abnormally low EOG responses. The disease is progressive and usually leads to decreased visual acuity later in life. In addition, many atypical cases occur, as the expressivity of the gene is variable. Monocular affection has been rarely reported.

The macular lesions have been noted to be present as early as one week after birth (88), or they may appear later. The classic macular lesions are frequently observed between the ages of 3 and 15 years, peaking around age 6 (9). Patients with a normal macula, who developed their first lesions later in life or later than 15 years, have also been observed. For descriptive and practical purposes, it is therefore feasible to divide the clinical appearance of the disease into stages (9,86,87) (Table 3; Fig. 14).

The visual acuity is normal or near normal in stages 0, 1, and 2. Almost 74% of all patients with BVMD are in these stages (86). It is only in stage 4, when atrophic changes take place, usually after age 40, that visual acuity may be drastically

Table 2 The Genetic Entities of Stargardt Disease

Name	Locus/ symbol	OMIM[a]	Chromosomal	Gene	Mutations and Remarks	References
Stargardt disease type I	STGD1	248200	1p21–pl3	ABCA4	Homozygous or compound heterozygous at least one severe mutation	(23,26)
Stargardt disease of late onset	STGD1	248200	1p21–pl3	ABCA4	Homozygous mild mutations or compound heterozygotes with mild mutation	(40)
Fundus flavimaculatus	FFM	248200	1p21–pl3	ABCA4	Mild mutations	(49)
AD Stargardt type 1	STGD1	248200	1p21–pl3	ABCA4	Heterozygous (one) severe mutation	(52)
AD Stargardt type 2	STGD2	600110	13q34	NK	Unknown	(53)
AD Stargardt type 3	STGD3	600110	6ql4	ELVL4	Truncated protein due to a 5 bp or two 1 bp deletions	(54,55)
AD Stargardt type 4	STGD4 MCDR2	603786	4pl5.2–pl6.3	NK	Unknown	(61,62)
Stargardt-like maculopathy	—	179605.0011	6p21.1-cen	RDS/peripherin	Various nonsense and missense mutations	(64)
Stargardt-like maculopathy	—	535000	Mitochondrial DNA, position 11778	Mitochon drial DNA	Together with LHON	(65)

[a]Reference 80.
Note: AD, autosomal dominant.

Table 3 Clinical Stages of BVMD

Stage			
No.	Name	Description	Percentage[a]
0	Normal	Normal fovea, abnormal EOG	33
1	Previtelliform	RPE defects in macula	20
2	Yellow cyst		10
2a	Vitelliform	Round smooth cyst filled with even yellow material	
2b	Scrambled egg	Uneven yellow material with irregular borders	
3	Pseudohypopyon	Yellow material accumulating in the bottom of the cyst	2
4	Atrophic		35
4a	Atrophy of RPE	Atrophic macula with hypopigmented RPE	
4b	Scar	Subretinal fibrous tissue in macular area	
4c	Neovascularization	Subretinal neovascularization in macular area	

[a]Percentages refer to the number of patients thus affected among 47 patients with BVMD studied by Godel et al. (86).
Source: Refs. 9, 87, and 86. [From Deutman (9), Mohler (87), and Godel et al. (86).]

reduced. In some instances, extramacular single or multiple lesions were described. They may be temporal to the macula, nasal, or superior to the disk (89).

In some patients, fluctuating vision with transient visual loss was reported (96). In cases of pseudohypopyon the fluid may be seen shifting when the head is turned sideways, indicating that the fluid is located between the RPE and the sensory retina (91).

The Clinical and Genetic Types

Classic BVMD

This is the classic disease, as described in (BVMD description and clinical findings). It is typified by the characteristic macular lesions, a persistent subnormal EOG, autosomal dominant heredity with variable expressivity, and progression through life. Hittner et al. (92) suggested calling this disease BVMD to distinguish it from two other types: atypical vitelliform macular dystrophy (AVMD) and pseudovitelliform macular dystrophy (PVMD).

The BVMD-causative gene was assigned in 1992 to chromosome 11q13 (93,94). Initially, the ROM1 gene seemed the most likely candidate, as it was found to be located at the same site 11q13. (95) However, it was later excluded (96) and the gene VMD2 with Best disease-causing mutations was identified (97,98). All 15 mutations initially reported were missense mutations, such as Tyr93Cys, Tyr85His, Gly299Glu, Tyr227Asp, Thr6Pro. Scientists found evidence that VMD2 mRNA is heavily and exclusively expressed in the RPE (97,98). The gene encodes a 585-amino acid protein of 68 kd. This protein was named bestrophin (99). It was found to be localized to the basolateral plasma membrane of the RPE (100). Its function is still unknown. A large number of mutations, predominantly missense mutations in the VMD2 gene, were identified and reported (101–103). By 2000, 40–48 mutations and several polymorphisms were identified (102,103).

In all affected individuals a heterozygous mutation was identified, thus confirming the autosomal dominant nature of the disease. One patient, carrying the same disease-bearing mutation as his affected family members, was asymptomatic and showed no objective sign of BVMD (104).

Atypical Vitelliform Macular Dystrophy (Adult-Onset Foveomacular Dystrophy)

Hittner et al. (92) described a large family with five generations affected by this condition. Initially, small yellow lesions are seen in the macular area, sometimes preceded by minimal fluorescein angiographic changes in the form of hypofluorescent spots. The lesions may show a continuum of appearances, from tiny dots to a single yellow lesion with a typical fluorescein angiographic finding (105). The single lesion is smaller than the one usually seen in BVMD (106). The single lesion is usually solitary, oval, slightly elevated, yellowish, and subretinal. Fluorescein is blocked in this area (107).

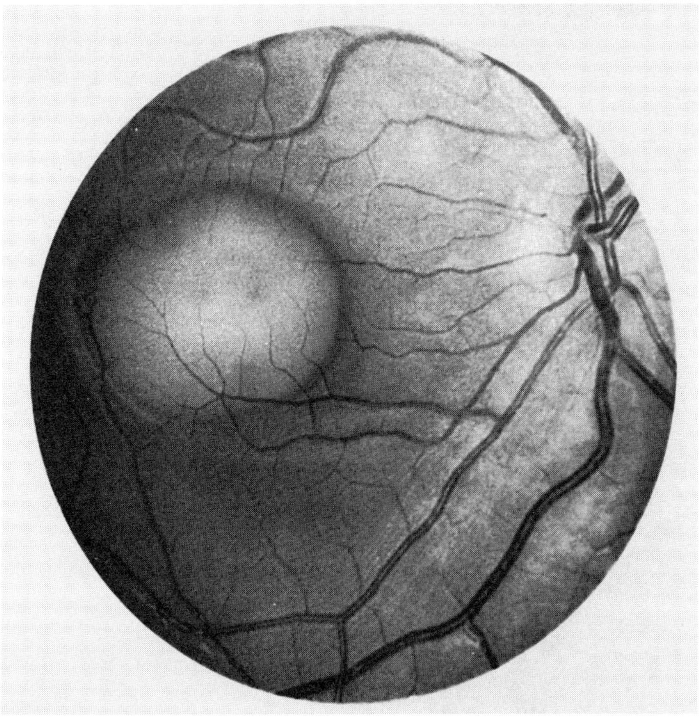

(a)

Figure 14 The yellow cyst stage of BVMD: (a) vitelliform stage: round smooth cyst filled with yellow material; (b) beginning of scrambled egg appearance—uneven distribution of yellow material; and (c) pseudohypopyon—yellow material at bottom of cyst and atrophy of RPE in center, (c) The same eye as (b), 1 year later. (Courtesy of GA. Fishman, MD, Illinois Eye and Ear Infirmary, Chicago.)

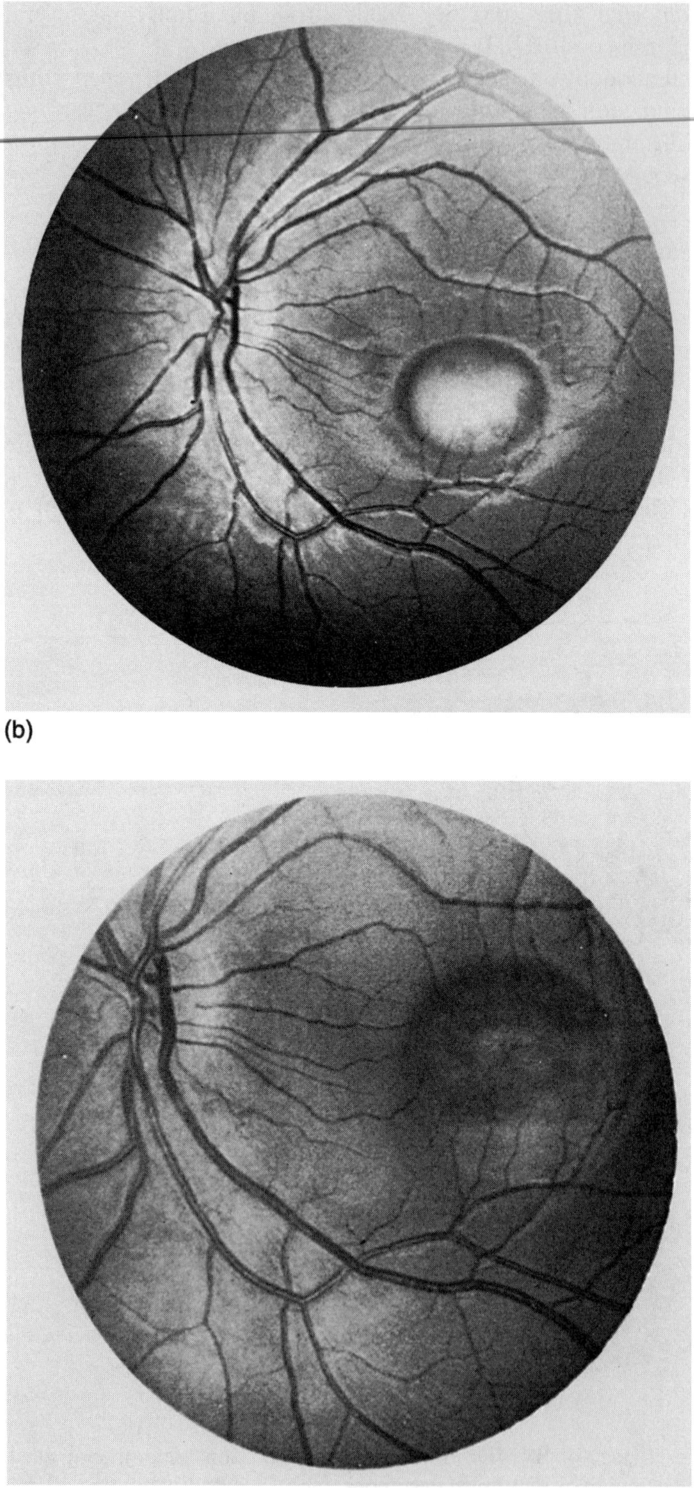

(b)

(c)

Figure 14 (*Continued*)

This condition was first reported by Gass, under the name of "peculiar foveomacular dystrophy" (106). Gass suggested that it is transmitted by the autosomal dominant mode. Various terms were used, such as pseudovitelliform macular degeneration, foveomacular dystrophy (105,106,108), and others. More recently, the terms used include AOFMD (109), adult-onset foveomacular pigment epithelial dystrophy (110), and adult-onset foveomacular vitelliform dystrophy (107).

The EOG of this atypical disease in contrast to that of BVMD, is normal or moderately reduced (111). The age of onset is variable, but much later than in BVMD, usually between 30 and 40 (106,108). The prognosis of final visual acuity seems poor (108), although the progression of the disease is variable. In one patient, this condition was found in one eye and a butterfly-shaped epithelial dystrophy was seen in the other eye (112). It was suggested that this condition may be more related to the pattern dystrophies than to BVMD (105,112).

Studies by optical coherence tomography showed thickening of the RPE layer and accumulation of hyperreflective material located between the RPE and the neural retina.

The autosomal dominant atypical VMD or AOFMD was initially found to be linked to the glutamate pyruvate transaminase locus (113), later localized to chromosome 8q24.3 and given the locus name of VMD1. Later, such linkage was excluded (114).

In some families and in sporadic cases of atypical VMD, a mutated gene cannot be detected. In other families, however, mutations in the VMD2 gene were identified (115). More frequently mutations were identified within the RDS/peripherin gene (109). It was suggested that this condition may be more related to the pattern dystrophies than to BVMD (105,109,112). Recently, optical coherence tomography (OCT) was used to distinguish between the two genotypes. The OCT manifested in all cases of AOFMD in a well-defined thickening of the RRE layer (278) and the location of the yellowish material above the RPE (279).

Pseudovitelliform Macular Dystrophy

The term PVMD should be used for one of two conditions: (1) a disease similar to atypical vitelliform macular dystrophy, but sporadic and nonhereditary in nature, and (2) a macular degeneration from different causes, which clinically mimics vitelliform macular dystrophy.

Cases of vitelliform dystrophy with normal EOGs were described as separate entities in sporadic cases (115,116), and rarely even in inherited cases (192,105,106,108). The clinical manifestation may be similar to those of typical BVMD. AOFMD is a term used for a heterogenous group of diseases caused by one of two or three mutated genes. In other cases, it is associated with age-related macular degeneration (ARMD).

Several maculopathies may mimic vitelliform dystrophy. The most frequent are macular drusen (117); serous detachment of RPE with lipid or protein deposition (117,118); subretinal neovascularization, especially in young persons (119) who tend to respond with a yellow deposit (Fig. 15); and basal laminar drusen, a recently defined clinical entity (120). As with AVMD, the resemblance to the pattern dystrophies is often striking (121,122).

The VMD2 Gene

A large number of various mutations in the VMD2 gene were identified in association with classic BVMD. Almost all were missense mutations and cause disease in

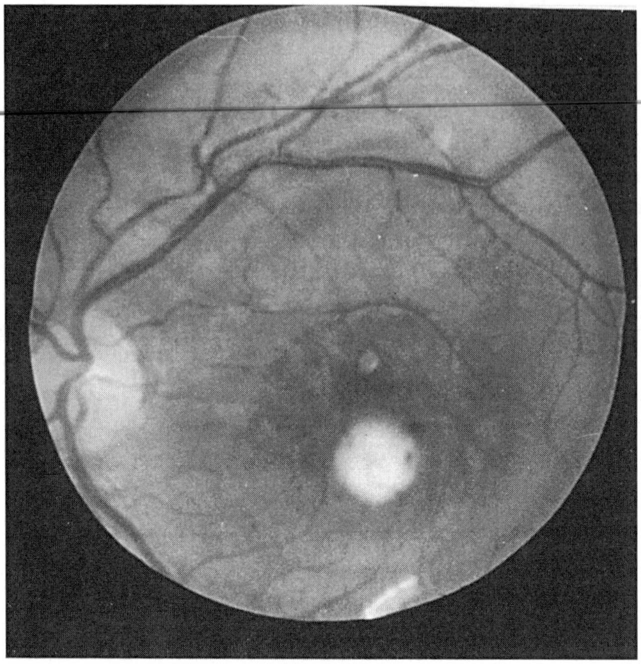

(a)

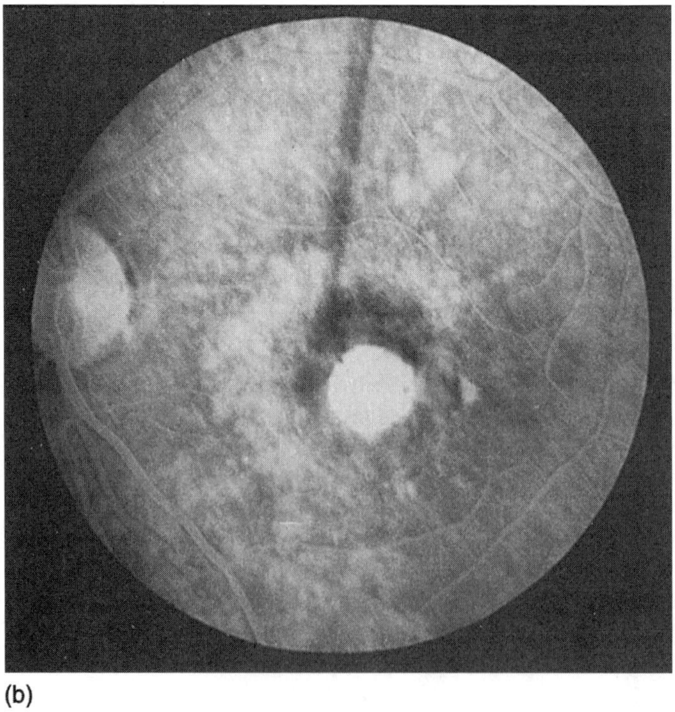

(b)

Figure 15 Pseudovitelliform macular dystrophy in a $4\frac{1}{2}$ year-old girl with congenital rubella syndrome: (a) clinical photograph of a macular cyst filled by a yellow material and; (b) fluorescein angiography showing subretinal neovascularization.

the heterozygous state (103). In some cases, in spite of the disease-causing haplotype, no clinical signs of BVMD were seen (104).

In many patients with AOFMD, a mutation in the VMD2 gene was detected (102,103). One of three cases of AOFMD had an associated mutation in the VMD2 gene (123). Bull's-eye maculopathy was also associated with a VMD2 mutation (99). A locus for autosomal dominant neovascular inflammatory vitreoretinopathy was mapped to chromosome 11q13 (124) and is likely linked to VMD2 mutation.

Diagnosis and Laboratory Tests

The diagnosis of BVMD is readily made by the combination of the typical ophthalmoscopic findings and an abnormally low EOG result. The diagnosis is confirmed by familial occurrence, with clear autosomal dominant transmission.

Fluorescein angiography is characteristic. The yellow material blocks choroidal fluorescence. When atrophy occurs, as in the stage of pseudohypopyon, defects in the RPE cause spots of hypofluorescence, with a mottling appearance (91). With progression of the disease, fluorescein angiography shows a sequence of changes that parallel the clinical developments. Initially, tiny spots of hypofluorescence (transmission defects) are seen. In the vitelliform cyst stage, blockage of the choroidal fluorescence is noted; later, with the atrophic changes occurring in the RPE, more and more transmission defects are seen. In the final stage of secondary changes, the typical appearance of a subretinal membrane of subretinal neovascularization with leakage is seen.

ERG was reported as normal. The foveal flicker fusion thresholds (foveal cone ERG) are abnormally elevated, even in patients with normal or near-normal vision (125).

EOG is the most important single test for BVMD, as it can distinguish between disease and the atypical or pseudovitelliform variants. In the hereditary cases, the light peak/dark trough ratio (Arden ratio) is abnormally low, usually less than 1.55 (87). The Arden ratio is low before any morphologic changes take place and in carriers of the gene who never develop the clinical signs of the disease (126).

In AVMD, the results of the tests are different. The EOG is usually normal, but sometimes moderately subnormal. Fluorescein angiography shows a characteristic picture, described as spots of hyperfluorescence (transmission defects) with a ring of hypofluorescence at the lesions (92) or spots of leakage from perifoveal capillaries around the macula, as in cystoid macular edema (108).

In PVMD, the results of the various tests vary with the cause of the disease, showing, for instance, a strong leakage ("hot spot") in cases of subretinal neovascularization (see Fig. 15).

Pathology and Pathogenesis

Several histopathologic studies were performed in BVMD and related diseases. These attempted to answer three questions as outlined by Cavender (127): What is the yellow material? Where is it located? Where does it originate? Kobrin et al. (128) examined an eye with relatively early BVMD and found that the RPE cells were engorged with cytosomes containing an abnormal unidentified substance. Such RPE cells may involute and become atrophic, with loss of central retinal function resulting later. Capillaries may invade the subretinal space through breaks in Bruch's membrane. Light and electron microscopic examination of an eye with the "scrambled-egg" lesion of a 28-year-old patient with BVMD, by Weingeist et al. (129), showed a heavy accumulation of lipofuscin granules within RPE cells (Fig. 16), within macrophages in the subretinal space, and within the choroid. These authors concluded that in the previtelliform stage the storage of lipofuscin in the RPE cells causes the decrease in the EOG; in the vitelliform stage, lipofuscin accumulates heavily in the RPE cells and partially in the subretinal space. In later stages, the disease may be predominately affected by alterations in the RPE, disruption of the "egg yolks," scar formation, and breaks in Bruch's membrane.

Frangieh et al. (130), after examining an eye of an 80-year-old woman with BVMD, similarly concluded that the most pronounced abnormality is the accumulation of an abnormal lipofuscin product. In the macular area, RPE cells were flattened, with an average height of 10 nm (normal range, 10–14 nm), and average diameter of 21.5 nm (normal 14 nm), and they contained a heavy deposition of an abnormal lipofuscin and melanolipofuscin granules. Abnormal granular material accumulated between neuroepithelium and RPE cells. An abnormal fibrillar material of unknown origin or nature was found underneath the RPE in the most affected

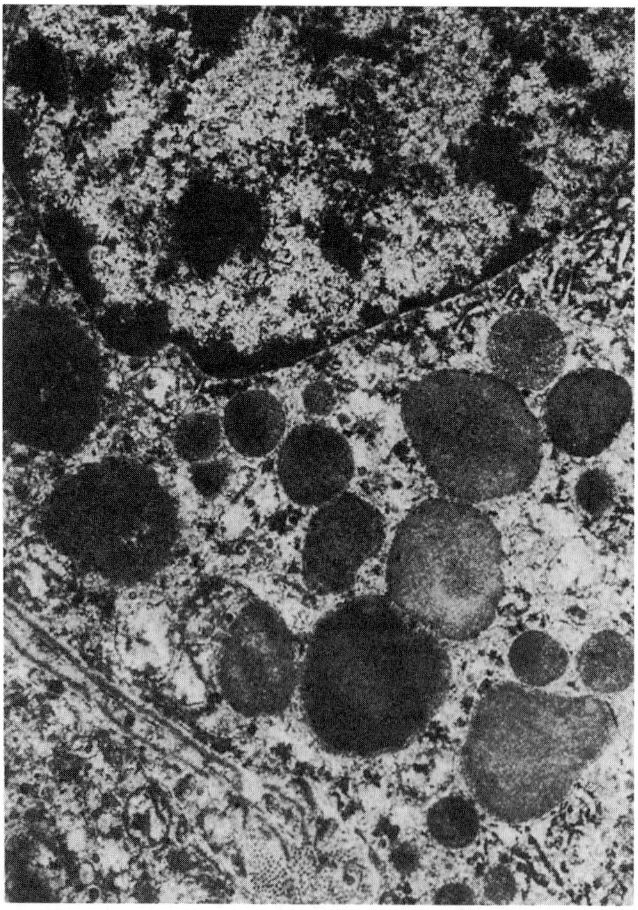

Figure 16 Electron micrograph of an eye of a 28-year-old patient with the scrambled-egg lesion diagnosed as BVMD: multiple lipofuscin granules are seen within the RPE cell (×18,000) (from Ref. 129).

areas. Bruch's membrane had breaks, with blood vessels crossing through them. The neural retina was severely affected, with most photoreceptor outer segments lost or degenerated and accumulation of acid mucopolysaccharides in the inner segments of the photoreceptors in the most affected areas.

These studies seem to indicate that the yellow material is mainly formed by lipofuscin or its products and, that it accumulates mainly within the RPE cells and later in the subretinal space. It did not answer the question of the origin of the disease, believed to be a malfunction of the RPE cells in one study (129) and a primary abnormality of the neuroepithelium in the other (130). One study confirmed the excessive amounts of lipofuscin accumulated in the RPE cells, a combination of regenerating RPE cells and lipofuscin granules producing the previtelliform lesion, and indicated the RPE layer as the primary site of the disorder (131). In fact, both clinical and pathologic studies confirmed the nature of the deposits between RPE cells and neuroepithelium to be lipofuscin (97,98,110). Lipofuscin accumulates within the RPE cells.

Different results were obtained in histopathologic studies of AVMD and PVMD. Gass, in the first reported such study (106), found that the yellow zone surrounding the central pigmented lesion corresponds to an area of thin and degenerated RPE cells separated from Bruch's membrane by an eosinophilic material. There was no intracellular deposit of any abnormal material. In contrast, in a later study of a condition they called "foveomacular vitelliform dystrophy, adult type," Patrinely and coauthors (132) found intracellular deposition of lipofuscin pigment, both in RPE cells and in intraretinal migratory macrophages. The size of RPE cells was abnormal, and these flat pigmented epithelial cells were surrounded by tall hypertrophied cells. These findings were much closer to the description of BVMD than those in the study by Gass (106). The variability of the pathologic findings in atypical vitelliform dystrophy stresses the heterogeneity of this condition.

Epidemiology and Genetics

The prevalence of BVMD is different in various populations, according to the prevalence of the gene. In Sweden 250 cases of BVMD were detected and traced to a single gene source in the 17th century (133). These authors present the clinical findings in a homozygous father whose 11 children were heterozygous and affected. There were great variations in the phenotypic presentation of the gene. The homozygous state did not seem different from the heterozygous state (133).

BVMD is transmitted by a single autosomal dominant gene, with high penetrance and very variable expressivity for age of onset, clinical findings, progression of the disease, and final outcome. This statement is true for both BVMD and AVMD. It was shown in the large family described by Nordström as the Vilhelmina type (134) and in many publications on smaller families.

The locus for AVMD was tentatively assigned to the short arm of chromosome 16 when linkage to the soluble glutamate pyruvate (GP) transaminase was suggested (113). A later study demonstrated tight linkage between *VMD-1,* the gene for AVMD and *GPD,* and a possible loose linkage between BVMD and GPD (135). The authors concluded that BVMD and atypical vitelliform dystrophy could be either allelic mutations or separate genetic disorders, and that atypical vitelliform dystrophy should provisionally be assigned to chromosome 16pter–p11 (135).

As mentioned earlier, both the locations and linkages were not confirmed and were, in fact, excluded. However, VMD2 mutations are the cause of classic BVMD and of some or many of the cases of AVMD or adult onset foveomacular dystrophy.

Management

Surgical and Medical Management

In the early stages of the disease the patient is asymptomatic. Later symptoms are mild, and there is a slight decrease in vision. It is usually only at a more advanced age, rarely before 40, that the central vision becomes substantially decreased. In that stage, low-vision aids for near and distance can be helpful. Subretinal neovascularization, if outside the foveal avascular zone, may be amenable to laser therapy and should be considered. Subfoveal CNV may be treated by photodynamic therapy.

Genetic Counseling

Genetic counseling should be based on the assumption that BVMD and AVMD are caused by an autosomal dominant gene, whereas PVMD is sporadic. If the transmission is in doubt, all available first-degree relatives should be examined and have an EOG test, as sometimes minor macular abnormalities or a subnormal EOG will be the proof for the dominant transmission. The variable expressivity and the prolonged course should be mentioned to the patient.

Identification of the causative gene and its mutation is important as VMD2 is not the only gene which may cause the disease.

Prenatal Diagnosis

Prenatal diagnosis is possible for vitelliform dystrophies once the mutated gene of the family is identified.

THE PATTERN DYSTROPHIES OF THE PIGMENT EPITHELIUM

Introduction

The pattern dystrophies of the pigment epithelium are a group of inherited diseases originating from a diffuse abnormality of the pigment epithelium and primarily affecting the macular area and the posterior pole. The visual acuity is only slightly affected, if at all.

Since Sjögren described the first of these pattern dystrophies, the reticular dystrophy (136), a series of families have been reported in whom different patterns of RPE involvement were manifested. These were presented each as a separate clinical entity. Later, reports on mixed manifestations of different patterns on intrafamilial variations and on two different expressions in the eyes of the same patient raised the possibility of one clinical entity with different manifestations. In addition, it is clear that some patients with pseudovitelliform dystrophy and with dominant drusen may display a typical pattern dystrophy.

The various pattern dystrophies will be described, bearing in mind that they may be different manifestations of the same disease. This discussion of pattern dystrophies is far from closed.

The Clinical and Genetic Types

Sjögren's Reticular Dystrophy of the Pigment Epithelium

Sjögren described the fundus findings in this rare reticular dystrophy as a fine network of pigmented lines, with a pigment dot (black point) at the junction (136). In its fully developed version, the pattern looks like a dark knotted fishing net (Fig. 17). The condition probably starts at the age of five (136) and progresses without affecting visual acuity. Sjögren suggested an autosomal recessive inheritance, as did Deutman and Rümke (132). The ERG, color vision, visual acuity, and visual fields are normal. The EOG may be normal or subnormal. The reticular figure can best be seen when photographing with a panchromatic film (9) or by red-free photography.

Mutations in the RDS/peripherin gene were reported in both autosomal recessive and autosomal dominant forms of pattern dystrophies (138). The authors cited unpublished data of Ed Stone that mutations in the RDS/peripherin gene were identified in 12.7% of 236 patients with pattern dystrophies.

Butterfly-Shaped Pigment Dystrophy

This condition, first described by Deutman et al. (139) has subsequently been described in other reports (140). The fundus displays a bilateral, symmetric, butterfly-shaped pigmentary lesion in the macula, in the deeper layer of the retina (Fig. 18). The typical pigmentation has been seen as early as eight years of age (140), but could have been present earlier. The pigmentation initially increases, and later slow depigmentation of the lesion occurs, with atrophic changes seen by

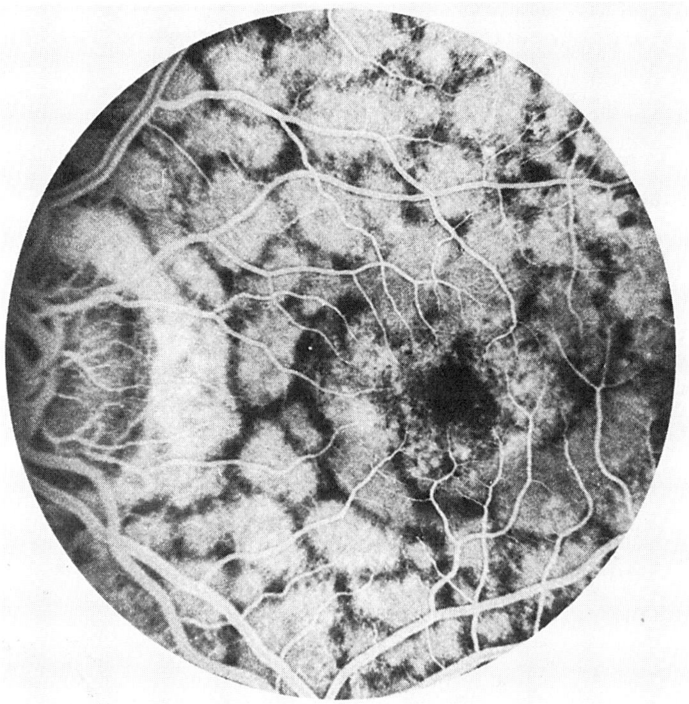

Figure 17 Sjögren's reticular dystrophy of the RPE. (Courtesy of Dr. A.F. Deutman, Nijmegen, Netherlands.)

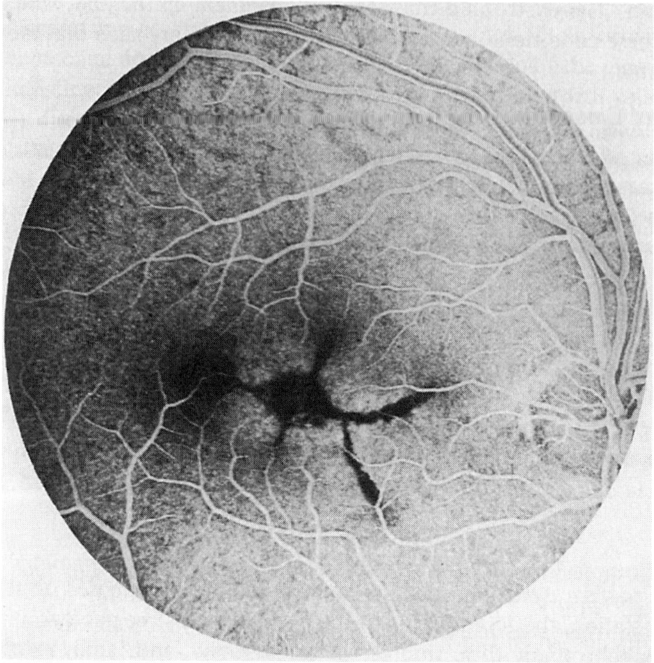

Figure 18 Butterfly-shaped pigment dystrophy. (Courtesy of Dr. A.F. Deutman, Nijmegen, Netherlands.)

window defects in fluorescein angiography. At this late stage, the visual acuity may become slightly decreased. Visual fields and color vision are normal. The ERG is normal, and EOG may be somewhat decreased.

Although a benign condition was assumed in the original reports, a chronic progressive course may occur in some patients with markedly reduced visual acuity in older individuals (141). Dark adaptation, color vision, ERG, and visual fields are normal but the EOG was in some cases very reduced (141).

The disease locus of butterfly-shaped pattern dystrophy has been mapped to chromosome 6p21.2 and mutations in the RDS/peripherin gene at that location were identified (142,143). Zhang and colleagues (141) summarized the reported mutations. These included a large deletion in exon 3, seven various missense mutations, two nonsense mutations, and one 2 bp deletion of codons 299 and 300. This last deletion was also linked to cases of retinitis pigmentosa and fundus flavimaculatus (141). A large deletion that removed exons 2 and 3 of the RDS gene was also associated with butterfly pattern dystrophy with yellow deposits and central choroidal atrophy in the elderly (144).

Macroreticular Pattern Dystrophy

A pattern of lines or network of partially butterfly-shaped pigmentation in the macular area has been described in several publications. These patterns were somewhat wider and larger than those in Sjögren's reticular dystrophy. In most, inheritance was clearly autosomal dominant. In spite of some differences among them, the article by Slezak and Hommer on fundus pulverulentus (145) and the articles by Mesker et al. (146), Benedikt and Werner (147), Marmor and Byers (148), and

O'Donnell et al. (149), possibly described the same clinical and genetic entity. Visual acuity is usually good, but slight decrease or metamorphopsia may occur (148). The ERG is normal and the EOG slightly subnormal. The fundus changes are seen as a pigmentary disturbance in the form of fragmented network in the macular area, a picture accentuated by red-free light or by fluorescein angiography (148).

Patterned Macular Dystrophy with Yellow Plaques

A condition in which a pattern figure of radiating lines of hyperpigmentation and yellow plaques are seen together with spots of depigmentation in the macular area was described under different names by several authors. It seems, despite individual clinical variations, to be the same disease. It includes dominant, slowly progressive macular dystrophy (150), pattern dystrophy of the retinal pigment epithelium (151), patterned macular dystrophy with yellow plaques and atrophic changes (121), and adult onset foveomacular vitelliform dystrophy (122,132).

The condition appears to be transmitted by an autosomal dominant gene. The yellow plaques radiating from the fovea, are one-third to one-half disk diameters in size, and are accompanied by hyperpigmentation and hypopigmentation of the pigment epithelium. Visual acuity is good, unless the fovea is affected by the plaques or by atrophy of the pigment epithelium. The ERG is normal, the EOG may be normal or subnormal, and there are indications for an abnormal deposition of lipofuscin in the RPE (151).

This disease has a difficult differential diagnosis with two other conditions: autosomal dominant AVMD and dominant drusen of the pigment epithelium. The dystrophic changes in the pigment epithelium, which accompany both of these conditions, may change the fundus such that they will be indistinguishable.

The association of mutations in the RDS/peripherin gene with autosomal dominant pattern dystrophy has been repeatedly reported. A 3 bp deletion of codon 153 or 154 was reported in one family in which each affected member had a different phenotype ranging from macular degeneration with fundus flavimaculatus through foveomacular pattern dystrophy to adult onset retinitis pigmentosa (84) A 4 bp insertion in codon 140 was associated with autosomal dominant pattern dystrophy (152), as was a nonsense mutation in codon 258 in another case of pattern dystrophy (152) and geographic atrophy of the RPE with pattern dystrophy in a further case (153). Twelve families showed extensive atrophy of the RPE and choriocapillaris in the center, mimicking phenotypically central areolar choroidal atrophy in association with mutations at codon 172 (154).

Mutations in the RDS/peripherin gene were associated with the clinical phenotype of AOFMD. These included missense mutations or nonsense mutations (182) and a splice site mutation (155). Finally, as mentioned earlier, AOFMD was associated also with mutations in the VMD2 gene (123). The RDS/peripherin gene is extensively discussed in the chapter on retinitis pigmentosa.

Mitochondrial Associated Pattern Dystrophy

In the differential diagnosis of pattern dystrophies, a new group of disorders must be accounted for. These are pattern dystrophies of the macula caused by mitochondrial DNA mutations.

Maternally inherited diabetes and deafness (MIDD) was reported in 1992 (156,157). The syndrome consists of adult onset (type II) diabetes mellitus, sensorineural hearing loss, and macular pattern dystrophy (158). The clinical manifestation of the macula resembles macroreticular pattern dystrophy (159) with speckled and patchy hyperpigmentation and hypopigmentation (160) (Fig. 19). The pattern dystrophy was present in the vast majority of affected patients, 77% in one study (160) and 86% in another (161). Visual acuity was only mildly affected, with 24 out of 30 patients having visual acuity of 20/25 or better (161).

One mutation associated with MIDD in all these studies was the mtA3243G mutation, the substitution of guanine for adenine in the mitochondrial position 3243 (156–161). Heteroplasmy occurs, meaning that within each cell normal and mutant mitochondria co-exist. The average percentage of mutant mitochondria in MIDD per cell (heteroplasia) was reported as 11–25% (159).

The syndrome is not rare. It causes, on average, 1.5% of all diabetes mellitus (range: 0.5–2.8%) (160,161).

Other mitochondrial-associated disorders, some of which may manifest a maculopathy as part of the syndrome, will be discussed separately.

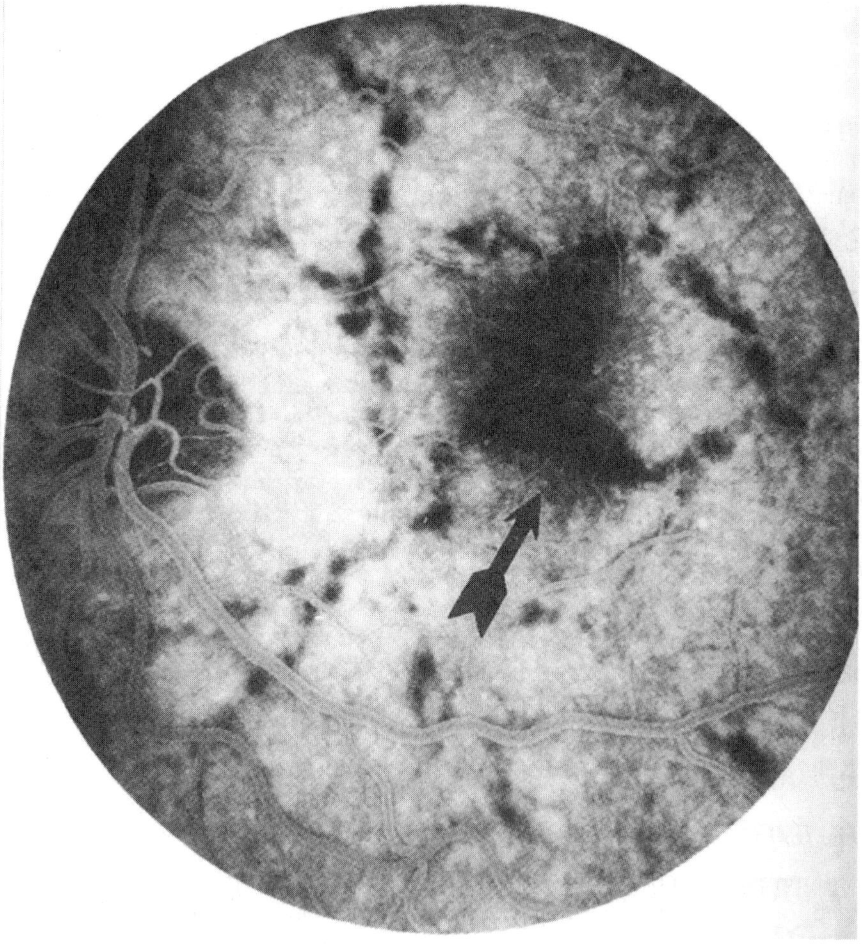

Figure 19 Fluorescein angiogram of the fundus of a patient with MIDD (MELAS) syndrome. Note the dark macula (arrow) and the radiating hypofluorescent lines, characteristic of pattern dystrophies (from Ref. 203).

A Unifying Concept of Classification

Several authors suggested that all pattern dystrophies of the pigment epithelium are one and the same disease, with different phenotypical expressions. Hsieh et al. (162) described three patients in the same family, each displaying a different one of three described entities: reticular dystrophy of Sjögren, macroreticular dystrophy, and butterfly-shaped pigment dystrophy. Guttman and coauthors (112) described a patient with the butterfly-shaped dystrophy in one eye and a vitelliform-like dystrophy in the other eye. Different manifestations of the various patterns in several members of the same family were also reported by DeJong and Delleman (163) and by Lodato and Giuffre (164).

Such articles suggest that all pattern dystrophies are one and the same disease, but this seems unlikely. In my opinion, based on the publications to date, the pattern dystrophies may best be classified under four different headings, as outlined in Table 4.

This classification is based on groups according to the clinical phenotype. The recent identification of genes and mutations showed that each may cause various maculopathies and, conversely, that the same maculopathy may be caused by different genes and certainly by different mutations of one gene. This statement particularly applies to the pattern dystrophies.

Diagnosis

The diagnosis of the pattern dystrophies of the pigment epithelium is based on the typical clinical manifestation, the accentuation of the picture by red-free photography or photography on panchromatic film, fluorescein angiography, and family examination. The electrophysiologic tests are not particularly helpful.

The differential diagnosis may sometimes be difficult, as it includes inherited diseases and several nongenetic diseases. AVMD, an autosomal dominant disease, and dominant drusen of the pigment epithelium may be indistinguishable from pattern macular dystrophy with yellow plaques. Nongenetic diseases include PVMD, acquired senile drusen with RPE dystrophy, cases of age-related macular degeneration, congenital rubella, and drug toxicity.

Management

The pattern dystrophies of the pigment epithelium are usually benign conditions and do not necessitate any particular treatment. Low-vision aids may be prescribed in advanced cases with decrease of vision.

In some cases, subretinal choroidal neovascularization occurs in older patients with pattern dystrophy. It is likely to be caused by the extensive RPE dystrophy associated with the pattern dystrophies. In such cases, laser retinal therapy or PDT should be considered (165).

Genetic counseling depends on the type of transmission in families with known inherited disorders. Autosomal dominant is the most common, followed by autosomal recessive and maternal (mitochondrial) inheritance. Identification of the causative mutated gene is possible and helpful for the management of the patient.

Table 4 The Clinical and Genetic Entities of the Pattern Dystrophies of the Pigment Epithelium

Entity No.	1	2	3	4
Name	Autosomal-recessive pattern dystrophy	Autosomal-dominant pattern dystrophy	Pattern macular dystrophy with yellow plaques	Mitochondrial-associated pattern dystrophy
Other names	Sjögren's reticular dystrophy of the RPE	Macroreticular dystrophy, butterfly-shaped dystrophy	Foveomacular vitelliform dystrophy AOFMD	MIDD
Fundus	Pigmented knotted fishing net	Fragmented irregular perimacular radiating pigmentation	Perimacular yellow radiating plaques, hyperpigmentation, and hypopigmentation lines	Macroreticular
Inheritance	Autosomal recessive	Autosomal dominant	Autosomal dominant	Mitochondrial
Visual acuity in young age	Normal	Normal	Normal	Normal
Visual acuity in advanced age	Normal: in some, reduction from CNV	Normal, slight to severe decrease	Normal, slight to severe decrease	Normal, slight to severe decrease
ERG	Normal	Normal or supernormal	Normal or slightly subnormal	Normal or slightly subnormal
EOG	Normal	Normal to moderately subnormal	Normal to severely subnormal (50%)	
Gene	RDS/peripherin	RDS/peripherin	RDS/peripherin VMD2	A3243G

DOMINANT DRUSEN AND THE EFEMP1 GENE

Introduction

Dominant drusen may well be the disease with the largest number of synonyms for one clinical entity in all of ophthalmology. The progressiveness of the disease, the multiple possible combinations between drusen of different size, forms, and distribution, and the accompanying variable atrophy of the RPE, result in different phenotypic manifestations. Hence, the interfamilial and intrafamilial differences caused many authors to give new names to "new" diseases often in a single family. The most common of these names were: Hutchinson–Tay choroiditis (166); Doyne's honeycomb dystrophy (167); macular degeneration of Holthouse–Batten (168); malattia leventinese, because it was found in a large family in the Levantine Valley in the Canton of Tessin in Switzerland (169); and dominant drusen of Bruch's membrane (170) and autosomal dominant radial drusen (171).

Little supports the view of separate diseases involving drusen, as suggested in some articles. The confusion resulted from the variable phenotypes both between families and within the family. In fact, the manifestation of the disorder in the fundus changes during life. Evidence supports Deutman, who stated that the dominantly inherited drusen is one single entity (170).

Description and Clinical Findings

The clinical findings in six families with 76 members found affected by dominant drusen were described by Pearce (172). The lesions were first observed between the ages of 20 and 30 years. Initially, small round drusen were observed in the peripapillary and macular areas. Drusen increased in number until around 40 or 50 years of age. They covered all of the posterior pole. Later, these spots coalesced, and the retina became atrophic. Pearce stressed the large variations between affected individuals and in the progression of the lesions. In about one-fourth of all affected, the lesions remained restricted to the peripapillary area.

Clinically, the disease is characterized by two findings: dispersed drusen in the posterior pole, and areas of RPE dystrophy, with variable combination of the two. Secondary changes may occur in the late stages. The disease is progressive. Drusen are seen in the third decade of life, although they may be found earlier, even in early childhood. Typically, drusen are seen in the macular area and around the disk, spreading into the nasal quadrants of the fundus. With time, they increase in number and extent of fundus involvement. Gradually and slowly, changes take place, which are characteristic of the evolutionary process of drusen in general, such as senile drusen. They change from hard pinpoint to semisolid, then soft serous, then become confluent, and finally regress and disappear with loss of RPE cells (173). Concurrently, changes in the layer of the pigment epithelium take place in the form of spots or larger areas of atrophy and spots of hyperpigmentation. With advancement of these changes, the characteristic picture of drusen becomes distorted and can hardly be recognized as drusen at all. Figure 20 illustrates the development of the changes in one patient with dominant drusen over several decades. The picture changed, becoming unrecognizable as the same condition. In the late stages, secondary changes in one of two forms may take place: (1) secondary atrophy of the choriocapillaris and the neural retina opposite areas of RPE atrophy and (2) eruption of subretinal neovascularization in the macular area, with fibrovascular membrane formation or hemorrhage.

Fluorescein angiography (Fig. 21) shows many more drusen than by clinical examination. They show hypofluorescence, which is sometimes accentuated (more than the choroidal background). In the macular area, spots of atrophy are seen as window defects, and hypofluorescent spots indicate hyperplasia or hyperpigmentation of the RPE.

Several articles that describe an autosomal dominant disease affecting the fundus, each with a different name, may well represent dominant drusen. In all of these, the combination of drusen and RPE dystrophy in different quantities, was the hallmark of each disease. These include the description of Lefler and coauthors (174) of a "hereditary macular degeneration and amino aciduria." The generalized aminoaciduria seemed, however, to segregate separately from the macular disease. Frank et al. (175) extended the description of the same family with 50 members affected by the disease and termed it "a new dominant progressive foveal dystrophy." The disease began earlier, with onset before 1 year of age in some patients and with multiple drusen in the macular area, which later turned into confluent drusen, followed by atrophy, sometimes as early as late puberty. The condition described by Singerman and his colleagues as "dominant slowly progressive macular dystrophy" (150) may also represent a variant of dominant drusen. Multiple drusen can clearly be seen in the fluorescein angiographic photographs of their patients. Members of the family described by Leveille and associates (176) also had multiple drusen in the periphery

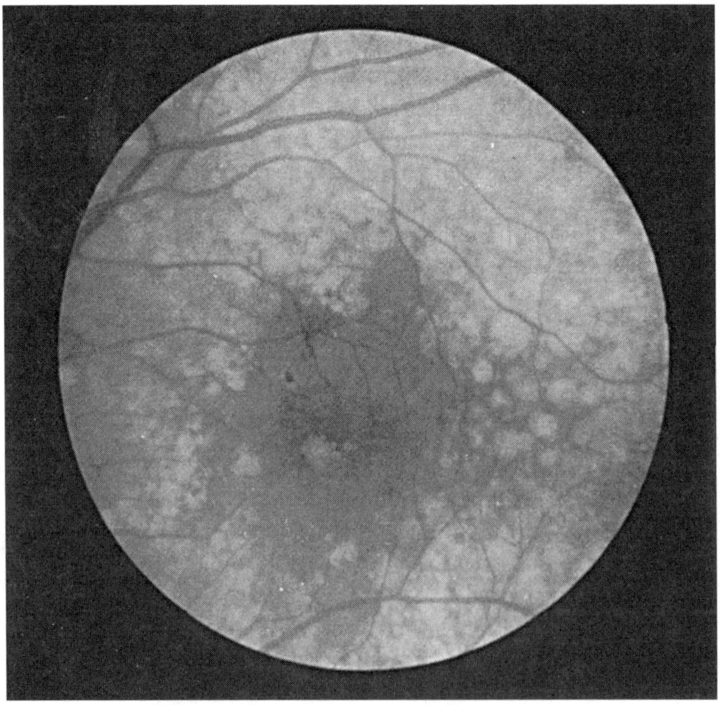

(a)

Figure 20 Evolution of changes of fundus in a patient with dominant drusen. (a) In 1976, when the patient is 44 years old, multiple drusen are seen in the posterior pole around the macula. (b) Ten years later, extensive atrophy of the RPE is the dominant finding. (c) More peripheral multiple drusen can still be found.

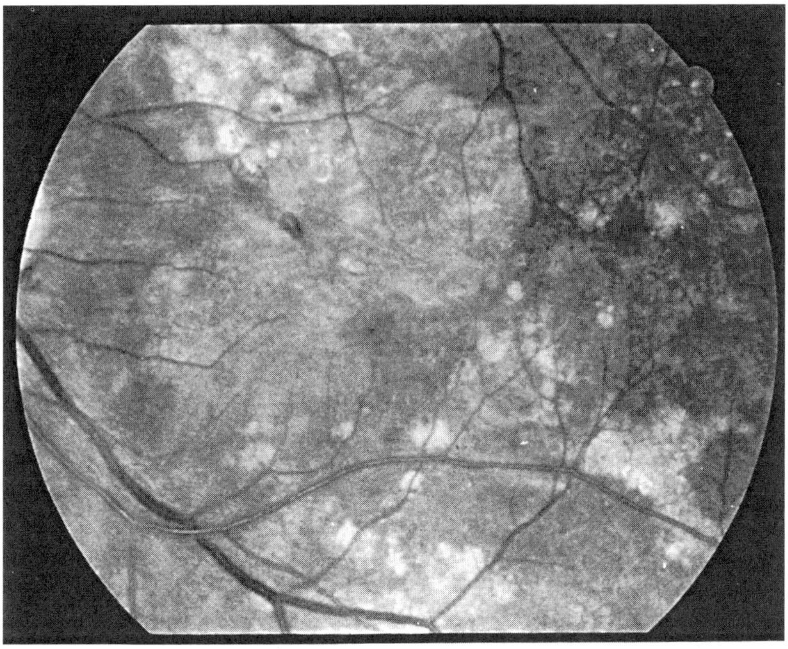

(b)

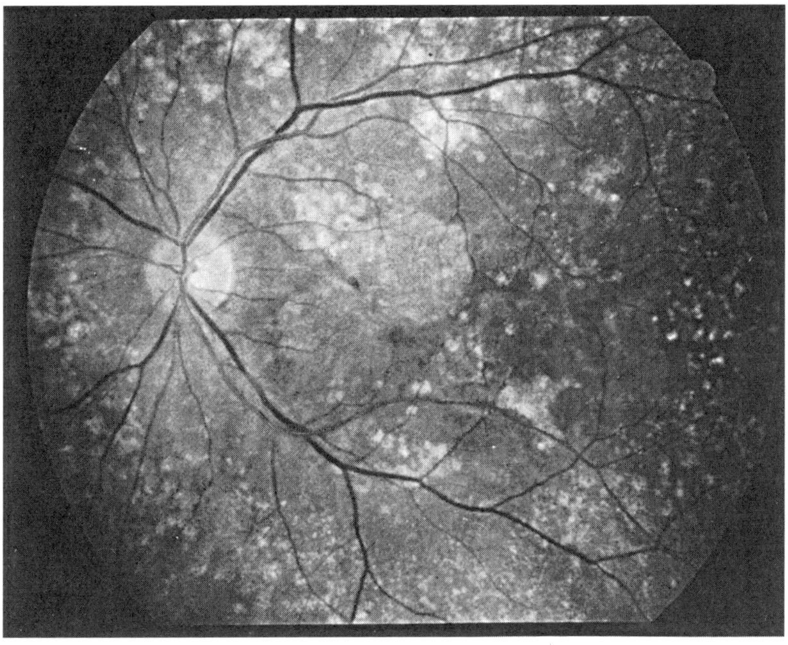

(c)

Figure 20 (*Continued*)

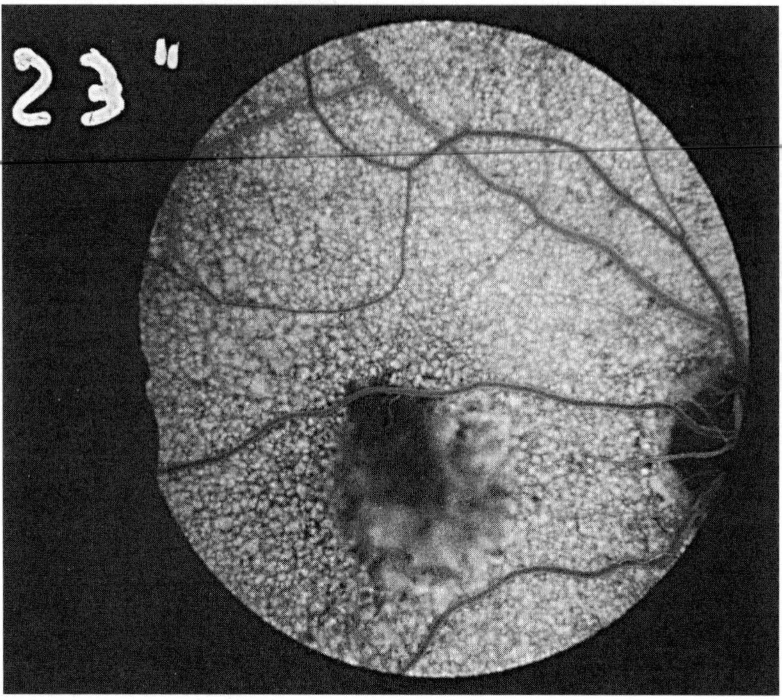

Figure 21 Patient with dominant drusen: fluorescein angiography shows numerous drusen along with RPE dystrophy.

and various forms of RPE atrophy in the center. They may represent an atypical appearance of dominant drusen.

In 1996, Heon and associates (171) reported the mapping of the locus malattia leventinese (autosomal dominant radial drusen) to chromosome 2p16–p21. In the same year, Gregory and associates (177) reported the mapping of the locus of Doyne's honeycomb retinal dystrophy to the same location (2p16). These authors examined a large family transmitting this autosomal dominant disorder and stressed the highly variable phenotype (178). A highly variable phenotype was also found in the study by Edwards and colleagues. They stressed that in elderly affected members the fundus manifestation may range from severe geographic atrophy, through subretinal fibrosis, to a single drusen (179)!

The gene was identified by Stone and associates in 1999 (180). The same single mutation of Arg345Trp was identified in both Doyne's honeycomb and malattia leventinese, thus confirming that the two disorders are in fact one clinical and genetic entity: the gene EFEMP1 [for: epithelial growth factor (EGF), containing fibrillin-like extracellular matrix protein]. The same mutation was identified in other North American families (181). In a study of several families in the United Kingdom and in North America, seven of the ten families studied carried the Arg345Trp mutation in the EFEMP1 gene, two other families showed linkage to a locus on 2p16 (182).

Three disorders, Doyne's honeycomb retinal dystrophy, malattia leventinese, and dominant radial drusen, seem therefore to be one clinical and genetic entity, associated in most cases with a single mutation Arg345Trp in the EFEMP1 gene on chromosome 2p16. This mutation is not associated with ARMD or any other known disease except dominant drusen. Another gene from the same group identified as EFEMP2 and mapped to chromosome 11q13 (183) was not found to be associated with a macular disorder. Another locus for dominant drusen was mapped to chromosome 6q14, the site of North Carolina macular dystrophy, and will be discussed with this disease.

Diagnosis

The diagnosis of dominant drusen is made when the combination of multiple drusen with RPE dystrophy is detected as a familial occurrence. The progressiveness of the disease and the variable manifestation in different-aged groups, in different families, and in different affected individuals within the same family, must be kept in mind. Fluorescein angiography accentuates the findings and should be routinely performed. Electrophysiologic tests are not particularly helpful; the ERG and the EOG, color vision, visual acuity, and visual fields are all normal in the early stages. Fishman and coauthors found a normal EOG in 12 patients with diffuse familial drusen (184). However, in advanced stages, all these tests may become abnormal. Visual acuity and color vision become abnormal with the involvement of the macula, the ERG becomes abnormal with the secondary involvement of the neural retina, and the EOG decreases because of the extensive atrophy of the RPE. The differential diagnosis of dominant drusen is with other causes: the flecked retina syndrome as described by Krill and Klein (185), flecked retina of Kandori (186), senile diffuse drusen, angioid streaks, and possibly other undefined causes of RPE atrophy.

Pathology

Light and electron microscopic investigations of eyes with diffuse drusen predominantly indicate that the pigment epithelial cells are likely to be the source of the material finally forming drusen. Controversy still exists about the questions of how and why this process is initiated (187–189). Dominant drusen, therefore, may be similar to senile drusen in the abnormal function, drusen formation, atrophic changes, and hyperpigmentation, occurring all in the RPE cells. In senile drusen, the cause is some aging phenomenon; in dominant drusen, the cause is an inherited abnormality of the RPE cells.

In one pathologic study of an eye of an 83-year-old woman with dominant drusen, membranous material including tubelike structures and vesicles accumulated between the basement membrane of the RPE and the inner collagenous layer of Bruchs membrane (190). These were similar to changes related to aging.

Marmorstein and associates (191) reported that the protein product of the mutated EFEMP1 gene behaves differently from the wild type. The function of the protein is unknown and the wild type is not found within drusen or nearby. The mutated protein is, however, misfolded and accumulated within RPE cells, and between RPE cells and drusen. This may be the cause of drusen formation (191).

SORSBY FUNDUS DYSTROPHY AND THE TIMP3 GENE

In 1949, five families reported by Sorsby et al. (192), who had a condition roughly similar to ARMD, became the basis of the recognition of this disorder as a separate entity. Sorsby and his colleagues described it as an autosomal dominant condition manifesting after age of 35. The disorder is not common and should be reserved for familial, autosomal dominant occurrence of subfoveal ingrowth of new vessels with progressive peripheral chorioretinal atrophy (193) or central RPE atrophy with peripheral widespread atrophy of the retina, RPE, and choroid (193,194). The differential diagnosis is with dominant drusen, vitelliform, atypical vitelliform, and ARMD. The term pseudo-inflammatory relates to the finding, in some patients with SFD, of heavy subretinal exudation.

Weber and colleagues mapped the Sorsby fundus dystrophy (SFD) locus to chromosome 22q13–qter (195) and later refined the location to 22q12.1–q13.2 (196). The same group identified a missense mutation in the TIMP3 gene associated with SFD (196). The gene tissue inhibitor of metalloproteinases 3 (TIMP3), plays an important role in extracellular matrix remodeling. One of its early manifestations is an abnormal accumulation of confluent, lipid-containing material in the inner portion of Bruch's membrane (196). Few mutations were identified in families. Ser181Cys mutation (196,197) was associated with intrafamilial variability of phenotype, ranging in affected family members from drusen, through exudative maculopathy, to frank choroidal neovascularization (197,198). This mutation was detected in the United Kingdom, Canada, United States, and South Africa (198). Other mutations, detected in Germany, Finland, Spain, Austria, and the United States, were all missense mutations of codons from 156 to 181 (198,199).

The gene TIMP3 plays no role in ARMD, vitelliform dystrophy, central areolar choroidal dystrophy, cone–rod dystrophy, or syndromic maculopathy (200). It is not related to a hemorrhagic macular dystrophy of older age (201).

A light and electron microscopic study of eyes with PFD revealed a striking finding of a 30 mm thick deposit within Bruchs' membrane that stained positive for lipids (202).

Patients with SFD frequently complain of reduced night vision. In fact, this is usually their first symptom before the reduction in visual acuity (203). Rod ERG is reduced in all SFD patients and becomes progressively worse. Jacobson and associates speculated that the TIMP3 gene mutations lead to disturbance of the normal balance between buildup and breakdown of extracellular matrix and result in abnormal subretinal deposits that form a barrier to diffusion of nutrients. Therefore, they treated their patient with oral vitamin A in the amount of 50,000 IU per day. After 1 month, the rod-ERG amplitudes were normal (203). Table 5 summarizes the findings in uncommon macular dystrophies.

NORTH CAROLINA MACULAR DYSTROPHY

This condition initially considered is now recognized rare and restricted to one large family in North Carolina in many countries and includes variable phenotypes including some cases diagnosed as central areolar pigment epithelial dystrophy (CAPED).

The disorder was probably reported first by Lefler et al. in 1971 under the term of hereditary macular degeneration (174). Frank et al. later expanded the description of the same family (175). Small and colleagues showed that several reports of macular dystrophies with different names, all relate, in fact, to North Carolina macular dystrophy.(204) These authors revealed that the large North Carolina family (counting now about 2000 members) stem from three Irish brothers who settled there in 1790 and exhibited the founder effect for the disorder (204). The disease was also

Table 5 Uncommon Macular Dystrophies

Name	Other names	Main fundus manifestations	Symbol/ locus	Inheritance	OMIM No.[a]	Chromosomal location	Gene	Mutations
Dominant drusen	Doyne's honeycomb; Malattia leventines and others	Drusen, RPE dystrophy	DHRD ML	AD	126600	2p16	EFEMP1	Arg345Trp
Sorsby fundus dystrophy	Sorsby pseudoinflammatory macular dystrophy	Drusen, exudative maculopathy CNV and hemorrhage	SFD	AD	136900	22q12.1–q13,2	TIMP3	Several missense
North Carolina macular dystrophy	Belize m.d.; central areolar pigment epithelium dystrophy	RPE dystrophy subretinal fibrosis	MCDR1 CAPED	AD	136550	6q14–q16.2	uk	uk
Dominant cystoid m.d.	—	Macular cyst angiographic leak	DCMD	AD	153880	7p15–p21	uk	uk
Dominant bull's-eye m.d.	Benign annular	Typical bull's-eye; late: pigmentary changes	—	AD	153870	11q13 4p15.2–p16.3	VMD2 STGD4(?)	Glu119Gln
Central areolar choroidal dystrophy		RPE dystrophy progresses to choriocapillaris atrophy	CACD	AR	215500	17p13 6p21.2	uk RDS	uk Arg142Trp
Progressive bifocal		Macular and nasal side atrophy	PBCRA	AD	600790	6q14–q16.2	uk	uk
Fenestrated sheen m.d.	FILM (familial inner limiting membrane dystrophy)	Yellowish refractile sheen	—	AD	153890	uk	uk	uk
Sjögren–Larsson		Macular glistening white spots	SLS	AR	270200	17q11.2	FALDH	Several

[a]Ref. 167.

Note: AD, autosomal dominant; AR, autosomal recessive; uk, unknown; m.d., macular dystrophy;

reported in Texas, Wisconsin, Canada, England, France, Spain, Belize, Mexico, and Germany (204–207).

Clinically, the disorder has early onset, and may even be congenital, as it was noticed at two months of life (207). It is characterized by the combined manifestation of drusen, RPE atrophy that turns into geographic atrophy in the elderly, and occasionally choroidal neovascularization. Subretinal fibrosis may be seen (Fig. 22). Visual acuity is extremely variable ranging from very good to poor.

The locus MCDR1 (for macular dystrophy retinal 1) was mapped to chromosome 6q14–q16 by Small and associates (208). A linkage to this locus was reported from other families in Belize and in Europe (207,209).

Histopathology performed on an eye of a 72-year-old individual showed a focal absence of photoreceptors and of RPE cells with attenuation of Bruch's membrane and focal atrophy of the choriocapillaris in the macular area (209).

In one family, phenotypically similar to North Carolina dystrophy, no linkage of the disease to chromosome 6q was found (210), possibly implying heterogeneity.

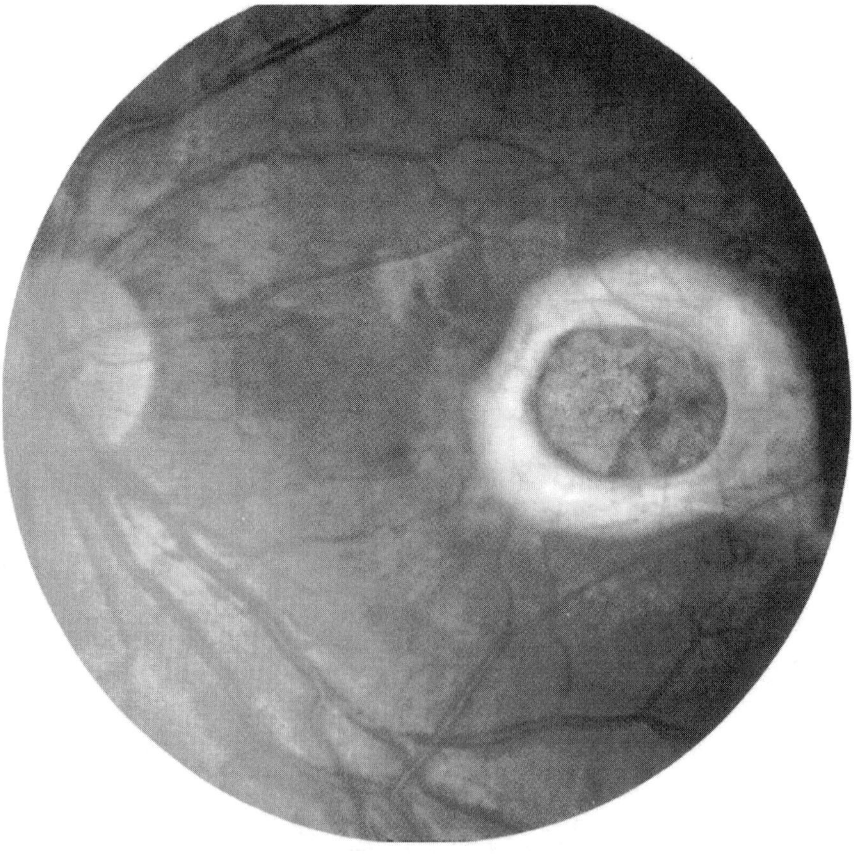

Figure 22 Fundus of a two year-old girl from a native Mayan family in Belize with the North Carolina phenotype found. [from: Rabb et al. Am J Ophthalmol 125, 502, 1998 (207).]

OTHER INHERITED MACULAR DISEASES

Dominantly Inherited Cystoid Macular Edema

This relatively rare inherited condition was first described in 1976 by Deutman and coauthors (211) and Deutman (212). Subsequent descriptions by Notting and Pinckers (213) and by Fishman et al. (214) delineate a uniform clinical picture of this disorder. Cystoid macular edema (CME) with leaking perifoveal capillaries is seen by fluorescein angiography in all affected patients. Onset is usually in the fourth decade of life (214) and may be earlier, but never in very young children. Visual acuity ranges from 6/7.5 to finger counting at 1–2 m. Typically, the patient is hyperopic, with a refractive error greater than +6.0 D, and a short axial length of 17.3–20.9 mm (213).

Color vision is abnormal in the direction of the red-green or the blue-yellow axis. In advanced cases, the CME may turn into an atrophy of the macula. The ERG is normal, the EOG is normal or subnormal, and fluorescein angiography displays a typical CME.

In families with dominant DCMD, affected members may go through three periods (215). In the first decade of life, only hyperopia and shortened axial length are noticed. From the second decade the EOG is reduced, visual acuity may be somewhat reduced, and leakage on fluorescein angiography can be seen. In later years atrophic changes occur at the macula and pericentral pigmentation in the form of bone corpuscles may be seen. Visual acuity may become very low (215,216).

DCMD is transmitted by an autosomal dominant gene, with full penetrance and similar expressivity, except for age of onset, in all affected members of the family.

Kremer and associates (215) mapped the DCMD locus to chromosome 7p15–p21. Previously, the RP7 locus was assigned to this location, and it became the candidate gene (215). However, this was excluded (217) and the gene has yet to be identified.

It is not clear whether focal laser, grid laser treatment, acetazolamide, or any other therapy is of any benefit in this condition.

The differential diagnosis is for acquired causes, such as ocular surgery, and hereditary diseases such as retinitis pigmentosa, which may display CME as an early finding (218,219).

Benign Concentric Annular Macular Dystrophy

This disorder, initially described by Deutman as a benign autosomal dominant disorder manifesting itself as a bull's-eye lesion in the macula, with minimal loss of visual acuity (220), was later re-evaluated and judged to be a cone–rod dystrophy (221). It will, therefore, be discussed in Chapter 9.

Ten years after the original description, patients with this benign condition were much worse, showing progression in the retinal manifestations and reduction in visual acuity and in night vision, and color vision disturbance. The ERG showed both rod and cone dysfunction (221).

It seems that autosomal dominant bull's-eye maculopathy, probably a better term, can be caused by a variety of mutated genes. Allikmets, Seddon, and associates (99,123) identified a missense mutation Glu119Gln, in exon 4 of the VMD2 gene (the gene associated with Best disease) in one patient with this disorder. In a large British family Michaelides et al. (62) mapped the locus for this disorder to chromosome 4p15.2–p16.3, the site of the STGD4 locus, which could be allelic. In other cases, a cone–rod dystrophy may be the cause for bull's-eye maculopathy.

Central Areolar Choroidal Dystrophy

This is one of the primary atrophies of the choroid and the choriocapillaris, manifesting itself as a round or oval lesion in the macular area. The condition is usually bilateral and symmetric. It is always related to decreased visual acuity. Most of these cases are sporadic, but familial cases of both autosomal dominant and autosomal recessive inheritance have been described (9). The condition will be described in detail in Chapter 11.

Central areolar choroidal dystrophy CACD is a progressive disease. Hoyng and Deutman studied 30 patients in 7 families and concluded that the disorder has four stages: stage 1, slight parafoveal RPE changes; stage 2, RPE mottling encircling the fovea; stage 3, atrophy of choriocapillaris sparing the fovea; and stage 4, visual acuity drastically reduced due to foveal involvement (222). CACD is an autosomal dominant disorder with established genetic heterogeneity. One mutation, Arg142Trp in the RDS/peripherin gene located on chromosome 6p21.2 was identified in several families (223,224). Another locus was mapped to chromosome 17p13, an area with several candidate genes but none yet identified (225,226).

Central Areolar Pigment Epithelial Dystrophy

First described by Fetkenhour and colleagues in 1976 (227), this condition relates to a familial condition of an atrophic lesion in the macula. The affected area varies in size. Contrary to central areolar choroidal dystrophy, the pigment epithelial layer is mainly affected. It is a benign condition. Visual acuity, ERG, EOG, dark adaptation, and color vision (except in one patient) were normal in all examined affected members of the family (227). The fundus displayed different macular changes, ranging from slight macular pigmentation to areas of depigmentation resembling a macular coloboma. In another family, described by Hermsen and Judisch, some patients had poor visual acuity (228). The inheritance was autosomal dominant, with full penetrance and variable expressivity.

It is now clear that the families described in the report of both Fetkenhour et al. (227) and Hermsen and Judisch (228) suffered from North Carolina macular dystrophy (80). It is not known if the large family described by Keithann and associates (229) also had North Carolina macular dystrophy. Future molecular studies will resolve the question of whether is a distinct entity in some cases or whether it is a manifestation of one or another macular dystrophies such as North Carolina, Sorsby fundus, Stargardt, or benign concentric (229).

Congenital Macular Coloboma

In this rather rare condition, a congenital macular coloboma is transmitted as a genetic trait.

The coloboma looks similar to congenital toxoplasmosis. It is symmetric, but differs in the various members of the family (Fig. 23). Visual acuity is severely reduced, usually around 3/60. In addition, nystagmus and photophobia are present.

The disorder was transmitted by an autosomal dominant gene in two families described by Sorsby (230,231). The mode of transmission was, however, autosomal recessive when in association with skeletal abnormalities (232) or in association with Leber's congenital amaurosis (233). In another family of congenital coloboma associated with apical dystrophy of hands and feet, the transmission was autosomal dominant (231).

I examined eight members of one affected family (Fig. 24). The mode of transmission is probably autosomal recessive, with pseudodominance owing to the high rate of consanguinity in this family. However, autosomal dominant inheritance cannot be excluded.

Progressive Bifocal Chorioretinal Atrophy

This rare condition is characterized by two separate areas of fundus involvement ("bifocal"), one in the macula and the other nasally. The macula manifests a large atrophic region, usually congenital, and subretinal deposits are seen nasally to the disk. In the second decade of life, the nasal lesion turns atrophic (234). Nystagmus, myopia, and poor vision from birth are the rule (235). The locus of this disorder, PBCRA, has been mapped to chromosome 6q14–q16.2, the site of MCDR1, the gene for North Carolina macular dystrophy, possibly an indication of allelic diseases or two closely located genes (234,235).

Fenestrated Sheen Macular Dystrophy

The name relates to a strange, rare, autosomal dominant disorder, in which a yellowish refractile sheen with red fenestration is seen in the fundus (236). Visual acuity is good till the third decade of life when RPE atrophy reduced vision with slow progression thereafter, sometimes to a typical bull's-eye maculopathy. Several families were described (237). A "familial internal limiting membrane dystrophy" (238) may be the same disease but a more severely expressed variance.

Ectodermal Dysplasia-Ectrodactyly-Macular Dystrophy Syndrome

In this autosomal recessive disease, a macular dystrophy sometimes resembling a coloboma is associated with systemic findings. The syndrome includes: (1) ectodermal dysplasia, in which the hair is thin and sparse, including the eyebrows and eyelashes, and the teeth are small and widely spaced; (2) ectrodactyly, various abnormalities of the fingers and toes; and (3) macular dystrophy in the form of a large or small area of chorioretinal atrophy, with or without pigmentary mottling. The macular changes seem progressive. In all three reported families (239–241), the transmission was clearly autosomal recessive.

Sjögren–Larsson syndrome

The hallmark of this disease is the triad of congenital ichthyosis, spastic diplegia or tetraplegia, and mental retardation. The ichthyosis affects the whole body but spares the face. Characteristic macular dystrophy consists of multiple crystalline deposits in the inner retina. The spots are white and glistening, their nature unknown (242,243).

Linkage to chromosome 17q11.2 was established (242,244), and mutations in the for fatty aldehydedehydrogenase (FALDH gene) were identified (244). The

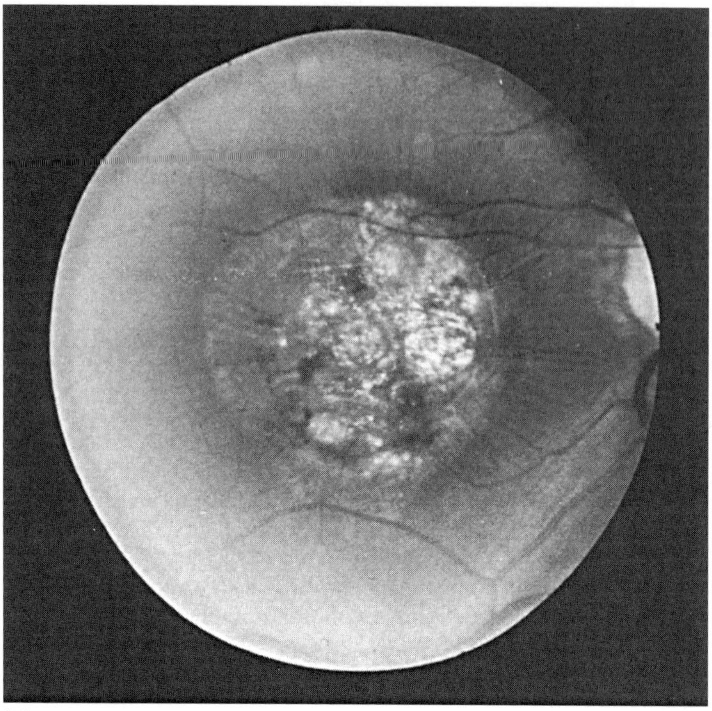

(a)

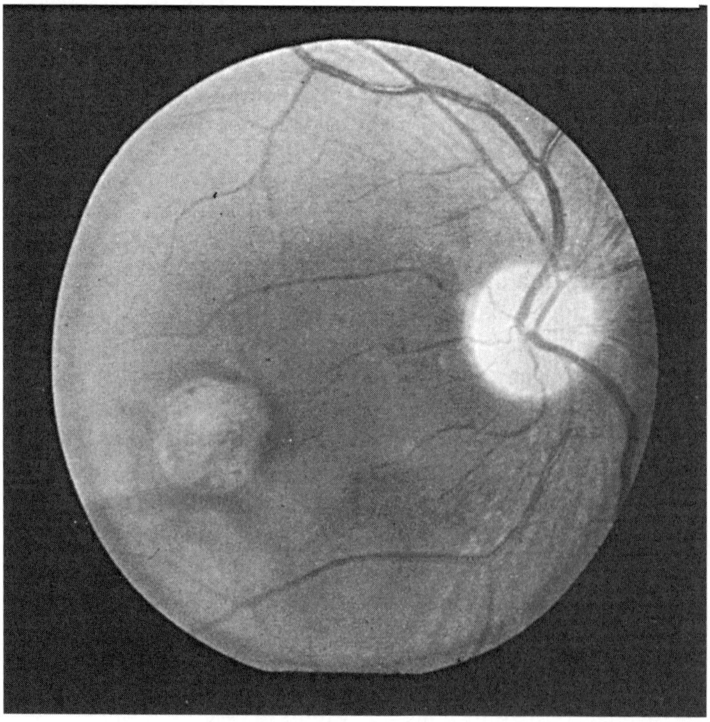

(b)

Figure 23 Congenital coloboma of the macula in two members of one family: (a) father and (b) son.

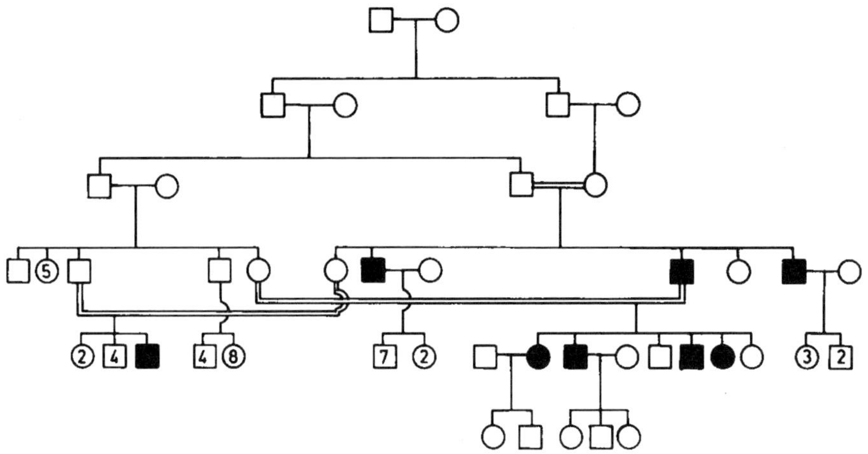

Figure 24 Pedigree of a family with congenital coloboma of the macula: the most likely mode of transmission is autosomal recessive, with pseudodominance owing to the high rate of consanguinity within the family.

gene consists of 10 exons, spans about 31 kb, and encodes a protein of 485 amino acids (243). This protein product, the enzyme FALDH catalyzes the oxidation of various medium-chain and long–chain fatty aldehydes into corresponding fatty acids (245).

AGE RELATED MACULAR DEGENERATION

ARMD is a common disease which has no clear pattern of inheritance and usually is not considered a genetic disease. However, it may be very difficult to confirm heredity in a disorder with such a late onset, when parents and other family members may not be available for examination. The importance of this disease stems from its being the prime cause of blindness. In England and Wales, ARMD is the cause of about 50% of all registered new blindness and its rate is increasing (246). A plethora of studies were performed on this subject in recent years. Several directions of research were taken.

One direction of research involves family studies. Hyman and coauthors compared 228 patients with 237 controls and found a positive family history in 21.6% of patients and 8.6% of controls (247). Prevalence of ARMD among first-degree relatives of affected individuals is greater than expected (248). Of 78 affected siblings, 20 were found to have ARMD while only 1 of 78 controls had this disease (249). The lifetime risk estimate of late ARMD, in relatives of patients was 50%, while in relatives of controls only 12% (250).

Another line of investigation nvolves twin studies. Isolated sporadic cases of monozygotic twins, when both of them developed exudative ARMD with or without choroidal neovascularization, were reported (251,252). Markedly similar fundus manifestations of ARMD-related changes were found in nine pairs of monozygotic (MZ) twins (253). Meyers and colleagues examined 134 twin pairs and found a 100% concordance regarding ARMD in MZ twins and only 42% concordance in dizygote

(DZ) twins (254). Hammond et al. (255) found a concordance of 0.37 in MZ twins and 0.19 in DZ twins, indicating heritability of 45%.

The third direction of research has been molecular studies. Several genes were excluded from being associated with ARMD. These included the EFEMP1 gene (causing dominant drusen) (183), the VMD2 gene (causing Best disease) (102,103), and the TIMP3 gene (causing Sorsby fundus dystrophy) (200,256). Controversy exists about the potential role of the ABCA4 gene (causing Stargardt disease) in ARMD (257). Some studies support this linkage, claiming a relatively high incidence of mutations in the ABCA4 gene in ARMD patients (258) and the existence of specific mutations (259,260). Other studies (261–266) claimed that the ABCA4 gene plays no role in ARMD, based on comparison of affected with controls and different methodology.

Fourth, linkage studies have been performed. Two possible linkage sites for loci of ARMD, at chromosome 1q31 and chromosome 17q25 were suggested (267,268), but not confirmed.

Finally, studies of environmental influence identified several risk factors for ARMD, such as cigarette smoking. The odds ratio was 3.6 for late ARMD in smokers in the POLA study (269), 2.4 for women smokers in the prospective large-scale nurses study (270), and a 6.6-fold increased risk of neovascular ARMD was found in smokers in the Rotterdam study (271). Lower risk of ARMD was found in individuals with higher intake of antioxidants (272–275).

A summary of all investigations indicates that ARMD is a multifactorial disease, in which multiple genetic factors and multiple environmental factors may play a role (246,276,277). The genetic factors are not yet known.

It may be safe to state that senile macular degeneration has some hereditary influence, but the pathogenesis is still unclear. Some risk factors identified in SMD may be genetic. These are a family history of SMD, blue or hazel-brown iris, race, light skin pigmentation, hypertension, and hyperopia (247,251). In addition, formation of drusen may have a genetic background.

REFERENCES

1. Bird HC. Retinal photoreceptor dystrophies (51st Edward Jackson Memorial Lecture). Am J Ophthalmol 1995; 119:543–562.
2. Van Driel MA, Maugeri A, Klevering BJ, et al. ABCR unites what ophthalmologists divide. Ophthalmic Genet 1998; 19:117–122.
3. Wells J, Wroblewski J, Keen J, et al. Mutations in the human retinal degeneration slow (RDS) gene can cause either retinitis pigmentosa or macular dystrophy. Nat Genet 1993; 3:213–218.
4. Stargardt K. Uber familiare, progressive Degeneration in der Maculagegend des Auges. Albrecht Von Graefes Arch Ophthalmol 1909; 71:534–550.
5. Stargardt K. Uber familiare, progressive Degeneration in der Makulagegend des Auges. Z Augenheilkd 1913; 30:95416.
6. Stargardt K. Zur Kasuistik der "familiaren, progressiven Degeneration in der Makulagegend des Auges" Z Augenheilkd 1916; 35:249–255.
7. Franceschetti A. Uber tapeto-retinale Degenerationen im Kindesalter. In: Sautter H ed. Entwicklung und Fortschritt in der Augenheilkunde. Stuttgart: Ferdinant Enke, 1963:107–120.
8. Franceschetti A, Francois J. Fundus flavimaculatus. Arch Ophthalmol (Paris) 1965; 25:505–530.

9. Deutman AF. The Hereditary Dystrophies of the Posterior Pole of the Eye. Asen, Netherlands: Van Gorcum, 1971.
10. Fishman GA, Buckman G, Van Every T. Fundus flavimaculatus: a clinical classification. Doc Ophthalmol Proc Ser 1977; 13:213–220.
11. Gelisken O, Delaey JJ. A clinical review of Stargardt disease and/or fundus flavimaculatus with follow-up. Int Ophthalmol 1985; 8:225–235.
12. Merin S. A new classification of juvenile hereditary macular dystrophy. In: XXIII Concilium Ophthalmologicum, kyoto, 1978. Amsterdam: Excerpta Medica, 1978: 751–754.
13. Fishman GA. Fundus flavimaculatus: A clinical classification. Arch Ophthalmol 1976; 94:2061–2067.
14. Noble KG, Carr RE. Stargardt disease and fundus flavimaculatus. Arch Ophthalmol 1979; 97:1281–1285.
15. Bonnin MP. Le signe du silence choroidien dans les dégénérescences tapeto-retiniennes centrales examinées sous fluorescéine. Bul Soc Ophthalmol Fr 1971; 71:348–351.
16. Fish G, Grey R, Sehmi KS, Bird AC. The dark choroid in posterior retinal dystrophies. Br J Ophthalmol 1981; 65:359–363.
17. Uliss AE, Moore AT, Bird AC. The dark choroid in posterior retinal dystrophies. Ophthalmology 1987; 94:1423–1427.
18. Fishman GA, Farber M, Patel BS, Derlacki DJ. Visual acuity loss in patients with Stargardt macular dystrophy. Ophthalmology 1987; 94:809–814.
19. Hadden OB, Gass JD. Fundus flavimaculatus and Stargardt disease. Am J Ophthalmol 1976; 82:527–539.
20. Moloney JBM, Mooney DJ, O'Connor MA. Retinal function in Stargardt disease and fundus flavimaculatus. Am J Ophthalmol 1983; 96:57–65.
21. Armstrong JD, Meyer D, Xu S, Elfervig JL. Long-term follow up of Stargardt disease and fundus flavimaculatus. Ophthalmology 1998; 105:448–458.
22. Zhang X, Hargitai J, Tammur J et al. Macular pigment and visual acuity in Stargardt macular dystrophy. Graefes Arch Clin Exp Ophthalmol 2002; 240:802–809.
23. Kaplan J, Gerber S, Larget-Piet D et al. A gene for Stargardt disease (fundus flavimaculatus) maps to the short arm of chromosome 1. Nat Genet 1993; 5:308–311.
24. Weleber RG. Stargardt macular dystrophy. Arch Ophthalmol 1999; 112:752–754.
25. Zhang K, Nguyen TH, Crandall A, Donoso LA. Genetic and molecular studies of macular dystrophies: recent developments. Surv Ophthalmol 1995; 40:51–60.
26. Allikmets R, Singh N, Sun H, et al. A photoreceptor cell-specific ATP-binding transporter gene (ABCR) is mutated in recessive Stargardt macular dystrophy. Nat Genet 1997; 15:236–246.
27. Sun H, Nathans J. Stargardt ABCR is localized to the disc membrane of retinal rod outer segments (correspondence). Nat Genet 1997; 17:15–16.
28. Gerber S, Rozet JM, van der Pol TJ, et al. Complete exon-intron structure of the retina-specific ATP binding transporter gene (ABCR) allows the identification of novel mutations underlying Stargardt disease. Genomics 1998; 48:139–142.
29. Molday LL, Rabin AR, Molday RS. ABCR expression in foveal cone photoreceptors and its role in Stargardt macular dystrophy. Nat Genet 2000; 25:257–258.
30. Nasonkin I, Illing M, Koehler MR, et al. Mapping of the red photoreceptor ABC transporter (ABCR) to 1p21-p22.1 and identification of novel mutations in Stargardt disease. Hum Genet 1998; 102:21–26.
31. Zhang K, Garibaldi DC, Kniazeva M, et al. A novel mutation in the ABCR gene in four patients with autosomal recessive Stargardt disease. Am J Ophthalmol 1999; 720–724.
32. Maugeri A, van Driel MA, van de Pol DJ, et al. The 2588G->C mutation in the ABCR gene is a mild frequent founder mutation in the Western European population and allows the classification of ABCR mutations in patients with Stargardt disease. Am J Hum Genet 1999; 64:1024–1035.

33. Webster AR, Heon E, Lotery AJ, et al. An analysis of allelic variation in the ABCA4 gene. Invest Ophthalmol Vis Sci 2001; 42:1179–1189.
34. Maugeri A, Klevering BJ, Rohrschneider K, et al. Mutations in the ABCA4 (ABCR) gene are the major cause of autosomal recessive cone-rod dystrophy. Am J Hum Genet 2000; 67:960–966.
35. Cremers FP, van de Pol DJ, van Driel M, et al. Autosomal recessive retinitis pigmentosa and cone-red dystrophy caused by splice site mutations in the Stargardt disease gene ABCR. Hum Mol Genet 1998; 7:355–362.
36. Klevering BJ, van Driel M, van de Pol DRJ, et al. Phenotypic variations in a family with retinal dystrophy as a result of different mutations in the ABCR gene. Br J Ophthalmol 1999; 83:914–918.
37. Martinez-Mir A, Paloma E, Allikmets R, et al. Retinitis pigmentosa caused by a homozygous mutation in the Stargardt disease gene ABCR. Nat Genet 1998; 18:11–12.
38. Klevering BJ, Blankenagel A, Maugeri A, et al. Phenotypic spectrum of autosomal recessive cone-rod dystrophies caused by mutations in the ABCA4 (ABCR) gene. Invest Ophthalmol Vis Sci 2002; 43:1980–1985.
39. Merin S, Auerbach E, Ivry M. The differential diagnosis of juvenile hereditary macular degeneration. Metab Ophthalmol 1978; 2:191–192.
40. Gerber S, Rozet JM, Bonneau D, et al. A gene for late-onset fundus flavimaculatus with macular dystrophy maps to chromosome 1pl3. Am J Hum Genet 1995; 56:396–399.
41. Yatsenko AN, Shroyer NF, Lewis RA, Lupski JR. Late-onset Stargardt disease is associated with missense mutations that map outside known functional regions of ABCR (ABCA4). Hum Genet 2001; 108:346–355.
42. Souied EH, Ducroq D, Rozet JM, et al. A novel ABCR nonsense mutation responsible for late-onset fundus flavimaculatus. Invest Ophthalmol Vis Sci 1999; 40:2740–2744.
43. Irvine AR, Wergeland FL. Stargardt hereditary progressive macular degeneration. Br J Ophthalmol 1972; 56:817–826.
44. Carpel EF, Kalina RE. A family study of fundus flavimaculatus. Am J Ophthalmol 1975; 80:238–241.
45. Aaberg TM. Stargardt disease and fundus flavimaculatus. Evaluation of morphologic progression and intrafamilial co-existence. Trans Am Ophthalmol Soc 1986; 84: 453–487.
46. Klien BA, Krill AE. Fundus flavimaculatus. Clinical, functional, and histopathologic observations. Am J Ophthalmol 1967; 64:3–23.
47. Merin S, Landau J. Abnormal findings in relatives of patients with juvenile hereditary rnacular degeneration. Ophthalmologica 1970; 161:1–10.
48. Deutman AF. Macular dystrophies. In: Goldberg MF, ed. Genetic and Metabolic Eye Disease. Boston: Little, Brown & Co, 1974:380–385.
49. Rozet JM, Gerber S, Souied E, et al. Spectrum of ABCR gene mutations in autosomal recessive macular dystrophies. Eur J Hum Genet 1998; 6:291–296.
50. Bloome MA, Garcia CA. Manual of Retinal and Choroidal Dystrophies. New York: Appleton-Century-Crofts, 1982.
51. Bithe PP, Berns LA. Dominant inheritance of Stargardt disease. J Am Optom Assoc 1988; 59:112–117.
52. Zhang K, Kniazeva M, Hutchinson A, et al. The ABCR gene in recessive and dominant Stargardt diseases: a genetic pathway in macular degeneration. Genomics 1999; 60: 234–237.
53. Zhang K, Bither PP, Park R, et al. A dominant Stargardt macular dystrophy locus maps to chromosome 13q34. Arch Ophthalmol 1994; 112:759–764.
54. Stone EM, Nichols BE, Kimura AE, et al. Clinical features of a Stargardt-like dominant progressive macular dystrophy with genetic linkage to chromosome 6q. Arch Ophthalmol 1994; 112:765–772.
55. Edwards AO, Miedziak A, Vrabec T, et al. Autosomal dominant Stargardt-like macular dystrophy: I. Clinical characterization, longitudinal follow-up, and evidence for a

common ancestry in families linked to chromosome 6q 14. Am J Ophthalmol 1999; 127: 426–435.
56. Lagali PS, MacDonald IM, Griesinger IB, et al. Autosomal dominant Stargardt-like macular dystrophy segregating in a large Canadian family. Can J Ophthalmol 2000; 35:315–324.
57. Griesinger IB, Sieving PA, Ayyagari R, et al. Autosomal dominant macular atrophy at 6ql4 excludes CORD7 and MCDR1/PBCRA loci. Invest Ophthalmol Vis Sci 2000; 41:248–255.
58. Donoso LA, Frost AT, Stone EM, et al. Autosomal dominant Stargardt-like macular dystrophy: founder effect and reassessment of genetic heterogeneity. Arch Ophthalmol 2001; 119:564–570.
59. Zhang K, Kniazeva M, Han M, et al. A 5-bp deletion in ELOVL4 is associated with two related forms of autosomal dominant macular dystrophy Nat Genet 27:89–93, 2001.
60. Bernstein PS, Tammur J, Singh N, et al. Diverse macular dystrophy phenotype caused by a novel complex mutation in the ELOVL4 gene. Invest Ophthalmol Vis Sci 2001; 42:3331–3336.
61. Kniazeva M, Chiang MF, Morgan B, et al. A new locus for autosomal dominant Stargardt-like disease maps to chromosome 4. Am J Hum Genet 1999; 64:1394–1399.
62. Michaelides M, Johnson S, Poulson A, et al. An autosomal dominant bull's-eye macular dystrophy (MCDR2) that maps to the short arm of chromosome 4. Invest Ophthalmol Vis Sci 2003; 44:1657–1662.
63. Weise EE, Yannuzzi LA. Ring maculopathies mimicking chloroquine retinopathy. Am J Ophthalmol 1974; 78:204–210.
64. Kohl S, Christ-Adler M, Apfelstedt-Sylla E, et al. RDS/peripherin gene mutations are frequent causes of central retinal dystrophies. J Med Genet 1997; 34:620–626.
65. Yen MY, Wei YH, Liu JH. Stargardt type maculopathy in a patient with 11778 Leber's optic neuropathy. J Neuro-Ophthalmol 1996; 16:120–123.
66. Harada T, Miyake Y, Natsume K. Atrophic macular degeneration in a patient with olivo-pontocerebellar atrophy. Ophthalmologica 1984; 188:259–265.
67. Cooles P, Michaud R, Best RV. A dominantly inherited progressive disease in a black family characterised by cerebellar and retinal degeneration, external ophthalmoplegia, and abnormal mitochondria. J Neurol Sci 1988; 87:275–288.
68. Gass DM, Pautler SE. Toxemia of pregnancy pigment epitheliopathy masquerading as heredomacular dystrophy. Trans Am Ophthalmol Soc 1985; 83:114–130.
69. von Ruckmann A, Fitzke FW, Bird AC. In vivo fundus autofluorescence in macular dystrophies. Arch Ophthalmol 1997; 115:609–615.
70. Wroblewski JJ, Gitter KA, Cohen G, Schomaker K. Indocyanine green angiography in Stargardt flavimaculatus. Am J Ophthalmol 1995; 120:208–218.
71. Merin S, Auerbach E. The central and peripheral retina in macular degeneration. Involvement as reflected by the electroretinogram. Arch Ophthalmol 1970; 84:710–718.
72. Fishman GA, Young RSL, Schall SP, Vasquez YA. Electro-oculogram testing in fundus flavimaculatus. Arch Ophthalmol 1979; 97:1896–1898.
73. Rover J, Bach M. The c-wave in hereditary degenerations of the ocular fundus. Doc Ophthalmol 1985; 60:127–132.
74. Van Meel GJ, Van Norren D. Foveal densitometry as a diagnostic technique in Stargardt disease. Am J Ophthalmol 1986; 102:353–362.
75. Fishman GA, Cunha-Vaz JG, Travassos AC. Vitreous fluorophotometry in patients with fundus flavimaculatus. Arch Ophthalmol 1982; 100:1086–1088.
76. Maumenee IH, Maumenee AE. Fundus flavimacuiatus. clinical, genetic, and pathologic observations. In: Francois J, ed. Fifth Congress of the European Society of Ophthalmology, Hamburg, 1976. Stuttgart: Ferdinant Enke, 1978:80–82.
77. Eagle RC, Lucier AC, Bernardino VB, Yanoff M. Retinal pigment epithelial abnormalities in fundus flavimacuiatus. Ophthalmology 1980; 87:1189–1200.

78. McDonnel PJ, Kivlin JD, Maumenee IH, Green WR. Fundus flavimaculatus without maculopathy. A clinicopathologic study. Ophthalmology 1986; 93:116–119.
79. Birnbach CD, Jarvelainen M, Possin DE, Milam AH. Histopathology and immunocytochemistry of the neurosensory retina in fundus flavimaculatus. Ophthalmology 1994; 101:1211–1219.
80. OMIM. http://www.ncbi.nlm.nih.gov/OMIM/.
81. Fonda B, Gardner LR. Characteristics and low vision corrections in Stargardt disease. Educational and vocational achievements enhanced by low vision corrections. Ophthalmology 1985; 92:1084–1091.
82. Schwartzenberg T, Merin S, Nawratzki I, Yanko L. Low vision aids in Stargardt disease. Ann Ophthalmol 1988; 20:428–430.
83. Fishman GA, Stone EM, Grover S, et al. Variation of clinical expression in patients with Stargardt dystrophy and sequence variations in the ABCR gene. Arch Ophthalmol 1999; 117:504–510.
84. Weleber RG, Carr RE, Murphey WH, et al. Phenotypic variation including retinitis pigmentosa, pattern dystrophy, and fundus flavimaculatus in a single family with a deletion of codon 153 or 154 of the peripherin/RDS gene. Arch Ophthalmol 1993; 111: 1531–1542.
85. Best F. Uber eine hereditare Makulaaffektion. Beitrage zur Vererbungslehre. Z Augenheilkd 1905; 13:199–212.
86. Godel V, Chaine G, Regenbogen L, Coscas G. Best's vitelliform macular dystrophy. Acta Ophthalmol 1986; 75(suppl):11–31.
87. Mohler CW, Fine SL. Long term evaluation of patients with Best's vitelltform dystrophy. Ophthalmology 1981; 88:688–691.
88. Barkman Y. A clinical study of a central TRD. Acta Ophthalmol 1961; 39:663–671.
89. Miller SAL. Multifocal Best's vitelliform dystrophy. Arch Ophthalmol 1977; 95: 984–990.
90. Park DW, Polk TD, Stone EM. Fluctuating vision in Best disease. Arch Ophthalmol 1997; 115:1469–1470.
91. Kraushar MF, Margolis S, Morse P, Nugent ME. Pseudohypopyon in Best's vitelliform macular dystrophy. Am J Ophthalmol 1983; 94:30–37.
92. Hittner HM, Ferrell RE, Borda RP, Justice J Jr. Atypical vitelliform macular dystrophy in a 5-generation family. Br J Ophthalmol 1984; 68:199–207.
93. Stone EM, Nichols BE, Streb LM, et al. Genetic linkage of vitelliform macular degeneration (Best's disease) to chromosome 11p13. Nat Genet 1992; 1:246–250.
94. Forsman K, Graff C, Nordstrom S, et al. The gene for Best's macular dystrophy is located at 11ql3 in a Swedish family. Clin Genet 1992; 42:156–159.
95. Nichols BE, Bascom R, Litt M, et al. Refining the locus for Best vitelliform macular dystrophy and mutation analysis of the candidate gene ROM1. Am J Hum Genet 1994; 54:95–103.
96. Hou YC, Richards JE, Bingham EL, et al. Linkage study of Best's vitelliform macular dystrophy (VMD2) in a large North American family. Hum Hered 1996; 46:211–220.
97. Marquardt A, Stohr H, Passmore LA, et al. Mutations in a novel gene, VMD2, encoding a protein of unknown properties cause juvenile-onset vitelliform macular dystrophy (Best's disease). Hum Mol Genet 1998; 7:1517–1525.
98. Petrukhin K, Koisti MJ, Bakall B, et al. Identification of the gene responsible for Best macular dystrophy. Nat Genet 1998; 19:241–247.
99. Allikmets R, Seddon JM, Bernstein PS, et al. Evaluation of the Best disease gene in patients with age-related macular degeneration and other maculopathies. Hum Genet 1999; 104:449–453.
100. Marmorstein AD, Marmorstein LY, Rayborn M, et al. Bestrophin, the product of the Best vitelliform macular dystrophy gene (VMD2), localizes to the basolateral plasma membrane of the retinal pigment epithelium. Proc Natl Acad Sci 2000; 97:12758–12763.

101. Palomba G, Rozzo C, Angius A, et al. A novel spontaneous missense mutation in VMD2 gene is a cause of a best macular dystrophy sporadic case. Am J Ophthalmol 2000; 129:260–262.
102. Lotery AJ, Munier FL, Fishman GA, et al. Allelic variation in the VMD2 gene in best disease and age-related macular degeneration. Invest Ophthalmol Vis Sci 2000; 41:1291–1296.
103. White K, Marquardt A, Weber BH. VMD2 mutations in vitelliform macular dystrophy (Best disease) and other maculopathies. Hum Mutat 2000; 15:301–308.
104. Weber BH, Walker D, Muller B. Molecular evidence for non-penetrance in Best's disease. J Med Genet 1994; 31:388–392.
105. Hodes BL, Feiner LA, Sherman SH, Cunningham D. Progression of pseudovitelliform macular dystrophy. Arch Ophthalmol 1984; 102:381–383.
106. Gass JDM. A clinicopathologic study of a peculiar foveomacular dystrophy. Trans Am Ophthalmol Soc 1974; 73:139–155.
107. Yamaguchi K, Yoshida M, Kano T, et al. Adult-onset foveomacular vitelliform dystrophy with retinal folds. Jpn J Ophthalmol 2001; 45:533–537.
108. Fishman GA, Trimble S, Rabb FM, Fishman M. Pseudovitelliform macular degeneration. Arch Ophthalmol 1977; 95:73–76.
109. Yang Z, Lin W, Moshfeghi DM, et al. A novel mutation in the RDS, peripherin gene causes adult-onset foveomacular dystrophy. Am J Ophthalmol 2003; 135:213–218.
110. Dubovy SR, Hairston RJ, Schatz H, et al. Adult-onset foveomacular pigment epithelial dystrophy: clinicopathologic correlation of three cases. Retina 2000; 20:638–649.
111. Theischen M, Schilling H, Steinhorst UH. EOG in adult vitelliform macular degeneration, butterfly-shaped pattern dystrophy, and Best disease. Der Ophthalmologe 1997; 94:230–233.
112. Guttman I, Walsh JB, Henkind P. Vitelliform macular dystrophy and butterfly-shaped epithelial dystrophy. A continuum? Br J Ophthalmol 1982; 66:170–173.
113. Ferrel RE, Hittner HM, Antoszyk JH. Linkage of atypical vitelliform macular dystrophy (VM-1) to the soluble glutamate pyruvate transaminase *(GPT1)* locus. Am J Hum Genet 1983; 35:78–84.
114. Sohocki MM, Sullivan LS, Mintz-Hittner HA, et al. Exclusion of atypical vitelliform macular dystrophy from 8q24.3 and from other known macular degenerative loci. Am J Hum Genet 1997; 61:239–241.
115. Arend O, Remky A, Dahlke C, Kirchhof B. Photo essay: normal electro-oculogram in a patient with vitelliruptive macular dystrophy and multiple vitelliform cysts. Arch Ophthalmol 2000; 118:1460–1461.
116. Kingham JD, Lochen GP. Vitelliform macular degeneration. Am J Ophthalmol 1977; 84:526–531.
117. Marmor MF. "Vitelliform" lesions in adults. Ann Ophthalmol 1979; 11:1705–1712.
118. Snyder DA, Fishman GA, Witteman G, Fishman M. Vitelliform lesions associated with retinal pigment epithelial detachment. Ann Ophthalmol 1978; 10:1711–1715.
119. Miller SA, Bresnick OH, Chandra SR. Choroidal neovascular membrane in Best's vitelliform macular dystrophy. Am J Ophthalmol 1976; 82:252–255.
120. Gass JDM, Jallow S, David B. Adult vitelliform macular detachment occurring in patients with basal laminar drusen. Am J Ophthalmol 1985; 99:445–459.
121. Cortin P, Archer D, Maumenee IH, et al. A patterned macular dystrophy with yellow plaques and atrophic changes. Br J Ophthalmol 1980; 64:127–134.
122. Burgess DB, Oik RJ, Uniat LM. Macular disease resembling adult foveomacular vitelliform dystrophy in older adults. Ophthalmology 1987; 94:362–366.
123. Seddon JM, Afshari MA, Sharma S, et al. Assessment of mutations in the Best macular dystrophy (VMD2) gene in patients with adult-onset foveomacular vitelliform dystrophy, age-related maculopathy, and bull's-eye maculopathy. Ophthalmology 2001; 108:2060–2067.

124. Stone EM, Kimura AE, Folk JC, et al. Genetic linkage of autosomal dominant neovascular inflammatory vitreoretinopathy to chromosome 11q13. Hum Mol Genet 1992; 1:685–689.
125. Massof RW, Fleischman JA, Fine SL, Yoder F. Flicker fusion thresholds in Best macular dystrophy. Arch Ophthalmol 1977; 95:991–994.
126. Francois J. Importance of electrophysiology in ophthalmogenetics. Ophthalmologica 1984; 188:14–27.
127. Cavender JC. Best's macular dystrophy. Arch Ophthalmol 1982; 100:1067.
128. Kobrin JL, Apple DJ, Hart WB. Vitelliform dystrophy. In: Rabb MF, ed. Macular Disease. Int Ophthalmol Clin 1981:2121(3):167–184.
129. Weingeist TA, Kobrin JL, Watzke RC. Histopathology of Best's macular dystrophy. Arch Ophthalmol 1982; 100:1108–1114.
130. Frangieh GT, Green R, Fine SL. A histopathologic study of Best's macular dystrophy. Arch Ophthalmol 1982; 100:1115–1121.
131. O'Gorman S, Flaherty WA, Fishman GA, Berson EL. Histopathologic findings in Best's vitelliform macular dystrophy. Arch Ophthalmol 1988; 106:1261–1268.
132. Patrinely OR, Lewis RA, Font RI. Foveomacular vitelliform dystrophy, adult type: a clinicopathologic study including electron microscopic observation. Ophthalmology 1985; 92:1712–1718.
133. Nordstrom S, Thorburn W. Dominantly inherited macular degeneration (Best's disease) in a homozygous father with 11 children. Clin Genet 1980; 18:211–216.
134. Nordstrom S. Hereditary macular degeneration—a population survey in the country of Vasterbotten, Sweden. Hereditas 1974; 78:41–62.
135. Yoder FE, Cross HE, Chase GA, et al. Linkage studies of Best's macular dystrophy. Clin Genet 1988; 34:26–30.
136. Sjögren H. Dystrophia reticularis laminae pigmentosae retinae. An earlier not described hereditary eye disease. Acta Ophthalmol 1950; 28:279–295.
137. Deutman AF, Rumke AML. Reticular dystrophy of the retinal pigment epithelium. Dystrophia reticularis laminae pigmentosae retinae of Sjögren. Arch Ophthalmol 1969; 82:4–9.
138. Grover S, Fishman GA, Stone EM. Atypical presentation of pattern dystrophy in two families with peripherin/RDS mutations. Ophthalmology 2002; 109:1110–1117.
139. Deutman AF, van Blommestein JDA, Henkes HE, et al. Butterfly-shaped pigment dystrophy of the fovea. Arch Ophthalmol 1970; 83:558–569.
140. Prensky JG, Bresnick GH. Butterfly-shaped macular dystrophy in four generations. Arch Ophthalmol 1983; 8:1198–1203.
141. Zhang K, Garibaldi DC, Li Y, et al. Butterfly-shaped pattern dystrophy: a genetic, clinical, and histopathological report. Arch Ophthalmol 2002; 120:485–490.
142. Nichols BE, Sheffield VC, Vandenburgh K, et al. Butterfly-shaped pigment dystrophy of the fovea caused by a point mutation in codon 167 of the RDS gene. Nat Genet 1993; 3:202–207.
143. Nichols BE, Drack AV, Vandenburgh K, et al. A 2 base pair deletion in the RDS gene associated with butterfly-shaped pigment dystrophy of the fovea. Hum Mol Genet 1993; 2:601–603.
144. Fossarello M, Bertini C, Galantuomo MS, et al. Deletion in the peripherin/RDS gene in two unrelated Sardinian families with autosomal dominant butterfly-shaped macular dystrophy. Arch Ophthalmol 1996; 114:448–456.
145. Slezak H, Hommer K. Fundus pulverulenlus. Graefes Arch Clin Exp Ophthalmol 1969; 178:177–182.
146. Mesker RP, Oosterhuis JA, Delleman JW. A retinal lesion resembling Sjogren dystrophia reticularis laminae pigmentosae retinae. Winkelman JE, Crone RA Perspectives of Ophthalmology. Vol. 2. Amsterdam: Excerpta Medica Foundation 1970:2:40–45.
147. Benedikt D, Werner W. Retikulare pigmentdystrophie der Netzhaut. Klin Monatsbl Augenheilkd 1971; 159:794–798.

148. Marmor MF, Byers B. Pattern dystrophy of the pigment epithelium. Am J Ophthalmol 1977; 84:32–44.
149. O'Donnell FE, Schatz H, Reid P, Green WR. Autosomal dominant dystrophy of the retinal pigment epithelium. Arch Ophthalmol 1979; 97:680–683.
150. Singerman LJ, Berkow JW, Patz A. Dominant slowly progressive macular dystrophy. Am J Ophthalmol 1977; 83:680–683.
151. Watzke RC, Folk JC, Lang RM. Pattern dystrophy of the retinal pigment epithelium. Ophthalmology 1982; 89:1400–1406.
152. Kim RY, Dollfus H, Keen TJ, et al. Autosomal dominant pattern dystrophy of the retina associated with a 4-base pair insertion at codon 140 in the peripherin/RDS gene. Arch Ophthalmol 1995; 113:451–455.
153. Marmor MF, McNamara JA. Pattern dystrophy of the retinal pigment epithelium and geographic atrophy of the macula. Am J Ophthalmol 1996; 122:382–392.
154. Downes SM, Fitzke FW, Holder GE, et al. Clinical features of codon 172 RDS macular dystrophy: similar phenotype in 12 families. Arch Ophthalmol 1999; 117:1373–1383.
155. Sears JE, Aaberg TA Sr, Daiger SP, Moshfeghi DM. Splice site mutation in the peripherin/RDS gene associated with pattern dystrophy of the retina. Am J Ophthalmol 2001; 132:693–699.
156. van den Ouweland JM, Lemkes HH, Ruitenbeek W, et al. Mutation in mitochondrial tRNA(Leu)(UUR) gene in a large pedigree with maternally transmitted type II diabetes mellitus and deafness. Nat Genet 1992; 1:368–371.
157. Ballinger SW, Shoffner JM, Hedaya EV, et al. Maternally transmitted diabetes and deafness associated with a 10.4 kb mitochondrial DNA deletion. Nat Genet 1992; 1:11–15.
158. Massin P, Guillausseau PJ, Vialettes B, et al. Macular pattern dystrophy associated with a mutation of mitochondrial DNA. Am J Ophthalmol 1995; 120:247–248.
159. Harrison TJ, Boles RG, Johnson DR, et al. Macular pattern retinal dystrophy, adult-onset diabetes, and deafness: a family study of A3243G mitochondrial heteroplasmy. Am J Ophthalmol 1997; 124:217–221.
160. Smith PR, Bain SC, Good PA, et al. Pigmentary retinal dystrophy and the syndrome of maternally inherited diabetes and deafness caused by the mitochondrial DNA 3243 tRNA(Leu) A to G mutation. Ophthalmology 1999; 106:1101–1108.
161. Massin P, Virally-Monod M, Vialettes B, et al. Prevalence of macular pattern dystrophy in maternally inherited diabetes and deafness. GEDIAM Group. Ophthalmology 1999; 106:1821–1827.
162. Hsieh RC, Fine BS, Lyons JS. Patterned dystrophies of the retinal pigment epithelium. Arch Ophthalmol 1977; 95:429–435.
163. De Jong PTVM, Delleman JW. Pigment epithelial pattern dystrophy: four different manifestations in a family. Arch Ophthalmol 1982; 100:1416–1421.
164. Lodato G, Giuffre G. Unusual associations of pattern dystrophies. J Fr Ophthamol 1985; 8:147–154.
165. Battaglia Parodi M, Da Pozzo S, Ravalico G. Photodynamic therapy for choroidal neovascularization associated with pattern dystrophy. Retina 2003; 23:171–176.
166. Hutchinson J, Tay W. Symmetrical chorio-retinal disease occurring in senile persons. R Lond Ophthalmol Hosp Rep 1875; 8:231.
167. Doyne RW. A note on family choroiditis. Trans Ophthalmol Soc UK 1910; 30:93–95.
168. Holthouse EH, Batten RD. A case of superficial choroido-retinitis of peculiar form and doubtful causation. Trans Ophthalmol Soc UK 1897; 17:62–63.
169. Klainguti E. Die tapeto-retinale degeneration im Kanton Tessin. Klin Monatsbl Augenheilkd 1932; 89:253–254.
170. Deutman AF, Jansen LMAA. Dominantly inherited drusen of Bruch's membrane. Br J Ophthalmol 1970; 54:373–382.

171. Heon E, Piguet B, Munier F, et al. Linkage of autosomal dominant radial drusen (malattia leventinese) to chromosome 2p16–21. Arch Ophthalmol 1996; 114: 193–198.
172. Pearce WG. Doyne's honeycomb retinal degeneration. Br J Ophthalmol 1968; 52:73–78.
173. Sarks SH. Drusen and their relationship to senile macular degeneration. Aust J Ophthalmol 1980; 8:117–130.
174. Lefler WH, Wadsworth JAC, Sidbury JB. Hereditary macular degeneration and amino aciduria. Am J Ophthalmol 1971; 71:224–230.
175. Frank HR, Landers MB, Williams RJ, Sidbury JB. A new dominant progressive foreal dystrophy. Am J Ophthalmol 1974; 78:903–916.
176. Leveille AS, Morse PH, Kiernan JP. Autosomal dominant central pigment epithelial and choroidal degeneration. Ophthalmology 1982; 89:1407–1413.
177. Gregory CY, Evans K, Wijesuriya SD, et al. The gene responsible for autosomal dominant Doyne's honeycomb retinal dystrophy (DHRD) maps to chromosome 2pl6. Hum-Mol Genet 1996; 5:1055–1059.
178. Evans K, Gregory CY, Wijesuriya SD, et al. Assessment of the phenotypic range seen in Doyne honeycomb retinal dystrophy. Arch Ophthalmol 1997; 115:904–910.
179. Edwards AO, Klein ML, Berselli CB, et al. Malattia leventinese. refinement of the genetic locus and phenotypic variability in autosomal dominant macular drusen. Am J Ophthalmol 1998; 126:417–424.
180. Stone EM, Lotery AJ, Munier FL, et al. A single EFEMP1 mutation associated with both Malattia leventinese and Doyne honeycomb retinal dystrophy. Nat Genet 1999; 22:199–202.
181. Matsumoto M, Traboulsi El. Dominant radial drusen and Arg345Trp EFEMP1 mutation. Am J Ophthalmol 2001; 131:810–812.
182. Tarttelin EE, Gregory-Evans CY, Bird AC, et al. Molecular genetic heterogeneity in autosomal dominant drusen. J Med Genet 2001; 38:381–384.
183. Katsanis N, Venable S, Smith JR, Lupski JR. Isolation of a paralog of the Doyne honeycomb retinal dystrophy gene from the multiple retinopathy critical region on 11ql3. Hum Genet 2000; 106:66–72.
184. Fishman GA, Carrasco C, Fishman M. The electrooculogram in diffuse (familial) drusen. Arch Ophthalmol 1976; 94:231–233.
185. Krill AE, Klien BA. Flecked retina syndrome. Arch Ophthalmol 1965; 74:496–508.
186. Kandori F, Tamai A, Kurimoto S, Fukunaga K. Fleck retina. Am J Ophthalmol 1972; 73:673–685.
187. Farkas TG, Sylvester V, Archer D. The ultrastructure of drusen. Am J Ophthalmol 1971; 71:1196–1205.
188. Kenyon KR, Maumenee AE, Ryan SJ, et al. Diffuse drusen and associated complications. Am J Ophthalmol 1985; 100:119–128.
189. Ishibashi T, Patterson R, Ohnishi Y, et al. Formation of drusen in the human eye. Am J Ophthalmol 1986; 101:342–353.
190. Holz FG, Owens SL, Marks J, et al. Ultrastructural findings in autosomal dominant drusen. Arch Ophthalmol 1997; 115:788–792.
191. Marmorstein LY, Munier FL, Arjenijevic Y, et al. Aberrant accumulation of EFEMP1 underlies drusen formation in malattia leventinese and age-related macular degeneration. Proc Natl Acad Sci USA 2002; 999:13067–13072.
192. Sorsby A, Mason J, Gardener N. A fundus dystrophy with unusual features. Br J Ophthalmol 1949; 33:67–97.
193. Capon MR, Polkinghorne PJ, Fitzke FW, Bird AC. Sorsby's pseudoinflammatory macula dystrophy—Sorsby's fundus dystrophies. Eye 1988; 2:114–122.
194. Dreyer RF, Hidayat AA. Pseudoinflammatory macular dystrophy. Am J Ophthalmol 1988; 106:154–161.
195. Weber BH, Vogt G, Wolz W, et al. Sorsby's fundus dystrophy is genetically linked to chromosome 22ql3-qter. Nat Genet 1994; 7:158–161.

196. Weber BHF, Vogt G, Pruett RC, et al. Mutations in the tissue inhibitor of metalloproteinases-3 (TIMP3) in patients with Sorsby's fundus dystrophy. Nat Genet 1994; 8: 352–356.
197. Carrero-Valenzuela RD, Klein ML, Weleber RG, et al. Sorsby fundus dystrophy. A family with the Serl81Cys mutation of the tissue inhibitor of metalloproteinase 3. Arch Ophthalmol 1996; 114:737–738.
198. Felbor U, Benkwitz C, Klein ML, et al. Sorsby fundus dystrophy: reevaluation of variable expressivity in patients carrying a TIMP3 founder mutation. Arch Ophthalmol 1997; 115:1569–1571.
199. Jacobson SG, Cideciyan AV, Bennett J, et al. Novel mutation in the TIMP3 gene causes Sorsby fundus dystrophy. Arch Ophthalmol 2002; 120:376–379.
200. Felbor U, Doepner D, Schneider U, et al. Evaluation of the gene encoding the tissue inhibitor of metalloproteinases-3 in various maculopathies. Invest Ophthalmol Vis Sci 1997; 38:1054–1059.
201. Ayyagari R, Griesinger IB, Bingham E, et al. Autosomal dominant hemorrhagic macular dystrophy not associated with the TIMP3 gene. Arch Ophthalmol 2000; 118:85–92.
202. Capon MR. Marshall J. Krafft JI, et al. Sorsby's fundus dystrophy. A light and electron microscopic study. Ophthalmology 1989; 96:1769–1777.
203. Jacobson SG, Cideciyan AV, Regunath G, et al. Night blindness in Sorsby's fundus dystrophy reversed by vitamin A. Nat Genet 1995; 11:27–32.
204. Small KW, Hermsen V, Gurney N, et al. North Carolina macular dystrophy and central areolar pigment epithelial dystrophy. One family, one disease. Arch Ophthalmol 1992; 110:515–518.
205. Small KW, Puech B, Mullen L, Yelchits S. North Carolina macular dystrophy phenotype in France maps to the MCDR1 locus. Mol Vis 1997; 3:1.
206. Pauleikhoff D, Sauer CG, Muller CR, et al. Clinical and genetic evidence for autosomal dominant North Carolina macular dystrophy in a German family. Am J Ophthalmol 1997; 124:412–415.
207. Rabb MF, Mullen L, Yelchits S, et al. A North Carolina macular dystrophy phenotype in a Belizean family maps to the MCDR1 locus. Am J Ophthalmol 1998; 125:502–508.
208. Small KW. Weber JL, Pericak-Vance MA. MCDRI (North Carolina macular dystrophy) maps to chromosome 6ql4-16. Ophthalmic Paediatr Genet 1993; 14:143–150.
209. Voo I, Glasgow BJ, Flannery J, et al. North Carolina macular dystrophy: clinicopathologic correlation. Am J Ophthalmol 2001; 132:933–935.
210. Holz FG, Evans K, Gregory CY, et al. Autosomal dominant macular dystrophy simulating North Carolina macular dystrophy. Arch Ophthalmol 1995; 113:178–184.
211. Deutman AF, Pinckers AJ, Aan de Kerk AL. Dominantly inherited cystoid macular edema. Am J Ophthalmol 1976; 82:540–548.
212. Deutman AF. Dominant macular dystrophies. Doc Ophthalmol Proc Soc 1976; 9: 415–430.
213. Notting JGA, Pinckers AJLG. Dominant cystoid macular dystrophy. Am J Ophthalmol 1977; 83:234–241.
214. Fishman GA, Goldberg MF, Trautman JG. Dominantly inherited cystoid macular edema. Ann Ophthalmol 1979; 11:21–27.
215. Kremer H, Pinckers A, van den Helm B, et al. Localization of the gene for dominant cystoid macular dystrophy on chromosome 7p. Hum Mol Genet 1999; 3:299–302.
216. Mendivil A. Bilateral cystoid macular edema in a 21-year-old woman. Surv Ophthalmol 1996; 40:407–412.
217. Inglehearn C, Keen TJ, al-Maghtheh M, Bhattacharya S. Loci for autosomal dominant retinitis pigmentosa and dominant cystoid macular dystrophy on chromosome 7p are not allelic. Am J Hum Genet 1994; 55:581–582.
218. Merin S. Macular cysts as an early sign of tapetoretinal degeneration. J Pediatr Ophthalmol 1970; 7:225–228.

219. Ffytche TJ. Cystoid maculopathy in retinitis pigmentosa. Trans Ophthalmol Soc UK 1972; 92:265–283.
220. Deutman AF. Benign concentric annular macular dystrophy. Am J Ophthalmol 1974; 78:384–396.
221. van den Biesen PR, Deutman AF, Pinckers AJLG. Evolution of benign concentric annular macular dystrophy. Am J Ophthalmol 1985; 100:73–78.
222. Hoyng CB and Deutman AF. The development of central areolar choroidal dystrophy. Graefes Arch Clin Exp Ophthalmol 1996; 234:87–93.
223. Hoyng CB, Heutink P, Testers L, et al. Autosomal dominant central areolar choroidal dystrophy caused by a mutation in codon 142 in the peripherin/RDS gene. Am J Ophthalmol 1996; 121:623–629.
224. Klevering BJ, van Driel M, van Hogerwou AJ, et al. Central areolar choroidal dystrophy associated with dominantly inherited drusen. Br J Ophthalmol 2002; 86: 91–96.
225. Lotery AJ, Ennis KT, Silvestri G, et al. Localization of a gene for central areolar choroidal dystrophy to chromosome 17p. Hum Genet 1996; 5:705–708.
226. Hughes AE, Lotery AJ, Silvestri G. Fine localisation of the gene for central areolar choroidal dystrophy on chromosome 17p. JMed Genet 1998; 35:770–772.
227. Fetkenhour CL, Gurney N, Dobbie JG, Choromokos E. Central areolar pigment epithelial dystrophy. Am J Ophthalmol 1976; 81:745–753.
228. Hermsen VM, Judisch GF. Central areolar pigment epithelial dystrophy. Ophthalmologica 1984; 189:69–72.
229. Keithahn MA, Huang M, Keltner JL, et al. The variable expressivity of a family with central areolar pigment epithelial dystrophy. Ophthalmology 1996; 103:406–415.
230. Sorsby A. The dystrophies of the macula. Br J Ophthalmol 1940; 24:469–529.
231. Sorsby A. Ophthalmic Genetics. 2nd ed. London: Butterworth & Co 1970:118.
232. Phillips CI, Griffiths DL. Macular coloboma and skeletal abnormality. Br J Ophthalmol 1969; 53:346–349.
233. Margolis S, Scher BM, Carr RE. Macular colobomas in Leber's congenital amaurosis. Am J Ophthalmol 1977; 83:27–31.
234. Godley BF, Tiffin PA, Evans K, et al. Clinical features of progressive bifocal chorioretinal atrophy: a retinal dystrophy linked to chromosome 6q. Ophthalmology 1996; 103:893–898.
235. Kelsell RE, Godley BF, Evans K, et al. Localization of the gene for progressive bifocal chorioretinal atrophy (PBCRA) to chromosome 6q. Hum Mol Genet 1995; 4: 1653–1656.
236. O'Donnell Jonnell FE Jr, Welch RB. Fenestrated sheen macular dystrophy. A new autosomal dominant maculopathy. Arch Ophthalmol 1979; 97:1292–1296.
237. Sneed SR, Sieving PA. Fenestrated sheen macular dystrophy. Am J Ophthalmol 1991; 112:1–7.
238. Polk TD, Gass JD, Green WR, et al. Familial internal limiting membrane dystrophy. A new sheen retinal dystrophy. Arch Ophthalmol 1997; 115:878–885.
239. Albrectsen B, Svendsen IB. Hypotrichosis, syndactyly, and retinal degeneration in two siblings. Acta Derm Venereol 1956; 1:96–101.
240. Hayakawa M, Kato K, Yamauchi Y. A case of central and pericentral retinopathia pigmentosa with abnormalities of hair, hands, and teeth. Nippon Ganka 1979; 21: 433–438.
241. Ohdo S, Hirayama K, Terawaki T. Association of ectodermal dysplasia, ectrodactyly, and macular dystrophy. the EEM syndrome. J Med Genet 1983; 20:52–54.
242. Pigg M, Jagell S, Sillen A, et al. The Sjogren-Larsson syndrome gene is close to D17S805 as determined by linkage analysis and allelic association. Nat Genet 1994; 8:361–364.

243. Willemsen MA, Ijlst L, Steijlen PML, et al. Clinical, biochemical, and molecular genetic characteristics of 19 patients with the Sjogren-Larsson syndrome. Brain 2001; 124: 1426–1437.
244. De Laurenzi V, Rogers GR, Hamrock DJ, et al. Sjogren-Larsson syndrome is caused by mutations in the fatty aldehyde dehydrogenase gene. Nat Genet 1996; 12:52–57.
245. Willemsen MA, Cruysberg JR, Rotteveel JJ, et al. Juvenile macular dystrophy associated with deficient activity of fatty aldehyde dehydrogenase in Sjogren-Larsson syndrome. Am J Ophthalmol 2000; 130:782–789.
246. Bird AC. What is the future of research in age-related macular disease?. Arch Ophthalmol 1997; 115:1311–1313.
247. Hyman LG, Lilienfeld AM, Ferris FL, Fine SL. Senile macular degeneration: a case-control study. Am J Epidemiol 1983; 118:213–227.
248. Seddon JM, Ajani UA, Mitchell BD. Familial aggregation of age-related maculopathy. Am J Ophthalmol 1997; 123:199–206.
249. Silvestri G, Johnston PB, Hughes AE. Is genetic predisposition an important risk factor in age-related macular degeneration? Eye 1994; 8:564–568.
250. Klaver CC, Wolfs RC, Assink JJ, et al. Genetic risk of age-related maculopathy. Population-based familial aggregation study. Arch Ophthalmol 1998; 116:1646–1651.
251. Melrose MA, Magargal LE, Lucier AC. Identical twins with subretinal neovascularization complicating senile macular degeneration. Ophthalmic Surg 1985; 16:648–651.
252. Meyers SM, Zalhary AA. Monozygotic twins with age-related macular degeneration. Arch Ophthalmol 1988; 106:651–653.
253. Klein ML, Mauldin WM, Stoumbos VD. Heredity and age-related macular degeneration. Observations in monozygotic twins. Arch Ophthalmol 1994; 112:932–937.
254. Meyers SM, Greene T, Gutman FA. A twin study of age-related macular degeneration. Am J Ophthalmol 1995; 120:757–766.
255. Hammond CJ, Webster AR, Snieder H, et al. Genetic influence on early age-related maculopathy: a twin study. Ophthalmology 2002; 109:730–736.
256. De La Paz MA, Pericak-Vance MA, Lennon F, et al. Exclusion of TIMP3 as a candidate locus in age-related macular degeneration. Invest Ophthalmol Vis Sci 1997; 38:1060–1065.
257. Gorin MB. The ABCA4 gene and age-related macular degeneration innocence or guilt by association. Arch Ophthalmol 2001; 119:752–753.
258. Allikmets R, Shroyer NF, Singh N, et al. Mutation of the Stargardt disease gene (ABCR) in age-related macular degeneration. Science 1997; 277:1805–1807.
259. Allikmets R. Further evidence for an association of ABCR alleles with age-related macular degeneration. The International ABCR Screening Consortium. Am J Hum Genet 2000; 67:487–491.
260. Souied EH, Ducroq D, Gerber S, et al. Age-related macular degeneration in grandparents of patients with Stargardt disease. genetic study. Am J Ophthalmol 1999; 128: 173–178.
261. Dryja TP, Briggs CE, Berson EL, et al. ABCR gene and age-related macular degeneration. Science 1998; 279:1107.
262. Stone EM, Webster AR, Vandenburgh K, et al. Allelic variation in ABCR associated with Stargardt disease but not age-related macular degeneration. Nat Genet 1998; 20:328–329.
263. Guymer RH, Heon E, Lotery AJ, et al. Variation of codons 1961 and 2177 of the Stargardt disease gene is not associated with age-related macular degeneration. Arch Ophthalmol 2001; 119:745–751.
264. De La Paz MA, Guy VK, Abou-Donia S, et al. Analysis of the Stargardt disease gene (ABCR) in age-related macular degeneration. Invest Ophthalmol Vis Sci 1998; 39(suppl):S915.
265. De La Paz MA, Guy VK, Abou-Donia S, et al. Analysis of the Stargardt disease gene (ABCR) in age-related macular degeneration. Ophthalmology 1999; 106:1531–1536.

266. Bernstein PS, Leppert M, Singh N, et al. Genotype-phenotype analysis of ABCR variants in macular degeneration probands and siblings. Invest Ophthalmol Vis Sci 2002; 43:466–473.
267. Klein ML, Schultz DW, Edwards A, et al. Age-related macular degeneration. Clinical features in a large family and linkage to chromosome lq. Arch Ophthalmol 1996; 116:1082–1088.
268. Weeks DE, Conley YP, Tsai HJ, et al. Age-related maculopathy: an expanded genome-wide scan with evidence of susceptibility loci within the 1q31 and 17q25 regions. Am J Ophthalmol 2001; 132:682–692.
269. Delcourt C, Diaz JL, Ponton-Sanchez A, Papoz L. Smoking and age-related macular degeneration. The POLA Study. Pathologies Oculaires Liees a l'Age. Arch Ophthalmol 1998; 116:1031–1035.
270. Seddon JM, Willett WC, Speizer FE, Hankinson SE. A prospective study of cigarette smoking and age-related macular degeneration in women. J AM Med Assoc 1996; 276:1141–1146.
271. Vingerling JR, Hofman A, Grobbee DE, de Jong PT. Age-related macular degeneration and smoking. The Rotterdam study. Arch Ophthalmol 1996; 114:1193–1196.
272. Seddon JM, Ajani UA, Sperduto RD, et al. Dietary carotenoids, vitamins A, C, and E, and advanced age-related macular degeneration. Eye Disease Case-Control Study Group. J AM Med Assoc 1994; 272:1413–1420.
273. Mares-Perlman JA, Brady WE, Klein R, et al. Serum antioxidants and age-related macular degeneration in a population-based case-control study. Arch Ophthalmol 1995; 113:1518–1523.
274. Mares-Perlman JA, Klein R, Klein BE, et al. Association of zinc and antioxidant nutrients with age-related maculopathy. Arch Ophthalmol 1996; 114:991–997.
275. Delcourt C, Cristol JP, Leger CL, et al. Associations of antioxidant enzymes with cataract and age-related macular degeneration. The POLA Study. Pathologies Oculaires Liees a l'Age. Ophthalmology 1999; 106:215–222.
276. Gorin MB, Breitner JC, De Jong PT, et al. The genetics of age-related macular degeneration. Mol Vis 1999; 5:29–43.
277. De la Paz MA, Pericak-Vance MA, Haines JL, Seddon JM. Phenotypic heterogeneity in families with age-related macular degeneration. Am J Ophthalmol 1997; 124:331–343.
278. Pierro L, Tremolada G, Introini U, et al. Optical coherence tomography findings in adult-onset foveomacular vitelliform dystrophy. Am J Ophthalmol 2002; 134:675–680.
279. Benhamou N, Souied EH, Zolf R, et al. Adult-onset foveomacular vitelliform dystrophy. a study by optical coherence tomography. Am J Ophthalmol 2003; 135:362–367.

9

The Cone Dystrophies and Color Vision Disorders

INTRODUCTION

This chapter deals with inherited disorders that exclusively, primarily, or predominantly affect the cones. These disorders include some with histopathologic abnormalities of the photoreceptors (the cone dystrophies) and others with normal cones, but with abnormal visual pigment content (the inborn color vision disorders or dyschromatopsias). In the cone dystrophies, the physical loss of cones is manifested by reduced visual acuity, in addition to the color vision abnormalities. The rods are often affected as well. In the inborn color vision disorders all retinal functions except color vision are normal or only minimally affected.

THE CONE DYSTROPHIES

Introduction

The cone dystrophies are a group of diseases frequently described in the literature under a confusing list of names. Sometimes, a cone dystrophy can even be found classified under altogether different headings, such as macular dystrophy, tapetoretinal degeneration, inherited optic atrophy, or inborn color vision disorders. In this chapter, a disorder is classified as a *cone dystrophy,* if it is inherited, if it affects predominantly the cones, if cones are diffusely affected all over the fundus, and if both color vision and other retinal functions are severely abnormal or absent. The cone dystrophies are further subclassified into separate clinical and genetic entities according to the quantity of cone function involvement (complete or incomplete), the amount of rod involvement (cone or cone-rod dystrophies), the presence or absence of progressiveness, and the genetic background.

The characteristic clinical findings, laboratory tests, and means of diagnosis of the various cone dystrophies are summarized in Table 1.

Table 1 Congential Cone Dystrophies

Name	Other names	Symbol/ locus and OMIM No.	Main clinical findings	Fundus	Cone function	Rod function	Heredity	Gene	Chromo-somal location	Mutations	Remarks
Congenital complete cone dystrophy type 2	Rod mono-chroma-tism, congenital achroma-topsia type 2	ACHM2 216900	Low v.a.: 20/200–20/400 in most; achro-matop-sia nystag-mus; photo-phobia	Normal or mild foveal dystro-phy	Absent or rudi-mentary	Normal	AR	CNGA3	2q11	Several missense	Rudimentary cone function may exist with milder mutations
Congenital complete cone dystrophy type 3	Same, type 3	ACHM3 262300	Same	Same	Same	Same	AR	CNGB3	8q21–q22	Frame-shift	Rudimentary cone function may exist with milder mutations
Congenital complete cone dystrophy type 4	Same, type 4	ACHM4	Same	Same	Same	Same	AR	GNAT2	1p13	Truncated protein	Rudimentary cone function may exist with milder mutations

Congenital incomplete X-linked cone dystrophy	Blue cone monochromacy X-linked incomplete achromatopsia	BCM 303700	Moderate–low v.a.: 20/80–20/200 in most; blue color vision; nystagmus photophobia	Normal or mild foveal dystrophy	Rudimentary cone function; absent red and green	Normal	XL	Red/green LCR or gene for red cone opsin	Xq28	Large deletion in LCR or missense mutation in red cone gene	
Congenital incomplete AR cone dystrophy	Congenital AR incomplete achromatopsia	ACHM 216900	Moderate–low v.a.; red or green partial color vision	Normal or mild foveal dystrophy	Rudimentary or moderate with reserved protan or deutan	Normal	AR	CNGA3	2q11	Mild missense	May exist also with other two ACHM genes

Note: AR—autosomal recessive; LCR—locus control region; XL—X-linked.

The Clinical and Genetic Types of Cone Dystrophies

Congenital Complete Cone Dystrophy

Various names have been given to this disease by different authors. Terms that have been used synonymously include rod-monochromatism, achromatopsia with amblyopia, congenital achromatopsia, congenital stationary form of cone dysfunction, day blindness, hemeralopia, total color blindness, and congenital complete achromatopsia. The other terms used were complete autosomal recessive achromatopsia (1), cone dysfunction syndrome group I (2), and typical π° monochromacy (3).

The clinical findings are typical: poor visual acuity in daylight, photophobia, congenital nystagmus, and color blindness. The fundus is normal or minor abnormalities are seen in patients with this disorder; Auerbach and Merin (4) found poor visual acuity in all patients. It ranged from 6/30 to 2/60, but in most patients it was 6/60–6/90. Definite nystagmus was seen in 29 of the 39 patients, and photophobia in 37. Nystagmus is probably invariably present in all complete achromats in early childhood, but may later decrease or even disappear. The visual acuity, which is always poor under photopic conditions, improves under mesopic conditions, and becomes normal under scotopic conditions.

Ophthalmoscopically, the fundus may be normal or may show macular abnormalities in the form of an absent foveal reflex or mild pigmentary changes in the macula. Tests for color vision show a lack of chromatic discrimination. Patients are unable to read Ishihara plates, although some patients can read one or several plates. The Farmsworth D-15 test usually shows a line of confusion in the middle, between the deutan and tritan lines (the scotopic line). The electroretinogram (ERG) shows no response to single-flash stimuli under photopic conditions. Under scotopic conditions, the ERG shows only, or predominantly, rod activity. In the aforementioned series, 10 of the 39 patients had some rudimentary cone activity. Psychophysical studies showed in three of five complete achromats, in addition to the scotopic plateau, the existence of three fast, high-intensity plateaus in their dark adaptation curve (5). These plateaus were photopic in the fast kinetics of their recovery and scotopic in their spectral luminosities, the lambda maximum (λ_{max}) being between 500 and 510 nm. Auerbach and Kripke (5) concluded that this indicates that patients with congenital achromatopsia have three types of receptors displaying cone kinetics (most probably cones), but containing rhodopsin, the visual pigment of the rods. Rhodopsin regenerates faster in cones than in rods, presumably because of the structure of the outer segments.

A curious phenomenon of a transient pupillary constriction to darkness was described by Price and colleagues in patients with congenital retinal diseases (6).

Congenital complete cone dystrophy is a stationary disease, with little change in clinical appearance and function during life, except for some improvement in nystagmus and possibly in photophobia.

The mode of inheritance of congenital complete cone dystrophy is autosomal recessive (2). Both sexes are equally affected; 20 of 39 in Auerbach and Merin's series (4) were males. The rate of consanguinity of parents is high, in about half of all in the aforementioned series. The largest pedigree was reported by Holm and Lodberg (7) in a Danish family with 19 affected members in four generations.

"Pingelapese blindness" is a curious autosomal recessive disorder, commonly found on the island of Pingelap and surrounding islands in the Caroline Islands of Southeast Asia. It was first described by Brody et al. (8) and the Pingelap people were extensively described in a book by Sacks, named *The Island of the Colorblind* (9).

Patients suffer from congenital complete cone dystrophy, stationary with complete achromatopsia associated with high myopia (8). Another population with a high incidence of congenital achromatopsia is the Jewish–Iranian community. Zlotogora (10) found a high rate of gene frequency coupled with a high degree of inbreeding.

By 2003, three loci for congenital complete cone dystrophy were identified (Table 1). Phenotypically it is one disease, as the result of all mutations seems to be the same in all three types: loss of function of cone transduction.

Arbour and colleagues (11) mapped the locus for congenital complete achromatopsia in a Jewish–Iranian family to chromosome 2 at centromere. The locus was termed ACHM2, as ACHM1 was already given to a phenotype of one single family which had a compound disorder (12) not yet defined as a distinct disorder. The location of ACHM2 locus at chromosome 2q11 was confirmed in another family by Wissinger and associates (13). The gene for ACHM2 was cloned the same year and identified as for cyclic nucleotide-gated channel, alpha 3 (CNGA3), by Kohl and associates (14). CNGA3 encodes the alpha-subunit of the cone photoreceptor cGMP gated cation channel, a key component in cone phototransduction. The rod photoreceptor uses another alpha-subunit gated channel for transduction, which, when mutated, results in night blindness. Kohl et al. (14) identified missense mutations in the CNGA3 gene in five families with rod monochromatism (congenital achromatopsia), two homozygous and three compound heterozygous. Wissinger et al. (15) studied 258 families with various cone disorders and detected disease-causing mutations in 53. Eighty five percent were various missense mutations, but four were common, comprising 42% of all cases: Arg277Cys, Arg283Trp, Arg436Trp, and Phe547Leu. The majority of CNGA3 mutations were associated with congenital complete cone dystrophy, some with the congenital incomplete form, and a few with progressive cone dystrophy (15). While studying families with congenital achromatopsia that was not linked to chromosome 2q11, Kohl and colleagues detected a new locus, ACHM3, mapped to chromosome 8q21 (16). The authors identified the gene CNGB3 and six different disease causing mutations (16). The CNGB3 gene encodes the beta-subunit of cGMP-gated channel of cone photoreceptors, another essential product of human cone phototransduction in all three classes of human cones. The gene is long, consists of 18 exons and a sequence of about 200 kb. The six identified mutations were stop codon mutations with the exception of one missense. Sundin et al. (17) identified a Ser322Phe mutation in the CNGB3 gene as causing the total achromatopsia with high myopia of Pingelapese blindness.

A third locus, which should probably be named ACHM4, was mapped to chromosome 1p13. Kohl and colleagues (18) identified protein-truncation mutations in the GNAT2 gene [guanine nucleotide-binding (G) protein, alpha subunit-transducing 2]. GNAT2 encodes the cone-photoreceptor specific alpha-subunit of transducin, another essential component of cone phototransduction (18). GNAT1 encodes the rod photoreceptor-specific transducin and its mutations are associated with autosomal dominant Nougaret–type night blindness.

All families with congenital achromatopsia had a similar phenotype, as described previously, of complete or almost complete cone deficiency. Of the families studied by molecular genetics, 20–30% were associated with CNGA3 mutations, 40–50% with CNGB3 mutations, and some with GNAT2 mutations (18). It is, therefore, possible that one additional locus for congenital achromatopsia exists.

Congenital Incomplete X-Linked Cone Dystrophy

The X-linked incomplete form of congenital cone dystrophy is less frequent than the complete form. It has been described under various names including atypical congenital achromatopsia (19), blue-cone monochromacy (19), π_1 cone monochromatism (20), X linked atypical monochromatism (21), atypical achromatopsia of sex-linked recessive inheritance (22), congenital X-linked achromatopsia (23), congenital X-linked incomplete achromatopsia (24), and rod-monochromatism, incomplete form (25). The characteristics of the disease were summarized by Smith and colleagues (26) and others. Visual acuity is reduced and ranges from 6/24 to 6/60. Photophobia and pendular nystagmus may be present, as in the complete form, but both are often absent. The short-wavelength sensitive (sws) cones ("blue cones") are functional, but there is absence of other functioning cones. There are minimal fundus changes, similar to those of the complete form, and associated myopia is common.

The disorder is transmitted by the X-linked mode: males are affected and females are carriers. In spite of functioning blue cones, color discrimination is extremely reduced, or nonexistent (19). The psychophysical dark adaptation curve shows the existence of a small knick on a higher plateau than usual (21), unlike in the complete form. The spectral sensitivity curve shows maximal sensitivity (λ_{max}) at about 440 nm, which fits the existence of one type of functioning cones, the blue cones or the π_1 cones (20). This spectral sensitivity is 500–510 nm.

The patients are unable to read the Ishihara charts, but are able to read HRR charts that relate to blue-yellow vision (27). The new plates, invented by Berson and colleagues, that use blue-green (491 nm) and purple-blue (468 nm) as dominant wavelengths can easily distinguish between the complete and incomplete forms (27). Patients with congenital incomplete cone dystrophy can read them, whereas patients with the complete form cannot.

The rod ERG is normal, whereas the cone ERG to 30 Hz white flicker is at least 97% below normal (27). The ERG to blue light is low under photopic conditions (27) and normal under scotopic conditions (25).

The fundus is normal or shows minimal changes in the form of macular mottling, with spots of hyper- and hypopigmentation (Fig. 1). In older persons, extensive retinal pigment epithelium (RPE) atrophy may be noted (24).

Female carriers can be recognized clinically. Some show mottling in the macular area (24). All obligate carriers had abnormal ERGs, which consisted of delayed cone b-wave implicit time, with subnormal responses to 30 Hz white flicker and loss of an oscillation in response to a single white flash under dark adaptation (28).

It is not clear whether or not a condition, termed by Heckenlively and Weleber (29) as "X-linked recessive cone dystrophy with tapetal-like sheen" is a separate entity. Slow progression of the functional abnormalities was previously described (24) and stressed again by these authors (29). In another family with "X-linked cone degeneration," a 15-year-old propositus had near-normal visual acuity, a protan deficiency, and diminished cone ERG responses (30). Two older patients in this family had both protan and deutan deficiency, poor visual acuity, signs of macular degeneration, and subnormal cone responses. All affected patients had an abnormality in the red cone pigment gene, by showing a 6.5 kb deletion in this gene. Early molecular genetics techniques did not reveal any apparent abnormality in the green cone pigment gene.

The disease is inherited on the X-chromosome. However, doubts exist whether one single gene transmits the disease. In fact, two contradicting theories could explain the heredity of this disorder (26). The "combination theory" states that

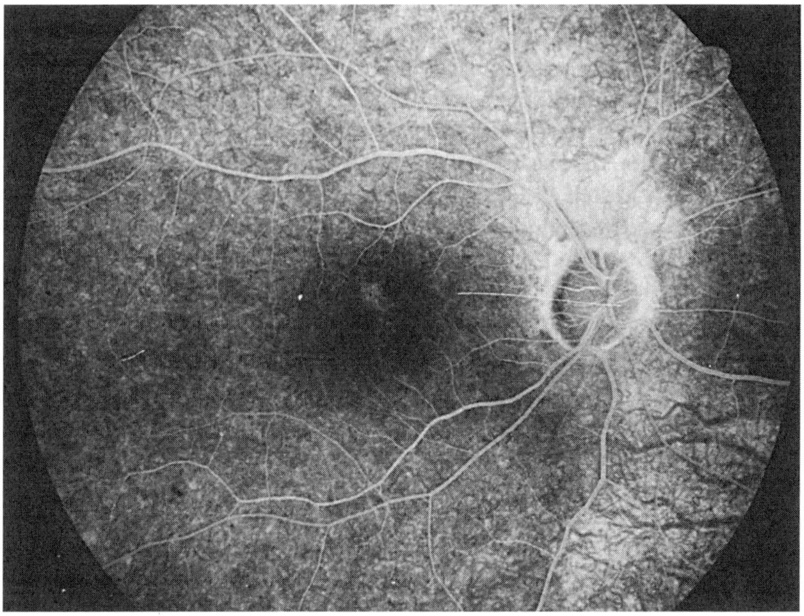

Figure 1 Fundus fluorescein angiography of an 18-year-old patient with congenital incomplete X-linked cone dystrophy. Note tiny spots of RPE atrophy in macular area. Ophthalmoscopy showed fine mottling in this area. Color vision tests showed the presence of blue vision. The photopic flicker ERG was extinct, whereas the ERG response to scotopic single-flash blue light was only slightly subnormal. There was no nystagmus, and visual acuity was 6/60.

the defect results from a combined presence of two mutations, one in each of the protan and the deutan genes. The "separate theory" claims that one single mutant gene causes the disease. Nathans and associates (31) studied 12 families with X-linked loss of both red and green cone pigments and claimed that both types exist. In some patients a two-step loss of function occurs. In a male who lost the function of one color pigment, a second mutation inactivates the remaining second gene. This was found to have occurred in six families. In another four families, one step loss of both red and green function occurred as a result of the deletion of a large segment upstream of the two genes (31). The human red and green genes are arranged in tandem, beginning upstream with a locus control region (LCR) of 600 bp, followed downstream by one "red gene" and further downstream by one or more "green genes." Ayyagari et al. (32) showed that in some families with blue cone monochromacy (BCM), the mutation is a large deletion in the LCR, and that loss of LCR function results in loss of function of both the red and green opsins (32). The mutations may mean small or large deletions of the LCR, or missense mutations in the red gene resulting in loss of function of the green gene as well (33,34). In approximately half of these cases the missense mutation was Cys203Arg (33).

Congenital Incomplete Cone Dystrophy—Autosomal Recessive Forms

In addition to the sex-linked congenital incomplete cone dystrophy, two forms of autosomal recessive congenital incomplete cone dystrophy have been described (35–37).

In these two, a protan mechanism or residual deutan mechanism was present, indicating the existence of functioning middle-wavelength (mws) cones in the first, and functioning long-wavelength (lws) cones in the second (35,36). Clinically, the patients resembled descriptions of patients with the complete form, except that they had somewhat better functions in both visual acuity and color discrimination.

The existence of congenital incomplete autosomal recessive cone dystrophy as a separate entity is still questionable. Two patients described by Young and Price with residual mws cone or lws cone function belonged to families with the complete form (37). Therefore, it is likely that such patients are patients with the genetic entity of congenital complete cone dystrophy (rod-monochromatism) with some residual cone function.

Molecular genetics of recent years confirmed the association between the complete and incomplete autosomal recessive forms of congenital achromatopsia (15). Allelic mutations in the same gene or modulating genes may cause the difference.

Progressive Dominant Cone Dystrophy

In sharp contrast with the congenital forms, which are basically stable, the late appearing cone dystrophies are all progressive. The onset is in the first decade of life (38) and thereafter the visual acuity slowly decreases. Color vision is initially normal and slowly becomes a red-green defect to total achromatopsia (38). Minimal macular pigmentary mottling can be seen. Occasionally, bull's-eye maculopathy develops (39). The ERG is similar to that of the congenital form. A reduced photopic single-flash response and absent photopic flicker response are coupled with a normal scotopic response. The electro-oculogram (EOG) is normal (40). The psychophysical dark adaptation curve is monophasic, with normal red thresholds (40). In the more advanced stages, the visual fields show an annular scotoma or a central or a paracentral scotoma (41). Visual acuity, initially 6/6, decreases slowly and gradually to 6/60 (26), 6/90 (40), or even less (42). The absent or grossly reduced cone ERG responses are found even in the early stages of the disease (43). They indicate an early widespread loss of cone function. Peripheral cones were affected earlier than the cones in the posterior pole (43).

The condition was probably first described by Sloan and Brown in 1962 (24), and 13 reports had been published by 1972 (45). However, in many articles, progressive cone dystrophy was confused with progressive cone-rod dystrophy, a different entity, with a much worse prognosis. Progressive cone dystrophy includes only patients with a normal or nearly normal rod function, but with cone function becoming progressively worse.

The disorder is most frequently transmitted by a single autosomal dominant gene, with full penetrance. It is not clear whether or not a similar disorder with autosomal recessive inheritance exists. Patients with a bull's-eye maculopathy and functional cone dysfunction, transmitted by an autosomal recessive gene, have been described. However, it seems similar to Stargardt disease, and, therefore, could be the same entity. On the other hand, there could also be a progressive cone dystrophy, autosomal recessive, separate from Stargardt disease. An X-linked cone dystrophy was also reported. Table 2 describes the major progressive cone dystrophies. Note that some of them may represent genetic entities which may have rods involved in the process, so that they actually represent a cone–rod dystrophy with minimal rod involvement. Cone-rod dystrophies are much more common than cone dystrophies (46).

The characteristic phenotype of autosomal dominant progressive cone dystrophy was described in a large family from Tennessee, by Small and Gehrs (47). First

Table 2 Progressive Cone Dystrophies

Symbol/locus	Heredity[a]	OMIM No.	Chromosome location	Gene	Mutations
RCD1	AD	180020	6q25–q26	uk[b]	—
RCD2	AD	601251	17p12–p13	RCV1[c]	—
COD3	AD	602093	6p21.1	GUCA1A	Tyr99Cys Pro59Leu
—	AD	—	6p21.1-cen	RDS/ peripherin	Pro210Arg Ser27Phe
COD1	XL	304020	Xp11.4	PRGR	Frameshift in ORF15
COD2	XL	300085	Xq27	uk	—
—	XL	—	Xp11.4–q13.1	uk	—

[a]AD—autosomal dominant; XL—X-linked.
[b]uk—Unknown.
[c]Candidate gene.

symptoms of reduced visual acuity and color vision disturbance occurred in the first decade of life and were slowly progressive. Later, photophobia, glare, and reduced visual acuity continued. The fundus manifested macular granularity or central macular atrophy. The photopic full-field ERG and the foveal ERG amplitudes became reduced. Photopic, light adapted 30 Hz flicker ERG amplitudes were extremely low. Variable and moderate to severe dyschromatopsia became worse (47).

Kellner and Foerster (46,48) described rare sporadic cases of progressive cone dystrophies with selected additional findings such as a "negative" ERG, blue cone hypersensitivity (S-cone syndrome), predominantly blue color vision affected, or predominantly red color vision affected. To this select group belongs a rare disorder, reported by Miyake et al. (49), in which the cone dystrophy involved only the macular cone system. No fundoscopic abnormal manifestations were apparent, but the focal macular ERG was abnormally low. A bull's-eye maculopathy was seen only much later in life.

Went and coauthors describe a large family with "late-onset dominant cone dystrophy with early blue cone involvement" (50). Visual acuity started to decline in the third decade of life but blue cone function was reduced earlier. This cone dystrophy is probably associated with locus RCD1 (for retinal cone dystrophy), OMIM number 180020, located at chromosome 6q25–q26 (51).

Another progressive cone dystrophy, locus RCD2, has been mapped to chromosome 17p12–p13. The main candidate gene in this region is RCV1, a retinally expressed gene, encoding recoverin, a calcium-binding protein that mediates the recovery from photoactivation of the retina (52,53).

A third locus marked COD3 (for cone dystrophy, no. 3) for autosomal dominant cone and cone–rod dystrophy, was mapped to chromosome 6p21.1 (54). Disease-bearing mutations in the guanylate cyclase activator (GUCA1A) were identified (54,55). Tyr99Cys mutation was associated with progressive cone dystrophy, including progressive loss of cone function and preserved rod function (54). Pro50Leu mutation resulted in minimal to severe progressive cone–rod dystrophy (55).

Mutations in the RDS/peripherin gene, located at chromosome 6p21.1-cen, are characteristically associated with retinitis pigmentosa. Some "mild mutations" are associated with progressive cone dystrophy. These included a Pro210Arg mutation (56) and a Ser27Phe mutation in another family (57).

Progressive X-Linked Cone Dystrophy

X-linked cone dystrophy may be more common than previously assumed (58). The earliest symptoms may occur in the first or second decade of life with abnormal color vision (pseudoprotanomaly), followed by mild reduction in visual acuity in the third decade of life (59). Visual acuity continues to decrease until the age of 30 to 20/25–20/50, until the age of 50 to 20/100, and later to 20/800 (60). Fundus manifestation includes macular granularity in the young and bull's-eye maculopathy in the old (60). Female carriers may show mild ophthalmoscopic changes, some mild color vision dysfunction, and mild visual acuity reduction (60). Eighty seven percent of carriers show mild color dysfunction (pseudoprotanomaly). Two or three mutated genes are associated with X-linked progressive cone dystrophy.

The locus COD1 was originally mapped to chromosome Xp11.3 (61). The phenotypic manifestation is as described, including progressive reduction in visual acuity, impaired color vision, photophobia, central scotoma and progressive macular abnormalities. In the elderly, rod dysfunction may also be noted (61–63). The localization was refined to Xp11.4 (64) and disease-causing mutations were identified in an open reading frame 15 (ORF 15) of the RPGR gene (65). The mutations, two nucleotide deletions or a nucleotide insertion, resulted in a frameshift with early termination. Similar frameshift mutations within ORF 15 of the RPGR gene were identified in two other families (66).

The locus COD2 associated with X-linked progressive cone dystrophy was mapped to chromosome Xq27 (67). The loss of visual acuity occurred earlier than with COD1.

A third locus was assigned to chromosome Xp11.4–q13.1 at the centromere, in a large Finnish family (68). This stresses the heterogeneity of X-linked progressive cone dystrophy.

Histologic and ultrastructural studies of a retina from a 73-year-old man with an unclassified type of retinal cone degeneration showed a wide spectrum of pathologic changes, ranging from minimal abnormalities, such as distortion and kinking of the outer segments, to areas of absent outer segments and few photoreceptor cell bodies (69).

To and associates studied the histopathology and immunohistochemistry of both dominant (70) and X-linked (71) cone dystrophy. In dominant progressive cone dystrophy, foveal cones were absent, a reduced number of cones were seen around the fovea, and they were preserved in the periphery at age 75. The RPE in the macular region was attenuated (70). In X-linked cone dystrophy, rod photoreceptors were also lost by age 71 (71).

Autosomal Dominant Cone-Rod Dystrophies

The term cone-rod degeneration was probably first used by Berson and coauthors to designate a disorder in three adults with progressively diminishing visual acuity, abnormal color vision, decreased or absent cone function, and reduced rod function (72). Probably most of the patients described by Krill and his colleagues (73) suffered from this disorder.

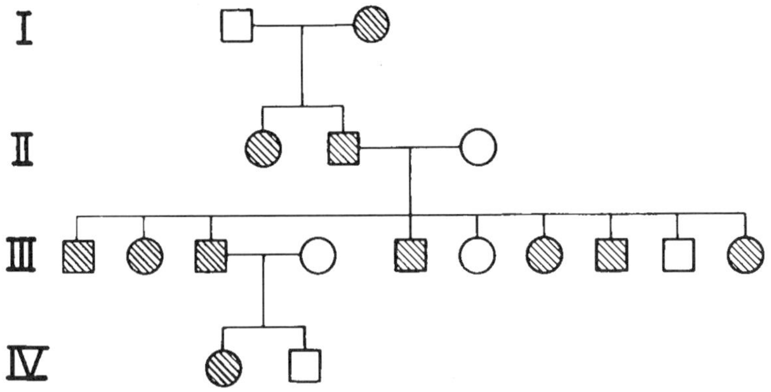

Figure 2 Pedigree of family with autosomal dominant progressive rod–cone dystrophy. The father in the second generation was blind, and his mother (first generation) died blind. The affected children of the third generation had various degrees of subnormal vision.

The age of onset is usually in the first or second decade of life, but may be later. Visual acuity decreases slowly and gradually from 6/6 or 6/7.5 in the first examinations to low or very low in old age. In the autosomal dominant form, it may advance to no light perception (74). The visual fields become progressively more constricted, in addition to a central scotoma that appears later in life.

The fundus changes are progressive and typical. I observed these in one family with autosomal dominant progressive cone-rod dystrophy (Fig. 2). The youngest patient had minimal macular pigmentary mottling; most affected members of the

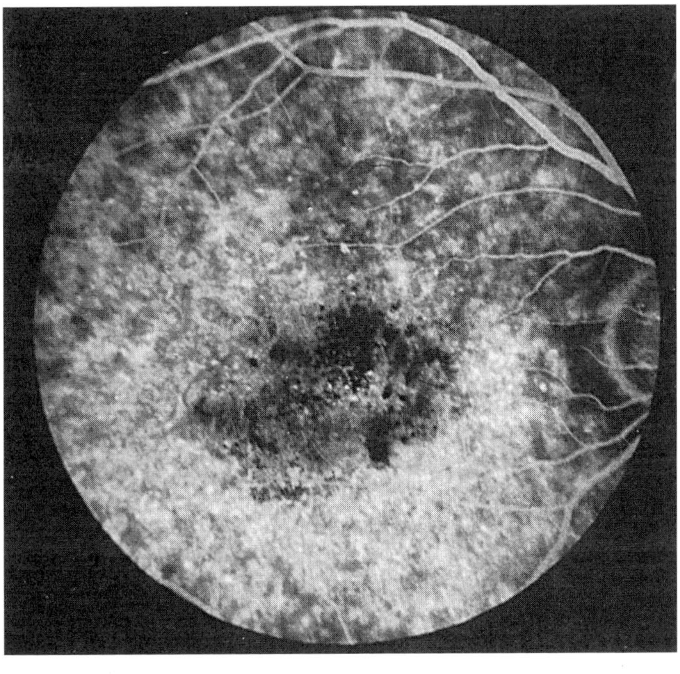

Figure 3 Fundus fluorescein angiography of a 22-year-old patient with autosomal dominant progressive cone–rod dystrophy showing partial bull's-eye maculopathy.

third generation had bull's-eye maculopathy (Fig. 3), and the father in the second generation was blind (no light perception) with multiple bone-corpuscular pigmentary changes in the periphery of the fundus. His mother was reported to have died blind. Figure 4 shows the typical fundus changes of a patient with advanced cone-rod dystrophy. Color vision tests indicate nonspecific errors in early stages and severe abnormalities in advanced stages (75). Photophobia and nystagmus may become progressively worse.

The psychophysical dark adaptation curve is monophasic. An abnormal cone threshold and a normal or near-normal rod threshold until increasing elevation occurs in older age. The ERG is always abnormal, with the photopic single-flash response extinguished and scotopic responses becoming progressively worse up to final extinction (75).

The few functional abnormalities of young patients with progressive cone-rod dystrophy, coupled with the slow and gradual progression of the disease, stand out in sharp contrast to the final poor visual prognosis. It is probably best illustrated by "benign concentric annular macular dystrophy," initially considered to be a functionally benign macular disease (76) and, finally, confirmed as a progressive cone-rod dystrophy (77).

Vitreous fluorophotometry shows a normal blood-retinal barrier in patients with early cone-rod dystrophy, in contrast with a breakdown of the blood-retinal barrier in patients with early rod-cone dystrophy (retinitis pigmentosa group) (78). A break down of the blood-retinal barrier was found in all patients with advanced cone-rod dystrophy (78,79), with clear correlation to peripheral pigmentary changes and reduction in scotopic b-wave (79).

It may be summarized, as did Kelsell et al. (80), that cone-rod dystrophies are a group of heterogenous disorders, characterized by the initial loss of cone photoreceptors, followed later by rod photoreceptor degeneration. Several attempts at classification were reported, such as the one by Szlyk and associates (81). However, with many of the causative genes now known, it makes sense to classify the cone-rod dystrophies according to their genetic background. The nomenclature review committee decided to use the symbol CORD for all the different cone-rod dystrophies. (80).

Rabb and associates (82) reported the light microscopic and electron microscopic findings of the eye of a 29-year-old patient with clinically documented cone-rod dystrophy. At the stage of bull's-eye maculopathy, a regional loss of cones and rods in the macular and peripheral areas occurred, with equatorial area preserved (Figs. 5 and 6). The percentage of degenerated cone cells was higher than the percentage of degenerated rod cells. The RPE cells in the macula had lipofuscin-like granules in their basal portions and some were atrophic.

Gregory-Evans et al. found, by histopathology, a reduced number of cone photoreceptors coupled with shortened enter segments of both cones and rods. In addition, they noted marked enlargement and distortion of the cone pedicles (83).

Progressive cone-rod dystrophy was usually described as an autosomal dominant disease (74) (Fig. 2). It shows full penetrance and some variation in expressivity, mainly in the age of onset and rapidity of progressiveness.

An autosomal recessive form has been described (82,84) (Fig. 7), which clinically behaves similarly to the autosomal dominant form, except that the rate of progression is slower and the final outcome better than in the autosomal dominant form. The fundus may show dispersed white spots (Fig. 8) in addition to the other signs of retinal dystrophy. The various cone-rod dystrophies are summarized in Table 3.

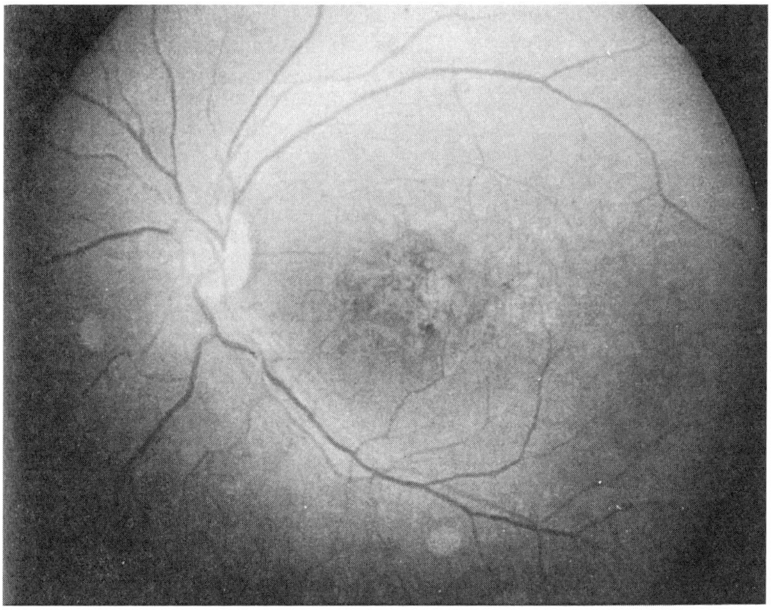

(a)

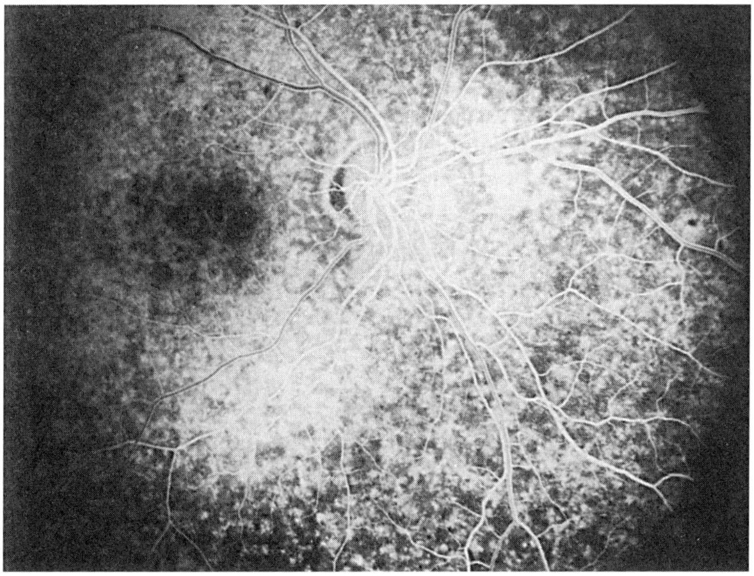

(b)

Figure 4 (a) Fundus and (b) fluorescein angiography of a 20-year-old patient with autosomal dominant progressive cone-rod dystrophy. Note the extensive retinal dystrophy in addition to the maculopathy. Visual acuity was 2/60. The visual fields showed a dense central scotoma and concentric constriction to 25° from the center.

Early linkage studies yielded negative results (85). In 1991, Warburg and colleagues (86) assigned a locus of retinal cone-rod dystrophy (C0RD1) to chromosome 18q21.1–q21.3. (86). In addition to the findings of cone-rod dystrophy,

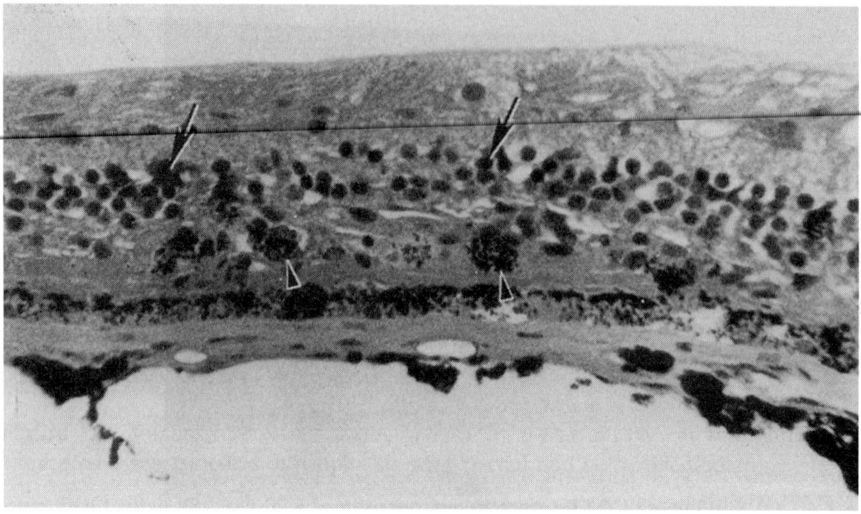

Figure 5 The posterior retina of a 29-year-old patient with progressive cone-rod dystrophy. Note the thin inner nuclear layer (arrows), the irregularly pigmented RPE layer, the absence of cone and rod outer segments, few cells in outer nuclear layer and in ganglion cell layer. Pigmented macrophages (arrowheads) invaded the retina (from Ref. 82).

and reduced cone and rod amplitudes of the ERG, the affected patients had mental retardation, hearing defect, and hypogonadism. These extraocular findings could result from the chromosomal deletion in this region. (86). CORD2 was assigned to chromosome 19q13.1–q13.2 in a 277-member family of Welsh origin in New England (87). The characteristic phenotype of CORD2-associated progressive cone-rod dystrophy included reduction in visual acuity in the first decade of life, night blindness after age 20 years and blindness at about 50 years (88). Cone losses were always more pronounced than rod photoreceptor losses (88). Later the

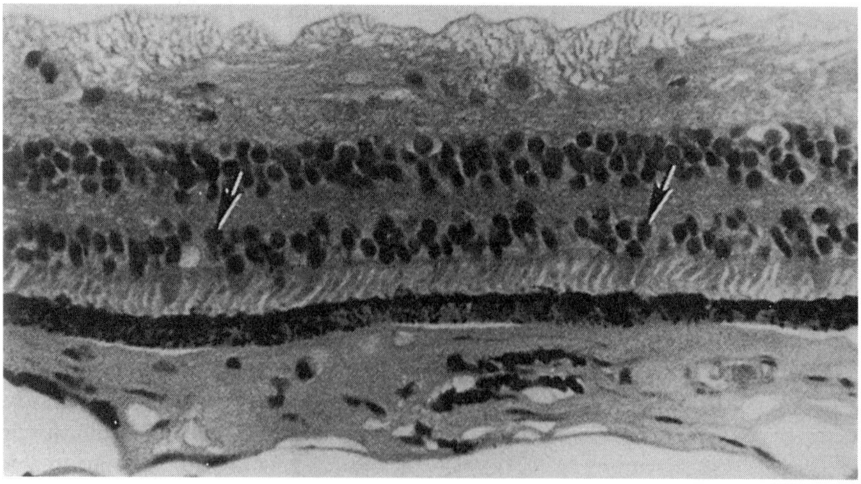

Figure 6 The equatorial retina of the same patient in Figure 5. The outer nuclear layer is thinner than normal (arrows) and the outer segments are preserved. The RPE contains lipofuscin-like granules (from Ref . 82).

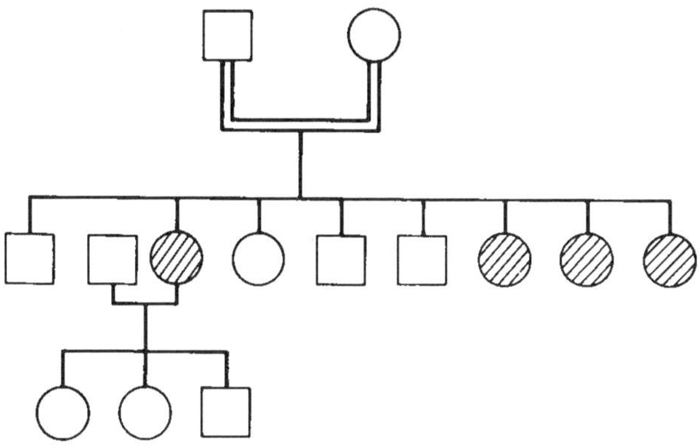

Figure 7 Pedigree of family with autosomal recessive progressive cone-rod dystrophy. The parents of the first generation were second cousins.

CORD2-causative gene was identified as CRX, a photoreceptor-specific homeobox gene (89,90). Disease-carrying mutations included nucleotide deletions, Glul68 (delta 1 bp) deletion (89) or a 4 bp deletion in codons 196–197 (90) and three missense mutations Arg41Trp, Arg41GIn, and Val42Met (90). CRX is a transcription factor for several retinal genes, including opsins and the gene for interphotoreceptor retinoid binding protein. Mutations may cause wide range of phenotypes, including autosomal dominant cone-rod dystrophy of variable severity, late-onset ADRP, early-onset ADRP, Leber congenital amaurosis, and benign variants (91). Truncation mutations, such as most nucleotide deletions, resulted in a severe phenotype (92).

The next locus for autosomal dominant cone-rod dystrophy, CORD6, was mapped to chromosome 17pl2–p13 in 1997 (93). The same group of investigators identified the causative gene as retinal specific guanylate cyclase gene (94). The gene was initially named RETGC-1 and later named GUCY2D. GUCY2D mutations were found to be associated with Leber congenital amaurosis, but cone-rod dystrophy of a milder phenotype with minimal rod involvement was associated with missense mutations in codons 837 and 838 of the GUCY2D gene (94–97).

CORD7, another locus for autosomal dominant cone-rod dystrophy has been mapped to chromosome 6cen-ql4 in one large British family (98). The gene was identified at this location as R1M1 (99). It is a large gene, contains at least 35 exons, spans 577 kb of genomic DNA, and encodes a protein of up to 1693 residues. One CORD7-associated mutation was identified as Arg844His, a missense mutation. (99) Clinically, CORD7-affected patients suffer from reduced visual acuity and dyschromatopsia from early childhood (99) and manifest characteristic macular abnormalities as described in Stargardt disease (100).

Autosomal dominant cone-rod dystrophy has also been reported in association with RDS/peripherin, a gene usually causative of some types of retinitis pigmentosa. In two Japanese families with ADCRD, missense mutations Asn244His and Tyrl84-Ser in the RDS/peripherin gene were identified. (101,102) The phenotype included early reduced visual acuity, maculopathy with peripheral retinal pigmentation and cone photoreceptors affected more than rod photoreceptors (101,102).

Autosomal Recessive Cone-Rod Dystrophies

Three distinct autosomal recessive cone-rod dystrophy (ARCRD) loci were recognized and reported until now. CORD3 symbol was applied (51) to an autosomal

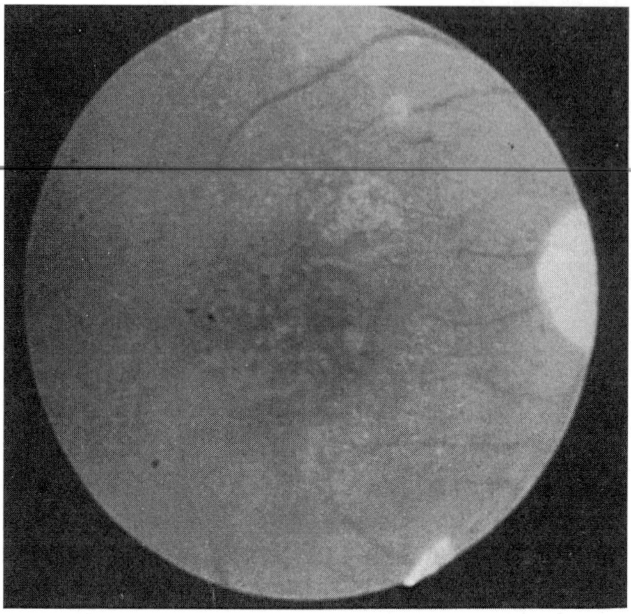

(a)

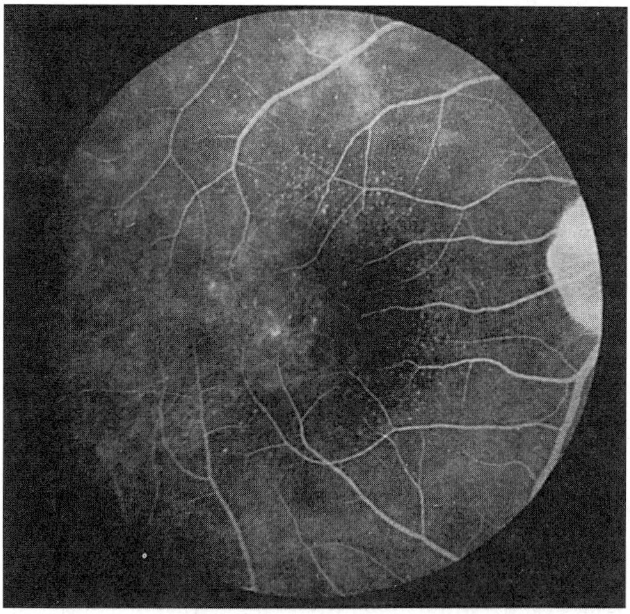

(b)

Figure 8 Progressive autosomal recessive cone-rod dystrophy: (a) fundus and (b) fluorescein angiography. Multiple white spots were seen in midperiphery in addition to the other signs of retinal dystrophy in the macular area and in midperiphery. This 32-year-old patient had a visual acuity of 0.25 m finger counting, a very low single-flash ERG response (10/100 μV), an extinct photopic flicker ERG, and a subnormal rod single-flash blue light ERO (about one-third of normal).

Table 3 Autosomal Dominant and Autosomal Recessive Cone-Rod Dystrophies

Symbol/locus	Heredity	OMIM No.	Chromosome location	Gene	Mutations
CORD1	AD	600624	18q21.1–q21.3	uk	—
CORD2	AD	602225	19q13.3	CRX	Nucleotide deletions and missense mutations
CORD6	AD	601777	17q13.1	GUCY2D	Missense in codons 837–838
CORD7	AD	603649	6cen-q14	uk	—
RDS gene associated	AD	—	6p21.1-cen	RDS/peripherin	Asn244His Tyr184Ser
CORD3	AR	604116	1p21–p13	ABCA4	Early termination or missense
CORD8	AR	605549	1q12–q24	uk	—
CORD9	AR	—	8p11	uk	—

Note: CORD—Cone-rod dystrophy; AD—autosomal dominant; uk—unknown; AR—autosomal recessive.

recessive cone-rod dystrophy associated with mutations in the ABCA4 (ABCR) gene, and mapped to chromosome Ip21–pl3 (103,104). Patients show clinical manifestations ranging from severe types of early loss of visual acuity, dyschromatopsia, central scotoma, and nonrecordable ERG, and milder types with cones affected more than rods (104). Pigmentary changes at the macula and in the periphery of the retina are seen to a large or small extent. Fishman and colleagues (105) showed that 53% of their 30 patients with suspected recessive cone-rod dystrophy had disease-carrying mutations in the ABCA4 gene. These authors and Maugeri et al. (106) concluded that mutations in the ABCA4 gene seem to be the major cause of ARCRD.

CORD8, a second locus for ARCRD, has been mapped, by Khaliq and associates, in one large Pakistani family, to chromosome Iql2–q24 (107). Patients suffered from reduction of visual acuity, photophobia, epiphora in bright light, color vision defects, macular degeneration, and later night blindness and attenuation of retinal blood vessels (107).

CORD9, the third locus for ARCRD, has been mapped to chromosome 8p11, distal but close to RP1 locus. (108) The family, of Brazilian origin, had a childhood onset of the disease (Table 3).

X-Linked Cone-Rod Dystrophies

The same genes implicated in causing X-linked cone dystrophy are also associated with XLCRD (see Table 2 and text). It is not clear whether different allelic mutations are the cause for these two distinct phenotypes.

Mitochondrial-Linked Cone-Rod Dystrophy

Mitochondrial DNA mutations are an uncommon cause of cone-rod dystrophies, as described by Chowers and colleagues (109). They are described separately in Chapter 23.

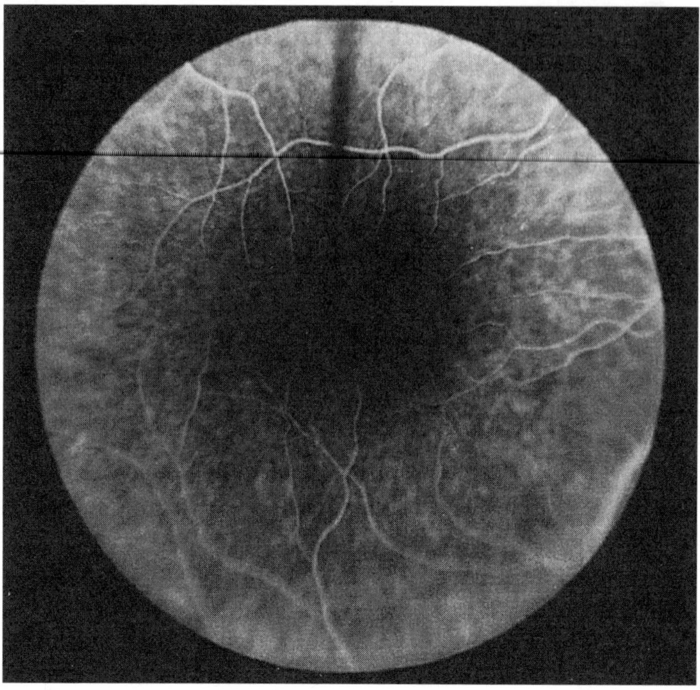

Figure 9 Fundus fluorescein angiography of a 15-year-old patient, with cone dystrophy with supernormal rod responses. Note the mild changes around the macular area in the form of tiny spots of RPE atrophy.

Cone Dystrophy with Supernormal Rod Responses

This curious condition was described by Gouras and coauthors (110) in two patients and by Alexander and Fishman (111) in three patients. Patients suffer from progressive loss of cone vision, including decreased visual acuity, progressive loss of color vision, photophobia and nystagmus, and central scotoma. The macula is abnormal, ranging from mild increased granularity with RPE defects to a full-blown bull's-eye phenomenon. The photopic ERG is mildly subnormal to extinct. Night vision is normal or subnormal, but the scotopic ERG is very supernormal, with a delayed implicit time of the positive wave. The inheritance seems to be autosomal recessive. Figure 9 shows the fundus of a patient with this disorder. This 15-year-old boy had mild mottling of the RPE in the macular area, barely noticed by opthalmoscopy but seen by fluorescein angiography. His visual acuity was 6/60. Color vision was severely impaired. He was hyperopic (+3.0 in each eye). The ERG was supernormal: 900 μV, about double the normal. The flicker cone response was very low, but rod response was normal. The EOG was normal. No change in visual acuity or any other visual function was noticed during three years of follow-up. His parents were first cousins, and the mode of inheritance was probably autosomal recessive.

Other Cone Dystrophies

Cone dystrophies that cannot be classified into one of the aforementioned entities also have been reported.

Progressive cone dystrophy with low α-L-fucosidase activity: Two patients suffered from slowly deteriorating visual acuity, progressive loss of color vision, decreasing photopic ERG responses, and had low activity of serum α-L-fucosidase (112). This is a separate entity as in all other forms of progressive cone dystrophy, normal α-L-fucosidase and other normal lysosomal enzyme activities were found (113).

Annular macular dystrophy: This autosomal dominant disorder in which dyschromatopsia is associated with abnormalities in the form of foveal hypergranularity or bull's-eye phenomenon (76,114) is now considered a stage in the development of progressive cone-rod dystrophy (79).

Management of Cone Dystrophies

No known medical or surgical method can improve the retinal function of patients with cone dystrophy, reverse the stable abnormal function of congenital cone dystrophies, or arrest the progressive loss of the late-occurring cone dystrophies. However, it is possible to improve the patients' condition by enabling the best possible function of the retina.

In complete cone dystrophy, the patients' macular vision is mediated by the rod mechanism. In normal eyes, the visual illumination approaches about 3-log scotopic troland, because of "rod saturation" (115). Young and coauthors (115) showed that the visual acuity and the visual field (size of the central scotoma) are best at intermediate-light levels at about 1-log scotopic troland, equal to 3.3-log photopic troland.

Ordinary sunglasses, which reduce transmission of light by 50–70%, can improve the photophobia and the dazzling effect of light, but they do not improve visual acuity. Berson and coauthors advised the use of gray-tinted lenses (20% transmission of light), with an additional front surface metallic coating to reduce transmission to only 4% (40). Such low-transmitting lenses are commercially available, for instance the NO-IR lenses. Fonda and Thomas (116) showed that low-vision aids are helpful in the management of patients with congenital cone dystrophy. The majority of their 43 patients were able to read regular-type print using low-vision aids.

A totally different way to reduce the amount of light reaching the retina in cone dystrophy was suggested by Schachar and associates (117) and used by Merin and colleagues (118). In these two studies, 1% or 2% pilocarpine was used to reduce the size of the pupil. Merin and colleagues (118) used 2% pilcarpine twice daily (morning and noon) and proved objective improvement in visual acuity in 11 of the 17 patients and subjective improvement in all but one.

THE CONGENITAL DYSCHROMATOPSIAS

Introduction

In the 19th century, two investigators formed the basis for the theory of normal color vision in humans (119–121), a theory still called the Young–Helmholtz trichromatic theory after these investigators. The theory claims that three independent light-sensitive mechanisms are responsible for the vision of the three colors that enable us to see the many hues of the visible spectrum. Several years earlier, Dalton accurately described the existence of human color blindness (122). Dalton himself was a dichromat. In the second half of the 20th century, studies showed that three different types of cones are responsible for the vision of the three independent colors and that dichromats lack one type of cone with its specific photopigment (123–125).

Normal color vision depends on the presence of three classes of cones, containing three different photopigments. Each photopigment contains a different cone opsin, an apoprotein, to which a similar derivative of vitamin A is bound: 11-*cis*-retinal, and each has a maximal absorption at a different wavelength of light (126). The three classes of cones are the long wavelength-sensitive (lws) cones for red or protan vision, the middle-wavelength-sensitive (mws) cones for green or deutan vision, and short-wavelength-sensitive (sws) cones for blue or tritan vision. Recently, a specialized color center was detected in the brain, in the region of the lingual and fusiform gyri, expressed much more in the left hemisphere (127).

The term *dyschromatopsia* is used for a color-defective vision in which all three types of cones function normally in their visual acuity, but the absence or anomaly of one photopigment causes an absence or anomaly of the color vision normally associated with one of the three classes of cones. Thus, defective color vision may be protanopia, deuteranopia, or tritanopia, when one photopigment is absent, or protanomaly, deuteranomaly, or tritanomaly, when one photopigment is anomalous in its function.

The Clinical Manifestation and Diagnosis of Color Vision Defects

Red-Green Color Vision Defects

The red-green defects are quite common in white populations, with about 8% of all white males affected, but are not rare in any other population or race (128,129) (Table 4). The normal vision of red and green and the associated protan and deutan color vision defects are transmitted on the X chromosome.

The pathophysiology of color vision defects is beyond the scope of this book, except for what is necessary for understanding the inheritance of such defects. It seems beyond doubt that in protanopia the "red cones" are replaced by "green cones" and vice versa in deuteranopia (123). In protanomaly and in deuteranomaly,

Table 4 Incidence of Red-Green Color Blindness

Population	% Male
Whites	8
Protanopia	1
Deuteranopia	1
Protanomaly	1
Deuteranomaly	5
Africans	2.3
Japanese	4
Australasians	2

Note: The figures are average and vary among the different populations of the same race. For instance, figures in whites range from 7% to 10% and in Africans, from less than 1% in South African tribes to 5% in North African countries. The relative frequency of deutan/protan defects varies in nonwhite populations. In some African populations deutan defects are more frequent, in others protan defects, and in some the ratio is about 1:1 (129).

the respective "red" or "green" cone exists, but carries an abnormal photopigment that absorbs light maximally somewhere between the normal red and green photopigments. The spectral sensitivity curve shows maximal absorption in the fovea at 555 nm in the normal persons, and a shift to 548 nm in protans, 566 nm in deutans, and 569 nm in tritans (123).

Several clinical tests are available for the clinician to fulfill his three aims: to screen for color vision defects, to diagnose and classify the type of defect, and to grade its severity (130). No single test fulfills all three aims (130). A good, simple screening test is the single-plate Farnsworth F-2 test (131). For diagnosis of red-green defects, Ishihara pseudoisochromatic plates are reliable, especially if used together with the simple Farnsworth panel D-15 dichotomous test (132). The American Optical H-R-R test adds also the capability of diagnosing blue-yellow defects and adds quantification to the qualitative diagnosis. It seems to me that the combination of the three tests (Ishihara plates, H-R-R test, and Farnsworth D-15) should fulfill all needs of the clinician for screening, diagnosis, and some quantification of congenital color vision defects. Tests such as the Farnsworth–Munsell 100-hue test (133) or color television display (134) are cumbersome and should be reserved for the expert and for research.

Standard pseudoisochromatic plates part 2 were constructed to detect blue-yellow defects and can be used in conjunction with Ishihara plates, instead of the H-R-R test (135). Objective measures to test red-green color vision defects are sparse and not in common use. Electroretinography under routine test circumstances usually yields normal results. However, spectral sensitivity of rapid off responses was shifted to the left in protans and had lower amplitudes (flatter curves) in deuteranopes (136). The ERG was abnormal in protanopes when long-wavelength stimuli were used (137). Also, the pupillary response to light, as measured by pupillometry, was abnormal in protanopes (138). The abnormal results of the last two tests probably stem from the fact that protanopes have a reduced spectrum of vision, in which the longest wavelengths of light are not seen at all. This occurs in addition to the abnormal color sensation within the visible spectrum.

Blue-Yellow Color Vision Defects

The existence of tritanopia, a defect of recognition of the blue-yellow color vision, transmitted by an autosomal dominant gene was confirmed by Wright (139) and is considered to be very rare. Its frequency was estimated as 1:20,000 (140), but it is probably much higher than this. In one study, the frequency of tritan disturbances was estimated as 1:500 (141). It seems that, in contrast with red-green defects, it is incorrect to subdivide between dichromasia (tritanopia) and anomalous trichomasia (tritanomaly) (141), a theory also suggested by recent research on the genetics of color vision defects. Electroretinography shows a marked reduction of the blue cone response to monochromatic light stimuli (142), thereby providing an objective measure for diagnosis of congenital tritanopia.

Differential Diagnosis of Congenital Dyschromatopsia

A series of diseases may cause acquired color vision defects, which may sometimes mimic the congenital forms. They include central nervous system diseases, such as multiple sclerosis (143), brain infarcts (144), optic atrophy of both the acquired and the inherited forms (145), aging phenomena such as cataract formation (146), iatrogenic causes such as digitalis toxicity (147,148), and others. Generally, the routine clinical tests can distinguish between congenital and acquired dyschromatopsia. In the congenital forms, the subjective responses of the subject are clear-cut and predictable lines, whereas, in the acquired forms, the responses are confused.

The Genetics of Normal Color Vision

The fact that congenital red-green dyschromatopsia is transmitted as an X-linked characteristic has been known for many years. Later, it became clear that congenital blue-yellow dyschromatopsia is transmitted as an autosomal dominant disorder. However, the exact mode of inheritance of deutan and protan anomalies remained unclear until recently. Several unexplained facts raised the discussion between supporters of a "one-locus" theory and supporters of a "two-locus" theory. First, the number of affected females in the general population was lower than expected. In most white populations, about 8% of males are affected. Therefore, the percentage of affected females should be 0.08×0.08, or 0.64%. The observation that it is much less supported the two-locus theory. Second, a double-hemizygote male, one who is both protanope and deuteranope, is an extremely rare phenomenon. If it does exist, it is certainly incomparably less frequent than expected if the two-locus theory, with two independent genes, is correct. This supported the one-locus theory, with interchanging allelic genes. Third, the relation of dichromasia (protanopia or deuteranopia) to anomalous trichomasia (protanomaly and deuteranomaly) was not clear. Are these allelic genes on several loci? Fourth, some dichromats show the existence of a third photopigment (149).

Waaler, who first supported the two-locus theory, finally concluded in 1968, that the two normal properties—protopia and deuteropia—depend on one locus in which these properties are located at two different places on the molecule of the one gene (150). Waaler described the gene in the form of a square when one missing side causes dichromasia and a missing part of another side causes anomalous trichromasia.

Linkage studies supported the two-locus theory and suggested the following order of the loci on the long arm of the X-chromosome: hypoxanthine-guanine phosphoribosyltransferase (HPRT), deutan, G6PD, protan, and Xq telomere (151), with all these genes tightly together.

More recently, Nathans and associates accomplished the isolation and sequencing of genomic and complementary DNA clones that encode the apoproteins (opsins) of the three photopigments of color vision (152). They showed an amazing similarity between the amino acid sequences in the two genes for red and green pigments. The mutual identity was 96%, whereas the identity of the amino acid sequence was only 43% for the blue photopigment and only 41% for rhodopsin (152), compared to red and green pigments. The genes for two cone pigments (red and green) are on the X chromosome, the gene for blue cone pigment on chromosome 7, and the gene for rod pigment on chromosome 3 (126). The rhodopsin gene is located at chromosome 3q21–q24; blue-cone pigment at 7q31-q32, and red and green cone pigments on chromosome X near the telomere of the long arm, Xq28 (153). The red and green opsin genes are arranged in a head to tail tandem array (153,154). The red and green genes are 98% homologous in their DNA sequence (154,155) and normal color vision individuals have one red gene followed by one, two, or three green genes (154). Sometimes the number of green genes may reach an extreme of eight (153,156). The number of the two types of genes was measured in Japanese males. 43% had a 1:1 ratio, 41% a 1:2 ratio, 6% a 1:3 ratio, and 9% had a ratio of more than 1 to 3 (157). The tandem array starts, on the telomeric edge of the long arm of chromosome X with a "pseudogene" called LCR, a sequence element of 3.1–3.7 kb followed downstream by one red pigment gene, and further downstream by one to eight green pigment gene(s), (153). Each gene consists of an approximate 15 kb segment and ≈24 kb intergenic sequence. The LCR controls the expression of both the red and the green genes in such a way that only one of each will be expressed (153).

In the retina the number of lws-cones is greater than the number of mws-cones by a factor range from 1.15:1 to 3.79:1 (158). This range variation applies to different normal individuals and to different areas of the retina. On average, lws-cones constitute 65% of the combined number of lws and mws cones, but the range varies widely from 15% to 80% in normal individuals (159). Normal exact peak absorptions for visual pigments are 498 nm for rhodopsin, 426 nm for sw pigment, 530 nm for mw pigment, and 558 nm for lw-pigment. (153).

Evolutionarily, the X-chromosome visual pigment genes are "young." A five-visual pigment system of one rod and four cone pigments has been known to exist for at least 350 million years in vertebrates. Mammals, however, had an rod-only dominated retina until about 35 million years ago, when in primates two new and distinct visual pigments produced the present-day trichromary in man (160).

The Inheritance of Congenital Dyschromatopsia

Nathans and colleagues studied the molecular genetics of inherited red-green color blindness by hybridization of genomic DNA for affected males with cloned red and green pigment genes as probes (161). They concluded that two tightly connected genes at the telomere of Xq are responsible for the normal red and green photopigments. In protanopes and in deuteranopes, only one of the two genes exists, the other one being replaced by the existing gene by one of two genetic mechanisms: homologous, but unequal, exchange, or by gene conversion. Anomalous trichromacy (protan or deutan) have one normal gene and one hybrid gene on the X chromosome and produce one normal photopigment and one abnormal photopigment, with spectral properties between red and green. This theory of the molecular biology may explain the evolution of color vision. In lower mammals only two cone pigments exist: sws cones, with a maximal absorption near 430 nm, on one autosome, and lws cone, with a maximal absorption between 510 and 570 nm, on the X chromosome (126). It was suggested that the hybrid gene found in anomalous trichromacy may indicate that a future human will have four color vision genes (162). It seems that the studies by Nathans and his colleagues explain the previous puzzles related to inheritance of color vision defects.

A later study from the same laboratory (163) indicated a head-to-tail tandem array of genes, with the red pigment gene at the end and a variable number of green pigment genes nearby, all at Xq28. Normal individuals possess one gene for red pigment and one to three genes for green pigment. Among 25 patients with red-green color blindness, 24 showed a gene deletion or a fusion of genes caused by rearrangement by homologous recombination (163).

Missense mutations causing dichromacy or anomalous trichromacy are uncommon. The substitution of cysteine by arginine in codon 203 of the green gene is probably the most frequent and may be the cause of deuteranomaly (160). Much more frequently, however, deuteranomaly or protanomaly are caused by hybridization of the defective gene and/or loss of function of one gene (164).

In protanopia and deuteranopia, the loss of function of one gene commonly occurs by the deletion of the whole gene or, less frequently, by point mutation. In protanomaly, the L-gene is missing and the M-gene changed to a hybrid gene, so as to somewhat express the red vision. In deuteranomaly, a normal L-gene is followed by a hybrid M-gene (165). In the retinal cones only one normal red cone and one hybrid pigment will be expressed (166), in addition to the unaffected blue cone. Several additional missense mutations were recently reported in both the red and green gene of Japanese males (167). While two out of 35 Japanese males with deutan deficiency were identified to have missense mutations, 32 others had a nucleotide substitution: A71C in the promoter region of the green gene in the second position (168). It is likely that mutant opsins are affected in the folding process, resulting in loss of function as a visual pigment (166).

Females suffering from full-blown color vision defects are rare and generally do not exceed 0.4% of the female population. However, this number increased in consanguineous families. In southern Iraq, 3.2% of all females were affected, an extremely high incidence, probably resulting from the fact that 60% were offspring of consanguineous marriages (169). The question of whether or not the asymptomatic female carrier can be detected by tests is still not fully solved. It seems that carriers of protanopia and protanomaly have a sensitivity loss of their color vision in the long-wavelength region (170). The situation is much less clear in carriers of deuteranopia and deuteranomaly, and many or most of these cannot be detected.

Tritanopia or blue blindness is an autosomal dominant disease with a frequency widely variable, ranging in extreme from 1:500 in some populations to 1:65,000 in others (153). The locus has been mapped to chromosome 7q31.3–32 (171) and three point mutations have been identified: Gly79Arg, Ser214Pro and Pro264Ser (153).

REFERENCES

1. Pokorny J, Smith VC, Pinckers AJLG, Cozijensen M. Classification of complete and incomplete autosomal recessive achromatopsia. Graefes Arch Clin Exp Ophthalmol 1982; 219:121–130.
2. Goodman G, Ripps H, Siegel IM. Cone dysfunction syndromes. Arch Ophthalmol 1963; 70:214–231.
3. Alpern M. What is it that confines in a world without color? Invest Ophthalmol 1974; 13:647–674.
4. Auerbach E, Merin S. Achromatopsia with amblyopia. A clinical and electroretinographic study of 39 cases. Doc Ophthalmol 1974; 37:79–117.
5. Auerbach E, Kripke B. Achromatopsia with amblyopia II. A psychophysical study of 5 cases. Doc Ophthalmol 1974; 37:119–144.
6. Price MJ, Thompson HS, Judisch GH, Corbett JJ. Pupillary constriction to darkness. Br J Ophthalmol 1985; 69:205–211.
7. Holm E, Lodberg CV. Family with total color-blindness. Acta Ophthalmol 1940; 18:224–258.
8. Brody JA, Hussels I, Brink E, Torres J. Hereditary blindness among Pingelapese people of eastern Carolina Islands. Lancet 1970; 1:1253–1257.
9. Sacks DW. The Island of the Colorblind. New York: Random House, 1996.
10. Zlotogora J. Hereditary disorders among Iranian Jews. Am J Med Genet 1995; 58:32–37.

11. Arbour NC, Zlotogora J, Knowlton RG, Merin S, et al. Homozygosity mapping of achromatopsia to chromosome 2 using DNA pooling. Hum Mol Genet 1997; 6:689–694.
12. Pentao L, Lewis RA, Ledbetter DH, et al. Maternal uniparental isodisomy of chromosome 14: association with autosomal recessive rod monochromacy. Am J Hum Genet 1992; 50:690–699.
13. Wissinger B, Jagle H, Kohl S, et al. Human rod monochromacy: linkage analysis and mapping of a cone photoreceptor expressed candidate gene on chromosome 2q11 Genomics 1998; 51:325–331.
14. Kohl S, Marx T, Giddings I, et al. Total colourblindness is caused by mutations in the gene encoding the alpha-subunit of the cone photoreceptor cGMP-gated cation channel. Nat Genet 1998; 19:257–259.
15. Wissinger B, Gamer D, Jagle H, et al. CNGA3 mutations in hereditary cone photoreceptor disorders. Am J Hum Genet 2001; 69:722–737.
16. Kohl S, Baumann B, Broghammer M, et al. Mutations in the CNGB3 gene encoding the beta-subunit of the cone photoreceptor cGMP-gated channel are responsible for achromatopsia (ACHM3) linked to chromosome 8qHum Mol Genet 2000; 9: 2107–2116.
17. Sundin OH, Yang JM, Li Y, et al. Genetic basis of total colourblindness among the Pingelapese islanders. Nat Genet 2000; 25:289–293.
18. Kohl S, Baumann B, Rosenberg T, et al. Mutations in the cone photoreceptor G-protein alpha-subunit gene GNAT2 in patients with achromatopsia. Am J Hum Genet 2002; 71:422–425.
19. Blackwell HR, Blackwell OM. Rod and cone receptor mechanisms in typical and atypical congenital achromatopsia. Vision Res 1961; 1:62–107.
20. Alpern M, Lee GB, Spivey BE. π_1 cone-monochromatism. Arch Ophthalmol 1965; 74:334–337.
21. Spivey BE. The X-linked recessive inheritance of atypical monochromatism. Arch Ophthalmol 1965; 74:327–333.
22. Francois J, Verriest G, Matton-van Leuven MT, et al. Atypical achromatopsia of sex-linked recessive inheritance. Am J Ophthalmol 1966; 61:1101–1108.
23. Spivey BE, Pearlman JT, Burian HM. Electroretinographic findings (including flicker) in carriers of congenital X-linked achromatopsia. Doc Ophthalmol 1964; 18:367–375.
24. Fleischman JA, O'Donnell FE Jr. Congenital X-linked incomplete achromatopsia: evidence for slow progression, carrier fundus findings, and possible genetic linkage with glucose-6-phosphate dehydrogenase locus. Arch Ophthalmol 1981; 99:468–472.
25. Godel V, Regenbogen L, Adam A, Stein R. Rod monochromatism—an incomplete form. J Pediatr Ophthalmol 1976; 13:211–225.
26. Smith VC, Pokorny J, Delleman JW, et al. X-linked incomplete achromatopsia with more than one class of functional cones. Invest Ophthalmol Vis Sci 1983; 24:451–457.
27. Berson EL, Sandberg MA, Rosner B, Sullivan PL. Color plates to help identify patients with blue cone monochromatism. Am J Ophthalmol 1983; 95:741–747.
28. Berson EL, Sandberg MA, Maguire A, et al. Electroretinograms in carriers of blue cone monochromatism. Arch Ophthalmol 1986; 102:254–261.
29. Heckenlively JR, Weleber RG. X-linked recessive cone dystrophy with tapetal-like sheen. A newly recognized entity with Mizuo-Nakamura phenomenon. Arch Ophthalmol 1986; 104:1322–1328.
30. Reichel E, Bruce AM, Sandberg MA, Berson EL. An electroretinographic and molecular genetic study of X-linked cone degeneration. Am J Ophthalmol 1989; 108:540–547.
31. Nathans J, Davenport CM, Maumenee IH, et al. Molecular genetics of human blue cone monochromacy. Science 1989; 245:831–838.
32. Ayyagari R, Kakuk LE, Coats CL, et al. Bilateral macular atrophy in blue cone monochromacy (BCM) with loss of the locus control region (LCR) and part of the red pigment gene. Mol Vis 5:13. 1999.

33. Nathans J, Maumenee IH, Zrenner E, et al. Genetic heterogeneity among blue-cone monochromats. Am J Hum Genet 1993; 53:987–1000.
34. Ayyagari R, Kakuk LE, Bingham EL, et al. Spectrum of color gene deletions and phenotype in patients with blue cone monochromacy. Hum Genet 2000; 107:75–82.
35. Smith VC, Pokorny J, Newell FW. Autosomal recessive incomplete achromatopsia with protan luminosity function. Ophthalmologica 1978; 177:197–207.
36. Smith VC, Pokorny J, Newell FW. Autosomal recessive incomplete achromatopsia with deutan luminosity function. Am J Ophthalmol 1979; 87:393–402.
37. Young RS, Price J. Wavelength discrimination deteriorates with illumination in blue cone monochromats. Invest Ophthalmol Vis Sci 1985; 26:1543–1549.
38. Pearlman JT, Owen WG, Brounley DW, Sheppard JJ. Cone dystrophy with dominant inheritance. Am J Ophthalmol 1974; 77:293–303.
39. Noble KG. Hereditary macular dystrophies. In: Renie WA, ed. Goldberg's Genetic and Metabolic Eye Disease. 2nd ed. Boston: Little, Brown & Co, 1986.
40. Berson EL, Gouras P, Gunkel RD. Progressive cone degeneration dominantly inherited. Arch Ophthalmol 1968; 80:77–83.
41. Gray RHB, Blach RK, Barnard WM. Bull's eye maculopathy with early cone degeneration. Br J Ophthalmol 1977; 61:702–718.
42. Francois J, De Rouck A, Verriest G, et al. Progressive generalized cone dysfunction. Ophthalmologica 1974; 169:255–284.
43. Ripps H, Noble KG, Greenstein VC, et al. Progressive cone dystrophy. Ophthalmology 1987; 94:1401–1409.
44. Sloan LL, Brown DJ. Progressive retinal degeneration with selective involvement of the cone mechanism. Am J Ophthalmol 1962; 54:629–641.
45. Krill AE, Deutman AF. Dominant macular degenerations: the cone dystrophies. Am J Ophthalmol 1972; 73:352–369.
46. Kellner U, Foerster MH. Pattern of dysfunction in progressive cone dystrophies—an extended classification. Ger J Ophthalmol 1993; 2:170–177.
47. Small KW, Gehrs K. Clinical study of a large family with autosomal dominant progressive cone degeneration. Am J Ophthalmol 1996; 121:1–12.
48. Kellner U, Foerster MH. Cone dystrophies with negative photopic electroretinogram. Br J Ophthalmol 1993; 77:404–409.
49. Miyake Y, Horiguchi M, Tomita N, et al. Occult macular dystrophy. Am J Ophthalmol 1996; 122:644–653.
50. Went LN, van Schooneveld MJ, Oosterhuis JA. Late onset dominant cone dystrophy with early blue cone involvement. J Med Genet 1992; 29:295–298.
51. OMIM at http://www.ncbi.nlm.nih.gov/omim/.
52. Balciuniene J, Johansson K, Sandgren O, et al. A gene for autosomal dominant progressive cone dystrophy (CORD5) maps to chromosome 17p12-p13. Genomics 1995; 30: 281–286.
53. Small KW, Syrquin M, Mullen L, et al. Mapping of autosomal dominant cone degeneration to chromosome 17p. Am J Ophthalmol 1996; 121:13–18.
54. Payne AM, Downes SM, Bessant DA, et al. A mutation in guanylate cyclase activator 1A (GUCA1A) in an autosomal dominant cone dystrophy pedigree mapping to a new locus on chromosome 6p21.1 Hum Mol Genet 1998; 7:273–277.
55. Downes SM, Holder GE, Fitzke FW, et al. Autosomal dominant cone and cone-rod dystrophy with mutations in the guanylate cyclase activator 1A gene-encoding guanylate cyclase activating protein-1. Arch Ophthalmol 2001; 119:96–105.
56. Gorin MB, Jackson KE, Ferrell RE, et al. A peripherin/retinal degeneration slow mutation (Pro-210-Arg) associated with macular and peripheral retinal degeneration. Ophthalmology 1995; 102:246–255.
57. Fishman GA, Stone EM, Alexander KR, et al. Serine-27-phenylalanine mutation within the peripherin/RDS gene in a family with cone dystrophy. Ophthalmology 1997; 104:299–306.

58. Pinckers A, Deutman AF. X-linked cone dystrophy. An overlooked diagnosis?. Int Ophthalmol 1987; 10:241–243.
59. van Everdingen JA, Went LN, Keunen JE, Oosterhuis JA. X linked progressive cone dystrophy with specific attention to carrier detection. J Med Genet 1992; 29:291–294.
60. Jacobson DM, Thompson HS, Bartley JA. X-linked progressive cone dystrophy. Clinical characteristics of affected males and female carriers. Ophthalmology 1989; 96: 885–895.
61. Hong HK, Ferrell RE, Gorin MB. Clinical diversity and chromosomal localization of X-linked cone dystrophy (COD1). Am J Hum Genet 1994; 55:1173–81.
62. Meire FM, Bergen AA, De Rouck A, et al. X linked progressive cone dystrophy. Localisation of the gene locus to Xp21-p11.1 by linkage analysis. Br J Ophthalmol 1994; 78:103–108.
63. Brown J Jr, Kimura AE, Gorin MB. Clinical and electroretinographic findings of female carriers and affected males in a progressive X-linked cone-rod dystrophy (COD-1) pedigree. Ophthalmology 2000; 107:1104–1110.
64. Seymour AB, Dash-Modi A, O'Connell JR, et al. Linkage analysis of X-linked cone-rod dystrophy: localization to Xp11.4 and definition of a locus distinct from RP2 and RP3Am J Hum Genet 1998; 62:122–129.
65. Demirci FY, Rigatti BW, Wen G, et al. X-linked cone-rod dystrophy (locus COD1): identification of mutations in RPGR exon ORF15 Am J Hum Genet 2002; 70: 1049–1053.
66. Yang Z, Peachey NS, Moshfeghi DM, et al. Mutations in the RPGR gene cause X-linked cone dystrophy. Hum Mol Genet 2002; 11:605–611.
67. Bergen AA, Pinckers AJ. Localization of a novel X-linked progressive cone dystrophy gene to Xq27: evidence for genetic heterogeneity. Am J Hum Genet 1997; 60:1468–1473.
68. Jalkanen R, Demirci FY, Tyynismaa H, et al. A new genetic locus for X linked progressive cone-rod dystrophy. J Med Genet 2003; 40:418–423.
69. Buchanan TAS, Gardiner TA, de Jesus V, et al. Retinal ultrastructural findings in cone degeneration. Am J Ophthalmol 1988; 106:405–413.
70. To K, Adamian M, Jakobiec FA, Berson EL. Histopathologic and immunohistochemical study of dominant cone degeneration. Am J Ophthalmol 1998; 126:140–142.
71. To KW, Adamian M, Jakobiec FA, Berson EL. Histopathologic and immunohistochemical study of an autopsy eye with X-linked cone degeneration. Arch Ophthalmol 1998; 116:100–103.
72. Berson EL, Gouras P, Gunkel RD. Progressive cone-rod degeneration. Arch Ophthalmol 1968; 80:68–76.
73. Krill AE, Deutman AF, Fishman M. The cone degenerations. Doc Ophthalmol 1973; 35:1–80.
74. Hittner HM, Murphree AL, Garcia CA, et al. Dominant cone-rod dystrophy. Doc Ophthalmol 1975; 39:29–52.
75. Krill AE, Deutman AF. Dominant macular degenerations: the cone dystrophies. Am J Ophthalmol 1972; 73:352–369.
76. Deutman AF. Benign concentric annular macular dystrophy. Am J Ophthalmol 1974; 78:384–396.
77. Van den Biesen PR, Deutman AF, Pinckers LG. Evolution of benign concentric annular macular dystrophy. Am J Ophthalmol 1985; 100:73–78.
78. Miyake Y, Goto S, Ota I, Ichikawa H. Vitreous fluorophotometry in patients with cone rod dystrophy. Br J Ophthalmol 1984; 68:489–494.
79. Fishman GA, Rhee AJ, Blair NP. Blood-retinal barrier function in patients with cone or cone-rod dystrophy. Arch Ophthalmol 1986; 104:545–548.
80. Kelsell RE, Gregory-Evans K, Gregory-Evans CY, et al. Localization of a gene (CORD7) for a dominant cone-rod dystrophy to chromosome 6q. Am J Hum Genet 1998; 63:274–279.

81. Szlyk JP, Fishman GA, Alexander KR, et al. Clinical subtypes of cone-rod dystrophy. Arch Ophthalmol 1993; 111:781–788.
82. Rabb MF, Tso MOM, Fishman GA. Cone-rod dystrophy. A clinical and histopathologic report. Ophthalmology 1986; 93:1443–1451.
83. Gregory-Evans K, Fariss RN, Possin DE, et al. Abnormal cone synapses in human cone-rod dystrophy. Ophthalmology 1998; 105:2306–2312.
84. Bloome MA, Garcia CA. Manual of Retinal and Choroidal Dystrophies. New York: Appleton-Century-Crofts, 1982.
85. Ferrell RE, Hittner HM, Chakravarti A. Autosomal dominant cone-rod dystrophy A linkage study with 17 biochemical and serological markers. Am J Med Genet New York 1981; 8:363–369.
86. Warburg M, Sjö O, Tranebjaerg L, Fledelius HC. Deletion mapping of a retinal cone-rod dystrophy: assignment to 18q211. Am J Med Genet 1991; 39:288–293.
87. Evans K, Fryer A, Inglehearn C, et al. Genetic linkage of cone-rod retinal dystrophy to chromosome 19q and evidence for segregation distortion. Nat Genet 1994; 6:210–213.
88. Evans K, Duvall-Young, J, Fitzke FW, et al. Chromosome 19q cone-rod retinal dystrophy. Ocular phenotype. Arch Opthalmol 1995; 113:195–201.
89. Freund CL, Gregory-Evans CY, Furukawa T, et al. Cone-rod dystrophy due to mutations in a novel photoreceptor-specific homeobox gene (CRX) essential for maintenance of the photoreceptor. Cell 1997; 91:543–553.
90. Swain PK, Chen S, Wang QL, et al. Mutations in the cone-rod homeobox gene are associated with the cone-rod dystrophy photoreceptor degeneration. Neuron 1997; 19: 1329–1336.
91. Sohocki MM, Sullivan LS, Mintz-Hittner HA, et al. A range of clinical phenotypes associated with mutations in CRX, a photoreceptor transcription-factor gene. Am J Hum Genet 1998; 63:1307–1315.
92. Jacobson SG, Cideciyan AV, Huang Y, et al. Retinal degenerations with truncation mutations in the cone-rod homeobox (CRX) gene. Invest Ophthalmol Vis Sci 1998; 39:2417–2426.
93. Kelsell RE, Evans K, Gregory CY, et al. Localisation of a gene for dominant cone-rod dystrophy (CORD6) to chromosome 17p. Hum Mol Genet 1997; 6:597–600.
94. Kelsell RE, Gregory-Evans K, Payne AM, et al. Mutations in the retinal guanylate cyclase (RETGC-1) gene in dominant cone-rod dystrophy. Hum Mol Genet 1998; 7:1179–1184.
95. Weigell-Weber M, Fokstuen S, Torok B, et al. Codons 837 and 838 in the retinal guanylate cyclase gene on chromosome 17p: hot spots for mutations in autosomal dominant cone-rod dystrophy? Arch Ophthalmol, 2000; 118:300.
96. Gregory-Evans K, Kelsell RE, Gregory-Evans CY, et al. Autosomal dominant cone-rod retinal dystrophy (CORD6) from heterozygous mutation of GUCY2D, which encodes retinal guanylate cyclase. Ophthalmology 2000; 107:55–61.
97. Downes SM, Payne AM, Kelsell RE, et al. Autosomal dominant cone-rod dystrophy with mutations in the guanylate cyclase 2D gene encoding retinal guanylate cyclase-1 Arch Ophthalmol 2001; 119:1667–1673.
98. Kelsell RE, Gregory-Evans K, Gregory-Evans CY, et al. Localization of a gene (CORD7) for a dominant cone-rod dystrophy to chromosome 6q. Am J Hum Genet 1998; 63:274–279.
99. Johnson S, Halford S, Morris AG, et al. Genomic organization and alternative splicing of human RIM1, a gene implicated in autosomal dominant cone-rod dystrophy (CORD7). Genomics 2003; 81:304–314.
100. Kniazeva MF, Chiang MF, Cutting GR, et al. Clinical and genetic studies of an autosomal dominant cone-rod dystrophy with features of Stargardt disease. Ophthalmic Genet 1999; 20:71–81.

101. Nakazawa M, Kikawa E, Chida Y, Tamai M. Asn244His mutation of the peripherin/RDS gene causing autosomal dominant cone-rod degeneration. Hum Mol Genet 1994; 3:1195–1196.
102. Nakazawa M, Kikawa E, Chida Y, et al. Autosomal dominant cone-rod dystrophy associated with mutations in codon 244 (Asn244His) and codon 184 (Tyr184Ser) of the peripherin/RDS gene. Arch Ophthalmol 1996; 114:72–78.
103. Cremers FP, van de Pol DJ, van Driel M, et al. Autosomal recessive retinitis pigmentosa and cone-rod dystrophy caused by splice site mutations in the Stargardt disease gene ABCR. Hum Mol Genet 1998; 7:355–362.
104. Klevering BJ, Blankenagel A, Maugeri A, et al. Phenotypic spectrum of autosomal recessive cone-rod dystrophies caused by mutations in the ABCA4 (ABCR) gene. Invest Ophthalmol Vis Sci 2002; 43:1980–1985.
105. Fishman GA, Stone EM, Eliason DA, et al. ABCA4 gene sequence variations in patients with autosomal recessive cone-rod dystrophy. Arch Ophthalmol 2003; 121:851–855.
106. Maugeri A, Klevering BJ, Rohrschneider K, et al. Mutations in the ABCA4 (ABCR) gene are the major cause of autosomal recessive cone-rod dystrophy. Am J Hum Genet 2000; 67:960–966.
107. Khaliq S, Hameed A, Ismail M, et al. Novel locus for autosomal recessive cone-rod dystrophy CORD8 mapping to chromosome 1q12–Q24 Invest Ophthalmol Vis Sci 2000; 41:3709–3712.
108. Danciger M, Hendrickson J, Lyon J, et al. CORD9 a new locus for arCRD: mapping to 8p11, estimation of frequency, evaluation of a candidate gene. Invest Ophthalmol Vis Sci 2001; 42:2458–2465.
109. Chowers I, Lerman-Sagie T, Elpeleg ON, et al. Cone and rod dysfunction in the NARP syndrome. Br J Ophthalmol 1999; 83:190–193.
110. Gouras P, Eggers HM, McKay CJ. Cone dystrophy, nyctalopia and supernormal rod responses. A new retinal degeneration. Arch Ophthalmol 1983; 101:718–724.
111. Alexander KR, Fishman GA. Supernormal scotopic ERG in cone dystrophy. Br J Ophthalmol 1984; 68:69–78.
112. Hayasaka S, Nakazawa M, Okabe H, et al. Progressive cone dystrophy associated with low alpha-L-fucosidase activity in serum and leukocytes. Am J Ophthalmol 1985; 99:681–685.
113. Stoumbos VD, Weleber RG, Kennaway NG. Normal α-L-fucosidase and other lysosomal enzyme activities in progressive cone dystrophy. Am J Ophthalmol 1988; 106:11–16.
114. Coppeto J, Ayazi S. Annular macular dystrophy. Am J Ophthalmol 1982; 93:278–284.
115. Young RSL, Krefman RA, Fishman GA. Visual improvements with, red-tinted glasses in a patient with cone dystrophy. Arch Ophthalmol 1982; 100:268–271.
116. Fonda G, Thomas H. Correction of low visual acuity in achromatopsia. Use of corrective lenses as an aid to educational and vocational placement. Arch Ophthalmol 1974; 91:20–23.
117. Schachar RA, Pokorny J, Krill AE. Use of miotics in patients with cone degeneration. Am J Ophthalmol 1973; 76:816–820.
118. Merin S, Ronen S, Nawaratzki I. Management of patients with congenital cone deficiency (achromatopsia with amblyopia). Doc Ophthalmol Proc Ser 1981; 25:241–245.
119. Young T. On the theory of light and colors. Phil Trans R Soc 1802; 12.
120. Young T. A Course of Lectures in Natural Philosophy. London, 1807.
121. Helmholtz H. Uber die Theorie der zusammengesetzten Farben. Poggendorff's Ann Physik Chemie 1852; 87:45–66.
122. Dalton J. Extraordinary facts relating to the vision of colours. Mem Lit Phil Soc Manchester 1798; 5:28.
123. Wald G. Defective color vision and its inheritance. Proc Natl Acad Sci USA 1966; 55:1347–1363.

124. Rushton WAH. Densitometry of pigments in rods and cones of normal and color defective subjects. Invest Opthalmol 1966; 5:233–241.
125. Alpern M, Wake T. Cone pigments in human deutan colour vision defects. J Physiol 1977; 266:595–612.
126. Mollon JD. Molecular genetics: understanding colour vision. Nature 1986; 321:12–13.
127. Lueck CJ, Zeki S, Friston KJ, et al. The colour centre in the cerebral cortex of man. Nature 1989; 340:386–389.
128. Kherumian R, Pickford RW. Hérédité et frequence des anomalies congenitales du senscromatique. Paris: Vigot Fréres, 1959.
129. Adam A. Colorblindness in Africa. Metab Pediatr Ophthalmol 1981; 5:181–185.
130. Birch J. A practical guide for colour-vision examination: Report of the Standardization Committee of the International Research Group on Colour-Vision Deficiencies. Ophthalmol Physiol Opt 1985; 5:265–285.
131. Adams AJ, Bailey JE, Harwood LW. Color vision screening: a comparison of the AOH-R-R and Farnsworth F-2 tests. Am J Optom Physiol Opt 1984; 61:1–9.
132. Aarnisalo E. Testing of colour vision for vocational purposes. Acta Ophthalmol Suppl 1984; 161:135–138.
133. Smith VC, Pokorny J, Pass AS. Color-axis determination on the Farnsworth-Munsell 100-hue test. Am J Ophthalmol 1985; 100:176–182.
134. Chioran GM, Sellers KL, Benes SC, et al. Color mixture thresholds measured on a color television—a new method for analysis, classification and diagnosis of neuroophthalmic disease. Doc Ophthalmol 1985; 61:119–135.
135. Pinckers A, Nabbe B, Vossen H. Standard pseudoisochromatic plates part 2. Ophthalmologica 1985; 190:118–124.
136. Kawasaki K, Yonemura D, Nakazato H. Empirical detection of congenital dyschromatopsia by electroretinography. Ophthalmic Res 1984; 16:329–333.
137. Ponte F, Anastasi M. Electroretinography as a diagnostic test in colour vision deficiencies. Mod Probl Ophthalmol 1978; 19:29–32.
138. Cohen GH, Saini VD. The human pupil response as an objective determination of colour vision deficiency. Med Probl Ophthalmol 1978; 19:197–200.
139. Wright WD. The characteristic of tritanopia. J Opt Soc Am 1952; 42:509–521.
140. Pokorny J, Smith VC, Verriest G, Pinckers AJLG. Congenital and Acquired Color Vision Defects. New York: Grune & Stratton 1979.
141. Went LN, Pronk N. The genetics of tritan disturbances. Hum Genet 1985; 69:255–262.
142. Shinzato K, Yokoyama M, Uji Y, Ichikawa H. The electroretinographic characteristics of congenital tritan defects. Doc Ophthalmol 1986; 62:19–24.
143. Frederikens J, Larsson H, Olesen J, Stigsby B. Evaluation of the visual system in multiple sclerosis. II. Color vision. Acta Neurol Scand 1986; 74:203–209.
144. Pearlman AL, Birch J, Meadows JC. Cerebral color blindness: an acquired defect in hue discrimination. Ann Neurol 1979; 5:253–261.
145. Miyake Y, Yagasaki K, Ichikawa H. Differential diagnosis of congenital tritanopia and dominantly inherited juvenile optic atrophy. Arch Ophthalmol 1985; 103:1496–1501.
146. Pinckers A. Color vision and age. Ophthalmologica 1980; 181:23–30.
147. Aronson JK, Ford AR. The use of colour vision measurement in the diagnosis of digoxin toxicity. Q J Med 1980; 49:273–282.
148. Chuman MA, Lesage J. Color vision deficiencies in two cases of digoxin toxicity. Am J Ophthalmol 1985; 100:682–685.
149. Frome FS, Piantanida TP, Kelly DH. Psychophysical evidence for more than two kinds of cone in dichromatic color blindness. Science 1982; 215:417–419.
150. Waaler GHM. The heredity of normal and defective color vision. Acta Ophthalmol 1968; 46:30–40.
151. Purrello M, Nussbaum R, Rinaldi A, et al. Old and new genetics help ordering loci at the telomere of the human X-chromosome long arm. Hum Genet 1984; 65:295–299.

152. Nathans J, Thomas D, Hogness DS. Molecular genetics of human color vision: the genes encoding blue, green and red pigments. Science 1986; 232:193–202.
153. Wissinger B, Sharpe LT. New aspects of an old theme: the genetic basis of human color vision. Am J Hum Genet 1998; 63:1257–1262.
154. Vollrath D, Nathans J, Davis RW. Tandem array of human visual pigment genes at Xq28. Science 1988; 240:1669–1672.
155. Feil R, Aubourg P, Heilig R, Mandel JL. A 195-kb cosmid walk encompassing the human Xq28 color vision pigment genes. Genomics 1990; 6:367–373.
156. Neitz M, Neitz J. Numbers and ratios of visual pigment genes for normal red-green color vision. Science 1995; 267:1013–1016.
157. Hayashi S, Ueyama H, Tanabe S, et al. Number and variations of the red and green visual pigment genes in Japanese men with normal color vision. Jpn J Ophthalmol 2001; 45:60–67.
158. Roorda A, Williams DR. The arrangement of the three cone classes in the living human eye. Nature 1999; 397:520–522.
159. Carroll J, Neitz J, Neitz M. Estimates of L:M cone ratio from ERG flicker photometry and genetics. J Vis 2002; 2:531–542.
160. Bowmaker JK. Evolution of colour vision in vertebrates. Eye 1998; 12:541–547.
161. Nathans J, Piantanida TP, Eddy RL, et al. Molecular genetics of inherited variation in human color vision. Science 1986; 232:203–210.
162. Botstein D. The molecular biology of color vision. Science 1986; 232:142–143.
163. Vollrath D, Nathans J, Davis RW. Tandem array of human visual pigment genes at Xq28. Science 1988; 240:1669–1672.
164. Neitz M, Neitz J. Molecular genetics of color vision and color vision defects. Arch Ophthalmol 2000; 118:691–700.
165. Winderickx J, Sanocki E, Lindsey DT, et al. Defective colour vision associated with a missense mutation in the human green visual pigment gene. Nat Genet 1992; 1:251–256.
166. Yamaguchi T, Motulsky AG, Deeb SS. Visual pigment gene structure and expression in human retinae. Hum Mol Genet 1997; 6:981–990.
167. Ueyama H, Kuwayama S, Imai H, et al. Novel missense mutations in red/green opsin genes in congenital color-vision deficiencies. Biochem Biophys Res Commun 2002; 294:205–209.
168. Ueyama H, Li YH, Fu GL, et al. An A-71C substitution in a green gene at the second position in the red/green visual-pigment gene array is associated with deutan color-vision deficiency. Proc Natl Acad Sci USA 2003; 100:3357–62.
169. Al-Amood WS, Mohammed SO, Al-Sanawi DA, et al. Incidence of colour blindness in Iraqi Arabs. Hum Heredity 1981; 31:122–123.
170. Yasuma T, Tokuda H, Ichikawa H. Abnormalities of cone photopigment in genetic carriers of protanomaly. Arch Ophthalmol 1984; 102:897–900.
171. Fitzgibbon J, Appukuttan B, Gayther S, et al. Localisation of the human blue cone pigment gene to chromosome band 7q31.3-Hum Genet 1994; 93:79–80.

10
Isolated (Non-Syndromic) Retinitis Pigmentosa

INTRODUCTION

In a review of retinitis pigmentosa (RP) written in 1976 (1), Merin and Auerbach mentioned that, in spite of voluminous literature on the subject, many questions about RP remained unanswered. In spite of extensive basic and clinical research, studies of experimentally induced and pathologic specimens of RP, symposia, books and thousands of articles devoted to RP, they remained so through the end of the 1980s (2). The breakthrough came with the advent of molecular genetics, and later, the detection of more and more genes associated with RP-causing mutations. The advance in the understanding of RP-related molecular genetics enabled a better understanding of the pathophysiology, biochemistry, electrophysiology, and clinical classifications of these diseases. In 1992, Humphries et al. marked the identification of two genes associated with RP (3). The discovery that both these genes encode transmembrane proteins of the rod outer segments indicated the important link between genetics, physiology and pathophysiology. In fact, in 1996 when 20 loci for RP were identified with seven genes cloned, Berson (4) considered the understanding of the effect of the mutation on the pathophysiology the most important contribution of the new developments in genetics. By the year 2000, 55 genes had been identified and 118 loci associated with photoreceptor degenerative diseases were known (5). By April 2004, the number of such known genes increased to 70, plus four mutations of the mitochondrial DNA (6). We are now not far from the point of recognizing all genes associated with RP. The 1990s marked the advent of a better understanding of mechanisms of normal function of photoreceptors (7) and of programmed cell death (apoptosis), a major factor in RP (8).

Retinitis pigmentosa has been defined as "a set" of progressive hereditary disorders that diffusely and primarily affect photoreceptor and pigment epithelial function (9). The term *rod-cone dystrophies* is often synonymously used to stress that rod function is affected earlier than cone function in most cases. The term *cone-rod dystrophies* relates to another group of diseases in which cone function is primarily and earlier affected, although in late stages rod function may be affected to such an extent that the disease is indistinguishable from RP. Therefore, the cone-rod dystrophies are dealt with in another chapter.

Because it consists of different genetic entities, RP must be subdivided into two major groups: (i) isolated (non-syndromic) RP, in which the retina and other ocular tissues may show abnormalities in structure and function; and (ii) associated syndromic RP, in which similar ocular findings are associated with extraocular abnormalities, which may involve one other organ or be part of multisystem disease. These two different groups of diseases may be subdivided into various clinical and genetic entities.

I will divide the two groups of RP diseases into two separate chapters. This chapter will discuss the isolated (non-syndromic) RP, while Chapter 11 will deal with syndromic RP. Thirty-four of the 70 genes known to be associated with RP are causative, when mutated, of isolated RP. As previously mentioned, the old dictum of "one gene, one protein, one disease" is no longer valid. Due to the subsequent explosion of research into molecular genetics, it has become clear that previous theories are invalid. It is now known that different mutations of one gene may cause different diseases, as may different combinations of mutated alleles in compound heterozygosity. One disease, in fact, may be caused by various combinations of two or more genes. Novel methods of genetic transmission, such as digenic or triallelic transmission may be responsible for a disease previously considered to be monogenic. Therefore, genetics cannot be dealt with separately and must be incorporated into the description of entities.

ISOLATED RETINITIS PIGMENTOSA

The term "retinitis pigmentosa" was applied in the 19th century when the now typical pigmentary bone corpuscles were seen in the retina of an affected patient. However, bone corpuscular pigment is a relatively late occurrence, and functional retinal abnormalities occur much earlier than these bone corpuscles. The term "atypical RP" was used for patients who had no pigmentary bone corpuscles in their fundus, but there is little justification to use the term for a disease with dynamic changes and progression in both function and structure.

Description and Clinical Findings

Symptomatology

Night blindness, increasing loss of side vision, and decrease in visual acuity are the three most important symptoms that initially bring the patient to the ophthalmologist. In a prospective study of 500 RP patients, Heckenlively et al. (10) showed that night vision was impaired in 86% of the patients and that the mean age at onset of night blindness was 19 years. However, if cone-rod dystrophies are excluded, then night blindness becomes practically universal in RP, with onset in childhood in some types and later in other types. About one patient out of four was not aware of visual field changes. Interestingly, about one-third of all patients complained of light flashes (10). In a large series of 670 patients, Boughman et al. found the symptom of night blindness in 96.5% and loss of peripheral vision in 94.5% (11).

Functional Abnormalities

Visual acuity, visual fields, color vision, threshold of light sense under photopic and scotopic conditions, and electroretinography (ERG) under different conditions are the standard tests used for RP patients. The loss of visual functions in RP is often strikingly symmetric, with a high degree of interocular congruence in visual acuity, visual field defects, color vision, and threshold profiles (12,13).

Visual acuity: Visual acuity was good in most patients with RP; 55% had vision better than 6/18, and 34% had visual acuity of 6/60 or better (14). Visual acuity was generally worse with advancing age and in certain types of RP, such as the X-linked recessive type (14). Pearlman et al. (15) showed that the average duration of night blindness was 13 years in the group with good visual acuity and 21 years in the group with poor visual acuity. The causes of decreased visual acuity, in order of frequency, were macular disease (by far the most common), cataract, myopia, and glaucoma.

Two studies by Grover et al. (16,17), found that the visual acuity of RP patients was not significantly affected by the disease. 73–75% of patients over the age of 45 had a visual acuity of better than 6/60. More than half saw better or equal to 20/40. The visual acuity of autosomal dominant RP patients was, on average, the best. However, patients with X-linked RP had, on average, the worst visual acuity and those with the autosomal recessive gene had acuity in an intermediate range (16).

Refractive error: Refractive errors are significantly more common in RP than in the general population. The RP patients are more myopic by −2.93 diopters (D) of spherical correction and are more astigmatic than the general population (18). Incidence and degree of myopia are higher in X-linked RP.

Visual fields: Visual fields are abnormal in early stages of the disease. The most common visual field defect is a concentric constriction of the field, with an invasion of the defect onto the inner area. The well-known typical ring scotoma is rare, but a partial annular defect is not uncommon.

The visual field defect increases with time, often to tubular vision or even light perception.

The rate of change of visual fields varies among patients (19). Loss of visual acuity did not correlate with loss of visual fields. In general, the loss of visual fields was generally greater (19). About half of all RP and choroideremia patients demonstrated progression even if the visual field was only 10 degrees in diameter (20). Using the Humphrey automated visual field apparatus, Swanson et al. observed that size V target was more useful in the detection of progression of the disease, while size III was more useful in the detection of any existing abnormality (21). The progression of visual field loss conformed to one of several patterns, but the end stage was in all patients residual tubular central visual field (22). Grover et al. (23) calculated that the average half-life value (indicating loss of half of the existing visual field) was about seven years, varying from about five to six years to about 9–9.5 year.

Color vision: Color vision is usually normal in children with RP, but defects in color vision become increasingly more common with advancing age (1) and with decrease in visual acuity (24). The two typical color vision defects are tritanopia (blue-blindness) and nonspecific (anarchic) (24).

Variability and progression in visual functions: Patients often complain of variability in their vision, both during the day and between different days (10); many express that they have"good days" and"bad days" of seeing. Ross et al. (25) showed that the mean variability in the area of the visual field between two visits or between two examiners testing on the same day is about 5% in normal subjects, but in RP patients, the mean was about three times as much, with a range of variability of 0–50%. With time, there is a general tendency for visual functions to decrease. In a three-year follow-up of 94 patients, Berson et al. (26) found a reduction, but not enough to become statistically significant, of the visual acuity. In contrast, the loss of visual field was significant, with an average of 4.6% of the area lost each year. The relative stability of visual acuity found in this study is probably the result of a different loss of these two functions in RP. Visual fields are progressively and gradually reduced, but, as Bird (27) pointed out, the loss of visual acuity occurs in a stepwise manner. Long periods of stability and arrest are followed by short periods of rapid loss of vision.

Ocular Abnormalities

The physical examination of the eye will reveal whether there are the characteristic abnormalities to diagnose or to suggest the diagnosis of RP.

Fundus: The fundus in more-advanced cases will show the typical triad of scattered pigment in the form of bone corpuscles, attenuated blood vessels, and a waxy pale disk. These advanced findings are usually bilateral and symmetric. In the very early stages, few abnormalities can be detected. Later, three types of fine changes at the level of the retinal pigment epithelium (RPE) can be seen (28) (Fig. 1): whitish spots, areas of reddish change, and areas of depigmentation. The RPE atrophy occurs initially in the postequatorial fundus (27). Later, pigmentary stippling and finally bone spicule pigmentation are seen. Michaelson and Yanco (29) divided the development of retinal pigmentation into five stages: (i) functional disability without fundal changes, (ii) pigmentary stippling, (iii) bone corpuscular pigment in the equatorial zone, (iv) vascular pigmentary sheathing in the midperiphery, and (v) vascular pigmentary sheathing up to the disk. It is now clear that the development of retinal pigmentation is dependent on both age and the genetic type of RP. Typical bone corpuscular pigment is seen more in autosomal dominant RP after the age of 20 (30,31). Bone corpuscular pigment increased in 54% of patients who were followed for three years (26).

Grunwald et al. measured major retinal veins using laser doppler velocimetry and laser monochromatic fundus photography (32). They demonstrated that retinal blood flow is significantly reduced in RP, probably as a result of vascular remodeling in response to reduced metabolic demand. However, in advanced stages, retinal vessels become attenuated together with a significant thinning of the retina.

Macula: Fishman and associates (33,34) drew attention to the high prevalence of macular lesions in RP patients. This reached 63% of patients in one series (34) and 74% in another (35). Cystoid maculopathy was one of the earliest macular changes described (36–38); bull's-eye maculopathy and atrophic maculopathy are the most common (39), but several different macular changes can be found (Table 1). These also include epiretinal membranes (40), which may be quite common and are responsible for the waxy pale color of the disk and exudative maculopathy, the result of the heavy leakage from abnormal retinal vessels (41).

Optical coherence tomography (OCT) may be the most accurate way to detect CME. The resulting findings correlated better than fluorescein angiography with the actual visual acuity of the patient (42). Heckenlively and colleagues (43) found that 90% of patients with both RP and CME manifested antiretinal protein antibody activity, while only 13% of RP patients without CME manifested such activity. Heckenlively considered, CME a possible immune process.

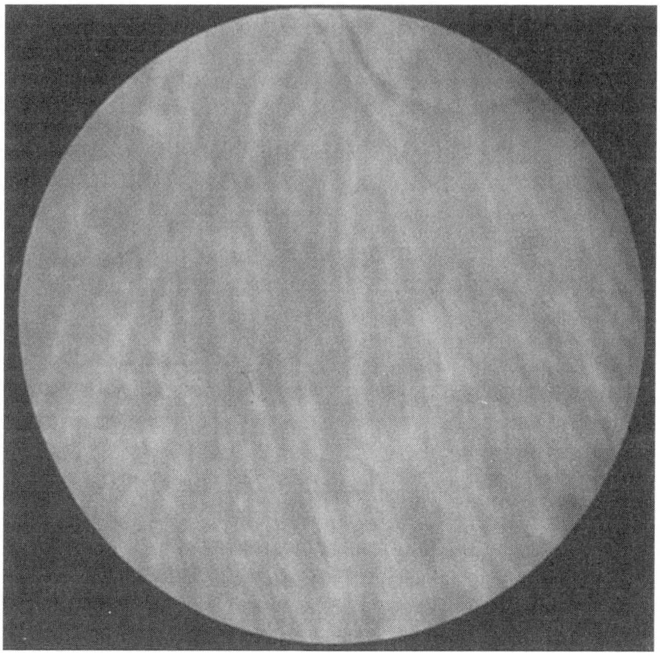

(a)

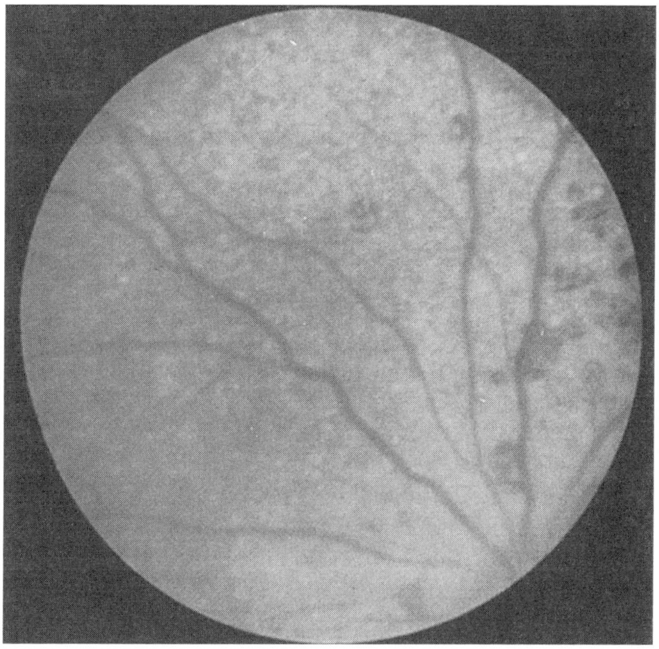

(b)

Figure 1 The different stages of retinal morphologic changes: (a) early changes of small, tiny white-gray dots, and spots of RPE atrophy; (b) salt-and-pepper fundus, RPE atrophy, and pigmentation; and (c) advanced stage with bone corpuscular pigment and attenuated blood vessels.

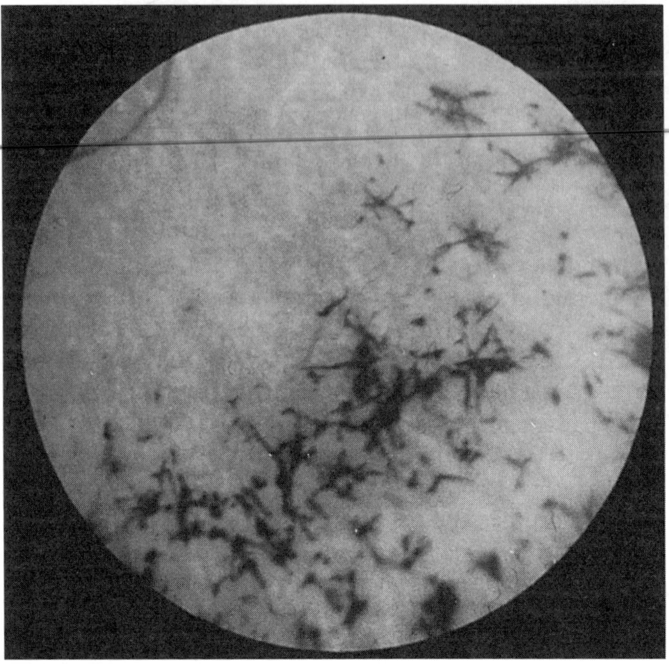

(c)

Figure 1 (*Continued*)

Optic disk: The optic disk may be abnormal in RP patients. In the early stage, the association of drusen of the optic disk and RP is probably not a coincidental occurrence (1). Histopathologic assessment confirms the excrescences to be drusen of the optic nerve (44,45), although the possible association of RP with hamartomas of the optic nervehead, in addition to drusen, was not ruled out (46,47). In advanced stages, the waxy pale disk may be the result of an epiretinal membrane covering the retina and the optic disk (48), combined with a loss of axons of the nerve fiber layer of the retina (49). The epiretinal membrane is a thin layer of fibrous astrocytes, with a thickness of up to 25 μm (48). The loss of the nerve fiber layer could be a result of transsynaptic degeneration or a primary disease of retinal cells, other than the photoreceptors (49).

Table 1 Macular Changes in RP

Maculopathy	Fluorescein angiography	Remarks
Atrophic	Window defects or typical bull's-eye	Most common maculopathy
Cystoid	Faint localized hyperfluorescence	
Cystoid edema	Multiple perifoveal spots of leakage	Leaking perifoveal capillaries
Preretinal gliosis	Traction on perifoveal vessels	May be very common
Exudative	Severe leakage	Rare

The incidence of optic nerve drusen is fairly equal in the three major types of isolated RP with an overall average 9.2% (50). The one exception seems to be RP with PPRPE (Retinitis pigmentosa with preserved para-arteriolar RPE): a strange, severe and rare disease in which the incidence of drusen is very high (50).

Retinal edema and Coats' disease: Retinal edema by biomicroscopy, with extensive leakage in the retina by fluorescein angiography, are not infrequently found in RP patients. It has no relation to any specific type of RP, and it was considered by Spalton et al. as a general response to actively degenerating photoreceptors (51). It is uncertain whether or not the retinal teleangiectasis, neovascularization, and Coats' disease are related to the same pathogenic mechanism. Coats' disease was repeatedly reported as being associated with RP (1,52–56). In fact, RP is the only disease in which Coats' disease is found both as a bilateral lesion without favoring either sex. Coats' disease was described in a brother and sister—two of three siblings (57). The usual retinal teleangiectasis found with Coats' disease in RP patients may be replaced by frank neovascularization on the disk or elsewhere, with recurrent vitreous hemorrhage (58). Treatment by laser may be effective despite absence of retinal ischemia (59). Heavy exudation in exceptional patients with RP may cause loss of vision from an exudative maculopathy (41) or from a frank papilledema (60).

Kim and Kearney described bilateral, exudative retinal telangiectasia (Coats' disease) in a 4-year-old child and claimed that Coats' disease may precede manifest RP (61). Chowers and associates (62), demonstrated a high frequency of Fuchs' heterochromic uveitis in patients with RP (62).

Other retinal changes can also be found in RP patients. Pruett (35) found retinal holes or retinal detachment, or both, in seven of 384 patients with RP, but this may be an underestimate. He also pointed out that microaneurysms and peripheral telean giectatic capillaries are not rare (35).

Vitreous abnormalities: Vitreous abnormalities are extremely common in RP and are possibly universal. Pruett (63) classified the vitreous changes into four stages: (i) fine, colorless, dustlike particles; (ii) posterior vitreous detachment; (iii) a matrix of coarse white interconnecting fibers appears on the posterior border of the gel; and (iv) the gel becomes collapsed and greatly reduced. Histologic examination showed the presence in the vitreous of isolated pigment granules, condensed collagen, and broken fibers (35).

Cataract: Cataract occurs frequently in all types of RP. Its usual form is a posterior subcapsular cataract (PSC), but less commonly, a nuclear cataract can be seen Its prevalence was 39% in one series (64), 41% in another (65), and 46% in a third (35), with no significant differences between various RP genetic types. The occurrence is age-related, but in all ages except the very young, cataract is much more common than in the general population. Seventy-four percent of RP patients over 40 years had PSC cataracts, and the youngest RP patient with cataract was 17 years old (64).

Fortuitous associations: It is likely that the association of RP with fundus flavimaculatus (66), myopathy (67), and hemoglobinopathies (52) is coincidental and not a true association. It is not clear whether pregnancy or the use of contraceptive pills have a deleterious effect on RP in women (68). It is also not clear whether RP patients manifest a high association with thyroid disease, as was suggested in one study (69).

Retinitis Pigmentosa Patients and Driving

It is interesting that a follow-up on the driving performance of 42 RP patients did not show any statistically significant difference in the rate of accidents compared with that of other drivers, except in a subgroup of young female RP patients (70). This is in contrast with a study performed on 20,000 volunteers, which showed that persons with visual field defects had a twice "normal" rate of accidents and convictions (71) This difference may be the result of the RP patients' greater awareness of their visual handicap, who consequently drive slower, more carefully, and only during daylight. Persons in the large study suffered from several different diseases and many were unaware of any handicap.

One other study did, however, find more traffic accidents in patients with RP and visual field loss (72). The researchers pointed out that the standard methods of visual field examination for drivers are not suitable for RP patients (73). The perceived difficulty in performing daily activities related to remaining visual acuity and visual fields, but the majority of their patients reported maintained ability to drive (74).

AUTOSOMAL DOMINANT NON-SYNDROMIC RP

Introduction

Retinitis pigmentosa as an isolated disease means that it clinically affects only the eye. Cells, such as ciliated cells outside the eye, may sometimes also be affected. Generally, it can be transmitted by the autosomal dominant (AD), autosomal recessive (AR) or the X-chromosome linked (XL) form. It can also occur in simplex or multiplex form, when a genetic background may not be obvious and defined. More recently the existence of digenic (two genes) and triallelic (three alleles) transmission was confirmed. As previously noted, 34 genes, about half of the known genes causative of RP, are now known to be associated with isolated RP. It is likely that their final number will reach about 50. The enormous number of identified mutations in some genes, such as the rhodopsin gene, where the number exceeds 100, indicate the complexity of the subject. On the one hand, different genes may be associated with RP of similar severity and progression; on the other hand, different mutations of the gene may be causative of RP of different severity.

In the following pages, I will describe the clinical findings and molecular genetics background of the many types of RP. Table 2 lists the clinical entities of siolated R.P.

Autosomal dominant RP (ADRP) is generally considered to be the mildest form; it has a later onset of the major symptoms, with longer preservation of central vision and visual field. However, different studies vary on the estimate of the differences in visual function among the types of RP and are often contradictory. The loss of visual acuity was mildest in ADRP and most extensive in X-linked recessive RP (XLRP) (14). All XLRP patients over 30 years old had a visual acuity of less than 6/60, whereas only one-third of patients with ADRP had such a visual acuity (Fig. 2). The visual field deteriorates later in autosomal dominant forms, compared with the other types of RP (31). Less myopia and more hyperopia are evident in ADRP than in other types (75). Other studies did not find differences in visual function among the different types of RP or in their rate of progression (76,77). Beaty and Boughman (78) were unable to build a representative "model choice" to identify the types of RP.

Mutations in many different genes may cause ADRP (Table 2). To date, at least 13 are identified. Different genes and different mutations within the same gene may or may not result in a somewhat different phenotype as to severity, age of onset and rate of progression. These differences are best perceived in intrafamilial similarities, compared with interfamilial differences or, for that matter, in the comparison of different studies. Such studies were usually performed on a large group of patients with ADRP, which were usually heterogeneous groups, possibly with milder and more severe disease entities mixed together. In a study performed on an isolate of Navajo Indians, Heckenlively et al. (30) identified two types of RP, an autosomal dominant and an autosomal recessive form, seemingly two distinct disease entities. Patients with ADRP had a more typical ophthalmoscopic picture, with pigmentary bone spicules developing with age, and they kept visual functions longer. Legal blindness occurred at 40–55 years of age. In contrast, patients with autosomal recessive RP (ARRP) showed a gray fundus and RPE dropout and developed clumps of pigment only in a very advanced stage. Legal blindness typically occurred at the age of 30 years (30).

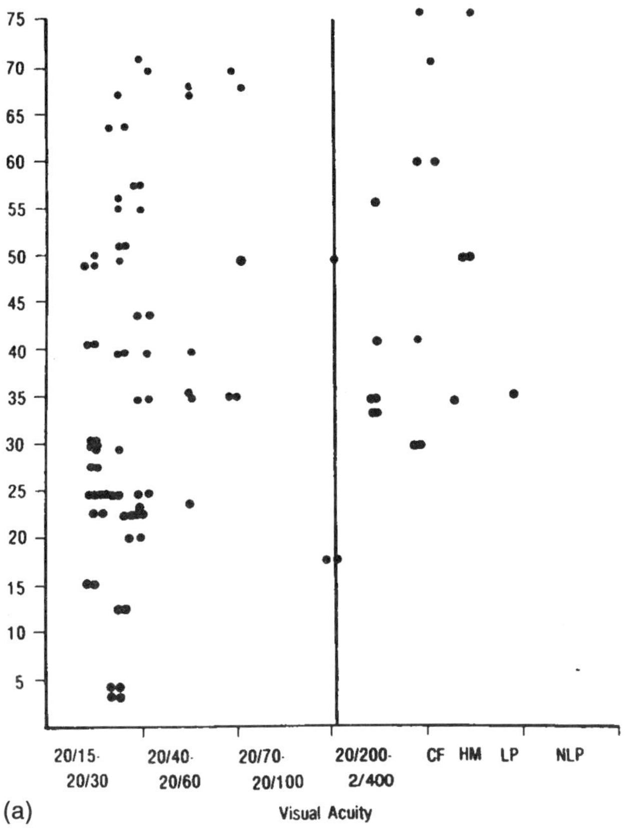

Figure 2 Visual acuity of patients with four types of isolated RP according to their age group: (a) autosomal dominant, (b) autosomal recessive, (c) X-linked recessive, and (d) simplex (sporadic). Note that over the age of 30, about one-third of ADRP patients (a), about one-half of ARRP patients (b), and all XLRP patients (c), had visual acuity of 6/60 (20/200). About one-fourth of simplex cases had poor visual acuity regardless of age (d) (from Ref. 14).

(b)

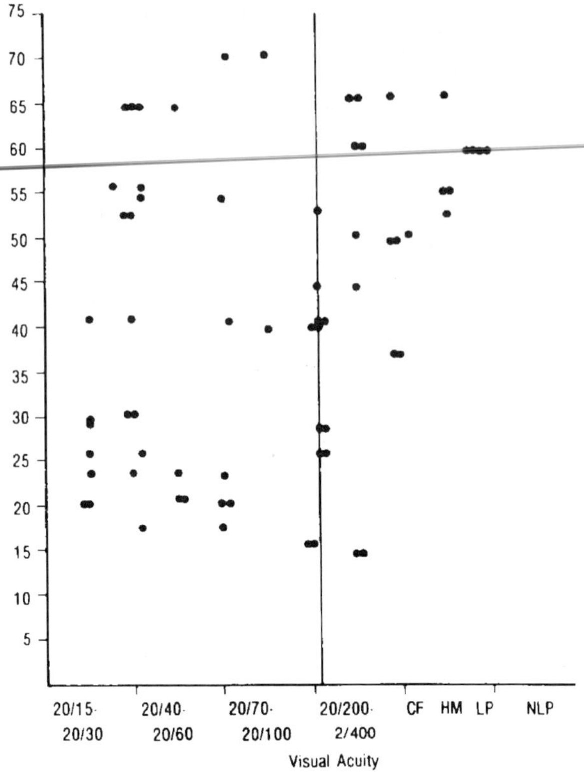

(c)

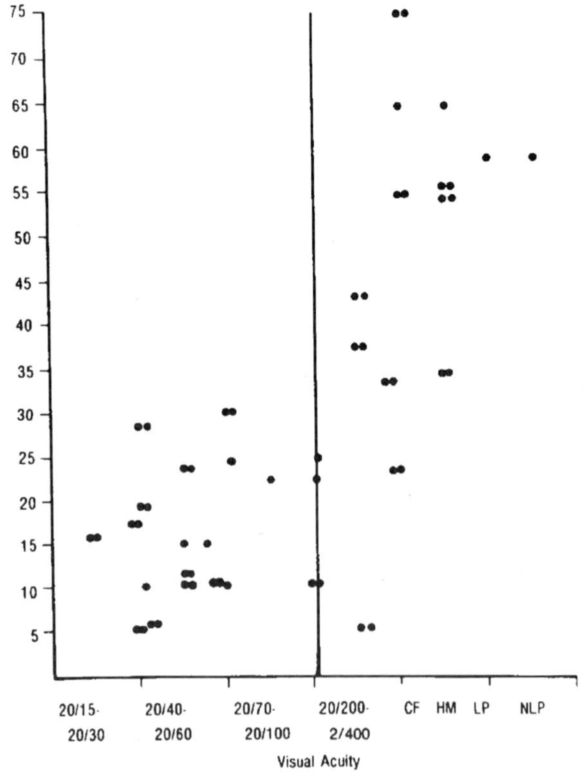

Figure 2 *(Continued)*

Attempts to identify the clinical and genetic entities of ADRP were made by several groups of investigators. Two types were suggested by Massof and Finkelstein (79), Massof et al. (80), Lyness et al. (81), and Kemp et al. (82); three types were suggested in another study by Massoff and Finkelstein (83); and four types were suggested by Fishman et al. (84). These four types ranged from the most severe, type I, in which onset of night blindness was early, visual fields were concentrically lost, and the retina was diffusely affected, to the mildest, type 4, which had only an annular ring scotoma (Table 3). Intrafamilial similarities in all cases support such classification as separate genetic and clinical entities. In the studies supporting two types of ADRP (79–81), there is a diffuse type in which loss of rod sensitivity throughout the visual field is coupled with relative conservation of cone activity. This is distinguished from a regional type in which a patchy loss of both rod and cone function coincide. The rod ERG is extinguished in the first type, but is detectable in the second type (79,81). This second type is probably similar to types 3 and 4 of Fishman's classification (84) and to the "delimited RP" identified by Marmor (77) in a subgroup of his patients. In this subgroup, closest to type 4 of Fishman's classification, night blindness occurs late, and visual functions decrease very slowly;

(d)

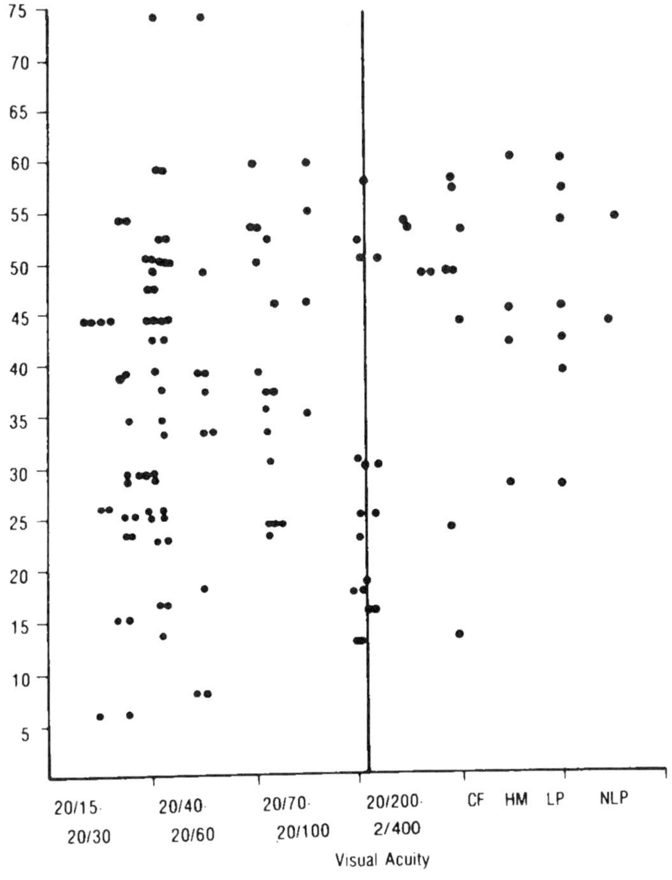

Figure 2 *(Continued)*

Table 2 Classification of Isolated RP into Clinical Entities

Classification	Clinical Characteristics	Inheritance
ADRP, severe and diffuse	Severe disease; rapid progression; legal blindness in second and third decades	AD
ADRP, moderate and regionalized	Lower retina more affected; slow progression	AD
ADRP, mild	Mild disease; slow or no progression; partial annular scotoma	AD
ADRP with reduced penetrance	Mild to moderate disease; slow progression	AD
Sector RP	One or two quadrants affected, usually stable, center not affected	AD
Sector RP with reduced Penetrance	Mild sector disease	AD
Sector RP with papilledema	Mild sector disease; optic nerve disease may be serious; hearing defect present	AD
Sector RP with optic atrophy	Mild sector disease; optic nerve disease may be serious	AD
ARRP, severe form	Severe disease, rapid progression; legal blindness in second and third decades	AR
ARRP, moderate form	Moderate disease, slower progression than in ARRP, severe form	AR
ARRP, mild form	Onset in old age; mild disease	AR
ARRP, early onset	Severe early onset; rapidly progressive; early legal blindness	AR
ARRP with preserved para-arteriolar RPE	Severe; rapidly progressive; early legal blindness	AR
Retinitis punctata albescens	Possibly a separate form of severe disease; could be the same entity as ARRP, severe form	AR
XLRP type 1	Severe disease; locus at Xp11	XL
XLRP type 2	Severe disease, metallic sheen reflex in fundus; locus at Xp21	XL
Leber amaurosis type 1	Congenital blindness or severe visual impairment	AR
Leber amaurosis type 2	Clinically similar to type 1, but caused by a different gene	AR

AD, autosomal dominant; AR, autosomal recessive; XL, X chromosomal-linked recessive.

gradually, rod and cone functions are detectable by ERG, and the flicker b-wave implicit time is normal.

Dominant retinitis pigmentosa, with reduced penetrance, was the name given by Berson et al. (85) to a familial occurrence of ADRP with skipped individuals, meaning that persons obviously carrying the gene did not show the disease. The existence of reduced penetrance in some families with ADRP was confirmed in a large study by Jay (86). In her series, 11.5% of families with autosomal dominant RP had reduced penetrance. Such families carry a different autosomal dominant gene. It is my impression that the disease is milder in these families, with later onset of symptoms and slower progression.

Table 3 Clinical and Genetic Types of ADRP

	Type 1	Type 2	Type 3	Type 4
Name[a]	Diffuse	Regionalized	Sectorial	Annular
Number of patients affected	23/80	46/80	10/80	5/80
Visual acuity < 6/60	44	11	5	
Visual fields	Concentric loss	Superior field	Superior field	Ring scotoma
ERG, rod amplitudes	Nondetectable	Nondetectable or minimal	Normal or subnormal	Normal or subnormal
ERG, cone amplitudes	Nondetectable	Normal or subnormal	Normal or subnormal	Normal or subnormal
ERG, cone implicit time	—	Prolonged	Normal	Normal

[a]Name indicates area of fundus affected by pigmentary clumping, but may conveniently serve as the name of the condition.
Source: Based on Ref. 84.

Molecular genetics of ADRP

Linkage studies in the 1980s and cloning of genes of the 1990s are the basis for the present knowledge of the molecular genetics of ADRP.

The suggestion by Botstein et al. in 1980 (87) to use restriction fragment length polymorphisms (RFLPs) to construct a genetic map in humans revolutionized the techniques for gene assignment.

Linkage studies of a large family with ADRP implied that the gene may be linked to the *Rh* locus, known to be located on the short arm of chromosome 1, with a lod score of 2.13 (suggestive) (88), but these studies were not confirmed (89). Possibly, different autosomal dominant genes were examined in these two separate studies. In a study performed on a large Irish family with ADRP, the authors concluded that the gene is most probably not located on the short arm of chromosome 1 (90).

The Rhodopsin (RHO) Gene

The isolation of the gene encoding human rhodopsin chromosome 3 has been known for several years (91–93). Later, a gene associated with one type of ADRP was also assigned to the long arm of chromosome 3 (94,95). In 1990, Dryja and associates (96) examined 148 unrelated patients with ADRP, searching for abnormalities in the rhodopsin gene and found 17 of them abnormal. In these patients, the mutant gene had a C→A base change in codon 23, corresponding to a proline→histidine substitution. Proline is an essential amino acid in all known rhodopsins and cone opsins, and its absence from the protein may cause the malfunction.

The same group of investigators identified four disease-bearing mutations on the rhodopsin gene. They also found that the first identified mutation, Pro23His, is by far the most common, comprising 12% of all ADRP patients thus far examined (97). Humphries et al. (98) pointed out that rhodopsin mutations were not found in their large Irish family with ADRP and stressed the existence of heterogeneity. The discovery of genetic heterogeneity including allelic heterogeneity became one of the most important and fundamental principles of molecular genetics of inherited eye disease.

The locus of the rhodopsin gene RHO was mapped to chromosome 3q22.1 (the long arm of chromosome 3). Disease-bearing mutations have been found in 30–40% of North American ADRP patients (6), far more than any other ADRP associated gene. More and more mutations have been subsequently identified. In 1991, five were known (99). By 1993, 32 were identified (100), 70 by 1996 (4), and more than 100 by 2004. Several of the mutations were noticeably characteristic. The rhodopsin gene includes five exons and encompasses seven Kb of DNA. Disease-bearing mutations are mostly missense mutations (100) with a minority of premature frame shift terminations. These last generally carry a more severe disease, but not always. In some cases, as with Glu344 stop mutation, symptomatology is minimal (99,101). Arg135Leu and Arg135Trp cause loss of rod function and variable reduction in cone function (99). Pro347Leu causes diffuse functional loss of variable severity (101). Four mutations at codon 347, Pro347Ala, Prp347Glu, Pro347Leu and Pro347Lys, produce a more severe phenotype than mutations at codon 23, Pro23Ala and Pro23-His (102). Table 4 outlines a list of mutations in the RHO gene and their resulting ADRP disease.

In some cases, a mutation in the RHO gene is associated with a distinct different phenotype than ADRP, such as retinitis punctata albescens, autosomal recessive RP, congenital stationary night blindness (CSNB) and sector RP (103–105).These will be discussed under the appropriate headings.

Mutations in the RHO gene cause RP because an abnormal opsin protein is produced. Some mutated opsin proteins cause totally misfolded, non-retinal binding opsin (4). Berson suggested that disk membranes with misfolded opsin are less compact, shed more easily and are slow to renew (4). Eighty percent of the protein of the rod outer segment is in form of rhodopsin and 10^8 molecules per rod photoreceptor are rhodopsin (7). As a rule, severity of RHO-associated ADRP depends on the position of the mutation within the rhodopsin molecule (106). Intradisc mutations, such as at codon 23, are the mildest, while cytoplasmic domains and retinol binding sites such as region flanking codon 135 are very severe (106). A mutation

Table 4 Mutations in RHO Gene and Severity of ADRP

Benign	Moderately benign	Moderately severe	Severe
Asn15Ser	Pro23His	Glu344ter (484)	Leu40Arg
Thr17Met (487)	FGlu64Ter (484)	T341–343del	Asp190Tyr
	Gly188Arg		Cys187Tyr (107)
Thr58Arg	Intr4 splice site ins (483,484)		Arg135Leu
Gly106Arg	255–6 36pdel		Arg135Trp (482)
Gly182Ser	Pro23Ala (106)		Lys296Glu
Asp190Asn	Cys110Tyr (486)		Val345Met
Pro267Leu			Val345Leu
			Pro347Leu
			Pro347Arg
			Pro347Ser
			Ter349Glu (485)

After Pannarale et al. (482).

at codon 187 disrupts a disulfide bond essential to normal rhodopsin function and results, therefore, in an early and severe retinal dysfunction (107).

The RDS/Peripherin

The second gene identified in association with ADRP, the RDS/peripherin gene, was detected on the short arm of chromosome 6, near the major histocompatibility locus (3,108,109). Mutations on the RDS /peripherin gene were second in frequency to the rhodopsin gene in causing RP. The two seem responsible for about a third of all ADRP cases (103). The term RDS comes from *retinal dystrophy slow* of mice and the term *peripherin* from the mutated protein in mice. The variability of resulting phenotypes from RDS/peripherin mutations is great (110). The ADRP may be milder, or of late onset with atrophic maculopathy (111) or peripheral retinal atrophy (112). Such a mild phenotype was described in a missense mutation (Pro216Ser) (111) and in a nonsense mutation (Arg46ter) (112).

By 1996, 43 different mutations had been reported (113), and 70 mutations were identified by 1993 (114). These may be associated with ADRP, progressive vascular dystrophy, pattern vascular dystrophy (113) and other entities. Retinitis punctata albescens, a more severe RP, was found to be associated with a frameshift mutation and premature termination at codon 43, caused by a 2-bp deletion in codon 25 (115). Subretinal, yellowish vascular deposits evolving into geographic atrophy and retinal hyper- and hypopigmentation are the phenotype of a nonsense mutation at codon 169 (116). Mutations of RDS/peripherin are responsible for 18% of adult-onset vitelliform macular dystrophy (AVMD) (117). Premature termination at codon 38 of RDS/peripherin associated with adult onset foveomacular dystrophy in four generations of a large family (118). Choroidal neovascularization and geographic atrophy were common in this family. Another macular dystrophy, autosomal dominant areolar choroidal dystrophy, was described with a missense mutation Arg195Leu. Impaired visual acuity occurred in the fifth decade of life (116).

The variability of phenotype associated with RDS/peripherin mutations is typical of this gene. It is responsible for 3–8% of all ADRP, but also for 7–10% of all macular dystrophies and 18% of all AVMD (114).

Another specific feature of the RDS/peripherin gene is the involvement in digenic inheritance. Kajiwara, Berson et al. (114) and Dryja et al. (117) pointed out that genes involved in polygenic disease are less recognized than genes involved in monogenic disease. They identified digenic inheritance in three families. Only members with heterozygotic mutations in both RDS/peripherin and ROM1 genes were affected by RP. In all families, RDS mutation Leu185Pro and one of several ROM1 mutations resulted in digenic inheritance of RP (120).

Other ADRP Genes

Table 5 describes, in short, genes confirmed to be associated with ADRP. The frequency of each varies among different populations and the genes are listed according to their roughly estimated universal frequency.

The rhodopsin gene is the most common RP-causative gene in North America, the United Kingdom (121) and in many other populations. Mutations in the RDS/peripherin gene follow in frequency, but many of these mutations are not RP-associated. RP11 was mapped to chromosome 19q13.4 in 1994 (322). A British study (121) found RP11 to be quite common (21%) in association with ADRP. The

Table 5 Genes and Loci Associated with ADRP

	Locus	Gene	Chromosome location	Remarks
1	RP4	RHO Rhodopsin	3q22.1 3q21-q24	30–40% of all ADRP
2	RP7	RDS/peripherin (retinal degeneration slow)	6p21.2	1. Large variability in phenotype 2. Digenic inheritance with ROM1 in some cases
3	RP11	PRPF 31 (precursor mRNA-processing factor) 31	19q 13.42	21% of ADRP in UK, variable severity (489,490)
4	RP13	PDRC8 precursor	17p13.3	Variable severity
5	RP17	CA4 Protein carbonic anhydrase type IV	17q22	Variable severity
6	RP9	PIM1-kinase associated protein 1	7p14.3	Variable severity
7	RP10	IMPDH1 (IMP dehydrogenase-like 1)	7q32.1	5–10% of ADRP variable severity
8	RP1	RP1 gene and protein	8q12.1	3–10% of ADRP RP1-photorecepter specific protein localized to connecting cilium variable severity
9	RP27	NRL (neural retina-specific leucine zipper)	14q11.2	NRL interacts with CRX to promote transcription of rhodopsin. 1% of ADRP (491,492)
10	RP30	FSCN2 (retinal fascin homolog 2	17q25	
11		ROM1 (rod outer segment protein 1)	11q12.3	Causes RP by digenic inheritance with RDS/peripherin
12	RP18	HPRP3 (precursor mRNA-processing factor 3)	1q21.2	

Based on RetNet (6), OMIM (488) and authors mentioned in text.

resulting disease is variable in expressivity and penetrance (122). It was suggested that penetrance and nonpenetrance depends on the haplotype inherited from the noncarrier parent (121). The carrier status was confirmed by molecular studies. The authors concluded that their results confirm the existence of a modifier locus near the RP11 locus (121).

The locus for RP13 was mapped to chromosome 17p in a large South African family (123). The gene recoverin was suggested as being implicated in the pathogenesis of ADRP (124) but another study could not confirm such association (123). McKie et al. (125) identified seven different missense mutations in the splicing factor PRPC8 in families diagnosed as RP13.

The locus for RP 17 was mapped to the long arm of chromosome 17 in a large South African family of German origin (126). It was later located on chromosome 17q22 (127) and recently the RP17-associated gene was identified by detection of the disease-bearing mutations as the gene encoding CA4, carbonic anhydrase IV protein (128). The phenotype is variable. Onset may be late, and in the third decade of life visual acuity ranges from 20/20 to 20/200, while the visual field may manifest a ring scotoma or be reduced to tubular vision (126,127). The identified protein is highly expressed in choriocapillaris. Rebello et al. (128) suggested that the high level of mutant protein expressed in the choriocapillaris leads to apoptosis of the photoreceptors. RP9 maps to chromosome 7p14.3 (129–131). Clinically, it is marked by great variability in expressivity, ranging from minimally affected to normal ERG and psychophysics, through moderate affection, to severely affected with extinguished ERG (130). More recently, Keen et al. (131) identified two disease-bearing missense mutations in the gene encoding Pim-1 kinase protein.

Phenotype variability is also characteristic of RP10, a type of ADRP found in American and Spanish families and localized at chromosome 7q32.1. While in the Spanish family the disease was severe, the ERG extinguished, and onset was of early age (132), in the American family the disease was mild with late onset (133). Recently the gene encoding inosine monophosphate dehydrogenase 1 was implicated in RP10, by comparative microarray analysis with mice (134) and by identifying RP-bearing mutations (135).

A locus for RP was mapped by linkage analysis to the pericentric region of human chromosome 8 as early as 1991 and termed RP1 (136). Pierce et al. (137) reported the identification of different mutations in a gene encoding an oxygen-regulated photoreceptor protein of unknown function. In all of four families the mutation led to frameshift and premature termination. Jacobson et al. (138) found an Arg677ter mutation in 13 of 17 families with RP1. The clinical expression of the disease was extremely variable, ranging from minimal symptoms and findings to severe retina-wide degeneration. The authors (138) concluded that in RP1 a modifier gene or environmental factors may play a role.

The chromosomal location and the causative gene for locus RP27 were determined in 1999 (139). The gene NRL encodes a basic motif - leucine zipper DNA-binding protein, that is expressed specifically in the retina (139). The locus was mapped to chromosome 14q11.2. Initially, only one mutation, Ser50Thr in exon 2 (of the three exons of the gene), was identified (140). Later, additional missense mutations were identified (141). The resulting retinitis pigmentosa is moderate to severe.

RP30 was first described in Japanese patients with ADRP and was mapped to chromosome 17q25. The four described Japanese families all had one mutation, 208del6 in FSCN2, the retinal fascin gene.

RP6 (retinitis pigmentosa of a rather mild variety) was described as linked to the short arm of chromosome 6 (142). As the authors pointed out, a tight linkage to the RDS gene exists and it is most likely that one and the same gene is involved in RP6 and RP7.

Locus RP18 was the ninth locus for ADRP. It was mapped to chromosome 1q21.2 by linkage analysis (143) and later by refinement. RP-bearing mutations were identified in 2002 in the HPRP3 gene (144). This turned out to be the third pre-mRNA splicing factor gene associated with RP, stressing the importance of photoreceptor degeneration due to defective splicing processes (144).

The ROM1 gene was mapped to human chromosome 11q13 (145). It encodes a retinal integral membrane protein that, together with the product of DRS/peripherin gene, defines a photoreceptor specific protein family. The gene was cloned as early as 1993 (146). Mutation analysis identified mutations potentially causing RP.

However it is more likely, as outlined above, that ROM1 mutations play a role in causing RP only by digenic inheritance together with RDS/peripherin gene mutations (147,148).

AUTOSOMAL DOMINANT SECTOR RETINITIS PIGMENTOSA

Sector RP is transmitted in an autosomal dominant manner, but it is likely that more than one gene is involved. The typical sector RP was described by Bietti (149) and, then, extensively reviewed by Bisantis (150) and again by Omphroy (151). The retina is affected bilaterally and symmetrically in almost all patients, but 15% have monocular involvement, and 7% have an asymmetric involvement (151). Both inferonasal quadrants are affected in about 50% of all patients, the inferonasal quadnant in 20%, and the two nasal quadrants, the superotemporal quadrant, or both superior quadrants in the rest of the patients (151). The affected retina manifests ophthalmoscopic signs of typical RP with diffuse atrophy of RPE, thinning of the retina, attenuation of blood vessels, and pigmentary clumping in the form of bone corpuscles or blots. Visual acuity is usually good, and the visual field is reduced, according to the affected area. Electroretinographic results reflect the size of the affected area.

Several subtypes of sector RP can be distinguished. Some of the patients of this group may belong to the ADRP described by Fishman et al. as type 3 (84). "Atypical sector pigmentary dystrophy" was the name given to a sector RP inherited by an autosomal dominant gene with reduced penetrance (152). Sector retinitis pigmentosa with chronic disk edema was described in a large family by Cope et al. (153). Patients with this entity may show chronic papilledema, with sector RP in childhood and reduction in visual acuity much later in life (153,154). A histopathologic study showed loss of photoreceptors, degenerated RPE and abnormal choriocapillaris in the affected quadrant, and absence of myelin in the optic nerve (154). All patients had elevated serum vitamin A levels and a depressed serum carotene concentration. All had a hearing defect (153).

We have also seen two families with sector RP and partial or complete optic atrophy (155). Patients were asymptomatic until the fifth or sixth decade of life, when visual functions failed as a result of the optic atrophy. Serum vitamin A levels were normal, and there was no hearing defect. Disk edema was not present in any stage. Therefore, it seems that this entity is different from the one described by Cope et al. (153).

Souied et al. (100) described a missense mutation within codon 15 of exon 1 of the RHO gene. This Ser15Asp mutation alters a glycolysation site in the intradiscal portion of the rhodopsin gene and results in sectorial RP that affects the inferior quadrants of the retina.

AUTOSOMAL RECESSIVE RETINITIS PIGMENTOSA

Description

Autosomal recessive RP (ARRP) is the most common form of isolated RP in some populations, whereas it is uncommon in others. The differences in ophthalmoscopic manifestations between ARRP and ADRP, as seen in the Navajo Indians (30), are probably a reflection of the typical differences of the two groups. In the typical case of ARRP, white-grayish dots diffusely seen initially in the fundus turn into a grayish fundus with a thin retina, a salt-and-pepper fundus (scattered dots of fine pigment and white-gray spots), atrophic RPE, and attenuated blood vessels. Bone corpuscular pigment occurs late and increases much slower than in ADRP. Loss of visual functions is faster than in ADRP (31) and slower than in XLRP (14); 78% have an undetectable ERG, compared with 60% of ADRP patients (31).

The smaller number of affected members in each family does not allow the same clinical investigation to recognize subtypes as is performed in ADRP. However, the existence of different subtypes is suggested by the variable severity of the disease in different isolates and populations. In addition, patients with ARRP show a higher intrafamilial correlation and a higher variability of their clinical progression and prognosis than do patients with ADRP (156).

Some clinical entities can be separated from the group. An autosomal recessive severe RP of early onset was described as mimicking Leber's congenital amaurosis (157). Preserved para-arteriolar retinal pigment epithelium RP is an aggressive and severe autosomal recessive form of RP described by Heckenlively (2,158). The disease starts in childhood and, characteristically, patients are hypermetropic (in contrast with the usual myopia in RP) and have preserved RPE along the retinal arterioles. On the other end, a mild form of ARRP, with onset of symptoms and signs in older age, was described by Grondahl (159).

"Retinitis punctata albescens" was the name given to an autosomal recessive condition that showed the typical functional abnormalities of RP, but in which no pigmentary bone corpuscles were seen ophthalmoscopically. Instead, whitish or yellow-white stippling of the retina was found, and the differential diagnosis with that of the stationary condition of night blindness with fundus albipunctatus should be made (160). With time, however, the spots fade and disappear, and RPE atrophy and retinal pigmentary changes develop (161). We have seen two sisters, the younger with a retinitis punctata albescens, the older with a typical RP. Nevertheless, the manifestation of retinitis punctata albescens may indicate a separate familial form of ARRP that is progressive. A similar picture of the fundus is described in vitamin A deficiency (162).

Molecular Genetics of ARRP

More genes and loci are associated with autosomal recessive RP than with ADRP. In addition, many of the mutations are family specific. In some families, the affected members are homozygotic for the mutated gene. In the majority, however, compound heterozygosity is the rule.

The TULP1 Gene and RP14

This locus was one of the first autosomal recessive loci to be recognized. It was identified on chromosome 6p, distinct and 20 cM telomeric from the RDS/peripherin gene (163). The locus named RP14 was mapped to chromosome 6p21.3 (164) then later refined to 6p21.31. The gene TULP1 encoding tubby-like protein 1 was also mapped to this area. In 1998, both missense and splice-site mutations were identified in TULP1 gene, associated with ARRP (164,165). The gene has 15 coding exons. The protein has an unknown function and is expressed exclusively in the retinal photoreceptors, predominantly in the inner segments (165,166). The defect in ULP 1(-/-) mice resides in the transport of opsins to the outer segment and it may well be the same in humans. By EM, massive accumulation of extracellular vesicles was seen in Tulp1 (-/-) mice in the interphotoreceptor matrix (166). RP14 is a severe phenotype with early onset and severe retinal degeneration involving both macular and peripheral cones and rods (167). Heretozygotes are normal but homozygotes have nystagmus (visual acuity of 20/200 or less), bull's eye maculopathy, extinguished ERG and progressive, rapid worsening of the visual fields (167).

The CRB1 Gene and RP12

RP12 is the locus of a severe retinitis pigmentosa morphologically manifesting RP with preserved para-arteriolar RPE. The disease onset is early in life. Maculopathy, visual field defects, and extinguished ERG are found in all patients (168). Hypermetropia was found in 96% of patients, optic nerve drusen in 38%, vascular sheathing in 46%, and yellow deposits in posterior pole in 38% (168). RP12 was assigned to chromosome1q31-q32.1 (169), and later refined to chromosome 1q31.3 (6). The gene was cloned and identified as CRB1 for crumbs homolog 1, as the protein is homologous to *Drosophila melanogaster* protein crumbs (170). CRB1 encodes an extracellular protein.

The RLBP1 Gene

RLBP1 is the gene encoding cellular retinalaldehyde-binding protein (CRALB) and was mapped to chromosome 15q26.1. It consists of eight exons with exons 1, 2, and 8 containing untranslated regions (171). The CRALBP protein is abundant in the RPE and in Muller cells, but not in photoreceptors. It normally carries 11-cis-retinol and 11-cis-retinaldehyde. The mutated protein cannot bind these products. Retinal degeneration occurs, therefore, from an RPE malfunction (171).

Most disease-bearing mutations are missense mutations, but frameshift, splice site mutations, and small deletions were also reported (171–173). Bothnia dystrophy, a unique RLBP1-associated phenotype seems to be a "relative" of retinitis punctata albescens (174).

The GMP Gated Channel Genes

Mutations in the gene encoding the alpha-subunit of the rod cGMP-gated channel are associated with ARRP (175). This protein participates in the rod phototransduction cascade. Five sequence variants were identified in four unrelated families with ARRP, including two missense, two nonsense mutations and one deletion truncating the last 32 amino acids. The gene CNGA1 was mapped to chromosome 4p12 (6).

The beta subunit of rod cGMP-gated channel is also associated with ARRP. The gene CNGB1 (cyclic nucleotide gated channel beta 1) was mapped to chromosome 16q13. Mutations causing severe retinitis pigmentosa were identified in a French family (176).

The cGMP-Phosphodiesterase Genes

Huang et al. (177) identified mutations leading to ARRP in PDEA, the gene encoding alpha subunit of cGMP-phosphodiesterase. The gene symbol was later changed to PDE6A. The gene PDE6A consists of 22 exons, spanning approximately 45–50 kb, on chromosome 5q33.1. The described mutations were all missense mutations (177). Mutated PDE6A gene accounts for about 3–4% of North American ARRP (178).

The beta subunit of cGMP-phosphodiesterase is required together with the alpha subunit for full phosphodiesterase activity. Mutations in the gene PDE6B, which encodes the beta subunit of rod cGMP phosphodiesterase, were found to be associated with ARRP (179) and sometimes with congenital stationary night blindness (autosomal dominant type). McLaughlin et al. (180) estimated that PDE6B gene mutations are responsible for about 4% of all ARRP in North America. The locus was mapped to chromosome 4p16.3.

The cyclic guanosine monophosphate (cGMP) phosphodiesterase enzymes are known to be involved in similar retinal degenerations in the mouse and in the Irish Setter dog (180).

Genes, whose products are implicated in the rod phototransduction cascade, may, when mutated, result in retinitis pigmentosa. These genes include rhodopsin, rod cGMP-gated cation channel alpha subunit, and both alpha and beta subunits of cGMP phosphodiesterase.

The gamma-subunit of rod cGM seems not to be involved in human retinitis pigmentosa (181) while in the mouse it may, when mutated, cause disease (182).

The Rhodopsin Gene

RHO, the gene encoding opsin 2, rod opsin, is implicated with a high proportion of ADRP cases (30–40% in North America). It is associated with ARRP in relatively uncommon cases. The described mutations are nonsense mutations (183) or missense mutations (184).

The ABCA4 Gene

Generally, ABCA4 gene mutations lead, when disease-associated, to Stargardt disease. In some cases, however, mutations in the ABCA4 gene, mapped to chromosome 1p22.1, lead to ARRP (185,186). The symbol of RP19 was given to this type of retinitis pigmentosa. Different members of the same family may be affected by Stargardt disease or by autosomal recessive RP. Frameshift mutations seem to cause ARRP.

The RPE65 Gene

The RPE65 gene encodes a 61-kDa protein that is RPE-tissue specific. The open reading frame encodes a 533 amino acid protein that contains 14 exons interrupted by 15 introns (187). It was mapped to chromosome 1p31.2. The protein may play a role in vitamin A metabolism through binding with both serum retinal-binding protein and with RPE-specific 11-cis retinal dehydrogenase (188). RPE65 protein is essential in the production of 11-cis vitamin A.

Mutations in the RPE65 gene were implicated in autosomal recessive RP (188–191). Mutations in RPE65 account for about 2% of ARRP and also for about 16% of Leber congenital amaurosis (LCA) (189). The ARRP, sometimes referred to as RP20, causes severe visual compromise with loss of rod and cone ERG before age 5. Blindness occurs by the second or third decade of life (191).

RP20 is one of the few examples in which photoreceptor degeneration stems from an RPE disease. In mice that are Rpe65-deficient, rod function is abolished after over-accumulation of all-trans-retinyl esters in the RPE took place. At the same time, 11-cis-retinyl esters are absent, not produced in the RPE (192).

Table 6 Genes and Loci associated with ARRP

	Locus/ Symbol	Gene	Chromosomal location	Remarks
1	RP14	TULP1 (tubby-like protein)	6p21.31	Early onset and severe disease
2	RP12	CRB1	1q31.3	Severe disease, preserved para-arterial RPE
3	RLBP1-assoc. RP	CRALBP (cellular-retinal aldehyde binding protein)	15q26.1	Retinitis punctata albescens
4	–	CNGA1 (cGMP-gated channel, sub alpha)	4p12	
5	–	CNGB1 (cGMP-gated channel, sub beta)	16q13	
6	–	PDEGA (cGMP-phosphodiesterase sub alpha)	5q33.1	3–4% of all North American ARRP
7	–	PDEGB (cGMP-phosphodiesterase sub beta)	4p16.3	4% of ARRP may cause ADCSNB
8	RP4/RP5	RHO (rhodopsin gene)	3q22.1	Uncommon ARRP associated with RHO mutations
9	RP19	ABCA4	1p22.1	Uncommon cases of ARRP associated with Stargardt disease gene
10	RP20	RPE65	1p31.2	Associated with 2% of ARRP
11	–	NR2E3 (nuclear receptor gene)	15q23	Implicated in crypto-Jews of Portugal
12	RP25	–	6cen-q15	10–20% of Spanish ARRP. Also Pakistani
13	RP29	–	4q32-q34	One Pakistani family
14	RP26	CERKL (ceramide kinase)	2q31.2-q32.3	Increased severity; later apoptosis
15	BCD	CYP4V2	4q35.2	Bietti corneo-retinal dystrophy
16	–	MERTK (tyrosine kinase)	2q13	Defective RPE function
17	–	LRAT (lecithin retinol acyltransferate)	4q32.1	Defective RPE function
18	–	RGR (RPE-G protein receptor)	10q23.1	Defective RPE function
19	–	RBP4 (retinol-binding protein 4)	10q23.33	Mild to moderate ARRP
20	RP22	–	16p12.1-p12.3	ARRP linkage in two Indian families (493)
21	RP28	–	2p11-p16	ARRP linkage in one Indian family

The NR2E3 Gene

This gene was formerly named PNR, for photoreceptor-specific nuclear receptor gene. The name was later changed to NR2E3 for *nuclear receptor family 2, group E, member 3*. It was mapped to chromosome 15q23. Mutations in the gene cause Goldmann-Favre syndrome, enhanced S-cone syndrome and clumped pigmentary retinal degeneration will be discussed under syndromic RP.

A missense mutation in the NR2E3 was implicated in ARRP of Crypto-Jews (Marranos), a highly consanguineous, endogamic population living in Portugal (193,194).

RP25

An autosomal recessive retinitis pigmentosa designated as RP25 was found, by linkage and homozygosity mapping, to be located at chromosome 6cen-q15. It is mapped to a region containing GABA receptor but the exact gene was not yet identified (6). Mutations were implicated in ARRP in Spanish (195) and Pakistani (196) families. It was suggested that 10%–20% of Spanish ARRP result from these mutations (195).

RP29

A novel locus for ARRP designated as RP29 was mapped by linkage analysis to chromosome 4q32-q34, in a Pakistani family (197). The RP was severe. After loss of night vision and peripheral visual fields by age of 20 and central vision by 25–30 years, complete blindness occurred between age of 40 and 50 (197).

The CERKL Gene and RP26

The locus of RP26, another autosomal recessive retinitis pigmentosa was mapped to the region of chromosome 2q31-q33 (198). Mapping was refined to chromosome 2q31.2-q32.3 and the gene was cloned by Tuson et al. (199). The gene encodes a ceramide kinase (CERKL) protein. It encompasses 13 exons. In a large family with ARRP, mutations that generate a premature termination codon were identified. The enzyme CK (ceramide kinase) converts sphingolipid ceramide into ceramide-1-phosphate. Both are considered key mediators of neuronal survival and apoptosis. The authors (199) suggested that CK deficiency could shift the relative levels of signaling sphingolipid metabolites and increase sensitivity of photoreceptors to apoptotic stimuli.

Bietti Crystalline Corneoretinal Dystrophy

Bietti dystrophy affects the retina, manifesting retinal degeneration and multiple glistening yellow-white refractive crystalline flecks. Its symptomatology is similar to any other ARRP with progressive reduction in visual fields and night blindness. Areas of blotchy pigment together with multiple fine yellow-white crystalline flecks can be seen in the retina (200). The cornea may be affected by crystalline deposits.

Linkage analysis mapped the locus BCD (for Bietti corneoretinal dystrophy) to chromosome 4q35-qtel (201) and later refined to chromosome 4q35.1 (202). The gene, CYP4V2 (for cytochrome P450, family 4, subfamily V, polypeptide 2), was cloned and BCD-causing mutations were identified. The authors (202) suggested that the gene might have a role in fatty acid and steroid metabolism.

The MERTK Gene and ARRP

The Mertk gene was found to be involved in the widely studied RP of RCS rats in which defective phagocytosis in RPE causes photoreceptor degeneration. Gal et al. (203) described three cases of MERTK, the human ortholog gene, and mutations among 328 samples of DNA of RP patients. The mutation consisted of a premature termination after codon 690, truncating a part of the MERTK protein.

MERTK, for *MER tyrosine kinase protooncogene,* was mapped to chromosome 2q14.1. The MERTK-associated ARRP seems to be another uncommon example of defective RPE causing photoreceptor degeneration.

The LRAT Gene

LRAT encoding lecithin retinol acyltransferase is an important gene for the production of 11-cis vitamin A in the retinal pigment epithelium, where it is derived from all-trans vitamin A (204). The gene was cloned; it consists of three exons and two introns and is rather small (205). It was localized to chromosome 4q31.2. Mutations were detected in three DNA samples out of 267 RP-associated blood samples. The mutations identified were Ser175Arg and 396delAA.

The LRAT-associated ARRP is yet another example of defective RPE and defective 11-cis vitamin A production leading to photoreceptor destruction.

The RGR Gene and ARRP

The human RGR gene (for *RPE-retinal G-protein-coupled receptor*) is a rhodopsin homolog found in RPE cells and Muller cells. Unlike rhodopsin, it binds all-trans retinal, on the way to converting it into11-cis retinal (206,207). The locus was mapped to chromosome 10q23.1. At least three different mutations were associated with ARRP of early onset and severe phenotype (207).

The RBP4 Gene

RBP4, a gene encoding retinol-binding protein was localized to chromosome 10q23.33. A family with a fundus disease manifesting RPE atrophy, reduced visual acuity, poor night vision, reduced rod and cone ERG (208), probably represent a mild to moderate ARRP. The affected members had a total absence of retinol binding protein in serum.

Other Genes and Loci

Mutations in the arrestin gene may cause Oguchi disease. It was suggested that in some cases mutations in this gene may cause ARRP (209), but such claims were not confirmed (210). RP28 was a locus for ARRP detected in one Indian family. Linkage analysis located RP28 to chromosome 2p11-p16 (211). Locus RP22 of ARRP was, by homozygosity mapping, mapped to chromosome 16p12.1-p12.3 in two large Indian families.

X-CHROMOSOME LINKED RP

Description

X-chromosome-linked RP (XLRP) is considered the most severe form of RP. Onset of night blindness in the first decade of life, progressive constriction of visual fields in the second decade, and legal blindness in the third decade are the rule rather than the exception. The disorder is relatively uncommon. In the British population, however, the frequency of XLRP was 21.5% of all RP families (212), and it was suggested that this form is probably underdiagnosed or incorrectly interpreted in many studies that indicated a low occurrence (212).

XLRP is transmitted in each specific family by one of several X-linked genes, and is recessive mode. The frequency of the involved genes varies in different populations (see Table 7 and Fig. 3).

The characteristic patient with XLRP has early onset of night blindness, constricted visual fields, a ring scotoma or a residual temporal field, reduced visual acuity by the fourth or fifth decade of life, myopia with a spherical error of at least - 3.0 D, and astigmatism with a vertical or oblique axis of cylinder of −2.0 D or more (75,213).

Male relatives of patients with XLRP have a higher risk for the disease if their visual acuity is 6/9 or less in the better eye, their astigmatic error is 1.0 D or more in the eye with less astigmatism, and the axis of the cylinder is vertical or oblique (75). As expected from Lyon's theory (214), most and possibly all female carriers of XLRP can be recognized by clinical or laboratory investigations. Ophthalmoscopy is the most sensitive single test (212,215). The studies by Bird (212) and by Fishman et al. (215) indicate the clinical characteristics of carriers of XLRP. The fundus (Fig. 4) shows a tapetal reflex or spots of RPE dropout, or both, which are well

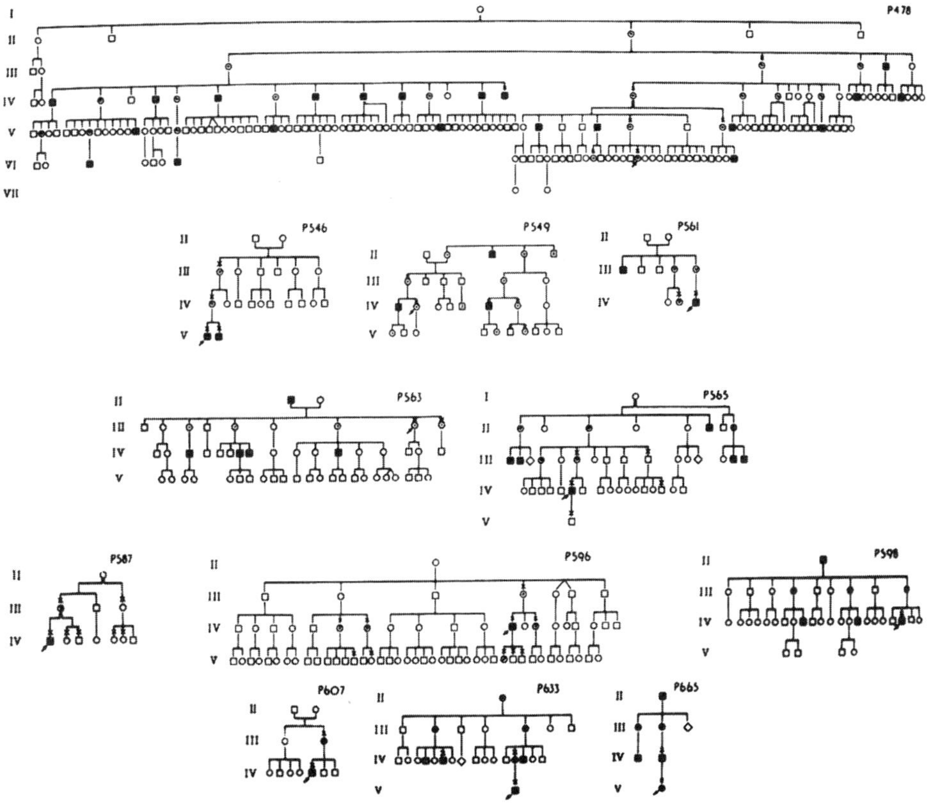

Figure 3 Pedigrees of 23 families with X chromosome-linked retinitis pigmentosa from the Moorfields study. Note that transmission is as expected (from Ref. 78). (*Figure continued on p. 308.*)

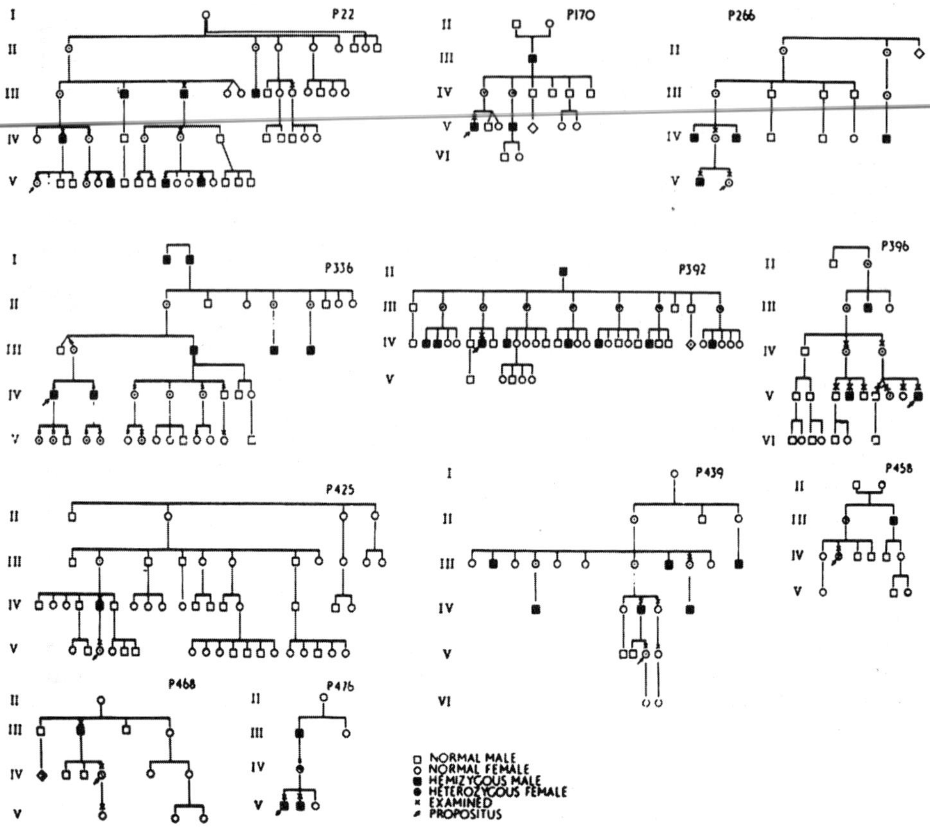

Figure 3 (*Continued*)

localized and patchy. Sometimes mild retinal pigmentation, localized choroidal atrophy, or peripheral pigmentary clumping in the form of blots or bone corpuscles can be seen. Most carriers have normal or almost normal visual acuity and normal visual fields, but either may be abnormal. A mild decrease in visual acuity is common. The majority of carriers have an abnormal psychophysical dark adaptation curve (212) and reduced ERG rod amplitudes (215). Carriers showed reduced rod sensitivity to

Table 7 Genes and Loci Associated with XLRP

	Locus/ symbol	Gene	Chromosal location	Remarks
1	RP2	RP2	Xp11.23	7–18% of all XLRP
2	RP3	RPGR (retinitis pigmentosa GTPase regulator)	Xp21.1	15–20% of all RP genes. 70% pfXLRP
3	RP15	RPGR	Xp21.1	Probably same as RP3
4	RP23	–	Xp22	One report
5	Rp24	–	Xq26-q27	One large family
6	RP6	–	Xp21.3-p21.2	Locus not yet confirmed

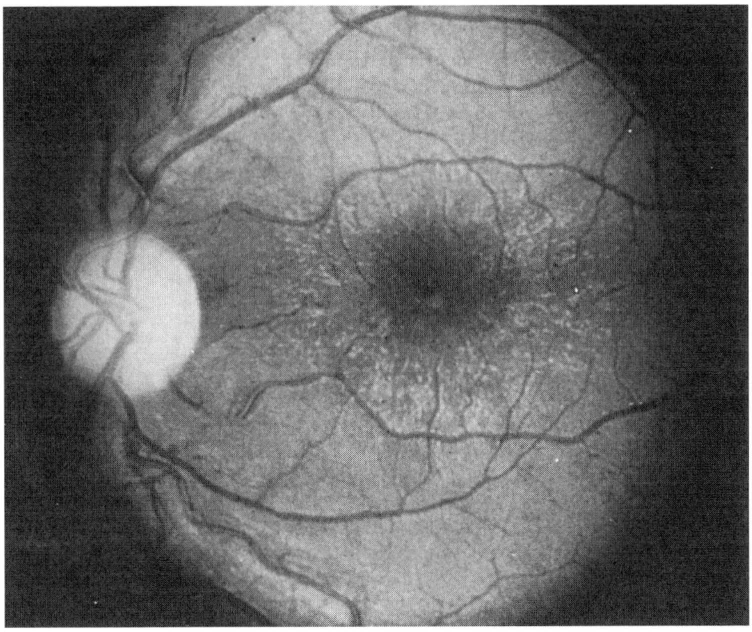

Figure 4 Fundus of a female carrier of XLRP. This 36-year-old black woman was an obligatory carrier and asymptomatic. Of her four children, three sons were affected, and the daughter was a carrier. Her brother also was affected by XLRP. Her visual acuity was 20/20 in each eye. Note the tapetal reflex and the RPE dropout (courtesy of G. A. Fishman, MD).

detect flicker over the whole frequency range (216) and had significantly higher threshold perimetry profiles than normals for both rod and cone systems (217).

It was suggested that disease manifestation of carriers varies with the specific gene association. A "tapetal reflex" was observed only or mainly in female carriers of RP3 (218). Grover et al. (219) grouped their carriers into three grades in order to establish their prognosis. Carriers of grade 1 (only tapetal reflex) showed no significant changes with time, carriers of grade 3 (diffuse peripheral pigmentary changes) manifested reduction in their visual fields and visual acuity with time. Grade 2 was in between. More recently, Vajaranant et al. (220) advised that multifocal ERG may be the best way to detect carriers of XLRP as most show reduced mfERG amplitudes and/or delayed implicit times.

Molecular Genetics of XLRP

Several loci and genes were confirmed to be associated with XLRP, thus manifesting significant heterogeneity although not to the extent of ADRP and certainly not to the extent of ARRP.

The RP2 Gene

Heterogeneity of XLRP has been known since the end of the 1980s. When the genes became known, Teague et al. (221) analyzed 40 kindreds with XLRP and found that 56% were RP3 associated and 26% were RP2 associated. Thiselton et al. (403) mapped RP2 to chromosome Xp11.3–11.23. Positional cloning of the gene was reported in 1998 (223). The location was later refined to Xp11.23 (6).

The predicted RP2 gene product shows significant homology with cofactor C, a protein involved in the folding of the beta-function molecule, which is the last step of biogenesis.(223). This protein carries 350 amino acids. Various mutations were identified including nonsense, missense, frameshift and small deletions. Schwahn et al. (224) considered the basis for photoreceptor degeneration in RP2 to be the loss of the protein or its intracellular distribution instead of localization to the cell membrane. It may also be that the accumulation of incorrectly folded photoreceptor or neuron-specific tubulin isoforms results in progressive cell death (6).

In their first study Schwahn et al. (223), found that 18% of XLRP cases are associated with RP2 mutations while this number is about double for RP3. Later Breuer et al. (225) found 10% for RP2 and 30% for RP3, while Sharon et al. (226) found 6.7% and 72.6%, respectively.

RP3 and the RPGR Gene

As mentioned before, the heterogeneity of XLRP was known from the end of the 1980s and was mentioned in the previous edition of this book. In 1992, Kaplan et al. reported evidence of linkage of an early onset XLRP with myopia which may be severe to RP2 locus. XLRP of later onset was generally associated with the RP3 locus (227). van Dorp et al. found several patients with RP3 that had recurrent respiratory infections because of abnormal cilia in the respiratory pathways, indistinguishable from the immobile cilia syndrome (228). Hearing impairment may also occur.

The gene was identified by two groups of investigators in 1996 using positional cloning (229–231). An earlier association of RP23 with the ETX1 gene at the same location was not confirmed (232).

The gene RPGR (*retinitis pigmentosa GTPase regulator*) was mapped to chromosome Xp21.1. In their first report, Meindl et al. (229) identified three missense mutations, two nonsense mutations, and two small intragenic mutations. Novel mutations were reported by many investigators following years (233–242). These included various missense mutations, various nonsense mutations, frameshifts, splice-site mutations, small deletions and small insertions leading to premature termination. Sharon et al. (226) pointed out the great variability of mutations in the RPGR gene, many of which are family-specific. In screening 135 patients with XLRP, they found 10 mutations in the RP2 gene, two of them novel, while among 80 mutations in the RPGR gene, 41 were novel. The expressivity of the disease may be different with different mutations. In the family with a missense mutation in exon 3, Fishman et al. found severe disease in hemizygotes and cone-rod dystrophy in heterozygotes (239). Two French Canadian families were studied. In one, a 2-bp deletion resulting in frameshift was associated with severe RP and preserved visual acuity with hearing loss, while in the other, a splice-site mutation was associated with early loss of central vision due to bull's eye maculopathy (242).

RP3 is the most frequent X-linked retinitis pigmentosa subtype. The percentage of mutated RPGR among XLRP patients may vary in different populations, but European figures seem to match American figures. Bader et al. in Germany found among 58 XLRP patients, 8% of mutations in the RP2 gene, and 71% of mutations in the RPGR gene (243). This is similar to the incidence of mutations found in American patients (226). Most of the RPGR disease-bearing mutations were detected in a 500-bp stretch in exon ORF15 (for open reading frame exon 15). These mutations were numerous. The in-frame sequence alterations in exon

ORF15 ranged from the deletion of 36 bp to the insertion of 75 bp (243), thus leading to premature termination. These authors considered the RPGR gene to be the most common gene causing RP with 15–20% of all cases of RP, regardless of mode of inheritance.

Mutations in exon ORF15 of the RPGR gene were reported to be, associated with diseases other than RP. Macular degeneration with normal ERG (244), and X-linked cone-rod dystrophy (245) were described. X-linked dominant RP was described in association with RP locus but no RPGR mutations were detected (246). Later, Rozet et al. presented 14 families with a dominant transmission of XLRP, all associated with an RPGR ORF15 mutation (247). In all dominant XLRP, heterozygotes were as severely affected as hemizygotes. As expected, the genetic transmission from father to daughters was seen.

Other X-linked Loci and Genes

RP15 was the term given to the locus of X-linked dominant cone-rod dystrophy that, when mapped, overlapped the region of both RP3 and RPGR (248,249). A disease-bearing mutation was identified in exon ORF15 (249).

RP23, a new locus for XLRP was reported in 2000 at the chromosome Xp22 location (250). *RP24*, another new XLRP locus, was reported in one large family (251). It is the first XLRP reported on the long arm of X chromosome at Xq26-q27. Affected hemizygotes showed an early onset of rod photoreceptor dysfunction while cone photoreceptor function, while initially normal, decreased gradually (251). *RP6,* a locus for XLRP, was mapped to chromosome Xp21.3-p21.2 and was suggested as another subtype of XLRP (252).

DIAGNOSTIC TESTS AND OTHER ASPECTS OF ISOLATED RETINITIS PIGMENTOSA

Introduction

The diagnosis of RP is usually easily established on clinical grounds, when the combination of typical symptoms and typical ophthalmoscopic changes in the fundus are observed. I also find that the vitreous abnormalities are helpful signs to establish the diagnosis. The diagnosis can then be confirmed by perimetry, which will show typical defects in the visual fields.

Unilateral RP was considered by us in a previous review (1) to be of a secondary, nonhereditary nature. Since then, this view has been strengthened by the absence of any report of inheritance of this form. Heckenlively (2) prefers the term "uniocular pigmentary retinopathy" and lists the causes as blunt trauma (most common), parasitic infection, retained foreign bodies, resolved exudative or rhegmatogenous retinal detachments, choroidal or retinal vascular occlusions, and chorioretinitis. This fits my own experience with such cases (Fig. 5).

Pseudo-RP is a bilateral condition in which acquired nonhereditary pigmentary retinopathy mimics RP by its ophthalmoscopic manifestation, but not necessarily by its functional disabilities. The causes are as listed for uniocular retinopathy, but the most common causes are congenital viral diseases, such as congenital rubella, or acquired viral diseases of childhood, such as measles. Visual acuity and visual field are usually, but not always, affected, The ERG may or may not be reduced. These secondary forms must be distinguished from inherited RP.

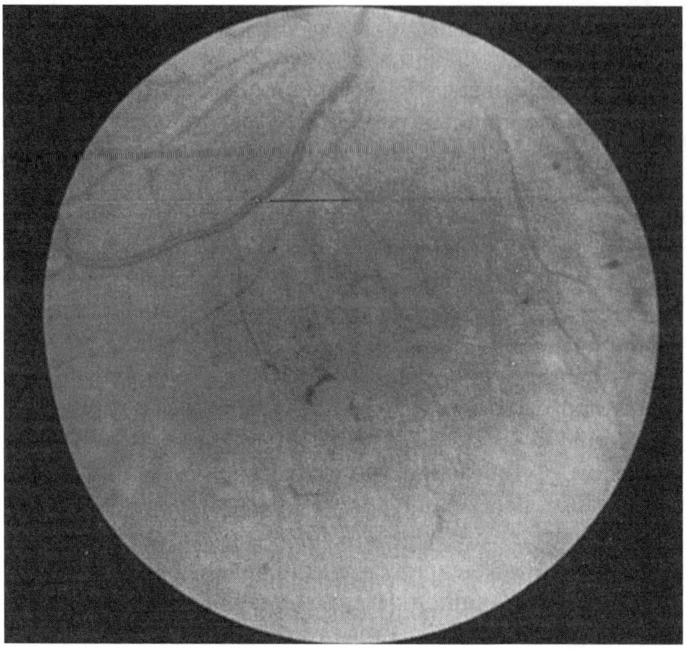

Figure 5 Fundus of a 35-year-old man with systemic lues and uniocular pigmentary retinopathy. The ophthalmoscopic picture is similar to the one of typical RP, except that the other eye was perfectly normal.

"Sporadic RP" or "RP, simplex type" are terms used for typical RP occurring as isolated cases without any familial history of a similar disease and without consanguinity of the parents. Most of these patients have some type of hereditary RP but some may have an acquired noninherited disease. As a group, the disease generally tends to be milder than in ARRP or XLRP, probably indicating a high percentage of autosomal dominant disease.

Retinitis pigmentosa may be misdiagnosed. In patients with early RP, before pigmentary changes occur in the fundus, the optic disk drusen or the visual field changes may be misinterpreted as a neurologic disease (253). In very early cases, especially in children, the diagnosis may be difficult to establish. It was suggested that an elevated pupil threshold (the retinal illuminance necessary to decrease the pupil diameter by 1 mm) may be an additional screening test (254) for children suspected of early RP. Once pigmentary changes are seen in the fundus, the differential diagnosis with other retinal dystrophies and degenerations must be ruled out. These include cone dystrophies, cone-rod dystrophies, which have a different prognosis; inherited macular dystrophies; primary choroidal dystrophies; and acquired nonhereditary diseases, such as pseudo-RP.

Laboratory tests should, be performed in every patient with suspected RP. The most important test is ERG.

Electroretinography

Since Karpe (255) showed that an undetectable ERG is the typical finding in RP, ERG has remained the basic laboratory test for RP. It is used today to confirm

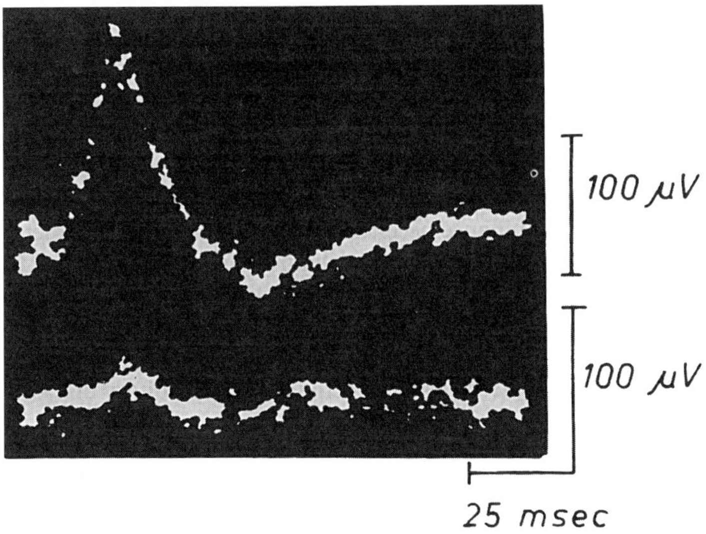

Figure 6 ERGs elicited by single-flash white light in early dark adaptation. A normal subject (above) and a 15-year-old RP patient (below) manifesting very abnormal b-wave amplitudes. Most patients with RP have an undetectable ERG.

the diagnosis, to follow the progression of the disease, to evaluate the patients' functional abnormalities, and for clinical research on the disease. Initially, the retinal responses to single flashes of white light (256), in light and during dark adaptation were measured (257) (Fig. 6). Full-field (Ganzfeld) ERG, with clear separation of the cone and rod components, was introduced and widely used by Berson (258) to distinguish between the different types of genetic RP. Normal or almost normal cone amplitudes with an increase in b-wave implicit time characterizes young patients with ADRP with reduced penetrance (259). In affected families, children with normal ERG amplitudes and normal cone and rod implicit times will not develop the disease (260). Widespread progressive forms of RP show reduced amplitudes and delays in cone or rod implicit times or both, whereas self-limited sector RP has reduced amplitudes and normal b-wave implicit times (260). Abnormal delays in b-wave implicit times can be seen in these patients before morphologic changes occur in the fundus and before rod amplitudes become reduced (261). A three-year follow-up of 94 patients with different forms of RP showed that the amplitudes were reduced in 77%, but only 44% of those with ADRP. Abnormal b-wave amplitudes or delayed cone b-wave implicit times, or both, were found in 96% of carriers of XLRP (262), making it an important adjunct for detection of the heterozygote state. The use of blue and sometimes red filters and of flicker light of 30 Hz to elicit separate cone and rod responses is now a standard practice in ERG.

As mentioned, the ERG may be used for the follow up of the natural course of RP to estimate the individual progression. Berson et al. found an average loss of 16–18.5% of remaining ERG per year (263), and to a 4.6% average loss of visual field area per year. Birch et al. (264) found an ERG loss of rod function of 64% and cone function of 60%, in four years.

Various modifications of the ERG technique were attempted. These include the relationship between scotopic b-wave amplitude and stimulus light intensity (265), the relationship between implicit time and intensity response (266), focal ERGs of the fovea and of the midperiphery (267,268), variable flicker frequency from 5 to 50 Hz (269), and the relationship between retinal illuminance and a specific b-wave implicit time (270). All of these, as well as a method in which very low amplitude cone ERGs elicited with 30-Hz white flicker are increased to be detectable by a narrowband electronic filter and computer averaging (271), are still research tools and are not used routinely in clinical laboratory practice.

Low frequency damped electroretinographic wavelets are obtained for 25–37 sec after very bright stimuli and are cone-generated. Lam et al. (272) showed their presence in young ADRP patients in whom the ERG was extinguished. Loss of multifocal ERG (mERG) response density was significant in all RP patient studies (243).

Other Electrophysiologic Tests

Two other tests are sometimes used in evaluating RP.

Electro-oculogram: The electro-oculogram (EOG) measures the standing potential generated by the RPE. Larger potentials generated in light (light peak) are divided into lower potentials generated in dark (dark trough). This fraction, called the Arden ratio, is normally above 1.8. Some laboratories multiply this number by 100 to give a percentage number (180% of light increase). In RP, this ratio is far lower than normal, sometimes reaching a ratio of 1.0 (no light rise of potentials).

Early receptor potential: The early receptor potential (ERP) is a very early electrical response elicited by strong light and generated by the photochemical events in the outer segments of the photoreceptors. It is not used as a routine clinical test.

Other Clinical Tests

Fluorescein angiography: Fluorescein angiography is used routinely by many ophthalmologists. It enables them to evaluate the macula, to quantitate the loss of RPE cells, to establish the competency of the retinal vasculature, and to detect abnormal capillaries and the presence of retinal leakage.

Fluorescein angiography together with color photographs of the fundus, also serve as basic tools to follow up the patient.

Dark adaptation: The dark adaptation test measures the increase in light sensitivity of both the cones and rods and their final thresholds. It measures and quantifies the amount of night blindness.

Dark adaptation, in spite of the important information it can supply, is not widely and routinely used for several reasons. It is a subjective (psychophysical) test that requires the patient's cooperation. It measures only one single point on the retina, which may not represent other areas. It is time-consuming (about an hour including preparation and initial light adaptation) and needs expensive specialized equipment. Finally, much of the information obtained can be found in the ERG.

Static perimetry: Static perimetry is sometimes used for clinical evaluation of the RP patient. It may supply some similar information on the dark adaptation of both cone and rod function. A comparison between ERG and dark adaptometry showed that the 57 patients tested by the two methods could be divided into three groups almost equally. In the first group, ERG and static perimetry showed the same results; in the second, the ERG showed only cone function, and static scotopic perimetry showed some residual rod function; whereas in the last group, ERG showed better results than static perimetry (274). Another study (275) found a very good concurrence between rod thresholds as found by static perimetry and full-field rod ERG thresholds. The widely used Humphrey "field-analyzer" has been modified to enable light-adapted and dark-adapted static perimetry in RP patients (276). It must be emphasized, however, that the ERG gives a general response of the whole retina, whereas static perimetry, like dark adaptation, gives information about selected areas of the retina. This is the source of the differences when the two methods are compared.

Other tests have been performed on patients with RP, but have not become clinical tools. Tests such as vitreous fluorophotometry, densitometry, spectral sensitivity and flicker testing, and diurnal rhythm are used for research and will be discussed.

Pathology

Donders was the first to report on a histopathologic specimen of an eye with RP (277). More than 40 histopathologic reports on the light microscopy and electron microscopy of RP in humans were published since then and recently reviewed by Mizuno et al. (278).

Several studies were performed on eyes of aged patients with advanced ADRP. Kolb and Gouras (279) found that all photoreceptors were absent, except the foveal cones, which had outer segments that were abnormally short and wide. Foveal RPE cells had excessive lipofuscin and reduced melanin, whereas extrafoveal RPE cells were abnormal and had excessive melanin. Szamier and Berson (280) found similar absence of photoreceptors, except for the foveal and perifoveal abnormal cones and abnormal RPE cells with apically displaced nuclei, some phagosomes, and large amounts of melanolysosomes.

Meyer et al. (281) described the eyes of two patients with ADRP. The retina could be divided into three different areas. Areas of bone spicule pigment had a total loss of photoreceptors with a partially preserved RPE and an intact outer limiting membrane (Fig. 7). In the inner retina, pigmentary deposits were found around small vessels and around hyalinized material. Areas of atrophic retina had no pigment but showed full-thickness retinal gliosis, which included the RPE layer and choriocapillaris. Intermediate areas showed retinal atrophy without scar formation. Photoreceptors were lost, but the outer limiting membrane and the choriocapillaris were

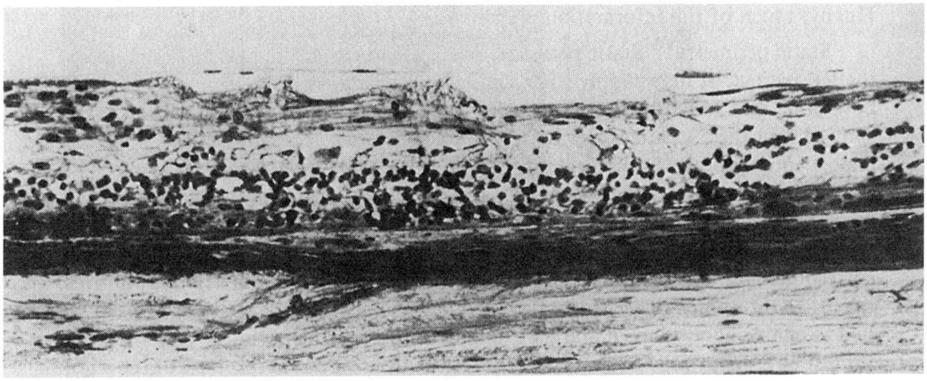

Figure 7 Epiretinal membrane in a patient with ADRP: note the extensive thinning of the retina, typical loss of photoreceptors, and the tangential traction on the retina exerted by the epiretinal membrane (from Ref. 281).

spared. Degenerative deposits in the form of a drusen-like material that stained positively with periodic acid-Schiff were seen at the level of Bruch's membrane. Amorphous material was found between basal infoldings of RPE cells.

Rodrigues et al. (282) also reported extensive gliosis, loss of photoreceptor cells, and occluded choriocapillaris. Santos-Anderson et al. (283) examined two cases of XLRP and one case of ADRP and did not find appreciable differences between these two genetic types. Photoreceptor degeneration took one of two forms: (i) mitochondrial swelling with "thin" cytoplasm around it and loss of other organelles or (ii) dense, shrunken cytoplasm with vacuolated mitochondria. The RPE layer was abnormal. Cells were focally absent, whereas in other areas RPE cells proliferated or were depigmented. The basal membrane of RPE cells was thickened. All six eyes showed an abnormal preretinal membrane, consisting of cellular elements that had characteristics of smooth muscle cells. The finding of a layer of a cellular amorphous material, between the RPE layer and Bruch's membrane was stressed by Duvall et al. (284), who examined four eyes of patients with advanced ADRP. Some patches of short and sparse photoreceptors remained.

The eyes of a 17-year-old boy with ADRP with reduced penetrance who died in a road accident were studied by Farber et al. (285). There were no rods in the equatorial area. Loss of rods (per mm^2) was greatest in the inferotemporal quadrant (99%) and was least in the inferonasal quadrant (89%). The superotemporal quadrant was best preserved (60% loss). Seventy-five percent of foveal cones were present. The RPE layer was preserved without intracellular visible morphologic changes, abnormal lipofuscin, or intercellular debris. By electron microscopy, these eyes were found to have phagocytic activity in areas of present photoreceptor outer segments (286). The authors concluded that, in the early phases, the choroid, RPE, and inner retina are normal. Shortened, disorganized, or absent segments were the earliest detectable abnormality. The primary disorder is likely to lie within the photoreceptor cell (286).

An eye of a 31-year-old patient with ARRP was removed because of a malignant melanoma and was examined by Bunt-Milam et al. (287). In some areas, outer segments of photoreceptors were missing, with inner segments reduced in numbers. In other areas, present outer segments were abnormally shortened and disorganized, whereas correlating cone inner segments were normal, and rod inner segments were abnormal with swollen mitochondria and granular inclusions. The RPE layer was abnormal. Reduplication of cells, loss of melanin, and increased melanolysosomes were noted and corresponded in size and location to clinically observed cream-colored deep retinal dots. Phagocytosed outer segments were found in RPE cells, indicating normal phagocytosis. The RPE protuberances enclosed individual outer segments of cones, but not of rods. Macrophages in the inner retina could be of local origin or arrive by hematogenous spread, or they could represent metaplasia of RPE cells.

The eyes of a 24-year-old patient with XLRP, who died of a malignancy, were studied by Szamier et al. (288). About half of the foveal cones were still present, but they had abnormally shortened and distorted outer segments. Their number decreased outward from the fovea, except in the far periphery where they were better preserved. The RPE cells had an abnormally large number of melanolysosomes.

Szamier and Berson (289) also studied the eyes of a 79-year-old XLRP heterozygote, who was asymptomatic most of her life. The posterior pole appeared normal, but in the midperiphery patches of photoreceptor degeneration were identified. Rods and cones were reduced in number. Some cones showed autophagic vacuoles in their inner segments, with shortened outer segments. The RPE was normal opposite normal neuroepithelium and abnormal in the affected patches.

Rodrigues et al. (290) found marked gliosis in outer retinal layers of a 79-year-old patient with sporadic RP. A localized nodule, with lipid infiltrates, found in the retina, and lipid accumulation found in the sub-RPE space may correspond to the clinical counterpart of Coats' disease.

Gartner and Henkind (291) examined 14 eyes of different types of RP and tried to draw conclusions about the sequence of pathologic events in RP. In their opinion, morphologic changes start with migration of nuclei from the outer nuclear layer to the rod and cone layer and to the outer plexiform layer as a result of degeneration of the whole-cell complex, causing shrinkage of the photoreceptors. Loss of photoreceptors, loss of connecting fibers in the outer plexiform layer, and partial loss of nuclei in the inner nuclear layer and ganglion cells in advanced cases follow in that order. The RPE cells remain normal, except in areas of loss of photoreceptors. The RPE cells may migrate into the neural retina or adhere to the outer limiting membrane. The equatorial zone is first affected; from here, the disease process extends centrally and peripherally.

Albert et al. (292) examined, by electron microscopy, six vitreous specimens of RP patients and found four types of intravitreal cells. These were heavily pigmented pigment epithelium cells, uveal melanocytes, retinal astrocytes, and macrophage-like cells. Loose pigment granules were also found. From this study and his own, Gouras (293) concluded that uveal melanocytes, and not RPE cells, compose the cellular pigment.

An ultrastructural study of a posterior subcapsular cataract from an RP patient did not show any unique features (294).

Milam and Jacobson found the loss of photoreceptors (particularly rods), and shortened foveal cone outer segments in a 76-year-old man with multiplex RP (295). Photoreceptors were arranged in rosettes and tubules (295,296). Histopathology of bone spicule pigmentation was studied by Li et al. (297). The pigment was found within pigment-containing cells derived from the RPE. Nearby vascular endothelial cells were thin and fenestrated, resembling choriocapillaris. Fariss et al. (298) demonstrated that rods, amacrine cells and horizontal cells, undergo neurite sprouting in human retinas with RP.

To et al. (299–301) compared the histopathological findings to the RP-associated mutations on the rhodopsin gene. In advanced RP of Glu181Lys mutation they found membranous swirls within the inner segments of macular cones, detected as electron-dense inclusion bodies by electronmicroscopy (EM) (299). Photoreceptor degeneration and bone corpuscular pigmentation was found in two retinas of Pro23His mutation. The younger patient was more severely affected, suggesting that factors other than genetic mutation may play a role (300). Similar pathologic findings were detected in RP patients when RHO mutations Pro23His, Cys110Arg, and Glu181Lys, were compared to RP13 gene mutation (301). In all, loss of rods and abnormality of remaining cones was apparent.

In summary, histopathologic studies of RP in humans shows that the outer layers of the retina degenerate totally in advanced cases. In early and moderate ADRP, cones are better preserved than rods, especially in the fovea. Initially, normal photoreceptors become abnormal, with wide and shortened outer segments, and they later degenerate and disappear. The disease process starts in the equatorial zone and spreads centrally and peripherally, the lower quadrants being more affected initially. The primary site of the disease has not been established, but some studies implicate the inner segments of the photoreceptors. Carriers of XLRP seem to have a patchy form of the disease.

Pathogenesis, Biochemistry, and Research of Retinitis Pigmentosa

Before 1990, we knew nothing about the structure of any one of the abnormal genes affecting the retina, let alone about their function. However this has changed, and by now most genes have been cloned: their structures known and in some cases their function and malfunction understood. Research on RP now consists of a voluminous and extensive body of literature. It can conveniently be divided into seven areas one of which, pathology, has already been discussed. The remaining areas are: (i) clinical study of the eye of RP patients; (ii) study of extraocular tissue in RP patients; (iii) study of immunology, biochemistry and metabolism of RP patients; (iv) immunologic and biochemical studies of enucleated RP eyes; and (v) study of molecular genetics and the function of normal and mutated genes.

Ocular Studies of Patients with Retinitis Pigmentosa

Vitreous fluorophotometry: Abnormally high concentrations of fluorescein within the vitreous cavity were detected in all 15 patients with various forms of RP who were examined by fluorophotometry (302). Such a high concentration of fluorescein indicates a break in the blood-retinal barrier (BRB) at the RPE level (outer BRB) or in the retinal vessels (inner BRB) (303). Carriers of XLRP always have abnormal vitreous fluorescein readings (304), hence, this method may be clinically used to confirm the heterozygote state. Kinetic vitreous fluorophotometry showed that inward permeability of fluorescein is increased and that outward permeability is decreased (305). The fluorescein has a rapid distribution inside the vitreous (306), probably implying an abnormal vitreous gel. Fluorescein concentrations in the vitreous are abnormal, even when fundus changes are minimal, and these concentrations increases with the progression of RP in the retina (307). In contrast, patients with cone-rod dystrophy have normal fluorophotometric readings, except in the advanced stages when rods are also affected (308). The clinical value of vitreous fluorophotometry in RP patients is not yet established. An abnormal BRB can also be found in most patients with RP by fluorescein angiography (309), but vitreous fluorophotometry seems to be abnormal in all RP patients, and in heterozygotes of XLRP.

Electrophysiology: Considerations of the intensity-amplitude functions for rod-isolated responses led Berson et al. to the conclusion that carriers of XLRP may have decreased visual pigment concentration in some rods, loss of some rods or both (262). The rods are involved in a patchy way. Focal cone ERGs performed in patients with ADRP with reduced penetrance, showed normal foveal cone function, but midperipheral cone ERGs were minimally reduced, with marked delay in b-wave implicit time (267). This may indicate a decreased state of adaptation of the cone system, which may be due to rod disease, at least in part (310).

Densitometry: Densitometry, or fundus reflectometry, is the method of measuring the amount of visual pigment in the photoreceptors (two-way or double-density values) and the regeneration time after bleaching. In RP patients, the reduction in light sensitivity has a linear relationship to the reduced rhodopsin found in the photoreceptor, which may indicate a reduced number of normal rods or a normal number of rods with shortened outer segments (27,311). However, in other cases, absolute thresholds may not be linearly related, but have a logarithmic relationship, as found in vitamin A deficiency (311). These two mechanisms may correspond to two different genetic and clinical entities of RP. In the first, a reduction in concentration of rhodopsin in each photoreceptor is found, as in vitamin A deficiency. In the second, a progressive shortening of the outer segments or a selective dropout of photoreceptors causes decrease in light sensitivity (311). Rhodopsin kinetics (regeneration of rhodopsin) is considered normal in human RP (311). Densitometric tests performed in four patients with sector RP showed that in dark-adapted eyes, threshold increases were not proportional to rhodopsin loss. This led to the conclusion that in sector RP, abnormalities of photoreceptor cell function central to the outer segment account for the increased thresholds (312). Foveal densitometry showed that disturbed foveal cones are an early feature of RP (313), but Kilbride et al. (314) found that the difference in cone pigment density (the change in light absorption before and after bleaching) is normal in most patients with ADRP, but is significantly reduced in patients with ARRP.

Psychophysical tests: Various psychophysical tests are used to study retinal function in RP patients. Foveal spectral sensitivity shows a significant reduction at only the lower wavelengths, for a reason yet unknown (315,316), but possibly related to a reduced cone directional sensitivity (317). The ability to detect flicker (a psychophysical test based on a pure cone phenomenon) becomes markedly worse with the dark adaptation of rods in normal subjects, indicating the normal rod–cone interaction. This rod–cone interaction was found to be absent or subnormal in RP (139). Arden (139) concluded that in mild cases of RP fewer rods are present—not normal numbers of rods with shorter outer segments.

Static perimetry of patients with early ADRP showed that light sensitivity thresholds were higher in the inferior and in the nasal retinal quadrants, compared with the temporal and upper retinal quadrants (140). It was suggested that this earlier reduction of function of the lower part of the retina may be the result of more light reaching this part (140).

Diurnal rhythm in the human rod electroretinogram: Birch et al. (141) showed that if a normal subject is entrained to a cyclic lighting of 14 hr of light and 10 hr of dark, full-field ERGs will manifest a significant increase in rod thresholds 1.5 hr after light onset, which will soon return to normal. This phenomenon may be associated with outer segment renewal. Patients with ADRP had a reduction of ERG amplitudes at 1.5 hr after light onset, but this was much larger than in normal subjects and remained reduced for many hours of the day (142). It may indicate an abnormal rod photoreceptor disk renewal mechanism (143).

Extraocular Studies of RP Patients

Arden and Fox (144) found that patients with RP have a significantly higher number of abnormal nasal cilia than normal controls. The range of abnormalities was 0–19% in controls and 6–37% in RP patients. Similar results were shown in Usher syndrome (145). Arden and Fox suggested that, similar to the abnormal microtubular structure of the axoneme in the nasal cilia, an abnormal photoreceptor axoneme could contribute to the pathogenesis of RP (144,145). These studies were confirmed by Finkelstein et al. (146) for all genetic forms of RP, but Lee et al. (147) doubted if the numbers had any significance.

Abnormal axonemes, significantly more than in normal controls, were also found in the sperm of patients with XLRP and Usher syndrome (148,149). The authors suggested that an inborn axoneme defect may also exist in the photoreceptor-connecting cilium causing decreased viability of photoreceptor outer segment (148).

Skeletal muscle investigations by electron microscopy and histochemistry and biochemical investigation of patients with RP yielded normal results (150).

Immunology, Biochemistry, and Metabolism in RP Patients

Studies intended to find the immune system abnormal in some or all RP patients failed to prove this point and remain controversial. Subnormal levels of interferon-γ, a lymphokine produced by the circulating lymphocytes, were found in 11 of 12 RP patients (151). Later studies showed that the production of the lymphokines, interferon-γ, interleukin-1, and interleukin-2 by peripheral blood lymphocytes in RP patients was not statistically different from that of normal controls (152,153).

The histocompatability HLA-DR antigens (class II antigens) were found to be abnormally-expressed in RPE cells of two patients with RP, in contrast with normal controls who have no such expression (154). This was not confirmed in another study that showed normal expression of HLA-DR antigens in circulating monocytes (155). No linkage was found between HLA antigens and RP in a third study (156). Newsome and Fishman (157), reviewing the subject of research on immunity and RP, concluded that the attempted four lines of study failed to prove such an association: studies on cellular immune alterations yielded results that were inconsistent; studies on lymphokine production gave controversial results: studies on an abnormal expression of class II antigens were unconfirmed; and studies on elevated serum IgM or IgG levels were unsubstantiated.

Abnormal metabolism of fatty acids in RP patients was identified in some studies. Reduced levels of docosahexaenoic acid (22:6) and arachidonic acid were found in the plasma of patients with ADRP (158), XLRP (159), and Usher syndrome (160). These two polyunsaturated fatty acids, normally found in the plasma, are phospholipids essential for the production of photoreceptor membranes. Significantly higher-than-normal plasma levels of apolipoprotein E isoforms (E_2/E_2; E_2/E_3) were found in 139 patients with RP (161). This could indicate that some forms of RP may be associated with an abnormal plasma lipoprotein metabolism.

Vitamin A and β-carotene serum levels are normal in patients with RP (162), but it was suggested that higher-than-normal serum levels after vitamin A intake in RP patients indicate an abnormal feedback mechanism, with less retention of vitamin A in the liver (163).

Taurine, implicated in animal experiments in one form of retinal dystrophy, is found in normal concentrations in human RP (164). However, one study found patients with ADRP type 3, who had an abnormally high concentration of taurine in the plasma, an abnormally low taurine uptake by platelets, and a significantly lower taurine intracellular concentration in lymphocytes (164).

Contradictory results were reported for plasma levels of copper and zinc in RP patients. To list just a few of the many reports, serum copper levels in RP patients were reported as abnormally low with low plasma ceruloplasmin levels (165), normal with low plasma ceruloplasmin levels and high urinary excretion (166), normal with normal plasma ceruloplasmin levels (167,168), and significantly higher than normal with high urinary excretion (169). Serum zinc levels were reported as abnormally high (169) or abnormally low (170). Different types of RP could show different results, however, these studies seem to yield conflicting results in all types of RP. They could be a reflection of the different populations studied, unrelated to RP.

Histochemical and Immunohistochemical Studies of Enucleated RP Eyes

Retinol (vitamin A), brought to the eye by the plasma retinol-binding protein, is bound to a specific receptor site on the RPE cell membrane, probably at the choroidal surface (171). Vitamin A, principally in the form of all-*trans*-retinol is further transported between RPE cells and photoreceptors by a large protein found only in the interphotoreceptor matrix, named interstitial retinol-binding protein (IRBP) (172). IRBP was reported as absent (109) or very low and found only in areas of preserved photoreceptors (117,173) in enucleated eyes of RP patients. These findings could indicate deficient synthesis of IRBP in RP patients (173), but could also be a secondary phenomenon, resulting from the degeneration of the neuroepithelium and pigment epithelium. A recent autopsy study on eyes of RP patients indicated that the reduction in proteins, including IRBP, is a consequence of photoreceptor loss and not of RPE loss (174). The human retina contains two distinct receptor species for retinol, 2s and 8s. One of the two, 8s, was absent in the retina of RP patients (175). A selective depletion of 11-*cis*-retinyl esters in the RPE cells was found in sector RP, possibly indicating an impaired ability of rod outer segments to isomerize retinol from all-*trans* to 11-*cis* (176). Cyclic guanosine monophosphate (cGMP) was significantly decreased in the affected retina of RP patients, probably indicating the loss of photoreceptors, which normally contain most of the cGMP (109,117). A significant elevation of cyclic adenosine monophosphate (cAMP) indicates its possible role in the pathogenesis of the disease (109). Abnormal glycoconjugates, both proteoglycans and glycosaminoglycans, were found in RPE cells of human RP eyes (177,178).

The major problem with the critical interpretation of the histochemical studies of the human retina afflicted by RP seems to be the lack of our present ability to distinguish between primary processes, which are the causative factors of the disease, and secondary processes, which result from the degeneration occurring as a result of the disease. Possibly culturing immature or embryonal photoreceptor cells from the human retina afflicted by RP will be useful for these studies (179).

Animal Models of RP

Retinal dystrophies, spontaneously occurring in mutant strains of animals are not infrequent. Retinal dystrophies may also be induced in experimental animals. All these serve as a model for human RP and may enable us to better understand the human disease. A vast literature is now available, and only some of it will be mentioned here.

Great enthusiasm was evoked in the 1970s by the discovery of a strain of rats with retinal dystrophy in which the pathogenesis of the disease seemed clear. The strain of RCS (for Royal College of Surgeons, where the strain was discovered) rats suffer from an aggressive, rapidly progressing retinal dystrophy that starts on day 18 of life and ends with death of all photoreceptors one to two months later. These rats show absence of the normal phagocytosis of shed particles of the rod outer segments by RPE cells (180). The shed rod outer segments accumulate between the shrinking outer segments and the RPE, until the outer segments become completely destroyed. It was clear that the RPE does not fulfill its normal phagocytic role in these animals (181), but only the production of rat chimeras solved the question of the primary site of the disease (182). These rat chimeras were produced by fusion of an albino RCS rat with a pigmented normal rat and have a mosaic of both normal and abnormal RPE cells and photoreceptors. Abnormal and degenerated photoreceptors were present only opposite patches of nonpigmented mutant RPE stemming from the RCS rats (182). It was later shown that it is the first step of the phagocytosis that is abnormal, so that the RPE cell cannot "recognize" the shed outer segments to start the process of phagocytosis. Cyclic lighting (12 hr dark, 12 hr light) provokes some detectable phagocytosis, amounting to 5% of the normal, about 1 hr after light onset (183). Opsin synthesized in the inner segments was normal until day 21 and then slowly declined, much slower than the rate of the degeneration of the outer segment (184), indicating that the photoreceptor abnormality is a secondary phenomenon. Starting on day 21, anatomic changes in the form of breaks in the tight junctions of the RPE were also noted and increased with time (185). It is probably a secondary phenomenon, and it may explain the rupture of the BRB seen in RP.

Transplantation of RPE cells from a mild strain of rats to the subretinal space of 25 RCS rats was successfully accomplished by Li and Turner (365). This was done at the age of 6–8 days, before structural degeneration occurs in the retina. Another attempt to treat the retinal dystrophy, by injecting RPE cells from a normal congenic pigmented strain of rats to the Bruch's membrane and subretinal space of RCS rats, was made by Lopez et al. (366). The transplantation seemed successful. Host and transplant cells formed close apposition with one another. Phagosomal material was found in the RPE cells within 48 hr of the implantation, implying photoreceptor survival and function.

The transplantations seemed to arrest the deterioration of the retina. The outer nuclear layer remained of normal thickness (365). Another, apparently successful transplantation of photoreceptors in rats was performed by Silverman and Hughes (367). Photoreceptors were destroyed by constant strong light, and photoreceptors of normal rats of the same strain were transplanted. Transplanted photoreceptors appeared to survive transplantation for at least six weeks.

Transplantation of RPE cells in RCS rats led to the rescue of photoreceptor cells (368,369). Retinal function was maintained in the transplant sites for long periods of time. Intraretinal ERGs were measured and found to be 59 μV in normal (wild type) rats, 2.5 μV in transplanted RCS rats and 0 in non-transplanted RCS rats (368). However, with time, a loss of photoreceptors was noted. Zhang and Bok (369) suggested that while there is no acute immune response to the transplanted RPE cells, a low-grade, chromic immune response causes reduction in function.

It was soon learned that the model of RCS rats with the primary site of disease in the RPE is not applicable to most types of human RP. In fact, another strain of rats, Wag/Rij, suffered from a retinal dystrophy with a different pathogenesis from RCS rats. The retinal degeneration was of early onset but of slow progression. The degeneration started in the photoreceptor cell body and only secondarily affected the outer segment, and the RPE phagocytic activity was preserved (370).

A similar, slowly progressive retinal photoreceptor cell dystrophy, found in albino rats with spontaneous hypertension, was treated by large amounts of D-galactose in their diet, which substantially reduced the prevalence and severity of the dystrophy (371). The mechanism of this effect is unknown.

A mutant strain of mice, homozygotic for the *rd/rd* gene, exhibits a rapidly progressive retinal dystrophy, with the primary site of the disease in the photoreceptors. In the early stages of development, a deficiency in cyclic nucleotide phosphodiesterase activity results in substantial accumulation of cGMP in the photoreceptors before they degenerate (372). Coinciding with the degeneration of the photoreceptors, retinal blood vessels become attenuated until, at 1 year, they are reduced to one-third of their normal size (373). The RPE appears normal, as shown by experiments with chimaeric mice (374).

Various dogs with retinal dystrophies were investigated. Irish setters with an autosomal recessive rod-cone dysplasia showed, similar to *rd* mice, a deficiency in cGMP phosphodiesterase activity and had elevated levels of cGMP in the photoreceptors in the early stages of the disease (375). These dogs showed a defect in the morphogenesis of the rod outer segment (376), possibly related to a deficiency in light-dependent opsin phosphorylation and a reduction in opsin synthesis (377).

In miniature poodles, a progressive rod-cone degeneration can be found. This disease has characteristics resembling human RP. The use of labeled leucine as an intravitreal injection and autoradiography enabled the investigators to conclude that the earliest recognizable abnormality is an abnormal renewal of the outer segments by a slow buildup of new disks (378). The renewal rate of outer segments was 0.99 μm/24 hr, in contrast with normal control dogs with a renewal rate of 2.35 μm/24 hr (379). No shed disk material accumulated between the neuroepithelium and pigment epithelium. The RPE showed normal ability for phagocytosis and contained phagosomes with shed material, in contrast with RCS rats.

Progressive retinal atrophy is inherited by the autosomal recessive mode in Abyssinian cats (380). Electron microscopic studies indicated that, initially, only rod outer segments are affected by disorganized disks or loss of outer segments; later, cones become similarly affected, especially in the equatorial area and, finally, at the age of six years, all rod and cone segments are lost (380).

Rhode Island red chickens, which suffer from a retinal dystrophy, have normal concentrations of IRBP, normal synthesis and storage of the 11-*cis* isomer of vitamin A, and normal production of rhodopsin (381).

Later, a gene, GC1, *cone-specific guanylate cyclase*, was found to be mutated by a null mutation, resulting in very low levels of cGMP. Absence of GC1 in the chicken rod retina prevents photo-transduction and leads to retinal degeneration (382). The human homolog gene for GC1 was mapped to chromosome 17p.

Various diet deficiencies may cause retinal dystrophy. Cats that are fed casein as their only protein, develop a retinal dystrophy associated with the low levels of taurine (383). In monkeys, a diet deficient in vitamin E, after two years, resulted in a macular degeneration caused by disruption of the photoreceptor outer segment (384). Vitamin A deficiency caused a diffuse retinal disease, with both photoreceptors affected (384).

Transgenic animals as models for human retinal disease were extensively studied in the last decade. Human defective genes were transfected into animal models and these animals studied. For example, RHO mutation Pro347Leu was transformed to produce a transgenic pig (385) and a human RDS/peripherin Pro216Leu to a transgenic mouse (386). Human genes were studied in the rescue of photoreceptors of affected animals. Genes such as the human rhodopsin transgene were introduced into RHO–/– mice (387).

In summary, studies of various animal models of retinal dystrophies indicate that different models may show different mechanisms for production of the disease. Such different pathogenetic mechanisms may be seen between species and even within the same species.

The last decade demonstrated a huge increase in animal studies in the field of molecular genetics. Researchers use animal modes of human diseases to study the molecular genetics, the structure and function of the 'wild type,' and the mutated genes. Extensive studies in rescue of photoreceptors and other therapies were performed in small and large animals. The homology of genes between humans and animals, particularly the mouse, is very helpful in this matter.

It is beyond the scope of this chapter to discuss all these studies. Studies on molecular genetics were discussed with the relevant subtypes of RP, and therapy will be discussed further on.

Epidemiology and Genetics

Prevalence of Retinitis Pigmentosa

Retinitis pigmentosa is a worldwide disease. It is known, to affect all races of mankind and can be found in every large population. Table 8 shows the prevalence of RP as calculated or estimated in the reported studies. There is a remarkable similarity of the prevalence rate in very different populations, ranging from about 1:3800 to about 1:4800, with a somewhat higher rate of incidence for the birth of a baby that will be affected by RP in the future. However, in isolates, such as the Navajo Indians or in communities with a high rate of consanguineous marriage, the figures are higher.

The Genetic Types of Retinitis Pigmentosa

An attempt to classify autosomal dominant, autosomal recessive, and sex-linked recessive types into subtypes was made in Table 2. It is based on the present knowledge of the clinical similarities and the genetic differences of the various types and subtypes. The prevalence of the various types and subtypes varies in different populations. It is important for the clinician to know, at least generally, the proportions of the different genetic types of the patient population he or she cares for. This information is important for genetic counseling of the sporadic case and for the individual prognosis. Table 9 lists the relative frequency of the genetic types of RP as reported for various populations. In spite of differences in the frequency of the various genotypes in different populations, it seems that, generally, ARRP is diagnosed in 24–28%, ADRP in 10–20%, and XLRP in 7–16%. It also seems from the table that, in Britain, autosomal dominant and sex-linked transmission is more common than in other populations (391).

Table 8 Retinitis Pigmentosa: Prevalence and Incidence

Country	Population	Prevalence	Incidence	Ref.
Switzerland		1:7000	NC	383
Israel		1:4500	NC	1
Israel	Communities with high consanguinity rate	1:2000	NC	1
United States			1:3700	11
United States	Navajo Indians	1:1878	NC	30
United States	Maine	1:4756	1:3544	388
United Kingdom	Birmingham	1:4869	NC	389
China		1:3784	NC	390

NC, not calculated.

Table 9 Relative Frequency of Genetic Types of RP

Country	Year reported	Autosomal dominant	Autosomal recessive	Sex-linked recessive	Simplex (sporadic)	Multiplex and undefined	Ref.
Finland	1964	37	20	4.5	38.5		399
Switzerland	1961	9	90[a]	1			400
Soviet Union	1961	12.7	27.9	1.1	41	17.3	401
United Kingdom	1972	39	15	25	21		402
United States	1978	26	19	16	38	1	403
United States	1980	10	84[a]	6			11
China	1982	11	33	7.7	48.3		414
United Kingdom	1982	24.4	6.8	15.7	41.1	12[a]	86
United States	1983	28.4	16.2	11.9	40.5	3	405
United Kingdom	1984	22	10 + 13[b]	14	37		406
China	1987	18	21	2	59		407

[a]Sporadic cases included in autosomal recessive.
[b]13% were autosomal recessive associated RP.

Epidemiologic studies of the last decade confirmed these earlier findings. A study in Denmark, where a nation-wide registration of diagnosed RP patients continuous since 1850 exists, reported a prevalence of 1 patient per 3943 (392).

The various identified RP-bearing mutations are listed both in the tables and with their appropriate subgroups of diseases. A short overview is suitable.

It is generally accepted that photoreceptor death in retinal degenerations of genetic origin is the result of an intrinsic "cell death program," or apoptosis (8). This was demonstrated in several RP animal models. Apoptosis plays a key role in RP. It may result from the poor functioning of a genetically defective photoreceptor or from mutations affecting nearby cells such as the RPE cells in RCS rats (393). Fragmentation of the cellular DNA is the hallmark of the programmed cell death. Malfunction is the beginning of the process.

Phototransduction is initially normal in most patients with RP. Subsequent degeneration of the rods results in reduction of transduction amplification (394).

Various mutations lead to abnormal function of photoreceptor. These were discussed in several reviews (395–397). They can be classified into several groups according to their pathophysiological effect.

In the first group are genes that encode proteins participating in the phototransduction cascade of the photoreceptor outer segment. These include rhodopsin (RHO), alpha subunit and beta subunit of cGMP-phosphodiesterase (PDE6A and PDE6B), and alpha and beta subunit of cGMP-gated channel.

The second group consists of genes encoding proteins of the visual cycle such as RPE65, a protein for isomerization of all-trans retinol to 11-cis retinol within the RPE cells (192,396); RBP4, retinol binding protein; CRALBP and RLBP1, both cellular-retinalaldehyde binding proteins; ABCA4, ATP-binding cassette transporter of rods; RGR, RPE retinal G-protein coupled receptor; and LRAT, lecithin retinol acyltransferase.

The third group consists of structural proteins of photoreceptors such as RDS/peripherin and ROM1. Both proteins are related and function together at the rim of the disks of the outer segment (396,398).

The fourth group consists of photoreceptor cell transcription factors such as NRL, the neural retina-specific leucine zipper, TULP1 involved in transportation of opsins and NR2E3 (PNR) a nuclear receptor.

The function of several other genes is unknown.

The concept of simplex RP emerged in the last 20 years or so. Although it relates to the same group of patients formerly referred to as sporadic or isolated, its meaning is different. Formerly, it was assumed that a patient with RP who has no family history of the disease is likely to have autosomal recessive RP, as his parents are asymptomatic heterozygotes. Thus, the chance of more-distant relatives manifesting RP is low because both parents of each patient must carry the gene in autosomal recessive disease, and the chance of any one of the patient's siblings having RP is only 25%. Therefore, an isolated case fits well into this autosomal recessive theory. It was assumed that autosomal dominant or sex-linked recessive transmisssion causes sporadic cases.

The simplex concept implies that we deal with a separate group of patients, although many or most cases are genetically induced. As a group, patients with simplex RP seem to suffer from the mildest disease of all groups. British patients with RP in the Birmingham study (406) had the following chances of being legally blind by age 40: 47% if in the ADRP group, 64% if ARRP, 84% if XLRP, and only 35% if in the RP simplex group. The latter figure is lower than for the presumed mildest group of ADRP. In addition, the frequency of simplex RP indicates an excess of such cases over the expected, which may not be explained by Mendelian laws (405).

Boughman and Fishman (405) listed several possibilities to explain the excessive number of simplex RP cases. These include autosomal dominant inheritance with incomplete penetrance; new mutation; or variable expressivity, with the parents only minimally affected. For others, non-Mendelian modes, such as multifactorial inheritance, unrecognized X chromosome-linked inheritance, or environmental phenocopïes, may be the cause. Of course, many and may be most of the simplex cases are autosomal recessive diseases, and this should be remembered in genetic counseling.

Management

Surgical and Medical

A wide discrepancy exists between the theoretical possibilities of future therapies based on extensive research being conducted and the meager therapeutic tools available to the practicing ophthalmologist. I have little doubt that this wide gap between practice and science will be closed in the future. I will discuss the present available managements and the studies being performed.

No treatment, medical or surgical, has proved itself effective for cure or amelioration of the diseased retina in isolated RP. A long list of various attempts at therapy is reviewed elsewhere (1,2,9,14). At the top of this list are various vitamins given in supplemental or therapeutic doses, vitamin derivatives, fatty acids and other chemical agents, RNA extracts, and surgical procedures such as placenta transplants. Often, initial enthusiasm for an effect of a treatment procedure was based on poor evaluation and lack of masking, as happened with the treatment by 11-*cis*-retinol (408).

Despite this general lack of effective therapy for the basic disease process, the patient with RP needs proper medical management. In practice, this management includes (i) evaluation of the ocular condition, such as the functional and anatomic office examinations, perimetry, and the routine laboratory tests, including color photography and fluorescein angiography; (ii) general medical evaluation to exclude associated RP, which may have different treatment; (iii) specialized examinations, when necessary, such as an audiogram if Usher syndrome is suspected; (iv) establishment of the diagnosis, including the genetic and clinical type; (v) provision of genetic counseling; (vi) discussion of the prognosis with the patient—it is important not to add to the despair of the patient but rather, point out the variable progression of the disease; (vii) advise to the patient about general behavior, such as limiting driving as needed, improving illumination at night, and wearing sunglasses in bright sunlight; (viii) evaluation of the possibility for using optical means such as low-vision aids; and (ix) evaluation of specific treatments the patient may need, such as cataract extraction.

Evidence is accumulating that the strong light of solar radiation may be damaging to the retina. This effect is most pronounced by the ultraviolet wavelengths, which reach the retina, and by the short wavelengths of visible light (409,410). This photic damage may be more pronounced in diseased retinas, such as found in age-related macular degeneration (410) and RP (411). Given the theoretical considerations, Berson (411) advised the use of a flush-fitting contact lens for light deprivation in RP patients, but results were negative—the disease process progressed despite the covered eye (412). However, this experiment does not rule out the deleterious effect of the short wavelengths of sunlight under normal conditions. Clinical evidence for such an effect is based both on the variability of the severity of the disease among siblings (the sibling more exposed to sunlight has worse retinal function than expected) and on patients' histories of visual deterioration after prolonged exposure to the sun. Therefore, until further evidence is available, patients should be advised to avoid exposure to strong sunlight by avoiding being outside during the brightest hours of the day or by wearing sunglasses. Sunglasses should at least eliminate all ultraviolet light and transmit 10–25% of visible light (413). In addition, more than 20 different manufacturers in the United States and several other countries produce "shield-sunglasses," which give extra protection by blocking the lower wavelengths of light, up to 500–550 nm, and by allowing transmission of a small percentage of the remaining wavelengths.

A large randomized study on vitamin A and vitamin E for patients with RP concluded that vitamin A supplementation (vitamin A palmitate 15,000 IU per day) may be effective in reducing loss of ERG response and, to some extent, also in reducing the loss of visual fields (414). The use of 400 IU vitamin E per day had an adverse effect in patients with RP. A beneficial effect was seen also in transgenic mice with two different rhodopsin mutations (414,415). The use of vitamin A was initially criticized (416), but it seems that with the years it is used by more ophthalmologists. Vitamin A should not be used in patients with liver problems and blood liver function tests should be performed before the treatment and periodically thereafter.

Reading may be helped with standard low-vision aids or by closed-circuit television (417) in patients with macular abnormalities. White print on a black background is preferred by RP patients (417).

Night vision can be aided by the use of a wide-field, high-intensity lantern (418) or somewhat helped by an ordinary strong light. Various instruments designed to help night vision by image amplification (419,420) did not prove their value in practice. Similarly, no good device to extend the visual fields is available.

Laser treatment is advised in selected patients with RP. Experiments with low-energy irradiation, by a pulsed ruby laser, of the retina of pigmented dystrophic rats showed a subsequent proliferation and repopulation of the irradiated area by RPE cells and a significant reduction in accumulation of debris (421). The ERG in the treated eye was significantly better than in the untreated eye for up to 25 days (422).

In patients with RP and Coats'-like disease, laser therapy, in the form of pan-retinal photocoagulation, was successfully used to treat neovascularization of the retina or disk (58,59,423). Cryotherapy may be used instead of, or in conjunction with, laser treatment (55).

Grid photocoagulation of the macula by laser was suggested as treatment for RP patients with angiographic evidence of cystoid macular edema (CME) and poor vision (424). The investigators claimed improvement or stabilization of the macular disease in all treated eyes, in contrast with untreated eyes (424). However, this treatment raises several concerns and remains controversial (425). The use of acetazolamide (Diamox) in daily dosages of about 250 mg as treatment of the macular edema in RP is still being investigated by several groups.

Ozone treatment for RP was advocated and widely used mainly in clinics in Cuba. Several reports of the treatment being useless and possibly causing harm (426–428) were published.

A yeast extract of RNA, widely used in Russia for treatment of RP, was also reported to be of no benefit (429).

Acetazolamide, by oral use in a rather small amount, was advocated for use in patients with RP and maculopathy, particularly macular edema. Fishman et al. (430) found in some patients both subjective and objective improvement. Orzalesi et al. also reported improved visual acuity and improved findings of the fluorescein angiography (431). Grover et al. reported similar improvement in fluorescein angiography and subjective improvement of visual acuity when dorzolamide eye drops were used instead of acetazolamide tablets in patients with RP and cystoid macular edema (432).

Retinitis pigmentosa patients with cataracts may have their cataracts removed without any worsening of the basic disease process. Most patients thus operated on reported satisfaction with the results of surgery, especially if an intraocular lens (IOL) (276) was implanted (433,434). This is also my own experience, and I routinely perform extracapsular cataract extraction with IOL implantation. Such an IOL should have an ultraviolet shield to eliminate short wavelengths of light, which can pass through an unshielded IOL (94).

Vitrectomy for troublesome vitreous opacities of RP resulted in the improved vision of a 36-year-old RP patient (432).

Treatment of RP by intramuscular injection of gangliosides was attempted (435). The reported marginal improvement in visual fields does not justify the clinical use of this substance.

Docosahexaenoic acid (DHA) is an omega 3-fatty acid of particular importance to photoreceptors. Fatty acids of the retinal photoreceptors consist of 30–40% of DHA, while other tissues have usually 3–5%. A recent study showed that supplementation with 400 mg per day for four years, elevated DHA plasma levels 2.5 times and was not associated with any identifiable risk (436). It seemed to be beneficial only in reducing rod ERG functional loss in patients under 12 years of age (437).

Investigative Therapies for RP

Several different approaches were studies in the last decade. These included retinal RPE transplantation, fetal tissue transplantation animal and human studies and more (438).

RPE Transplants. RPE transplantation techniques were started in the beginning of the 1990s principally to find a solution for age related macular degeneration (AMD). Autologous or homologous grafts were used to replace the missing RPE cells (439). The subretinal neovascular membranes were surgically removed and fetal (15–17 weeks of gestational age) RPE cells were transplanted (440). The transplant in humans survived but severe cystoid macular edema occurred (440–442).

Similar animal experiments with RPE cell transplantation for retinal dystrophies took place. Transplantation of RPE cells from wild-type rats into RCS dystrophic rats seemed an effective treatment (443). Transplanted healthy RPE cells seemed to rescue the degenerating photoreceptors (444–446). The photoreceptors manifested normal renewal rates, normal shedding of disks, normal metabolic rates and normal interaction with RPE cells (444). An outer nuclear layer started to form four weeks after the transplant (445) and good fusion between RPE and outer retina developed (446). Other experiments showed that human fetal RPE was rejected in the rabbit after one month (447), but it survives better in the monkey (448). However, transplants from same wild type animal of RPE cells and photoreceptors, were able to rescue degenerating photoreceptor cells in the dystrophic animal (449).

RPE cells were transplanted in cell suspension, in patches, grown on artificial substrates or grown as microspheres on cross-linked fibrinogen (450). The reattachment of RPE cells to a substrate is of crucial importance to prevent apoptosis (451).

Transplantation of autologous iris pigment epithelium into the subretinal space was successfully performed in rabbits (452) and in humans (453). In RCS rat iris pigment epithelium transplants rescued the photoreceptors (454).

Photoreceptor Transplantation. Photoreceptor transplantation started with animal experiments. Photoreceptor layers from normal-sighted mice were graphed into the subretinal space of retinal degeneration (rd) mice, lacking rod photoreceptors. The short-term results were good with a mean of 38% of transplanted surviving cones at two weeks (455). The *rd* mice lose all their rods at about five weeks of age. Transplantation of rods increases cone survival (456). A similar effect was seen in cultures when normal rods were added (457).

Human photoreceptors were transplanted into the eye of several RP patients in the form of a sheet of photoreceptor cells taken from a cadaver (458,459) or intact sheets of fetal retina (14–18 week of gestational age) (460–462). In all cases a vitrectomy was performed, a retinotomy and the sheet of cells was implanted into the subretinal space. The studies performed and published between 1996 and 2003 were safety studies. No serious complications were seen with either method and there was no sign of rejection (458,460,461). No immunosuppresives were used. However, no improvement of visual functions of significance could be detected in the operated

RP patients. In spite of some claims to the contrary, it appears that there is no evidence that neural cell transplantation in humans is effective (463).

Another method of transplantation was used by Humayun et al. (464). Human fetal retinal microaggregate suspensions were injected into the subretinal space. No improvement was demonstrated but it was well tolerated (464).

Ribozyme Use. Animal experiments are being conducted. Ribozymes may promote a variety of reactions mainly through their RNA molecules. They can be helpful in both pathways leading to degeneration in RP, namely the reduced production of an essential molecule needed for normal function, and the building up of toxic proteins interfering with normal function (465). Ribozymes may be used for the delivery of genes or may provide mutation-independent methods of treating RP (466,467).

Many other experiments have been performed in animals, such as intraocularly injected survival factors like CNTF (ciliary neurotrophic factor) that protected photoreceptors from degeneration (468), or calcium-channel blockers to rescue photoreceptors of the *rd/rd* mouse (469). We are still far from applying these results to the treatment of patients.

Gene Therapy. Animal experiments with gene transfer for replacement of the defective gene were started about ten years ago. Transfection of the wild type gene linked to an adenovirus by subretinal injection in *rd/rd* mice, which lack cGMP PDE-beta was obtained without complications (470). PDE activity increased and delayed photoreceptor death by six weeks. In other experiments with the *rd/rd* mouse, a successful vector was HIV virus. Photoreceptor nuclei were still observed at the age of six months (471). Successful use of HIV as a vector for the wild type gene in retinal degeneration of rats and of AAV (adeno-associated virus) for *RPE−/−* dogs, was also reported (472,473).

Retinal Prosthesis. Human experiments with a retinal prosthesis are being performed by several groups of investigators, mainly in the United States. By the year 2001, five American teams, two German teams, one Belgian and one Japanese team had studied this subject (474).

A retinal implant may be useful only for patients who have a relative sparing of the inner retinal neurons (474,475). It is not known how many bipolar cells and especially how many ganglion cells are needed for a retinal implant to function. We know that cochlear implants can be used successfully when only 10% of ganglion cells remain (475). In RP inner retinal nuclear cells deteriorate with time, although it may take years for all ganglion cells to disappear. When remaining outer nuclear cells are 0–28% of normal, inner nuclear layer cells were 40–88% of normal and ganglion cells were 20–48% of normal (475).

Devices were implanted either in front of the retina (476) or subretinally (477). The preretinal device needs one tack to afix it to the retina (476). Figure 8 and table 10, both from Loewenstein et al. (475) explain the various implant approaches. The optic nerve implant and the cortical implant were studied by other groups of investigators.

By now, both the epiretinal implant and subretinal implant have been successfully implanted without rejection, infection, erosion or inflammation. The subretinal implant was named ASR or artificial silicone retina. It seems that it is simpler to use. Efficacy studies have not been yet performed.

Genetic Counseling. The rapid and large increase in identification of the involved genes associated with isolated RP raises expectations for full knowledge of all disease-causing genes. Almost all X-linked RP genes, most ADRP genes and

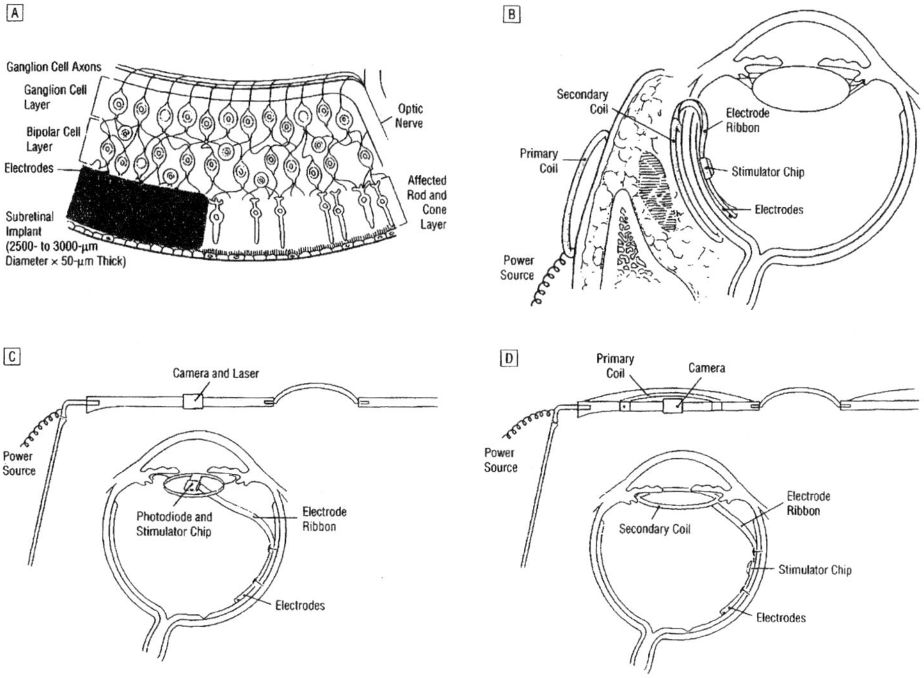

Figure 8 Retinal implants: A. subretinal implants; B. epiretinal implants with extraocular components; C and D. epiretinal implants with intraocular components from Loewenstein et al. (475).

many of the ARRP genes are known. We are not far from identifying them all. In his daily practice, the ophthalmologist would wish to have easy access to laboratories to study the molecular genetics of his or her individual patient in order to identify the involved mutation. This can be done today for many patients with hereditary retinal dystrophies and hopefully will be available for all such patients in the near future.

In patients with known mutations, the prognosis, risks of offspring, and sometimes even therapeutic approach can be individually tailored. Otherwise, genetic counseling should be based on the diagnosis after evaluation of the clinical and family data. Patients with ADRP may have reduced penetrance and this should be considered in genetic counseling. In the British series (86), 11.5% of such families showed reduced penetrance. This was radically lower in the American series (405).

Autosomal recessive RP seems also to have reduced segregation ratios, estimated as 19% (instead of 25%) (405). It is likely that more than one autosomal recessive gene may cause RP. From calculations of the prevalence of RP in China and consanguinity rates, Hu (404) estimated the number of autosomal recessive genes to be between 11 and 41. This estimate seems to be based on insufficient data, but the figure of about 40 seems quite possible.

Each patient with simplex RP must be evaluated individually according to gender and severity of disease. Jay (86) estimated that males with severe disease have a 21% chance to have XLRP, and the rest will have ARRP. Males or females with mild disease may have a fresh dominant mutation or ADRP, with reduced penetrance, or they may be phenocopies. Females with severe disease should be considered to have ARRP (86). Bundey and Crews (478) followed up 12 affected males with simplex RP

Table 10 Characteristics of Retinal Implants

Implant type	Viable cells needed	Stimulated threshold	Signal encoding	Power requirements	Bioompatibility
Epiretinal	Retinal ganglion cells	High in diseased eyes	Likely to be moderately complex	Moderate: will limit number of electrodes	Seems good
Subretinal	Retional ganglion cells, possibly bipolar cells	Probably lower than epiretinal	May be simpler than spiretinal	Probably lower than epiretinal	More problems than epiretinal
Cortical	No retinal cells needed	Lower than retina	Most complex	May be lower, probably easier to deliver	Seems good, though brian surgery required
Optic nerve	Retinal ganglion cells	Similar to or lower than retina	Complex and difficult to localize	Low to moderate; probably easler to deliver	Seems good, though neurosurgical approach used

From Loewenstein et al. (475).

and severe disease and found that 50% have XLRP. In males suspected with simplex RP, obligatory carriers, such as daughters and mothers, should be examined.

Prenatal Diagnosis. Identification of many disease-bearing mutated genes enables us, in many cases, to perform a prenatal diagnosis by the use of amniocentesis, chorionic villus sampling (CVS) or pre-implantation genetic diagnosis (PGD). Amniocentesis was successfully used to prenatally check the DNA of a potential XLRP carrier (479). More recently, PGD was performed to detect ADRP mutations (480).

In the future, it will be possible to predict the presence of RP in an unborn child. The results of a study performed in Germany on the acceptability of prenatal diagnosis by patients with RP are interesting. The authors received responses from 414 patients (481) and found that 85% would terminate the pregnancy if the child is predicted to be blind and mentally retarded; 68% if the child is predicted to be blind in childhood; and 29% would terminate pregnancy if the child is predicted to be blind in adulthood.

REFERENCES

1. Merin S, Auerbach E. Retinitis pigmentosa. Surv Ophthalmol 1976; 20:303–346.
2. Heckenlively JR. Retinitis Pigmentosa. Philadelphia: JB Lippincott, 1988.
3. Humphries P, Kenna P, Farrar GJ. On the molecular genetics of retinitis pigmentosa. Science 1992; 256:804–808.
4. Berson EL. Retinitis pigmentosa: unfolding its mystery. Proc Nat Acad Sci USA 1996; 93:4526–4528.
5. Clarke G, Heon E, McInnes RR. Recent advances in the molecular basis of inherited photoreceptor degeneration. Clin Genet 2000; 57:313–329.
6. RetNet, http: //www.sph.uth.tmc.edu/retnet/.
7. Yau KW. Phototransduction mechanism in retinal rods and cones. The Friedenwald Lecture. Invest Ophthalmol Vis Sci 1994; 35:9–32.
8. Adler R. Mechanisms of photoreceptor death in retinal degenerations. From the cell biology of the 1990s to the ophthalmology of the 21st century? Arch Ophthalmol 1996; 114:79–83.
9. Marmor MF, Aguirre G, Arden G, et al. Retinitis pigmentosa; a symposium on terminology and methods of examinations. Ophthalmology 1983; 90:126–131.
10. Heckenlively JR, Yoser SL, Friedman SL, Oversier JJ. Clinical findings and common symptoms in retinitis pigmentosa. Am J Ophthalmol 1988; 105:504–511.
11. Boughman AJ, Conneally PM, Nance WE. Population genetic studies of retinitis pigmentosa. Am J Hum Genet 1980; 32:223–235.
12. Massof RW, Finkelsteiri O, Starr SJ, Kenyon KR, et al. Bilateral symmetry of vision disorders in typical retinitis pigmentosa. Br J Ophthalmol 1979; 63:90–96.
13. Jiang M, Thompson HS. Pupillary defects in retinitis pigmentosa. Am J Ophthalmol 1985; 99:607–608.
14. Fishman GA. Retinitis pigmentosa: Visual loss. Arch Ophthalmol 1978; 96:1185–1188.
15. Pearlman JT, Axelrod RN, Tom A. Frequency of central visual impairment in retinitis pigmentosa. Arch Ophthalmol 1977; 95:894.
16. Grover S, Fishman GA, Alexander KR, Anderson RJ, Derlacki DJ. Visual acuity impairment in patients with retinitis pigmentosa. Ophthalmology 1996; 103:1593–1600.
17. Grover S, Fishman GA, Anderson RJ, Tozatti MS, Heckenlively JR, Weleber RG, Edwards AO, Brown J Jr. Visual acuity impairment in patients with retinitis pigmentosa at age 45 years or older. Ophthalmology. 1999; 106:1780–1785.
18. Sieving PA, Fishman GA. Refractive errors of retinitis pigmentosa patients. Br J Ophthalmol 1978; 62:163–167.

19. Holopigian K, Greenstein V, Seiple W, Carr RE. Rates of change differ among measures of visual function in patients with retinitis pigmentosa. Ophthalmology 1996; 103:398–405.
20. Hirakawa H, Iijima H, Gohdo T, Imai M, Tsukahara S. Progression of defects in the central 10-degree visual field of patients with retinitis pigmentosa and choroideremia. Am J Ophthalmol 1999; 127:436–442.
21. Swanson WH, Felius J, Birch DG. Effect of stimulus size on static visual fields in patients with retinitis pigmentosa. Ophthalmology 2000; 107:1950–1954.
22. Grover S, Fishman GA, Brown J Jr. Patterns of visual field progression in patients with retinitis pigmentosa. Ophthalmology 1998; 105:1069–1075.
23. Grover S, Fishman GA, Anderson RJ, Alexander KR, Derlacki DJ. Rate of visual field loss in retinitis pigmentosa. Ophthalmology 1997; 104:460–465.
24. Fishman GA. Color vision defects in retinitis pigmentosa. Ann Ophthalmol 1981; 13:609–618.
25. Ross DF, Fishman GA, Gilbert LS, et al. Variability of visual field measurements in normal subjects and patients with retinitis pigmentosa. Arch Ophthalmol 1984; 102:1004–1010.
26. Berson EL, Sandberg MA, Rosner B, et al. Natural course of retinitis pigmentosa over a three-year interval. Am J Ophthalmol 1985; 99:240–251.
27. Bird AC. Clinical investigation of retinitis pigmentosa. Prog Clin Biol Res 1987; 247: 3–20.
28. Adams A, Aspinall P, Hayreh SS. Primary retinal pigmentary degeneration. Trans Ophthalmol Soc UK 1972; 92:233–249.
29. Michaelson IC, Yanko L. Histo-ophthalmoscopy: the use of ophthalmoscope in histology. In: Bellows JG, ed. Contemporary Ophthalmology. Baltimore: Williams & Wilkins, 1972.
30. Heckenlively J, Friederich R, Farson C, Pabatis G. Retinitis pigmentosa in the Navajo. Metab Pediatr Ophthalmol 1981; 5:201–206.
31. DeRouck A, de Bie S, Kayembe D. Statistical evaluation of visual functions in dominant and recessive autosomal pigmentary retinopathy. Doc Ophthalmol 1986; 62: 265–280.
32. Grunwald JE, Maguire AM, Dupont J. Retinal hemodynamics in retinitis pigmentosa. Am J Ophthalmol 1996; 122:502–508.
33. Fishman GA, Fishman M, Maggiano J. Macuiar lesions associated with retinitis pigmentosa. Arch Ophthalmol 1977; 95:798–803.
34. Fishman GA, Maggiano JM, Fishman M. Foveal lesions seen in retinitis pigmentosa. Arch Ophthalmol 1977; 95:1993–1996.
35. Pruett RC. Retinitis pigmentosa: Clinical observations and correlations. Trans Am Ophthalmol Soc 1983; 81:693–735.
36. Merin S. Macular cysts as an early sign of tapetoretinal degeneration. J Pediatr Ophthalmol 1970; 7:225–228.
37. Ffytche TJ. Cystoid maculopathy in retinitis pigmentosa. Trans Ophthalmol Soc UK 1972; 92:265–283.
38. Fetkenhour CL, Choromokos E, Weinstein J, Schoch D. Cystoid macular edema in retinitis pigmentosa. Trans Am Acad Ophthalmol Otolaryngol 1977; 83:515–521.
39. Chachia N, Combes AM, Romdane K, Bee P. La maculopathie dans la retinopathie pigmentaise typique. J Fr Ophtalmol 1987; 10:381–386.
40. Hansen RT, Friedman AH, Gartner S, Henkind P. The association of retinitis pigmentosa with preretinal macular gliosis. Br J Ophthalmol 1977; 61:597–600.
41. Schubert HD, Shields JA. Isolated exudative maculopathy in retinitis pigmentosa. Am J Ophthalmol 1987; 103:834–835.
42. Hirakawa H, Iijima H, Gohdo T, Tsukahara S. Optical coherence tomography of cystoid macular edema associated with retinitis pigmentosa. Am J Ophthalmol 1999; 128:185–191.

43. Heckenlively JR, Jordan BL, Aptsiauri N. Association of antiretinal antibodies and cystoid macular edema in patients with retinitis pigmentosa. Am J Ophthalmol 1999; 127:565–573.
44. Puck A, Tso MOM, Fishman GA. Drusen of the optic nerve associated with retinitis pigmentosa. Arch Ophthalmol 1986; 103:231–234.
45. Novack RL, Foos RY. Drusen of the optic disk in retinitis pigmentosa. Am J Ophthalmol 1987; 103:44–47.
46. DeBustros S, Miller NR, Finkelstein D, et al. Bilateral astrocytic hamartoma of the optic nerve heads in retinitis pigmentosa. Retina 1983; 3:21–23.
47. Pillai S, Limaye SR, Saimovici LB. Optic disk hamartoma associated with RP. Retina 1983; 3:24–26.
48. Szamier RB. Ultrastructure of the preretinal membrane in retinitis pigmentosa [Abstract]. Invest Ophthalmol Vis Sci 1979; 18(suppl):206.
49. Newman NM, Stevens RA, Heckenlively JR. Nerve fiber layer loss in diseases of the outer retinal layer. Br J Ophthalmol 1987; 71:21–26.
50. Grover S, Fishman GA, Brown J Jr. Frequency of optic disk or parapapillary nerve fiber layer drusen in retinitis pigmentosa Ophthalmology. 1997; 104:295–298.
51. Spalton DJ, Bird AE, Cleary PE. Retinitis pigmentosa and retinal oedema. Br J Ophthalmol 1978; 62:174–182.
52. Heckenlively JR. Retinitis pigmentosa, unilateral Coats' disease and thalassemia minor: a case report. Metab Ophthalmol 1981; 5:67–72.
53. Heckenlively JR. The hereditary retinal and choroidal degenerations. In: Emery AEG, Kimoin DL, eds. Principles and Practice of Medical Genetics. Edinburgh: Churchill-Livingstone, 1983:522–538.
54. Hammerstein W, Leide E. Netzhautdystrophie mit Coats-Syndrome. Klin Monatsbl Augenheilkd 1987; 190:527–529.
55. Lodato G, Giuffre G, Anastasi M. Télangiectasies rétiniennes périphériques dan la rétinopathie pigmentaire. J Fr Ophthalmol 1987; 10:777–782.
56. Ide CH, Khan JA, Podolsky TL, et al. Morbus Coats Typus Retinopathia pigmentosa. Klin Monatsbl Augenheilkd 1987; 190:205–206.
57. Spallone A, Carlevaro G, Ridling P. Autosomal dominant retinitis pigmentosa and Coats'-like disease. Int Ophthalmol 1985; 8:147–151.
58. Uliss AE, Gregor ZJ, Bird AC. Retinitis pigmentosa and retinal neovascularization. Ophthalmology 1986; 93:1599–1603.
59. Bressler NM, Gragoudas ES. Retinitis pigmentosa and retinal neovascularization. Ophthalmology 1987; 94:895.
60. Sachdev MS, Verma L, Garg SP, et al. Bilateral disk oedema in retinitis pigmentosa: an unusual sign. Jpn J Ophthalmol 1987; 31:621–626.
61. Kim RY, Kearney JJ. Coats-type retinitis pigmentosa in a 4-year-old child. Am J Ophthalmol 1997; 124:846–848.
62. Chowers I, Zamir E, Banin E, Merin S. Retinitis pigmentosa associated with Fuchs' heterochromic uveitis. Arch Ophthalmol 2000; 118:800–802.
63. Pruett RC. Retinitis pigmentosa: a biomicroscopical study of vitreous abnormalities. Arch Ophthalmol 1975; 93:603–608.
64. Merin S. Cataract formation in retinitis pigmentosa. Birth Defects 1982; 18:187–191.
65. Heckenlively JR. The frequency of posterior subcapsular cataract in the hereditary retinal degenerations. Am J Ophthalmol 1982; 93:733–738.
66. Fiore C, Santoni G, Lupidi G, Ricci AL. Associated retinitis pigmentosa and fundus flavimaculatus. Ophthalmologica 1987; 194:111–118.
67. Gadoth N, Treves T, Kuritzky A, Shapira Y. Retinitis pigmentosa and early onset myopathy: a case report. Metab Pediatr Syst Ophthalmol 1985; 8:37–38.
68. Pearlman J, Saxton J. Retinitis pigmentosa and birth control pills. JAMA 1975; 331:810.

69. Whitcup SM, Iwata F, Podgor MJ, Valle D, Sran PK, Kaiser-Kupfer MI. Association of thyroid disease with retinitis pigmentosa and gyrate atrophy. Am J Ophthalmol 1996; 122:903–935.
70. Fishman GA, Anderson RJ, Stinson L, Haque A. Driving performance of retinitis pigmentosa patients. Br J Ophthalmol 1981; 65:122–126.
71. Johnson CA, Keltner JL. Incidence of visual field loss in 20,000 eyes and its relationship to driving performance. Arch Ophthalmol 1983; 101:371–375.
72. Szlyk JP, Alexander KR, Severing K, Fishman GA. Assessment of driving performance in patients with retinitis pigmentosa. Arch Ophthalmol 1992; 110:1709–1713.
73. Szlyk JP, Fishman GA, Master SP, Alexander KR. Peripheral vision screening for driving in retinitis pigmentosa patients. Ophthalmology 1991; 98:612–618.
74. Szlyk JP, Fishman GA, Alexander KR, Revelins BI, Derlacki DJ, Anderson RJ. Relationship between difficulty in performing daily activities and clinical measures of visual function in patients with retinitis pigmentosa. Arch Ophthalmol 1997; 115:53–59.
75. Berson EL, Rosner B, Simonoff E. Risk factors for genetic typing and detection in retinitis pigmentosa. Am J Ophthalmol 1980; 89:763–775.
76. Pearlman JT. Mathematical models of retinitis pigmentosa: a study of the rate of progress in the different genetic forms. Trans Am Ophthalmol Soc 1979; 77:643–656.
77. Marmor MF. The electroretinogram in retinitis pigmentosa. Arch Ophthalmol 1979; 97:1300–1304.
78. Beaty TH, Boughman JA. Problems in detecting etiological heterogeneity in genetic disease illustrated with retinitis pigmentosa. Am J Med Genet 1986; 24:493–504.
79. Massof RW, Finkelstein D. Two forms of autosomal dominant primary retinitis pigmentosa. Doc Ophthalmol 1981; 51:289–346.
80. Massof RW, Johnson MA, Finkelstein D. Peripheral absolute threshold spectral sensitivity in RP. Br J Ophthalmol 1981; 65:112–121.
81. Lyness AL, Ernst W, Quinlan MP, et al. A clinical, psychophysical and electroretinographic survey of patients with abnormal dominant retinitis pigmentosa. Br J Ophthalmol 1985; 69:326–339.
82. Kemp CM, Jacobson SG, Faulkner DJ. Two types of visual dysfunction in autosomal dominant retinitis pigmentosa. Invest Ophthalmol Vis Sci 1988; 29:1235–1241.
83. Massoff RW, Finkelstein D. Rod sensitivity relative to cone sensitivity in retinitis pigmentosa. Invest Ophthalmol 1979; 18:263–272.
84. Fishman GA, Alexander KR, Anderson RJ. Autosomal dominant retinitis pigmentosa: a method of classification. Arch Ophthalmol 1985; 103:366–374.
85. Berson EL, Gouras P, Gunkel RD, Myrianthopoulos N. Dominant retinitis pigmentosa with reduced penetrance. Arch Ophthaimol 1969; 81:226–234.
86. Jay M. On the heredity of retinitis pigmentosa. Br J Ophthalmol 1982; 66:405–416.
87. Botstein D, White RL, Skolnick M, Davis RW. Construction of a genetic map in man using restriction fragment length polymorphisms. Am J Hum Genet 1980; 32:314–331.
88. Heckenlively J, Pearlman TJ, Sparkes RS, et al. Possible assignment of a dominant RP gene to chromosome 1. Ophthalmic Res 1982; 14:46–53.
89. Goode ME, Daiger SP, Lewis RA, Rogers WB. Linkage of autosomal dominant retinitis pigmentosa (ADRP) to the Rh blood group. Am J Hum Genet 1985; 37:A196.
90. Bradley DG, Farrar GJ, Sharp EM, et al. Autosomal dominant retinitis pigmentosa: Exclusion of the gene from the short arm of chromosome I including the region surrounding the rhesus locus. Am J Hum Genet 1989; 44:570–576.
91. Nathans J, Hogness DS. Isolation and nucleotide sequence of the gene encoding human rhodopsin. Proc Natl Acad Sci USA 1984; 81:4851–4855.
92. Sparkes RS, Mohandas T, Newman SL, et al. Assignment of the rhodopsin gene to human chromosome 3. Invest Ophthalmol Vis Sci 1986; 27:1170–1172.
93. Nathans J, Piantanida TP, Eddy RL, et al. Molecular genetics of inherited variation in human color vision. Science 1986; 232:203–210.

94. Donis-Keller H, Green P, Helms C, et al. A genetic linkage map of the human genome. Cell 1987; 51:319–337.
95. McWilliam P, Farrar GJ, Kenna P, et al. Autosomal dominant retinitis pigmentosa (ADRP): Localization of an ADRP gene to the long arm of chromosome 3. Genomics 1989; 5:619–622.
96. Dryja TP, McGee TL, Reichel E, et al. A point mutation of the rhodopsin gene in one form of retinitis pigmentosa. Nature 1990; 343:364–366.
97. Dryja TP, McGee TL, Hahn LB, Cowley GS, Olsson JE, Reichel E, Sandberg MA, Berson EL. Mutations within the rhodopsin gene in patients with autosomal dominant retinitis pigmentosa. New Engl J Med 1990; 323:1302–1307.
98. Humphries P, Farrar GJ, Kenna P, McWilliam P. Retinitis pigmentosa: genetic mapping in X-linked and autosomal forms of the disease. Clin Genet 1990; 38:1–13.
99. Jacobson SG, Kemp CM, Sung CH, Nathans J. Retinal function and rhodopsin levels in autosomal dominant retinitis pigmentosa with rhodopsin mutations. Am J Ophthalmol 1991; 112:256–271.
100. Souied E, Gerber S, Rozet JM, Bonneau D, Dufier JL, Ghazi I, Philip N, Soubrane G, Coscas G, Munnich A, et al. Five novel missense mutations of the rhodopsin gene in autosomal dominant retinitis pigmentosa. Hum Mol Genet 1994; 3:1433–1434.
101. Kim RY, al-Maghtheh M, Fitzke FW, Arden GB, Jay M, Bhattacharya SS, Bird AC. Dominant retinitis pigmentosa associated with two rhodopsin gene mutations. Leu-40-Arg and an insertion disrupting the 5′-splice junction of exon 5. Arch Ophthalmol 1993; 111:1518–1524.
102. Oh KT, Longmuir R, Oh DM, Stone EM, Kopp K, Brown J, Fishman GA, Sonkin P, Gehrs KM, Weleber RG. Comparison of the clinical expression of retinitis pigmentosa associated with rhodopsin mutations at codon 347 and codon 23. Am J Ophthalmol 2003; 136:306–313.
103. Souied E, Soubrane G, Benlian P, Coscas GJ, Gerber S, Munnich A, Kaplan J. Retinitis punctata albescens associated with the Arg135Trp mutation in the rhodopsin gene. Am J Ophthalmol 1996; 121:19–25.
104. Sullivan LJ, Makris GS, Dickinson P, Mulhall LE, Forrest S, Cotton RG, Loughnan MS. A new codon 15 rhodopsin gene mutation in autosomal dominant retinitis pigmentosa is associated with sectorial disease. Arch Ophthalmol 1993; 111:1512–1517.
105. Shastry BS. Retinitis pigmentosa and related disorders: phenotypes of rhodopsin and peripherin/RDS mutations. Am J Med Genet 1994; 52:467–474.
106. Oh KT, Weleber RG, Lotery A, Oh DM, Billingslea AM, Stone EM. Description of a new mutation in rhodopsin, Pro23Ala, and comparison with electroretinographic and clinical characteristics of the Pro23His mutation. Arch Ophthalmol 2000; 118: 1269–1276.
107. Richards JE, Scott KM, Sieving PA. Disruption of conserved rhodopsin disulfide bond by Cys187Tyr mutation causes early and severe autosomal dominant retinitis pigmentosa. Ophthalmology 1995; 102:669–677.
108. Farrar GJ, Kenna P, Jordan SA, Kumar-Singh R, Humphries MM, Sharp EM, Sheils DM, Humphries P. A three-base-pair deletion in the peripherin-RDS gene in one form of retinitis pigmentosa. Nature 1991; 354:478–480.
109. Kajiwara K, Hahn LB, Mukai S, Travis GH, Berson EL, Dryja TP. Mutations in the human retinal degeneration slow gene in autosomal dominant retinitis pigmentosa. Nature 1991; 354:480–483.
110. Jacobson SG, Cideciyan AV, Kemp CM, Sheffield VC, Stone EM. Photoreceptor function in heterozygotes with insertion or deletion mutations in the RDS gene. Invest Ophthalmol Vis Sci 1996; 37:1662–1674.
111. Fishman GA, Stone E, Gilbert LD, Vandenburgh K, Sheffield VC, Heckenlively JR. Clinical features of a previously undescribed codon 216 (proline to serine) mutation in the peripherin/retinal degeneration slow gene in autosomal dominant retinitis pigmentosa. Ophthalmology 1994; 101:1409–1421.

112. Lam BL, Vandenburgh K, Sheffield VC, Stone EM. Retinitis pigmentosa associated with a dominant mutation in codon 46 of the peripherin/RDS gene (arginine-46-stop). Am J Ophthalmol 1995; 119:65–71.
113. Keen TJ, Inglehearn CF. Mutations and polymorphisms in the human peripherin-RDS gene and their involvement in inherited retinal degeneration. Hum Mutat 1996; 8: 297–303.
114. van Lith-Verhoeven JJ, van den Helm B, Deutman AF, Bergen AA, Cremers FP, Hoyng CB, de Jong PT. A peculiar autosomal dominant macular dystrophy caused by an asparagine deletion at codon 169 in the peripherin/RDS gene. Arch Ophthalmol 2003; 121:1452–1457.
115. Kajiwara K, Sandberg MA, Berson EL, Dryja TP. A null mutation in the human peripherin/RDS gene in a family with autosomal dominant retinitis punctata albescens. Nat Genet 1993; 3:208–212.
116. Yanagihashi S, Nakazawa M, Kurotaki J, Sato M, Miyagawa Y, Ohguro H. Autosomal dominant central areolar choroidal dystrophy and a novel Arg195Leu mutation in the peripherin/RDS gene. Arch Ophthalmol 2003; 121:1458–1461.
117. Dryja TP, Hahn LB, Kajiwara K, Berson EL. Dominant and digenic mutations in the peripherin/RDS and ROM1 genes in retinitis pigmentosa. Invest Ophthalmol Vis Sci 1997; 38:1972–1982.
118. Yang Z, Lin W, Moshfeghi DM, Thirumalaichary S, Li X, Jiang L, Zhang H, Zhang S, Kaiser PK, Traboulsi EI, Zhang K. A novel mutation in the RDS/peripherin gene causes adult-onset foveomacular dystrophy. Am J Ophthalmol 2003; 135:213–218.
119. Kajiwara K, Berson EL, Dryja TP. Digenic retinitis pigmentosa due to mutations at the unlinked peripherin/RDS and ROM1 loci. Science 1994; 264:1604–1608.
120. van Soest S, Westerveld A, de Jong PT, Bleeker-Wagemakers EM, Bergen AA. Retinitis pigmentosa: defined from a molecular point of view [Review]. Sur Ophthalmol 1999; 43:321–334.
121. Inglehearn CF, Tarttelin EE, Plant C, Peacock RE, al-Maghtheh M, Vithana E, Bird AC, Bhattacharya SS. A linkage survey of 20 dominant retinitis pigmentosa families: frequencies of the nine known loci and evidence for further heterogeneity. J Med Genet 1998; 35:1–5.
122. Nakazawa M, Xu S, Gal A, Wada Y, Tamai M. Variable expressivity in a Japanese family with autosomal dominant retinitis pigmentosa closely linked to chromosome 19q. Arch Ophthalmol 1996; 114:318–322.
123. Greenberg J, Goliath R, Beighton P, Ramesar R. A new locus for autosomal dominant retinitis pigmentosa on the short arm of chromosome 17. Hum Mol Genet 1994; 3: 915–918.
124. Parminder AH, Murakami A, Inana G, Berson EL, Dryja TP. Evaluation of the human gene encoding recoverin in patients with retinitis pigmentosa or an allied disease. Invest Ophthalmol Vis Sci 1997; 38:704–709.
125. McKie AB, McHale JC, Keen TJ, Tarttelin EE, Goliath R, van Lith-Verhoeven JJ, Greenberg J, Ramesar RS, Hoyng CB, Cremers FP, Mackey DA, Bhattacharya SS, Bird AC, Markham AF, Inglehearn CF. Mutations in the pre–mRNA splicing factor gene PRPC8 in autosomal dominant retinitis pigmentosa (RP13). Hum Mol Genet 2001; 10:1555–1562.
126. Bardien S, Ebenezer N, Greenberg J, Inglehearn CF, Bartmann L, Goliath R, Beighton P, Ramesar R, Bhattacharya SS. An eighth locus for autosomal dominant retinitis pigmentosa is linked to chromosome 17q. Hum Mol Genet 1995; 4:1459–1462.
127. den Hollander AI, van der Velde-Visser SD, Pinckers AJ, Hoyng CB, Brunner HG, Cremers FP. Refined mapping of the gene for autosomal dominant retinitis pigmentosa (RP17) on chromosome 17q22. Hum Genet 1999; 104:73–76.
128. Rebello G, Ramesar R, Vorster A, Roberts L, Ehrenreich L, Oppon E, Gama D, Bardien S, Greenberg J, Bonapace G, Waheed A, Shah GN, Sly WS. Apoptosis-

inducing signal sequence mutation in carbonic anhydrase IV identified in patients with the RP17 form of retinitis pigmentosa. Proc Nat Acad Sci USA 2004; 101:6617–6622.
129. Inglehearn CF, Carter SA, Keen TJ, Lindsey J, Stephenson AM, Bashir R, al-Maghtheh M, Moore AT, Jay M, Bird AC, et al. A new locus for autosomal dominant retinitis pigmentosa on chromosome 7p. Nat Genet 1993; 4:51–53.
130. Kim RY, Fitzke FW, Moore AT, Jay M, Inglehearn C, Arden GB, Bhattacharya SS, Bird AC. Autosomal dominant retinitis pigmentosa mapping to chromosome 7p exhibits variable expression. Br J Ophthalmol 1995; 79:23–27.
131. Keen TJ, Hims MM, McKie AB, Moore AT, Doran RM, Mackey DA, Mansfield DC, Mueller RF, Bhattacharya SS, Bird AC, Markham AF, Inglehearn CF. Mutations in a protein target of the Pim-1 kinase associated with the RP9 form of autosomal dominant retinitis pigmentosa. Eur J Hum Genet 2002; 10:245–249.
132. Jordan SA, Farrar GJ, Kenna P, Humphries MM, Sheils DM, Kumar-Singh R, Sharp EM, Soriano N, Ayuso C, Benitez J, et al. Localization of an autosomal dominant retinitis pigmentosa gene to chromosome 7q. Nat Genet 1993; 4:54–58.
133. McGuire RE, Gannon AM, Sullivan LS, Rodriguez JA, Daiger SP. Evidence for a major gene (RP10) for autosomal dominant retinitis pigmentosa on chromosome 7q: linkage mapping in a second, unrelated family. Hum Genet 1995; 95:71–74.
134. Kennan A, Aherne A, Palfi A, Humphries M, McKee A, Stitt A, Simpson DA, Demtroder K, Orntoft T, Ayuso C, Kenna PF, Farrar GJ, Humphries P. Identification of an IMPDH1 mutation in autosomal dominant retinitis pigmentosa (RP10) revealed following comparative microarray analysis of transcripts derived from retinas of wild-type and Rho (−/−) mice. Hum Mol Genet 2002; 11:547–557.
135. Bowne SJ, Sullivan LS, Blanton SH, Cepko CL, Blackshaw S, Birch DG, Hughbanks-Wheaton D, Heckenlively JR, Daiger SP. Mutations in the inosine monophosphate dehydrogenase 1 gene (IMPDH1) cause the RP10 form of autosomal dominant retinitis pigmentosa. Hum Mol Genet 2002; 11:559–568.
136. Blanton SH, Heckenlively JR, Cottingham AW, Friedman J, Sadler LA, Wagner M, Friedman LH, Daiger SP. Linkage mapping of autosomal dominant retinitis pigmentosa (RP1) to the pericentric region of human chromosome 8. Genomics 1991; 11: 857–869.
137. Pierce EA, Quinn T, Meehan T, McGee TL, Berson EL, Dryja TP. Mutations in a gene encoding a new oxygen-regulated photoreceptor protein cause dominant retinitis pigmentosa. Nat Genet 1999; 22:248–254.
138. Jacobson SG, Cideciyan AV, Iannaccone A, Weleber RG, Fishman GA, Maguire AM, Affatigato LM, Bennett J, Pierce EA, Danciger M, Farber DB, Stone EM. Disease expression of RP1 mutations causing autosomal dominant retinitis pigmentosa. Invest Ophthalmol Vis Sci 2000; 41:1898–1908.
139. Swaroop A, Xu JZ, Pawar H, et al. A conserved retina-specific gene encodes a basic motif/leucine zipper domain. Proc Natl Acad Sci USA 1992; 89:266–270.
140. Bessant DA, Payne AM, Mitton KP, Wang QL, Swain PK, Plant C, Bird AC, Zack DJ, Swaroop A, Bhattacharya SS. A mutation in NRL is associated with autosomal dominant retinitis pigmentosa. Nat Genet 1999; 21:355–356.
141. DeAngelis MM, Grimsby JL, Sandberg MA, Berson EL, Dryja TP. Novel mutations in the NRL gene and associated clinical findings in patients with dominant retinitis pigmentosa. Arch of Ophthalmol 2002; 120:369–375.
142. Farrar GJ, Jordan SA, Kenna P, Humphries MM, Kumar-Singh R, McWilliam P, Allamand V, Sharp E, Humphries P. Autosomal dominant retinitis pigmentosa: localization of a disease gene (RP6) to the short arm of chromosome 6. [erratum appears in Genomics 1992; 13:1384]. Genomics 1991; 11:870–874.
143. Xu SY, Schwartz M, Rosenberg T, Gal A. A ninth locus (RP18) for autosomal dominant retinitis pigmentosa maps in the pericentromeric region of chromosome 1. Hum Mol Genet 1996; 5:1193–1197.

144. Chakarova CF, Hims MM, Bolz H, Abu-Safieh L, Patel RJ, Papaioannou MG, Inglehearn CF, Keen TJ, Willis C, Moore AT, Rosenberg T, Webster AR, Bird AC, Gal A, Hunt D, Vithana EN, Bhattacharya SS. Mutations in HPRP3, a third member of pre-mRNA splicing factor genes implicated in autosomal dominant retinitis pigmentosa. Hum Mol Genet 2002; 11:87–92.
145. Bascom RA, Garcia-Heras J, Hsieh CL, Gerhard DS, Jones C, Francke U, Willard HF, Ledbetter DH, McInnes RR. Localization of the photoreceptor gene ROM1 to human chromosome 11 and mouse chromosome 19: sublocalization to human 11q13 between PGA and PYGM. Am J Hum Genet 1992; 51:1028–1035.
146. Bascom RA, Schappert K, McInnes RR. Cloning of the human and murine ROM1 genes: genomic organization and sequence conservation. Hum Mol Genet 1993; 2:385–391.
147. Bascom RA, Liu L, Heckenlively JR, Stone EM, McInnes RR. Mutation analysis of the ROM1 gene in retinitis pigmentosa. Hum Mol Genet 1995; 4:1895–1902.
148. Martinez-Mir A, Vilela C, Bayes M, Valverde D, Dain L, Beneyto M, Marco M, Baiget M, Grinberg D, Balcells S, Gonzalez-Duarte R, Vilageliu L. Putative association of a mutant ROM1 allele with retinitis pigmentosa. Hum Genet 1997; 99:827–830.
149. Bietti GB. Su alcune forme atipiche o rare di degenerazione retinica. Bull Ocul 1937; 16:1159–1244.
150. Bisantis CL. La rétiopathie pigmentaire en secteur de G. B. Bietti. Contribution a la connaisance de ses divers aspects cliniques. Ann Oculist 1971; 204:907–954.
151. Omphroy CA. Sector retinitis pigmentosa and chronic angle-closure glaucoma: a new association. Ophthalmologica 1984; 189:12–20.
152. Pinckers A, Greydanus J, Deutman AF, Duinkerke-Eerola KU. Atypical sector pigmentary dystrophy. Int Ophthalmol 1986; 9:143–149.
153. Cope LA, Teeters VW, Borda RP, McCrary JA. Sector retinitis pigmentosa with chronic disk edema. Doc Ophthaimol Proc Ser 1976; 9:431–437.
154. Rauborn ME, Moorhead LC, Hollyfield JG. A dominantly inherited chorio-retinal degeneration resembling sectoral retinitis pigmentosa. Ophthalmology 1982; 89: 1441–1454.
155. Merin S, Palmer D. Sector retinitis pigmentosa with optic nerve atrophy: An autosomal dominant entity unpublished data.
156. Grondahl J. Estimation of prognosis and prevalence of retinitis pigmentosa and Usher syndrome in Norway. Clin Genet 1987; 31:255–264.
157. Foxman SG, Heckenlively JR, Bateman JB, Wirtschafter JD. Classification of congenital and early onset retinitis pigmentosa. Arch Ophthalmol 1985; 103:1502–1506.
158. Heckenlively JR. Preserved para-arteriolar retinal pigment epithelium (PPRPE) in retinitis pigmentosa. Br J Ophthalmol 1982; 66:26–30.
159. Grondahl J. Autosomal recessive inheritance in "senile" retinitis pigmentosa. Acta Ophthalmol 1987; 65:231–236.
160. Lauber H. Die sogenannte Retinitis punctata albescens. Klin Monatsbl Augenheilkd 1910; 48:133.
161. Ellis DS, Heckenlively JR. Retinitis punctata albescens: fundus appearance and functional abnormalities. Retina 1983; 3:27–31.
162. Levy NS, Toskes PP. Fundus albipunctatus and vitamin A deficiency. Am J Ophthalmol 1974; 78:926–929.
163. Knowles JA, Shugart Y, Banerjee P, Gilliam TC, Lewis CA, Jacobson SG, Ott J. Identification of a locus, distinct from RDS-peripherin, for autosomal recessive retinitis pigmentosa on chromosome 6p. Hum Mol Genet 1994; 3:1401–1403.
164. Banerjee P, Kleyn PW, Knowles JA, Lewis CA, Ross BM, Parano E, Kovats SG, Lee JJ, Penchaszadeh GK, Ott J, Jacobson SG, Gilliam TC. TULP1 mutation in two extended Dominican kindreds with autosomal recessive retinitis pigmentosa. Nat Gene 1998; 18:177–179.

165. Hagstrom SA, North MA, Nishina PL, Berson EL, Dryja TP. Recessive mutations in the gene encoding the tubby-like protein TULP1 in patients with retinitis pigmentosa. Nat Genet 1998; 18:174–176.
166. Hagstrom SA, Duyao M, North MA, Li T. Retinal degeneration in tulp1 −/− mice: vesicular accumulation in the interphotoreceptor matrix. Invest Ophthalmol Vis Sci 1999; 40:2795–2802.
167. Lewis CA, Batlle IR, Batlle KG, Banerjee P, Cideciyan AV, Huang J, Aleman TS, Huang Y, Ott J, Gilliam TC, Knowles JA, Jacobson SG. Tubby-like protein 1 homozygous splice-site mutation causes early-onset severe retinal degeneration. Invest Ophthalmol Vis Sci 1999; 40:2106–2114.
168. van den Born LI, van Soest S, van Schooneveld MJ, Riemslag FC, de Jong PT, Bleeker-Wagemakers EM. Autosomal recessive retinitis pigmentosa with preserved para-arteriolar retinal pigment epithelium. Am J Ophthalmol 1994; 118:430–439.
169. van Soest S, Ingeborgh van den Born L, Gal A, Farrar GJ, Bleeker-Wagemakers LM, Westerveld A, Humphries P, Sandkuijl LA, Bergen AA. Assignment of a gene for autosomal recessive retinitis pigmentosa (RP12) to chromosome 1q31-q32.1 in an inbred genetically heterogeneous disease population. Genomics 1994; 22:499–504.
170. den Hollander AI, ten Brink JB, de Kok YJ, van Soest S, van den Born LI, van Driel MA, van de Pol DJ, Payne AM, Bhattacharya SS, Kellner U, Hoyng CB, Westerveld A, Brunner HG, Bleeker-Wagemakers EM, Deutman AF, Heckenlively JR, Cremers FP, Bergen AA. Mutations in a human homologue of Drosophila crumbs cause retinitis pigmentosa (RP12). Nat Genet 1999; 23:217–221.
171. Maw MA, Kennedy B, Knight A, Bridges R, Roth KE, Mani EJ, Mukkadan JK, Nancarrow D, Crabb JW, Denton MJ. Mutation of the gene encoding cellular retinaldehyde-binding protein in autosomal recessive retinitis pigmentosa. Nat Genet 1997; 17:198–200.
172. Morimura H, Berson EL, Dryja TP. Recessive mutations in the RLBP1 gene encoding cellular retinaldehyde-binding protein in a form of retinitis punctata albescens. Invest Ophthalmol Vis Sci 1999; 40:1000–1004.
173. Fishman GA, Roberts MF, Derlacki DJ, Grimsby JL, Yamamoto H, Sharon D, Nishiguchi KM, Dryja TP. Novel mutations in the cellular retinaldehyde-binding protein gene (RLBP1) associated with retinitis punctata albescens: evidence of interfamilial genetic heterogeneity and fundus changes in heterozygotes. Arch Ophthalmol 2004; 122:70–75.
174. Burstedt MS, Forsman-Semb K, Golovleva I, Janunger T, Wachtmeister L, Sandgren O. Ocular phenotype of bothnia dystrophy, an autosomal recessive retinitis pigmentosa associated with an R234W mutation in the RLBP1 gene. Arch Ophthalmol 2001; 119:260–267.
175. Dryja TP, Finn JT, Peng YW, McGee TL, Berson EL, Yau KW. Mutations in the gene encoding the alpha subunit of the rod cGMP-gated channel in autosomal recessive retinitis pigmentosa. Proc Natl Acad Sci USA 1995; 92:10177–10181.
176. Bareil C, Hamel CP, Delague V, Arnaud B, Demaille J, Claustres M. Segregation of a mutation in CNGB1 encoding the beta-subunit of the rod cGMP–gated channel in a family with autosomal recessive retinitis pigmentosa. Hum Genet 2001; 108:328–334.
177. Huang SH, Pittler SJ, Huang X, Oliveira L, Berson EL, Dryja TP. Autosomal recessive retinitis pigmentosa caused by mutations in the alpha subunit of rod cGMP phosphodiesterase. Nat Genet 1995; 11:468–471.
178. Dryja TP, Rucinski DE, Chen SH, Berson EL. Frequency of mutations in the gene encoding the alpha subunit of rod cGMP-phosphodiesterase in autosomal recessive retinitis pigmentosa. Invest Ophthalmol Vis Sci 1999; 40:1859–1865.
179. McLaughlin ME, Sandberg MA, Berson EL, Dryja TP. Recessive mutations in the gene encoding the beta-subunit of rod phosphodiesterase in patients with retinitis pigmentosa. Nat Genet 1993; 4:130–134.

180. McLaughlin ME, Ehrhart TL, Berson EL, Dryja TP. Mutation spectrum of the gene encoding the beta subunit of rod phosphodiesterase among patients with autosomal recessive retinitis pigmentosa. Proc Natl Acad Sci USA 1995; 92:3249–3253.
181. Hahn LB, Berson EL, Dryja TP. Evaluation of the gene encoding the gamma subunit of rod phosphodiesterase in retinitis pigmentosa. Invest Ophthalmol Vis Sci 1994; 35: 1077 1082.
182. Tsang SH, Gouras P, Yamashita CK, Kjeldbye H, Fisher J, Farber DB, Goff SP. Retinal degeneration in mice lacking the gamma subunit of the rod cGMP phosphodiesterase. Science 1996; 272:1026–1029.
183. Rosenfeld PJ, Cowley GS, McGee TL, Sandberg MA, Berson EL, Dryja TP. A null mutation in the rhodopsin gene causes rod photoreceptor dysfunction and autosomal recessive retinitis pigmentosa. Nat Genet 1992; 1:209–213.
184. Kumaramanickavel G, Maw M, Denton MJ, John S, Srikumari CR, Orth U, Oehlmann R, Gal A. Missense rhodopsin mutation in a family with recessive RP. Nat Genet 1994; 8:10–11.
185. Cremers FP, van de Pol DJ, van Driel M, den Hollander AI, van Haren FJ, Knoers NV, Tijmes N, Bergen AA, Rohrschneider K, Blankenagel A, Pinckers AJ, Deutman AF, Hoyng CB. Autosomal recessive retinitis pigmentosa and cone-rod dystrophy caused by splice site mutations in the Stargardt disease gene ABCR. Hum Mol Genet 1998; 7:355–362.
186. Rozet JM, Gerber S, Ghazi I, Perrault I, Ducroq D, Souied E, Cabot A, Dufier JL, Munnich A, Kaplan J. Mutations of the retinal specific ATP binding transporter gene (ABCR) in a single family segregating both autosomal recessive retinitis pigmentosa RP19 and Stargardt disease: evidence of clinical heterogeneity at this locus. J Med Genet 1999; 36:447–451.
187. Nicoletti A, Wong DJ, Kawase K, Gibson LH, Yang-Feng TL, Richards JE, Thompson DA. Molecular characterization of the human gene encoding an abundant 61 kDa protein specific to the retinal pigment epithelium. Hum Mol Genet 1995; 4:641–649.
188. Gu SM, Thompson DA, Srikumari CR, Lorenz B, Finckh U, Nicoletti A, Murthy KR, Rathmann M, Kumaramanickavel G, Denton MJ, Gal A. Mutations in RPE65 cause autosomal recessive childhood-onset severe retinal dystrophy. Nat Genet 1997; 17:194–197.
189. Morimura H, Fishman GA, Grover SA, Fulton AB, Berson EL, Dryja TP. Mutations in the RPE65 gene in patients with autosomal recessive retinitis pigmentosa or leber congenital amaurosis. Proc Natl Acad Sci USA 1998; 95:3088–3093.
190. Wada Y, Nakazawa M, Abe T. Clinical variability of patients associated with gene mutations of visual cycle protein, arrestin RPE65 and RDH5 genes [ARVO Abstract no. 327]. Invest Ophthalmol Vis Sci 2000; 41:s617.
191. Felius J, Thompson DA, Khan NW, Bingham EL, Jamison JA, Kemp JA, Sieving PA. Clinical course and visual function in a family with mutations in the RPE65 gene. Arch Ophthalmol 2002; 120:55–61.
192. Redmond TM, Yu S, Lee E, Bok D, Hamasaki D, Chen N, Goletz P, Ma JX, Crouch RK, Pfeifer K. Rpe65 is necessary for production of 11-cis-vitamin A in the retinal visual cycle. Nat Genet 1998; 20:344–351.
193. Kaplan J, Gerber S, Rozet JM. The survival of persecuted Jews in Spain and Portugal in the 15th century lad to endogamic preservation and emergence of ARRP mapped to chromosome 15q22 [ASHG Abstract No. 113]. Am J Hum Genet 1999; 65:A206.
194. Gerber S, Rozet JM, Takezawa SI, dos Santos LC, Lopes L, Gribouval O, Penet C, Perrault I, Ducroq D, Souied E, Jeanpierre M, Romana S, Frezal J, Ferraz F, Yu-Umesono R, Munnich A, Kaplan J. The photoreceptor cell-specific nuclear receptor gene (PNR) accounts for retinitis pigmentosa in the Crypto-Jews from Portugal (Marranos), survivors from the Spanish Inquisition. Hum Genet 2000; 107:276–284.
195. Ruiz A, Borrego S, Marcos I, Antinolo G. A major locus for autosomal recessive retinitis pigmentosa on 6q, determined by homozygosity mapping of chromosomal regions

that contain gamma-aminobutyric acid-receptor clusters. Am J Hum Genet 1998; 62:1452–1459.
196. Khaliq S, Hameed A, Ismail M, Mehdi SQ, Bessant DA, Payne AM, Bhattacharya SS. Refinement of the locus for autosomal recessive retinitis pigmentosa (RP25) linked to chromosome 6q in a family of Pakistani origin. Am J Hum Genet 1999; 65:571–574.
197. Hameed A, Khaliq S, Ismail M, Anwar K, Mehdi SQ, Bessant D, Payne AM, Bhattacharya SS. A new locus for autosomal recessive RP (RP29) mapping to chromosome 4q32-q34 in a Pakistani family. Invest Ophthalmol Vis Sci 2001; 42:1436–1438.
198. Bayes M, Goldaracena B, Martinez-Mir A, Iragui-Madoz MI, Solans T, Chivelet P, Bussaglia E, Ramos-Arroyo MA, Baiget M, Vilageliu L, Balcells S, Gonzalez-Duarte R, Grinberg D. A new autosomal recessive retinitis pigmentosa locus maps on chromosome 2q31-q33. J Med Genet 1998; 35:141–145.
199. Tuson M, Marfany G, Gonzalez-Duarte R. Mutation of CERKL a novel human ceramide kinase gene causes autosomal recessive retinitis pigmentosa (RP26). Am J Hum Genet 2004; 74:128–138.
200. Chan WM, Pang CP, Leung AT, Fan DS, Cheng AC, Lam DS. Bietti crystalline retinopathy affecting all 3 male siblings in a family. Arch Ophthalmol 2000; 118:129–131.
201. Jiao X, Munier FL, Iwata F, Hayakawa M, Kanai A, Lee J, Schorderet DF, Chen MS, Kaiser-Kupfer M, Hejtmancik JF. Genetic linkage of Bietti crystallin corneoretinal dystrophy to chromosome 4q35. Am J Hum Genet 2000; 67:1309–1313.
202. Li A, Jiao X, Munier FL, Schorderet DF, Yao W, Iwata F, Hayakawa M, Kanai A, Shy Chen M, Alan Lewis R, Heckenlively J, Weleber RG, Traboulsi EI, Zhang Q, Xiao X, Kaiser-Kupfer M, Sergeev YV, Hejtmancik JF. Bietti crystalline corneoretinal dystrophy is caused by mutations in the novel gene CYP4V2. Am J Hum Genet 2004; 74:817–826.
203. Gal A, Li Y, Thompson DA, Weir J, Orth U, Jacobson SG, Apfelstedt-Sylla E, Vollrath D. Mutations in MERTK, the human orthologue of the RCS rat retinal dystrophy gene, cause retinitis pigmentosa. Nat Genet 2000; 26:270–271.
204. Thompson DA, Li Y, McHenry CL, Carlson TJ, Ding X, Sieving PA, Apfelstedt-Sylla E, Gal A. Mutations in the gene encoding lecithin retinol acyltransferase are associated with early-onset severe retinal dystrophy. Nat Genet 2001; 28:123–124.
205. Ruiz A, Kuehn MH, Andorf JL, Stone E, Hageman GS, Bok D. Genomic organization and mutation analysis of the gene encoding lecithin retinol acyltransferase in human retinal pigment epithelium. Invest Ophthalmol Vis Sci 2001; 42:31–37.
206. Chen XN, Korenberg JR, Jiang M, Shen D, Fong HK. Localization of the human RGR opsin gene to chromosome 10q23. Hum Genet 1996; 97:720–722.
207. Morimura H, Saindelle-Ribeaudeau F, Berson EL, Dryja TP. Mutations in RGR, encoding a light-sensitive opsin homologue, in patients with retinitis pigmentosa. Nat Genet 1999; 23:393–394.
208. Seeliger MW, Biesalski HK, Wissinger B, Gollnick H, Gielen S, Frank J, Beck S, Zrenner E. Phenotype in retinol deficiency due to a hereditary defect in retinol binding protein synthesis. Invest Ophthalmol Vis Sci 1999; 40:3–11.
209. Nakazawa M, Wada Y, Tamai M. Arrestin gene mutations in autosomal recessive retinitis pigmentosa. Arch Ophthalmol 1998; 116:498–501.
210. Sippel KC, DeStefano JD, Berson EL, Dryja TP. Evaluation of the human arrestin gene in patients with retinitis pigmentosa and stationary night blindness. Invest Ophthalmol Vis Sci 1998; 39:665–670.
211. Gu S, Kumaramanickavel G, Srikumari CR, Denton MJ, Gal A. Autosomal recessive retinitis pigmentosa locus RP28 maps between D2S1337 and D2S286 on chromosome 2p11-p15 in an Indian family. J Med Genet 1999; 36:705–707.
212. Bird AC. X-linked retinitis pigmentosa. Br J Ophthalmol 1975; 59:177–199.
213. Fishman GA, Farber MD, Derlacki DJ. X-linked retinitis pigmentosa: profile of clinical findings. Arch Ophthalmol 1988; 106:369–375.

214. Lyon MF. Gene action in the X-chromosome of the mouse (Mus musculus). Nature 1961; 190:372.
215. Fishman GA, Weinberg AB, McMahon T. X-linked recessive retinitis pigmentosa: clinical characteristics of carriers. Arch Ophthalmol 1986; 104:1329–1335.
216. Ernst W, Clover G, Falukner DJ. X-linked retinitis pigmentosa; reduced rod flicker sensitivity in heterozygous females. Invest Ophthalmol Vis Sci 1981; 20:812–816.
217. Peachey NS, Fishman GA, Derlacki DJ, Alexander KE. Rod and cone dysfunction in carriers of X-linked retinitis pigmentosa. Ophthalmology 1985; 95:677–685.
218. Bergen AA, Van den Born LI, Schuurman EJ, Pinckers AJ, Van Ommen GJ, Bleekers-Wagemakers EM, Sandkuijl LA. Multipoint linkage analysis and homogeneity tests in 15 Dutch X-linked retinitis pigmentosa families. Ophthalmic Genet 1995; 16:63–70.
219. Grover S, Fishman GA, Anderson RJ, Lindeman M. A longitudinal study of visual function in carriers of X-linked recessive retinitis pigmentosa. Ophthalmology 2000; 107:386–396.
220. Vajaranant TS, Seiple W, Szlyk JP, Fishman GA. Detection using the multifocal electroretinogram of mosaic retinal dysfunction in carriers of X-linked retinitis pigmentosa. Ophthalmology 2002; 109:560–568.
221. Teague PW, Aldred MA, Jay M, Dempster M, Harrison C, Carothers AD, Hardwick LJ, Evans HJ, Strain L, Brock DJ, et al. Heterogeneity analysis in 40 X-linked retinitis pigmentosa families. Am J Hum Genet 1994; 55:105–111.
222. Thiselton DL, Hampson RM, Nayudu M, Van Maldergem L, Wolf ML, Saha BK, Bhattacharya SS, Hardcastle AJ. Mapping the RP2 locus for X-linked retinitis pigmentosa on proximal Xp: a genetically defined 5-cM critical region and exclusion of candidate genes by physical mapping. Genome Res 1996; 6:1093–1102.
223. Schwahn U, Lenzner S, Dong J, Feil S, Hinzmann B, van Duijnhoven G, Kirschner R, Hemberger M, Bergen AA, Rosenberg T, Pinckers AJ, Fundele R, Rosenthal A, Cremers FP, Ropers HH, Berger W. Positional cloning of the gene for X-linked retinitis pigmentosa 2. Nat Genet 1998; 19:327–332.
224. Schwahn U, Paland N, Techritz S, Lenzner S, Berger W. Mutations in the X-linked RP2 gene cause intracellular misrouting loss of the protein. Hum Mol Genet 2001; 10: 1177–1183.
225. Breuer DK, Yashar BM, Filippova E, Hiriyanna S, Lyons RH, Mears AJ, Asaye B, Acar C, Vervoort R, Wright AF, Musarella MA, Wheeler P, MacDonald I, Iannaccone A, Birch D, Hoffman DR, Fishman GA, Heckenlively JR, Jacobson SG, Sieving PA, Swaroop A. A comprehensive mutation analysis of RP2 and RPGR in a North American cohort of families with X-linked retinitis pigmentosa. Am J Hum Genet 2002; 70:1545–1554.
226. Sharon D, Sandberg MA, Rabe VW, Stillberger M, Dryja TP, Berson EL. RP2 and RPGR mutations and clinical correlations in patients with X-linked retinitis pigmentosa. Am J Hum Genet 2003; 73:1131–1146.
227. Kaplan J, Pelet A, Martin C, Delrieu O, Ayme S, Bonneau D, Briard ML, Hanauer A, Larget-Piet L, Lefrancois P, et al. Phenotype-genotype correlations in X-linked retinitis pigmentosa. J Med Genet 1992; 29:615–623.
228. van Dorp DB, Wright AF, Carothers AD, Bleeker-Wagemakers EM. A family with RP3 type of X-linked retinitis pigmentosa: an association with ciliary abnormalities. Hum Genet 1992; 88:331–334.
229. Meindl A, Dry K, Herrmann K, Manson F, Ciccodicola A, Edgar A, Carvalho MR, Achatz H, Hellebrand H, Lennon A, Migliaccio C, Porter K, Zrenner E, Bird A, Jay M, Lorenz B, Wittwer B, D'Urso M, Meitinger T, Wright A. A gene (RPGR) with homology to the RCC1 guanine nucleotide exchange factor is mutated in X-linked retinitis pigmentosa (RP3). Nat Genet 1996; 13:35–42.
230. Roepman R, van Duijnhoven G, Rosenberg T, Pinckers AJ, Bleeker-Wagemakers LM, Bergen AA, Post J, Beck A, Reinhardt R, Ropers HH, Cremers FP, Berger W.

Positional cloning of the gene for X-linked retinitis pigmentosa 3: homology with the guanine-nucleotide-exchange factor RCC1. Hum Mol Genet 1996; 5:1035–1041.
231. Fujita R, Swaroop A. RPGR: part one of the X-linked retinitis pigmentosa story. Mol Vis 1996; 2:4.
232. Dry KL, Aldred MA, Edgar AJ, Brown J, Manson FD, Ho MF, Prosser J, Hardwick LJ, Lennon AA, Thomson K, et al. Identification of a novel gene, ETX1 from Xp21.1, a candidate gene for X-linked retintis pigmentosa (RP3). Hum Mol Genet. 1995; 4: 2347–2353.
233. Fujita R, Buraczynska M, Gieser L, Wu W, Forsythe P, Abrahamson M, Jacobson SG, Sieving PA, Andreasson S, Swaroop A. Analysis of the RPGR gene in 11 pedigrees with the retinitis pigmentosa type 3 genotype: paucity of mutations in the coding region but splice defects in two families. Am J Hum Genet 1997; 61:571–580.
234. Weleber RG, Butler NS, Murphey WH, Sheffield VC, Stone EM. X-linked retinitis pigmentosa associated with a 2-base pair insertion in codon 99 of the RP3 gene RPGR. Arch Ophthalmol 1997; 115:1429–1435.
235. Andreasson S, Ponjavic V, Abrahamson M, Ehinger B, Wu W, Fujita R, Buraczynska M, Swaroop A. Phenotypes in three Swedish families with X-linked retinitis pigmentosa caused by different mutations in the RPGR gene. Am J Ophthalmol 1997; 124:95–102.
236. Buraczynska M, Wu W, Fujita R, Buraczynska K, Phelps E, Andreasson S, Bennett J, Birch DG, Fishman GA, Hoffman DR, Inana G, Jacobson SG, Musarella MA, Sieving PA, Swaroop A. Spectrum of mutations in the RPGR gene that are identified in 20% of families with X-linked retinitis pigmentosa. Am J Hum Genet 1997; 61:1287–1292.
237. Jacobson SG, Buraczynska M, Milam AH, Chen C, Jarvalainen M, Fujita R, Wu W, Huang Y, Cideciyan AV, Swaroop A. Disease expression in X-linked retinitis pigmentosa caused by a putative null mutation in the RPGR gene. Invest Ophthalmol Vis Sci 1997; 38:1983–1997.
238. Fishman GA, Grover S, Buraczynska M, Wu W, Swaroop A. A new 2-base pair deletion in the RPGR gene in a black family with X-linked retinitis pigmentosa. Arch Ophthalmol 1998; 116:213–218.
239. Fishman GA, Grover S, Jacobson SG, Alexander KR, Derlacki DJ, Wu W, Buraczynska M, Swaroop A. X-linked retinitis pigmentosa in two families with a missense mutation in the RPGR gene and putative change of glycine to valine at codon 60. Ophthalmology 1998; 105:2286–2296.
240. Guevara-Fujita M, Fahrner S, Buraczynska K, Cook J, Wheaton D, Cortes F, Vicencio C, Pena M, Fishman G, Mintz-Hittner H, Birch D, Hoffman D, Mears A, Fujita R, Swaroop A. Five novel RPGR mutations in families with X-linked retinitis pigmentosa. Hum Mutat 2001; 17:151.
241. Vervoort R, Wright AF. Mutations of RPGR in X-linked retinitis pigmentosa (RP3). Hum Mutat 2002; 19:486–500.
242. Koenekoop RK, Loyer M, Hand CK, Al Mahdi H, Dembinska O, Beneish R, Racine J, Rouleau GA. Novel RPGR mutations with distinct retinitis pigmentosa phenotypes in French-Canadian families. Am J Ophthalmol 2003; 136:678–687.
243. Bader I, Brandau O, Achatz H, Apfelstedt-Sylla E, Hergersberg M, Lorenz B, Wissinger B, Wittwer B, Rudolph G, Meindl A, Meitinger T. X-linked retinitis pigmentosa: RPGR mutations in most families with definite X linkage and clustering of mutations in a short sequence stretch of exon ORF15. Invest Ophthalmol Vis Sci 2003; 44: 1458–1463.
244. Ayyagari R, Demirci FY, Liu J, Bingham EL, Stringham H, Kakuk LE, Boehnke M, Gorin MB, Richards JE, Sieving PA. X-linked recessive atrophic macular degeneration from RPGR mutation. Genomics 2002; 80:166–171.
245. Demirci FY, Rigatti BW, Wen G, Radak AL, Mah TS, Baic CL, Traboulsi EI, Alitalo T, Ramser J, Gorin MB. X-linked cone-rod dystrophy (locus COD1): identification of mutations in RPGR exon ORF15. Am J Hum Genet 2002; 70:1049–1053.

246. Souied E, Segues B, Ghazi I, Rozet JM, Chatelin S, Gerber S, Perrault I, Michel-Awad A, Briard ML, Plessis G, Dufier JL, Munnich A, Kaplan J. Severe manifestations in carrier females in X linked retinitis pigmentosa. J Med Genet 1997; 34:793–797.
247. Rozet JM, Perrault I, Gigarel N, Souied E, Ghazi I, Gerber S, Dufier JL, Munnich A, Kaplan J. Dominant X linked retinitis pigmentosa is frequently accounted for by truncating mutations in exon ORF15 of the RPGR gene. J Med Genet 2002; 39:284–285.
248. McGuire RE, Sullivan LS, Blanton SH, Church MW, Heckenlively JR, Daiger SP. X-linked dominant cone-rod degeneration: linkage mapping of a new locus for retinitis pigmentosa (RP 15) to Xp22.13-p22.11. Am J Hum Genet 1995; 57:87–94.
249. Mears AJ, Hiriyanna S, Vervoort R, Yashar B, Gieser L, Fahrner S, Daiger SP, Heckenlively JR, Sieving PA, Wright AF, Swaroop A. Remapping of the RP15 locus for X-linked cone-rod degeneration to Xp11.4-p21.1, and identification of a de novo insertion in the RPGR exon ORF15. Am J Hum Genet 2000; 67:1000–1003.
250. Hardcastle AJ, Thiselton DL, Zito I, Ebenezer N, Mah TS, Gorin MB, Bhattacharya SS, Evidence for a new locus for X-linked retinitis pigmentosa (RP23). Invest Ophthalmol Vis Sci 2000; 41:2080–2086.
251. Gieser L, Fujita R, Goring HH, Ott J, Hoffman DR, Cideciyan AV, Birch DG, Jacobson SG, Swaroop A. A novel locus (RP24) for X-linked retinitis pigmentosa maps to Xq26–27. Am J Hum Genet 1998; 63:1439–1447.
252. Ott J, Bhattacharya S, Chen JD, Denton MJ, Donald J, Dubay C, Farrar GJ, Fishman GA, Frey D, Gal A, et al. Localizing multiple X chromosome-linked retinitis pigmentosa loci using multilocus homogeneity tests. Proc Natl Acad Sci USA 1990; 87: 701–704.
253. Heidemann DG, Beck RW. Retinitis pigmentosa: a mimic of neurologic disease. Surv Ophthalmol 1987; 32:445–451.
254. Birch EE, Birch DG. Pupillometric measures of retinal sensitivity in infants and adults with retinitis pigmentosa. Vision Res 1987; 27:499–505.
255. Karpe G. Basis of clinical electroretinography. Acta Ophthalmol 1945; 23:Suppl 24.
256. Goodman G, Ripps H. Electroretinography in the differential diagnosis of visual loss in children. Arch Ophthalmol 1960; 64:221–235.
257. Auerbach E. The human electroretinogram in the light and during dark adaptation. Doc Ophthalmol 1967; 22:1–71.
258. Berson EL. Retinitis pigmentosa and allied retinal diseases: electrophysiological findings. Trans Am Acad Ophthalmol Otolaryngol 1976; 81:659–666.
259. Berson EL, Simonoff EA. Dominant retinitis pigmentosa with reduced penetrance: further studies of the electroretinogram. Arch Ophthalmol 1979; 97:1286–1291.
260. Berson EL. Retinitis pigmentosa and allied diseases: applications of electroretinographic testing. Int Ophthalmol 1981; 4:7–22.
261. Berson EL. Electroretinographic findings in retinitis pigmentosa. Jpn J Ophthalmol 1987; 31:327–348.
262. Berson EL, Rosen JB, Simonoff EA. Electroretinographic testing as an aid in detection of carriers of X-chromosome linked RP. Am J Ophthalmol 1979; 87:460–468.
263. Berson EL, Sandberg MA, Rosner B, Birch DG, Hanson AH. Natural course of retinitis pigmentosa over a three-year interval. Am J Ophthalmol 1985; 99:240–251.
264. Birch DG, Anderson JL, Fish GE. Yearly rates of rod cone functional loss in retinitis pigmentosa cone-rod dystrophy. Ophthalmology 1999; 106:258–268.
265. Arden GB, Carter RM, Hogg CR. A modified ERG technique and the results obtained in X-linked RP. Br J Ophthalmol 1983; 67:419–430.
266. Massof RW, Wu L, Finkelstein D, et al. Properties of electroretinographic intensity: response functions in retinitis pigmentosa. Doc Ophthalmol 1984; 57:279–296.
267. Sandberg MA, Effron MH, Berson EC. Focal cone electroretinograms in dominant retinitis pigmentosa with reduced penetrance. Invest Ophthalmol Vis Sci 1978; 17: 1096–1101.

268. Seiple WH, Siegel IM, Carr RE, Mayron C. Evaluating macular function using the focal ERG. Invest Ophthalmol Vis Sci 1986; 27:1123–1130.
269. Massof RW, Johnson MA, Sunness JS, et al. Flicker electroretinogram in retinitis pigmentosa. Doc Ophthalmol 1986; 31:231–245.
270. Birch DG, Fish GE. Rod ERGs in retinitis pigmentosa and cone-rod degeneration. Invest Ophthalmol Vis Sci 1987; 28:140–150.
271. Andreasson S, Sandberg MA, Berson EL. Narrow-band filtering for monitoring low-amplitude cone electroretinograms in retinitis pigmentosa. Am J Ophthalmol 1988; 105:500–503.
272. Lam BL, Liu M, Hamasaki DI. Low-frequency damped electroretinographic wavelets in young asymptomatic patients with dominant retinitis pigmentosa: a new electroretinographic finding. Ophthalmology 1999; 106:1109–1113.
273. Seeliger M, Kretschmann U, Apfelstedt-Sylla E, Ruther K, Zrenner E. Multifocal electroretinography in retinitis pigmentosa. Am J Ophthalmol 1998; 125:214–226.
274. Arden GB, Carter RM, Hogg CR, et al. Rod and cone activity in patients with dominantly inherited retinitis pigmentosa: comparisons between psychophysical and electroretinographic measurements. Br J Ophthalmol 1983; 67:405–418.
275. Birch DG, Herman WK, deFaller JM, et al. The relationship between rod perimetric thresholds and full-field rod ERGs in retinitis pigmentosa. Invest Ophthalmol Vis Sci 1987; 28:954–965.
276. Jacobson SG, Voigt WJ, Parel JM. Automated light- and dark-adapted perimetry for evaluating retinitis pigmentosa. Ophthalmology 1986; 93:1604–1611.
277. Donders FC. Beiträge zur pathologischen Anatomie des Auges: 2. Pigmentbildung in der Netzhaut. Graefes Arch Clin Exp Ophthalmol 1957; 3:139–150.
278. Mizuno K, Nishida S, Takei Y. Pathology of human retinal dystrophy. Prog Clin Biol Res 1987; 247:21–33.
279. Kolb H, Gouras P. Electron microscopic observation of human retinitis pigmentosa, dominantly inherited. Invest Ophthalmol Vis Sci 1974; 13:487–498.
280. Szamier RB, Berson EL. Retinal ultrastructure in advanced RP. Invest Ophthalmol Vis Sci 1977; 16:947–962.
281. Meyer KT, Heckenlively JR, Spitznas M, Foos RY. Dominant retinitis pigmentosa: a clinicopathologic correlation. Ophthalmology 1982; 89:1414–1424.
282. Rodrigues MM, Wiggert B, Hacket J, et al. Dominantly inherited retinitis pigmentosa: Ultrastructure and biochemical analysis. Ophthalmology 1985; 92:1165–1172.
283. Santos-Anderson RM, Tso MOM, Fishman GA. A histopathologic study of retinitis pigmentosa. Ophthalmic Paediatr Genet 1982; 1:151–168.
284. Duvall J, McKechnie NM, Lee WR, et al. Extensive subretinal pigment epithelial deposit in two brothers suffering from dominant retinitis pigmentosa: a histopathological study. Graefes Arch Clin Exp Ophthalmol 1986; 224:299–309.
285. Farber DB, Flannery JG, Bird AC et al: Histopathological and biochemical studies on donor eyes affected with retinitis pigmentosa. Prog Clin Biol Res 1987; 247:53–67.
286. Flannery JG, Farber DB, Bird AL, Bok O. Degenerative changes in a retina affected with autosomal dominant retinitis pigmentosa. Invest Ophthalmol Vis Sci 1989; 30:191–211.
287. Bunt-Milam AH, Kalina RE, Pagon RA. Clinical-ultrastructural study of a retinal dystrophy. Invest Ophthalmol Vis Sci 1983; 24:458–469.
288. Szamier RB, Berson EL, Klein R, Meyers S. Sex-linked retinitis pigmentosa: ultrastructure of photoreceptors and pigment epithelium. Invest Ophthalmol Vis Sci 1979; 18: 145–160.
289. Szamier RB, Berson EL. Retinal histopathology of a carrier of X-chromosome-linked retinitis pigmentosa. Ophthalmology 1985; 92:271–278.
290. Rodrigues MM, Bardenstein D, Wiggert B, et al. Retinitis pigmentosa with segmental massive retinal gliosis. An immunohistochemical, biochemical, and ultrastructural study. Ophthalmology 1987; 94:180–186.

291. Gartner S, Henkind P. Pathology of retinitis pigmentosa. Ophthalmology 1982; 89: 1425–1432.
292. Albert DM, Pruett RC, Carft JL. Transmission electron microscopic observations of vitreous abnormalities in retinitis pigmentosa. Am J Ophthalmol 1986; 101:665–672.
293. Gouras P. Transmission electron microscopic observations of vitreous abnormalities in retinitis pigmentosa. Am J Ophthalmol 1987; 103:345.
294. Eshaghian J, Rafferty NS, Goossens W. Ultrastructure of human cataract in retinitis pigmentosa. Arch Ophthalmol 1980; 98:2227–2230.
295. Milam AH, Jacobson SG. Photoreceptor rosettes with blue cone opsin immunoreactivity in retinitis pigmentosa. Ophthalmology 1990; 97:1620–1631.
296. Tulvatana W, Adamian M, Berson EL, Dryja TP. Photoreceptor rosettes in autosomal dominant retinitis pigmentosa with reduced penetrance. Arch Ophthalmol 1999; 117:399–402.
297. Li ZY, Possin DE, Milam AH. Histopathology of bone spicule pigmentation in retinitis pigmentosa. Ophthalmology 1995; 102:805–816.
298. Fariss RN, Li ZY, Milam AH. Abnormalities in rod photoreceptors, amacrine cells, and horizontal cells in human retinas with retinitis pigmentosa. Am J Ophthalmol 2000; 129:215–223.
299. To K, Adamian M, Dryja TP, Berson EL. Retinal histopathology of an autopsy eye with advanced retinitis pigmentosa in a family with rhodopsin Glu181Lys. Am J Ophthalmol 2000; 130:790–792.
300. To K, Adamian M, Dryja TP, Berson EL. Histopathologic study of variation in severity of retinitis pigmentosa due to the dominant rhodopsin mutation Pro23His. Am J Ophthalmol 2002; 134:290–293.
301. To K, Adamian M, Berson EL. Histologic study of retinitis pigmentosa due to a mutation in the RP13 gene (PRPC8): comparison with rhodopsin Pro23His, Cys110Arg, and Glu181Lys. Am J Ophthalmol 2004; 137:946–948.
302. Fishman GA, Cunha-Vaz J, Salzano T. Vitreous fluorophotometry in patients with retinitis pigmentosa. Arch Ophthalmol 1981; 99:1202–1207.
303. Gieser DK, Fishman GA, Cunha-Vaz J. X-linked recessive retinitis pigmentosa and vitreous fluorophotometry. Arch Ophthalmol 1980; 98:307–310.
304. Fishman GA, Cunha-Vaz JE. Carriers of X-linked recessive retinitis pigmentosa: Investigation by vitreous fluorophotometry. Int Ophthalmol 1981; 4:37–44.
305. Mallick KS, Zeimer RC, Fishman GA, et al. Transport of fluorescein in the ocular posterior segment in retinitis pigmentosa. Arch Ophthalmol 1984; 102:691–696.
306. Ogura Y, Cunha-Vaz JG, Zeimer RC. Evaluation of vitreous body integrity in retinitis pigmentosa by vitreous fluorophotometry. Arch Ophthalmol 1987; 105:517–519.
307. Travassos A, Fishman G, Cunha-Vaz JG. Vitreous fluorophotometry studies in retinitis pigmentosa. Graefes Arch Glin Exp Ophthalmol 1985; 222:237–240.
308. Miyakae Y, Goto S, Ota I, Ichikawa H. Vitreous fluorophotometry in patients with cone-rod dystrophy. Br J Ophthalmol 1984; 68:489–493.
309. Newsome DA. Retinal fluorescein leakage in retinitis pigmentosa. Am J Ophthalmol 1986; 101:354–360.
310. Birch DG, Sandberg MA. Dependence of cone b-wave implicit time on rod amplitude in retinitis pigmentosa. Vision Res 1987; 27:1105–1112.
311. Ripps H, Brin KP, Weale RA. Rhodopsin and visual threshold in retinitis pigmentosa. Invest Ophthalmol Vis Sci 1978; 17:735–745.
312. Fulton AB, Hansen RM. The relation of rhodopsin and scoptopic retinal sensitivity in sector retinitis pigmentosa. Am J Ophthalmol 1988; 105:132–140.
313. Van Meel GH, Van Nooren D. Foveal densitometry in retinitis pigmentosa. Invest Ophthalmol Vis Sci 1983; 24:1123–1130.
314. Kilbride PE, Fishman M, Fishman GA, Hutman LP. Foveal cone pigment density difference and reflectance in retinitis pigmentosa. Arch Ophthalmol 1986; 104:220–224.

315. Alexander KR, Hutman LP, Fishman GA. Abnormal foveal spectral sensitivity in retinitis pigmentosa. Invest Ophthalmol Vis Sci 1987; 28:725–730.
316. Alexander KR, Kilbride PE, Fishman GA, Fishman M. Macular pigment and reduced foveal short-wavelength sensitivity in retinitis pigmentosa. Vision Res 1987; 27: 1077–1083.
317. Birch DG, Sandberg MA, Bersion EL. The Stiles-Crawford effect in retinitis pigmentosa. Invest Ophthalmol Vis Sci 1982; 22:157–164.
318. Arden GB. Rod-cone interactions in night-blinding disease. Jpn J Ophthalmol 1987; 31:6–19.
319. Merin S, Maggiano JM, Fishman GA. Retinal sensitivity under photopic conditions in patients with retinitis pigmentosa and carriers of the X-linked recessive form. Metab Ophthalmol 1978; 2:225–229.
320. Birch DG, Sandberg MA, Berson EL. Diurnal rhythm in the human rod ERG. Relationship to cyclic lighting. Invest Ophthalmol Vis Sci 1986; 27:268–270.
321. Sandberg MA, Baruzzi CM, Hanson AH, Berson EL. Rod ERG diurnal rhythm in some patients with dominant retinitis pigmentosa. Invest Ophthalmol Vis Sci 1988; 29:494–498.
322. Birch DG. Diurnal rhythm in the human rod ERG: retinitis pigmentosa. Invest Ophthalmol Vis Sci 1987; 28:2042–2048.
323. Arden GB, Fox B. Increased incidence of abnormal nasal cilia in patients with retinitis pigmentosa. Nature 1979; 279:534–536.
324. Arden GB, Fox B. Retinitis pigmentosa. a generalized disease of cilia [Abstract] Invest Ophthalmol Vis Sci 1979; 18(suppl) 206.
325. Finkelstein D, Reissig M, Kashima U, et al. Nasal cilia in retinitis pigmentosa. Birth Defects 1982; 18:197–206.
326. Lee RMKW, Rossman CM, Forrest JB, et al. No evidence for pathological ciliary structure in retinitis pigmentosa. J Clin Dysmorphol 1983; 1:29–30.
327. Hunter DG, Fishman GA, Mehta RS, et al. Abnormal sperm and photoreceptor axonemes in Usher's syndrome. Arch Ophthalmol 1986; 104:385–389.
328. Hunter DG, Fishman GA, Kretzer FL. Abnormal axonemes in X-linked retinitis pigmentosa. Arch Ophthalmol 1988; 106:362–368.
329. Bastiaensen LA, Ruitenbeek W, Stadhouders AM, et al. Neuromuscular investigations in retinitis pigmentosa. Ophthalmologica 1987; 194:185–187.
330. Hooks JJ, Detrick-Hooks B, Geis S, Newsome DA. Retinitis pigmentosa associated with a defect in the production of interferon-gamma. Am J Ophthalmol 1983; 96:755–758.
331. Ben-Ezra D, Gery I, Chan C, et al. Cellular and humoral immune parameters among patients with RP and other retinal disorders. Ophthalmic Paediatr Genet 1984; 4: 193–197.
332. Hendricks RL, Fishman GA. Cellular immune function of patients with retinitis pigmentosa. Invest Ophthalmol Vis Sci 1986; 27:356–363.
333. Detrick B, Rodrigues MM, Chan CC, et al. Expression of HLA-DR antigen on retinal pigment epithelial cells in retinitis pigmentosa. Am J Ophthalmol 1986; 101:584–590.
334. Hendricks RL, Fishman GA. Interferon-gamma production and HLA-DR expression in patients with retinitis pigmentosa. Exp Eye Res 1987; 45:923–931.
335. Chen MC, Marak GE, Pilkerton AR. The incidence of HLA-SD antigens in recessive retinitis pigmentosa. Br J Ophthalmol 1978; 62:172–173.
336. Newsome DA, Fishman GA. Research update: report on retinitis pigmentosa and the immune system workshop 7–8 November 1985. Exp Eye Res 1986; 43:1–5.
337. Anderson RE, Maude MB, Lewis RA, et al. Abnormal plasma levels of polyunsaturated fatty acid in autosomal dominant retinitis pigmentosa. Exp Eye Res 1987; 44:155–159.
338. Converse CA, McLachlan T, Bow AC et al. Lipid metabolism in retinitis pigmentosa. Prog Clin Biol Res 1987; 247:93–101..

339. Bazan NG, Scott BL, Reddy TS, Pelias HZ. Decreased content of docosahexaenoate and arachidonate in plasma phospholipids in Usher's syndrome. Biochem Biophys Res Comm 1986; 141:600–604.
340. Jahn CE, Oette K, Esser A, et al. Increased prevalence of apolipoprotein E2 in patients with retinitis pigmentosa. Ophthalmic Res 1987; 19:285–288.
341. Massoud WH, Bird AC, Perkins ES. Plasma vitamin A and beta-carotene in retinitis pigmentosa. Br J Ophthalmol 1975; 59:200–204.
342. Zheng JZ, Xiao WJ, Liu SL, et al. Vitamin A metabolism in primary retinitis pigmentosa. Metab Pediatr Syst Ophthalmol 1987; 10:99–102.
343. Hussain AA, Voaden MJ. Some observations on taurine homeostasis in patients with retinitis pigmentosa. Prog Clin Biol Res 1987; 247:119–129.
344. Silverstone B, Berson D, Eilat W, Kuperman O. Copper metabolism changes in pigmentary retinopathies and high myopia. Metab Pediatr Syst Ophthalmol 1981; 5:49–53.
345. Ghalot DK, Khosla PK, Makashir PD, et al. Copper metabolism in retinitis pigmentosa. Br J Ophthalmol 1976; 60:770–774.
346. Ehlers N, Bulow N. Clinical copper metabolism parameters in patients with retinitis pigmentosa and other tapeto-retinal degenerations. Br J Ophthalmol 1977; 61:595–596.
347. Marmor MF, Nelson JW, Levin AS. Cooper metabolism in American retinitis pigmentosa patients. Br J Ophthalmol 1978; 62:168–171.
348. Tsata-Voyatzoglou V, Voyatzogluo B, Roussos I. Cu, Zn and SOD determination in patients with retinitis pigmentosa. Trans Ophthalmol Soc UK 1986; 105:345–347.
349. Silverstone B, Berson D, Seelenfreund MH. Plasma zinc levels in high myopia and retinitis pigmentosa. Metab Ophthalmol 1981; 5:187–190.
350. Heller J, Bok D. A specific receptor for retinol binding protein as detected by the binding of human and bovine retinol binding protein to pigment epithelial cells. Am J Ophthalmol 1976; 81:93–97.
351. Liou GI, Bridges CDB, Fong SL. Vitamin A transport between retina and pigment epithelium: an interphotoreceptor matrix protein carrying endogenous retinal (IRBP). Invest Ophthalmol Vis Sci 1982; 22(suppl):65.
352. Rodrigues MM, Wiggert B, Tso MOM, Chader GJ. Retinitis pigmentosa: immunihistochemical and biochemical studies of the retina. Can J Ophthalmol 1986; 21:79–83.
353. Schmidt SY, Heth CA, Edwards RB, et al. Identification of proteins in retinas and IPM from eyes with retinitis pigmentosa. Invest Ophthalmol Vis Sci 1988; 29:1585–1593.
354. Bergsma DR, Wiggert BN, Funahash M, et al. Vitamin A receptors in normal and dystrophic human retina. Nature 1977; 265:66–67.
355. Bridges CDB, Alvarez RA. Selective loss of 11-*cis* vitamin A in an eye with hereditary chorioretinal degeneration similar to sector RP. Retina 1982; 2:256–260.
356. Hewitt AT, Newsome DA. Altered glycoconjugates in cultures of retinitis pigmentosa retinal pigment epithelium. Prog Clin Biol Res 1987; 247:79–92.
357. Hewitt AT, Newsome DA. Altered proteoglycans in cultured human retinitis pigmentosa retinal pigment epithelium. Invest Ophthalmol Vis Sci 1988; 29:720–726.
358. Springer M. Tissue culture method sheds light on retinitis pigmentosa. Arch Ophthalmol 1986; 104:1758.
359. Herron WL, Riegel BW, Myers OE, Rubin ML. Retinal dystrophy in the rat: a pigment epithelial disease. Invest Ophthalmol 1969; 8:595–604.
360. Bok D, Hall MO. The role of pigment epithelium in the etiology of inherited retinal dystrophy in the rat. J Cell Biol 1971; 49:664–682.
361. Mullen RJ, La Vail MM. Inherited retinal dystrophy: primary defect in pigment epithelium determined with experiemtnal rat chimeras. Science 1976; 192:799–801.
362. Goldman AI, O'Brien PJ. Phagocytosis in the retinal pigment epithelium of the RCS rat. Science 1978; 201:1023–1025.
363. Batelle BA, La Vail MM. Protein synthesis in retinas of rats with inherited retinal dystrophy. Exp Eye Res 1980; 31:251–269.

364. Caldwell RB, McLaughlin BJ, Boykins LG. Intramembrane changes in retinal pigment epithelial cell junctions of the dystrophic rat retina. Invest Ophthalmol Vis Sci 1982; 23:305–318.
365. Li X, Turner JE. Inherited retinal dystrophy in the RCS rat: prevention of photoreceptor degeneration by pigment epithelial cell transplantation. Exp Eye Res 1988; 47: 911–917.
366. Lopez R, Gouras P, Kielbye H, et al. Transplanted retinal pigment epithelium modifies the retinal degeneration in the RCS rat. Invest Ophthalmol Vis Sci 1989; 30:586–588.
367. Silverman MS, Hughes SE. Transplantation of photoreceptors to light-damaged retina. Invest Ophthalmol Vis Sci 1989; 30:1684–1690.
368. Yamamoto S, Du J, Gouras P, Kjeldbye H. Retinal pigment epithelial transplants and retinal function in RCS rats. Invest Ophthalmol Vis Sci 1993; 34:3068–3075.
369. Zhang X, Bok D. Transplantation of retinal pigment epithelial cells and immune response in the subretinal space. Invest Ophthalmol Vis Sci 1998; 39:1021–1027.
370. Lai YL, Jacoby RO, Jonas AM, Papermaster DS. A new form of hereditary retinal degeneration in Wag/Rij rats. Invest Ophthalmol 1975; 14:62–67.
371. Frank RN, Keirn RJ, Keirn GV, et al. Retinal dystrophy: development retarded by galactose feeding in spontaneously hypertensive rats. Science 1986; 231:376–378.
372. Farber DB, Lolley RN. Cyclic guanosine monophosphate: elevation in degenerating photoreceptor cells of the C3H mouse retina. Science 1984; 186:449–451.
373. Matthes MT, Bok D. Blood vascular abnormalities in the degenerative mouse retina. Invest Ophthalmol Vis Sci 1984; 25:364–369.
374. Sanyal S, Hawkins RK, Zeilmaker GH. Development and degeneration of retina in rds mutant mice; analysis of interphotoreceptor matrix staining in chimaeric retina. Curr Eye Res 1988; 7:1183–1190.
375. Aguirre G, Farber D, Lolley R, et al. Rod-cone dysplasia in Irish setters: a defect in cyclic GMP metabolism in visual cells. Science 1978; 201:1133–1134.
376. Bujyukmich N, Aguirre G, Marshall J. Retinal degenerations in the dog: II. Development of the retina in rod-cone dysplasia. Exp Eye Res 1980; 30:575–591.
377. Schmidt SY, Andley UP, Heth CA, Miller J. Deficiency in light-dependent opsin phosphorylation in Irish setters with rod-cone dysplasia. Invest Ophthalmol Vis Sci 1986; 27:1551–1559.
378. Aguirre G, Alligood J, O'Brien P, Buyukmichi N. Pathogenesis of progressive rod-cone degeneration in miniature poodles. Invest Ophthalmol Vis Sci 1982; 23:610–630.
379. Aguirre G, O'Brien P. Morphological and biochemical studies of canine progressive rod-cone degeneration. Invest Ophthalmol Vis Sci 1986; 27:635–655.
380. Narfstrom K, Nilsson SE. Progressive retinal atrophy in the Abyssinian cat: electron microscopy. Invest Ophthalmol Vis Sci 1986; 27:1569–1576.
381. Bridges CDB, Alvarez RA, Fong SL, et al. Rhodopsin, vitamin A and interstitial retinol-binding protein in the *rd* chicken. Invest Ophthalmol Vis Sci 1987; 28:613–617.
382. Semple-Rowland SL, Lee NR, Van Hooser JP, Palczewski K, Baehr W. A null mutation in the photoreceptor guanylate cyclase gene causes the retinal degeneration chicken phenotype. Proc Natl Acad Sci USA 1998; 95:1271–1276.
383. Hayes KC, Carey RE, Schmidt SY. Retinal degeneration associated with taurine deficiency in the cat. Science 1975; 188:949–951.
384. Hayes KC. Retinal degeneration in monkeys induced by deficiencies of vitamin E or A. Invest Ophthalmol 1974; 13:499–510.
385. Li ZY, Wong F, Chang JH, Possin DE, Hao Y, Petters RM, Milam AH. Rhodopsin transgenic pigs as a model for human retinitis pigmentosa. Invest Ophthalmol Vis Sci 1998; 39:808–819.
386. Kedzierski W, Lloyd M, Birch DG, Bok D, Travis GH. Generation and analysis of transgenic mice expressing P216L-substituted rds/peripherin in rod photoreceptors. Invest Ophthalmol Vis Sci 1997; 38:498–509.

387. McNally N, Kenna P, Humphries MM, Hobson AH, Khan NW, Bush RA, Sieving PA, Humphries P, Farrar GJ. Structural and functional rescue of murine rod photoreceptors by human rhodopsin transgene. Hum Mol Genet 1999; 8:1309–1312.
388. Bunker CH, Berson EL, Bromley WC, et al. Prevalence of retinitis pigmentosa in Maine. Am J Ophthalmol 1984; 97:357–365.
389. Bundey S, Crews SJ. A study of retinitis pigmentosa in the city of Birmingham. J Med Genet 1984; 21:417–420.
390. Hu DN. Prevalence and mode of inheritance of major genetic eye diseases in China. J Med Genet 1987; 24:584–588.
391. Philips CI, Stokoe NL, Hughes HE. An ophthalmic genetics clinic. Trans Ophthalmol Soc UK 1975; 95:472–476.
392. Haim M. Epidemiology of retinitis pigmentosa in Denmark. Acta Ophthalmol Scand Suppl 2002; 233:1–34.
393. Wong F. Photoreceptor apoptosis in animal models. Implications for retinitis pigmentosa research. Arch Ophthalmol 1995; 113:1245–1247.
394. Shady S, Hood DC, Birch DG. Rod phototransduction in retinitis pigmentosa. Distinguishing alternative mechanisms of degeneration. Invest Ophthalmol Vis Sci 1995; 36:1027–1037.
395. Dryja TP, Li T. Molecular genetics of retinitis pigmentosa. Hum Mol Gene 1995; 4 Spec No:1739–1743.
396. Phelan JK, Bok D. A brief review of retinitis pigmentosa and the identified retinitis pigmentosa genes. Mol Vis 2000; 6:116–124.
397. Bessant DA, Ali RR, Bhattacharya SS. Molecular genetics prospects for therapy of the inherited retinal dystrophies. Curr Opin Genet Dev 2001; 11:307–316.
398. Travis GH, Hepler JE. A medley of retinal dystrophies. Nat Genet 1993; 3:191–192.
399. Voipio H, Grippenburg U, Raitta C, Horsmanheimo A. Retinitis pigmentosa: a preliminary report. Hereditas 1964; 52:247.
400. Amman F, Klein D, Franceschetti A. Genetic and epidemiological investigations on pigmentary degeneration of the retina and allied disorders in Switzerland. J Neurol Sci 1965; 2:183–196.
401. Panteleeva OA. On hereditary tapeto-retinal degenerations. Vestn Oftalmol 1969; 82:53–56.
402. Jay B. Hereditary aspects of pigmentary retinopathy. Trans Ophthalmol Soc UK 1972; 92:173–178.
403. Fishman GA. Retinitis pigmentosa: genetic percentages. Arch Ophthalmol 1978; 96:822–826.
404. Hu DN. Genetic aspects of retinitis pigmentosa in China. Am J Med Genet 1982; 12: 51–56.
405. Boughman JA, Fishman GA. A genetic analysis of retinitis pigmentosa. Br J Ophthalmol 1983; 67:449–454.
406. Bundey S, Crews SJ. A study of retinitis pigmentosa in the city of Birmingham. II. Clinical and genetic heterogeneity. J Med Genet 1984; 21:421–428.
407. Zeng LH, Wu DZ, Ma QY, Wu LH. Genetic study of retinitis pigmentosa in China. Ophthalmologica 1987; 194:34–39.
408. Havener WH. Evaluation of therapeutic response. In New Orleans Academy of Ophthalmology Symposium on Ocular Pharmacology and Therapeutics. St Louis, CV Mosby 1970:18–19.
409. Ham WT, Mueller HA, Sliney D. Nature of retinal radiation damage: Dependence on wavelength, power level and exposure time. Vis Res 1980; 20:1105–1111.
410. Young RW. Solar radiation and age-related macular degeneration. Surv Ophthalmol 1988; 32:252–269.
411. Berson EL. Experimental and therapeutic aspects of photic damage to the retina. Invest Ophthalmol 1973; 12:35–44.
412. Berson EL. Light deprivation and retinitis pigmentosa. Vision Res 1980; 20:1179–1184.

413. Miller D. The effect of sunglasses on the visual mechanism. Surv Ophthalmol 1974; 19:38–44.
414. Berson EL, Rosner B, Sandberg MA, Hayes KC, Nicholson BW, Weigel-DiFranco C, Willett W. A randomized trial of vitamin A and vitamin E supplementation for retinitis pigmentosa. Arch Ophthalmol 1993; 111:761–772.
415. Li T, Sandberg MA, Pawlyk BS, Rosner B, Hayes KC, Dryja TP, Berson EL. Effect of vitamin A supplementation on rhodopsin mutants threonine-17 –> methionine and proline-347 –> serine in transgenic mice and in cell cultures. Proc Natl Acad Sci USA 1998; 95:11933–11938.
416. Massof RW, Finkelstein D. Supplemental vitamin A retards loss of ERG amplitude in retinitis pigmentosa. Arch Ophthalmol 1993; 111:751–754.
417. Ehrlich D. A comparative study in the use of closed-circuit television reading machines and optical aids by patients with retinitis pigmentosa and maculopathy. Ophthalmic Physiol Opt 1987; 7:293–302.
418. Marmor MF. The management of retinitis pigmentosa and allied diseases. Ophthalmol Digest 1979; 41:13–29.
419. Berson EL, Mehaffey L, Rabin AR. A night vision pocketscope for patients with retinitis pigmentosa: Design considerations. Arch Ophthalmol 1974; 91:495–500.
420. Alaux F, Chauveau N, Bee P, Morucci JP. Aide visuelle electronique par amplificateur de luminance dans les alterations de la vision nocturne. J Fr Ophthalmol 1986; 9: 191–197.
421. Ansell PL, Marshall J. Laser induced phagocytosis in the pigment epithelium of the Hunter dystrophic rat. Br J Ophthalmol 1976; 60:819–828.
422. Behbehani MM, Bowyer DW, Ruffolo JJ, Kranias G. Preservation of retinal function in the RCS rat by laser treatment. Retina 1984; 4(4):257–263.
423. Spallone A. Retinal fluorescein leakage in retinitis pigmentosa. Am J Ophthalmol 1986; 102:408–409.
424. Newsome DA, Blacharski PA. Grid photocoagulation for macular edema in patients with retinitis pigmentosa. Am J Ophthalmol 1987; 103:161–166.
425. Heckenlively JR. Grid photocoagulation for macular edema in patients with retinitis pigmentosa. Am J Ophthalmol 1987; 104:94–95.
426. Berson EL, Remulla JF, Rosner B, Sandberg MA, Weigel-DiFranco C. Evaluation of patients with retinitis pigmentosa receiving electric stimulation, ozonated blood, and ocular surgery in Cuba. Arch Ophthalmol 1997; 115:1215–1216.
427. Gerding H. Evaluation of patients with retinitis pigmentosa receiving electric stimulation, ozonated blood, ocular surgery in Cuba. Arch Ophthalmol 1997; 115:1215–1216.
428. Bacal DA, Rousta S, Hertle RW, Maguire A. Restrictive strabismus after ocular surgery for retinitis pigmentosa in Cuba. Arch Ophthalmol 1997; 115:930–931.
429. Weleber RG. The Cuban experience. False hope for a cure for retinitis pigmentosa. Arch Ophthalmol 1996; 114:606–607.
430. Fishman GA, Gilbert LD, Fiscella RG, Kimura AE, Jampol LM. Acetazolamide for treatment of chronic macular edema in retinitis pigmentosa. Arch Ophthalmol 1989; 107:1445–1452.
431. Orzalesi N, Pierrottet C, Porta A, Aschero M. Long-term treatment of retinitis pigmentosa with acetazolamide. A pilot study. Graefes Arch Clin Exp Ophthalmol 1993; 231:254–256.
432. Grover S, Fishman GA, Fiscella RG, Adelman AE. Efficacy of dorzolamide hydrochloride in the management of chronic cystoid macular edema in patients with retinitis pigmentosa. Retina 1997; 17:222–231.
433. Baster JV, Heckenlively JR, Straatsma BR. Cataract surgery in retinitis pigmentosa patients. Ophthalmology 1982; 89:880–884.
434. Newsome DA, Stark WJ, Maumenne IH. Cataract extraction and intraocular lens implantation in patients with retinitis pigmentosa or Usher's syndrome. Arch Ophthalmol 1986; 104:852–854.

435. Newsome DA, Dorsey FC, May JG, et al. Ganglioside administration in retinitis pigmentosa. J Ocular Pharmacol 1987; 3:323–332.
436. Wheaton DH, Hoffman DR, Locke KG, Watkins RB, Birch DG. Biological safety assessment of docosahexaenoic acid supplementation in a randomized clinical trial for X-linked retinitis pigmentosa. Arch Ophthalmol 2003; 121:1269–1278.
437. Hoffman DR, Locke KG, Wheaton DH, Fish GE, Spencer R, Birch DG. A randomized, placebo-controlled clinical trial of docosahexaenoic acid supplementation for X-linked retinitis pigmentosa. Am J Ophthalmol 2004; 137:704–718.
438. del Cerro M, Lazar ES, Diloreto D Jr. The first decade of continuous progress in retinal transplantation. Microsc Res Tech 1997; 36:130–41.
439. Peyman GA, Blinder KJ, Paris CL, Alturki W, Nelson NC Jr, Desai U. A technique for retinal pigment epithelium transplantation for age-related macular degeneration secondary to extensive subfoveal scarring. Ophthalmic Surg 1991; 22:102–108.
440. Algvere PV, Berglin L, Gouras P, Sheng Y. Transplantation of fetal retinal pigment epithelium in age-related macular degeneration with subfoveal neovascularization. Graefes Arch Clin Exp Ophthalmol 1994; 232:707–716.
441. Gouras P, Algvere P. Retinal cell transplantation in the macula: new techniques. Vis Res 1996; 36:4121–4125.
442. Algvere PV, Berglin L, Gouras P, Sheng Y, Kopp ED. Transplantation of RPE in age-related macular degeneration: observations in diskiform lesions and dry RPE atrophy. Graefes Arch Clin Exp Ophthalmol 1997; 235:149–158.
443. Li LX, Sheedlo HJ, Gaur V, Turner JE. Effects of macrophage and retinal pigment epithelial cell transplants on photoreceptor cell rescue in RCS rats. Curr Eye Res 1991; 10:947–958.
444. Lavail MM, Li L, Turner JE, Yasumura D. Retinal pigment epithelial cell transplantation in RCS rats: normal metabolism in rescued photoreceptors. Exp Eye Res 1992; 55:555–562.
445. Little CW, Castillo B, DiLoreto DA, Cox C, Wyatt J, del Cerro C, del Cerro M. Transplantation of human fetal retinal pigment epithelium rescues photoreceptor cells from degeneration in the Royal College of Surgeons rat retina. Invest Ophthalmol Vis Sci 1996; 37:204–211.
446. Seiler MJ, Aramant RB. Intact sheets of fetal retina transplanted to restore damaged rat retinas. Invest Ophthalmol Vis Sci 1998; 39:2121–2131.
447. Sheng Y, Gouras P, Cao H, Berglin L, Kjeldbye H, Lopez R, Rosskothen H. Patch transplants of human fetal retinal pigment epithelium in rabbit and monkey retina. Invest Ophthalmol Vis Sci 1995; 36:381–390.
448. Berglin L, Gouras P, Sheng Y, Lavid J, Lin PK, Cao H, Kjeldbye H. Tolerance of human fetal retinal pigment epithelium xenografts in monkey retina. Graefes Arch Clin Exp Ophthalmol 1997; 235:103–110.
449. Litchfield TM, Whiteley SJ, Lund RD. Transplantation of retinal pigment epithelial, photoreceptor and other cells as treatment for retinal degeneration. Exp Eye Res 1997; 64:655–666.
450. Oganesian A, Gabrielian K, Ernest JT, Patel SC. A new model of retinal pigment epithelium transplantation with microspheres. Arch Ophthalmol 1999; 117:1192–1200.
451. Tezel TH, Del Priore LV. Reattachment to a substrate prevents apoptosis of human retinal pigment epithelium. Graefes Arch Clin Exp Ophthalmol 1997; 235:41–47.
452. Thumann G, Bartz-Schmidt KU, El Bakri H, Schraermeyer U, Spee C, Cui JZ, Hinton DR, Ryan SJ, Heimann K. Transplantation of autologous iris pigment epithelium to the subretinal space in rabbits. Transplantation 1999; 68:195–201.
453. Thumann G, Aisenbrey S, Schraermeyer U, Lafaut B, Esser P, Walter P, Bartz-Schmidt KU. Transplantation of autologous iris pigment epithelium after removal of choroidal neovascular membranes. Arch Ophthalmol 2000; 118:1350–1355.
454. Schraermeyer U, Kayatz P, Thumann G, Luther TT, Szurman P, Kociok N, Bartz-Schmidt KU. Transplantation of iris pigment epithelium into the choroid slows down

the degeneration of photoreceptors in the RCS rat. Graefes Arch Clin Exp Ophthalmol 2000; 238:979–984.
455. Mohand-Said S, Hicks D, Simonutti M, Tran-Minh D, Deudon-Combe A, Dreyfus H, Silverman MS, Ogilvie JM, Tenkova T, Sahel J. Photoreceptor transplants increase host cone survival in the retinal degeneration (rd) mouse. Ophthalmic Res 1997; 29:290–297.
456. Mohand-Said S, Hicks D, Dreyfus H, Sahel JA. Selective transplantation of rods delays cone loss in a retinitis pigmentosa model. Arch Ophthalmol 2000; 118:807–811.
457. Mohand-Said S, Deudon-Combe A, Hicks D, Simonutti M, Forster V, Fintz AC, Leveillard T, Dreyfus H, Sahel JA. Normal retina releases a diffusible factor stimulating cone survival in the retinal degeneration mouse. Proc Nat Acad Sci USA 1998; 95: 8357–8362.
458. Kaplan HJ, Tezel TH, Berger AS, Wolf ML, Del Priore LV. Human photoreceptor transplantation in retinitis pigmentosa. A safety study. Arch Ophthalmol 1997; 115: 1168–1172.
459. Berger AS, Tezel TH, Del Priore LV, Kaplan HJ. Photoreceptor transplantation in retinitis pigmentosa: short-term follow-up. Ophthalmology 2003; 110:383–391.
460. Das T, del Cerro M, Jalali S, Rao VS, Gullapalli VK, Little C, Loreto DA, Sharma S, Sreedharan A, del Cerro C, Rao GN. The transplantation of human fetal neuroretinal cells in advanced retinitis pigmentosa patients: results of a long-term safety study. Exp Neurol 1999; 157:58–68.
461. Radtke ND, Aramant RB, Seiler M, Petry HM. Preliminary report: indications of improved visual function after retinal sheet transplantation in retinitis pigmentosa patients. Am J Ophthalmol 1999; 128:384–387.
462. Radtke ND, Seiler MJ, Aramant RB, Petry HM, Pidwell DJ. Transplantation of intact sheets of fetal neural retina with its retinal pigment epithelium in retinitis pigmentosa patients. Am J Ophthalmol 2002; 133:544–550.
463. Berson EL, Jakobiec FA. Neural retinal cell transplantation: ideal versus reality. Ophthalmology 1999; 106:445–446.
464. Humayun MS, de Juan E Jr, del Cerro M, Dagnelie G, Radner W, Sadda SR, del Cerro C. Human neural retinal transplantation. Invest Ophthalmol Vis Sci 2000; 41:3100–3106.
465. Hauswirth WW, Lewin AS. Ribozyme uses in retinal gene therapy. Prog Retin Eye Res 2000; 19:689–710.
466. Lewin AS, Drenser KA, Hauswirth WW, Nishikawa S, Yasumura D, Flannery JG, LaVail MM. Ribozyme rescue of photoreceptor cells in a transgenic rat model of autosomal dominant retinitis pigmentosa. Nat Med 1998; 4:967–971.
467. O'Neill B, Millington-Ward S, O'Reilly M, Tuohy G, Kiang AS, Kenna PF, Humphries P, Farrar GJ. Ribozyme-based therapeutic approaches for autosomal dominant retinitis pigmentosa. Invest Ophthalmol Vis Sci 2000; 41:2863–2869.
468. LaVail MM, Yasumura D, Matthes MT, Lau-Villacorta C, Unoki K, Sung CH, Steinberg RH. Protection of mouse photoreceptors by survival factors in retinal degenerations. Invest Ophthalmol Vis Sci 1998; 39:592–602.
469. Frasson M, Sahel JA, Fabre M, Simonutti M, Dreyfus H, Picaud S. Retinitis pigmentosa: rod photoreceptor rescue by a calcium-channel blocker in the rd mouse. Nat Med 1999; 5:1183–1187.
470. Bennett J, Tanabe T, Sun D, Zeng Y, Kjeldbye H, Gouras P, Maguire AM. Photoreceptor cell rescue in retinal degeneration (rd) mice by in vivo gene therapy. Nat Med 1996; 2:649–654.
471. Takahashi M, Miyoshi H, Verma IM, Gage FH. Rescue from photoreceptor degeneration in the rd mouse by human immunodeficiency virus vector-mediated gene transfer. J Virol 1999; 73:7812–7816.
472. Miyoshi H, Takahashi M, Gage FH, Verma IM. Stable and efficient gene transfer into the retina using an HIV-based lentiviral vector. Proc Nat Acad Sci USA 1997; 94: 10319–10323.

473. Acland GM, Aguirre GD, Ray J, Zhang Q, Aleman TS, Cideciyan AV, Pearce-Kelling SE, Anand V, Zeng Y, Maguire AM, Jacobson SG, Hauswirth WW, Bennett J. Gene therapy restores vision in a canine model of childhood blindness. Nat Genet 2001; 28: 92–95.
474. Rizzo JF III, Wyatt J, Humayun M, de Juan E, Liu W, Chow A, Eckmiller R, Zrenner E, Yagi T, Abrams G. Retinal prosthesis: an encouraging first decade with major challenges ahead. Ophthalmology 2001; 108:13–14.
475. Loewenstein JI, Montezuma SR, Rizzo JF III. Outer retinal degeneration: an electronic retinal prosthesis as a treatment strategy. Arch Ophthalmol 2004; 122:587–596.
476. Humayun MS, Weiland JD, Fujii GY, Greenberg R, Williamson R, Little J, Mech B, Cimmarusti V, Van Boemel G, Dagnelie G, de Juan E. Visual perception in a blind subject with a chronic microelectronic retinal prosthesis. Vis Res 2003; 43:2573–2581.
477. Chow AY, Chow VY, Packo KH, Pollack JS, Peyman GA, Schuchard R. The artificial silicon retina microchip for the treatment of vision loss from retinitis pigmentosa. Arch Ophthalmol 2004; 122:460–469.
478. Bundey S, Crews SJ. A study of retinitis pigmentosa in the city of Birmingham. J Med Genet 1986; 23:188.
479. Hogenkamp T, Wienker TF, Majewski F, Gal A. Molekulargenetische Diagnostik bei X-chromosomal vererbter Retinitis pigmentosa. Klin Monatsbl Augenheilkd 1987; 191:307–309.
480. Strom CM, Rechitsky S, Wolf G, Cieslak J, Kuliev A, Verlinsky Y. Preimplantation diagnosis of autosomal dominant retinitis pigmentosum using two simultaneous single cell assays for a point mutation in the rhodopsin gene. Mol Hum Reprod 1998; 4: 351–355.
481. Pawlowitzki IH, Ruther K, Brunsmann F, von Gizycki R. Acceptability of prenatal diagnosis for retinitis pigmentosa. Lancet 1986; 2:1394–1395.
482. Pannarale MR, Grammatico B, Iannaccone A, Forte R, DeBernardo C, Flagiello L, Vingolo EM, Del Porto G. Autosomal-dominant retinitis pigmentosa associated with an Arg-135-Trp point mutation of the rhodopsin gene. Clinical features and longitudinal observations. Ophthalmology 1996; 103:1443–1452.
483. al-Maghtheh M, Kim RY, Hardcastle A, Inglehearn C, Bhattacharya SS. A 150 bp insertion in the rhodopsin gene of an autosomal dominant retinitis pigmentosa family. Hum Mol Genet 1994; 3:205–206.
484. Jacobson SG, Kemp CM, Cideciyan AV, Macke JP, Sung CH, Nathans J. Phenotypes of stop codon and splice site rhodopsin mutations causing retinitis pigmentosa. Invest Ophthalmol Vis Sci 1994; 35:2521–2534.
485. Bessant DA, Khaliq S, Hameed A, Anwar K, Payne AM, Mehdi SQ, Bhattacharya SS. Severe autosomal dominant retinitis pigmentosa caused by a novel rhodopsin mutation (Ter349Glu). Mutations in Brief no. 208. Online. Hum Mutat 1999; 13:83.
486. Milla E, Heon E, Grounauer PA, Piguet B, Ducrey N, Stone EM, Schorderet DF, Munier FL. Rhodopsin C110Y mutation causes a type 2 autosomal dominant retinitis pigmentosa. Ophthalmic Genet 1998; 19:131–139.
487. Hayakawa M, Hotta Y, Imai Y, Fujiki K, Nakamura A, Yanashima K, Kanai A. Clinical features of autosomal dominant retinitis pigmentosa with rhodopsin gene codon 17 mutation and retinal neovascularization in a Japanese patient. Am J Ophthalmol 1993; 115:168–173.
488. OMIM, http: //www.ncbi.nlm.nih.gov/omim/.
489. al-Maghtheh M, Inglehearn CF, Keen TJ, Evans K, Moore AT, Jay M, Bird AC, Bhattacharya SS. Identification of a sixth locus for autosomal dominant retinitis pigmentosa on chromosome 19. Hum Mol Genet 1994; 3:351–354.
490. McGee TL, Devoto M, Ott J, Berson EL, Dryja TP. Evidence that the penetrance of mutations at the RP11 locus causing dominant retinitis pigmentosa is influenced by a gene linked to the homologous RP11 allele. Am J Hum Genet 1997; 61:1059–1066.

491. Wada Y, Abe T, Takeshita T, Sato H, Yanashima K, Tamai M. Mutation of human retinal fascin gene (FSCN2) causes autosomal dominant retinitis pigmentosa. Invest Ophthalmol Vis Sci 2001; 42:2395–2400.
492. Wada Y, Abe T, Itabashi T, Sato H, Kawamura M, Tamai M. Autosomal dominant macular degeneration associated with 208delG mutation in the FSCN2 gene. Arch Ophthalmol 2003; 121:1613–1620.
493. Finckh U, Xu S, Kumaramanickavel G, Schurmann M, Mukkadan JK, Fernandez ST, John S, Weber JL, Denton MJ, Gal A. Homozygosity mapping of autosomal recessive retinitis pigmentosa locus (RP22) on chromosome 16p12.1-p12.3. Genomics 1998; 48:341–345.

11
Syndromic Retinitis Pigmentosa

INTRODUCTION

For many years, ophthalmologists were well aware of the fact that in some cases, retinitis pigmentosa is associated with extraocular abnormalities. Well-known examples were the polydactyly and other abnormalities of what is now called Bardet–Biedl syndrome or the hearing impairment of Usher syndrome. Mutational analysis will detect that some syndromic retinitis pigmentosa (RP) entities and isolated RP are all caused by mutations of the same genes. These will usually be mutation-specific, meaning that the same gene with a different disease-bearing mutation will cause isolated RP, while another mutation will cause a disease included in syndromic RP. In other entities, the disease results from a specific, distinct gene.

RP is the hallmark of these ocular diseases, sometimes associated with other ocular or extraocular abnormalities. Leber congenital amaurosis (LCA), the congenital form of RP, is introduced in this chapter because extraocular abnormalities are often found.

LEBER CONGENITAL AMAUROSIS

LCA is a separate entity from isolated or syndromic RP. Due to its varied clinical manifestations and several subtypes, it may be considered to be a combination of both isolated and syndromic RP. The genes that determine LCA are usually different from those that cause nonsyndromic RP, but in some cases the same gene exists, mutated differently in each of the two groups of diseases.

LCA was considered rare and was not well recognized until two population studies, one from Sweden (1) and the other from Holland (2), proved that it is not.

Description and Clinical Findings

The child with LCA is usually born blind. During the first two three months of life, most parents notice that the child does not follow objects or light, and this is when they seek medical assistance. Connatal blindness was noted in 95% of the cases in one series (3). Nystagmus of the pendular type can be seen in the first months of life. The ERG is markedly subnormal or extinguished, even if performed early in life (4). A few patients have some preserved vision, with visual acuities reaching, in exceptional cases, the 6/60–6/15 range. In one series (3), 94% of the patients had a visual acuity of 6/60 or less, and 6% had 6/30–6/15. The fundus is initially normal, but abnormal changes always develop. These include salt-and-pepper pigmentation, bone corpuscular pigment, attenuation of retinal vessels, atrophy of the RPE and choriocapillaris, and, less commonly, multiple, irregular, yellowish white flecks deep in the peripheral and midperipheral retina (5,6). The fundus changes are progressive, as in late-onset RP, but, in contrast, the functional changes are usually non-progressive. Visual acuity, visual fields, and ERG tend to remain unchanged from what they were at birth. Other ocular abnormalities are commonly found. Hyperopia seems to be a common feature, possibly characteristic of all cases. It is the result of a shortened axial length of the globe, as in microphthalmos without microcornea (7). Keratoconus develops with time; in one series 57% of the patients had keratoconus after 15 years of age. In another study, 10 out of 35 children blind due to LCA (29%) had keratoconus and 3% had keratoglobus (8).

About half of all LCA patients suffer from absolute blindness (no light perception), while median vision in one study was 20/500 (9). Vision was stable in the majority of seeing patients. In rare cases optic disk neovascularization may occur with resulting vitreous hemorrhage (10). This is similar to complications that rarely occur in nonsyndromic RP.

LCA may be associated with macular colobomas, neurologic abnormalities, mental retardation, or renal disease, but all these may be separate entities as well.

The Clinical Types of LCA

Isolated Leber Congenital Amaurosis

This is the most common form of Leber amaurosis. It is transmitted by the autosomal recessive mode. At least two different genes may cause this disease (11). As even this form is rare, its frequency is highest in populations with a high consanguinity rate (4). Foxman and coworkers (12) classified LCA into two groups: (1) uncomplicated and (2) complicated (with a syndrome or neurologic abnormalities). They stressed the differential diagnosis with early onset or juvenile RP. Henkes and Verduin (13) tried to distinguish between Leber amaurosis, in which the EOG is abnormal, and Waardenburg dysgenesis neuroepithelialis, in which the EOG is normal. However, such a differentiation is not substantiated.

LCA Associated with Central Nervous System Abnormalities

Up to 30% of patients with LCA have CNS abnormalities (3). Spastic hyperreflexia, paraparesis, and tetraparesis, decreased gross and fine muscular ability, mental retardation, and deafness, all have been reported (3,12). In addition, markedly delayed milestones and mild mental retardation may be secondary to the severe intellectual impairment resulting from the congenital blindness of these patients (14). Computed tomographic (CT) scan is usually reported to be normal, but hypoplasia of the cerebellar vermis has been reported in Leber amaurosis (14).

Table 1 Clinical Types of Leber Congenital Amaurosis (LCA)

Classification	Clinical characteristics	Inheritance[a]
Isolated LCA	Congenital blindness or severe visual impairment; no extra-ocular abnormalities.	AR
LCA with CNS abnormalities	Congenital blindness or severe visual impairment with neurologic symptoms or mental retardation or deafness	AR Not clear whether or not same as isolated LCA gene(s)
Senior–Loken syndrome	Congenital blindness or severe visual impairment with nephronophthisis	AR
LCA with macular coloboma	Congenital blindness and bilateral macular coloboma	Not yet established as a separate entity
LCA with hyperthreoninemia	Congenital blindness with increased plasma threonine	AR Not yet established as a separate entity
LCA, AD	Congenital severe impairment of vision, with progression to blindness	AD Not yet established as a separate entity

[a]AR—autosomal recessive; AD—autosomal dominant.

It is not clear if Leber amaurosis with neurologic abnormalities is genetically a separate entity from isolated Leber amaurosis, but this is likely. If so, more than one gene may be active in this group (Table 1).

Other Associations of LCA

LCA may be associated with nephronophthisis in the Senior–Loken's syndrome (15). (See under RP with Lipid Disorders.) Isolated reports of LCA associated with macular colobomas may indicate a separate gene (16). Leber amaurosis and hyperthreoninemia was reported in two siblings of one family, possibly indicating a separate genetic entity (17).

A rare autosomal dominant type of Leber congenital amaurosis was reported by Heckenlively as the fifth family known to have this disease. The disease started with a maculopathy and progressed to light perception in adulthood, possibly indicating that it is an aggressive type of cone–rod dystrophy and not Leber amaurosis (18).

The Genetic Types of LCA

With the identification of the first gene associated with LCA in 1995 (19), it became clear that LCA is a heterogenous disorder. Later, the number of genes involved turned out to be unexpectedly high. (Table 2).

LCA1 and the GUCY2D Gene

Initially, LCAl was mapped to chromosome 17pl3.1 (19,20) in families of Tunisian origin. It was later identified in British, Finnish, and other families. GUCY2D is a retinal-specific guanylate cyclase, a transmembrane enzyme involved in the production

Table 2 The Genetic Types of LCA

Locus/ symbol	Gene/Protein	Chromosomal location	Remarks
LCA1	GUCY2D/guanylate cyclase	17p13.1	6.3–21.2% of all LCA, 7% of ADCORD
LCA2	RPE65	1p31.2	Other mutations cause RP2D
LCA3	—	14q24	In Saudi Arabia
LCA4	A1PL1/aryl hydrocarbon-interacting receptor protein-like	17p13.2	5% of all LCA
LCA5	—	6q11–q16	
LCA6	RPGRIP1/RPGTPase regulator interacting protein 1	14q11.2	6% of all LCA
LCA9	—	1p36	One Pakistani family
—	CRX/cone–rod homeobox	19q13.32	0.6–3% of LCA, AD lCA
—	CRB1 crumbs homolog	1q31.3	9–13% of LCA Coats-like disease
—	TULP1/tubby-like	6p21.3	1.7% of LCA

of intracellular cGMP. The gene consists of 20 exons. In 1996, Perrault and coworkers reported finding (21) mutations in this gene associated with LCAl. Many mutations were family-specific. Other mutations were associated with autosomal recessive or autosomal dominant cone–rod dystrophy, or rod–cone dystrophy.

GUCY2D encodes a transmembrane enzyme found in the outer segments of both rods and cones that is located in the disk membrane. Mutated GUCY2D results in abnormally low levels of cGMP, which induces permanent closure of the cGMP-gated ion channels, corresponding to permanent light exposure (22).

Koenekoop et al. (22) also claimed that, unlike other genetic types of LCA, in GUCY2D-associated LCA, ERG characteristic changes are found in obligatory carriers.

Lotery and associates (23) and Hanein and associates (24) calculated the frequency of the different genetic subtypes of LCA in 176 and 179 LCA patients, respectively. Mutations were identified in about half the LCA patients (24). GUCY2D mutations were identified in 6.3% in one study (23) and 21.2% in another (24).

LCA2 and the RPE65 Gene

In LCA2 mutations in RPE65, an RPE specific protein of unknown function was identified (25). The gene was mapped to chromosome lp31. It contains 14 coding exons and encodes a 65 kD protein (hence its name). An RPE65-associated mutation was detected in 6.1–6.8% of LCA patients (23,24).

LCA3

The locus LCA3 was mapped to chromosome 14q24 in a single Saudi-Arabian family by Stockton and associates (26). The gene is unknown and it is not known whether more affected families exist.

LCA4 and the AIPL1 Gene

LCA4 locus was mapped within the area of GUCY2D but no mutations were identified in this gene (27). Mutations were later identified in the gene encoding aryl hydrocarbon receptor interacting protein-like 1 (AIPL1). It probably involves about 5% of LCA patients (28).

LCA5

A novel locus for LCA, named LCA5, was mapped to chromosome 6qll–ql6 in a large family of Swiss origin (29). Several candidate genes in this area were checked but no LCA-associated mutations have been identified.

LCA6 and RPGRIPl Gene

RPGRIP1, a newly identified gene (named for RPGR-interacting-protein 1) interacts with RPGR, a gene known to be associated, when mutated, with X-linked retinitis pigmentosa (30). It was mapped to chromosome 14qll. The gene encodes a protein of 1259 ammo acids (30). Mutations comprise about 6% of LCA patients.

LCA9

The locus termed LCA9 was mapped to chromosome lp36 in one large and consanguineous Pakistani family (31). This location is near the telomene, and in spite of careful search, the disease-bearing gene has not been not identified.

The CRX Gene

The CRX or cone–rod homeobox-containing gene encodes a protein named cone–rod otx-like photoreceptor homeobox transcription, which is essential for normal maintenance of photoreceptors and for early photoreceptor development (32). It is found in both cones and rods. Generally, premature termination, codon mutations, and less frequently, missense mutations were identified in families with autosomal dominant cone–rod dystrophy (ADCORD), and in families with autosomal dominant LCA (32–34).

The mutation locus was mapped to chromosome 19ql3.32. About 3% of all LCA cases are associated with CRX mutations (23).

The CRBl Gene

Mutations in the CRB1 gene are known to be associated with RP12, an especially severe type of RP. The most common mutation resulting in RP12 was a missense mutation, Cys948Tyr (35). CRB1 mutations leading to LCA were identified in 9% of 190 LCA patients in one study (35), 13% in another study (36), and 10% in a third (24). The gene, a crumbs homolog of *Drosophila*, was mapped to chromosome lq31.3. Both CRB1-associated RP and LCA were found to be affected by a very severe complication of their retinal dystrophy, Coats-like exudative retinopathy (37).

The TULPl Gene

LCA was associated with a tubby-like protein 1 TULP1 gene mutation in one Dominican family (35). Later, a TULP1 mutation was identified in 1.7% of patients with LCA (24). The protein is well known to be associated with nonsyndromic autosomal recessive RP. It was mapped to chromosome 6p21.3.

Pathology of Leber Amaurosis

A pathologic study by Mizuno and coworkers on the eyes of a 16-year-old Japanese girl with Leber amaurosis showed that the subretinal deposits, corresponding to ophthalmoscopically seen white spots, consisted of loose outer segments, apical processes of RPE, and macrophages. Rod outer segments were missing, the few cones that were seen were abnormal, and other cells resembled undifferentiated photoreceptors and embryonal RPE cells (38). These findings imply an immaturity and undifferentiation of both photoreceptors and RPE cells as the cause of the disease. A study of the eye of a 6-month-old baby with Leber amaurosis, associated with neurologic abnormalities, also revealed apparently normal inner segments and shortened and abnormal outer segments (3).

USHER SYNDROME

Usher syndrome is the most common disease associated with RP. Usher described the syndrome at the beginning of the century in several patients who suffered from RP and deafness (39).

Sensorineural hearing loss, in general, is not uncommon in patients with RP. Audiologic testing in 45 patients with RP revealed that 10 (22%) had a hearing loss that varied from mild to severe (40). Probably not all of these represent actual cases of Usher syndrome, which should be diagnosed only if deafness and RP coincide or if progresive sensorineural hearing loss coincides with RP in affected members of the family.

Clinical Aspects of Usher Syndrome

The prevalence of Usher syndrome was estimated as ranging between 1.8:100,000 and 3.5:100,000 on the basis of a series of studies from different countries (4). If the higher figure is true for most populations, as is likely, then about 15% of all RP patients have Usher syndrome. It was estimated that two–thirds of deaf–blind people in the United States suffer from Usher syndrome (41).

Four clinical types of Usher syndrome can be distinguished and may be termed types I–IV (42). The first two types are definite separate genetic entities. Although the last two types differ clinically, they are not necessarily caused by different genes (Table 3). In order to avoid confusion, I will use the current method of classification which divides Usher syndrome into three subtypes. In a recent study on prevalence and clinical classification, Hope and coworkers (43) found a prevalence of Usher syndrome of 6.2 per 100,000 people in Birmingham, which is higher than previous figures. The division of the subtypes was 33% for type I, 47% for type II, and 20% for type III (43).

In Usher syndrome type I, both hearing loss and retinal function loss are more severe, and are found earlier than in type II. The neurosensory deafness is congenital and complete (about 100 dB or more), vestibular functions are absent or abnormal, and visual fields become tubular in the second decade of life (42). In another series, patients complained of night blindness in the first decade of life, had nonrecordable

Table 3 The Clinical Types

Type	Decade of onset of night blindness	Visual fields 20° or less in decade	Hearing loss	Speech	Vestibular function	Vestibular ataxia
I	First	Second	Congenital, profound loss of 100 dB	Unintelligible	Absent or present	Absent or present
II	Second to third	Third or fourth	Congenital, moderate 30–40 dB loss variable	Intelligible	Absent	Absent
III	Second to third	Third or fourth	Initially normal, progressive loss of 40–60 dB in third decade	Intelligible	Absent	Absent

ERGs and unintelligible speech. Intrafamilial similarities were the rule. At the age of 29, 11% had a visual acuity of 6/30 or less (44).

In some patients with Usher type I, ataxia of vestibular source is apparent. This type was described as common in a large series of patients in Sweden studied by Hallgren (45). It was described as relatively common among Usher syndrome patients in Sweden but it is rather rare in other populations (4,46). Mental retardation may sometimes be found in Usher type I patients. In some populations Usher type I is the most common subtype (4,47). In other populations type II is more common (44,43).

In Usher syndrome type II, congenital hearing impairment is much less than in type I. Audiograms indicate a reduction in hearing by 30–40 dB compared to 90–100 dB in type I. Night blindness may appear in the second year of life along with a reduction in visual fields. Speech is often, but not always, intelligible. Vestibular function is normal.

In Usher syndrome type III, newborns have normal vision and auditory functions. Gradual and slow reductions in night and day vision occur, along with progressive impairment of hearing. Speech is usually normal. The hearing loss is of varying degrees, with interfamilial variability often encountered (42), and is generally of late occurrence (48).

Visual acuity is also variable. Both visual acuity and visual fields are less affected than in type I and may remain quite good during the third and fourth decades of life (36). In one study only 2% of patients had a visual acuity of 20/100 or less (49).

Reduction in visual acuity results from foveal lesions (50). In one study, 62% of Usher type I patients had atrophic or cystic foveal lesions, while 34% of Usher type II patients had a similar finding (51).

Drusen of the optic nervehead was found in 35% of Usher type I, in 8% of Usher type II, in 1.4% of RP patients without Usher, and in 0.34% of the general population (52). Abnormal regeneration kinetics for visual pigments was found in the fovea of three patients with Usher syndrome, in spite of normal foveal light sensitivity (53).

Why should one gene cause a disease of the eye, inducing blindness, and of the ear, inducing deafness? This question has generated various speculations.

One theory about a common origin of both the RPE and the organ of Corti (54) has not been confirmed. Another theory, a possible connecting cilium in the photoreceptor as part of a genetically induced widespread disease of ciliated cells (such as the nasal cilia sperm, hair cells in the organ of Corti, and also retinal photoreceptors) was confirmed and discussed in the previous chapter. However, while being accurate for one or more of the genetic subtypes of Usher syndrome, it may be incorrect for other subtypes. Generally, an abnormality of the axoneme structure may be present in all patients with Usher syndrome. Photoreceptors, auditory hair cells, vestibular hair cells, nasal cilia, and spermatozoa all develop from ciliated progenitors (55).

Computed tomography scans detected a sizable proportion of patients with Usher syndrome having abnormalities such as cerebellar atrophy, occipital lobe atrophy, cavum septum pellucidum, cavum vergae, or diminished cerebellar circulation (46,56). The meaning of these findings is not clear, as the abnormalities seem to be nonprogressive and do not cause detectable clinical symptoms (56). Also, magnetic resonance imaging (MRI) revealed abnormal high-signal intensity lesions from the midbrain and cerebellum of patients with Usher syndrome (57), but, again, their meaning is poorly understood.

A histopathologic study of the inner ear of a 52-year-old patient with Usher syndrome type II (58) demonstrated loss of hair cells in the basal turn, severe loss of spiral ganglion cells, neural degeneration in the cochlea, and degenerating supporting cells in the organ of Corti. As in pathologic studies of ocular tissues, it was difficult to distinguish primary from secondary abnormalities in this ear specimen. Almost total degeneration of the organ of Corti and the cochlear neurons was found in another study (59).

The Genetic Types of Usher Syndrome

DNA linkage studies to detect chromosomal localization of Usher syndrome started in the 1980s and were unsuccessful (60,61). By now, 11 genetic loci are known, seven in Usher syndrome type I, three in type II, and one in type III (see Table 4).

The USH1A Locus

Linkage analysis performed on 10 French families mapped the first gene for Usher syndrome to the long arm of chromosome 14. USH1A was mapped to chromosome 14q by Kaplan and associates (62). Eight families originated from one place in western France, suggesting a founder effect. The gene has not yet been identified. The localization, however, has been refined to chromosome 14q32.

The USH1B Locus and the MYO7A

The gene for USH1B locus was mapped to chromosome 11q (63), and later refined to 11q13.5. Disease-bearing mutations associated with Usher syndrome were identified

Table 4 The Genetic Types of Usher Syndrome

Locus/symbol	Gene/protein	Chromosomal location	Remarks
USH1A		14q32	
USH1B	MY07A; myosin vlla	11q13.5	May cause congenital deafness without RP
USH1C	USH1C; harmonin	11p15.1	Implicated in USH1C or deafness alone; recessive or dominant
USH1D	CDH 23; cadherin-like	10q22.1	Implicated in USH1D or deafness alone
USH1E		21q21	
USH1F	PCDH15 protocadherin 15	10q21.1	Implicated in USH1F or deafness alone
USH1G	SANS	17q24–q25	
USH2A	USH2A usherin	1q41	Also isolated ARRP; 4.5% of all ARRP
USH2B	—	3p24–p23	Also isolated deafness
USH2C	MASS1/VLGR1	5q14.3	
USH3A	USH3A; Clarin 1	3q15.1	40% of Usher syndrome in Finland

on the gene encoding myosin VIIA (64,65), a cytoskeletal protein forming one type of myosin involved in formation and activity of the cilium in photoreceptors, cochlear, and vestibular hair cells. The myosin unconventional family VII, memberA (MYO7A) gene was found to be large. It consists of 49 coding exons and is expressed in both RPE cells and photoreceptors (65,66) but is preferentially expressed in the connecting cilium (67).

A great variety of various mutations have been identified to be associated with USH1B including missense, nonsense, small deletions, splice site mutations, and others (68–70). Different mutated alleles were associated with Usher syndrome type IB and others were associated with deafness and variable vestibular dysfunction without RP (71). In some populations USH1B is the most common subtype (70). It is common in Morocco, Algeria, and Tunisia (69), and has been identified in the Samaritans, an inbred isolated population (72,73).

The USH1C Locus and Gene

The gene encodes a PDZ domain-containing protein, harmonin (74), which forms a protein complex with CDHZ3, (implicated with USH1D) to become a transmembrane complex that connects stereocilia into a bundle (75). They are expressed in the ear and in photoreceptors.

USH1C mutations were identified in a large Louisiana cohort whose ancestors emigrated from Acadia in Nova Scotia to southwestern Louisiana. A different mutation was identified in patients of Lebanese origin (76).

The USH1D Locus and CDH23 Gene

The locus USH1D was mapped to chromosome l0q (77,78), later refined to 10q22.1. The locus was found in families of Moroccan, Pakistani, and Turkish origin (77).

Bolz and colleagues (79) identified the gene in patients of a Cuban family using a positional candidate approach. They identified a missense mutation (Argl746Gln) associated with a mild retinal disease and a truncating splice site mutation associated with a severe retinal disease. Hearing loss was profound in both types. In another study, missense mutations of the CDH23 (for cadherin-like 23 or otocadherin) were associated with nonsyndromic deafness without retinal affection. Other truncating mutations (nonsense and frameshift) were associated with Usher syndrome type ID (80).

The three proteins, myosin VII A, harmonin, and cadherin 23, when defective, are associated with an abnormality of the axoneme structures.

The USH1E Locus

This locus was identified in a large consanguineous Moroccan family and mapped to chromosome 21q21 (81). The gene has not yet been identified and currently no other family has been described with this condition.

The USH1F Locus and PCDH15 Gene

A study by Ahmed and coworkers refined the mapping of this locus to chromosome 10q21.1 (82). These investigators studied 120 families with Usher syndrome, all of Pakistani origin, and found eight families suffering from Usher type ID and three families suffering from Usher type IF. In these three families they identified mutations associated with USH1F on PCDH15, protocadherin 15, a gene that belongs to the cadherin super family (82). Recessive splice site and nonsense mutations of PCDH15 were demonstrated (82,83). Milder mutations were shown to cause only nonsyndromic deafness (DFNB23). The protein product of PCDH15, protocadherin, was localized to inner ear hair cell stereocilia and to retinal photoreceptors by immunocytochemistry (83).

The USH1G Locus and SANS Gene

This locus was mapped to chromosome 17q24–q25 by Mustapha and associates (84). Mutations in the SANS gene were identified in families of Jordanian, Tunisian, and German origin by Weil and colleagues (85). The gene encodes the scaffold protein containing ankyrin repeats and SAM domain (SANS protein), a protein that interacts with harmonin in maintenance of stereocilia bundles in the ear. Various mutations were identified, most truncating due to small (one or two) base pair deletions (85).

The USH2A Locus and Gene

Variability of phenotype expression marks type 2 in general and type 2A in particular (86). Hearing loss may be stable or progressive. The RP may be milder or more severe. Hearing defects without RP, or autosomal recessive retinitis pigmentosa (ARRP) without hearing defect have been rarely reported as the clinical expression of USH2A.

The gene was mapped to chromosome lq (86), and later refined to chromosome 1q41 (87). Eudy et al. (87,88) isolated the gene, a member of the nuclear receptor superfamily. It encodes a putative extracellular matrix protein, unique to this disease and later termed usherin (89). The gene contains 21 exons and spans a length of 105 kb (89). The protein usherin contains 1546 amino acids and preserves domains observed in basal lamina in extracellular matrix and in cell adhesion molecules (90,91).

Many different mutations have been identified. Most are single- or double-nucleotide deletions (87–92). The most common is probably the 2299delG mutation (89). The great majority of mutations lead to premature termination (92).

Usher type 2 is the most common of the three types. Among 560 families with Usher syndrome, Eudy and associates (88) found 59% with type 2. USH2A is the most common subtype of type 2. USH2B has been reported in many European countries including Britain, Sweden, Holland, Germany (88), Denmark, Norway (92) and others. It has been reported in Pakistan (91), the United States (88), and in Israel in Jewish people of various origins (90). A milder missense mutation (Cys759Phe) in the USH2A gene was associated with ARRP without hearing impairment (93). Rivolta et al. (93) described the same USH2A mutation, which is 4.5% of all ARRP. In a later article, these authors described an ARRP patient who inherited two copies of the mutated gene from her heterozygotic father (partial iso-disomy) (94). Zlotogora (95) stressed the importance of such uniparental disomy in genetic counseling.

The USH2B Locus

Hmani and colleagues mapped this locus to chromosome 3p23–24.2, after studying a large consanguineous Tunisian family (96). The phenotype may be milder than in Usher type IIA.

The USH2C Locus and MASS1/VLGR1 Gene

The third locus of type 2, USH2C was mapped in nine families to chromosome 5q (97) and later refined to location 5ql4.3. Weston and colleagues (98) identified the USH2C associated gene as monogenic, audiogenic, seizure susceptiblity 1 (MASS 1). The same gene is also named VLGR1 (very large G protein-coupled receptor 1). Usher II type C seems a milder disease than type A.

The USH3A Locus and CLARIN1 Gene

This locus was mapped to chromosome 3q24–q25 in an Italian family and two Finnish families (99). Mutations were found in a novel gene with transmembrane domain. In the Italian family a 3 bp deletion and in the Finnish families a nonsense mutation (Tyrl00shop) (100) were identified. Adato and associates demonstrated that the gene encodes clarin-1, a four-transmembrane-domain protein with a role in hair cell and photoreceptor cell synapses (101).

Liu and coworkers described two families with Usher syndrome type III associated with missense mutations (Leu651Pro, Argl602Gln) of the myosinVIIA gene usually associated with USH1B (102).

BARDET–BIEDL SYNDROME

The Bardet–Biedl syndrome (BBS), formerly referred to as the Laurence–Moon–Bardet–Biedl (LMBB) syndrome, consists of five principal signs: RP, obesity, hypogonadism, polydactyly or syndactyly, and mental retardation. It was later suggested that the Laurence–Moon syndrome is a separate entity and that Laurence and Moon, in their original article described a condition in which RP is associated with severe neurologic abnormalities, mental retardation, and hypogonadism, but without polydactyly (103). In contrast, the articles by Bardet (104) and by Biedl (105) stressed polydactyly and obesity. The two, therefore, seem to be separate clinical and genetic entities (106,107) (see Table 5).

Clinical Description

BBS syndrome is rare. Most patients show all five principal signs, but others do not have one or more of these signs. In adulthood, a typical RP is found, with bone corpuscles in the retina, but in childhood and adolescence a salt-and-pepper fundus, with atrophic retina and attenuated vessels, is seen and slowly progresses (108). Often a bull's-eye maculopathy is seen in early cases, and a diffuse atrophy of the RPE and choriocapillaris is seen in late cases (107). The visual acuity is low, and the ERG is unrecordable or extremely low (108). The obesity is typically generalized, and stature is often shorter than normal. Mental retardation is usually mild, but intelligence may also be normal or, sometimes, severely abnormal.

A description of a patient who manifested RP with both neurological signs and polydactyly (109) stressed the likelihood for heterogeneity and variable expressivity.

The visual prognosis for patients with BBS is variable and depends on the genetic subtype of the disease (see later). In the study of 21 nonclassified BBS patients, visual acuity loss was 0.09 log unit per year. The ERGs were attenuated early in life (110).

Death occurs at a considerably younger age than in the general population (111). Renal disease is the main cause of the reduction in life expectancy.

BBS must be differentiated from several differential diagnoses (112) (see Table 6). A histopathologic study (113) suggested that the photoreceptors are the primary affected tissue in BBS, but this has not been confirmed.

Table 5 The Genetic Types of Bardet-Biedl Syndrome

Locus/ symbol	Gene/protein	Chromosal location	Remarks
BBS1	BBS 1 protein	11q13	40% of all BBS families common:Met390Arg
BBS2	BBS 2 protein	16q12.2	20% of all BBS families; triallelic inheritance
BBS3	Canadian family mild phenotype; 3–6% of all BBS; also implicated in triallelic in heritance	3p13–p12	
BBS4	BBS 4 protein, similar to O-linked, *N*-acetylglucosamine transferase	15q24.1	
BBS5		2q31	
BBS6	MKKS; McKusick–Kaufman protein	20p12.2	Also implicated in triallelic inheritance
BBS7	BBS 7 protein	4q27	
BBS8	TTC8; tetratricopeptide repeat domain 8	14q32.11	

Table 6 Associated RP Syndromes

Disease or syndrome	Gene	Chromosomal location	RP	Obesity	Neurologic abnormalities	Mental retardation	Hypogenitalism	Deafness	Renal disease	Characteristic findings
Abetalipoproteinemia	MTP	4q22–q24	Progressive; moderate	No	Variable	No	No	No	No	Absence of β-lipoproteins in plasma; acanthocytosis
Refsum I	PHYH/PAHX	6q22–q24	Progressive	No	Yes	No	No	Some-times	No	Typical ataxia; phytanic acid in plasma
Refsum II	PHYH/PAHX	6q22–q24	Mild to moderate	No	Yes	No	No	Some-times	No	Typical ataxia; phytanic acid in plasma
Cockayne	CSA	5	Progressive; mild to moderate	No	Yes	Severe	No	Yes	No	Dwarfism; typical female apperance
Juvenile Batten	CLN3	16p12.1–p11.2	Starts in macula; progressive	No	Yes	Progressive	No	No	No	Vacuolized lymphocytes
Cohen	COH1	8q22	Starts in macula; progressive	Yes	Mild	Mild	No	No	No	Facial and oral abnormalities

(*Continued*)

Table 6 Associated RP Syndromes (*Continued*)

Disease or syndrome	Gene	Chromosomal location	RP	Obesity	Neurologic abnormalities	Mental retardation	Hypogenitalism	Deafness	Renal disease	Characteristic findings
Hallervorden–Spatz	PANK2	20p13–p12.2	Flecked retina maculopathy; progressive	No	Yes	Variable	No	No	No	Ataxia choreoathetoid movements
Laurence–Moon			Progressive	Yes	Yes	Severe	Yes	No	No	Short stature
Alstrom	ALMS1	2p13.1	Congenital; severe and progressive	Yes	No	No	No	Yes	Frequent	Diabetes mellitus; baldness
Biemond II			Progressive; moderate to severe	Yes	Variable	Yes	Yes	No (?)	No	Iris coloboma, may not exist as a separate nosology (136).
Zellweger	PEX1 and others	7q21–q22 and others	Occasionally	No	Yes	Variable	No	No	Yes	Cerebrohepatorenal abnormalities

BBS and the allied syndromes are all transmitted by the autosomal recessive mode.

Subtypes of BBS and Molecular Genetics

Introduction

With the advent of linkage studies, it became obvious that BBS is a heterogenous disease transmitted by a number of genes. The first linkage to chromosome 16q (now termed BBS2 locus) was reported in 1993 (114). By 1994, four genetic loci were identified and by 2004, eight distinct loci were mapped. Phenotype variability occurs, and will also be described.

BBS1

This locus was mapped to chromosome 11ql3 by Leppert and associates in 1994 (115) in 31 families of Northern European ancestry. The BBS1 gene was identified by Mykytyn and associates in 2000 (116). It is composed of 17 exons and spans approximately 23 kb.

BBSl is the most common of the genetic subtypes of BBS. It comprises about half of the affected families ensure 44% in one study, 36–56% in another study (117). The second most common subtype varies among different populations. It was reported as BBS2 with 17% in one study (118), and as BBS4 with 32% in another study (117). Approximately 80% of all BBS1 gene mutations were Met390Arg missense mutations (119). The inheritance is a regular autosomal inheritance. Complex triallelic inheritance, described for other subtypes of BBS, is not found in BBS1. The phenotype is similar in all types, and includes increased risk of diabetes mellitus, hypertension, and congenital heart disease (119). Apparently, BBS1 is the major gene for BBS (120).

BBS2

In a large family of Israeli Bedouins living in the Negev desert, locus BBS2, linked to chromosome 16q, was identified as early as 1993 (114). This was later refined to chromosome 16q21 (121) and to 16ql2.2 (28). Three large Bedouin families in the Negev desert suffer from BBS, each associated with a different gene (118,122). Carmi and associates (122) compared phenotypes and demonstrated that polydactyly in BBS3 usually affects all four limbs, while in BBS4 mostly hands are affected. Obesity is notable in BBS4, not seen in BBS2, and intermediate in BBS3.

The gene was cloned by Nishimura and colleagues in 2001 (121). It comprises of 17 exons. The authors identified five different mutations in the affected families, some homozygous and other compound heterozygous.

Katsanis and coworkers (123) claimed that 47% of patients with mutations of the BBS2 gene, additionally showed mutations of the BBS6 gene. They assumed that in a large proportion, BBS is a triallelic disease transmitted by two mutated alleles on one gene, and one mutated allele on another gene.

BBS3

BBS3 was mapped to chromosome 3pl3–pl2. It was identified in a large Bedouin family (124), in a Newfoundland family of North European descent (125), and in seven affected members of an Iranian family (126). The variability of phenotypes was not great, expressed mainly in variable polydactyly.

BBS4

As mentioned, BBS4 was the third gene identified in a Bedouin family in the Negev desert (127), and later in three families in Norway (128). Obesity was reported. Intelligence can be variable. Renal dysfunction, hypertension, and cardiovascular diseases are common. Mykytyn and associates reported the positional cloning and mutations of the BBS4 gene (129).

BBS5

This rare gene was mapped by Young and associates to chromosome 2q31 in a family detected by a population study in Newfoundland (130,131). The family was of European ancestry, and suffered from a very severe visual impairment leading to no light perception, vision of counting fingers, or light perception only in most patients.

BBS6

The sixth BBS locus was described as associated with McKusick-Kaufman syndrome (MKKS) gene, by Katsanis and colleagues (132). MKKS bears similarities to BBS by developmental anomalies, polydactyly, and congenital heart disease. The gene was mapped to chromosome 20pl2.2. Many different mutations were identified, most leading to loss of function of MKKS protein (132). The identified mutations were missense, nonsense, or small deletions and showed homozygosity or compound heterozygosity (133). As mentioned before, Katsanis and colleagues suggested that triallelic inheritance is common in patients with BBS2 and BBS6. Forty seven percent of BBS2 patients carried an additional mutation on the gene for BBS6, and 37% of BBS6 patients carried a mutation on the BBS2 gene (123). It was also suggested that BBS4 may, in some cases, participate in this triallelic inheritance.

BBS7

The BBS7 gene maps to chromosome 4q27 (134). It was the seventh BBS gene to be identified and the fifth to be cloned. The gene has 19 exons. The gene product shows great similarity to the BBS1 and BBS2 proteins (134). About 3.5% of BBS patients are of subtype. The mutations were missense or small deletions.

BBS8

In 2003, Ansley and coworkers reported the association between mutations in the gene tetratricopeptide repeat domain 8 (TTC8) and BBS8 (135). The locus maps to chromosome 14q32.11. The authors suggested that BBS is caused by a defect in the basal body of ciliated cells. The cloned BBS8 gene encodes a protein pilF that is involved in pilus formation and twitching mobility (135).

This is the first BBS-associated protein with a known function, and it presents an insight into the malfunction of the mutated protein.

RETINITIS PIGMENTOSA ASSOCIATED WITH OTHER DISORDERS

RP with Lipid Disorders

Various syndromes make up this group of disorders, which also includes the only treatable forms of RP (Table 6).

The Syndrome of Bassen and Korzweig

The syndrome of Bassen and Kornzweig (137) consists of malabsorption, neurologic abnormalities, and RP. Because the basic biochemical abnormality of absence of β-lipoproteins in the plasma became known, the term *abetalipoproteinemia* has been used. The disease starts in early childhood, with some similarities to celiac syndrome. Neurologic abnormalities include ataxia, tremor, absence of deep reflexes, and pathologic pyramidal reflexes. Retinal changes progress very slowly, displaying, after the early period of a normal fundus, an "atypical RP" until finally bone corpuscular pigment appears (4). The ERG is abnormal before any visible changes in the fundus occur and is progressively reduced, until it finally becomes undetectable.

A pathologic study of an eye of a 40-year-old patient with abetalipoproteinemia showed loss of both photoreceptors and RPE cells, except in the far periphery, where the cells were normal, and in the macular area, where RPE cells were preserved, but abnormally filled by lipofuscin and trilaminar structures. The authors were impressed by the similarities with experimental vitamin A and E deficiency (138).

Lipoproteins containing apoprotein-β are absent from the plasma of patients with abetalipoproteinemia. The plasma contains no chylomicrons, very low density liproproteins, or low-density lipoproteins. Erythrocytes show acanthocytosis, a peculiar anomaly which they appear "thorny." Both vitamin A and E are transported in the plasma by lipoproteins. Levels of circulating vitamin A and vitamin E are very low in untreated patients, probably because of the absence of the transporting agent. Therefore, it was conceivable to treat patients with abetalipoproteinemia with large doses of vitamin A and vitamin E. Such treatment was shown to prevent the deterioration of the ERG, (139), and to prevent the retinal and neurologic lesions (140). No progression of the disturbed visual function was detected in any of the eight treated patients who were followed for two to eight years (139). In our series (139), the treatment dose was monitored so that blood concentration of vitamin A reached normal levels and that of vitamin E reached one–third of normal levels.

A recent study demonstrated that combined vitamin A and vitamin E therapy is effective even in the long term, but must start before the age of two years (141).

The gene associated with Bassen–Kornzweig syndrome or abetalipoproteinemia (ABL) was cloned and mapped to chromosome 4q22–q24. It is known that in ABL, the production of apoB-containing lipoproteins is abolished but studies have demonstrated no abnormality of the apoB gene (142). Narcisi and associates characterized the gene microsomal triglyceride transfer protein (MTP), that encodes a large polypeptide of 88 kDa. They identified mutations of this gene in all eight ABL patients examined. Each mutant allele identified was predicted to encode a truncated form of MTP. They concluded that an intact carboxyl terminus is necessary for normal MTP activity (142).

Refsum Disease

In Refsum disease, first described by the Norwegian neurologist Refsum (143), RP is associated with chronic polyneuritis, albuminocytologic dissociation (high albumin and a small number of cells in the cerebrospinal fluid), ataxia, and other cerebellar phenomena. The disease is transmitted by the autosomal recessive mode. Refsum syndrome is rare, but is probably most common in Scandinavian countries and has been reported in many other populations.

Night blindness occurs early, but the pigmentary retinopathy appears milder than in the average case of RP. Visual fields and visual acuity may be preserved for many years (144), and pigmentary bone corpuscles appear late in life (4). The ERG may be extinguished or subnormal.

An abnormal enzyme causes an unusual fatty acid to accumulate in the plasma and in various tissues of the body (145). It is called phytanic or 3,7,11,15-tetramethyl-hexadecanoic acid. It is probable that the same substance is accumulating in the RPE and in other cells of the neural retina (146), and, therefore, the pigment epithelium may be the primary site of the disease through an early dysfunction of its cells.

Exogenous phytol is readily converted into phytanic acid in these patients. Therefore, it was suggested that the accumulation of phytanic acid can be reduced in patients with Refsum syndrome by a diet low in phytol and phytanic acid. Several studies performed on patients receiving such a diet for a prolonged time indicated arrest of the ocular and neurologic abnormalities (148,149).

Beneficial results were also reported from periodic treatment by plasmapheresis, which removes the phytanic acid from the plasma (148,149).

A disease that clinically resembles Refsum disease, except that the patients did not have any detectable biochemical abnormalities, was described in one family by Tuck and McLead (150). It seems to be a separate entity.

The locus for Refsum disease was mapped to chromosome l0pter–p11.2 by Nadal and coworkers (151). The gene was identified and cloned by Mihalik and associates (152) as the gene encoding phytanoyl-CoA hydroxylase (PAHX/PHYH). In the patients with Refsum disease, these researchers identified homozygous inactivating mutations. The pronounced accumulation of phytanic acid seems to result from selective loss of peroxisomal dioxygenase required for alpha-hydroxylation of phytanoyl CoA (152). The first step of the metabolism, the activation of phytanic acid to its CoA ester by phytanoyl CoA hydroxylase, does not occur (153,154).

Van den Brink and associates (155), who investigated a minority of patients with Refsum disease who had no mutation in the PHYH gene, recently reported a second locus for Refsum disease. They identified disease-associated mutations in the PEX7 gene at chromosome 6q22–q24. The mutations result in elevated levels of phytanic acid, RP, ataxia, and polyneuropathy, but the expression may range from a severe (rhizomelic chondrodysplasia punctata) to mild disease (155)). Dietary restriction of both phytanic acid and phytol may prevent the progressive visual loss (156).

Retinitis Pigmentosa with CNS Disorders

Cockayne Syndrome

Cockayne syndrome is characterized by RP associated with very short stature (dwarfism), mental retardation with or without microcephaly, deafness, and premature aging phenomena (4). Ocular abnormalities consist of a slowly progressive atypical RP, an early developing senile cataract, alacrima, and a band keratopathy with recurrent corneal ulcers, probably related to the lack of tears. A hyperlipoproteinemia was described in some cases, but a special sensitivity to UV radiation is the hallmark of the disease and was used to make a positive prenatal diagnosis (157).

A histopathologic study of an eye from a patient with Cockayne syndrome showed abnormalities consistent with RP, such as loss of photoreceptors, excessive lipofuscin deposition in abnormal RPE, and pigment-bearing cells in the neural retina and in the subretinal space (158). No accumulation of any abnormal material could be detected.

A major problem in Cockayne syndrome is the increased sensitivity of all cells exposed to UV light, specifically the lack of recovery of the ability to synthesize RNA following exposure to UV light (159). The exact causes are still speculative. The cells are defective in transcriptionally active genes (160). The gene associated with Cockayne syndrome was cloned by Henning and associates (160). It encodes a protein that is one component of a transcriptional regulator. The gene is located on chromosome 5 and was named Cockayne syndrome A (CSA).

Neuronal Ceroid Lipofuscinosis

"Batten disease" or "neuronal ceroid lipofuscinosis" is the name given to a group of disorders characterized by intracellular accumulation of ceroid and lipofuscin, mainly in the neurons. Four subtypes are distinguished, and they relate approximately to their age of onset. The infantile Batten disease (Haltia–Sanatavuori) starts in infancy, with severe neurologic signs, and is rapidly progressive. Optic atrophy occurs early as a result of a degeneration of the retinal ganglion cells (161). The late infantile form (Jansky–Bielschowsky) has its onset at the age of two to four years, with a rapidly progressive course of the neurologic signs. Optic atrophy occurs. The juvenile form (Spielmeyer–Vogt) begins at aged six to eight years and is associated with RP, which is slowly progressive, as are the neurologic findings. The adult form (Kufs) starts much later, is milder than the other types, and is slowly progressive (161).

A deficiency of a peroxidase enzyme is probably the cause for the accumulation of lipofuscin and ceroid; both pigments contain a polymerized, unsaturated fatty acid. The subtypes can also be distinguished by electron microscopy; the abnormally accumulating material is in the form of snowballs in the infantile type, curvilinear bodies in the late infantile type, and fingerprint bodies in the juvenile form.

Juvenile Batten disease is of particular interest to ophthalmologists. Spalton and coworkers (162) studied the ocular findings in a group of 26 patients with this subtype. Visual loss starts at age six to seven years, followed by abnormal findings in the macular region in the form of a bull's-eye maculopathy or macular pigmentation. Later, retinal atrophy and bone corpuscular pigment occur. In parallel, mental abilities decrease, and grand mal seizures occur spasticity, pyramidal signs, and cerebral dysfunction become progressively worse. Patients show typically vacuolated lymphocytes in the peripheral blood, which should make the diagnosis easy. Early death occurs, as in other subtypes of Batten disease.

A histopathologic study revealed that both ceroid and lipofuscin are abnormally accumulating in the pigment epithelium, cones and rods, inner segments, and ganglion cells (163). Zeman (161) assumed that in this disease a primary degeneration of the outer segments is followed by degeneration of the RPE. The disease seems to be much more common in the Scandinavian population.

Batten disease, the juvenile form of neuronal ceroid lipofuscinosis, in which pigmentary retinal dystrophy occurs, is a lysosomal disease. The protein ceroid lipofuscinosis, neuronal type 3 (CLN3) is localized to the lysosomal compartment. The CLN3 gene was identified. It contains 15 exons, an open reading frame of 1314 bp, and encodes a 438 amino acid protein (164), which probably represents an integral transmembrane protein of unknown function. It was mapped to chromosome 16p11.2–p12.1 (164,165).

A recent histopatholgic study of the ocular tissues of a 22-year-old man with juvenile neuronal ceroid lipofuscinosis revealed RP-like changes. Cones and rods were degenerated with short outer segments in the surviving photoreceptors. Lipopigment granules were found in the ganglion cells, while RPE cells had fewer than normal lipofuscin granules (166).

Cohen Syndrome

Cohen syndrome also starts with visual reduction owing to a maculopathy, which later progresses into a typical RP with constricted fields, attenuated retinal vessels, pigmentary bone corpuscles, and an unrecordable ERG (167). The RP is associated with mental retardation; obesity of the trunk; hypotonia; facial, oral, and limb anomalies in the form of malar hypoplasia, micrognathia, high-arched palate, and other abnormalities (167). The differential diagnoses of Bardet-Biedl's, Laurence-Moon's, and Alstrom's syndromes should be considered. The syndrome is unusually common in Israel (168). It is caused by an autosomal recessive gene.

The ocular findings of Cohen syndrome resemble RP. Clinical examination of 22 patients with Cohen syndrome, aged 2–57 years revealed impaired vision and loss of visual fields, retinal spicule-like pigment that increased with time, and bull's-eye maculopathy (169). Night blindness was an early symptom. Systemically, typical craniofacial features, microcephaly, and mental retardation were seen. The syndrome seems to be more frequent in Finland (169).

The gene was characterized and mapped by Kholehainen and coworkers. The gene COH1 is very large, contains 62 exons, spans 864 kb and encodes a protein of 4022 amino acids. The protein has a role in intracellular protein transportation (170,171). It was mapped to chromosome 8q22 (171).

Hallervorden–Spatz Syndrome

In the Hallervorden–Spatz syndrome, RP is associated with severe extrapyramidal neurologic abnormalities with dystonic posture, ataxia and choreoathetoid movements, hyperreflexia and spasticity, and a progressive mental deficiency (172). A rusty brown discoloration of the globus pallidus and the substantia nigra is the hallmark of pathologic identification (172,173). Inheritance is autosomal recessive. Ocular findings include atrophy of the RPE and the neural retina, attenuation of blood vessels, pigmentary bone corpuscles, and peculiar yellowish white globular masses in the fundi (173). Nystagmus and gaze palsies may be present. Flecked retina and bull's-eye maculopathy were early findings in two other reported cases (174). Diagnosis can be made by conjunctival fibrocytes, which contained single membrane-bound lipofuscin granules (174). Histopathologic study of an eye showed loss of the photoreceptor cell layers and abnormal RPE cells with accumulation of round aggregates, which by electron microscopy seemed to be giant single membrane-bound melanolipofuscin granules embedded in membranous lipofuscin (174). This may indicate a primary inability of the RPE cells to hydrolyze melanolipofuscin intralysosomally.

Hallervorden–Spatz syndrome has been mapped to chromosome 20p13–pl2.3 and mutations were identified in the PANK2 gene at this location (175,176). The pantothenate kinase-associated neuro-degeneration (PANK2) gene carries mutations associated with all cases of classic Hallervorden–Spatz syndrome (175,176).

Laurence-Moon Syndrome

In the Laurence-Moon syndrome, RP is found with obesity, hypogonadism mental retardation, spastic paraparesis, and markedly short stature. It is very rare. The gene and its location are unknown.

Alstrom Syndrome

Loss of photoreceptors is gradual but rapid. Cones are lost earlier; rods initially remain relatively preserved (177,178). The ERG is attenuated and usually becomes undetectable toward the second half of the first decade of life (177). Cardiomyopathy occurs in the vast majority of children with Alstrom syndrome and diabetes mellitus is diagnosed in the second or third decade of life (178).

Alstrom disease is also included in differential diagnosis of BBS. Retinitis pigmentosa is associated with diabetes, obesity, sensorineural deafness, and normal intelligence (179). Impaired vision is found in the first year of life and decreases to finger counting during the first decade of life. Nystagmus, photophobia, a salt-and-pepper fundus, progressing to retinal and choroidal atrophy, with attenuation of retinal vessels are the rule (179). Substantial hair loss is characteristic, and renal failure may be the cause of death.

Collin and coworkers mapped the locus of Alstrom syndrome to chromosome 2pl2–pl4 in a large French–Acadian family (180). The disease seems to have a higher concentration in Nova Scotia, where French-Acadians live. The localization was later refined to chromosome 2p13.1.

The gene for ALMSl (or ALSSl, both stand for Alstrom syndrome 1) was identified in 2002 by two groups of investigators (181,182). The gene was found to be relatively large and consist of 23 exons. Six different mutations were identified in seven families. All carried nonsense or frameshift mutations. The protein ALMS-1 has an unknown function. The mutated gene codes for a truncated protein with 34 imperfect repetitions of 47 amino acids (181). The mutated gene was associated with childhood obesity, hyperinsulinemia, chronic hyperglycemia, and neurosensory deficits. Additional clinical abnormalities may occur as a result of interaction between this mutated gene and other genetic modifiers (182).

Zellweger Syndrome

Zellweger syndrome or cerebrohepatorenal syndrome affects three organs and the retina. RP with an extinguished ERG was reported (183). Zellweger syndrome is a peroxisome biogenesis disorder caused by a defective single enzyme. However, several different genes may be associated with this disease. These are PEXl at chromosome 7q21, PEX2 at chromosome 8q, PEX3 at chromosome 6q, PEX5 at chromosome 12, PEX6 at chromosome 6p, and an additional locus at chromosome 7q11 (55). The most common association seems to be with PEXl (184).

RP with Renal Disease

Retinitis pigmentosa associated with a juvenile familial nephropathy (Juvenile nephronophthisis) is usually referred to as the Senior–Loken syndrome after the first two descriptions of this association (15,174), although other synonyms, such as renal dysplasia and retinal aplasia, hereditary renal–retinal dysplasia, or familial renal-retinal dystrophy, are also used. The retinal disease starts at birth and is usually evident in the first year of life (15). The renal disease is characterized by juvenile nephronophthisis or medullary cystic disease (185) with polydypsia, polyuria, renal salt-wasting, anemia, hypertension (186), and usually progressive renal failure. About 4% of patients who underwent kidney transplantation suffered from the Senior–Loken syndrome (187).

The ocular fundus may show white flakes, have a salt-and-pepper appearance, and later show typical bone corpuscles (188), as in patients with LCA. The retinal function is, however, much better preserved than in Leber amaurosis, in spite of an extinguished or very subnormal ERG (189).

The disease is transmitted by an autosomal recessive gene. It was suggested, that asymptomatic heterozygotes also have an abnormal ERG, a subnormal EOG, or both (188).

Friedlaender and colleagues (190) described a family with late-occurring visual symptoms and renal failure. Vision was preserved in the fifth decade of life. The renal lesion was also different from the Senior–Loken syndrome by the absence of salt-wasting and by marked hypertension. It seems that late-occurring RP with renal disease, as described by Friedlaender et al., and mentioned by others (191), is a separate genetic entity and not the result of the action of a pleiotropic gene, as has been suggested (191). Intrafamilial similarities are the rule, rather than the exception.

Four loci for nephronophthisis named NPHP I-IV are now known (Table 7). NPHP1, juvenile nephronophthisis, was mapped to chromosome 2ql3. The NPHP1 gene was identified (192) and its product named nephrocystin (193). The NPHP2 gene and locus was found associated with infantile nephronophthisis and mapped to chromosome 9q22–q31. Type 3 nephronophthisis NPHP3 associated with adolescent occurrence was mapped to chromosome 3q21–q22 (194). Type 4 nephronophthisis was mapped to chromosome 1p36 (195). The gene for NPHP4 was identified. It contains 30 exons and encodes a protein termed nephroretinin (196). Two loss-of-function mutations were identified in the NPHP4 gene in association with SLS. The major clinical manifestation regarding the nephronophthisis is renal malfunction which varies from mild to renal failure. RP may be found in any one of the four types, or be absent. Otto and colleagues (196) suggested that modifier genes might be responsible for occurrence or nonoccurrence of RP. RP is mild, and of late occurrence in type 1, and is congenital in NPHP2 (195) and NPHP3. In all reported

Table 7 The Senior-Loken Syndromes

Type	Name	Symbol	Gene	Protein	Chromosomal location	RP
1	Juvenile nephronophthisis	SLSN1	NPHP1	Nephrocystin	2q13	Mild late
2	Infantile nephronophthisis	SLSN2	NPHP2	Inversin	9q22–q31	Congenital (LCA)
3	Adolescent nephronophthisis	SLSN3	NPHP3	NPHP3 protein	3q21–q22	Congenital (LCA)
4	Nephronophthisis (wide range of onset)	SLSN4	NPHP4	Nephroretinin	1p36	Late-onset

Notes: Renal histology is similar in all types: interstitial fibrosis and renal tubular cell atrophy. ARRP may occur or not in association with any of the four types onset.

cases the transmission was autosomal recessive. The NPHP3 gene has been recently identified (197). It encodes a 1330 amino acid protein that interacts with nephrocystin. INVS, a gene mutated in NPHP2 encodes inversin, a protein that interacts with nephrocystin (198).

RP has also been described as being associated with mesangio-proliferative glomerulonephritis (199), with Alport's syndrome (186), and with polycystic kidneys, and cerebral malformation (200), but these may be fortuitous associations.

RP with External Ophthalmoplegia

Retinitis Pigmentosa with External Ophthalmoplegia

The triad of RP associated with external opthalmoplegia of the chronic progressive ocular myopathy variety and complete atrioventricular block was described by Kearns and Sayre, in 1958, and usually called after their names (201). The vast literature on this syndrome reflects confusion among the many associated RP syndromes. These include external ophthalmoplegia as outlined by Drachmann (202), a possible additional disease in which progressive ophthalmoplegia is associated with benign retinal pigmentation (203), and a possible heterogenous disease, with several clinical subgroups as outlined by Mitsumoto (204). Heterogeneity is also emphasized by many nonfamilial cases (205,206), autosomal dominant transmittance (207), autosomal recessive transmittance (208), and mitochondrial inheritance (211). Marked variability in expressivity of the autosomal dominant form also occurs. Out of nine patients with Kearns–Sayre syndrome, seven had external ophthalmoplegia; six, limb weakness; five, rhythm cardiac disturbance; four, pigmentary retinopathy; three, ptosis; two, a cardiac conduction disturbance, and one, dysphagia (208).

The cardiomyopathy, which involves only 20% of the affected, may become progressively worse (210). Death occurred from severe metabolic dysfunction (hyperglycemic coma) in two patients who received oral corticosteroids for a brief period (211). Muscle biopsy reveals ragged-red fibers, lipid accumulation, and variation in muscle fiber size, whereas electron microscopy reveals enlarged mitochondria containing inclusions (207) Pathologic specimens of an eye suggested that the RPE may be the site of the primary retinal affection, as the RPE cells were atrophic and flattened and rod outer segments were absent or, in other places, normal (212,213). In another study, marked degeneration of RPE cells was coupled with focal loss of photoreceptors (214). The abnormal function of mitochondria was expressed in declining cytochrome C oxidase activity (215) and abnormal protein synthesis (216).

No known therapy is available, Thiamine or vitamin E (207) and coenzyme Q10 (217) have been suggested, but their therapeutic value is still not confirmed.

Mitochondrial diseases affecting the eye will be discussed separately.

RP Associated Mucopolysaccharidoses

Retinitis pigmentosa is associated with the first three of the mucopolysaccharidoses (MPSs), which include Hurler syndrome, both variants of Hunter's syndrome, and both variants of Sanfilippo's syndrome. The combination of corneal cloudiness and retinal findings can assist with the clinical distinction of the different syndromes of MPS and is important for determining their prognosis (Table 8). Electrophysiologic studies may establish the retinal condition (218), even when the retina cannot be ophthalmoscopically examined because of a cloudy cornea. It is important to

Table 8 Ocular Involvement in the Mucopolysaccharidoses

Mucopolysaccharidoses								
Type	Name	Gene	Chromosome location	Deficient enzyme	Cornea	Retinal involvement	Systemic	Inheritance
IH	Hurler	IDUA	4p16.3	α-L-Iduronidase	Severe	RP frequent	Severe	AR
IS	Scheie	IDUA	4p16.3	α-L-Iduronidase	Severe	RP frequent	Mild	AR
II, Mild	Hunter, mild variant	IDS	xq28	Iduronate sulfatase	No	Normal or mildly affected	Moderate to severe	XL
II, Severe	Hunter, severe variant	IDS	xq28	Iduronate sulfatase	Moderate	RP frequent	Severe	XL
III A	Sanfilippo A	SGSH	17q25.3	Heparan sulfate sulfatase	No	RP frequent	Mild	AR
III B	Sanfilippo B	NAGLU	17q21	α-Acetylglucosamidase	No	RP frequent	Mild (?)	AR
IV A	Morquio A	GALNS	16q24.4	Galactosamine-6-sulfatase	Mild to severe	No	Severe	AR
IV B	Morquio B			β-Galactosidase	Mild to severe	No	Severe	AR
VI, Mild	Maroteaux-Lamy, mild variant	ARSB	5q1–q13	Arylsulfatase B	Moderate to severe	No	Moderate	AR
VI, Severe	Maroteaux-Lamy, severe variant	ARSB	5q1–q13	Arylsulfatase B	Severe	No	Severe	AR

AR—autosomal recessive; XL—X chromosomal-linked recessive.

perform an ERG before making a decision on keratoplasty. Rod-mediated responses were found to be more affected than cone-mediated responses (218). The ERG becomes progressively worse (219). Carriers of the sex-linked Hunter's syndrome may show night blindness and abnormal psychophysical and ERG dark adaptation (219).

In Morquio syndrome, the ERG is normal, but mild impairment of rod function can be found by psychophysical dark adaptation (220).

Table 8 describes the ocular involvement in mucopolysaccharidoses, most of their subtypes, and the genes involved and their chromosomal locations (55). Mild and severe forms with their variable clinical manifestations are determined by the variable mutations. Generally, large deletions in the mutated gene or premature termination lead to severe forms, while missense mutations are mostly associated with a milder form. Various forms of therapy such as enzyme replacement, bone marrow transplantation, and gene therapy are currently in the stage of advanced clinical investigation.

Other RP Associations

Isolated reports about the association of RP with a multitude of syndromes and multisystem diseases can also be found. These include RP with von Hippel's tumors described in three siblings (221), RP with congenital trichomegaly and short stature (222), RP with a neurodegenerative condition and decreased levels of fucosidase (223), RP with myotonic dystrophy (1), and RP with olivopontocerebellar degeneration (224). Some of these associations, such as the last one, are separate nosologic entities, whereas others have yet to be confirmed as separate genetic and clinical entities.

Olivopontocerebellar degeneration is also named autosomal dominant cerebellar ataxia type II (ADCA2) or spinocerebellar ataxia type 7 (SCA7). The three types of ADCA carry variable clinical expression ranging from mild to severe. ADCAl is associated with optic atrophy, ADCA2 is associated with retinal dystrophy, and ADCA3 manifests cerebellar ataxia without ocular involvement. The causative gene SCA7/ADCA2 encodes ataxin-7, an 892 aminoacid protein (225). Retinal dysfunction may be mild or severe with both cones and rods equally affected (225). The gene has been mapped to chromosome 3pl4.1.

An autosomal recessive ataxia affects the CNS posterior columns and causes proprioceptive loss, sensory ataxia, and areflexia (226). The eye manifests typical RP with ring scotoma, pigmentary bone spicules in the retina, and usually macular sparing. The locus, AXPC1 for ataxia, posterior column, type l, has been mapped to chromosome 1q31–q32 (226).

Two additional rare diseases may be amenable to efficient treatment. Friedrich-like ataxia with RP is caused by a missense mutation (Hisl01glu) in the alpha-tocopherol transfer protein gene. The gene TTPA was mapped to chromosome 8ql2.3 (227). The product, a cytosolic liver protein, functions in intracellular transportation of alpha-tocopherol, the active form of vitamin E deficiency. Ataxia may be autosomal recessive. Oral vitamin E supplementation may halt the progression of the disease (227).

Another possible treatable disease results from a mutation in RBP4, the gene encoding retinol-binding protein. No retinol-binding protein can be detected in the serum and retinol levels are 20% or less than normal. Epithelial cells are affected, and in the eye RPE cells are severely affected with progressive RP-like changes

(228). Compound missense mutations of the RBP4 gene were reported to be associated with RP. Supplementation with vitamin A may halt the progression of visual loss.

REFERENCES

1. Alstrom CH, Olson O. Heredo-retinopathia congenitalis monohybrida recessiva autosomalis. Hereditas 1957; 43:1–178.
2. Schappert-Kimmijser J, Henkes HE, van de Bosch J. Amaurosis congenita (Leber). Arch Ophthalmol 1959; 61:211–218.
3. Noble KC, Carr RE. Leber's congenital amaurosis. A retrospective study of 33 cases and a histopathological study of one case. Arch Ophthalmol 1978; 96:818–821.
4. Merin S, Auerbach E. Retinitis pigmentosa. Surv Ophthalmol 1976; 20(5):303–346.
5. Edwards WC, Price WD, MacDonald R. Congenital amaurosis of retinal origin (Leber). Am J Ophthalmol 1971; 72:724–728.
6. Chew E, Deutman A, Pinckers A, DeKerk A. Yellowish flecks in Leber's congenital amaurosis. Br J Ophthalmol 1984; 68:727–731.
7. Wagner RS, Caputo AR, Nelson LB, Zanoni D. High hyperopia in Leber's congenital amaurosis. Arch Ophthalmol 1985; 103:1507–1509.
8. Elder MJ. Leber congenital amaurosis and its association with keratoconus and keratoglobus. J Pediatr Ophthalmol Strabismus. 1994; 31(1):38–40.
9. Fulton AB, Hansen RM, Mayer DL. Vision in Leber congenital amaurosis. Arch Ophthalmol 1996; 114(6):698–703.
10. Kurz D, Ciulla TA. Leber congenital amaurosis associated with optic disk neovascularization and vitreous hemorrhage. Am J Ophthalmol 2003; 135(5):723–725.
11. Waardenburg P, Schappert-Kimmijser J. On various recessive biotypes of Leber's congenital amaurosis. Acta Ophthalmol 1963; 41:317–320.
12. Foxman SG, Heckenlively JR, Bateman JB, Wirtschafter JD. Classification of congenital and early onset retinitis pigmentosa. Arch Ophthalmol. 1985; 103(10):1502–1506.
13. Henkes HE, Verduin PC. Dysgenesis or abiotrophy? A differentiation with the help of the ERG and EOG in Leber's congenital amaurosis. Ophthalmologica 1963; 145:144–160.
14. Nickel B, Hoyt CS. Leber's congenital amaurosis: is mental retardation a frequent associated defect? Arch Ophthalmol 1982; 100:1089–1092.
15. Senior B, Friedman AE, Braudo JL. Juvenile familial nephronopathy with tapetoretinal degeneration in a new ocular-renal dystrophy. Am J Ophthalmol 1961; 52:625–633.
16. Margolis S, Scher BM, Carr RE. Macular colobomas in Leber's congenital amaurosis. Am J Ophthalmol 1977; 83:27–31.
17. Hayasaka S, Hara S, Mizuno K, et al. Leber's congenital amaurosis associated with hyperthreoninemia. Am J Ophthalmol 1986; 101:475–479.
18. Heckenlively JR. Retinitis pigmentosa. Philadelphia: Lippincott, 1988.
19. Camuzat A, Dollfus H, Rozet JM, Gerber S, Bonneau D, Bonnemaison M, Briard ML, Dufier JL, Ghazi I, Leowski C, et al. A gene for Leber's congenital amaurosis maps to chromosome 17p. Hum Mol Genet 1995; 4(8):1447–1452.
20. Camuzat A, Rozet JM, Dollfus H, Gerber S, Perrault I, Weissenbach J, Munnich A, Kaplan J. Evidence of genetic heterogeneity of Leber's congenital amaurosis (LCA) and mapping of LCA1 to chromosome 17pl3. Hum Genet 1996; 97(6):798–801.
21. Perrault I, Rozet JM, Calvas P, Gerber S, Camuzat A, Dollfus H, Chatelin S, Souied E, Ghazi I, Leowski C, Bonnemaison M, Le Paslier D, Frezal J, Dufier JL, Pittler S, Munnich A, Kaplan J. Retinal-specific guanylate cyclase gene mutations in Leber's congenital amaurosis. Nat Genet 1996; 14(4):461–464.
22. Koenekoop RK, Fishman GA, Lannaccone A, Ezzeldin H, Ciccarelli ML, Baldi A, Sunness JS, Lotery AJ, Jablonski MM, Pittler SJ, Maumenee I. Electroretinographic

abnormalities in parents of patients with Leber congenital amaurosis who have heterozygous GUCY2D mutations. Arch Ophthalmol 2002; 120(10):1325–1330.
23. Lotery AJ, Namperumalsamy P, Jacobson SG, Weleber RG, Fishman GA, Musarella MA, Hoyt CS, Heon E, Levin A, Jan J, Lam B, Carr RE, Franklin A, Radha S, Andorf JL, Sheffield VC, Stone EM. Mutation analysis of 3 genes in patients with Leber congenital amaurosis. Arch Ophthalmo 2000; 118(4):538–543.
24. Hanein S, Perrault I, Gerber S, Tanguy G, Barbet F, Ducroq D, Calvas P, Dollfus H, Hamel C, Lopponen T, Munier F, Santos L, Shalev S, Zafeiriou D, Dufier JL, Munnich A, Rozet JM, Kaplan J. Leber congenital amaurosis: comprehensive survey of the genetic heterogeneity, refinement of the clinical definition, and genotype-phenotype correlations as a strategy for molecular diagnosis. Hum Mutat 2004; 23(4):306–317.
25. Marlhens F, Bareil C, Griffoin JM, Zrenner E, Amalric P, Eliaou C, Liu SY, Harris E, Redmond TM, Arnaud B, Claustres M, Hamel CP. Mutations in RPE65 cause Leber's congenital amaurosis. Nat Genet 1997; 17(2):139–141.
26. Stockton DW, Lewis RA, Abboud EB, Al-Rajhi A, Jabak M, Anderson KL, Lupski JR. A novel locus for Leber congenital amaurosis on chromosome 14q24. Hum Genet 1998; 103(3):328–333.
27. Hameed A, Khaliq S, Ismail M, Anwar K, Ebenezer ND, Jordan T, Mehdi SQ, Payne AM, Bhattacharya SS. A novel locus for Leber congenital amaurosis (LCA4) with anterior keratoconus mapping to chromosome 17p13. Invest Ophthalmol Vis Sci 2000; 41(3):629–633.
28. Retnet. http: //www.sph.uth.tmc.edu/retnet/disease.htm.
29. Dharmaraj S, Li Y, Robitaille JM, Silva E, Zhu D, Mitchell TN, Maltby LP, Baffoe-Bonnie AB, Maumenee IH. A novel locus for Leber congenital amaurosis maps to chromosome 6q. Am J Hum Genet 2000; 66(1):319–326.
30. Dryja TP, Adams SM, Grimsby JL, McGee TL, Hong DH, Li T, Andreasson S, Berson EL. Null RPGRIP1 alleles in patients with Leber congenital amaurosis. Am J Hum Genet 2001; 68(5):1295–1298.
31. Keen TJ, Mohamed MD, McKibbin M, Rashid Y, Jafri H, Maumenee IH, Inglehearn CF. Identification of a locus (LCA9) for Leber's congenital amaurosis on chromosome 1p36. Eur J Hum Genet 2003; 11(5):420–423.
32. Freund CL, Wang QL, Chen S, Muskat BL, Wiles CD, Sheffield VC, Jacobson SG, McInnes RR, Zack DJ, Stone EM. De novo mutations in the CRX homeobox gene associated with Leber congenital amaurosis. Nat Genet 1998; 18(4):311–312.
33. Swaroop A, Wang QL, Wu W, Cook J, Coats C, Xu S, Chen S, Zack DJ, Sieving PA. Leber congenital amaurosis caused by a homozygous mutation (R90W) in the homeodomain of the retinal transcription factor CRX: direct evidence for the involvement of CRX in the development of photoreceptor function. Hum Mol Genet 1999; 8(2):299–305.
34. Perrault I, Hanein S, Gerber S, Barbet F, Dufier JL, Munnich A, Rozet JM, Kaplan J. Evidence of autosomal dominant Leber congenital amaurosis (LCA) underlain by a CRX heterozygous null allele. J Med Genet 2003; 40(7):e90.
35. Lotery AJ, Jacobson SG, Fishman GA, Webber RG, Fulton AB, Namperumalsamy P, Heon E, Levin AV, Grover S, Rosenow JR, Kopp KK, Sheffield VC, Stone EM. Mutations in the CRB1 gene cause Leber congenital amaurosis. Arch Ophthalmol 2001; 119(3):415–420.
36. Edwards A, Fishman GA, Anderson RJ, Grover S, Derlacki DJ. Visual acuity and visual field impairment in Usher syndrome. Arch Ophthalmol 1998; 116:165–168.
37. den Hollander AI, Heckenlively JR, van den Born LI, de Kok YJ, van der Velde-Visser SD, Kellner U, Jurklies B, van Schooneveld MJ, Blankenagel A, Rohrschneider K, Wissinger B, Cruysberg JR, Deutman AF, Brunner HG, Apfelstedt-Sylla E, Hoyng CB, Cremers FP. Leber congenital amaurosis and retinitis pigmentosa with Coats-like exudative vasculopathy are associated with mutations in the crumbs homologue 1 (CRB1) gene. Am J Hum Genet 2001; 69(1):198–203.

38. Mizuno K, Takei Y, Sears ML, et al. Leber's congenital amaurosis. Am J Ophthalmol 1967; 83:32–42.
39. Usher CH. On the inheritance of retinitis pigmentosa with notes of cases. R Lond Ophthalmol Hosp Rep 1914; 19:130.
40. McDonald JM, Newsome DA, Rintelmann WF. Sensorineural hearing loss in patients with typical retinitis pigmentosa. Am J Ophthalmol 1988; 105:125–131.
41. Vernon M. Usher's syndrome-deafness and progressive blindness. Clinical cases, prevention, theory and literature survey. J Chronic Dis 1969; 22:13–151.
42. Merin S, Abraham FA, Auerbach E. Usher's and Hallgren's syndromes. Acta Genet Med Gemellol 1973; 23:49–55.
43. Hope CI, Bundey S, Proops D, Fielder AR. Usher syndrome in the city of Birmingham-prevalence and clinical classification. Br J Ophthalmol 1997; 81(1):46–53.
44. Piazza L, Fishman GA, Farber M, et al. Visual acuity loss in patients with Usher's syndrome. Arch Ophthalmol 1986; 104:1336–1339.
45. Hallgren B. Retinitis pigmentosa combined with congenital deafness; with vestibular cerebellar ataxia and mental abnormality in a proportion of cases. A clinical and genetico-statistical study. Acta Psychiat Neurol Scand Suppl 1959; 34:138.
46. Kumar A, Fishman G, Torok N. Vestibular and auditory function in Usher's syndrome. Ann Otol Rhinol Laryngol 1984; 93:600–608.
47. Kloepfer HW, Laguaite JK, McLaurin JW. The hereditary syndrome of congenital deafness and retinitis pigmentosa (Usher's syndrome). Laryngoscope 1966; 76:850–862.
48. Karp A, Santore F. Retinitis pigmentosa and progressive hearing loss. J Speech Hear Disord 1985; 48:308–314.
49. Fishman GA, Kumar A, Joseph ME, et al. Usher's syndrome. Ophthalmic and neuro-otologic findings suggesting genetic heterogeneity. Arch Ophthalmol 1983; 101:1367–1374.
50. Fishman GA, Vasquez V, Fishman M, et al. Visual loss and foveal lesions in Usher's syndrome. Br J Ophthalmol 1979; 63:484–488.
51. Fishman GA, Anderson RJ, Lam BL, Derlacki DJ. Prevalence of foveal lesions in type 1 and type 2 Usher's syndrome. Arch Ophthalmol 1995; 113(6):770–773.
52. Edwards A, Grover S, Fishman GA. Frequency of photographically apparent optic disc and parapapillary nerve fiber layer drusen in Usher syndrome. Retina 1996; 16(5):388–392.
53. Fulton AB, Hansen RM. Foveal cone pigments and sensitivity in young patients with Usher's syndrome. Am J Ophthalmol 1987; 103:150–160.
54. Mills RP, Calver DM. Retinitis pigmentosa and deafness. J R Soc Med 1987; 80:17–20.
55. OMIM. http: //www.ncbi.nlm.nih.gov/omim/.
56. Bloom TD, Fishman GA, Mafee MF. Usher's syndrome: CNS defects determined by computed tomography. Retina 1983; 3:108–113.
57. Piazza L, Fishman GA, Kaplan RD, et al. Magnetic resonance imaging of central nervous system defects in Usher's syndrome. Retina 1987; 7:241–245.
58. Shinkawa H, Nadol JB. Histopathology of the inner ear in Usher's syndrome as observed by light and electron microscopy. Ann Otol Rhinol Laryngol 1986; 95:313–318.
59. Cremers CW, Delleman WJ. Usher's syndrome, temporal bone pathology. Int J Pediatr Otol 1988; 16:23–30.
60. Diager SP, Heckenlively JR, Lewis RA, Pelias MZ. DNA linkage studies of degenerative retinal diseases. Prog Clin Biol Res 1987; 247:147–162.
61. Pelias MZ, Lemoine DR, Kossar AL, et al. Linkage studies of Usher syndrome: analysis of an Acadian kindred in Louisiana. Cytogenet Cell Genet 1988; 47:111–112.
62. Kaplan J, Gerber S, Bonneau D, Rozet JM, Delrieu O, Briard ML, Dollfus H, Ghazi I, Dufier JL, Frezal J, et al. A gene for Usher syndrome type I (USH1A) maps to chromosome 14q. Genomics 1992; 14(4):979–987.
63. Kimberling WJ, Moller CG, Davenport S, Priluck IA, Beighton PH, Greenberg J, Reardon W, Weston MD, Kenyon JB, Grunkemeyer JA, et al. Linkage of Usher syndrome type I gene (USH1B) to the long arm of chromosome 11. Genomics 1992; 14(4):988–994.

64. Weil D, Blanchard S, Kaplan J, Guilford P, Gibson F, Walsh J, Mburu P, Varela A, Levilliers J, Weston MD, et al. Defective myosin VIIA gene responsible for Usher syndrome type IB. Nature 1995; 374(6517):60–61.
65. Weil D, Levy G, Sahly I, Levi-Acobas F, Blanchard S, El-Amraoui A, Crozet F, Philippe H, Abitbol M, Petit C. Human myosin VIIA responsible for the Usher IB syndrome: a predicted membrane-associated motor protein expressed in developing sensory epithelia. Proc Natl Acad Sci USA 1996; 93(8):3232–3237.
66. Kelley PM, Weston MD, Chen ZY, Orten DJ, Hasson T, Overbeck LD, Pinnt J, Talmadge CB, Ing P, Mooseker MS, Corey D, Sumegi J, Kimberling WJ. The genomic structure of the gene defective in Usher syndrome type IB (MYO7A). Genomics 1997; 40(1):73–79.
67. Kubota R, Noda S, Wang Y, Minoshima S, Asakawa S, Kudoh J, Mashima Y, Oguchi Y, Shimizu N. A novel myosin-like protein (myocilin) expressed in the connecting cilium of the photoreceptor: molecular cloning, tissue expression, and chromosomal mapping. Genomics 1997; 41(3):360–369.
68. Levy G, Levi-Acobas F, Blanchard S, Gerber S, Larget-Piet D, Chenal V, Liu XZ, Newton V, Steel KP, Brown SD, Munnich A, Kaplan J, Petit C, Weil D. Myosin VIIA gene: heterogeneity of the mutations responsible for Usher syndrome type IB. Hum Mol Genet 1997; 6(1):111–116.
69. Adato A, Weil D, Kalinski H, Pel-Or Y, Ayadi H, Petit C, Korostishevsky M, Bonne-Tamir B. Mutation profile of all 49 exons of the human myosin VIIA gene, and haplotype analysis, in Usher IB families from diverse origins. Am J Hum Genet 1997; 61(4):813–821.
70. Astuto LM, Weston MD, Carney CA, Hoover DM, Cremers CW, Wagenaar M, Moller C, Smith RJ, Pieke-Dahl S, Greenberg J, Ramesar R, Jacobson SG, Ayuso C, Heckenlively JR, Tamayo M, Gorin MB, Reardon W, Kimberling WJ. Genetic heterogeneity of Usher syndrome: analysis of 151 families with Usher type I. Am J Hum Genet 2000; 67(6):1569–1574.
71. Weil D, Kussel P, Blanchard S, Levy G, Levi-Acobas F, Drira M, Ayadi H, Petit C. The autosomal recessive isolated deafness, DFNB2, and the Usher IB syndrome are allelic defects of the myosin-VIIA gene. Nat Genet 1997l; 16(2):191–193.
72. Bonne-Tamir B, Nystuen A, Seroussi E, Kalinsky H, Kwitek-Black AE, Korostishevsky M, Adato A, Sheffield VC. Usher syndrome in the Samaritans: strengths and limitations of using inbred isolated populations to identify genes causing recessive disorders. Am J Phys Anthropol 1997; 104(2):193–200.
73. Bonne-Tamir B, Korostishevsky M, Kalinsky H, Seroussi E, Beker R, Weiss S, Godel V. Genetic mapping of the gene for Usher syndrome: linkage analysis in a large Samaritan kindred. Genomics 1994; 20(1):36–42.
74. Verpy E, Leibovici M, Zwaenepoel I, Liu XZ, Gal A, Salem N, Mansour A, Blanchard S, Kobayashi I, Keats BJ, Slim R, Petit C. A defect in harmonin, a PDZ domain-containing protein expressed in the inner ear sensory hair cells, underlies Usher syndrome type 1C. Nat Genet 2000; 26(1):51–55.
75. Siemens J, Kazmierczak P, Reynolds A, Sticker M, Littlewood-Evans A, Muller U. The Usher syndrome proteins cadherin 23 and harmonin form a complex by means of PDZ-domain interactions. Proc Natl Acad Sci USA 2002; 99(23):14946–14951.
76. DeAngelis MM, McGee TL, Keats BJ, Slim R, Berson EL, Dryja TP. Two families from New England with usher syndrome type IC with distinct haplotypes. Am J Ophthalmol 2001; 131(3):355–358.
77. Gerber S, Larget-Piet D, Rozet JM, Bonneau D, Mathieu M, Der Kaloustian V, Munnich A, Kaplan J. Evidence for a fourth locus in Usher syndrome type I. J Med Genet 1996; 33(1):77–79.
78. Wayne S, Der Kaloustian VM, Schloss M, Polomeno R, Scott DA, Hejtmancik JF, Sheffield VC, Smith RJ. Localization of the Usher syndrome type ID gene (Ush1D) to chromosome 10. Hum Mol Genet 1996; 5(10):1689–1692.

79. Bolz H, von Brederlow B, Ramirez A, Bryda EC, Kutsche K, Nothwang HG, Seeliger M, del C-Salcedo Cabrera M, Vila MC, Molina OP, Gal A, Kubisch C. Mutation of CDH23, encoding a new member of the cadherin gene family, causes Usher syndrome type ID. Nat Genet 2001; 27(1):108–112.
80. Bork JM, Peters LM, Riazuddin S, Bernstein SL, Ahmed ZM, Ness SL, Polomeno R, Ramesh A, Schloss M, Srisailpathy CR, Wayne S, Bellman S, Desmukh D, Ahmed Z, Khan SN, Kaloustian VM, Li XC, Lalwani A, Riazuddin S, Bitner-Glindzicz M, Nance WE, Liu XZ, Wistow G, Smith RJ, Griffith AJ, Wilcox ER, Friedman TB, Morell RJ. Usher syndrome ID and nonsyndromic autosomal recessive deafness DFNB12 are caused by allelic mutations of the novel cadherin-like gene CDH23. Am J Hum Genet 2001; 68(1):26–37.
81. Chaib H, Kaplan J, Gerber S, Vincent C, Ayadi H, Slim R, Munnich A, Weissenbach J, Petit C. A newly identified locus for Usher syndrome type I, USH1E, maps to chromosome 21q21. Hum Mol Genet 1997; 6(1):27–31.
82. Ahmed ZM, Riazuddin S, Bernstein SL, Ahmed Z, Khan S, Griffith AJ, Morell RJ, Friedman TB, Riazuddin S, Wilcox ER. Mutations of the protocadherin gene PCDH15 cause Usher syndrome type IF. Am J Hum Genet 2001; 69(1):25–34.
83. Ahmed ZM, Riazuddin S, Ahmad J, Bernstein SL, Guo Y, Sabar MF, Sieving P, Riazuddin S, Griffith AJ, Friedman TB, Belyantseva IA, Wilcox ER. PCDH15 is expressed in the neurosensory epithelium of the eye and ear and mutant alleles are responsible for both USH1F and DFNB23. Hum Mol Genet 2003; 12(24):3215–3223.
84. Mustapha M, Chouery E, Torchard-Pagnez D, Nouaille S, Khrais A, Sayegh FN, Megarbane A, Loiselet J, Lathrop M, Petit C, Weil D. A novel locus for Usher syndrome type I, USH1G, maps to chromosome 17q24–25. Hum Genet 2002; 110(4):348–350.
85. Weil D, El-Amraoui A, Masmoudi S, Mustapha M, Kikkawa Y, Laine S, Delmaghani S, Adato A, Nadifi S, Zina ZB, Hamel C, Gal A, Ayadi H, Yonekawa H, Petit C. Usher syndrome type I G (USH1G) is caused by mutations in the gene encoding SANS, a protein that associates with the USH1C protein, harmonin. Hum Mol Genet 2003; 12(5):463–471.
86. van Aarem A, Pinckers AJ, Kimberling WJ, Huygen PL, Bleeker-Wagemakers EM, Cremers CW. Stable and progressive hearing loss in type 2A Usher's syndrome. Ann Otol Rhinol Laryngol 1996; 105(12):962–927.
87. Eudy JD, Yao S, Weston MD, Ma-Edmonds M, Talmadge CB, Cheng JJ, Kimberling WJ, Sumegi J. Isolation of a gene encoding a novel member of the nuclear receptor superfamily from the critical region of Usher syndrome type IIa at Iq41. Genomics 1998; 50(3):382–384.
88. Eudy JD, Weston MD, Yao S, Hoover DM, Rehm HL, Ma-Edmonds M, Yan D, Ahmad I, Cheng JJ, Ayuso C, Cremers C, Davenport S, Moller C, Talmadge CB, Beisel KW, Tamayo M, Morton CC, Swaroop A, Kimberling WJ, Sumegi J. Mutation of a gene encoding a protein with extracellular matrix motifs in Usher syndrome type IIa. Science 1998; 280(5370):1753–1757.
89. Weston MD, Eudy JD, Fujita S, Yao S-F, Usami, S, Cremers C, Greenburg J, Ramesar R, Martini A, Moller C, Smith RJ, Sumegi J, Kimberling William J. Genomic structure and identification of novel mutations in usherin, the gene responsible for Usher syndrome Type IIa. Am J Hum Genet 2000; 66(4):1199–11210.
90. Adato A, Weston MD, Berry A, Kimberling WJ, Bonne-Tamir A. Three novel mutations and twelve polymorphisms identified in the USH2A gene in Israeli USH2 families. Hum Mutat 2000; 15(4):388.
91. Leroy BP, Aragon-Martin JA, Weston MD, Bessant DA, Willis C, Webster AR, Bird AC, Kimberling WJ, Payne AM, Bhattacharya SS. Spectrum of mutations in USU2A in British patients with Usher syndrome type II. Exp Eye Res 2001; 72(5):503–509.

92. Dreyer B, Tranebjaerg L, Rosenberg T, Weston MD, Kimberling WJ, Nilssen O. Identification of novel USH2A mutations: implications for the structure of USH2A protein. Eur J Hum Genet 2000; 8(7):500–506.
93. Rivolta C, Sweklo EA, Berson EL, Dryja TP. Missense mutation in the USH2A gene: association with recessive retinitis pigmentosa without hearing loss. Am J Hum Genet 2000; 66(6):1975–1978.
94. Rivolta C, Berson EL, Dryja TP. Paternal uniparental heterodisomy with partial isodisomy of chromosome 1 in a patient with retinitis pigmentosa without hearing loss and a missense mutation in the Usher syndrome type II gene USH2A. Arch Ophthalmol 2002; 120(11):1566–1571.
95. Zlotogora J. Parents of children with autosomal recessive diseases are not always carriers of the respective mutant alleles. Hum Genet 2004; 114:521–526.
96. Hmani M, Ghorbel A, Boulila-Elgaied A, Ben Zina Z, Kammoun W, Drira M, Chaabouni M, Petit C, Ayadi H. A novel locus for Usher syndrome type II, USH2B, maps to chromosome 3 at p23–24.2. Eur J Hum Genet 1999; 7(3):363–367.
97. Pieke-Dahl S, Moller CG, Kelley PM, Astuto LM, Cremers CW, Gorin MB, Kimberling WJ. Genetic heterogeneity of Usher syndrome type II localisation to chromosome 5q. J Med Genet 2000; 37(4):256–262.
98. Weston MD, Luijendijk MW, Humphrey KD, Moller C, Kimberling WJ. Mutations in the VLGR1 gene implicate G-protein signaling in the pathogenesis of Usher syndrome type II. Am J Hum Genet 2004; 74(2):357–366.
99. Gasparini P, De Fazio A, Croce AI, Stanziale P, Zelante L. Usher syndrome type III (USH3) linked to chromosome 3q in an Italian family. J Med Genet 1998; 35(8):666–667.
100. Joensuu T, Hamalainen R, Yuan B, Johnson C, Tegelberg S, Gasparini P, Zelante L, Pirvola U, Pakarinen L, Lehesjoki AE, de la Chapelle A, Sankila EM. Mutations in a novel gene with transmembrane domains underlie Usher syndrome type 3. Erratum appears in Am J Hum Genet 2001; 69(4): 673–684. 2001; 69(5):1160.
101. Adato A, Vreugde S, Joensuu T, Avidan N, Hamalainen R, Belenkiy O, Olender T, Bonne-Tamir B, Ben-Asher E, Espinos C, Millan JM, Lehesjoki AE, Flannery JG, Avraham KB, Pietrokovski S, Sankila EM, Beckmann JS, Lancet D. USH3A transcripts encode clarin-1, a four-transmembrane-domain protein with a possible role in sensory synapses. Eur J Hum Genet 2002; 10(6):339–350.
102. Liu XZ, Hope C, Walsh J, Newton V, Ke XM, Liang CY, Xu LR, Zhou JM, Trump D, Steel KP, Bundey S, Brown SD. Mutations in the myosin VIIA gene cause a wide phenotypic spectrum, including atypical Usher syndrome. Am J Hum Genet 1998; 63(3):909–912.
103. Laurence JZ, Moon RC. Four cases of retinitis pigmentosa, occurring in the same family, and accompanied by general imperfections of development. Ophthalmic Rev 1866; 2:32–34.
104. Bardet G. Sur un syndrome d'obésité congenitale avec polydactylie et rétinite pigjrnentaire. Thesis, Paris, 1920.
105. Biedl A. Ein Geschwisterpaar mit adiposo-genitaler dystrophie. Dtsch Med Wochenschr 1922; 48:1630.
106. Schachat AP, Maumenee IH. Bardet-Biedl syndrome and related disorders. Arch Ophthalmol 1982; 100:285–288.
107. Campo RV, Aaberg TM. Ocular and systemic manifestations of the Bardet-Biedl syndrome. Am J Ophthalmol 1982; 34:750–756.
108. Ehrenfeld EN, Rowe H, Auerbach E. Laurence-Moon-Bardet-Biedl syndrome in Israel. Am J Ophthalmol 1970; 70:524–532.
109. Rizzo JF, Berson EL, Lessell S. Retinal and neurologic findings in the Laurence-Moon-Bardet-Biedl phenotype. Ophthalmology 1986; 93:1452–1456.
110. Fulton AB, Hansen RM, Glynn RJ. Natural course of visual functions in the Bardet-Biedl syndrome. Arch Ophthalmol 1993; 111(11):1500–1506.

111. Riise R. The cause of death in Laurence-Moon-Bardet-Biedl syndrome. Acta Ophthalmol Scand Suppl 1996; 219:45–47.
112. Cantani A, Bellioni P, Bamonte G, et al. Severe hereditary syndromes with pigmentary retinopathy: a review and differential diagnosis. Clin Pediatr 1985; 24:578–583.
113. Runge P, Calver D, Marshall J, Taylor O. Histopathology of mitochondrial cytopathy and the Laurence-Moon-Biedl syndrome. Br J Ophthalmol 1986; 70:782–796.
114. Kwitek-Black AE, Carmi R, Duyk GM, Buetow KH, Elbedour K, Parvari R, Yandava CN, Stone EM, Sheffield VC. Linkage of Bardet-Biedl syndrome to chromosome 16q and evidence for non-allelic genetic heterogeneity. Nat Genet 1993; 5(4):392–396.
115. Leppert M, Baird L, Anderson KL, Otterud B, Lupski JR, Lewis RA. Bardet-Biedl syndrome is linked to DNA markers on chromosome 1 lq and is genetically heterogeneous. Nat Genet 1994; 7(1):108–112.
116. Mykytyn K, Nishimura DY, Searby CC, Shastri M, Yen HJ, Beck JS, Braun T, Streb LM, Cornier AS, Cox GF, Fulton AB, Carmi R, Luleci G, Chandrasekharappa SC, Collins FS, Jacobson SG, Heckenlively JR, Weleber RG, Stone EM, Sheffield VC. Identification of the gene (BBSl) most commonly involved in Bardet-Biedl syndrome, a complex human obesity syndrome. Nat Genet 2002; 31(4):435–438.
117. Bruford EA, Riise R, Teague PW, Porter K, Thomson KL, Moore AT, Jay M, Warburg M, Schinzel A, Tommerup N, Tornqvist K, Rosenberg T, Patton M, Mansfield DC, Wright AF. Linkage mapping in 29 Bardet-Biedl syndrome families confirms loci in chromosomal regions 11ql3, 15q22.3-q23 and 16q21. Genomics 1997; 41(1):93–99.
118. Beales PL, Warner AM, Hitman GA, Thakker R, Flinter FA. Bardet-Biedl syndrome: a molecular and phenotypic study of 18 families. J Med Genet 1997; 34(2):92–98.
119. Mykytyn K, Nishimura DY, Searby CC, Beck G, Bugge K, Haines HL, Cornier AS, Cox GF, Fulton AB, Carmi R, Iannaccone A, Jacobson SG, Weleber RG, Wright AF, Riise R, Hennekam RC, Luleci G, Berker-Karauzum S, Biesecker LG, Stone EM, Sheffield VC. Evaluation of complex inheritance involving the most common Bardet-Biedl syndrome locus (BBS1). Am J Hum Genet 2003; 72(2):429–437.
120. Koenekoop R. The major gene for Bardet-Biedl syndrome is BBS1. Ophthalmic Genet 2003; 24(2):127.
121. Nishimura DY, Searby CC, Carmi R, Elbedour K, Van Maldergem L, Fulton AB, Lam BL, Powell BR, Swiderski RE, Bugge KE, Haider NB, Kwitek-Black AE, Ying L, Duhl DM, Gorman SW, Heon E, Lannaccone A, Bonneau D, Biesecker LG, Jacobson SG, Stone EM, Sheffield VC. Positional cloning of a novel gene on chromosome 16q causing Bardet-Biedl syndrome (BBS2). Hum Mol Genet 2001; 10(8):865–874.
122. Carmi R, Elbedour K, Stone EM, Sheffield VC. Phenotypic differences among patients with Bardet-Biedl syndrome linked to three different chromosome loci. Am J Med Genet 1995; 59(2):199–203.
123. Katsanis N, Ansley SJ, Badano JL, Eichers ER, Lewis RA, Hoskins BE, Scambler PJ, Davidson WS, Beales PL, Lupski JR. Triallelic inheritance in Bardet-Biedl syndrome, a Mendelian recessive disorder. Science 2001; 293(5538):2256–2259.
124. Sheffield VC, Carmi R, Kwitek-Black A, Rokhlina T, Nishimura D, Duyk GM, Elbedour K, Sunden SL, Stone EM. Identification of a Bardet-Biedl syndrome locus on chromosome 3 and evaluation of an efficient approach to homozygosity mapping. Hum Mol Genet 1994; 3(8):1331–1335.
125. Young TL, Woods MO, Parfrey PS, Green JS, O'Leary E, Hefferton D, Davidson WS. Canadian Bardet-Biedl syndrome family reduces the critical region of BBS3 (3p) and presents with a variable phenotype. Am J Med Genet 1998; 78(5):461–467.
126. Ghadami M, Tomita HA, Najafi MT, Damavandi E, Farahvash MS, Yamada K, Majidzadeh-A K, Niikawa N. Bardet-Biedl syndrome type 3 in an Iranian family: clinical study and confirmation of disease localization. Am J Med Genet. 2000; 94(5):433–437.
127. Carmi R, Rokhlina T, Kwitek-Black AE, Elbedour K, Nishimura D, Stone EM, Sheffield VC. Use of a DNA pooling strategy to identify a human obesity syndrome locus on chromosome 15. Hum Mol Genet 1995; 4(1):9–13.

128. Riise R, Tornqvist K, Wright AF, Mykytyn K, Sheffield VC. The phenotype in Norwegian patients with Bardet-Biedl syndrome with mutations in the BBS4 gene. Arch Ophthalmol 2002; 120(10):1364–1367.
129. Mykytyn K, Braun T, Carmi R, Haider NB, Searby CC, Shastri M, Beck G, Wright AF, Iannaccone A, Elbedour K, Riise R, Baldi A, Raas-Rothschild A, Gorman SW, Duhl DM, Jacobson SG, Casavant T, Stone EM, Sheffield VC. Identification of the gene that, when mutated, causes the human obesity syndrome BBS4. Nat Genet 2001; 28(2):188–191.
130. Young TL, Penney L, Woods MO, Parfrey PS, Green JS, Hefferton D, Davidson WS. A fifth locus for Bardet-Biedl syndrome maps to chromosome 2q31. Am J Hum Genet 1999; 64(3):900–904.
131. Woods MO, Young TL, Parfrey PS, Hefferton D, Green JS, Davidson WS. Genetic heterogeneity of Bardet-Biedl syndrome in a distinct Canadian population: evidence for a fifth locus. Genomics 1999; 55(1):2–9.
132. Katsanis N, Beales PL, Woods MO, Lewis RA, Green JS, Parfrey PS, Ansley SJ, Davidson WS, Lupski JR. Mutations in MKKS cause obesity, retinal dystrophy and renal malformations associated with Bardet-Biedl syndrome. Nat Genet 2000; 26(1):67–70.
133. Slavotinek AM, Stone EM, Mykytyn K, Heckenlively JR, Green JS, Heon E, Musarella MA, Parfrey PS, Sheffield VC, Biesecker LG. Mutations in MKKS cause Bardet-Biedl syndrome. Nat Genet 2000; 26(1):15–16.
134. Badano JL, Ansley SJ, Leitch CC, Lewis RA, Lupski JR, Katsanis N. Identification of a novel Bardet-Biedl syndrome protein, BBS7, that shares structural features with BBS1 and BBS2. Am J Hum Genet 2003; 72(3):650–658.
135. Ansley SJ, Badano JL, Blacque OE, Hill J, Hoskins BE, Leitch CC, Kim JC, Ross AJ, Eichers ER, Teslovich TM, Mah AK, Johnsen RC, Cavender JC, Lewis RA, Leroux MR, Beales PL, Katsanis N. Basal body dysfunction is a likely cause of pleiotropic Bardet-Biedl syndrome. Nature 2003; 425(6958):628–633.
136. Verloes A, Temple IK, Bonnet S, Bottani A. Coloboma, mental retardation, hypogonadism, and obesity: critical review of the so-called Biemond syndrome type 2, updated nosology, and delineation of three "new" syndromes. Am J Med Genet 1997; 69(4):370–379.
137. Bassen FA, Kornzweig AL. Malformations of the erythrocytes in a case of atypical retinitis pigmentosa. Blood 1950; 5:381–387.
138. Cogan DG, Rodrigues MM, Chu FC, Schaefer EJ. Ocular abnormalities in abetalipoproteinemia: a clinicopathologic correlation. Ophthalmology 1984; 91:991–998.
139. Bishara S, Merin S, Cooper M, et al. Combined vitamin A and E therapy prevents retinal electrophysiological deterioration in abetalipoproteinemia. Br J Ophthalmol 1982; 66:767–770.
140. Runge P, Muller DPR, McAllister J, et al. Oral vitamin E supplements can prevent the retinopathy of abetalipoproteinemia. Br J Ophthalmol 1986; 70:166–173.
141. Chowers I, Banin E, Merin S, Cooper M, Granot E. Long-term assessment of combined vitamin A and E treatment for the prevention of retinal degeneration in abetalipoproteinaemia and hypobetalipoproteinaemia patients. Eye 2001; 15(Pt 4):525–530.
142. Narcisi TM, Shoulders CC, Chester SA, Read J, Brett DJ, Harrison GB, Grantham TT, Fox MF, Povey S, de Bruin TW, et al. Mutations of the microsomal triglyceride-transfer-protein gene in abetalipoproteinemia. Am J Hum Genet 1995; 57(6):1298–1310.
143. Refsum S. Heredopathia atactica polyneuritiformis: a familial syndrome not hitherto described. Acta Psychiatr Scand Suppl 1946; 38.
144. Hansen E, Bachen Nl, Flage T. Refsum's disease: eye manifestations in a patient treated with low phytol low phytanic acid diet. Acta Ophthalmol 1979; 57:899–913.
145. Klenk E, Kahlke W. Ueber das Vorkommen der 3.7.11.15-tetramethyl hexadecansaeure (Phytansaeure) in der cholesterinestern und anderen Lipoidfraktionen der Organe beieinem Krankheitsfall unbekannter Genese (Verdacht aus heredopathia atactica polyneuritiformis Refsum-syndrom). Hoppe Seyler Z Physiol Chem 1963; 333:133–142.

146. Toussaint D, Danis P. An ocular pathologic study of Refsum's syndrome. Am J Ophthalmol 1971; 72:342–347.
147. Elojarn L, Stokke O, Try K. Biochemical aspects of Refsum's disease and principles for the dietary treatment. In: Vinken PJ, Bruyn GW, eds. Handbook of Clinical Neurology, Amsterdam: Elsevier North-Holland 1977; Vol. 27:519–541.
148. Gibbard FB, Page NGR, Billimoria JD, Retsas S. Heredopathia atactica polyneuritiformis (Refsum's disease) treated by diet and plasma exchange. Lancet 1979; 1:575–578.
149. Moser HW, Braine H, Peyritz RE, et al. Therapeutic trial of plasmapheresis in Refsum disease and in Fabry disease. Birth Defects 1980; 16:491–497.
150. Tuck RR, McLeod JG. Retinitis pigmentosa, ataxia and peripheral neuropathy. J Neurol Neurosurg Psychiatry 1983; 46:206–213.
151. Nadal N, Rolland MO, Tranchant C, Reutenauer L, Gyapay G, Warter JM, Mandel JL, Koenig M. Localization of Refsum disease with increased pipecolic acidaemia to chromosome l0p by homozygosity mapping and carrier testing in a single nuclear family. Hum Mol Genet 1995; 4(10):1963–1966.
152. Mihalik SJ, Morrell JC, Kim D, Sacksteder KA, Watkins PA, Gould SJ. Identification of PAHX, a Refsum disease gene. Nat Genet 1997; 17(2):185–189.
153. Jansen GA, Ofman R, Ferdinandusse S, Ijlst L, Muijsers AO, Skjeldal OH, Stokke OH, Jakobs C, Besley GT, Wraith JE, Wanders RJ. Refsum disease is caused by mutations in the phytanoyl-CoA hydroxylase gene. Nat Genet 1997; 17(2):190–193.
154. Jansen GA, Wanders RJ, Watkins PA, Mihalik SJ. Phytanoyl-coenzyme A hydroxylase deficiency-the enzyme defect in Refsum's disease. N Engl J Med 1997; 337(2):133–134.
155. van den Brink DM, Brites P, Haasjes J, Wierzbicki AS, Mitchell J, Lambert-Hamill M, de Belleroche J, Jansen GA, Waterham HR, Wanders RJ. Identification of PEX7 as the second gene involved in Refsum disease. Am J Hum Genet 2003; 72(2):471–477.
156. Grant CA, Berson EL. Treatable forms of retinitis pigmentosa associated with systemic neurological disorders. Int Ophthalmol Clin. 2001; 41(1):103–110.
157. Lehmann AR, Francis AJ, Gianneli F. Prenatal diagnosis of Cockayne's syndrome. Lancet 1985; 1:486–488.
158. Levin PS, Green R, Victor DI, McLean AL. Histopathology of the eye in Cockayne's syndrome. Arch Ophthalmol 1985; 101:1093–1097.
159. van Oosterwijk MF, Versteeg A, Filon R, van Zeeland AA, Mullenders LH. The sensitivity of Cockayne's syndrome cells to DNA-damaging agents is not due to defective transcription-coupled repair of active genes. Mol Cell Biol 1996; 16(8):4436–4444.
160. Henning KA, Li L, Iyer N, McDaniel LD, Reagan MS, Legerski R, Schultz RA, Stefanini M, Lehmann AR, Mayne LV, et al. The Cockayne syndrome group A gene encodes a WD repeat protein that interacts with CSB protein and a subunit of RNA polymerase II TFIIH. Cell 1995; 82(4):555–564.
161. Zeman W. Batten disease. ocular features differential diagnosis and diagnosis by enzyme analysis. Birth Defects 1976; 12:441–453.
162. Spalton DJ, Taylor DSI, Sanders MD. Juvenile Batten's disease: an ophthalmological assessment of 26 patients. Br J Ophthalmol 1980; 69:726–732.
163. Goebel HH, Fix JD, Zeman W. Retina in ceroid lipofuscinosis. Am J Ophthalmol 1977; 77:25–39.
164. Jarvela I, Sainio M, Rantamaki T, Olkkonen VM, Carpen O, Peltonen L, Jalanko A. Biosynthesis and intracellular targeting of the CLN3 protein defective in Batten disease. Hum Mol Genet 1998; 7(1):85–90.
165. Goebel HH. The neuronal ceroid-lipofuscinoses. J Child Neurol 1995; 10(6):424–437.
166. Bensaoula T, Shibuya H, Katz ML, Smith JE, Johnson GS, John SK, Milam AH. Histopathologic and immunocytochemical analysis of the retina and ocular tissues in Batten disease. Ophthalmology 2000; 107(9):1746–1753.
167. Resnick K, Zuckerman J, Cotlier E. Cohen syndrome with bull's eye macular lesion. Ophthalmic Paediatr Genet 1986; 7:1–8.

168. Sack J, Friedman G. The Cohen syndrome in Israel. Isr J Med Sci 1986; 22:766–770.
169. Kivitie-Kallio S, Summanen P, Raitta C, Norio R, Ophthalmologic findings in Cohen syndrome. A long-term follow-up. Ophthalmology 2000; 107(9):1737–1745.
170. Kolehmainen J, Norio R, Kivitie-Kallio S, Tahvanainen E, de la Chapelle A, Lehesjoki AE. Refined mapping of the Cohen syndrome gene by linkage disequilibrium. Eur J Hum Genet 1997; 5(4):206–213.
171. Kolehmainen J, Black GC, Saarinen A, Chandler K, Clayton-Smith J, Traskelin AL, Perveen R, Kivitie-Kallio S, Norio R, Warburg M, Fryns JP, de la Chapelle A, Lehesjoki AE. Cohen syndrome is caused by mutations in a novel gene, COH1, encoding a transmembrane protein with a presumed role in vesicle-mediated sorting and intracellular protein transport. Am J Hum Genet 2003; 72(6):1359–1369.
172. Dooling EC, Schoene WC, Richardson EP. Hallervorden-Spatz syndrome. Arch Neurol 1974; 30:70–83.
173. Newell FW, Johnson RD, Huttenlocher PR. Pigmentary degeneration of the retina in the Hallervorden-Spatz syndrome. Am J Ophthalmol 1979; 88:467–471.
174. Luckenbach MW, Green WR, Miller NR, et al. Ocular clinicopathologic correlation of Hallervorden-Spatz syndrome with acenthocytosis and pigmentary retinopathy. Am J Ophthalmol 1983; 95:369–382.
175. Zhou B, Westaway SK, Levinson B, Johnson MA, Gitschier J, Hayflick SJ. A novel pantothenate kinase gene (PANK2) is defective in Hallervorden-Spatz syndrome. Nat Genet 2001; 28(4):345–349.
176. Hayflick SJ, Westaway SK, Levinson B, Zhou B, Johnson MA, Ching KH, Gitschier J. Genetic, clinical, and radiographic delineation of Hallervorden-Spatz syndrome. N Engl J Med 2003; 348(1):33–40.
177. Tremblay F, LaRoche RG, Shea SE, Ludman MD. Longitudinal study of the early electroretinographic changes in Alstrom's syndrome. Am J Ophthalmol 1993; 115(5):657–665.
178. Russell-Eggitt IM, Clayton PT, Coffey R, Kriss A, Taylor DS, Taylor JF. Alstrom syndrome. Report of 22 cases and literature review. Ophthalmology 1998; 105(7):1274–1280.
179. Millay RH, Weleber RG, Heckenlively JR. Ophthalmologic and systemic manifestations of Alstrom's disease. Am J Ophthalmol 1986; 102:482–490.
180. Collin GB, Marshall JD, Cardon LR, Nishina PM. Homozygosity mapping at Alstrom syndrome to chromosome 2p. Hum Mol Genet 1997; 6(2):213–219.
181. Hearn T, Renforth GL, Spalluto C, Hanley NA, Piper K, Brickwood S, White C, Connolly V, Taylor JF, Russeli-Eggitt I, Bonneau D, Walker M, Wilson DI. Mutation of ALMSl, a large gene with a tandem repeat encoding 47 amino acids, causes Alstrom syndrome. Nat Genet 2002; 31(1):79–83.
182. Collin GB, Marshall JD, Ikeda A, So WV, Russell-Eggitt I, Maffei P, Beck S, Boerkoel CF, Sicolo N, Martin M, Nishina PM, Naggert JK. Mutations in ALMSl cause obesity, type 2 diabetes and neurosensory degeneration in Alstrom syndrome. Nat Genet 2002; 31(1):74–78.
183. Stanesu-Segal B, Evrard P. Zellweger syndrome, retinal involvement. Metab Pediatr Syst Ophthalmol 1989; 12(4):96–99.
184. Reuber BE, Germain-Lee E, Collins CS, Morrell JC, Ameritunga R, Moser HW, Valle D, Gould SJ. Mutations in PEX1 are the most common cause of peroxisome biogenesis disorders. Nat Genet 1997; 17(4):445–448.
185. Loken AC, Hanssen O, Halvorsen S, Jolster NJ. Hereditary renal dysplasia and blindness. Acta Paediatr Scand 1961; 50:177–184.
186. Peterson WS, Albert DM. Fundus changes in the hereditary nephropathies. Trans Am Acad Ophthalmol Otolaryngol 1974; 78:762–771.
187. Polak BCP, Hogewind BL, van Lith HM. Tapetoretinal degeneration associated with recessively inherited medullary cystic disease. Am J Ophthalmol 1977; 84:645–651.

188. Polak BCP, van Lith FHM, Delleman JW, van Ballen TM. Carrier detection in tapetoretinal degeneration in association with medullary cystic disease. Am J Ophthalmol 1983; 95:487–494.
189. Abraham FA, Yanko L, Licht A, Viskoper RJ. Electrophysiologic study of the visual system in familial juvenile nephronophthisis and tapetoretinal dystrophy. Am J Ophthalmol 1974; 78:591–597.
190. Friedlaender MM, Rubinger D, Silver J, et al. A family with retinitis pigmentosa and ESRD with late presentation, hypertension and absence of polyuria or salt wasting. Clin Nephrol 1986; 25:202–206.
191. Godel V, Iaina A, Nemet P, Lazar M. Retinal manifestations in familial juvenile nephronophthisis. Clin Genet 1979; 16:277–281.
192. Hildebrandt F, Otto E, Rensing C, Nothwang HG, Vollmer M, Adolphs J, Hanusch H, Brandis M. A novel gene encoding an SH3 domain protein is mutated in nephronophthisis type 1. Nat Genet 1997; 17(2):149–153.
193. Otto E, Kispert A, Schatzle, Lescher B, Rensing C, Hildebrandt F. Nephrocystin: gene expression and sequence conservation between human, mouse, and Caenorhabditis elegans. J Am Soc Nephrol 2000; 11(2):270–282.
194. Omran H, Sasmaz G, Haffner K, Volz A, Olbrich H, Melkaoui R, Otto E, Wienker TF, Korinthenberg R, Brandis M, Antignac C, Hildebrandt F. Identification of a gene locus for Senior-Loken syndrome in the region of the nephronophthisis type 3 gene. J Am Soc Nephrol 2002; 13(1):75–79.
195. Schuermann MJ, Otto E, Becker A, Saar K, Ruschendorf F, Polak BC, Ala-Mello S, Hoefele J, Wiedensohler A, Haller M, Omran H, Nurnberg P, Hildebrandt F. Mapping of gene loci for nephronophthisis type 4 and Senior-Loken syndrome, to chromosome 1p36. Am J Hum Genet 2002; 70(5):1240–1246.
196. Otto E, Hoefele I, Ruf R, Mueller AM, Hiller KS, Wolf MT, Schuermann MJ, Becker A, Birkenhager R, Sudbrak R, Hennies HC, Nurnberg P, Hildebrandt F. A gene mutated in nephronophthisis and retinitis pigmentosa encodes a novel protein, nephroretinin, conserved in evolution. Am J Hum Genet 2002; 71(5):1161–1167.
197. Olbrich H, Fliegauf M, Hoefele J, Kispert A, Otto E, Volz A, Wolf MT, Sasmaz G, Trauer U, Reinhardt R, Sudbrak R, Antignac C, Gretz N, Walz G, Schermer B, Benzing T, Hildebrandt F, Omran H. Mutations in a novel gene, NPHP3, cause adolescent nephronophthisis, tapeto-retinal degeneration and hepatic fibrosis. Nat Genet 2003; 34(4):455–459.
198. Otto EA, Schermer B, Obara T, O'Toole JF, Hiller KS, Mueller AM, Ruf RG, Hoefele J, Beekmann F, Landau D, Foreman JW, Goodship JA, Strachan T, Kispert A, Wolf MT, Gagnadoux MF, Nivet H, Antignac C, Walz G, Drummond IA, Benzing T, Hildebrandt F. Mutations in INVS encoding inversin cause nephronophthisis type 2, linking renal cystic disease to the function of primary cilia and left-right axis determination. Nat Genet 2003; 34(4):413–420.
199. Kalra PA, Turney JH. Mesangioproliferative glomerulonephritis associated with retinitis pigmentosa. Br J Ophthalmol 1988; 72:210–211.
200. Dekaban AS. Hereditary syndrome of congenital retinal blindness (Leber), polycystic kidneys and maldevelopment of the brain. Am J Ophthalmol 1969; 68: 1029–1037.
201. Kearns TP, Sayre GP. Retinitis pigmentosa, external ophthalmoplegia and complete heart block. Arch Ophthalmol 1958; 60:280–289.
202. Drachmann DA. Ophthalmoplegia plus: the neurodegenerative disorders associated with progressive external ophthalmoplegia. Arch Neurol 1968; 18:654–674.
203. Beckerman BL, Henkind P. Progressive external ophthalmoplegia and benign retinal pigmentation. Am J Ophthalmol 1976; 81:89–92.
204. Mitsumoto H, Aprille JR, Wray SH, et al. Chronic progressive external ophthalmoplegia (CPEO): clinical morphologic and biochemical studies. Neurology 1983; 33: 452–461.

205. Butler IJ, Gadoth N. Kearns-Sayre syndrome: a review of a multisystem disorder of children and young adults. Arch Intern Med 1976; 136:1290–1293.
206. Yorifuji S, Nishikawa Y, Takahashi M, Tarui S. Mitochondrial function in Kearns-Sayre syndrome. Neurology 1988; 38:999–1000.
207. Leveille AS, Newell FW. Autosomal dominant Kearns-Sayre syndrome. Ophthalmology 1980; 87:99–108.
208. Bernal JE, Winz O, Tamayo M. The Kearns-Sayre syndrome in three members of a consanguineous Colombian family. Seventh International Congress on Human Genetics, Berlin, 1986: p280.
209. Egger J, Wilson J. Mitochonrial inheritance in a mitochondrially mediated disease. N Engl J Med 1983; 309:142–146.
210. Channer KS, Channer JL, Campbell MJ, Rees JR. Cardiomyopathy in the Kearns-Sayre syndrome. Br Heart J 1988; 59:486–490.
211. Bachynski BN, Flynn JT, Rodigues MM, et al. Hyperglycemic acidotic coma and death in Kearns-Sayre syndrome. Ophthalmology 1986; 193:391–396.
212. Eagle RC, Hedges TR, Yanoff M. The atypical pigmentary retinopathy of Kearns-Sayre syndrome. A light and electron microscopic study. Ophthalmology 1982; 89:1433–1440.
213. Eagle RC, Hedges TR, Yanoff M. The Kearns-Sayre syndrome: a light and electron microscopic study. Trans Am Ophthalmol Soc 1982; 80:218–232.
214. Flynn JT, Bachynski BN, Rodrigues MM, et al. Hyperglycemic acidotic coma and death in Kearns-Sayre syndrome. Trans Am Ophthalmol Soc 1985; 83:131–161.
215. Bresolin N, Moggio M, Bet L, et al. Progressive cytochrome c oxidase deficiency in a case of Kearns-Sayre syndrome: morphological, immunological, and biochemical studies in muscle biopsies and autopsy tissues. Ann Neurol 1987; 21:564–572.
216. Byrae E, Marzuki S, Sattayasai N, et al. Mitochondrial studies in Kearns-Sayre syndrome: Normal respiratory chain function with absence of a mitochondrial translation product. Neurology 1987; 37:1530–1534.
217. Ogasahara S, Nishikawa Y, Yorifuji S, et al. Treatment of Kearns-Sayre syndrome with coenzyme Q10. Neurology 1986; 36:45–53.
218. Baruso RC, Kaiser-Kupfer MI, Muenzer J, et al. Electroretinographic findings in the mucopolysaccharidoses. Ophthalmology 1986; 93:1612–1616.
219. Abraham FA, Yatziv S, Russell A, Auerbach E. Electrophysiological and psychophysical findings in Hunter syndrome. Arch Ophthalmol 1974; 91:181–186.
220. Abraham FA, Yatziv S, Russell A, Auerbach E. A family with two siblings affected by Morquio syndrome (MPS IV). Electrophysiological and psychophysical findings in the visual system. Arch Ophthalmol 1977; 91:265–269.
221. Kollarits CR, Mehelas TJ, Shealy TR, Zahn JR. Von Hippel tumors in siblings with retinitis pigmentosa. Ann Ophthalmol 1982; 14:256–259.
222. Patton MA, Harding AE, Baraitser M. Congenital trichomegaly, pigmentary retinal degeneration and short stature. Am J Ophthalmol 1986; 101:490–492.
223. Portoian-Shuhaiber S, Gumaa K, Hamalawi H, et al. Siblings with a progressive neurodegenerative condition associated with basal ganglia calcifications, retinitis pigmentosa and decreased levels of fucosidase: a new presentation? J Inherited Metab Dis 1987; 10:397–398.
224. Ryan SJ, Smith RE. Retinopathy associated with olivopontocerebellar degeneration. Am J Ophthalmol 1971; 71:838–843.
225. Aleman TS, Cideciyan AV, Volpe NJ, Stevanin G, Brice A, Jacobson SG. Spinocerebellar ataxia type 7 (SCA7) shows a cone-rod dystrophy phenotype. Exp Eye Res 2002; 74(6):737–745.
226. Higgins JJ, Morton DH, Loveless JM. Posterior column ataxia with retinitis pigmentosa (AXPC1) maps to chromosome 1q31-q32. Neurology 1999; 52(1):146–150.
227. Yokota T, Shiojiri T, Gotoda T, Arita M, Arai H, Ohga T, Kanda T, Suzuki J, Imai T, Matsumoto H, Harino S, Kiyosawa M, Mizusawa H, Inoue K. Friedreich-like ataxia

with retinitis pigmentosa caused by the His101Gln mutation of the alpha-tocopherol transfer protein gene. Ann Neurol 1997; 41(6):826–832.

228. Seeliger MW, Biesalski HK, Wissinger B, Gollnick H, Gielen S, Frank J, Beck S, Zrenner E. Phenotype in retinol deficiency due to a hereditary defect in retinol binding protein synthesis. Invest Ophthalmol Vis Sci 1999; 40(1):3–11.

12

Vitreous and Hyaloideoretinal Degeneration

INTRODUCTION

To the examining physician, the vitreous displays such an inert appearance that it is difficult to consider the possibility of serious pathologic activity occurring in its low-metabolic-activity, low-cellularity, sticky fluid. However, about a decade after Jules Gonin discovered the role of retinal holes in causing retinal detachments, the first report of an inherited vitreoretinal degeneration was published (1). Wagner (1) described an autosomal dominant disease affecting the vitreous, retina, and lens in a Swiss family and named it hyaloideoretinal degeneration. Later, it became apparent that three different hereditary forms of hyaloideoretinal degenerations occur, namely, autosomal dominant, autosomal recessive, and sex-linked (2). Still later, the occasional association with extraocular abnormalities such as abnormalities of the joints and skeleton (3), cleft palate (4), and generalized connective tissue disease was found (5). In fact, the autosomal dominant isolated form of Wagner (1) seemed to be much less common than the autosomal dominant form associated with a generalized connective tissue disorder. In addition, several "new" forms of an isolated vitreoretinal degeneration were described, which did not fit into any of the known forms.

In this chapter, the inherited vitreoretinopathies or, as they were usually called by the previous generation, the hereditary hyaloideoretinal degenerations will be discussed under two separate headings: the isolated forms (Table 1) and the associated forms, or as they are now frequently named the nonsyndromic and syndromic types, respectively. A large number of mutations in genes associated with collagen metabolism have been identified found to be associated with vitreo–retinal degenerations.

VITREORETINAL NONSYNDROMIC DEGENERATION AS AN ISOLATED DISORDER

Description

This group of disorders involves several clinical entities, each with a clear genetic background and abnormalities of both the vitreous and the retina (see Table 1).

Table 1 The Isolated (Nonsyndromic) Inherited Vitreoretinal Degenerations

			Main clinical characteristics					
Name	Synonyms	Inheritance	Early	Late complications	Myopia	ERG	Gene/locus	Chromosomal location
Wagner disease	Dominant hyaloideo-retinal dystrophy	AD	Optical empty vitreous with circumferential membrane and retinal pigmentation	Cataract; retinal vascular sheathing; retinal detachment	Usually mild	Subnormal	WGN1 WGN2/ COL2A1	5q13–14 12q13.11
Jansen disease	Wagner disease[a]	AD	Fibrillar degeneration of vitreous white-with-pressure; chorioretinal atrophy	Giant breaks; retinal detachment	Often high	Mild to severe reduction	As above	As above
Erosive vitreo-retinopathy	Wagner disease[a]	AD	RPE atrophy	Progressive RPE and retinal atrophy	Variable	Mild to severe reduction	As above	As above
GFS Goldmann-Favre	Recessive hyaloideo-retinal dystrophy; ESCS	AR	Night blindness; retinoschisis; retinal pigmentation and atrophy	Retinal detach-ment; cystoid edema or maculo-schisis	Variable; hyperopia common	Often unrecord-able or very low	NR2E3	15q23
Familial exudative vitreoreti-nopathy	AD-FEVR	AD	Fibrillar degeneration of vitreous; leaky retinal vasculature; dragged macula	Massive periretinal exudation and retinal detachment	Variable	Normal or mildly reduced	EVR1/FADH	11q13–23

FEVR X-linked	XL-FEVR	XL	Falciform fold	Retinal exudate, avascularity, and neovascularization	Variable	Mild to severe reduction	EVR3/LRP5 EVR2/NDP	11p12–13 Xp11.4–11.3
Hereditary snowflake vitreoretinal degeneration	—	AD	Fibrillar degeneration of vitreous; white-with-pressure; white or yellowish retinal flakes	Retinal detachment	Variable	Normal or mildly reduced	—	—
Autosomal dominant vitreoretinochoroidopathy	ADVIRC	AD	Annular midperipheral retina; pigmentation	Usually nonprogressive; cystold macular edema	Variable	Normal or mildly reduced	—	—
Autosomal recessive vitreo-retinopathy		AR	Vitreous liquefaction	RP-like retinal dystrophy	High	Moderate to severe reduction	—	22q13

Note: AD, autosomal dominant; AR, autosomal recessive; XL, X-linked recessive; ESCS, enhanced S-cone syndrome.

[a]Used as a synonym by those who have a wider classification of Wagner disease; Wagner and Jansen diseases and erosive vitreoretinopathy seem to be one entity of different severity.

One or more additional ocular tissues may be affected by the disease, but no apparent extraocular involvement can be detected. The primary site of the disorder may be the retina or the vitreous, but the vitreous always plays a major role in the pathogenesis of the ocular abnormalities.

The Clinical and Genetic Types of Isolated Vitreoretinal Degeneration

Wagner Disease

In 1938, Wagner described an autosomal dominant vitreoretinal degeneration in 13 of 26 members of a Swiss family he examined (1). In 1960, Boehringer and associates (6) reported 10 additional cases in the same family. Ricci (2) named it the dominant hyaloideoretinal dystrophy of Wagner. Maumenee and coworkers (7) reexamined five members of the same family.

In their childhood, the affected family members suffered from night blindness and progressively constricted visual fields, although the condition never progressed to tubular vision and complete loss of vision, as occurs in retinitis pigmentosa. Visual acuity often became reduced in adulthood owing to presenile cataracts. Most patients had mild myopia, but a few had moderate or severe myopia. An eye examination displayed affected liquefaction of the vitreous or an optical empty space in the vitreous cavity, preretinal vitreous membranes with breaks in some areas, a characteristic dense whitish circumferential membrane at the equator, a normal macula, and in the retinal periphery, sheathing of the blood vessels, pigmented lattice degeneration and pigmentation in the form of clumps (Fig. 1) (1). Boehringer and coauthors (6) assumed that the primary source of the disease is in the vitreous and that it results from an abnormal development of the secondary vitreous. They concluded that both the retinal pigmentary changes and the cataracts are secondary phenomena occurring no earlier than the second to fourth decades of life.

Wagner disease or Wagner hereditary vitreoretinal degeneration became, thereafter, a synonym for the autosomal dominant form of vitreoretinal degeneration. Numerous articles were published stressing that many affected members had retinal detachments with frequent loss of vision in early life.

Other authors had doubts (5,7). In 1995, Graemiger and coauthors (8) published an updated follow-up of the original pedigree of Wagner disease. Now, the affected members were older. The authors demonstrated that chorioretinal atrophy progressed and increased with age, and was found in all patients over 45. In addition, any existing cataract progressed. Glaucoma was diagnosed in 25% of all affected. Fifty-five percent of affected family members manifested a peripheral retinal detachment of the tractional type. At the age of 20 years, only one in four had such a detachment. The electroretinogram was attenuated (8).

In 1962, Jansen described two Dutch families in whom 30 members were affected by an autosomal dominant vitreoretinopathy, which he called Wagner disease (9). The vitreal and retinal changes were similar to those described by Wagner, but retinal detachment occurred very frequently, at a young age, and bilaterally. All affected individuals had high myopia and astigmatism, and the electroretinogram (ERG) was subnormal in light and in dark. Lens opacities were found in all affected members in the second decade of life, and open-angle glaucoma was frequently found after the third decade of life.

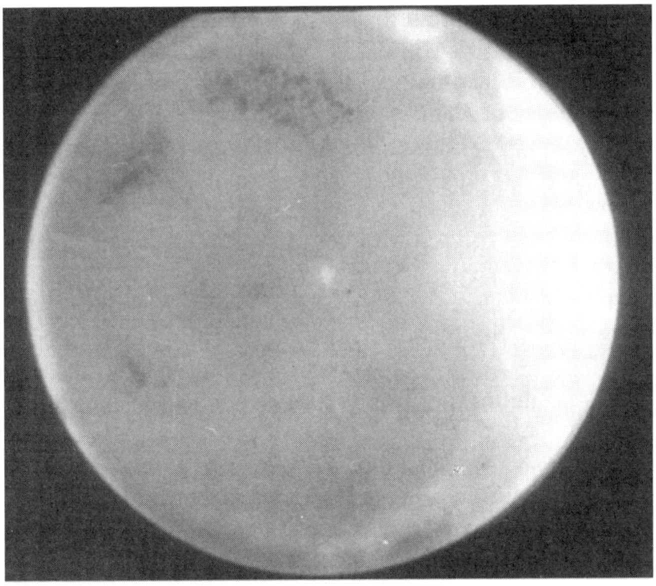

(a)

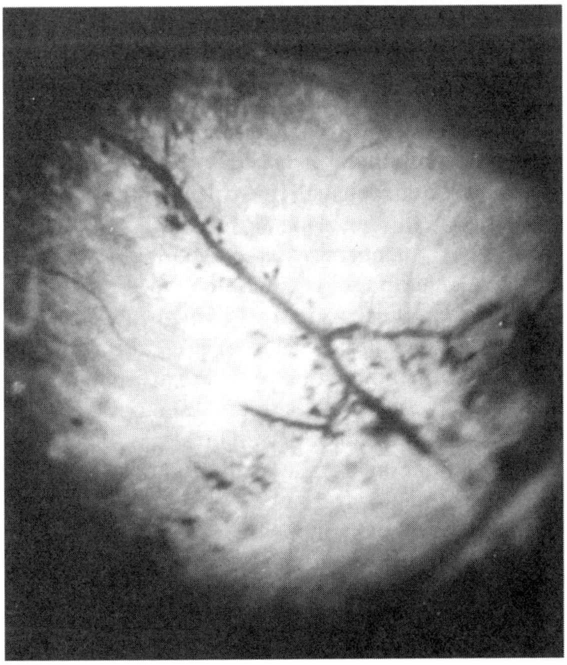

(b)

Figure 1 Autosomal dominant hyaloideoretinopathy: a similar picture can be found in Wagner and Jansen diseases and in Stickler syndrome. (a) Wide-angle fundus photography showing peripheral retinal pigmentation and chorioretinal atrophy and (b) chorioretinal atrophy and pigmentation along retinal vessels. (Courtesy of N. Blair, MD.)

Two families with similar findings were followed by Alexander and Shea (10) for many years. The atrophy and pigmentation of the retina and choroid occurred early in life. The myopia progressed, but usually not to extreme degrees.

Hirose and coworkers (11) examined 41 patients, most of whom had the entity. They stressed the abnormal vitreoretinal adhesions, with concurrent white-with-pressure, lattice degenerations, chorioretinal atrophy, and retinal breaks. Retinal breaks were found in 75% of the patients, even at a young age. Most patients had more than one break, and one patient had 15 breaks. Almost half had retinal detachments. A high rate of failure (50%) of retinal surgery in these patients was reported (11,12).

Other findings included a high incidence of myopia (84%), especially of high myopia (54%), cataract (41% in patients older than 40), and retinal pigmentation in different forms (61%) (11). The ERG was normal or moderately reduced.

Lisch (13) describes five possibilities for vitreoretinal attachment in these cases of vitreoretinopathy: (1) single-filament insertion, (2) arcuate insertion, (3) A-shaped insertion, (4) V-shaped insertion, and (5) linear or band-shaped insertion. These different attachments may constitute different risks for the development of a retinal detachment.

In 1994, Brown and colleagues (14) described a "new" clinical entity, which they named erosive vitreoretinopathy. Progressive RPE atrophy ("thinning") with diffuse rod–cone dysfunction was found. Retinal detachment was common among affected family members. Marked vitreous syneresis existed but myopia was low. Later, the authors confirmed that erosive vitreoretinopathy is allelic to Wagner (15).

Black and associates studied 23 members of one family with vitreous pathology, early-onset retinal detachment, and additional ocular abnormalities, including congenital glaucoma, iris hyperplasia, congenital cataract, ectopia lentis, microphthalmus, and persistent hyperplastic primary vitreous (PHPV) (16). Linkage to the locus for Wagner disease was also detected. The locus for Wagner disease, WGN1, and for erosive vitreoretinopathy, ERVR, was mapped to chromosome 5q13–q14 (15,16), or chromosome 5q14.3 (17). The gene has not yet been identified.

In 2000, Richards and associates demonstrated that mutations in exon 2 of the COL2A1 gene, the gene associated with Stickler disease type I, cause a predominantly ocular phenotype (without the systemic involvement) (18). Gupta and coworkers (19) reported a family with autosomal dominant vitreoretinopathy characteristic of Wagner disease but without the systemic involvement of Stickler disease. The large family, with 32 affected members, showed linkage to COL2A1. The gene for Stickler and a frame shift mutation (Cys57stop), leading to a truncated protein, were identified. The authors concluded that Wagner disease might be one of two types: type 1 at 5q13–q14 and type 2 with mutations in exon 2 of COL2A1 gene, at chromosome 12q13.11 (19).

In summary, Wagner disease seems to be associated with at least two genes: Wagner type I at chromosome 5q13–q14 in the majority of cases, and Wagner type II, with mutations in exon 2 in the COL2A1 gene at chromosome 12q13.11 in the minority. The large variability of phenotypes is a result of different mutations in the respective genes.

Goldmann–Favre Syndrome

A vitreoretinal degeneration transmitted by the autosomal recessive mode was described by Goldmann in 1957 (20) and by Favre in 1958 (21) and was then termed the recessive hyaloideoretinal degeneration of Goldmann–Favre by Ricci (2). Patients complained of night blindness early in childhood and suffered from progressive loss

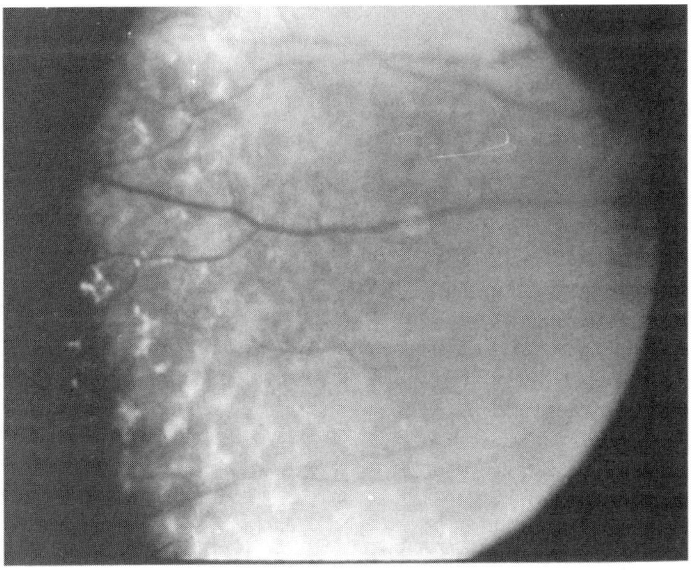

(a)

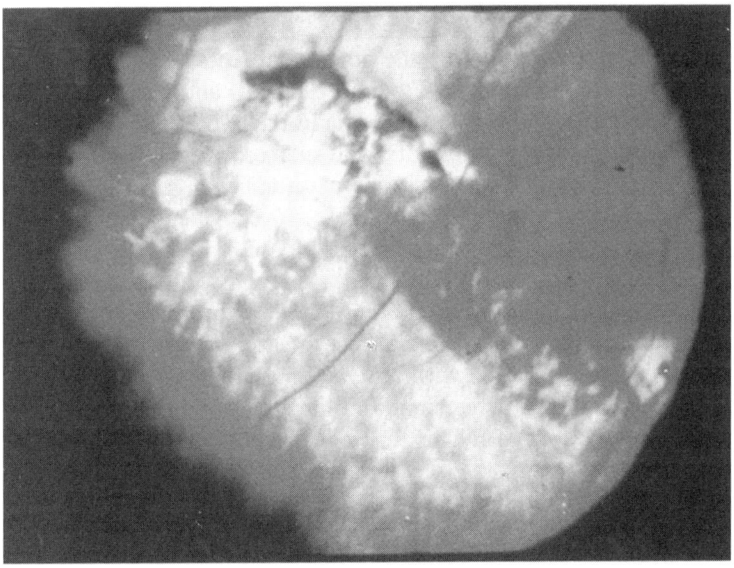

(b)

Figure 2 Goldmann–Favre syndrome: peripheral retina showing localized retinoschisis (a) and diffuse chorioretinal atrophy and pigmentation (b).

of visual fields. Vitreous abnormalities and peripheral retinal changes in the form of retinoschisis with retinal pigmentation were noted (Fig. 2). Macular retinoschisis ("maculoschisis") was also seen (Fig. 3). The dark adaptation curve was monophasic (21), and the ERG was extinct (2). Subsequent electrophysiologic studies demonstrated an unrecordable ERG in most patients with Goldmann–Favre disease (22). In one family, which could be of the autosomal recessive type or of the sex-linked type, the night blindness was associated with a Schubert–Bornschein ERG (23). In another family, the ERG displayed subnormal and identical responses under light and dark

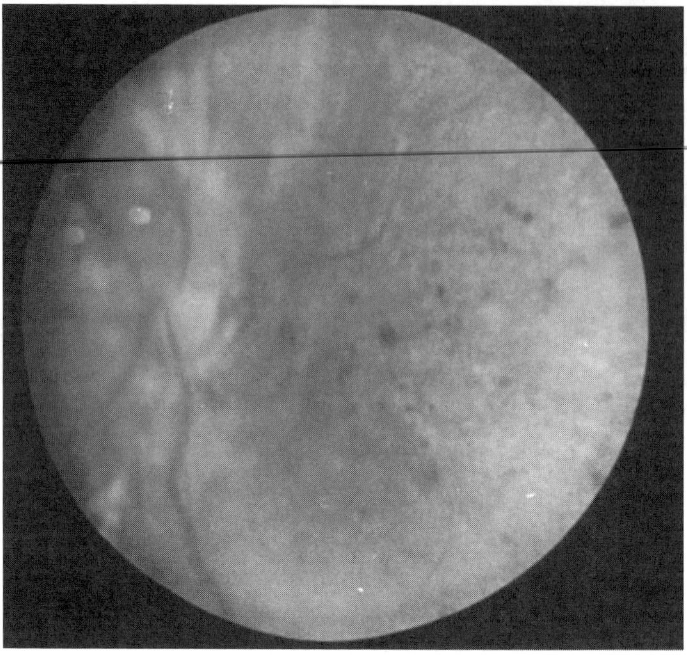

Figure 3 Goldmann–Favre syndrome: abnormal macula.

conditions and an abnormal flicker fusion in the presence of normal cone amplitudes (24). In contrast, a 4-year-old girl with this disease showed an almost nonrecordable ERG under scotopic conditions and marked reduction of the b-wave under photopic conditions (25).

Typically, a patient with Goldmann–Favre syndrome will display signs of the disease in early childhood. Night blindness is the earliest symptom and hyperopia can be found. Later, an atypical pigmentary retinopathy, diffuse chorioretinal atrophy, and peripheral or central retinoschisis are found. By fluorescein angiography, Fishman and associates (24) demonstrated large areas of peripheral nonperfused retina with heavy leakage from abnormal capillaries at the edge of the retinoschisis and the nonperfused areas, in the posterior pole, and from perifoveal capillaries. They suggested that this heavy leakage may be the source of the fluid causing the retinoschisis. A similar leakage from abnormal retinal vessels had already been demonstrated in childhood (25).

The vitreous is abnormal, displaying posterior vitreous detachment, liquefaction, microfibrillar strands, and membranes. It is possible, however, that these changes are mild in childhood (25), and progress with time. Cataracts are frequent, and optic atrophy seems rare (13).

In 1991, Jacobson and associates (26) found, in four patients with Goldmann–Favre syndrome (GFS) a relatively higher sensitivity to S (blue) cones, compared to midspectral (green) cones, throughout the visual field. They suggested that GFS and the enhanced S-cone syndrome (ESCS) are linked by a common pattern of retinal dysfunction. In 2000, Haider and colleagues described the clinical findings of ESCS and identified disease-causing mutations in the NR2E3/PNR gene (27). In 2003, Sharon and coworkers identified mutations in the NR2E3/PNR gene in three retinal dystrophies, the ESCS, the Goldmann–Favre syndrome, and clumped pigmentary retinal degeneration (28). The gene NR2E3 (for nuclear receptor subfamily 2, group E, member 3) encodes a photoreceptor-specific nuclear receptor. The previous name was therefore PNR. It consists of eight exons and was mapped to chromosome 15q23 (29). Sharon and coworkers (28) found a mutation in the NR2E3 in association with GFS in one patient. It is not yet known if the clinical entity of GFS can also be associated with mutations in other genes.

X-Linked Juvenile Retinoschisis

Traditionally, this disorder, once termed congenital veils of the vitreous, is classified together with the hereditary vitreoretinal degenerations. However, in this book it is discussed with "other retinal diseases" in Chapter 13 for several reasons: (1) the main pathology lies in the periphery of the retina (retinoschisis) and in the macula, (2) the vitreous has only mild changes, (3) the "veils" represent the inner layer of the retina and not vitreous membranes, and, finally, (4) recent evidence indicates that the primary site of the disease lies within the retina, and the vitreous plays no role in the development of the disease. An autosomal dominant juvenile retinoschisis is also described in Chapter 13 (30).

Familial Exudative Vitreoretinopathy

Six members of two families suffered from a vitreoretinopathy, which resembled the one described by Wagner. They occasionally had a retinal detachment, as described by Jansen, but also displayed severe peripheral exudative changes, as are found in Coats' disease or retinopathy of prematurity (31). Criswick and Schepens (31) reported these families in 1969 and called the disease familial exudative vitreoretinopathy (FEVR), a term still used.

Gow and Oliver (32) demonstrated that the inheritance of the disease is autosomal dominant.

Characteristically, the onset of FEVR is congenital or in early childhood, with slow progression during life (31). The vitreous is abnormal, with organized membranes in all quadrants, localized areas of traction on the retina, and snowflake-like exudates in the periphery. Subretinal and intraretinal exudation is common. Abnormal vasculature, with occasional neovascularization, can be seen in the periphery. Retinal breaks are seen. Retinal detachment can be localized or total. The macula is occasionally dragged and heterotopic.

Three stages are distinguished in the development of FEVR (32). First, vitreoretinal interface abnormalities are associated with vitreous bands and membranes as well as retinal degenerative peripheral changes; second, dilated tortuous and pathologic retinal vessels may be associated with extensive vitreal, intraretinal, and sub-retinal exudation, elevated fibrovascular masses, localized retinal detachments, and dragging of the disk and macula (Figs. 4 and 5); third, massive subretinal exudates and vitreous membranes are associated with a total retinal detachment.

Fluorescein angiography reveals abrupt cessation of the retinal capillary network at the equator, just posterior to the fibrovascular tissue (Fig. 6), severe circulatory abnormalities in both the retina and the choroid, and heavy leakage (Fig. 7) (33).

Since then, numerous families with FEVR have been reported (33–42). The clinical picture generally fits the foregoing description and its various stages. However, many patients did not ever reach the second and third stages of the disease (33,34,36), whereas others showed an advanced disease at a young age (34).

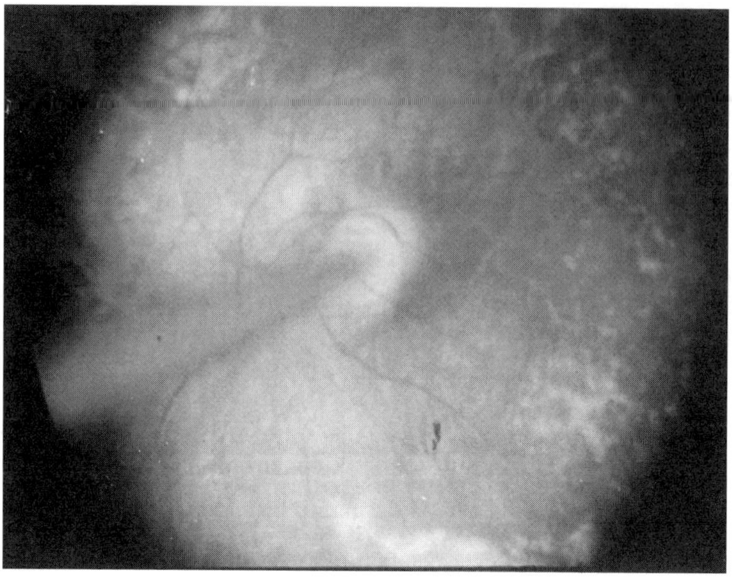

Figure 4 Familial exudative vitreoretinopathy: a characteristic temporal vitreoretinal fold dragging the disk. Yellow-white spots, lines, and flakes can be seen. (Courtesy of M.F. Goldberg, MD.)

The disorder is bilateral, but unilateral cases may occur (42). Great variability of gene expression can be found, both between and within affected families (35,36,40,42).

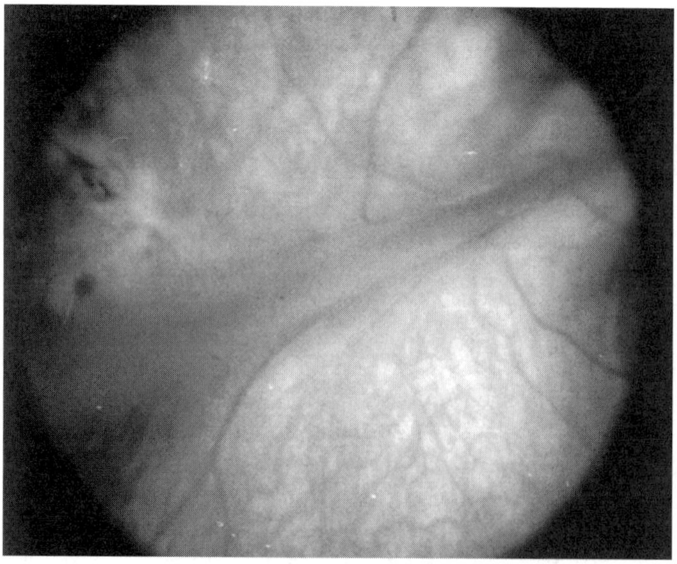

Figure 5 Familial exudative vitreoretinopathy: the characteristic fold or band and a peripheral area of chorioretinal atrophy and pigmentation can be seen. (Courtesy of M.F. Goldberg, MD.)

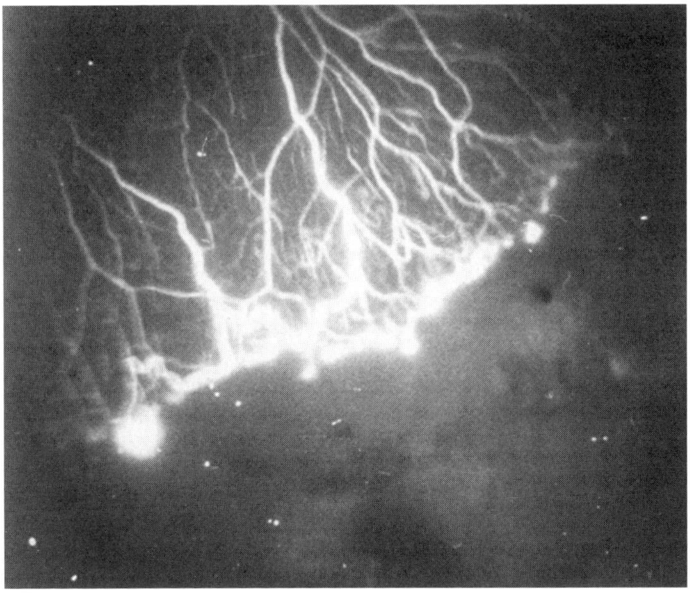

Figure 6 Familial exudative vitreoretinopathy: fluorescein angiography in the early stage shows a peripheral zone of capillary nonperfusion.

The vitreous abnormalities vary from minimal or even nonexistent in some individuals (36) to severe membrane formation, exudation, and fibrovascular masses. Most patients show intermediate changes in the vitreous, including early and prominent posterior vitreous detachment; thickened posterior vitreous face; dot-like opacities;

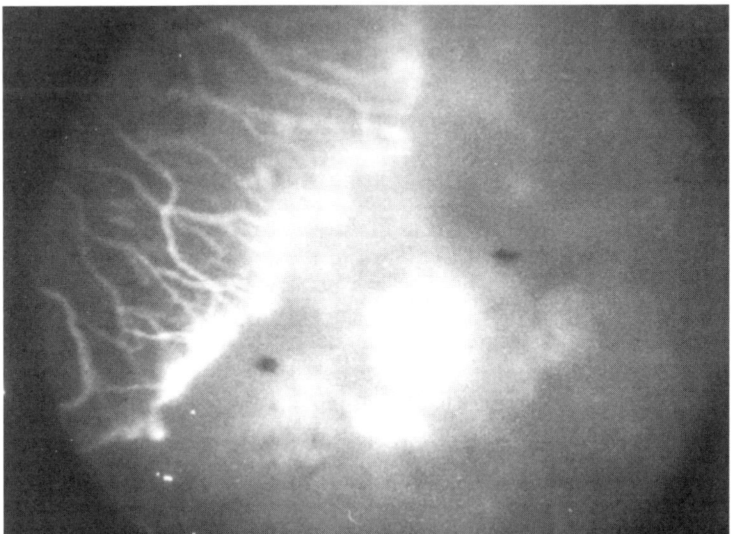

Figure 7 Familial exudative vitreoretinopathy: fluorescein angiography in late stage displays extensive leakage from abnormal retinal vasculature posterior to the zone of capillary nonperfusion.

white-with-pressure, white-without-pressure, and membranes of variable density exerting traction on the retina (37).

Vision may be lost because of retinal detachment. In one study, 19 of 28 eyes developed retinal detachment; in 11 of these, the detachment was rhegmatogenous and in 7 it was the traction type (38). Other patients may have reduced vision from a vitreous hemorrhage, stemming from the neovascular tissue (40) or from massive edema of the retina from the heavy leakage of the abnormal capillaries (39).

In the early 1990s, several new facts came to light: first, that the disorder may be genetically transmitted either by an autosomal dominant gene or by an X-linked gene or by the autosomal recessive mode; second, that in many cases the phenotypic manifestation is indistinguishable from Norrie's disease or retinopathy of prematurity (ROP); third, some clinical signs are found in a percentage of cases in each mode of transmission; and fourth, that the severity of the disease is associated with the age of onset. Neonatal appearance is rare but is the most severe (43). The prognosis is better with later onset, but only 2 out 28 FEVR patients with disease onset before three years of age have vision of 20/200 or better (44). Patients with stable condition are not immune from progression through retinal detachment, massive exudation, retinal neovascularization, or dragging of the macula by a falciform fold. Results of surgery are often poor (45), and treatment will be discussed later.

Autosomal dominant is the most common mode of transmission of FEVR (46). In 1992, Li and colleagues mapped the locus for AD FEVR, later termed EVR1, to chromosome 11q13–q23. (47,48). In a large family of German origin, the disorder manifested the typical retinal peripheral avascular zone, neovascularization and ectopic macula. Blindness occurred from vitreous hemorrhage or from retinal detachment (48).

The search for the mutated gene at chromosomal location 11q13–q23 continued. No mutations associated with AD FEVR were detected in the ROM1 gene (49). In 2002, Robitaille and associates (50) identified FEVR-causing mutation in the FZD4 (for frizzled homolog of *Drosophila* 4) gene, that encodes the alleged Wnt receptor frizzled-4. This protein is assumed to have a function in retinal angiogenesis. The authors showed, in animal experiments, that in the mutant subcellular trafficking is defective, resulting in the defective vascularization of the retina (50). Recently, Toomes and colleagues (51) described mutations in another gene in the same EVR1 locus associated with AD FEVR. The gene, LRP5 (for low-density-lipoprotein receptor-related protein 5) is a Wnt-coreceptor, also involved in signaling in retinal vascularization.

Bamashmus and associates reported a large family with AD FEVR without any association with the EVR1 gene (52). Downey and colleagues (53) mapped the second locus for AD FEVR at chromosome 11p12–p13, now termed VER3. In 1992 and 1993 it was shown that FEVR might be transmitted by the X-linked recessive mode, in addition to the autosomal dominant mode (54,55). Clinically it has similar abnormalities as the AD mode, but it tends to be more severe. The differential diagnosis had to be one of the following: ROP, PHPV, Coats' disease, Norrie disease, and retinoblastoma (54). Linkage studies mapped the locus now named EVR2 to chromosome Xp11.4–11.3 (56,57), and a missense mutation (Leu124Phe) was identified in the NDP gene, the gene associated with Norrie disease or pseudoglioma (57). A summary of reported cases showed that XL FEVR carries a worse prognosis than AD FEVR (58), and carried more similarities to Norrie disease. The NDP gene consists of three exons and encodes a protein, norrin, of 133 amino acids,

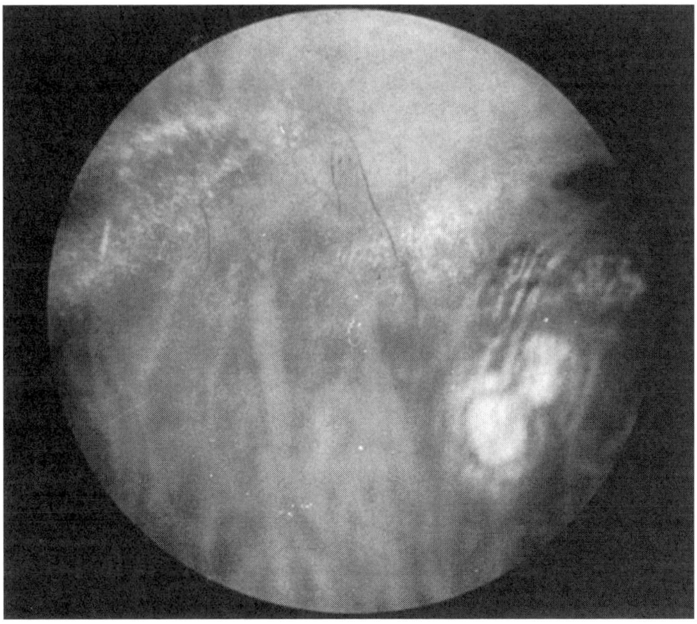

Figure 8 Hereditary snowflake vitreoretinal degeneration: fundus photography demonstrates abnormal retinal vasculature treated by xenon arc photocoagulation and the characteristic snowflakes, two or three rows of glistening, whitish dots. (Courtesy of A. Polack, MD.)

encoded by a portion of exon 2 and a portion of exon 3 (59). Shastry and associates found a series of mutations associated with EVR2 (46,60,61). All were missense mutations, most in exon 3. The most common mutation was Arg121Trp.

The NDP gene encodes norrin, a protein of unknown biochemical function. A recent study showed norrin and F-4 (the frizzled-4 protein) function as a ligand–receptor pair in the signaling system of the cell. This pair plays a central role in the development of the vascular system in the eye and ear (62).

Are Norrie disease and XLFEVR the same disease? In spite of many clinical similarities, these should probably be approached as two distinct diseases. Genetically, allelic heterogeneity exists, with EVR2 mutations being missense in all cases, while in Norrie disease some are deletions and others are various mutations.

Autosomal recessive transmission of FEVR was suggested for two families (63). The disease was congenital and severe.

Hereditary Snowflake Vitreoretinal Degeneration

Hirose and coauthors described this autosomal dominant disorder in 1974 (64). A large family had affected members who suffered from frequent retinal detachment and extensive vitreal and retinal abnormalities. The vitreous displayed a thickened posterior cortex, strands and fibrillary degeneration, and liquefaction of the gel. Characteristic changes were seen in the retinal periphery. Extensive white-with-pressure was seen together with multiple, minute, white or yellow-white flakes or spots (Fig. 8). More posteriorly, sheathing of retinal vessels, increased pigmentary clumping, and chorioretinal atrophy were noted. Myopia and presenile cataracts were common.

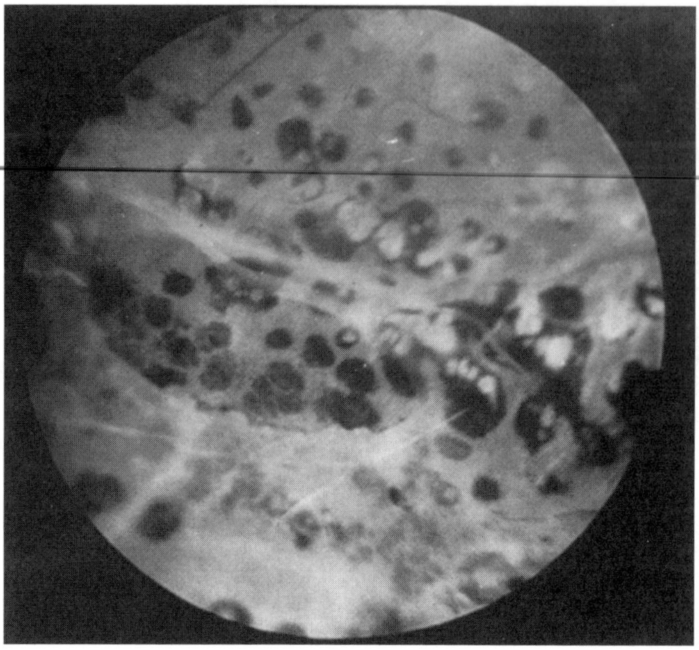

Figure 9 Hereditary snowflake vitreoretinal degeneration: retinal tear treated by argon laser.

Few families with hereditary snowflake vitreoretinal degeneration have been reported (65–67). Variability in expressivity occurs. This degeneration ranges from a mild, innocent, and stable condition of numerous tiny "snowflake" deposits in the retinal periphery, without posterior pigmentation (66), to a serious disease, with pigmentation, retinal breaks, severe vitreous abnormalities, and retinal detachment that may not be amenable to treatment (Fig. 9) (64,67).

In 2003, Lee and colleagues reported a follow-up of the original family (68). Six patients were examined. All showed fibrillar degeneration of the vitreous and most had the crystallin-like deposits in the retinal periphery (the "snowflake"). Other findings included cornea guttata, early-onset cataract, and retinal detachment. The transmission was autosomal dominant with full penetrance and with variable expressivity, in five generations of this family (68).

Autosomal Dominant Vitreoretinochoroidopathy

This autosomal dominant vitreoretinopathy was first described by Kaufman and associates in 1982 (69) as a disorder distinct from FEV and from hereditary snowflake vitreoretinal degeneration. Six members of three generations were affected. All around, the peripheral fundus displayed abnormal chorioretinal hyperpigmentation and hypopigmentation with minute punctate yellow-white opacities (Fig. 10). Retinal arterioles were sometimes narrowed or occluded. Fluorescein angiography demonstrated peripheral areas of capillary nonperfusion (Fig. 11), and a preretinal neovascular frond in one patient. The vitreous showed fibrillar condensation and degeneration with occasional dark cells. Moderate myopia and presenile cataracts were noted.

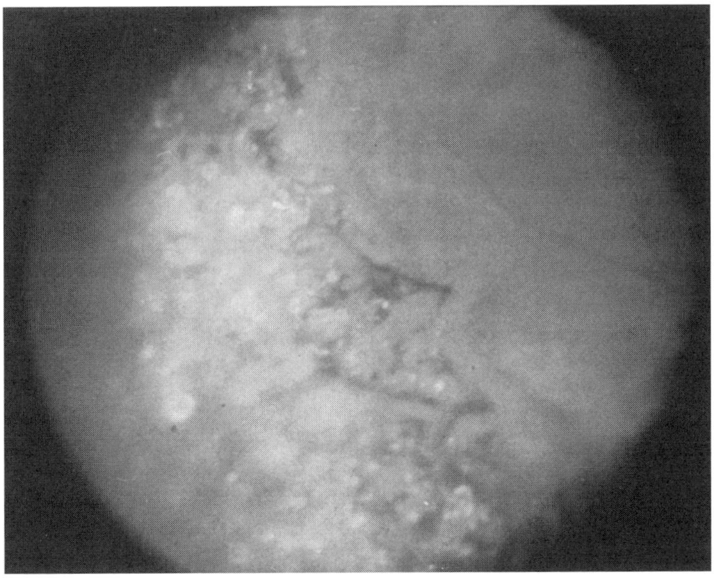

Figure 10 Autosomal dominant vitreoretinochoroidopathy (ADVIRC): the typical wide ring of pigmentation can be seen. (Courtesy of M. F. Goldberg, MD.)

A second family was reported in 1984 (70), and a pathologic report was published in 1989 (71). The characteristic finding of all those affected was the broad pigmentary ring in the periphery of the fundus, for which the name peripheral annular pigmentary dystrophy of the retina was suggested (71).

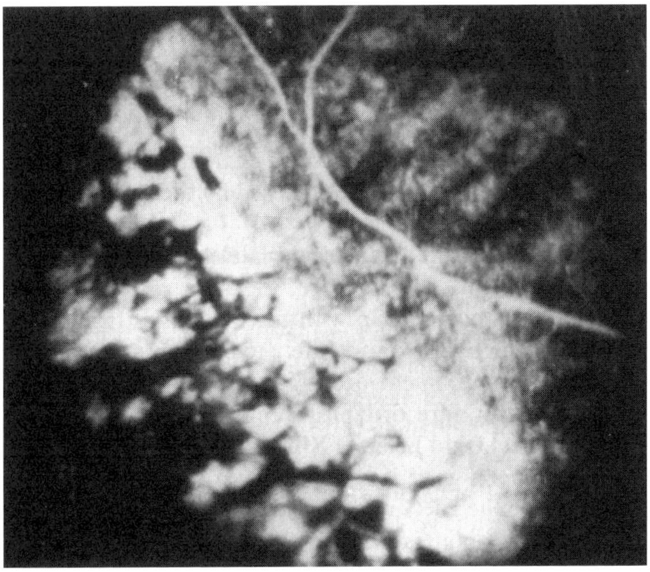

Figure 11 ADVIRC, fluorescein angiography: leakage from retinal vessels posterior to the pigmented annular area.

Six families with ADVIRC have been reported (72,73). The most striking findings were the circumferential retinochoroidal dystrophy with vitreous liquefaction and occasional early cataract, occasional glaucoma, and occasional retinal detachment.

The ERG is frequently reduced but the EOG was found normal (73). The location of the gene is not known.

Other Isolated (Nonsyndromic) Vitreoretinopathies

Other autosomal dominant vitreoretinopathies were described but not confirmed as distinct clinical and genetic entities. These include the "dominantly inherited peripheral retinal neovascularization" in a family reported by Gitter and coworkers (74), and "autosomal dominant juvenile vitreoretinal degeneration and retinal detachment" described by Saari (75). The vitreoretinopathy seen in the first family could be FEVR and the second Wagner disease.

The disorder described by Stone and associates (76) and named autosomal dominant neovascular inflammatory vitreoretinopathy (ADNIV), was mapped to chromosome 11q13, and could represent an allelic variant to the EVR1 locus of FEVR.

More recently, an autosomal recessive vitreoretinopathy with similar clinical features to the common autosomal dominant types was reported (77,78). High myopia, vitreous liquification, RP-like degeneration of the retina, RPE atrophy, macular staphyloma, and premature cataracts were frequently found (77). The locus was mapped to chromosome 22q13, but no mutations were identified in FBLN1, the gene-encoding fibulin at this location (78).

The gene responsible for GFS may, when mutated, be associated with other diseases as demonstrated by Sharon and colleagues (28). These include the enhanced S-cone syndrome (ESCS), clumped pigmentary retinal degeneration (CPRO), and night-blindness. As these are presumed to be retinal diseases, they will be discussed in Chapter 13.

Diagnosis

The diagnosis of an isolated vitreoretinal degeneration is based on the characteristic clinical findings. Many patients who present with juvenile retinal detachment with giant tears probably suffer from an inherited vitreoretinopathy that is not diagnosed. This is particularly true of Wagner disease, which may be much more common than has been diagnosed if the vitreous abnormalities are not noted.

FEVR should be distinguished from a series of inherited and noninherited conditions. The most important differential diagnosis is with retinopathy of prematurity (ROP), as both ROP (in its cicatridal stage II) and FEVR may demonstrate the typical dragging of the disk and macula (32,79). Other possible differential diagnoses are peripheral uveitis, Coats' disease, congenital heterotopia of the macula, congenital retinal septa, angiomatosis retinae, Eales disease, Norrie disease, incontinentia pigmenti, and X-linked primary retinal dysplasia. All typical findings for FEVR, such as vitreous abnormalities, retinal neovascularization and exudation, retinal falciform folds, and retinal detachment, can also occasionally be found in the other disorders (45). Two families with FEVR also showed absent platelet aggregation with arachidonic acid (41), but this was not found in another family (45).

Hereditary snowflake degeneration displays the characteristic flakes and spots, and vascular abnormalities. The presence of the characteristic ring of pigmentation assists in the diagnosis of ADVIRC.

Electrophysiologic tests may be of help with the diagnosis. In both Wagner disease and Jansen's disease, the ERG is moderately to severely subnormal, but not unrecordable (unless retinal detachment occurred). In Goldmann–Favre syndrome, the ERG is extinguished or almost unrecordable, even in patients with minimal clinical abnormality of the fundus (80). In juvenile X-linked retinoschisis, the ERG may be unrecordable, but usually the a-wave is characteristically preserved and the b-wave is absent (24). In FEVR, the ERG has been reported as normal (42) or reduced in all components (81). Variable responses may be obtained in different members of the same family and in the different stages of progression of the disease. The EOG is sometimes normal and sometimes reduced (81). In hereditary snowflake degeneration, the scotopic b-wave is subnormal in amplitude in all patients, whereas the photoptic b-wave is subnormal in some (82). In ADVIRC the ERG is normal in young individuals (70) and moderately subnormal in older persons (71).

Pathology and Pathogenesis

Histopathologic studies on eyes of patients from the original family described by Wagner were reported by Boehringer and associates (6) and by Manschott (83). Starting near the equator, an epiretinal membrane was found to be adherent to the retina over its whole posterior surface, including the disk. Variable areas of retinal atrophy were seen. The choroid was generally normal.

In Wagner disease, when retinal detachment was present, atrophy and pigmentation of both the retina and the choroid were found (10).

Material obtained from a full-thickness eye wall biopsy in a 27-year-old woman with Goldmann–Favre syndrome demonstrated diffuse degenerative changes in the sensory retinal layers and a relatively normal retinal pigment epithelium (RPE) and choroid (84). The retinal vessels were occluded in some areas and showed thickened basement membrane in other areas. The authors suggested that these findings indicate a primary disorder of the retinal vasculature and of the photoreceptors (84).

In FEVR, an acellular, prominent, thick, amorphous vitreous membrane was found to be attached to the internal limiting membrane in multiple areas, producing retinal folds. A superimposed fibrous cellular membrane could be of RPE origin (37).

No pathological description of snowflake degeneration is available. In ADVIRC, disorganization of the peripheral retina, with focal atrophy of the RPE, migration of the RPE cells into the neural retina, and extensive preretinal membranes were found (71). In addition, a unique loss of photoreceptors in isolated foci was noted. The primary site of the disease seems to be the retina (71).

Another histopathologic study of ADVIRC suggested that in ADVIRC, intraretinal migration of RPE cells and deposition of extracellular matrix of pigment, occurs (85).

Genetics

The isolated inherited vitreoretinal degenerations are all transmitted by the autosomal dominant mode, except Goldmann–Favre syndrome, which is autosomal recessive, and X-linked juvenile retinoschisis, not included here. The gene penetrance in all of these disorders is reported as complete or almost complete, such as 90% (36)

or 80% (65). Occasionally, autosomal recessive inheritance has been reported. Table 1 describes the known isolated (nonsyndromic) vitreoretinopathies.

For patients with Goldmann–Favre syndrome, regular autosomal recessive inheritance occurs. The risk for each subsequent sibling is 25%.

For all autosomal dominant disorders of the isolated vitreoretinal degenerations, a penetrance of 80–100% should be considered, with an extremely variable gene expressivity.

Mutations can be identified in the known disease-causative genes: in some cases of Wagner disease (locus WGN1 and WGN2), GFS (NR2E3 gene), and in the three genes associated with FEVR: FZD4, LRP5, and NDP.

Prenatal diagnosis should be considered in families with severe disease.

Management

In patients with a vitreoretinopathy threatened by a retinal detachment, prophylactic treatment by cryoapplication or photocoagulation has been suggested (11,86). Also, a preventive circular band to indent the sclera at the equator can be applied. However, none of these measures have been confirmed as being effective. Surgical repair of the retinal detachment in vitreoretinal degenerations carries an extremely high risk of failure. By conventional surgical methods, including the various buckling procedures, the reported failures ranged from 36 to 52% (12), incomparably higher than in routine rhegmatogenous detachment. A successful use of vitrectomy as an adjunct to retinal surgery in such cases was first reported by Brown and Tasman (12). The use of buckling procedures, along with vitrectomy and fluid–gas exchange, should significantly reduce the number of surgical failures. However, even with these methods, the results are not good (45). In milder cases when retinal detachment does not involve the macula, surgery consisting of vitreotomy with membrane peeling may improve vision in most patients (87,88). In more extensive cases the surgical outcome remains poor. Of eight eyes operated, one was enucleated and all the others had vision from hand movements to finger counting (89). Preventive laser yields poor results. Of 15 eyes treated, 7 developed retinal detachment after the laser (88). In another study, the surgeons reported very strong vitreoretinal adhesions in the peripheral avascular zone. Of 28 operations, iatrogenic breaks occurred in 22 (90). These authors advised dissection of the posterior vitreous membranes, using a bimanual technique of scissors and forceps.

Cataract extraction by phacoemulsification for the premature cataract almost always seen in Wagner disease generally has good results.

Preventive cryopexy to induce atrophy of the peripheral vascular tissue in patients with familial exudative vitreoretinopathy was performed and advised by Gow and Oliver (32). However, others are doubtful of the value of such prophylactic treatment (35,39).

Prophylactic treatment by laser photocoagulation was successfully performed in eight eyes of patients with hereditary snowflake vitreoretinal degeneration (67).

Patients with FEVR or snowflake degeneration and retinal detachment have poor results with conventional retinal surgery (67). Vitrectomy and fluid–gas exchange with a buckling procedure is probably the treatment of choice.

No treatment is usually needed in patients with ADVIRC.

INHERITED VITREORETINAL DEGENERATIONS ASSOCIATED WITH A GENERALIZED DISEASE (SYNDROMIC VITREORETINAL DEGENERATIONS)

Description and Clinical Findings

Several years after the vitreoretinopathies became widely known as distinct genetic and clinical entities, the association of such ocular abnormalities in some families with a generalized disease became clear. Stickler and colleagues (3) were the first to report a family in which over five generations of affected members suffered from congenital high myopia, chorioretinal degeneration, and frequent retinal detachment in 1965. This ocular disorder was associated with deformities of the joints and skeleton and occasionally with cleft palate. The authors called this entity hereditary progressive arthro-ophthalmopathy (3), a term occasionally used today. However, Stickler syndrome or hereditary arthro-ophthalmopathy of Stickler are more often-used terms. This syndrome seems to be very common. Hermannn and coworkers studied 64 patients and concluded that Stickler syndrome is the most common autosomal dominant connective tissue dysplasia in the North American Midwest, exceeding Marfan syndrome and all others (91). Tasman pointed out that many cases previously reported as Wagner disease were in fact Stickler syndrome (7, discussion section). Some ophthalmologists believe that all patients with a diagnosis of Wagner or Jansen's disease actually have a generalized disease of the Stickler type, but often the extra-ocular findings are minimal or limited to radiologic signs only.

When it became apparent that Stickler syndrome may represent several different disorders of connective tissue associated with an ocular disorder of the type of vitreoretinal degenerations, Maumenee attempted to clarify the subject. She classified the possible connective tissue disorders associated with the ocular disease into six types (5). Later, Lisch (13) suggested eight subtypes, and, in a recent review article, Temple (92) described 9 or 10 different entities.

Some authors consider that the different syndromes are extremes of the same disease spectrum, and they suggested that one pleiotropic gene has a different and varying expressivity (93). Another study, however, indicated that the Marshall and Stickler syndromes are phenotypically two distinct entities (94).

The group of associated vitreoretinopathies has been therefore classified into subtypes according to the phenotypic manifestation of the connective tissue generalized disorder. However, it was usually stressed, as in the previous edition, that it is not known whether the different clinical entities are also distinct genetic entities. Ten years later, most of the disease-bearing genes associated with syndromic vitreoretinopathies were known. The number of genes involved was surprisingly small and the variability of clinical expression surprisingly large.

The ocular disorder in all subtypes is similar. It is actually indistinguishable from the described clinical manifestation of Wagner disease. Patients have congenital myopia, which may or may not progress; vitreous with veils; microfibrillar degeneration; and posterior vitreous detachment. The retina shows peripheral degenerative changes, such as lattice formation, pigmentation, white-with-pressure, and often, retinal breaks. Myopia is common and ranges from moderate to severe. Retinal detachment occurs frequently, probably in about 50% of all patients.

All these disorders are transmitted by the autosomal dominant mode, with a high penetrance, but variable expressivity.

The Clinical and Genetic Types of Associated Vitreoretinopathies

The majority of patients with a syndromic vitreoretinopathy suffer from Stickler disease, with most, by far, from Stickler disease type I. All types of Stickler disease are associated with a mutated gene that normally encodes a collagen protein.

Stickler syndrome, Stickler disease, or hereditary progressive arthro-ophthalmopathy of Stickler are different terms used for the same connective tissue disease. Maumenee thought that the term Stickler syndrome and "hereditary arthro-ophthalmopathy, marfanoid variety" (5) should be used for patients with normal height, loose joints, flat epiphyses, and commonly cleft palate or high-arched palate and micrognathia.

The ocular disorder in Stickler syndrome is the same as that found for the whole group. Incurable retinal detachment is common (95), and progression of peripheral white-with-pressure over a period of 18 months was reported (96). This increase in white-with-pressure is the best indicator of the progressive increase in vitreous traction and of the increasing risk of giant tear formation (96). Abnormal anterior chamber angles were described (95) and occurred in about 26% of patients in one study (97). Elevated intraocular pressure, ectopia lentis, and early cataracts were other findings (97). Marfanoid features, laxity, and hyperextensibility of joints and wide joints were each found in 21–23% of all patients with skeletal abnormalities (97).

Hearing loss, caused by a sensorineural hearing defect, is commonly found in patients with Stickler syndrome (98).

The frequent occurrence of a cleft palate, together with a characteristic physiognomy in association with the ocular and joint abnormalities of Stickler syndrome was termed "the clefting syndrome" by Knobloch and Layer (98). The cleft palate may be of different degrees, including only a posterior cleft (99). Flat facies, a broad and depressed nasal bridge, and hypoplasia of the maxilla are characteristic changes (99). Hyperextensibility of joints was found in all four affected members of one family (100). Roentgenograms indicated generalized epiphyseal dysplasia in 20 of 21 examined patients (101). The ocular abnormalities were as described for the other associated vitreoretinal degenerations and for Jansen's disease (previously called Wagner disease) (101), including the extremely high risk of inoperable retinal detachment (102,103).

Of the four main abnormalities of Stickler syndrome, namely, ocular changes, flat midface, cleft palate, and arthropathy, all the 21 affected members in 8 families had at least two findings (104). This indicates the variable expressivity of the gene. However, the authors found facial expressivity extremely useful for the diagnosis. By facial measurements they could correctly identify 90% of their patients (104).

The three large families described by Van Balen and Falger in 1970 (4) as having a vitreoretinopathy associated with cleft palate and, in some, genu valgum, probably suffered from the same Stickler syndrome. Similarly, the Cervenka or Cohen syndrome (105) of vitreoretinal degeneration, cleft palate, and maxillary hypoplasia seems to be a variant of Stickler syndrome.

Lisch (13) separates this Stickler syndrome group into four phenotypic entities, all with vitreoretinal degeneration and tendency to retinal detachment and the following: (1) flat face and cleft palate, (2) Eskimo-like face, (3) hyperextensibility of joints and cleft palate, and (4) progressive arthro-ophthalmopathy.

Stickler Syndrome Type I and the COL2A1 Gene

Type II collagen is the major collagen of vitreous, nucleus pulposus, and cartilage. It is made up of three α_1 (II) collagen chains. A structural defect in this protein could explain the defects in the eye and in the cartilagenous and bony structures (91). Recently, close linkage was established between *COL2A1,* the structural gene for type II collagen, assigned to chromosome 12 and a spectrum of disorders with defects of type II collagen, such as type II achondrogenesis, hypochondrogenesis, spondyloepiphyseal dysplasia congenita, and Kniest and Stickler syndromes (91,106,107).

The identification of the gene associated with Stickler type I verified the assumption that the phenotypic variability is not due to separate disease entities, but due to several allelic mutations. The clinical manifestation of the vitreoretinopathy depends on the mutation present in each case. The ocular findings are relatively similar; the extraocular findings vary substantially.

Variability is mainly interfamilial with less intrafamilial variability (108). The disorder is congenital with many ocular abnormalities detected early in life. In one study of 17 children, the mean age of diagnosis was 1.5 years (range: newborn to 5.5 years). Follow-up at 15 years of age detected few changes in refractive error, cataract, and vitreoretinal abnormalities (109).

The gene COL2A1 encodes collagen type II, alpha-1 chain, the collagen of the vitreous, and cartilage. Mutations associated with Stickler disease cause premature termination (110–114). Ocular findings included vitreous abnormalities (syneresis and bands), retinal perivascular pigmentation, common retinal detachment due to breaks, and peripheral cortical cataracts (112). Glaucoma and giant tears occur (113). Brown and associates (114) suggested that the vitreous gel normally contains a matrix primarily composed of collagen type II, alpha-1 chain fibrils as a scaffold for hyaluronic acid macromolecules. This scaffold is collapsed in Stickler disease (114). Extraocular findings included abnormalities of the soft palate, epiphyseal dysplasia with severe joint pain (112), mandibular hypoplasia, hypermobility or reduced mobility of joints with osteoarthritis-like changes (113). Progressive sensorineural hearing loss is frequent (113). Donoso and colleagues (115) pointed out that the COL2A1 gene undergoes alternation splicing of exon 2 resulting either in a short form of collagen, preferentially expressed in cartilage, or in a long form, preferentially expressed in the vitreous. They described a large family with a truncating mutation, Cys86Stop, in exon 2 of the COL2A1 gene. The family suffered from a severe ocular disease with 57% of affected manifesting retinal detachment but with uncommon extraocular abnormalities (115). The gene COL2A1 is large and consists of 53 coding exons. When premature termination occurs in exon 2, the long collagen fibers, predominantly found in the vitreous, are defective and may therefore be expressed mainly or only in the eye (18,116). Stickler and associates (116) and Donoso and associates (117) reviewed the literature and reported the wide range of eye manifestations, including optically empty vitreous, vitreous veils and bands, myopia in more than 90%, retinal detachment in about 60%, common glaucoma, and giant retinal breaks; 4% were blind. Perivascular pigmentation was detected in all families with an exon 2 mutation (116).

In addition, mutations outside exon 2 were associated with extraocular abnormalities. These included arthropathy in 90%, usually loose joints, or facial structure abnormalities such as a flat midface, small mandible, and cleft palate in 84% and hearing loss in 70% (116,117).

Table 2 Syndromic (Associated) Vitreoretinopathies

Name	Locus/symbol	Gene	Chromosomal location	Vitreous	Retina	Remarks
Stickler type I	STL1	COL2A1	12q13.11–q13.2	Membranous appearance	Giant tears, RD, pigmentation	70% of all vitreoretinopathies
Stickler type II	STL2	COL11A1	1p21	"Beaded" appearance	Tears, RD, pigmentation	
Stickler type III	STL3	COL11A2	6p21.3	Normal	Normal	

Note: Congential spondyloepiphyseal dysplasia, congenital spondyloepimetaphyseal dysplasia, and Kniest disease are allelic to STL1. Ocular findings as in Stickler type 1. Marshall syndrome is allelic to STL2. Ocular findings as in Stickler type II. Weissenbacher–Zweymueller syndrome is allelic to STL3. Vitreous is normal but hypertelorism and refractive disorders occur.

The great interfamilial variability and to a lesser degree, but still great, intrafamilial variability make it difficult to predict the phenotype from the genotype (118). In some families, both clinical associated vitreoretinopathy (Stickler syndrome) and clinical isolated vitreoretinopathy (Wagner disease) may occur (119). In typical Stickler syndrome the mutated COL2A1 gene produces a truncated collagen. Wilkin and associates recommend a rapid way of analyzing potential premature terminations codons (120).

The locus for Stickler syndrome type 1, STL 1, maps to chromosome 12q13.11-q13.2 (121).

Following is a long list of various clinical phenotypes, known by various names, subsequently found to be associated with mutations in the COL2A1 gene.

Several mutations not in exon 2 were described. Cole and associates describe a heterozygous missense mutation in exon 48 of COL2A1 gene, associated with *congenital spondyloepiphyseal dysplasia* (124).

In congenital spondyloepiphyseal dysplasia, dwarfism is associated with dysplasia of the epiphyses of the long bones and vertebrae, short trunk, kyphoscoliosis, normal head, hands, and feet (122,123). The ocular condition is typical of all vitreoretinopathies, with myopia, abnormal vitreous, and the tendency to retinal detachment (13). Hearing was reported to be normal.

In the diastrophic variant, dwarfism is associated with flat epiphyses, wide metaphyses, loose ligaments and joints, normal face, and common deafness (5).

Missense mutations in the COL2A1 gene were reported (125).

In *Kniest syndrome*, dwarfism occurs in conjunction with deformed epiphyses and broad metaphyses. As in Stickler syndrome, a flat face, depressed nasal bridge, and marked joint limitation was noted. A short trunk, kyphoscoliosis, and clubfoot also occur. Sensorineural deafness is common. The vitreoretinal degeneration is severe and high myopia, cataract, and retinal detachment occur frequently (86,91,126). Mutations in the COL2A1 gene were identified (126).

Different types of spondyloepiphyseal and spondylometaphyseal dysplasia of varying severity ranging from mild to severe were described is association with typical vitreoretinopathy of Stickler (91,127,128). Mutations in the COL2A1 gene were identified (128).

Stickler Syndrome Type II and the COL11A1 Gene

Studies of mutations in the COL2A1 gene revealed that Stickler syndrome is a heterogenous disease (118,129) and that Stickler type 1 comprises only 70% of all Stickler phenotypes. The second locus for Stickler syndrome, STL2, was mapped to chromosome 1p21 and mutations in COL11A1, the gene encoding collagen type XI, alpha-1, were identified (130).

In all cases, the clinical expression consisted of congenital, nonprogressive myopia of a high degree along with vitreous abnormalities (130). Snead and Yates (131), and Richards et al. (132) claimed that slit lamp biomicroscopy provides a mechanism to distinguish between the vitreous of Stickler type I, which is optically empty or has membranous appearance, and the vitreous of Stickler type II, which has a beaded appearance ("irregularly thickened fibers giving a string of pearls appearance"). As in Stickler type 1, phenotypic variability was great. In the same family, Bonaventure and colleagues found affected members with both ocular and extraocular diseases and members with only the ocular disease (129).

Marshall Syndrome

The autosomal dominant transmission of a disorder characterized by the association of vitreoretinal degeneration, early cataracts, marked midfacial hypoplasia, short stature, cleft palate, spondyloepiphyseal dysplasia, and frequently deafness was reported by Marshall (133) and later by O'Donnell and coauthors (134).

Winter and coworkers suggested that the Stickler and Marshall syndromes and another syndrome of short stature with the Pierre-Robin sequence of findings and chondrodysplasia (Weissenbacher–Zweymüller syndrome) are one identical entity (135).

The controversy whether these were distinct conditions or variations of Stickler syndrome continued for several years (136,137). It now seems that these are just allelic variants of the same STL2 locus, which includes Stickler syndrome type 2 and Marshall syndrome (136–138). Weissenbacher–Zweymüller syndrome is allelic to Stickler syndrome type III (nonocular Stickler syndrome) (139).

Annunen and colleagues characterized the COL11A1 gene (138). It is very large, consists of 68 exons and spans 150 kb. Most reported mutations were small deletions. The locus was mapped to chromosome 1p21.

Stickler Syndrome Type III

Stickler syndrome type III is characterized by various extraocular skeletal abnormalities similar to other Stickler syndromes. However, the eye is not affected and it was termed the nonocular type. The locus STL3 was mapped to chromosome 6p21.3 (121). Linkage of Stickler syndrome, later defined a type III, was reported in 1994 (140). The vitreous appears normal (117). As mentioned, mutations at the STL3 locus were identified in Weissenbacher–Zweymüeller syndrome. The mutated gene is COL11A2.

Hereditary Vitreoretinopathies Associated with Other Syndromes

Three rare conditions were described in which a vitreoretinal degeneration was associated with an extraocular, generalized disease of an autosomal recessive inheritance. These include the association of vitreoretinopathy with occipital encephalocele (13), vitreoretinopathy with diverticula of the gut and multiple inguinal and femoral hernias (13), and vitreoretinopathy with skeletal dysplasia (13,91,141). The last disorder, termed the *Nance–Sweeney syndrome* or *Nance–Astley syndrome*, manifests a vitreoretinopathy associated with skeletal anomalies, short long bones, large epiphyses, flat facies, and cleft palate.

The association of a Stickler-like vitreoretinopathy with occipital encephalocele became known as *Knobloch syndrome* (142). Sertie and associates (143) identified a homozygous mutation in COL18A1, the gene encoding collagen type 18, alpha 1. The mutation resulted in a stop codon in exon 4. The locus was mapped to chromosome 21q22.3. Additional mutations of the COL18A1 associated with Knobloch syndrome were identified in the last year. Knobloch syndrome was confirmed as a rare autosomal recessive syndromic vitreoretinopathy.

In Weissenbacher–Zweymüller syndrome, ocular abnormalities include hypertelorism, protruding eyes in all patients, and refractive errors from hyperopia to high myopia, and strabismus (144). No vitreoretinopathy was encountered.

Diagnosis, Pathology, and Pathogenesis

The diagnosis of the associated vitreoretinopathies is based on the clinical manifestations of the different varieties. The subdivision into the various entities is certainly not yet final. Even the separation into isolated and associated forms is often clinically not apparent. Many patients diagnosed with Wagner disease may manifest the generalized involvement of the joints if roentgenograms of the epiphyses are taken. Identification of the implicated mutation in the collagen genes is an extremely important step in the diagnosis of syndromic vitreoretinopathy. It enables more accurate decisions as to prognosis, genetic counseling, and preventive measures.

The histopathologic appearance of eyes with Stickler syndrome may reveal a detached retina, calcification, and bone formation (4), or detached retina with folding, disorganization, preretinal vitreous membranes, and adherent vitreous at the edge of retinal break (95).

Many animal studies regarding syndromic vitreoretinopathy were performed. Several studies used transgenic mice. Human collagen genes such as the COL2A1 gene were transfected into mice. Disastrous effects on the skeleton were studied (145), but the effects on the eyes were minor.

Labrador retrievers were found to have a disorder of associated ocular and skeletal dysplasia, and a breeding colony was established (146–148). The disorder was amazingly similar to the human disease. The ocular lesions included vitreous strands, persistent hyaloid remnants, retinal folds, and rhegmatogenous retinal detachment. The skeletal lesions were recognized as shorter-than-normal forelimbs, with an abnormal ulna and radius. The human disease may thus be studied on a feasible animal model.

Management

The medical and surgical approach to the associated disorders is, from the ocular point of view, identical with the approach to the isolated vitreoretinopathies. Some authors strongly advocate prophylactic treatment to avoid the disastrous effects of a retinal detachment (100). see page 414.

Prenatal diagnosis can be performed in familial cases once the mutation is identified (149).

OTHER INHERITED ABNORMALITIES OF THE VITREOUS

Excluding the inherited vitreoretinal degeneration, other inherited abnormalities affecting the vitreous are extremely rare.

Persistent hyperplastic primary vitreous occurs in the total or posterior type and can be either unilateral or bilateral; it is usually a sporadic, noninherited disorder (150–152). However, several reports indicated a familial occurrence, most probably of an X-linked recessive mode of transmission (153).

An abnormal vitreous and giant retinal tears in association with a coloboma of the lens were reported in eight bilateral cases. No positive family history was reported (154).

Vitreous amyloidosis may occur in familial amyloidotic polyneuropathy (155).

White spots or patches were reported to occur at the vitreoretinal surface in patients with the juvenile form of Gaucher's disease (156,157). They are thought to be Gaucher foam cells.

REFERENCES

1. Wagner H. Ein bisher unbekanntes Erbleiden des Auges (Degeneratio hyalideo-retinalis hereditaria) beobachtet im Kanton Zürich. Klin Monatsbl Augenheilkd 1938; 100: 840–857.
2. Rici A. Clinique et transmission génétique des differentes formes de dégénérescences vitreoretiniennes. Ophthalmologica 1960; 139:338–343.
3. Stickler GB, Belau PG, Farrell FJ, et al. Hereditary progressive arthtro-ophthalmopathy. Mayo Clin Proc 1965; 40:433–455.
4. Van Balen AT, Falger ELF. Hereditary hyaloideoretinal degeneration and palatoschisis. Arch Ophthalmol 1920; 83:152–162.
5. Maumenee IH. Vitreoretinal degeneration as a sign of generalized connective tissue diseases. Am J Ophthalmol 1979; 88:432–449.
6. Boehringer HR, Dieterle P, Landolt E. Zur Kiinik und Pathologie der degeneratio hyalloideo-retinalis hereditaria (Wagner). Ophthalmologica 1960; 139:330–338.
7. Maumenee IH, Stoll HU, Mets MB. The Wagner syndrome versus hereditary arthroophthalmopathy. Trans Am Ophthalmol Soc 1982; 80:349–365.
8. Graemiger RA, Niemeyer G, Schneeberger SA, Messmer EP. Wagner vitreoretinal degeneration. Follow-up of the original pedigree. Ophthalmology 1995; 102(12):1830–1839.
9. Jansen LMAA. Degeneratio hyaloideo-retinalis hereditaria. Ophthalmologica 1962; 144:458–464.
10. Alexander RL, Shea M. Wagner's disease. Arch Ophthalmol 1965; 74:310–318.
11. Hirose T, Lee K, Schepens CL. Wagner's hereditary vitreoretinal degeneration and retinal detachment. Arch Ophthalmol 1973; 89:176–185.
12. Brown GC, Tasman WS. Vitrectomy and Wagner's vitreoretinal degeneration. Am J Ophthalmol 1978; 86:485–488.
13. Lisch W. Hereditary vitreoretinal degenerations. Dev Ophthalmol 1983; 8:1–90.
14. Brown DM, Kimura AE, Weingeist TA, Stone EM. Erosive vitreoretinopathy. A new clinical entity. Ophthalmology 1994; 101(4):694–704.
15. Brown DM, Graemiger RA, Hergersberg M, Schinzel A, Messmer EP, Niemeyer G, Schneeberger SA, Streb LM, Taylor CM, Kimura AE, et al. Genetic linkage of Wagner disease and erosive vitreoretinopathy to chromosome 5q13–14. Arch Ophthalmol 1995; 113(5):671–675.
16. Black GC, Perveen R, Wiszniewski W, Dodd CL, Donnai D, McLeod D. A novel hereditary developmental vitreoretinopathy with multiple ocular abnormalities localizing to a 5-cM region of chromosome 5q13-q14. Ophthalmology 1999; 106(11):2074–2081.
17. Perveen R, Hart-Holden N, Dixon MJ, Wiszniewski W, Fryer AE, Brunner HG, Pinkners AJ, van Beersum SE, Black GC. Refined genetic and physical localization of the Wagner disease (WGN1) locus and the genes CRTL1 and CSPG2 to a 2- to 2.5-cM region of chromosome 5q14.3. Genomics 1999; 57(2):219–226.
18. Richards AJ, Martin S, Yates JR, Scott JD, Baguley DM, Pope FM, Snead MP. COL2A1 exon 2 mutations: relevance to the Stickler and Wagner syndromes. Br J Ophthalmol 2000; 84(4):364–371.
19. Gupta SK, Leonard BC, Damji KF, Bulman DE. A frame shift mutation in a tissue-specific alternatively spliced exon of collagen 2A1 in Wagner's vitreoretinal degeneration. Am J Ophthalmol 2002; 133(2):203–210.
20. Goldmann H. Biomicroscopie du corps vitre et du fond de l'oeil. Bull Mem Soc Fr Ophthalmol 1957; 70:265.
21. Favre M. A propos de deux cas de dégénérescence hyaloidéoretinienne. Ophthalmologica 1958; 135:604–609.
22. Carr RE, Siegel IM. The vitreo-tapeto-retinal degenerations. Arch Ophthalmol 1970; 84:436–445.
23. Feiler-Ofry V, Adams A, Regenbogen L. Hereditary vitreoretinal degeneration and night blindness. Am J Ophthalmol 1969; 67:553–558.

24. Fishman GA, Jampol LM, Goldberg MF. Diagnostic features of Favre-Goldmann syndrome. Br J Ophthalmol 1976; 60:345–353.
25. Izumi K, Matsuhashi M. Goldmann-Favre syndrome in a four-year-old-girl. Doc Ophthalmol 1987; 66:219–226.
26. Jacobson SG, Roman AJ, Roman MI, Gass JD, Parker JA. Relatively enhanced S cone function in the Goldmann-Favre syndrome. Am J Ophthalmol 1991; 111(4):446–453.
27. Haider NB, Jacobson SG, Cideciyan AV, Swiderski R, Streb LM, Searby C, Beck G, Hockey R, Hanna DB, Gorman S, Duhl D, Carmi R, Bennett J, Weleber RG, Fishman GA, Wright AF, Stone EM, Sheffield VC. Mutation of a nuclear receptor gene, NR2E3, causes enhanced S cone syndrome, a disorder of retinal cell fate. Nat Genet 2000; 24(2):127–131.
28. Sharon D, Sandberg MA, Caruso RC, Berson EL, Dryja TP. Shared mutations in NR2E3 in enhanced S-cone syndrome, Goldmann-Favre syndrome, and many cases of clumped pigmentary retinal degeneration. Arch Ophthalmol 2003; 121(9):1316–1323.
29. RetNet (retrieval system on the internet). Texas: The University of Texas Health Science Center. C1996–2004 (cited Jun 11 2004). Avaliable from: http://www.sph.uth.tmc.edu/retnet/.
30. Yassur Y, Nissenkorn I, Ben-Sira I, et al. Autosomal dominant inheritance of retinoschisis. Am J Ophthalmol 1982; 94:338–343.
31. Criswick VG, Schepens CL. Familial exudative vitreoretinopathy. Am J Ophthalmol 1969; 68:578–594.
32. Gow J, Oliver GL. Familial exudative vitreoretinopathy: An expanded view. Arch Ophthalmol 1971; 86:150–155.
33. Canny CL, Oliver GL. Fluorescein angiographic findings in familial exudative vitreoretinopathy. Arch Ophthalmol 1976; 94:1114–1120.
34. Slusher MM, Hutton WE. Familial exudative vitreoretinopathy. Am J Ophthalmol 1979; 87:152–156.
35. Ober RR, Bird AC, Hamilton AM, et al. Autosomal dominant exudative vitreoretinopathy. Br J Ophthalmol 1980; 64:112–120.
36. Van Nouhuys CE. Dominant exudative vitreoretinopathy and other vascular development disorders of the peripheral retina. Monogr Ophthalmol 1982; 5:1–413.
37. Brochhurst RJ, Albert DM, Zakov N. Pathologic findings in familial exudative vitreoretinopathy. Arch Ophthalmol 1981; 99:2143–2146.
38. Miyakubo H, Inohara N, Hashimoto K. Retinal involvement in familial exudative vitreoretinopathy. Ophthalmologica 1982; 185:125–135.
39. Swanson D, Rush P, Bird AL. Visual loss from retinal oedema in autosomal dominant exudative vitreoretinopathy. Br J Ophthalmol 1982; 66:627–629.
40. Bergen RL, Glassman R. Familial exudative vitreoretinopathy. Ann Ophthalmol 1983; 15:275–276.
41. Chaudhuri PR, Rosenthal AR, Goulstine DB, et al. Familial exudative vitreoretinopathy associated with familial thrombocytopathy. Br J Ophthalmol 1983; 67:755–758.
42. Feldman EL, Norris JL, Cleasby GW. Autosomal dominant exudative vitreoretinopathy. Arch Ophthalmol 1983; 101:1532–1535.
43. Chang-Godinich A, Paysse EA, Coats DK, Holz ER. Familial exudative vitreoretinopathy mimicking persistent hyperplastic primary vitreous. Am J Ophthalmol 1999; 127(4):469–471.
44. Benson WE. Familial exudative vitreoretinopathy. Trans Am Ophthalmol Soc 1995; 93:473–521.
45. van Nouhuys CE. Signs, complications, and platelet aggregation in familial exudative vitreoretinopathy. Am J Ophthalmol 1991; 111(1):34–41.
46. Shastry BS, Hejtmancik JF, Plager DA, Hartzer MK, Trese MT. Linkage and candidate gene analysis of X-linked familial exudative vitreoretinopathy. Genomics 1995; 27(2):341–344.

47. Li Y, Muller B, Fuhrmann C, van Nouhuys CE, Laqua H, Humphries P, Schwinger E, Gal A. The autosomal dominant familial exudative vitreoretinopathy locus maps on 11q and is closely linked to D11S533. Am J Hum Genet 1992; 51(4):749–754.
48. Li Y, Fuhrmann C, Schwinger E, Gal A, Laqua H. The gene for autosomal dominant familial exudative vitreoretinopathy (Criswick-Schepens) on the long arm of chromosome 11. Am J Ophthalmol 1992; 113(6):712–713.
49. Shastry BS, Hejtmancik JF, Hiraoka M, Ibaraki N, Okubo Y, Okubo A, Han DP, Trese MT. Linkage and candidate gene analysis of autosomal-dominant familial exudative vitreoretinopathy. Clin Genet 2000; 58(4):329–332.
50. Robitaille J, MacDonald ML, Kaykas A, Sheldahl LC, Zeisler J, Dube MP, Zhang LH, Singaraja RR, Guernsey DL, Zheng B, Siebert LF, Hoskin-Mott A, Trese MT, Pimstone SN, Shastry BS, Moon RT, Hayden MR, Goldberg YP, Samuels ME. Mutant frizzled-4 disrupts retinal angiogenesis in familial exudative vitreoretinopathy. Nat Genet 2002; 32(2):326–330.
51. Toomes C, Bottomley HM, Jackson RM, Towns KV, Scott S, Mackey DA, Craig JE, Jiang L, Yang Z, Trembath R, Woodruff G, Gregory-Evans CY, Gregory-Evans K, Parker MJ, Black GC, Downey LM, Zhang K, Inglehearn CF. Mutations in LRP5 or FZD4 underlie the common familial exudative vitreoretinopathy locus on chromosome 11q. Am J Hum Genet 2004; 74(4):721–730.
52. Bamashmus MA, Downey LM, Inglehearn CF, Gupta SR, Mansfield DC. Genetic heterogeneity in familial exudative vitreoretinopathy; exclusion of the EVR1 locus on chromosome 11q in a large autosomal dominant pedigree. Br J Ophthalmol 2000; 84(4): 358–363.
53. Downey LM, Keen TJ, Roberts E, Mansfield DC, Bamashmus M, Inglehearn CF. A new locus for autosomal dominant familial exudative vitreoretinopathy maps to chromosome 11p12–13. Am J Hum Genet 2001; 68(3):778–781.
54. Plager DA, Orgel IK, Ellis FD, Hartzer M, Trese MT, Shastry BS. X-linked recessive familial exudative vitreoretinopathy. Am J Ophthalmol 1992; 114(2):145–148.
55. Shastry BS, Trese MT. X-linked familial exudative vitreoretinopathy (FEVR): results of DNA analysis with candidate genes. Am J Med Genet 1993; 45(1):111–113.
56. Fullwood P, Jones J, Bundey S, Dudgeon J, Fielder AR, Kilpatrick MW. X linked exudative vitreoretinopathy: clinical features and genetic linkage analysis. Br J Ophthalmol 1993; 77(3):168–170.
57. Chen ZY, Battinelli EM, Fielder A, Bundey S, Sims K, Breakefield XO, Craig IW. A mutation in the Norrie disease gene (NDP) associated with X-linked familial exudative vitreoretinopathy. Nat Genet 1993; 5(2):180–183.
58. Clement F, Beckford CA, Corral A, Jimenez R. X-linked familial exudative vitreoretinopathy. Report of one family. Retina 1995; 15(2):141–145.
59. Mintz-Hittner HA, Ferrell RE, Sims KB, Fernandez KM, Gemmell BS, Satriano DR, Caster J, Kretzer FL. Peripheral retinopathy in offspring of carriers of Norrie disease gene mutations. Possible transplacental effect of abnormal norrin. Ophthalmology 1996; 103(12):2128–2134.
60. Shastry BS, Trese MT. Identification of a polymorphic missense (G338D) and silent (106V and 121L) mutations within the coding region of the peripherin/RDS gene in a patient with retinitis punctata albescens. Biochem Biophys Res Commun 1997; 231(1):103–105.
61. Shastry BS, Hejtmancik JF, Trese MT. Identification of novel missense mutations in the Norrie disease gene associated with one X-linked and four sporadic cases of familial exudative vitreoretinopathy. Hum Mutat 1997; 9(5):396–401.
62. Xu Q, Wang Y, Dabdoub A, Smallwood PM, Williams J, Woods C, Kelley MW, Jiang L, Tasman W, Zhang K, Nathans J. Vascular development in the retina and inner ear: control by norrin and frizzled-4, a high-affinity ligand-receptor pair. Cell 2004; 116(6):883–895.

63. de Crecchio G, Simonelli F, Nunziata G, Mazzeo S, Greco GM, Rinaldi E, Ventruto V, Ciccodicola A, Miano MG, Testa F, Curci A, D'Urso M, Rinaldi MM, Cavaliere ML, Castelluccio P. Autosomal recessive familial exudative vitreoretinopathy: evidence for genetic heterogeneity. Clin Genet 1998; 54(4):315–320.
64. Hirose T, Lee KY, Schepens CL. Snowflake degeneration in hereditary vitreoretinal degeneration. Am J Ophthalmol 1974; 77:143–153.
65. Gheiler M, Pollack A, Uchenik D, et al. Hereditary snowflake vitreoretinal degeneration. Birth Defects 1982; 18:577–580..
66. Robertson DM, Link TP, Rostvold JA. Snowflake degeneration of the retina. Ophthalmology 1982; 89:1513–1517.
67. Pollack A, Uchenik D, Chemke J, Oliver M. Prophylactic laser photocoagulation in hereditary snowflake vitreoretinal degeneration. A family report. Arch Ophthalmol 1983; 101:1536–1539.
68. Lee MM, Ritter R 3rd, Hirose T, Vu CD, Edwards AO. Snowflake vitreoretinal degeneration: follow-up of the original family. Ophthalmology 2003; 110(12):2418–2426.
69. Kaufman SJ, Goldberg MF, Orth DH, et al. Autosomal dominant vitreoretinochroidopathy. Arch Ophthalmol 1982; 100:272–278.
70. Blair NP, Goldberg MF, Fishman GA, Salzano T. Autosomal dominant vitreoretinochoroidopathy (ADVIRC). Br J Ophthalmol 1984; 68:2–9.
71. Goldberg MF, Lee FL, Tso MOM, Fishman GA. Histopathologic study of autosomal dominant vitreoretinochoroidopathy (peripheral annular pigmentary dystrophy of the retina). Ophthalmol 1989; 96:1736–1746.
72. Traboulsi EI, Payne JW. Autosomal dominant vitreoretinochoroidopathy. Report of the third family. Arch Ophthalmol 1993; 111(2):194–196.
73. Kellner U, Jandeck C, Kraus H, Foerster MH. Autosomal dominant vitreoretinochoroidopathy with normal electrooculogram in a German family. Graefes Arch Clin Exp Ophthalmol 1998; 236(2):109–114.
74. Fitter KA, Rothschild H, Waltman DD, et al. Dominantly inherited peripheral retinal neovascularization. Arch Ophthalmol 1978; 96:1601–1605.
75. Saari KM. Autosomal dominant juvenile vitreoretinal degeneration and retinal detachment. Int Ophthalmol 1986; 9:45–60.
76. Stone EM, Kimura AE, Folk JC, Bennett SR, Nichols BE, Streb LM, Sheffield VC. Genetic linkage of autosomal dominant neovascular inflammatory vitreoretinopathy to chromosome 11q13. Hum Mol Genet 1992; 1(9):685–689.
77. Sarra GM, Weigell-Weber M, Kotzot D, Niemeyer G, Messmer E, Hergersberg M. Clinical description and exclusion of candidate genes in a novel autosomal recessively inherited vitreoretinal dystrophy. Arch Ophthalmol 2003; 121(8):1109–1116.
78. Weigell-Weber M, Sarra GM, Kotzot D, Sandkuijl L, Messmer E, Hergersberg M. Genomewide homozygosity mapping and molecular analysis of a candidate gene located on 22q13 (fibulin-1) in a previously undescribed vitreoretinal dystrophy. Arch Ophthalmol 2003; 121(8):1184–1188.
79. Campo RV. Similarity of familial exudative vitreoretinopathy and retinopathy of prematurity. Arch Ophthalmol 1983; 101:821.
80. Hirose T, Schepens CL, Brockhurst RJ, et al. Congenital retinoschisis with night blindness in two girls. Ann Ophthalmol 1980; 12:848–856.
81. Ohkubo H, Tanino T. Electrophysiology findings in familial exudative vitreoretinopathy. Doc Ophthalmol 1987; 65:461–469.
82. Hirose T, Wolf E, Schepens CL. Retinal functions in snowflake degeneration. Ann Ophthalmol 1980; 12:1135–1146.
83. Manschot WA. Pathology of hereditary conditions related to retinal detachment. Ophthalmologica 1971; 162:223–234.
84. Peyman GA, Fishman GA, Sanders DR, Vlchek J. Histopathology of Goldmann-Favre syndrome obtained by full-thickness eye-wall biopsy. Ann Ophthalmol 1977; 9:479–484.

85. Han DP, Burke JM, Blair JR, Simons KB. Histopathologic study of autosomal dominant vitreoretinochoroidopathy in a 26-year-old woman. Arch Ophthalmol 1995; 113(12):1561–1566.
86. Hagler WS, Crosswell HH. Radial perivascular chorioretinal degeneration and retinal detachment. Trans Am Acad Ophthalmol Otolaryngol 1968; 72:203–216.
87. Glazer LC, Maguire A, Blumenkranz MS, Trese MT, Green WR. Improved surgical treatment of familial exudative vitreoretinopathy in children. Am J Ophthalmol 1995; 120(4):471–479.
88. Pendergast SD, Trese MT. Familial exudative vitreoretinopathy. Results of surgical management. Ophthalmology 1998; 105(6):1015–1023.
89. Shubert A, Tasman W. Familial exudative vitreoretinopathy: surgical intervention and visual acuity outcomes. Graefes Arch Clin Exp Ophthalmol 1997; 235(8):490–493.
90. Ikeda T, Fujikado T, Tano Y, Tsujikawa K, Koizumi K, Sawa H, Yasuhara T, Maeda K, Kinoshita S. Vitrectomy for rhegmatogenous or tractional retinal detachment with familial exudative vitreoretinopathy. Ophthalmology 1999; 106(6):1081–1085.
91. Herrmann J, France T, Spranger J, et al. The Stickler syndrome (hereditary arthroophthalmopathy). Birth Defects 1975; 11:76–103..
92. Temple IK. Stickler's syndrome. J Med Genet 1989; 26:119–126.
93. Godel V, Regenbogen L, Feiler-Ofry V, Lazar M. Clinical variability in vitreoretinal degeneration. Hum Heredity 1983; 33:153–159.
94. Aymes S, Preus M. The Marshall and Stickler syndromes: objective rejection of lumping. J Med Genet 1984; 21:34–38.
95. Nielsen CE. Stickler's syndrome. Acta Ophthalmol 1981; 59:286–295.
96. Blair NP, Albert DM, Liberfarb RM, et al. Hereditary progressive arthro-ophthalmopathy of Stickler. Am J Ophthalmol 1979; 88:876–888.
97. Spallone A. Stickler's syndrome: a study of 12 families. Br J Ophthalmol 1987; 71: 504–509.
98. Vallat M, Fritsch D, Van Coppenolle F, et al. Le syndrome de Stickler ou arthroophthalmopathie progressive hereditaire. J Fr Ophtalmol 1985; 8:301–307.
99. Knobloch WH, Layer JM. Clefting syndromes associated with retinal detachment. Am J Ophthalmol 1972; 73:517–530.
100. Daniel R, Kanski JJ, Glasspool MG. Hyaloretinopathy in the clefting syndrome. Br J Ophthalmol 1974; 58:96–102.
101. Knobloch WH. Inherited hyaloideoretinopathy and skeletal dysplasia. Trans Am Ophthalmol Soc 1976; 73:413–451.
102. Feiler-Ofry V, Godel V, Nemet P, Lazar M. Retinal detachment in median cleft-face syndrome. Br J Ophthalmol 1980; 64:121–123.
103. Godel V, Regenbogen L, Feiler-Ofry V, Lazar M. Vitreoretinal degeneration in facial clefting syndrome. Birth Defects 1982; 18:581–586.
104. Saksena SS, Bixler D, Yu PI. Stickler syndrome: a cephalometric study of the face. J Craniofac Genet Dev Biol 1983; 3:19–28.
105. Cohen MM, Knobloch WH, Gorlin RJ. A dominantly inherited syndrome of hyaloideoretinal degeneration, cleft palate, and maxillary hypoplasia. Birth Defects 1971; 7:83–86.
106. Francomano CA, Liberfarb RM, Hirose T, et al. The Stickler syndrome in closely linked to *COL2AI,* the structural gene for type II collagen. Pathol Immunopathol Res 1988; 7:104–106.
107. Godfrey M, Hoolister DW. Type II achondrogenesis-hypochondrogenesis: identification of abnormal type II collagen. Am J Hum Genet 1988; 43:904–913.
108. Zlotogora J, Sagi M, Schuper A, Leiba H, Merin S. Variability of Stickler syndrome. Am J Med Genet 1992; 42(3):337–339.
109. Wilson MC, McDonald-McGinn DM, Quinn GE, Markowitz GD, LaRossa D, Pacuraru AD, Zhu X, Zackai EH. Long-term follow-up of ocular findings in children with Stickler's syndrome. Am J Ophthalmol 1996; 122(5):727–728.

110. Ahmad NN, Ala-Kokko L, Knowlton RG, Jimenez SA, Weaver EJ, Maguire JI, Tasman W, Prockop DJ. Stop codon in the procollagen II gene (COL2A1) in a family with the Stickler syndrome (arthro-ophthalmopathy). Proc Natl Acad Sci USA 1991; 88(15):6624–6627.
111. Ahmad NN, McDonald-McGinn DM, Zackai EH, Knowlton RG, LaRossa D, Di-Mascio J, Prockop DJ. A second mutation in the type II procollagen gene (COL2AI) causing stickler syndrome (arthro-ophthalmopathy) is also a premature termination codon. Am J Hum Genet 1993; 52(l):39–45.
112. Brown DM, Nichols BE, Weingeist TA, Sheffield VC, Kimura AE, Stone EM. Procollagen II gene mutation in Stickler syndrome. Arch Ophthalmol 1992; 110(11):1589–1593.
113. Ahmad NN, Dimascio J, Knowlton RG, Tasman WS. Stickler syndrome. A mutation in the nonhelical 3′ end of type II procollagen gene. Arch Ophthalmol 1995; 113(11): 1454–1457.
114. Brown DM, Vandenburgh K, Kimura AE, Weingeist TA, Sheffield VC, Stone EM. Novel frameshift mutations in the procollagen 2 gene (COL2A1) associated with Stickler syndrome (hereditary arthro-ophthahnopathy). Hum Mol Genet 1995; 4(1):141–142.
115. Donoso LA, Edwards AO, Frost AT, Ritter R, Ahmad NN, Vrabec T, Rogers J, Meyer D. Identification of a stop codon mutation in exon 2 of the collagen 2A1 gene in a large Stickler syndrome family. Am J Ophthalmol 2002; 134(5):720–727.
116. Stickler GB, Hughes W, Houchin P. Clinical features of hereditary progressive arthro-ophthalmopathy (Stickler syndrome): a survey. Genet Med 2001; 3(3):192–196.
117. Donoso LA, Edwards AO, Frost AT, Ritter R 3rd, Ahmad N, Vrabec T, Rogers J, Meyer D, Parma S. Clinical variability of Stickler syndrome: role of exon 2 of the collagen COL2A1 gene. Surv Ophthalmol 2003; 48(2):191–203.
118. Liberfarb RM, Levy HP, Rose PS, Wilkin DJ, Davis J, Balog JZ, Griffith AJ, Szymko-Bennett YM, Johnston JJ, Francomano CA, Tsilou E, Rubin BI. The Stickler syndrome: genotype/phenotype correlation in 10 families with Stickler syndrome resulting from seven mutations in the type II collagen gene locus COL2A1. Genet Med 2003; 5(l):21–27.
119. Vu CD, Brown J Jr, Korkko J, Ritter R 3rd, Edwards AO. Posterior chorioretinal atrophy and vitreous phenotype in a family with Stickler syndrome from a mutation in the COL2A1 gene. Ophthalmology 2003; 110(1):70–77.
120. Wilkin DJ, Liberfarb R, Davis J, Levy HP, Cole WG, Francomano CA, Cohn DH. Rapid determination of COL2A1 mutations in individuals with Stickler syndrome: analysis of potential premature termination codons. Am J Med Genet 2000; 94(2):141–148.
121. OMIM. http://www.ncbi.nlm.nih.gov/omim/.
122. Spranger JW, Langer LO Jr. Spondyloepiphyseal dysplasia congenita. Radiology 1970; 94:313–322.
123. Hamidi-Toosi S, Maumenee IH. Vitreoretinal degeneration in spondyloepiphyseal dysplasia congenita. Arch Ophthalmol 1982; 100:1104–1107.
124. Cole WG, Hall RK, Rogers JG. The clinical features of spondyloepiphyseal dysplasia congenita resulting from the substitution of glycine 997 by serine in the alpha 1(II) chain of type II collagen. J Med Genet 1993; 30(1):27–35.
125. Vikkula M, Ritvaniemi P, Vuorio AF, Kaitila I, Ala-Kokko L, Peltonen L. A mutation in the amino-terminal end of the triple helix of type II collagen causing severe osteochondrodysplasia. Genomics 1993; 16(1):282–285.
126. Yokoyama T, Nakatani S, Murakami A. A case of Kniest dysplasia with retinal detachment and the mutation analysis. Am J Ophthalmol 2003; 136(6):1186–1188.
127. Godel V, Lazar M. Wagner's vitreoretinal degeneration with generalized epiphyseal dysplasia. Acta Ophthalmol 1982; 60:469–474.
128. Williams CJ, Considine EL, Knowlton RG, Reginato A, Neumann G, Harrison D, Buxton P, Jimenez S, Prockop DJ. Spondyloepiphyseal dysplasia and precocious osteoarthritis in a family with an Arg75–>Cys mutation in the procollagen type II gene (COL2A1). Hum Genet 1993; 92(5):499–505.

129. Bonaventure J, Philippe C, Plessis G, Vigneron J, Lasselin C, Maroteaux P, Gilgenkrantz S. Linkage study in a large pedigree with Stickler syndrome: exclusion of COL2A1 as the mutant gene. Hum Genet 1992; 90(1–2):164–168.
130. Richards AJ, Yates JR, Williams R, Payne SJ, Pope FM, Scott JD, Snead MP. A family with Stickler syndrome type 2 has a mutation in the COL11A1 gene resulting in the substitution of glycine 97 by valine in alpha 1 (XI) collagen. Hum Mol Genet 1996; 5(9):1339–1343.
131. Snead MP, Yates JR. Clinical and molecular genetics of Stickler syndrome. J Med Genet 1999; 36(5):353–359.
132. Richards AJ, Baguley DM, Yates JR, Lane C, Nicol M, Harper PS, Scott JD, Snead MP. Variation in the vitreous phenotype of Stickler syndrome can be caused by different amino acid substitutions in the X position of the type II collagen Gly-X-Y triple helix. Am J Hum Genet 2000; 67(5):1083–1094.
133. Marshall D. Ectodermal dysplasia. Report of a kindred with ocular deformities and hearing defect. Am J Ophthalmol 1958; 45:143–156.
134. O'Donnell JJ, Sirkin S, Hall BD. Generalized osseous abnormalities in the Marshall syndrome. Birth Defects 1976; 12:299–314.
135. Winter RM, Baraitser M, Laurence KM, et al. The Weissenbacher-Zweymuller, Stickler and Marshall syndromes: further evidence for their identity. Am J Med Genet 1983; 16:189–199.
136. Griffith AJ, Sprunger LK, Sirko-Osadsa DA, Tiller GE, Meisler MH, Warman ML. Marshall syndrome associated with a splicing defect at the COL11A1 locus. Am J Hum Genet 1998; 62(4):816–823.
137. Shanske A, Bogdanow A, Shprintzen RJ, Marion RW. Marshall syndrome and a defect at the COL11A1 locus. Am J Hum Genet 1998; 63(5):1558–1561.
138. Annunen S, Korkko J, Czarny M, Warman ML, Brunner HG, Kaariainen H, Mulliken JB, Tranebjaerg L, Brooks DG, Cox GF, Cruysberg JR, Curtis MA, Davenport SL, Friedrich CA, Kaitila I, Krawczynski MR, Latos-Bielenska A, Mukai S, Olsen BR, Shinno N, Somer M, Vikkula M, Zlotogora J, Prockop DJ, Ala-Kokko L. Splicing mutations of 54-bp exons in the COL11A1 gene cause Marshall syndrome, but other mutations cause overlapping Marshall/Stickler phenotypes. Am J Hum Genet 1999; 65(4):974–983.
139. Pihlajamaa T, Prockop DJ, Faber J, Winterpacht A, Zabel B, Giedion A, Wiesbauer P, Spranger J, Ala-Kokko L. Heterozygous glycine substitution in the COL11A2 gene in the original patient with the Weissenbacher-Zweymüller syndrome demonstrates its identity with heterozygous OSMED (nonocular Stickler syndrome). Am J Med Genet 1998; 80(2):115–120.
140. Brunner HG, van Beersum SE, Warman ML, Olsen BR, Ropers HH, Mariman EC. A Stickler syndrome gene is linked to chromosome 6 near the COL11A2 gene. Hum Mol Genet 1994; 3(9):1561–1564.
141. Miny P, Lenz W. Autosomal recessive deafness with skeletal dysplasia and facial appearance of Marshall syndrome. Am J Med Genet 1985; 21:317–324.
142. Knobloch WH, Layer JM. Retinal detachment and encephalocele. J Pediatr Ophthal 1971; 8:181–184.
143. Sertie AL, Sossi V, Camargo AA, Zatz M, Brahe C, Passos-Bueno MR. Collagen XVIII, containing an endogenous inhibitor of angiogenesis and tumor growth, plays a critical role in the maintenance of retinal structure and in neural tube closure (Knobloch syndrome). Hum Mol Genet 2000; 9(13):2051–2058.
144. Rabinowitz R, Gradstein L, Galil A, Levy L, Lifshitz T. The ocular manifestations of Weissenbacher-Zweymuller syndrome. Eye 2004; 18:1258–1263.
145. Li SW, Prockop DJ, Helminen H, Fassler R, Lapvetelainen T, Kiraly K, Peltarri A, Arokoski J, Lui H, Arita M. et al. Transgenic mice with targeted inactivation of the Col2 alpha 1 gene for collagen II develop a skeleton with membranous and periosteal bone but no endochondral bone. Genes Dev 1995; 9(22):2821–2830.

146. Blair NP, Dodge JT, Schmidt GM. Rhegmatogenous retinal detachment in labrador retrievers. I. Development of retinal tears and detachment. Arch Ophthalmol 1985; 103:842–847.
147. Blair NP, Dodge JT, Schmidt GM. Rhegmatogenous retinal detachment in labrador retrievers. II. Proliferative vitreoretinopathy. Arch Ophthalmol 1985; 103:848–854.
148. Carrig CB, Sponnenberg DP, Schmidt GM, Tvedten HW. Inheritance of associated ocular and skeletal dysplasia in labrador retrievers. J Am Vet Med Assoc 1988; 193: 1269–1272.
149. Lisi V, Guala A, Lopez A, Vitali M, Spadoni E, Olivieri C, Danesino C, Mottes M. Linkage analysis for prenatal diagnosis in a familial case of Stickler syndrome. Genet Couns 2002; 13(2):163–170.
150. Chaudhuri PR, Rosenthal AR. Posterior hyperplastic primary vitreous. Trans Ophthalmol Soc UK 1982; 102:237–240.
151. Sneed PJ, Augsburger JJ, Shields JA, et al. Bilateral retinal vascular hypoplasia associated with persistence of the primary vitreous: a new clinical entity? J Pediatr Ophthalmol Strabismus 1988; 25:77–85.
152. Haddad R, Font RL, Reeser F. Persistent hyperplastic primary vitreous. A clinicopathologic study of 62 cases and review of the literature. Surv Ophthalmol 1978; 23:123–134.
153. Menchini U, Pece A, Alberti M, et al. Vitre′ primitif hyperplastique avec persistance de l'artère hyaloide, chez deux fréres non jumeaux. J Fr Ophtalmol 1987; 10:241–245.
154. Hovland KR, Schepens CL, Freeman HM. Developmental giant retinal tears associated with lens coloboma. Arch Ophthalmol 1968; 80:325–331.
155. Sandgren O, Holmgren G, Lundgren E, Steen L. Restriction fragment length polymorphism analysis of mutated transthyretin in vitreous amyloidosis. Arch Ophthalmol 1988; 106:790–792.
156. Ueno H, Veno S, Kajitani T, et al. Clinical and histopathological studies of a case with juvenile form of Gaucher's disease. Jpn J Ophthalmol 1977; 21:98–108.
157. Cogan DG, Chu FC, Gittinger J, Tychsen L. Fundal abnormalities of Gaucher's disease. Arch Ophthalmol 1980; 98:2202–2203.

13
Other Inherited Retinal Diseases

INTRODUCTION

Ocular diseases affecting the retina constitute a substantial portion of inherited eye diseases. In this book, retinitis pigmentosa (RP), the large group of retinal blinding diseases was discussed separately in Chapter 10 and syndromic RP was discussed in Chapter 11. Macular diseases were considered in Chapter 8, primary cone photoreceptor disorders in Chapter 9 and inherited vitreo-retinopathies in Chapter 12. Night blindness and albinism, both affecting the retina, will be discussed in Chapters 15 and 22, respectively. In this chapter, diseases that affect primarily the retina and were not included in these previous chapters will be described. Some overlapping must exist, therefore a specific disorder may be discussed in two chapters.

X-LINKED JUVENILE RETINOSCHISIS

Historically, X-linked juvenile retinoschisis (XLJRS, XLRS) was classified as one of the vitreoretinopathies. However, recently, more and more evidence seems to support the view that XLJRS is a primary disease of the retina itself, with little involvement of the vitreous. It is difficult to draw a line between the vitreoretinopathies and retinal diseases. It seems to me that vitreoretinopathies should include all diseases in which the vitreous is primarily affected or plays a major role in the development of the disease, including traction on the retina; otherwise, a disorder remains a retinal disorder.

Various terms have been used for XLJRS. Initially, terms such as vitreous veils or congenital vascular veils in the vitreous were used, when the inner layer of the schitic retina was mistaken for vitreous bands or veils. Later, the term congenital retinoschisis, X-linked recessive (1) was used, after the congenital nature of the disorder and its heredity became clear. However, juvenile retinoschisis was probably used most, to distinguish this disease from senile retinoschisis. The name XLJRS will be used here to distinguish this disorder from hereditary retinoschisis transmitted by another mode of genetic transmission and from noninherited senile retinoschisis. The term is abbreviated by some as XLRS.

Description and Clinical Findings

There are three presenting symptoms of XLJRS (2). In infancy or early childhood, strabismus or nystagmus come to the attention of the parents. Later, a school vision test or other eye examination may detect poor visual acuity.

George et al. described five patients with infantile presentation of the disorder (3). All presented with nystagmus or strabismus or both and manifested bullous retinoschisis.

The visual acuity is almost always lower than normal in the affected males. It varies from 6/7.5 to 6/60 in most cases (2), but most patients have a visual acuity of less than 6/15 in their better eye, so they are unable to drive (4).

Visual fields are often restricted in the upper field in patients with retinoschisis (2). The extent of the defect reflects the size of the retinoschisis. Color vision may be normal, or there may be a tendency toward tritanopia or deuteranopia (5).

Macular lesions are the typical finding of XLJRS (Fig. 1). In fact, they are found in all patients (2,4,5) and are the only finding in about half of all patients (6). The macular lesions may be in the form of small cysts, with fine radial folds, a peri-macular reticular pattern, pigmentation of the macula, and foveal retinoschisis (2). Harris and Yeung (5) claimed that progressive changes occur in the macula, and that six stages can be distinguished. These changes start in stage 1 as small cysts arranged in a radial pattern toward the fovea, with yellowish intraretinal septa. In stage 2, a breakdown of the radial septa happens with a central cyst formation, which continues to enlarge in stage 3, together with formation of a honeycomb pattern. In stage 4, the intraretinal septa are broken and the retina forms two layers, the anterior lamina being very thin (foveal retinoschisis). In stage 5, regression starts

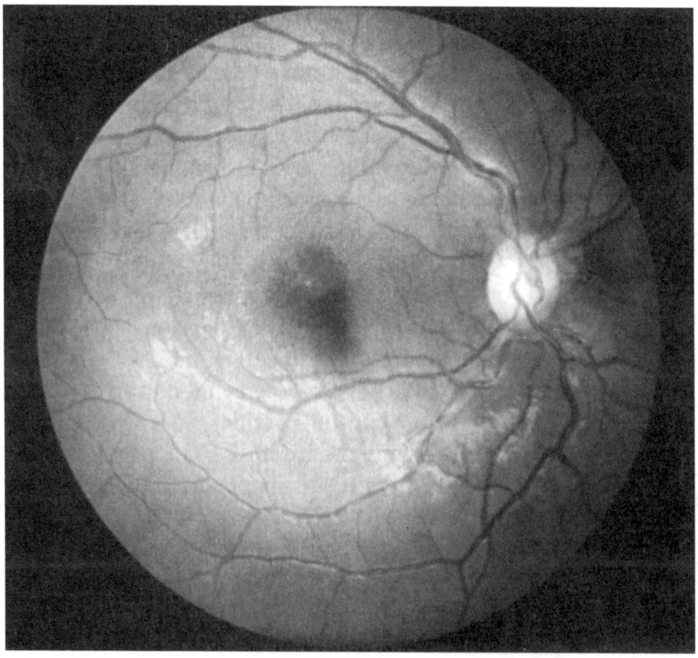

Figure 1 The macula of a 13-year-old boy with XLJRS. Note the central cyst and the typical radial pattern around the fovea.

with a collapse of the central cyst and continues in stage 6 with flattening of the fovea, pigmentation, atrophy, and yellow deposits.

Foveal schisis occurs in 83–100% of patients (7,8). Most commonly it is cystic spoke-wheel maculopathy (9). In older males absent foveal reflex, macular pigmentation or atrophic lesions are more common (7,10).

About half of the patients with XLJRS have a retinoschisis in one or, more often, both eyes. This is usually symmetric, starts at approximately the equator, and spreads peripherally, but may also start more posteriorly up to the macula, or more anteriorly. The lower temporal quadrant is mostly affected, but the retinoschisis may be much milder and involve other quadrants or another area (Fig. 2).

Kawano et al. (11) reported on two male infants who had tremendously elevated retinoschisis in both the foveal and equatorial-peripheral locations. This later regressed and flattened out. From a survey of 201 affected eyes with XLJRS reported in the literature, these authors claimed that ballooning or bullous retinoschisis is significantly more frequent in young patients, particularly those younger than age five years (11), indicating a pattern of regression with age.

The inner layer of the retinoschisis is extremely thin and, frequently, shows white lacquer-like glistening lines of dendritic and sclerotic vessels, which may extend into the nonelevated retina and, less frequently, become retinal breaks (Fig. 2). The inner layer, which most likely constitutes only a part of the nerve fiber layer, is so thin that it tends to tear and fold on itself, become loose in the vitreous (vitreous veils) or cause baring of the retinal vessels (2), with or without accompanying hemorrhage. The vitreous is not universally affected, as previously suggested (2). If abnormalities of the vitreous occur, they will be in the form of posterior vitreous detachment, liquefaction, veils from the inner layer of the schisis, or changes secondary to the vitreous hemorrhage.

Most patients feel that the disease is stable after school years (4), although some patients show continuing decrease in visual acuity (5). Several complications

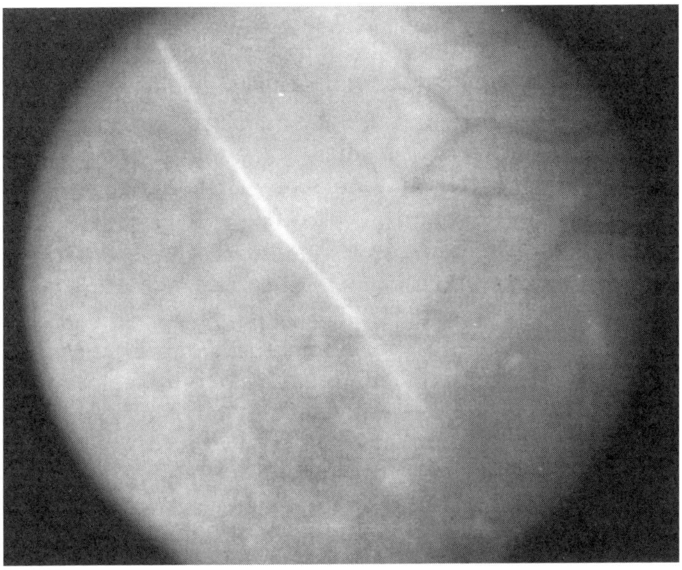

Figure 2 Peripheral retinoschisis in a 13-year-old boy with XLJRS. Note the characteristic demarcation line.

may occur. Vitreous hemorrhage may result from bleeding of torn retinal vessels or from the development of new vessels. Arkfeld and Brockhurst (12) followed up a male infant who showed, together with the typical striate maculopathy, a posterior vitreous detachment. This posterior surface became the "scaffold" for development of neovascularization, which later shrunk, leaving an intravitreal free-floating membrane. Both disk and retinal neovascularization developed in a young boy with XLJRS and resulted in vitreous hemorrhage (13).

Retinal detachment may develop in patients with XLJRS if the outer, thick layer of retina has a hole or tear. The incidence of retinal detachment is probably much less common than the 22% found in one group of 40 patients (14). Retinal detachment poses a serious problem in early childhood, when it is very difficult to diagnose and may be misdiagnosed as retinoblastoma (15).

In another study (7), peripheral retinoschisis was reported in 71%, retinal detachment in 16% and vitreous hemorrhage in 21%. Out of 56 male patients, four eyes were blind. Refractive errors ranged from −7.50 to +7.75 diopters (7). The peripheral retina manifested lattice degeneration, pigmentation and retinal holes, in addition to the retinoschisis (16). Twenty-nine to 50% had no peripheral schisis and the foveal changes were their only abnormality (8).

Vitreous hemorrhage and retinal detachment are the most frequent complications of XLJRS. Other reported complications are rare and include neovascular glaucoma, optic atrophy, iridocorneal angle anomalies, and hemorrhagic or exudative retinal cysts (1).

In contrast to other X-linked diseases, the female carrier of XLJRS does not show any obvious manifestations of the disease. Most clinical investigators were unable to distinguish carriers from normal relatives (5,6). It is possible that the rare cases of women with a maculopathy typical of XLJRS and with retinoschisis is actually a manifesting carrier, but this has never been proven. Recently, Arden et al. (17) suggested that heterozygotes for XLJRS demonstrate a complete absence of normal rod-cone interaction. They examined 11 obligate carriers from different families by testing the relationship of cone flicker threshold to changing background intensities. In normal subjects, the ability of the photopic system to detect flicker becomes impaired as rods dark-adapt, and it improves when rods are exposed to light. This did not happen in the heterozygous carriers they examined.

George et al. (18) agree with most other studies by claiming that there are no pathognomonic features of the carrier state of XLJRS. They studied the ERG of female carriers, including oscillatory potentials and scotopic threshold response (STR) and found all their results to be normal (18). Girls may be affected when they are homozygous for the gene, as in a family with an affected father and a hemizygous mother (19).

Clinical and Genetic Types of Congenital Retinoschisis

X-linked juvenile retinoschisis is, by far, the most common type of congenital retinoschisis (Fig. 3). However, several families were reported in which a different mode of inheritance could be possible. Autosomal recessive inheritance was suggested in one family with three affected women (20). The autosomal dominant mode seemed likely in two other families with a father-to-son (21) or mother-to-daughter (14) transmission of the disease. In all three families (20–22) the clinical findings were similar to those of typical XLJRS.

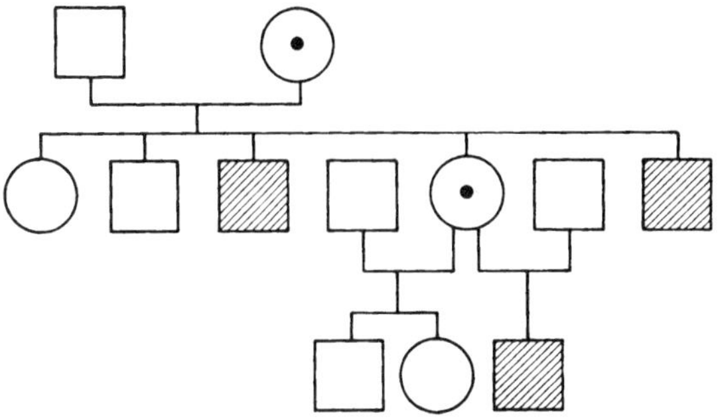

Figure 3 A family with XLJRS displays a typical X-linked transmission of the disease. Female obligatory carriers are marked by a central dot, but do not show any clinical abnormality.

It is possible, although rare, that a female patient with retinoschisis is a manifesting heterozygous carrier or a homozygous affected female, as suggested by Forssius et al. in their report of one family (23), and by Ali et al. in another family (19).

Diagnosis, Pathology, and Pathogenesis

Molecular genetics will be discussed below. It is possible to make a definite diagnosis by gene identification. In practice, the diagnosis of XLJRS is based on clinical findings, especially the foveal changes, and on a positive family history. Fluorescein angiography is usually not helpful. It may show a normal vascular pattern in the posterior pole or, in older patients, spots of retinal pigment epithelium (RPE) atrophy, such as window defects (5). In one study, Green and Jampol (24) found, by fluorescein angiography, sluggish retinal circulation, with areas of capillary nonperfusion and leakage, even in areas without schisis.

Patterns of retinal thickness and structure can be measured by one of two methods. Scanning retinal thickness analysis (RTA) was effctively used to demonstrate the extent and structural details of the foveal schisis (8) Optical coherence tomography (OCT) revealed the retinal cleavage into two layers. The two layers were connected by thin-walled vertical pallisades, separated by cystoid spaces and more prominent in the foveal area (25).

The electroretinogram (ERG) to single-flash white light stimulation characterically shows a normal a-wave and a significally reduced b-wave in all affected males (26) and in the affected females (22). In addition, oscillatory potentials are reduced. In spite of this, psychophysical tests performed by static perimetry yielded normal or only slightly elevated thresholds (26). Peachey et al. (26) theorized that in XLJRS a primary defect in Muller's cells would result in a markedly reduced ERG b-wave but normal absolute thresholds. In advanced cases photoreceptors also become involved, possibly secondary to Muller's cell disease, and the a-wave is reduced as well. By pattern ERG, b-waves are also significantly smaller than normal, indicating abnormality in the inner layers, such as in the bipolar cells or Muller's cells (27).

The ERG manifests a characteristic pattern of a greater reduction in cone-photoreceptor responses. The rod responses were often normal. This was obtained in studies using Ganzfeld ERG, multifocal ERG and ERG on/off responses (28–30).

The ERG may help with the differential diagnosis between XLJRS and retinoschisis of the senile type or Goldman-Favre syndrome. In senile retinoschisis, the inner layer is much thicker, as the split is in the outer plexiform layer, and both a-waves and b-waves are reduced according to the size of the retinoschisis. In Goldman-Favre syndrome, the vitreous is severely affected, the retina shows pigmentary changes, and the ERG is extinct. In young infants with retinoschisis and retinal detachment, XLJRS must be differentiated from retinoblastoma (15,31), retinal dysplasia, congenital retinal folds, retinal nonattachment, and retinopathy of prematurity. The electro-oculogram (EOG) varies from normal to abnormally low in different patients with XLJRS.

Several histopathologic studies were performed on eyes with XLJRS. Splitting between the two layers was found within the nerve fiber layer (31–33). Veil formations in the vitreous were of retinal origin (31). The inner thin layer of the schitic cavity frequently had holes (31). An inherent abnormality of Muller fibers (31) or of the inner nerve fiber layer (32) could cause the condition. Amorphous material was found in the retina adjacent to the schitic cavity, which by electron microscopy was shown to be extracellular filaments measuring approximately 11 nm in diameter (33). Condon et al. (33) suggested that these filaments are produced by defective Muller's cells, and that degeneration of Muller's fibers may cause the schisis formation. Using immunohistochemical techniques in a severe case with retinal detachment, the retina was found disorganized with tightly packed retinal folds fused together by fibrovascular tissue (15). Mooy et al. concluded that photoreceptors are the primarily involved cells in XLRS (9).

Epidemiology and Genetics

XLRS has been reported in many countries as a disease that is neither common nor rare. Its prevalence varies in different reports ranging from 1:5000 to 1: 25,000 (9). It is probably much more common in the Finnish population (34,35).

Linkage studies published in 1987 and 1988 located the locus for XLRS on the short arm of chromosome X near Xp22 (36–39). The locus for XLRS was mapped in 1995 to chromosome Xp22.2 (or Xp22.2–p22.1) and used for carrier detection (40). Sauer et al. (41) cloned the gene XLRS1 (or RS1). The RS1 gene consists of six exons. It encodes a protein, retinoschisin, which contains a discoidin domain implicated in cell-to-cell adhesion and phospholipid binding. Sauer et al. (41) suggested therefore that the defective protein function might be implicated in the splitting of the retina. The gene is expressed exclusively in the retina and when defective may also result in abnormal function of Muller fibers. Sauer et al. found mutations in the RS1 gene in nine families with juvenile retinoschisis (41). In 1998, the Retinoschisis Consortium reported the identification of mutations in the RS1 gene in 214 of 234 examined patients diagnosed as XLJRS (42). Eighty two different mutations were identified; of these 51 were private mutations, seen only in one family. The majority were loss-of-function mutations (42). By 1999, 300 patients with mutations, including point mutations, small deletions and re-arrangements, were reported worldwide (43). Hot spots concentrated in exons 4–6 (43). Huopaniemi et al. (44) studied Finnish families and reported that 95% had one of three mutations, all in exons 4–6, thereby identifying three ancestors of founder effect. The three mutations were missense, Glu72Lys (70% of all), Gly74Val (6% of all), and Glyl09Arg (19% of all). No mutations were found in 5%, indicating possible heterogeneity (44). Different point mutations, missense, nonsense and frameshift were detected in 10 Japanese patients (45). Various other mutations were reported, including missense mutations (10), a 4-base pair insertion at codon 55 (46) and a 4-base pair deletion in exon 5 (16). Phenotype/genotype correlation was not impressive. A great variability in severity of the disease exists but it is not associated with specific mutations. By the year 2000 about 100 different mutations were reported. By 2004, the Retinoschisis Consortium was aware of 128 different disease-causing mutations in the RS1 gene (47).

Management

Medical and Surgical

Patients with XLJRS who develop neovascularization on the disk or elsewhere may be treated by panretinal laser photocoagulation. Such treatment has successfully caused regression of new bleeding vessels (13). However, such new vessels may shrink spontaneously without treatment (12). The use of laser photocoagulation in retinoschisis without neovascularization is controversial. It is advised by some (5,48), but objected to by others (44). It seems that most ophthalmologists would not treat the majority of cases in whom the schisis is stationary. Treatment by laser or xenon-arc photocoagulation or by cryopexy should be considered in very high or rapidly advancing retinoschisis. In some cases, especially if retinal detachment develops, buckling procedures, fluid aspiration, and sometimes vitrectomy may be performed (1).

Genetic Counseling

X-linked juvenile retinoschisis is considered to be one clinical and genetic entity caused by a single gene, and the patient should be thus advised. The risk that an obligatory carrier's son will be affected is 50%, that a daughter will be a carrier is 50%, that a daughter of an affected man will be a carrier is 100%, and that the son of an affected man will be affected is zero. It may be possible to detect carriers heterozygote carriers by the method advised by Arden (17), but this has yet to be confirmed for all heterozygotes.

The identification of disease-bearing mutations at the RS1 gene facilitates genetic counseling. It is the most reliable method to detect the heterozygous carrier and identify the existence of the mutation (43).

Prenatal Diagnosis

A distinction between a boy and girl can, of course, be made prenatally, leaving the chance of 50% that a son of a carrier woman will be affected. Identification of the mutation enables more accurate prenatal diagnosis.

FAMILIAL RETINAL DETACHMENT

Many articles on the familial occurrence of retinal detachment have been published in the older literature. However, most of these studies related to families with high myopia, families with congenital cataract who developed retinal detachment in aphakic eyes after cataract extraction, or families with a hereditary vitreoretinopathy not recognized at the time (50,51). Other associations reported were the Ehlers-Danlos syndrome (52), optic disk anomalies (53), and lattice degeneration (54,55). The pedigrees reported did not show any clear pattern of transmission in most cases, therefore, both autosomal recessive and autosomal dominant transmission, with a reduced penetrance, were suggested. Even multifactorial inheritance was considered (55).

One strange case of identical twins was reported in which each developed a giant retinal tear in one eye without any external cause (56).

Retinal detachment as an inherited phenomenon has, in my opinion, not been shown to exist. However, some families may display a much higher-than-normal tendency to develop a retinal detachment. The most frequent cause of such a familial occurrence is one of the inherited vitreoretinopathies, followed by the pathologic myopias. These conditions are discussed in separate chapters.

NORRIE DISEASE AND ALLIED DISORDERS (PSEUDOGLIOMA)

Pseudoglioma is a general term used to describe a vitreoretinal condition similar to "glioma" (retinoblastoma) in appearance, but not retinoblastoma itself. Some causes of pseudoglioma are sporadic and nonfamilial, such as retinopathy of prematurity (ROP), unilateral persistent hyperplastic vitreous (PHPV), and various congenital ocular anomalies of embryogenesis. Others are clearly inherited. The hallmark of these is the pathologic finding of retinal dysplasia (Fig. 4). The retina is not normally differentiated into regular layers and shows rosettes of immature retinal cells embedded in a vascular connective tissue of a hyperplastic primary vitreous. Various disorders were included in this group and the nosology of these diseases was quite confusing. After the identification of the NDP gene as associated with Norrie disease, subsequent studies clarified the picture. Several clinical entities are allelic

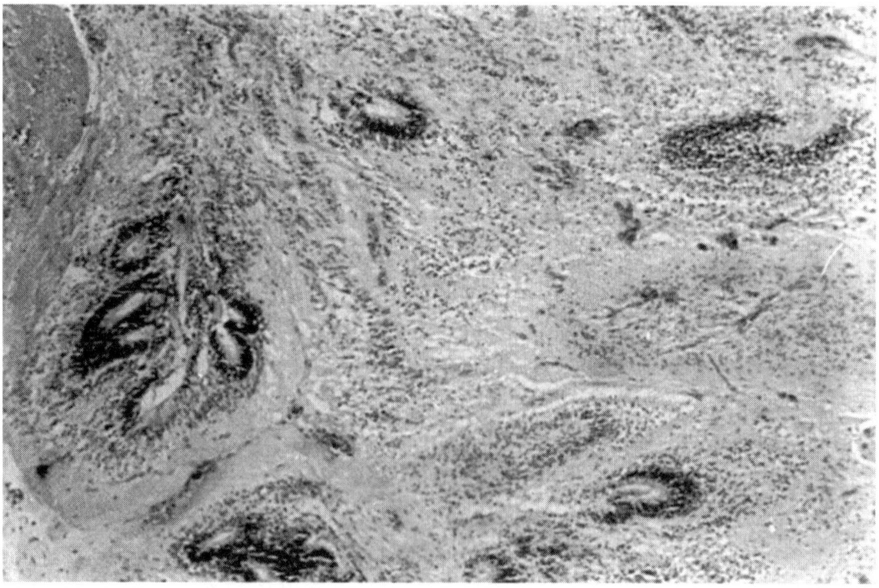

Figure 4 Histopathologic appearance of an eye of a one-year-old infant with retinal dysplasia. Note the typical rosettes embedded in fibrovascular tissue.

mutations of the NDP gene and these include Norrie disease, X-linked pseudoglioma and X-linked familial exudative vitreoretinopathy (XL-FEVR).

The Clinical Types of Inherited Pseudoglioma

Norrie Disease

Norrie disease was first reported in 1927 by Norrie (57). In a report on 25 years of activity as an ophthalmic surgeon for the Royal Danish Institutes for the Blind, Norrie mentioned two families with nine affected blind boys (56). The disease was further investigated by Warburg, who described the clinical findings in 35 male patients in six Danish families and gave the disease by its present name: Norrie disease (58). The disease is transmitted by an X chromosome-linked gene. All of the affected have the ocular condition, about two-thirds are mentally retarded and about one-third are deaf (the oculoacousticocerebral degeneration) (58). The ocular condition can usually be noted at birth by the presence of retinal nonattachment, falciform detachment, or pseudoglioma—a mass of fibrovascular tissue in the vitreous mixed with retinal tissue (59). I have seen boys born with a flat retina, but hazy vitreous with hemorrhage, who developed inoperable retinal detachment in the first or second month of life. During the first year of life, a cataract develops, the cornea becomes opaque, and usually phthisis bulbi occurs (Fig. 5).

Warburg collected and listed the cases described in the literature. By 1975, she found 43 described families with 243 affected members. Of these, 26 families had associated mental retardation, two had no retardation, and 13 probably had no retardation (59).

The female carrier of Norrie disease is usually asymptomatic. However, symptomatic female carriers have been described. One such female carrier suffered from congenital blindness, leukocoria and bilateral total retinal detachment, associated with a missense (Ilel23Asn) mutation in the NDP gene (60). Mintz-Hittner et al. studied the female status in seven families with Norrie disease and detected peripheral retinal changes in three carrier women (61). Three healthy, noncarrier female members of the families and one healthy male member also had abnormal peripheral retinal changes. This could indicate that the defective product of the mutated gene (the mutated protein norrin) is transmitted transplacentally to the fetus, thus affecting inner retinal vasculogenesis (61).

Many histologic studies were reported (54,62). These usually showed the fibrovascular retrolental tissue embedding abnormal undifferentiated retinal cells,

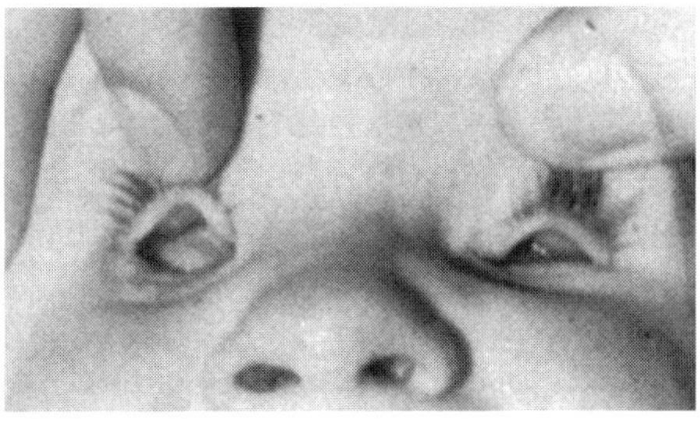

Figure 5 Bilateral phthisis bulbi in a boy with Norrie disease from the Canadian island Manitoulin.

including rosettes. Chynn et al. described a thickened, hemorrhagic detached retina with large retrolental vessels, retinal dysplasia and gliosis (62).

X-Linked Pseudoglioma

This disease has ocular findings that may be identical with those of Norrie disease, and, like Norrie disease, it is also transmitted by the X-linked mode and affects males. However, there is absence of the two other findings of Norrie disease, namely, mental retardation and hearing loss. In fact, the three families I examined, one in Cyprus (63) and two in Israel, had a milder ocular disease. The disease is well described by Godel and associates (64–66). The onset is congenital or in early childhood, when strabismus, nystagmus, head posture, and poor vision are noted. The ocular findings (Fig. 6) vary and may consist of any of the following: a vascularized retinal fold extending from the disc through the macula into the inferotemporal periphery (quite similar to cicatricial ROP stage II), white fibrous tissue over posterior pole, a tumorlike protrusion into the vitreous, or diffuse pigmentation. Congenital glaucoma was found in one eye, and one eye was normal in one case (65). Obligate heterozygote carriers are usually normal, but a paramacular fold, a veil-like retinal fold, and peripheral dysplastic tissue were noted in three carriers, respectively (66).

One female with a chromosomal translocation (X chromosome-autosome) showed a full-blown picture of X-linked pseudoglioma, probably because of loss of a gene and preferential (nonrandom) inactivation of the normal X chromosome (67).

X-linked pseudoglioma or X-linked recessive primary retinal dysplasia was previously presumed a separate disease from Norrie (68). Currently it seems that these two different phenotypes are genetically associated with different allelic mutations of the NDP gene. Table 1 describes the different diseases associated with mutations of the NDP gene.

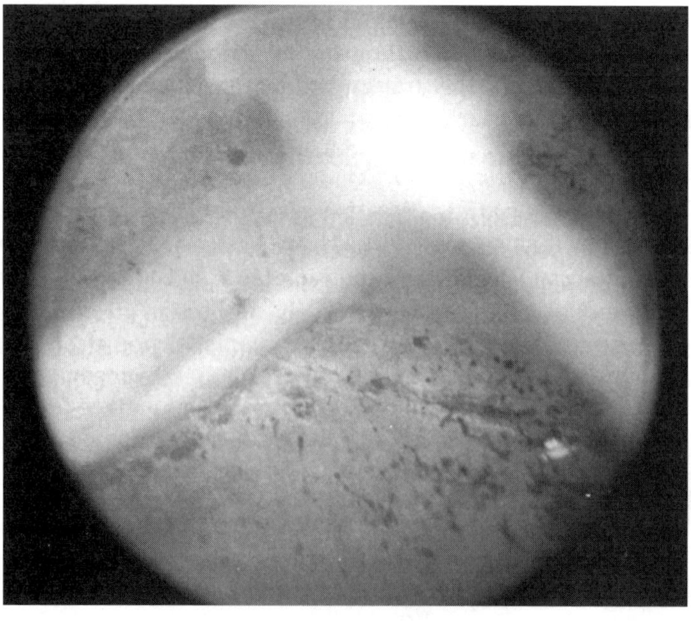

Figure 6 X-linked pseudoglioma: the fundus displays a large retinal fold. Clinically, the disease is usually milder than in Norrie disease, in which phthisis bulbi is common.

Table 1 Norrie and Allied Diseases and the NDP Gene[a]

Disease	Gene/protein/mutations	Chromosomal location	Major ocular abnormality	Extraocular abnormal	Remarks
Norrie	NDP/norrin/majority: nonfunctioning gene	Xp11.3–11.4	Retinal dysplasia, neovascularization detachment	Mental retardation, hearing impairment	Near-by genes MAOA and MAOB may be mutated
X-linked pseudoglioma	NDP/norrin/majority: missense mutations	Same as above	Same as above	None	
X-linked FEVR	NDP/norrin/majority: missense mutations	Same as above	Same as above	None	
ROP (retinopathy of prematurity)	In some cases: NDP/truncating mutations	Same as above	Same as above	Variable CNS abnormalities. None to severe	
Bloch-Sulzberger	NEMO/NF-Kappa essential modulator	Xq28	Various congenital retinal detachment	Skin, hair, nails, teeth and CNS	X-linked dominant transmission

[a]Other disorders to be considered in differential diagnosis: X-linked retinoschisis; autosomal dominant and autosomal recessive FEVR; severe cases of Stickler syndrome and retinal dysplasia in severe CNS abnormalities.

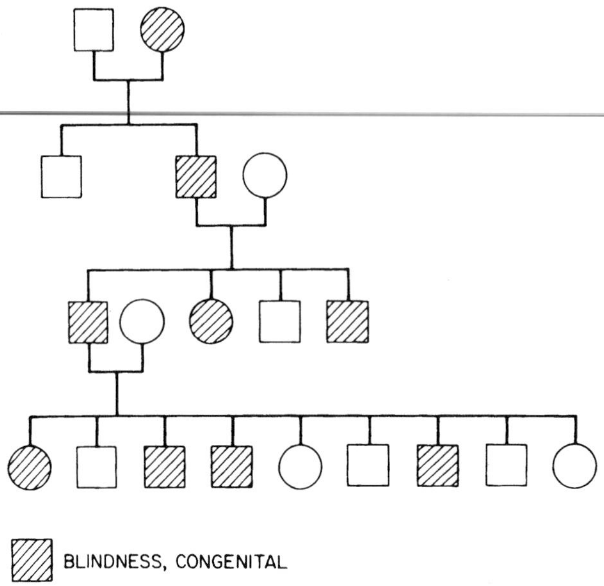

Figure 7 A Greek family with congenital pseudoglioma and blindness transmitted by the autosomal dominant mode. (Courtesy of G. Sgouros, MD, Athens)

Other Inherited Pseudogliomas

Several other entities may present a pseudoglioma-like entity, including leukocoria. Isolated reports on inherited pseudoglioma transmitted by the autosomal dominant or autosomal recessive mode can be found, but these have not been confirmed, and their existence was reported as being doubtful (69). However, I examined one family with congenital pseudoglioma and blindness transmitted by the autosomal dominant mode (Fig. 7). Such cases may well represent autosomal recessive or autosomal dominant FEVR (familial exudative vitreoretinopathy), which are associated with genes different from those associated with X-linked FEVR. A mutated NDP gene transmits X-linked FEVR, while the former diseases are associated with other genes.

Congenital non-attachment of the retina or falciform congenital detachment of the retina may be associated with various extraocular abnormalities (69–71). These include the association of these retinal abnormalities with mental retardation, osteoporosis, microphthalmus, microcephaly, encephalocele, cleft palate, and polydactyly (Meckel syndrome). Autosomal recessive inheritance was confirmed in some cases.

Bloch-Sulzberger syndrome (incontinentia pigmenti) pseudoglioma may be associated with a variety of systemic abnormalities (72). Different forms of retinal detachment may occur (73). The disease is transmitted by the X-linked dominant mode and is usually lethal in males, causing abortions of male offspring (74). In affected females, variable abnormalities may occur in the eyes, skin, hair, nails, teeth and CNS. The locus IP (for incontinentia pigmenti) is linked to chromosome Xq28, near the telomere of the long arm of this chromosome. The disease-causative gene was identified as NEMO (for NF-KappaB essential modulator) or otherwise named

IKK gamma (for I Kappa B Kinase-gamma) (74). Rarely, affected male individuals are born and carry similar abnormalities (75).

The retinal dysplasia described by Reese (76) also includes pseudoglioma with various abnormalities of the CNS and seems to be transmitted by the autosomal recessive mode.

Genetics

In 1955, linkage analysis with polymorphic DNA markers led to the discovery of a close linkage between *NDP* (the gene for Norrie disease) and the *DXS7* locus (L1.28 probe) located at Xp11.3, the same location as the gene for X-linked retinitis pigmentosa (77). Gal et al. (78) also found a family in whom an affected male and several obligatory heterozygotes had a small submicroscopic deletion at Xp11.3. The affected boy had phthisis bulbi and severe mental retardation, hypogonadism, growth disturbance, and increased susceptibility to infections. In another family, Ohba and Yamashita (67) found a translocation between the X chromosome at Xp11 and an autosome, with a possible loss of some genes. The affected female had pseudoglioma.

Sims et al., using positional mapping, mapped the locus for Norrie disease to chromosome Xp11 (79), near the loci for RP2, CSNB and Åland Island eye disease. In 1992, Chen et al. (80) and Berger et al. (81) isolated and cloned the gene associated with Norrie disease. The gene NDP (for Norrie disease protein) consists of three exons and two introns, and spans 27 kb (82). Of the three exons, the first is not translated. DNA sequence predicts a protein of 133 amino acids that is expressed only in the brain and in the eyes (82). The function of the protein, norrin, is unknown.

By 2003, about 70 disease-causing sequence variants in the NDP gene were identified. These include small intragenic deletions, nonsense mutations, deletions of the whole gene, and insertions and missense mutations in the vicinity of codon 60 (83–86). Wong et al. (82) stressed that the normal ND protein has a relatively large number of cysteine-containing amino acids and their mutation alters the function of the protein.

Chen et al. (86) demonstrated that in the same band Xp11.4–Xp11.3 the genes are located in this order: telomere . . . MAOA-MAOB-NDP-centromere. MAO (monoamine oxidase) plays a critical role in degeneration of biogenic amines. If the gene MAOA is deleted or defective, mental retardation occurs. If MAOB and NDP are deleted, congenital blindness is associated with abnormal metabolism of certain biogenic amines, but intelligence is normal (86).

In some patients with typical Norrie disease, no mutation in the NDP gene was identified. This was reported in 8% of patients in one study (84) and 33% of families (7 of 21) in another study (87).

Mutations in the NDP genes were associated with X-linked FEVR and X-linked pseudoglioma (X-linked retinal dysplasia). Chynn et al. (62) pointed out that the mutations associated with Norrie disease are usually deletions or nonsense mutations leading to a non-functioning protein, while XL-FEVR is associated with milder, missense mutations. In addition, X-linked pseudoglioma (without the extra-ocular abnormalities of Norrie disease) is associated with milder missense mutations (62,83,85).

Mutations in the NDP gene may explain why, in some cases, retinopathy of prematurity (ROP) progresses to a severe disease and in other cases does not.

Several studies detected such mutations in premature infants with severe ROP (88,89).

Management

No effective treatment is available for the majority of cases of Norrie disease and allied diseases. For some patients with vitreous changes or total retinal detachment, pars plana vitrectomy can be considered. Dass and Trese reported 35 eyes of 27 patients diagnosed as PHPV (persistent hyperplastic primary vitreous) operated by pars plana vitrectomy. Functional vision was obtained in some but the results depended on the degree of ocular malformation (90). The results in cases of retinal dysplasia as in Norrie disease are consistently poor.

Genetic counseling must be based on family history. In the majority of families, a clear X-chromosome inheritance will be noted.

Prenatal diagnosis can be made in several ways. In appropriate cases, an interruption of pregnancy has been suggested for a male embryo with a 50% chance of being affected. In some cases, an attempt to detect ocular abnormalities of the fetus by prenatal ultrasound can be attempted (91). Finally, an attempt to detect the mutated gene can be taken. Such prenatal tests have been successfully performed, initially using primitive genetic methods, since the end of the 1980s (77,78,92–94).

INHERITED RETINAL VASCULAR ABNORMALITIES

Several uncommon inherited diseases, unrelated to each other, may affect the retinal vasculature. These are transmitted as isolated disorders or in association with other affected tissues.

The Clinical and Genetic Types

Familial Retinal Arteriolar Tortuosity

Beyer first described this condition in a father and son (95) and later elaborated in a large family with 12 affected members by Goldberg et al. (96). Most patients are asymptomatic, but an ophthalmoscopic examination will reveal a marked tortuosity of the small arterioles. The condition is not congenital; the tortuosity increases dramatically in the teens (97,98). Arterioles of the second and third order are affected, whereas veins are usually unaffected (98). Most patients show no progression after reaching a certain stage of tortuosity. Retinal bleeding in the inner layers (Fig. 8)—round, splinter, or preretinal—is common and may occur spontaneously or after exercise (96,99). Visual acuity may drop suddenly when the macula is affected by bleeding (100). One reported pathologic study (96) did not reveal any abnormalities, even when a trypsin-digested retina was studied.

The transmission of the disorder is by the autosomal dominant mode (95,96,98,100), but sporadic cases have also been described (101). Usually no other abnormality is detected, but nose bleeding (95) and intracerebral bleeding (100) have been described in patients

Sears et al. described a family with autosomal dominant arteriolar tortuosity with retinal hemorrhages (102). In spite of extensive systemic examinations, no

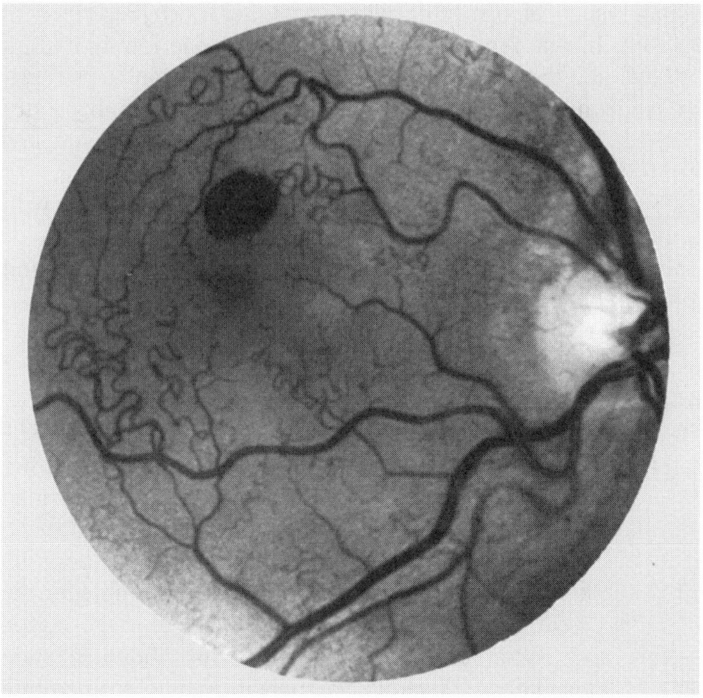

Figure 8 Fundus of a 53-year-old woman with familial retinal arteriolar tortuosity. Note the tortuosity of the small arterioles and the mild tortuosity of some small venules. The dark blot above the fovea is a retinal hemorrhage, typical in size and appearance. (Courtesy of M. F. Goldberg, MD)

similar vascular abnormality was detected in any other organ or tissue, except that all affected suffered from hypertension.

The pathogenesis of the disorder is not known (96), but it was suggested (98) that retinal arterioles become tortuous in response to increased capillary resistance. This is strengthened by the fact that hemorrhages may precede the arteriolar tortuosity (97). The disorder should be suspected when only arterioles are tortuous, whereas veins are normal. However, systemic abnormalities affecting the small blood vessels should be ruled out, such as Osler-Weber-Rendu (hereditary hemorrhagic teleangiectasia) (103) and other hematologic disorders (polycythemia, leukemia, macroglobulinemia, and sickle cell disease); storage diseases, such as Maroteau-Lamy and Fabry; and systemic hypertension or hyperlipidemia (96,98).

Retinal Vascular Teleangiectasis

Paramacular teleangiectatic capillaries are described in three members of one family by Ehlers and Jensen (104). Tortuous arterioles, ectatic capillaries, microaneurysms, small retinal hemorrhages, and tiny white dots are present and resembled the intraretinal vascular abnormalities often found in diabetic retinopathy. The condition may be asymptomatic or become symptomatic in middle life (105). Autosomal dominant inheritance was suggested. The disease may be the same or separate from Osler-Weber-Rendu, an autosomal dominant disease manifested in skin; palpebral, conjunctival, and retinal teleangiectases; and bleeding (103). Teleangiectatic retinal capillaries with microaneurysms, bleeding, or white dots were also described in Alport syndrome (106–108). In one report, four generations of one family had an unusual beading or sausage-like configuration of the veins, in addition to the teleangiectasis and Alport syndrome transmitted (108). A family with probably autosomal dominant venous beading, varying degree of arterioral tortuosity, and low to normal leukocyte count was also recently reported (109).

Teleangiectasis of retinal capillaries was also described in most patients with facioscapulohumeral muscular dystrophy (110).

A single family with a prepapillary vascular loop that affected mother and daughter has been reported (111).

INHERITED THROMBOPHILIA

Several inherited hematologic disorders increase the risk of retinal thrombosis, either arterial or venous. The group of diseases associated with such a tendency is termed thrombophilia. A multitude of publications referred to this subject in the last decade. Only a proportion of retinal vascular events are associated with a thrombophilia state. The exact figure is not known and even controversial, but undoubtedly the percentage of thrombophilia as causative of retinal vascular events is much higher in younger patients. Vine and Samama concluded that a thrombophilic state accounts for 15%–28% of unexplained systemic vascular thrombosis in young patients (112).

The Clinical and Genetic Entities

Several clinical entities may lead to thrombophilia and an increased tendency to retinal vascular occlusions.

Hyperhomocysteinemia

Hyperhomocysteinemia is an independent risk factor for vascular occlusions. The causes for elevated blood homocysteine may be genetic or acquired. Welch and Loscalzo, in an excellent review of the subject (113) discussed these issues. Two genetic causes included a severe disease in the homozygous state of cystathionine (beta)-synthase deficiency resulting in a severe increase in blood homocysteine levels. Patients suffering from this type of homocystinuria manifest the typical ocular abnormalities of ectopia lentis in association with systemic abnormalities including a much-increased rate of vascular thrombosis. In the heterozygous state a mild increase in blood homocysteine is found. The second enzyme involved is MTHFR, which, if defective, results in a mild increase in blood homocysteine levels. (see below).

Acquired causes for hyperhomocysteinemia also cause a mild increase in blood homocysteine levels. These are nutritional deficiencies such as vitamin B6, vitamin B12, or folate deficiencies. Likewise, certain diseases increase the homocysteine plasma level. These include renal failure, hypothyroidism, various malignant tumors, pernicious anemia and certain drugs (113).

At least five percent of the general population have mild hyperhomocysteinemia and usually have no clinical signs until the fourth decade of life, while thereafter an increased incidence of atherosclerosis and atheromatosis occurs (113).

Homocysteine is a sulfur containing amino acids. How and why it increases the risk for thrombosis is unknown (114), but it seems to be associated with vascular endothelial cell dysfunction (113).

Mean total plasma homocysteine is increased in patients with retinal vein occlusion (RVO), both central (CRVO) and branch vein occlusion (BRVO). Brown et al. (114) found a value of 18.4 ± 6.6 μmol/L in RVO patients, 8.2 ± 4.2 in diabetics and 7.0 ± 4.5 in controls. Weger et al. (115) found 11.4 ± 4.3 μmol/L in BRVO patients and 9.9 ± 2.8 in controls. Weger et al. (116) found 12.2 ± 4.8 μmol/L in patients with retinal artery occlusion (RAO) and 10.3 ± 3.4 in controls, and Vine (117) found 11.58 ± 4.67 for CRVO patients and 9.49 ± 2.65 μmol/L for controls. All these studies showed statistically significant differences of mean homocysteine value between RVO or RAO patients and controls. Pianka et al. (118) demonstrated hyperhomocysteinemia in 45% of their patients with NAION (non-arteritic ischemic anterior neuropathy), 61.5% of their CRAO patients, 14.4% of their CRVO patients, and 9.8% of their controls.

MTHFR

MTHFR (for 5,10-methylenetetrahydrofolate reductase) catalyzes the conversion of 5,10-methylenetetrahydrofolate to 5-methylenetetrahydrofolate, a substrate for homocysteine remethylation to methionine (119). The enzyme, when defective, results in an increase of homocysteine in the plasma. Goyette et al. (120) mapped the MTHFR gene to chromosome 1p36.3. Frosst et al. (121) identified a common mutation, a C to T substitution at nucleotide 677, which correlated with reduced enzyme activity and increased thermolability. Loewenstein and associates demonstrated an increased risk of CRVO and BRVO in homozygous C677T substitution, and possibly also in the heterozygous state (120,122) Salomon et al. (123) found an odds ratio of 1.9 retinal vein thrombosis patients homozygous for C677T transition in the MTHFR gene, while the odds ratio for hypertension was 2.12 and for family history of stroke was 3.25.

The C-T transition at nucleotide 677 of the MTHFR gene, resulting in Ala222Val mutation, is the most common polymorphism of this gene. It is found in all populations but it is uncommon in Africans (119). Other mutations may rarely result in the much more severe disease, homocystinuria (119).

Factor V Leiden and APC Resistance

Factor V is one of the factors of normal blood clotting. Mutations of the gene may lead to increased tendency for bleeding and to thrombophilia. The gene F5 was mapped to chromosome 1q23. Bertina et al. (124) identified a mutation, G-A substitution at nucleotide 1691 of F5, leading to Arg506Gln missense mutation. The authors described that individuals carrying homozygous or heterozygous mutations show APC resistance (activated protein C resistance). Activated protein C limits clot formation by proteolytic inactivation of factors Va and VIIIa in normal hemostasis. Individuals with the described mutation show resistance to APC associated with a seven-fold increase in risk of deep vein thrombosis (124). Dhar-Munshi et al. demonstrated that the risk for thromboembolic events is 7-fold in heterozygotes and 20-fold in homozygotes (125).

The single point mutation (GA transition at nucleotide 1691) is responsible for more than 90% of cases of APC resistance (APCR) (126). It is often referred to as the thermolabile mutation (126) for the laboratory method to detect its existence.

Many studies have demonstrated an increased risk for retinal vascular occlusions in individuals with this mutation. These included CRVO (127–130), BRVO (131), CRAO (132) and Eale's disease (133). Thrombophilia (increased risk of thrombosis) is particularly high in younger patients (128,130).

Some studies do not agree with these results and claim that factor V Leiden mutation plays a minor role in thrombophilia (134–136).

The distribution of this mutation is population-specific. Among Europeans, the average prevalence is 4.4% with the highest among Greeks (7%) (137). It is not found or is rare in Aboriginals, American-Indians, and natives of Indonesia, Taiwan, Pakistan, India, Africa, and Australia (137). In white populations the range is from 1% to 7.7% (138).

It is not clear why clotting time tests for APCR are more sensitive than mutation tests (138).

Other mutations in factor V were described and they carry various names of cities such as factor V, Hong Kong, Casablanca, Cambridge, Seoul, and Liverpool. No ophthalmic vascular complications were reported.

Primary Antiphospholipid Syndrome

Antiphospholipid syndrome is often a familial condition in which antiphospholipid antibodies are detected in the plasma. The clinical presentation includes fetal loss, CNS vascular involvement and vein thrombosis (139). One-third of the patients with antipholipid syndrome have visual symptoms, many of them transient (139). The presence of antiphospholipid antibodies increases the risk for retinal vascular occlusions including CRVO, BRVO, vasculitis, RAO, NAION (nonarteritic ischemic optic neuropathy) and multiple retinal arteriolar occlusions in both eyes (140–143). The associated antibodies, which should be tested for, are anticardiolipin antibodies and lupus anticoagulants (140–142). The ELISA test can be used for IgG and IgM of anticardiolipin antibodies and the Russel viper venom time assay for lupus anticoagulant activity (144).

Protein C and Protein S Deficiencies

Deficiency of protein C and deficiency of protein S, both normally anticoagulant factors, are familial disorders, transmitted by the autosomal dominant mode (145). The locus for PC (protein C) is linked to chromosome 2q13-q14. Protein C, a serine protease zymogen, has an important anticoagulant role. More than 160 mutations were reported to be associated with PC (146). Increased risk for CRVO, BRVO, BRAO, vitreous hemorrhage, and retinal detachment, was reported (146,147). The locus for PS (protein S) was mapped to chromosome 3p11.1–q11.2 (near the centromere). PS plays a role in the normal clotting process by serving as a cofactor for APC. More than 65 mutations were reported in protein S deficiency and tendency to thrombosis. Occlusions of retinal arteries or ischemic optic neuropathy and systemic thromboembolic phenomena or cardiac valvular disease were reported (145,146). In one family with congenital PS deficiency, bilateral PHPV with tractional retinal detachment was reported (146).

Thrombophilia Associated with Other Factors

Hereditary thrombophilia was described in association with other hematologic factors. ATIII (anthithrombin III factor).

- AT III (anthithrombin III factor)
  The AT3 gene was mapped to chromosome 1q23-q25 (146). A large number of different mutations, including missense and nonsense mutations, were reported. Thromboembolic phenomena are not uncommon but retinal vascular occlusion has not been confirmed.
- Factor II
  Coagulation factor II, associated with prothrombin or thrombin, was mapped to chromosome 11p11-q12 (near centromere). A substitution G-A in nt.20210 of the prothrombin gene was associated with a significantly increased risk for cerebral vein thrombosis (148). Retinal vein thrombosis was reported (149).
- Factor XII
  Factor XII or Hageman factor was mapped to chromosome 5q33-qter (119). Factor XII deficiency has been implicated in major thromboembolic phenomena, as it is normally involved in the intrinsic pathway of fibrinolysis. A recent study demonstrated a significant association between factor XII deficiency and retinal vein occlusion. Factor XII deficiency was found in 9.3% of 150 RVO patients and in 0.7% of 135 controls (150).
- Factor XIII
  Patients with factor XIII Val34Leu mutation in the homozygous state have a reduced risk of stroke and an increased risk of intracerebral hemorrhage. Weger et al. report a low prevalence of the homozygotic Val34Leu state in patients with retinal artery occlusion (151). In addition, Incorvaia et al. (152) report a high recurrence of unexplained subconjunctival hemorrhage in these patients.

Thrombophilia Associated with Several Factors

Several studies pointed out the significantly higher risk of thrombotic events in patients with more than one defect of the clotting mechanisms. Primary antiphospholipid syndrome, factor V Leiden (143), homozygous MTHFR G1691A mutation with vascular risk factors hypertension, diabetes, and hypercholesterolemia (153), factor V Leiden with these systemic factors (154), systemic factors alone (155), and other combinations, all carry an increased risk for vascular thrombotic events.

Management of Thrombophilia

Patients with hyperhomocysteinemia after a retinal vascular event should be treated by daily supplementation of folic acid (156), as it was found to lower the elevated plasma homocysteine, often to normal levels. Other studies recommend daily supplementation with folic acid, vitamin B6 (pyridoxine) and betaine (118). A combined therapy of folic acid, vitamin B6, and vitamin B12 (157) is also commonly used. This therapy was confirmed to reduce plasma homocysteine and to decrease the rate of coronary restenosis (157).

In thrombophilias in which factors of the normal clotting mechanisms are involved, anticoagulants are used as preventive treatment. This applies to the primary antiphospholipid syndrome, protein C or protein S deficiency, and factor XII deficiency. The decision to use anticoagulants should be individually decided for each patient with factor V Leiden mutation.

In the antiphospholipid syndrome, long-term anticoagulant therapy should be recommended. The international normalized ratio (INR) should be kept at 3 or above

(158). However, in all cases a hematologist experienced in such treatment must make the final decision of anticoagulation, determining its effectiveness, and follow-up.

FLECKED RETINA

Flecked retina is a loose term introduced by Krill (159) as an outline for a heterogeneous group of diseases manifested in various spots or flecks in the retina. Most of these are discussed in other chapters of this book. Fundus flavimaculatus and inherited drusen are discussed in Chapter 8 on the macula, fundus albipunctatus and flecked retina of Kandori with disorders of night vision (Chapter 15), and retinitis punctata albescens with retinitis pigmentosa (RP) in Chapter 10.

Bietti described a crystalline retinopathy, in 1937, that looked like "punctata albescens" and was associated with a marginal corneal dystrophy (160). The symptomatology may be similar to that of RP, such as decrease in central vision and progressive constriction of the visual fields (161). The fundus demonstrates yellowish white spots, deep in the retina or at the retinal pigment epithelial (RPE) level, together with marked loss of RPE cells and choriocapillaris, with pigment clumps in the macula and elsewhere (162,163). The spots look like glistening crystals, one-half to one-third the size of a vessel at the disk (163). The EOG is flat, whereas the ERG is normal (163) or is slightly reduced in rod function and somewhat more reduced in cone function (162). The disease is rare in Western countries, but much more common in China and Japan (162–165). It is most probably transmitted by an autosomal recessive gene (162–164). The locus BCD, for Bietti crystalline corneoretinal dystrophy, was mapped by linkage analysis to chromosome 4q35-qter (166), later refined to chromosome 4q35.1 (167). Li et al. identified BCD-causing mutations in the CYP4V2 gene in 23 of 25 patients with this disorder (167). The gene CYP4V2, for cytochrome p450, family 4, subfamily V, polypeptide 2, contains 11 exons spanning 19 Kb, encodes a protein which may play a role in fatty acid and steroid metabolism (167).

The disease shows variability in expression and progresses in stages (168). The cornea shows crystalline deposits at the limbus, but these may be absent, especially in early stages of the disease. The ERG may be normal, but may also be severely subnormal in amplitude.

The pathogenesis of the disorder is unknown. However, Welch (162) performed both conjunctival and corneal biopsies and found lipid accumulation in the conjunctival fibroblasts, as well as lipid inclusion bodies in the corneal epithelium. Clinically, it seems to be a primary disease of the RPE—choriocapillaris complex (168). This is strengthened by the electrophysiologic findings of a normal (or mildly reduced) ERG, with a flat EOG.

Fundus pulverulentus was the name given by Slezak and Hommer (169) to a disorder found in several patients, including a father and two daughters. White-yellow spots with dark pigmented spots were dispersed in the fundus. The patients were asymptomatic and had normal visual functions, ERG, and dark adaptation curves.

These conditions must be differentially diagnosed from cystinosis and oxalosis. Cystinosis, an autosomal recessive disease of several forms, with ocular manifestations, may affect the eye, the conjunctiva, cornea, and retina. Ophthalmoscopy reveals yellow mottling of the macula, with widespread pigmentary changes (170). In oxalosis, an acquired disease described as resulting from methoxyflurane anesthesia, calcium oxalate crystals accumulate in the RPE and in the neural retina (171,172). Clinically, numerous yellow-white punctate lesions are seen in the posterior pole.

PIGMENTED PARAVENOUS RETINOCHOROIDAL ATROPHY

This condition has been described most often as a sporadic acquired entity (173–175), but hereditary, familial cases do occur (176,177). Typically, patients show areas of chorioretinal atrophy, with pigmentary clumps or bone corpuscles in a paravenous (along retinal veins) distribution. The differential diagnosis is with conditions such as RP, angioid streaks, hellicoid chorioretinal atrophy; and proliferating choroiditis (173). The fundus changes may be stationary (178,179), rapidly progressive (180), or slowly progressive (173,174). In one case, a microangiopathy was found (181). The ERG is normal or mildly reduced, and the EOG is normal or flat (178,180), indicating, in these cases, a widespread RPE-choriocapillaris complex disease, although the paravenous distribution of the choriocapillaris atrophy is not well understood. In the inherited cases, the severity of the chorioretinal atrophy is variable, signs of vitreoretinal degeneration are present, and hyperopia with esotropia is common (177). The inheritance was suggested to be Y chromosome-linked (176), autosomal dominant, or X chromosome-linked (177). Most of the described cases, both familial and sporadic, were in males.

Macular involvement is the cause of the reduction in vision in PPRCA (pigmented paravenous retinochoroidal atrophy) (182–184). In familial cases, affected females always show a mild manifestation while males show the full-blown disorder (183), which supports the probability of an x-linked mode of transmission.

The etiology of the sporadic cases is usually not known, but systemic infections, such as syphilis, tuberculosis, sarcoidosis, and rubeola, have been suggested (185). In one patient, Heckenlively (186) found high levels of blood ornithine and a higher-than-normal activity of fibroblast ornithine aminotransferase.

CONGENITAL HYPERTROPHY OF THE RETINAL PIGMENT EPITHELIUM

Congenital hypertrophy of the retinal pigment epithelium (CHRPE) occurs not uncommonly as an isolated dark area of hyperpigmented, well-delineated RPE (Fig. 9). It has probably no clinical importance and does not change through life. However, in 1980, Blair and Trempe (187) pointed out that CHRPE occurs as one sign of Gardner syndrome, an autosomal dominant disease.

In such inherited cases, CHRPE is found bilaterally, witn multiple lesions in each eye (187). CHRPE is an additional finding to the triad of Gardner syndrome: polyposis of large and small intestines (100 or more polyps are common), hamartomata of the skeleton, and tumors of various soft tissues. The risk of carcinoma of the colon developing from a polyp when the patient is aged 40–50 is essentially 100% (188). Practically all patients with Gardner syndrome also have CHRPE (188–190) and, therefore, this finding can serve as a genetic marker. In fact, CHRPE is congenital, and can indicate the future affected member of the family with Gardner syndrome and distinguish between an affected and an unaffected member before any other sign of the disease is found (189). CHRPE is both a congenital marker and the most powerful marker of all phenotypic features of Gardner syndrome (190,191).

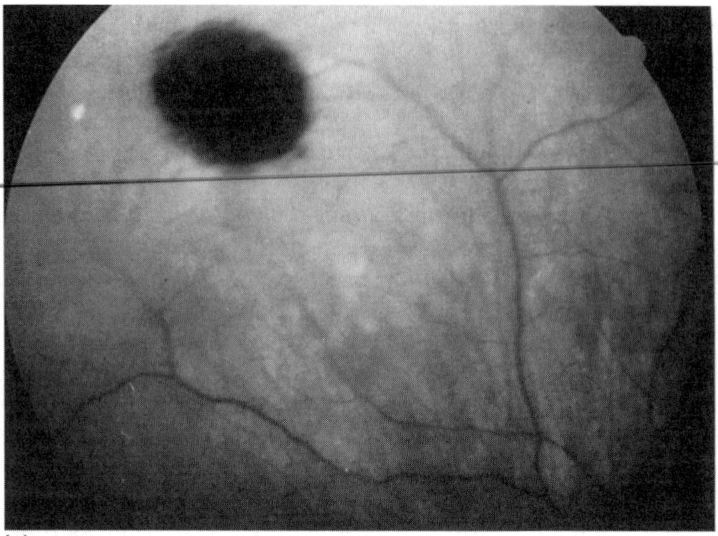

(a)

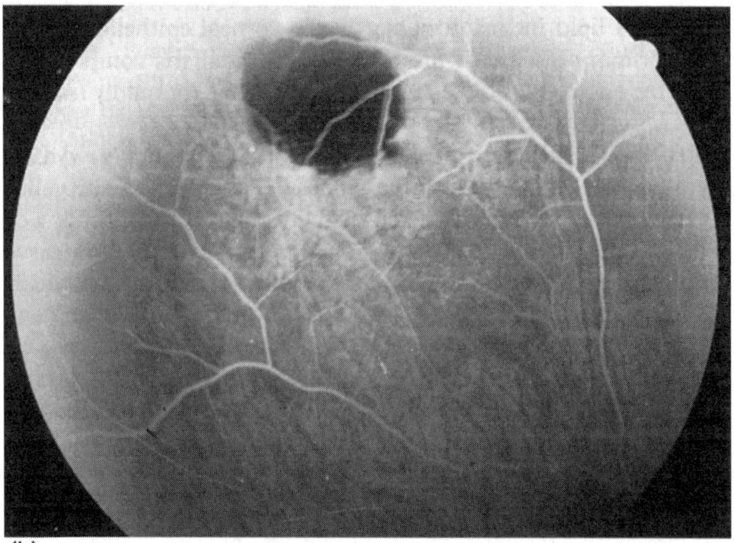

(b)

Figure 9 Congenital hypertrophy of RPE: The fundus shows a dark area consisting of enlarged RPE cells. (a) clinical appearance; (b) fluorescein angiography.

Gardner syndrome, described in the 1950s as a multi-system disease, is now usually referred to as FAP familial adenomatous polyposis (FAP) (192). Ruhswurm et al. examined 16 FAP families with 20 affected members, and 19 nonaffected relatives. The mean number of pigmented ocular lesions was 10.9, while the minimal number to diagnose positively was decided as four lesions. Out of 19 asymptomatic relatives, five showed positive CHRPE (192).

Gardner syndrome is not rare. Its incidence in Sweden is 1:7500 and in England or Japan is 1:22,500 (188), with an average incidence of 1:14,000 live births (190). The gene assignment to chromosome 5 at 5q21-q22 was achieved with restriction fragment length polymorphism markers by two groups of investigators (193,194).

Caspari et al. pointed out that more than 100 mutations were known on the adenomatous polyposis coli (APC) gene (195). They described a novel mutation, a 5-bp detection at codon 1309 in exon 15 of the APC gene, which, on average, causes earlier development of intestinal cancer.

ANGIOID STREAKS

Radiating lines from the disk outward or in the posterior pole, which are wider than normal choroidal vessels with an irregular pathway, are known as *angioid streaks* (Fig. 10). Their color varies from red, to brown, to maroon, to gray, according to the background pigmentation (196). Angioid streaks are probably not congenital, but most often develop in the second or third decade of life and gradually become wider, followed by other changes in the fundus, such as drusen of the posterior pole and pigmentary mottling (leopard-skin fundus) (196). The RPE yellowish speckled mottling known also as "peau d'orange" may predate the onset of angioid streaks (197). Drusen of the optic nerve are found in a higher frequency than in the general population (198,199). The pigmentary mottling may take a peculiar form of small, round pigment dots arranged in a reticular (fishnet) fashion in the posterior pole (200). All these findings indicate a generalized disease of the RPE, and this may be a secondary phenomenon to the angioid streaks, which are considered to be a disorder of Bruch's membrane.

In more advanced age, usually around the fifth or sixth decade of life, subretinal neovascularization of choroidal origin may occur and form an exudative or hemorrhagic maculopathy, similar in appearance to age-onset maculopathy (196–200), with subsequent drastic loss of visual acuity.

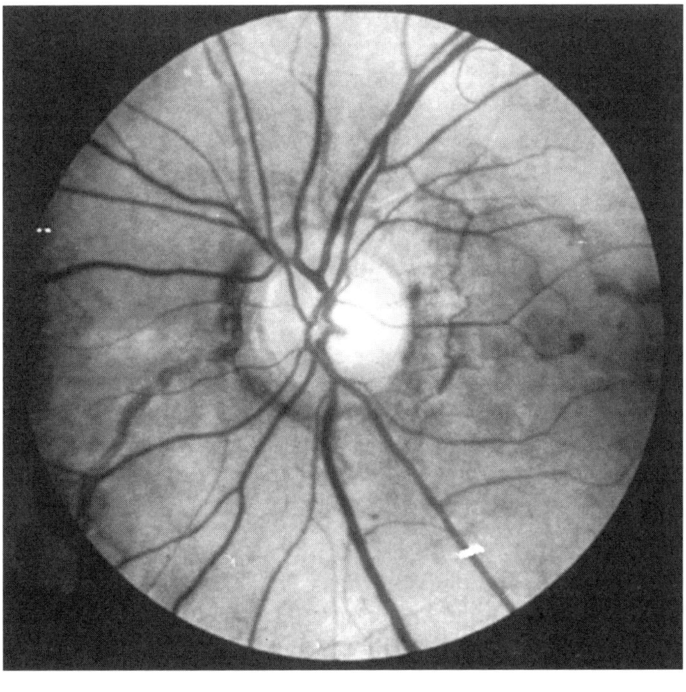

Figure 10 Angioid streaks.

The most common association of angioid streaks is with pseudoxanthoma elasticum (PXE), an association named Grönblad-Standberg's syndrome. Pseudoxanthoma elasticum is a hereditary disorder of the connective tissue that probably affects all elastic membranes and includes calcification of elastic membranes (199). At least 53% of patients with angioid streaks have PXE, but this percentage may be much higher, as some PXE patients may not manifest the skin disease (196). On the other hand, 87% of patients with PXE show angioid streaks of the fundus (196).

The triad of abnormalities found in PXE are the ocular changes (angioid streaks) and their complications, skin changes, and the vascular changes. The cutaneous lesions consist of small yellow infiltrative papules, which are linearly arranged and may coalesce into an elevated plaque (the plucked chicken sign) (196,197,201). The most affected area is the neck, followed by the axilla, groin, antecubital and popliteal spaces. The vascular changes consist of increased arterial calcifications, resulting in reduction in pulses, premature occlusion of vessels, renal hypertension, and solitary or recurrent gastrointestinal hemorrhage (197).

The diagnosis of Grönblad-Strandberg syndrome (PXE with angioid streaks) is confirmed by the typical skin changes, by biopsy of the skin, or by biopsy of a scar. Skin biopsy displays an increase in elastic staining material in the dermis together with frayed, curled, and disintegrated fibers (elastorrhexis) (196,201). Scar biopsy is the most sensitive method and yields the highest percentage of positive results (202).

Pseudoxanthoma elasticum is usually transmitted as an autosomal recessive disorder (196,199,200), but an autosomal dominant form has also been described (203).

The locus for PXE was mapped to chromosome 16pl3.1 (204). In the year 2000, three groups of investigators identified the gene as ABCC6, for ATP-binding cassette, subfamily C, member 6. Mutations of these genes were identified to cause both autosomal recessive (most common) and autosomal dominant PXE (205–207).

Other disorders, some hereditary and others not, were also found to be associated with angioid streaks, although much less commonly than PXE. These include sickle cell hemoglobinopathies, Paget disease of bone, senile elastosis, Marfan syndrome, Ehlers-Danlos syndrome (194,197), and familial polyposis (208). The management of the patient with angioid streaks, from the ophthalmologist's point of view, consists of properly diagnosing the disorder and following the macular condition. In some cases, successful eradication of subretinal neovascularization by laser may save the patient's central vision.

CHORIORETINAL DEGENERATIONS WITH CENTRAL NERVOUS SYSTEM ANOMALIES

A variety of rare disorders affecting the retina and choroid, together with anomalies of the central nervous system, which have not been described elsewhere in this book, will be mentioned here.

Chorioretinopathy, with hereditary microcephaly, was originally described by McKusick et al. in 1966 (209) as an autosomal recessive disease. Since then, it has been reported in other families (210,211) and given the catalog number McK 251270 (212). The ocular findings consist of localized areas of chorioretinal atrophy and pigmentation with localized absence of choriocapillaris, microcornea, and microphthalmos, with high hyperopia and nystagmus (209,210). Microcephaly is associated with mental retardation. The pigmentary clumps are usually seen at the fovea or around the disk (209) and may resemble patches of congenital hypertrophy of the RPE (211). The retinal vessels may become narrow (210).

A similar disorder of microcephaly, with mild mental retardation and chorioretinal hypopigmentation and hyperpigmentation, transmitted by the autosomal dominant mode, was reported in three families (213).

Olivopontocerebellar atrophy (OPCA) occurs as one of five different hereditary disorders designated as types I–V (212). Type II OPCA is an autosomal recessive disease; the rest are autosomal dominant disorders. Only OPCA type III is associated with ocular abnormalities. The disease often starts as a macular RPE disease, with macular pigmentary mottling and, later, beaten-bronze appearance or epiretinal membrane, but spreads to involve most of the retina in the form of a severe chorioretinal atrophy (214,215). Neurologic symptoms and signs usually occur some years after the maculopathy in form of cerebellar, pyramidal, extrapyramidal, and brain stem dysfunction, expressed in ataxia, intentional tremor, choreoathetotic movements, spontaneous nystagmus, and other signs (215,216).

The disease is described in Chapter 11.

A histopathologic study on two eyes of twins with OPCA type III was performed by Traboulsi et al. (216), who found degenerated photoreceptors, especially in the macula, and hypopigmented and hyperpigmented RPE cells. Electron microscopy showed osmiophilic, multimembranous, complex lipofuscin inclusions in various ocular cells, including RPE. The authors noted similarities to the neuronal ceroid lipofuscinoses.

PIGMENTARY RETINOPATHY ASSOCIATED WITH THE ENHANCED S-CONE SYNDROME (ESCS)

Clinical Entities

Three entities compose this group of retinal disorders.

The Enhanced S-cone Syndrome

In 1996, Marmor et al. (217) described a "new" syndrome of maculopathy, night blindness and enhanced S-cone sensitivity. Eight patients manifested degenerative changes in the region of the vascular perimacular arcades and in the macula. Visual fields were mildly narrowed. The ERG was characteristic of this new disorder. No retinal responses were obtained to low-intensity stimuli, in the scotopic range. Large slow responses were obtained in the photopic range, with greater sensitivity of the short-wavelength cones. The authors proposed the term enhanced S-cone syndrome (ESCS) (217). Jacobson et al. (218) demonstrated that in ESCS patients, the rod mechanism was reduced in sensitivity by at least 3 log units. No measurable rhodopsin could be detected by fundus reflectometry. However, ERG responses were obtained for cone function due to supernormal responses of the blue cones (SWS, short wavelength-sensitive cones) in the range of 420–460 nm (218).

Clumped Pigmentary Retinal Degeneration

To et al. (219) described this condition as a distinct entity in 24 patients. Clinically, thee patients suffered from night blindness of variable severity. Visual acuity ranged from 20/25 to no light perception. Onset of disease was variable with a mean of 17 years. Fundus examination manifested clumps of pigment in midperiphery, very different from classic retinitis pigmentosa. A histopathological study performed by the same group demonstrated extensive photoreceptor degeneration and fleurette- and rosette-like formations in the inner retina. Striking was the excessive accumulation of melanin pigment in the RPE. This accumulation was expressed in the clinical finding of pigment clumps (219).

Goldmann-Favre Syndrome (GFS)

In 1991 Jacobson et al. found an increased sensitivity of the S-cones [compared to midspectral (green) cones] throughout the visual field in GFS patients. They suggested that ESCS and GFS are linked by a common pattern of retinal dysfunction (220). GFS is described in Chapter 12.

Genetics and Molecular Genetics

Haider et al. identified mutations in the NR2E3/PNR gene in patients with ESCS (221). Sharon et al. (222) demonstrated that mutations in NR2E3 gene are associated with all three clinical entities of this group. They identified homozygous or compound heterozygous mutations in nine CPRD patients, one GFS patient and one ESCS patient (222).

The gene, NR2E3, for nuclear receptor subfamily 2, group E, member 3, was mapped to chromosome 15q23. It encodes a transcription factor, which may indicate that it is a disorder of retinal cell fate (221,222). Mutations in the same gene were reported in the Crypto-Jews (Marranos) of Portugal, associated with a typical retinitis pigmentosa (See Chapter 10).

REFERENCES

1. Schulman J, Merin S. Hereditary vitreoretinal degenerations. In: Newsome DA, ed. Retinal Dystrophies and Degenerations. New York: Raven Press, 1988:85–88.
2. Lisch W. Sex-linked juvenile retinoschisis. Dev Ophthalmol 1983; 8:19–31.
3. George ND, Yates JR, Moore AT. X-linked retinoschisis. Br J Ophthalmol 1995; 79:697–702.
4. Ewing CC, Ives EJ. Juvenile hereditary retinoschisis. Trans Ophthalmol Soc UK 1969; 89:29–39.
5. Harris S, Yeung JWS. Maculopathy of sex-linked juvenile retinoschisis. Can J Ophthalmol 1976; 11:1–10.
6. Deutman AF. The Hereditary Dystrophies of the Posterior Pole of the Eye. Assen, Netherlands: Van Gorcum, 1971.
7. George ND, Yates JR, Moore AT. Clinical features in affected males with X-linked retinoschisis. Arch Ophthalmol 1996; 114:274–280.
8. Tanna AP, Asrani S, Zeimer R, Zou S, Goldberg MF. Optical cross-sectional imaging of the macula with the retinal thickness analyzer in X-linked retinoschisis. Arch Ophthalmol 1998; 116:1036–1041.
9. Mooy CM, Van Den Born LI, Baarsma S, Paridaens DA, Kraaijenbrink T, Bergen A, Weber BH. Hereditary X-linked juvenile retinoschisis: a review of the role of Muller cells. Arch Ophthalmol 2002; 120:979–984.
10. Nakamura M, Ito S, Terasaki H, Miyake Y. Japanese X-linked juvenile retinoschisis: conflict of phenotype and genotype with novel mutations in the XLRSl gene. Arch Ophthalmol 2001; 119:1553–1554.

11. Kawano N, Tanaka K, Murakami F, Ohba N. Congenital hereditary retinoschisis: evolution at the initial stage. Graefes Arch Clin Exp Ophthalmol 1981; 217:315–323.
12. Arkfeld DF, Brockhurst RJ. Vascularized vitreous membranes in congenital retinoschisis. Retina 1987; 7:20–23.
13. Brancato R, Menchini U, Pece A. Idiopathic macular retinoschisis in the young subject associated with preretinal and prepapillary neovessels. J Fr Ophthalmol 1984; 7: 685–688.
14. Krausher MF, Schepens CL, Kaplan JA, Freeman H. Congenital retinoschisis. In: Bellows JG, ed. Contemporary Ophthalmology Honoring Sir Steward Duke-Elder. Baltimore: Williams & Wilkins, 1972: 265–290.
15. Laatikainen L, Tarkkanene A, Saksela T. Hereditary X-linked retinoschisis and bilateral congenital retinal detachment. Retina 1987; 7:24–27.
16. Tantri A, Vrabec TR, Cu-Unjieng A, Frost A, Annesley WH Jr, Donoso LA. X-linked retinoschisis: report of a family with a rare deletion in the XLRSl gene. Am J Ophthalmol 2003; 136:547–549.
17. Arden GB, Gorin MB, Polkinghorne PJ et al. Detection of the carrier state of X-linked retinoschisis. Am J Ophthalmol 1988; 105:590–595.
18. George ND, Yates JR, Moore AT. X linked retinoschisis. Br J Ophthalmol 1995; 79:697–702.
19. Ali A, Feroze AH, Rizvi ZH, Rehman TU. Consanguineous marriage resulting in homozygous occurrence of X-linked retinoschisis in girls. Am J Ophthalmol 2003; 136:767–769.
20. Lewis RA, Lee GB, Martonyi CL et al. Familial foveal retinoschisis. Arch Ophthalmol 1977; 95:1190–1196.
21. Yassur Y, Nissenkorn I, Ben-Sira I et al. Autosomal dominant inheritance of retinoschisis. Am J Ophthalmol 1982; 94:338–343.
22. Shimazaki J, Matsuhashi M. Familial retinoschisis in female patients. Doc Ophthalmol 1987; 65:393–400.
23. Forsius H, Eriksson AW, Vainio-Mattila BA. Geschlechtgebundene erbliche Retinoschisis in zwei Familien in Finland. Klin Monatsbl Augenheilkd 1969; 143:806–816.
24. Green JL, Jampol LM. Vascular opacification and leakage in X-linked juvenile retinoschisis. Br J Ophthalmol 1979; 63:368–373.
25. Eriksson U, Larsson E, Holmstrom G. Optical coherence tomography in the diagnosis of juvenile X-linked retinoschisis. Ada Ophthalmol Scand 2004; 82:218–223.
26. Peachey NS, Fishman GA, Derlacki DJ, Brigell MG. Psychophysical and electroretinographic findings in X-linked juvenile retinoschisis. Arch Ophthalmol 1987; 105: 513–516.
27. Papst N, Bopp M, Remler B. Muster-ERG bei X-chromosomaler juveniler retinoschisis. Klin Monatsbl Augenheilkd 1986; 188:150–152.
28. Sieving PA, Bingham EL, Kemp J, Richards J, Hiriyanna K. Juvenile X-linked retinoschisis from XLRS1 Arg213Trp mutation with preservation of the electroretinogram scotopic b-wave. Am J Ophthalmol 1999; 128:179–184.
29. Alexander KR, Barnes CS, Fishman GA. High-frequency attenuation of the cone ERG and ON-response deficits in X-linked retinoschisis. Invest Ophthalmol Vis Sci 2001; 42:2094–2101.
30. Piao CH, Kondo M, Nakamura M, Terasaki H, Miyake Y. Multifocal electroretinograms in X-linked retinoschisis. Invest Ophthalmol Vis Sci 2003; 44:4920–4930.
31. Yanoff M, Rahn EH, Zimmerman LE. Histopathology of juvenile retinoschisis. Arch Ophthalmol 1968; 79:49–53.
32. Manschot WA. Pathology of hereditary juvenile retinoschisis. Arch Ophthalmol 1972; 88:131–138.
33. Condon GP, Brownstein S, Wang NS et al. Congenital hereditary (juvenile X-linked) retinoschisis. Histopathologic and ultrastructural findings in three eyes. Arch Ophthalmol 1986; 104:576–583.

34. Forsius HR, Eriksson AW. Population Structure and Genetic Disorders. New York: Academic Press, 1980.
35. Peltonen L, Jalanko A, Varilo T. Molecular genetics of the Finnish disease heritage. Hum Mol Genet 1999; 8:1913–1923.
36. Alitalo T, Koarnoa J, Forsuis H, de la Chapelle A. X-linked retinoschisis is closely linked to *DXS41* and *DXS16* but not *DXS85*. Clin Genet 1987; 32:192–195.
37. Gal A. X-linked retinoschisis and linkage. Clin Genet 1988; 33:143.
38. Dahl N, Goonewardena P, Chotai J, et al. DNA linkage analysis of X-linked retinoschisis. Hum Genet 1988; 78:228–232.
39. Gellert G, Peterson J, Krawczak M, Zoll B. Linkage relationship between retinoschisis and four marker loci. Hum Genet 1988; 79:382–384.
40. Bergen AA, ten Brink JB, van Schooneveld MJ. Efficient DNA carrier detection in X linked juvenile retinoschisis. Br J Ophthalmol 1995; 79:683–686.
41. Sauer CG, Gehrig A, Warneke-Wittstock R, Marquardt A, Ewing CC, Gibson A, Lorenz B, Jurklies B, Weber BH. Positional cloning of the gene associated with X-linked juvenile retinoschisis. Nat Genet 1997; 17:164–170.
42. Anonymous. Functional implications of the spectrum of mutations found in 234 cases with X-linked juvenile retinoschisis. The Retinoschisis Consortium. Hum Mol Genet 1998; 7:1185–1192.
43. Sieving PA, Yashar BM, Ayyagari R, Juvenile retinoschisis: a model for molecular diagnostic testing of X-linked ophthalmic disease. Trans Am Ophthalmol Soc 1999; 97: 451–464; discussion 464–469.
44. Huopaniemi L, Rantala A, Forsius H, Somer M, de la Chapelle A, Alitalo T. Three widespread founder mutations contribute to high incidence of X-linked juvenile retinoschisis in Finland. Eur J Hum Genet 1999; 7:368–376.
45. Inoue Y, Yamamoto S, Okada M, Tsujikawa M, Inoue T, Okada AA, Kusaka S, Saito Y, Wakabayashi K, Miyake Y, Fujikado T, Tano Y. X-linked retinoschisis with point mutations in the XLRSl gene. Arch Ophthalmol 2000; 118:93–96.
46. Hiraoka M, Trese MT, Shastry BS. X-Linked juvenile retinoschisis associated with a 4-base pair insertion at codon 55 of the XLRSl gene. Biochem Biophys Res Commun 2000; 268:370–372.
47. Tantri A, Vrabec TR, Cu-Unjieng A, Frost A, Annesley WH Jr, Donoso LA. X-linked retinoschisis: a clinical and molecular genetic review. Sur Ophthalmol 2004; 49: 214–230.
48. Harris GS. Retinoschisis: Pathogenesis and treatment. Can J Ophthalmol 1968; 3: 312–317.
49. Brockhurst RJ. Photocoagulation in congenital retinoschisis. Arch Ophthalmol 1970; 84:158–165.
50. Edmund J. Familial retinal detachment. Acta Ophthalmol 1961; 39:644–654.
51. Van Den Bergh J. Hereditary disposition to retinal detachment in two families. Ophthalmologica 1965; 149:236–240.
52. Pemberton JW, Freeman HM, Schepens LL. Familial retinal detachment and the Ehlers-Danlos syndrome. Arch Ophthalmol 1966; 76:817–824.
53. Hamada S, Ellsworth RM. Congenital retinal detachment and the optic disk anomaly. Am J Ophthalmol 1971; 71:460–464.
54. Everett WG. Study of family with lattice degeneration and retinal detachment. Am J Ophthalmol 1968; 65:229–232.
55. Murakami F, Ohba N. Genetics of lattice degeneration of the retina. Ophthalmologica 1982; 185:136–140.
56. Chaudhry NA, Flynn HW Jr, Tabandeh H. Idiopathic giant retinal tears in identical twins. Am J Ophthalmol 1999; 127:96–99.
57. Norrie G. Cases of blindness in children. Acta Ophthalmol 1927; 5:357–386.
58. Warburg M. Norrie's disease. A congenital progressive oculo-acoustico-cerebral degeneration. Acta Ophthalmol Suppl 1966; 89:1–147.

59. Warburg M. Norrie's disease: differential diagnosis and treatment. Acta Ophthalmol 1975; 53:217–236.
60. Sims KB, Irvine AR, Good WV. Norrie's disease in a family with a manifesting female carrier. Arch Ophthalmol 1997; 115:517–519.
61. Mintz-Hittner HA, Ferrell RE, Sims KB, Fernandez KM, Gemmell BS, Satriano DR, Caster J, Kretzer FL. Peripheral retinopathy in offspring of carriers of Norrie disease gene mutations. Possible transplacental effect of abnormal norrin. Ophthalmology 1996; 103:2128–234.
62. Chynn EW, Walton DS, Hahn LB, Dryja TP. Norrie disease. Diagnosis of a simplex case by DNA analysis. Arch Ophthalmol 1996; 114:1136–1138.
63. Merin S, Lapithis AG, Horowitz D, Michaelson IC. Childhood blindness in Cyprus. Am J Ophthalmol 1972; 74:538–542.
64. Godel V, Romano A, Stein R, et al. Primary retinal dysplasia transmitted as X-chromosome linked recessive disorder. Am J Ophthalmol 1978; 86:221–227.
65. Godel V, Goodman RM. X-linked recessive primary retinal dysplasia: clinical findings in affected males and carrier females. Clin Genet 1981; 20:260–266.
66. Godel V, Goodman RM. The heterozygote female in X-linked recessive primary retinal dysplasia. Birth Defects 1982; 18:587–591.
67. Ohba N, Yamashita T. Primary vitreoretinal dysplasia resembling Norrie's disease in a female: association with X autosome chromosomal translocation. Br J Ophthalmol 1986; 70:64–71.
68. Ravia Y, Braier-Goldstein O, Bat-Miriam KM, Erlich S, Barkai G, Goldman B. X-linked recessive primary retinal dysplasia is linked to the Norrie disease locus. Hum Mol Genet 1993; 2:1295–1297.
69. Warburg M. Retinal malformations: aetiological heterogeneity and morphological similarity in congenital retinal non-attachment and falciform folds [Doyne Memorial Lecture, 1979]. Trans Ophthalmol Soc UK 1979; 99:272–283.
70. Warburg M. Heterogeneity of congenital retinal nonattachment falciform folds and retinal dysplasia. Hum Hered 1976; 26:137–148.
71. Hittner HM. Retinal and central nervous system abnormalities: syndromes which resemble retrolental fibroplasia. Metab Pediatr Syst Ophthalmol 1985; 8:5–10.
72. Scott JG, Friedmann AI, Chitters M, Pepler WJ. Ocular changes in the Bloch-Sulzberger syndrome (incontinentia pigmenti). Br J Ophthalmol 1955; 39:276.
73. Goldberg MF. The blinding mechanisms of incontinentia pigmenti. Trans Am Ophthalmol Soc 1994; 92:167–176; discussion 176–179.
74. Smahi A, Courtois G, Vabres P, Yamaoka S, Heuertz S, Munnich A, Israel A, Heiss NS, Klauck SM, Kioschis P, Wiemann S, Poustka A, Esposito T, Bardaro T, Gianfrancesco F, Ciccodicola A, D'Urso M, Woffendin H, Jakins T, Donnai D, Stewart H, Kenwrick SJ, Aradhya S, Yamagata T, Levy M, Lewis RA, Nelson DL. Genomic rearrangement in NEMO impairs NF-kappaB activation and is a cause of incontinentia pigmenti. The International Incontinentia Pigmenti (IP) Consortium. Nature 2000; 405:466–472.
75. Cho SY, Lee CK, Drummond BK. Surviving male with incontinentia pigmenti: a case report. Int J Paediatr Dent 2004; 14:69–72.
76. Reese AB, Blodi FC. Retinal dysplasia. Am J Ophthalmol 1950; 33:23–32.
77. Bleeker-Wagemakers LM, Friedrich U, Gal A, et al. Close linkage between Norrie disease, a cloned DNA sequence from the proximal short arm and the centromere of the X chromosome. Hum Genet 1985; 71:211–214.
78. Gal A, Wieringa B, Smeets DF, et al. Submicroscopic interstitial deletion of the X chromosome explains a complex genetic syndrome dominated by Norrie's disease. Cytogenet Cell Genet 1986; 42:219–224.
79. Sims KB, Lebo RV, Benson G, Shalish C, Schuback D, Chen ZY, Brans G, Craig IW, Golbus MS, Breakefield XO. The Norrie disease gene maps to a 150 kb region on chromosome Xp11.3. Hum Mol Genet 1992; 1:83–89.

80. Chen ZY, Hendriks RW, Jobling MA, Powell JF, Breakefield XO, Sims KB, Craig IW. Isolation and characterization of a candidate gene for Norrie disease. Nat Genet 1992; 1:204–208.
81. Berger W, Meindl A, van de Pol TJ, Cremers FP, Ropers HH, Doerner C, Monaco A, Bergen AA, Lebo R, Warburgh M, et al. Isolation of a candidate gene for Norrie disease by positional cloning. Nat Genet 1992; 2:84.
82. Wong F, Goldberg MF, Hao Y. Identification of a nonsense mutation at codon 128 of the Norrie's disease gene in a male infant. Arch Ophthalmol 1993; 111: 1553–1557.
83. Fuchs S, Xu SY, Caballero M, Salcedo M, La OA, Wedemann H, Gal A. A missense point mutation (Leul3Arg) of the Norrie disease gene in a large Cuban kindred with Norrie disease. Hum Mol Genet 1994; 3:655–656.
84. Schuback DE, Chen ZY, Craig IW, Breakefield XO, Sims KB. Mutations in the Norrie disease gene. Hum Mutat 1995; 5:285–292.
85. Meindl A, Lorenz B, Achatz H, Hellebrand H, Schmitz-Valckenberg P, Meitinger T. Missense mutations in the NDP gene in patients with a less severe course of Norrie disease. Hum Mol Genet 1995; 4:489–490.
86. Chen ZY, Denney RM, Breakefield XO. Norrie disease and MAO genes: nearest neighbors. Hum Mol Genet 1995:1729–1737.
87. Royer G, Hanein S, Raclin V, Gigarel N, Rozet JM, Munnich A, Steffann J, Dufier JL, Kaplan J, Bonnefont JP. NDP gene mutations in 14 French families with Norrie disease. Hum Mutat 2003; 22:499.
88. Talks SJ, Ebenezer N, Hykin P, Adams G, Yang F, Schulenberg E, Gregory-Evans K, Gregory-Evans CY. De novo mutations in the 5′ regulatory region of the Norrie disease gene in retinopathy of prematurity. J Med Genet 2001; 38:E46.
89. Hiraoka M, Berinstein DM, Trese MT, Shastry BS. Insertion and deletion mutations in the dinucleotide repeat region of the Norrie disease gene in patients with advanced retinopathy of prematurity. J Hum Genet 2001; 46:178–181.
90. Dass AB, Trese MT. Surgical results of persistent hyperplastic primary vitreous. Ophthalmology 1999; 106:280–284.
91. Redmond RM, Vaughan JI, Jay M, Jay B, In-utero diagnosis of Norrie disease by ultrasonography. Ophthalmic Paediatr Genet. 1993; 14:1–3.
92. Ngo JT, Spence MA, Cortessis V, et al. Recombinational event between Norrie disease and *DXS7* loci. Clin Genet 1988; 34:43–47.
93. Gal A, Uhlhass S, Glaser D, Grimm T. Prenatal exclusion of Norrie disease with flanking DNA markers. Am J Med Genet 1988; 31:449–453.
94. Curtis D, Blank CE, Parsons MA, Hughes HN. Carrier detection and prenatal diagnosis in Norrie disease. Prenat Diagn 1989; 9:735–740.
95. Beyer EM. Familiare Tortuositas der kleinen Netzhautarterien mit Makulablutung. Klin Monatsbl Augenheilkd 1958; 132:532–539.
96. Goldberg MF, Pollack IP, Green WR. Familial retinal arteriolar tortuosity with retinal hemorrhage. Am J Ophthalmol 1972; 73:183–191.
97. Wells CG, Kalina MD. Progressive inherited retinal arteriolar tortuosity with spontaneous retinal hemorrhage. Ophthalmology 1985; 92:1015–1021.
98. Clearkin IG, Rose H, Patterson A, Mody CH. Development of retinal arteriolar tortuosity in previously unaffected family members. Trans Ophthalmol Soc UK 1986; 105:568–574.
99. Goldberg MF. Discussion of paper by Wells and Kalina. Ophthalmology 1985; 92:1021–1024.
100. Bartlett WJ, Price J. Familial retinal arteriolar tortuosity with retinal hemorrhage. Am J Ophthalmol 1983; 95:556–557.
101. Pau H. Extreme Tortuositas der kleinen Netzhautarterien. Klin Monatsbl Augenheilkd 1987; 190:517–518.

102. Sears J, Gilman J, Steinberg P Jr. Inherited retinal arteriolar tortuosity with retinal hemorrhages. Arch Ophthalmol 1998; 116:1185–1188.
103. Brant AM, Schachat AP, White RI. Ocular manifestations in hereditary hemorrhagic telangiectases (Rendu-Osler-Weber disease). Am J Ophthalmol 1989; 107:642–646.
104. Ehlers N, Jensen VA. Hereditary central retinal angiopathy. Acta Ophthalmol 1973; 51:171–178.
105. Hutton WL, Snyder WF, Fuller D, Vaiser A. Focal parafoveal retinal teleangiectasis. Arch Ophthalmol 1978; 96:1362–1367.
106. Polak BCB, Hogewind BL. Macular lesions in Alport's disease. Am J Ophthalmol 1977; 84:532–535.
107. Kondra L, Cangemi FE, Pitta CG. Alport's syndrome and retinal teleangiectasia. Ann Ophthalmol 1983; 15:550–551.
108. Meredith TA. Inherited retinal venous beading. Arch Ophthalmol 1987; 105:949–953.
109. Stewart MW, Gitter KA. Inherited retinal venous beading. Am J Ophthalmol 1988; 106:675–681.
110. Fitzsimons RB, Gurwin EB, Bird AC. Retinal vascular abnormalities in facioscapulohumeral muscular dystrophy. A general association with genetic and therapeutic implications. Brain 1987; 110:631–648.
111. Grossniklaus H, Thall E, Annable W. Familial prepapillary vascular loops. Arch Ophthalmol 1986; 104:1755–1756.
112. Vine AK, Samama MM. The role of abnormalities in the anticoagulant and fibrinolytic systems in retinal vascular occlusions. Surv Ophthalmol 1993; 37:283–292.
113. Welch GN, Loscalzo J. Homocysteine and atherothrombosis. New Engl J Med 1998; 338:1042–1050.
114. Brown BA, Marx JL, Ward TP, Hollifield RD, Dick JS, Brozetti JJ, Howard RS, Thach AB. Homocysteine: a risk factor for retinal venous occlusive disease. Ophthalmology. 2002; 109:287–290.
115. Weger M, Stanger O, Deutschmann H, Temmel W, Renner W, Schmut O, Quehenberger F, Semmelrock J, Haas A. Hyperhomocyst(e)inemia, but not methylenetetrahydrofolate reductase C677T mutation, as a risk factor in branch retinal vein occlusion. Ophthalmology 2002; 109:1105–1109.
116. Weger M, Stanger O, Deutschmann H, Leitner FJ, Renner W, Schmut O, Semmelrock J, Haas A. The role of hyperhomocysteinemia and methylenetetrahydrofolate reductase (MTHFR) C677T mutation in patients with retinal artery occlusion. Am J Ophthalmol 2002; 134:57–61.
117. Vine AK. Hyperhomocysteinemia: a risk factor for central retinal vein occlusion. Am J Ophthalmol 2000; 129:640–644.
118. Pianka P, Almog Y, Man O, Goldstein M, Sela BA, Loewenstein A. Hyperhomocystinemia in patients with nonarteritic anterior ischemic optic neuropathy, central retinal artery occlusion, and central retinal vein occlusion. Ophthalmology 2000; 107:1588–1592.
119. Online Mendelian Inheritance in Man, OMIM (TM). McKusick-Nathans Institute for Genetic Medicine, Johns Hopkins University (Baltimore, MD) and National Center for Biotechnology Information, National Library of Medicine (Bethesda, MD), 2000. World Wide Web URL: http://www.ncbi.nlm.nih.gov/omim/
120. Goyette P, Sumner JS, Milos R, Duncan AM, Rosenblatt DS, Matthews RG, Rozen R. Human methylenetetrahydrofolate reductase: isolation of cDNA, mapping and mutation identification. Nat Genet 1994; 7:195–200.
121. Frosst P, Blom HJ, Milos R, Goyette P, Sheppard CA, Matthews RG, Boers Gl, den Heijer M, Kluijtmans LA, van den Heuvel LP, et al. A candidate genetic risk factor for vascular disease: a common mutation in methylenetetrahydrofolate reductase. Nat Gene 1995; 10:111-113 1995.
122. Loewenstein A, Goldstein M, Roth A, Lazar M. Cilioretinal artery occlusion during coronary catheterization. Acta Ophthalmol Scand 1999; 77:717–718.

123. Salomon O, Moisseiev J, Rosenberg N, Vidne O, Yassur I, Zivelin A, Treister G, Steinberg DM, Seligsohn U. Analysis of genetic polymorphisms related to thrombosis and other risk factors in patients with retinal vein occlusion. Blood Coagul Fibrinolysis 1998; 9:617–622.
124. Bertina RM, Koeleman BP, Koster T, Rosendaal FR, Dirven RJ, de Ronde H, van der Velden PA, Reitsma PH. Mutation in blood coagulation factor V associated with resistance to activated protein C. Nature 1994; 369:64–67.
125. Dhar-Munshi S, Ayliffe WH, Jayne D. Branch retinal arteriolar occlusion associated with familial factor V Leiden polymorphism and positive rheumatoid factor. Arch Ophthalmol 1999; 117:971–973.
126. Talmon T, Scharf J, Mayer E, Lanir N, Miller B, Brenner B. Retinal arterial occlusion in a child with factor V Leiden and thermolabile methylene tetrahydrofolate reductase mutations. Am J Ophthalmol 1997; 124:689–691.
127. Hunt BJ. Activated protein C and retinal vein occlusion. Br J Ophthalmol 1996; 80:194.
128. Larsson J, Olafsdottir E, Bauer B. Activated protein C resistance in young adults with central retinal vein occlusion. Br J Ophthalmol 1996; 80:200–202.
129. Williamson TH, Rumley A, Lowe GD. Blood viscosity, coagulation, and activated protein C resistance in central retinal vein occlusion: a population controlled study. Br J Ophthalmol 1996; 80:203–208.
130. Gottlieb JL, Blice JP, Mestichelli B, Konkle BA, Benson WE. Activated protein C resistance, factor V Leiden, and central retinal vein occlusion in young adults. Arch Ophthalmol 1998; 116:577–579.
131. Greven CM, Wall AB. Peripheral retinal neovascularization and retinal vascular occlusion associated with activated protein C resistance. Am J Ophthalmol 1997; 124: 687–689.
132. Larsson J. Central retinal artery occlusion in a patient homozygous for factor V Leiden. Am J Ophthalmol 2000; 129:816–817.
133. Eller AW, Bontempo FA, Faruki H, Hassett AC. Peripheral retinal neovascularization (Eales disease) associated with the factor V Leiden mutation. Am J Ophthalmol 1998; 126:146–149.
134. Hodgkins PR, Perry DJ, Sawcer SJ, Keast-Butler J. Factor V and antithrombin gene mutations in patients with idiopathic central retinal vein occlusion. Eye 1995; 9: 760–762.
135. Ciardella AP, Yannuzzi LA, Freund KB, DiMichele D, Nejat M, De Rosa JT, Daly JR, Sisco L. Factor V Leiden, activated protein C resistance, and retinal vein occlusion. Retina 1998; 18:308–315.
136. Vine AK. Retinal vascular occlusion and deficiencies in the protein C pathway. Am J Ophthalmol 2000; 129:113–115.
137. Rees DC, Cox M, Clegg JB. World distribution of factor V Leiden. Lancet 1995; 346:1133–1134.
138. Vine AK, Samama MM. Screening for resistance to activated protein C and the mutant gene for factor V: Q506 in patients with central retinal vein occlusion. Am J Ophthalmol 1997; 124:673–676.
139. Gelfand YA, Dori D, Miller B, Brenner B. Visual disturbances and pathologic ocular findings in primary antiphospholipid syndrome. Ophthalmology 1999; 106:1537–1540.
140. Glacet-Bernard A, Bayani N, Chretien P, Cochard C, Lelong F, Coscas G. Antiphospholipid antibodies in retinal vascular occlusions A prospective study of 75 patients. Arch Ophthalmol 1994; 112:790–795.
141. Cobo-Soriano R, Sanchez-Ramon S, Aparicio MJ, Teijeiro MA, Vidal P, Suarez-Leoz M, Rodriguez-Mahou M, Rodriguez-Huerta A, Fernandez-Cruz E, Cortes C. Antiphospholipid antibodies and retinal thrombosis in patients without risk factors: a prospective case-control study. Am J Ophthalmol 1999; 128:725–732.
142. Srinivasan S, Fern AI, Wilson K. Orbital apex syndrome as a presenting sign of maxillary sinus carcinoma. Eye 2001; 15:343–345.

143. Dori D, Beiran I, Gelfand Y, Lanir N, Scharf J, Miller B, Brenner B. Multiple retinal arteriolar occlusions associated with coexisting primary antiphospholipid syndrome and factor V Leiden mutation. Am J Ophthalmol 2000; 129:106–108.
144. Glueck CJ, Bell H, Vadlamani L, Gupta A, Fontaine RN, Wang P, Stroop D, Gruppo R. Heritable thrombophilia and hypofibrinolysis. Possible causes of retinal vein occlusion Arch Ophthalmol 1999; 117:43–44.
145. Greven CM, Slusher MM, Weaver RG. Retinal arterial occlusions in young adults. Am J Ophthalmol 1995; 120:776–783.
146. Mintz-Hittner HA, Miyashiro MJ, Knight-Nanan DM, O'Malley RE, Marlar RA. Vitreoretinal findings similar to retinopathy of prematurity in infants with compound heterozygous protein S deficiency. Ophthalmology 1999; 106:1525–1530.
147. Greiner K, Hafner G, Dick B, Peetz D, Prellwitz W, Pfeiffer N. Retinal vascular occlusion and deficiencies in the protein C pathway. Am J Ophthalmol 1999; 128:69–74.
148. Martinelli I, Sacchi E, Landi G, Taioli E, Duca F, Mannucci PM. High risk of cerebral-vein thrombosis in carriers of a prothrombin-gene mutation and in users of oral contraceptives. New Engl J Med 1998; 338:1793–1797.
149. Incorvaia C, Lamberti G, Parmeggiani F, Ferraresi P, Calzolari E, Bemardi F, Sebastiani A. Idiopathic central retinal vein occlusion in a thrombophilic patient with the heterozygous 20210 G/A prothrombin genotype. Am J Ophthalmol 1999; 128:247–148.
150. Kuhli C, Scharrer I, Koch F, Ohrloff C, Hattenbach LO. Factor XII deficiency: a thrombophilic risk factor for retinal vein occlusion. Am J Ophthalmol 2004; 137: 459–464.
151. Weger M, Renner W, Stanger O, Schmut O, Deutschmann H, Wascher TC, Haas A. Role of factor XIII Val34Leu polymorphism in retinal artery occlusion. Stroke 2001; 32:2759–2761.
152. Incorvaia C, Costagliola C, Parmeggiani F, Gemmati D, Scapoli GL, Sebastiani A. Recurrent episodes of spontaneous subconjunctival hemorrhage in patients with factor XIII Val34Leu mutation. Am J Ophthalmol 2002; 134:927–929.
153. Salomon O, Huna-Baron R, Moisseiev J, Rosenberg N, Rubovitz A, Steinberg DM, Davidson J, Sela BA, Seligsohn U. Thrombophilia as a cause for central and branch retinal artery occlusion in patients without an apparent embolic source. Eye 2001; 15:511–514.
154. Bertina RM, Rosendaal FR. Venous thrombosis—the interaction of genes and environment. New Engl J Med 1998; 338:1840–1841.
155. Hayreh SS, Zimmerman B, McCarthy MJ, Podhajsky P. Systemic diseases associated with various types of retinal vein occlusion. Am J Ophthalmol 2001; 131:61–77.
156. Loewenstein A, Winder A, Goldstein M, Lazar M, Eldor A. Bilateral retinal vein occlusion associated with 5,10-methylenetetrahydrofolate reductase mutation. Am J Ophthalmol 1997; 124:840–841.
157. Schnyder G, Roffi M, Pin R, Flammer Y, Lange H, Eberli FR, Meier B, Turi ZG, Hess OM. Decreased rate of coronary restenosis after lowering of plasma homocysteine levels. New Engl J Med 2001; 345:1593–600.
158. Khamashta MA, Cuadrado MJ, Mujic F, Taub NA, Hunt BJ, Hughes GR. The management of thrombosis in the antiphospholipid-antibody syndrome. New Engl J Med. 1995; 332:993–997.
159. Krill AE. Hereditary Retinal and Choroidal Diseases. Vol. 2. Hagerstown, Harper and Row, MD: 1977; 739–819.
160. Bietti G. Ueber familiares Vorkommen von "Retinitis punctata albescens" (Verbundenmit "Dystrophia marginalis cristallinae corneae"), Glitzern des Glaskörpers and anderen degenerativen Augenveränderungen. Klin Monatsbl Augenheilkd 1937; 99:737–757.
161. Bagolini B, Ioli-Spada G. Bietti's tapetoretinal degeneration with marginal corneal dystrophy. Am J Ophthalmol 1968; 65:53–60.
162. Welch RB. Bietti's tapetoretinal degeneration with marginal corneal dystrophy: crystalline retinopathy. Trans Am Ophthalmol Soc 1977; 75:164–179.

163. Grizzard WS, Deutman AF, Nijhuis F, De Kerk AA. Crystalline retinopathy. Am J Ophthalmol 1978; 86:81–88.
164. Hu DN. Ophthalmic genetics in China. Ophthalmic Pediatr Genet 1983; 2:39–45.
165. Chan WM, Pang CP, Leung AT, Fan DS, Cheng AC, Lam DS. Bietti crystalline retinopathy affecting all 3 male siblings in a family. Arch Ophthalmol 2000; 118:129–131.
166. Jiao X, Munier FL, Iwata F, Hayakawa M, Kanai A, Lee J, Schorderet DF, Chen MS, Kaiser-Kupfer M, Hejtmancik JF. Genetic linkage of Bietti crystallin corneoretinal dystrophy to chromosome 4q35. Am J Hum Genet 2000; 67:1309–1313.
167. Li A, Jiao X, Munier FL, Schorderet DF, Yao W, Iwata F, Hayakawa M, Kanai A, Shy Chen M, Alan Lewis R, Heckenlively J, Weleber RG, Traboulsi EL, Zhang Q, Xiao X, Kaiser-Kupfer M, Sergeev YV, Hejtmancik JF. Bietti crystalline corneoretinal dystrophy is caused by mutations in the novel gene CYP4V2. Am J Hum Genet 2004; 74:817–826.
168. Yuzawa M, Mae Y, Matsui M. Bietti's crystalline retinopathy. Ophthalmic Paediatr Genet 1986; 7:9–20.
169. Slezak H, Hommer K. Fundus pulverulentus. Albrecht von Graefes Arch Klin Ophthalmol 1969; 178:177–182.
170. Sanderson PO, Kuwabara T, Stark WJ, et al. Cystinosis: a clinical, histologic and ultra structure study. Arch Ophthalmol 1974; 91:270–274.
171. Bullock J, Albert DM. Flecked retina, appearance secondary to oxalate crystals from methoxyflurane anaesthesia. Arch Ophthalmol 1975; 93:26–31.
172. Albert DM, Bullock JD, Lahav M, Caine R. Flecked retina secondary to oxalate crystals from methoxyflurane anaesthesia. Clinical and experimental studies. Trans Am Acad Ophthalmol 1975; 79:817–826.
173. Pearlman JT, Kamin DF, Kopelow SM, Saxton J. Pigmented paravenous retinochoroidal atrophy. Am J Ophthalmol 1975; 80:630–635.
174. Pearlman JT, Heckenlively JR, Bastek JV. Progressive nature of pigmented paravenous retinochoroidal atrophy. Am J Ophthalmol 1978; 85:215–217.
175. Noble KG, Carr RE. Peripapillary pigmentary retinal degeneration. Am J Ophthalmol 1978; 86:65–75.
176. Skalka HW. Hereditary pigmented paravenous retinochoroidal atrophy. Am J Ophthalmol 1979; 87:286.
177. Traboulsi El, Maumenee IH. Hereditary pigmented paravenous chorioretinal atrophy. Arch Ophthalmol 1986; 104:1636–1640.
178. Noble KG, Carr RE. Pigmented paravenous chorioretinal atrophy. Am J Ophthalmol 1983; 96:338–344.
179. Kenneth G, Noble MD. Hereditary pigmented paravenous chorioretinal atrophy. Am J Ophthalmol 1989; 108:365–369.
180. Lessel MR, Thaler A, Heilig P. ERG and EOG in progressive paravenous retinochoroidal atrophy. Doc Ophthalmol 1986; 62:25–29.
181. Limaye SR, Mahmood MA. Retinal microangiopathy in pigmented paravenous chorioretinal atrophy. Br J Ophthalmol 1987; 71:757–761.
182. Nucci P, Manitto MP, Piantanida A, Brancato R. Macular dysplasia and pigmented paravenous retino-choroidal atrophy. Ophthalmic Genet 1994; 15:161–164.
183. Bozkurt N, Bavbek T, Kazokoglu H. Hereditary pigmented paravenous chorioretinal atrophy. Ophthalmic Genet 1998; 19:99–104.
184. Murray AT, Kirkby GR. Pigmented paravenous retinochoroidal atrophy: a literature review supported by a unique case and insight. Eye 2000; 5:711–716.
185. Foxman SG, Heckenlively JR, Sinclair SH. Rubeola retinopathy and pigmented paravenous retinochoroidal atrophy. Am J Ophthalmol 1985; 99:605–606.
186. Heckenlively JR. Possible syndrome of high myopia with retinal degeneration, cataract, manic depression and elevated plasma amino acids. Metab Pediatr Ophthalmol 1980; 4:155–160.

187. Blair NP, Trempe CL. Hypertrophy of the retinal pigment epithelium associated with Gardner's syndrome. Am J Ophtalmol 1987; 103:235–236.
188. Lewis RA, Crowder WE, Eierman LA, et al: The Gardner syndrome. Significance of ocular features. Ophthalmology 1984; 91:916–925.
189. Diaz Llopis M, Menezo JL. Congenital hypertrophy of the retinal pigment epithelium and familial polyposis of the colon. Am J Ophthalmol 1987; 103:235–236.
190. Lyons LA, Lewis RA, Strong LC, et al. A genetic study of Gardner syndrome and congenital hypertrophy of the retinal pigment epithelium. Am J Hum Genet 1988; 42: 290–296.
191. Traboulsi EI, Maumenee IH, Krush AJ, et al. Pigmented ocular fundus lesions in the inherited gastrointestinal polyposis syndromes and in hereditary nonpolyposis colorectal cancer Ophthalmology 1988; 95:964–969.
192. Ruhswurm I, Zehetmayer M, Dejaco C, Wolf B, Karner-Hanusch J. Ophthalmic and genetic screening in pedigrees with familial adenomatous polyposis. Am J Ophthalmol 1998; 125:680–686.
193. Bodmer WF, Bailey CJ, Bodmer J, et al. Localization of the gene for familial adenomatous polyposis on chromosome. Nature 1987; 328:614–616.
194. Leppert M, Dobbs M, Scambler P et al. The gene for familial polyposis coli maps to the long arm of chromosome. Science 1987; 238:1411–1413.
195. Caspari R, Friedl W, Mandl M, Moslein G, Kadmon M, Knapp M, Jacobasch KH, Ecker KW, Kreissler-Haag D, Timmermanns G, et al. Familial adenomatous polyposis: mutation at codon 1309 and early onset of colon cancer. Lancet 1994; 343:629–632.
196. Paton D. The Relation of Angioid Streaks to Systemic Disease. Springfield, I: Charles C Thomas, 1972.
197. Grand MG, Isserman MJ, Miller CW. Angioid streaks associated with pseudoxanthoma elasticum in a 13-year-old patient. Ophthalmology 1987; 94:197–200.
198. Meislik J, Neldner K, Reeve EB, Ellis PP. Atypical drusen in pseudoxanthoma elasticum. Ann Ophthalmol 1979; 11:653–656.
199. Erkkila H, Raitta C, Niemi KM. Ocular findings in four siblings with pseudoxanthoma elasticum. Acta Ophthalmol 1983; 61:589–599.
200. McDonald HR, Schatz H, Aaberg TM. Reticular like pigmentary patterns in pseudoxanthoma elasticum. Ophthalmology 1988; 95:306–311.
201. Neldner KH. Pseudoxanthoma elasticum. Clin Dermatol 1988; 6:1–159.
202. Lebwohl M, Phelps RG, Yannuzzi L, et al. Diagnosis of pseudoxanthoma elasticum by scar biopsy in patients without characteristic skin lesions. N Engl J Med 1987; 317: 347–350.
203. Pope FM. Autosomal dominant pseudoxanthoma elasticum. J Med Genet 1974; 11:152–157.
204. Struk B, Neldner KH, Rao VS, St Jean P, Lindpaintner K. Mapping of both autosomal recessive and dominant variants of pseudoxanthoma elasticum to chromosome 16pl3.l. Hum Mol Genet 1997; 6:1823–1828.
205. Ringpfeil F, Lebwohl MG, Christiano AM, Uitto J. Pseudoxanthoma elasticum: mutations in the MRP6 gene encoding a transmembrane ATP-binding cassette (ABC) transporter. Proc Nat Acad Sci USA 2000; 97:6001–6006.
206. Bergen AA, Plomp AS, Schuurman EJ, Terry S, Breuning M, Dauwerse H, Swart J, Kool M, van Soest S, Baas F, ten Brink JB, de Jong PT. Mutations in ABCC6 cause pseudoxanthoma elasticum. Nat Genet 2000; 25:228–231.
207. Le Saux O, Urban Z, Tschuch C, Csiszar K, Bacchelli B, Quaglino D, Pasquali-Ronchetti I, Pope FM, Richards A, Terry S, Bercovitch L, de Paepe A, Boyd CD. Mutations in a gene encoding an ABC transporter cause pseudoxanthoma elasticum. Nat Genet 2000; 25:223–227.
208. Awan KJ. Familial polyposis and angioid streaks in the ocular fundus. Am J Ophthalmol 1977; 83:123–125.

209. McKusick VA, Stauffer M, Knox DL, Clark DB. Chorioretinopathy with hereditary microcephaly. Arch Ophthalmol 1966; 75:597–600.
210. Cantu JM, Rojas JA, Garcia-Cruz D, et al. Autosomal recessive microcephaly associated with chorioretinopathy. Hum Genet 1977; 36:243–247.
211. Parke JT, Riccardi VM, Lewis RA, Ferrell RE. A syndrome of microcephaly and pigmentary abnormalities without mental retardation in a family with coincidental autosomal dominant hyperreflexia. Am J Med Genet 1984; 17:585–594.
212. McKusick VA. Mendelian Inheritance in Man. 8th ed. Baltimore: Johns Hopkins University Press, 1988.
213. Warburg M, Heuer HE. Autosomal dominant microcephaly with lacunar retinal hypopigmentations. In: XXIV Int Cong Ophthalmol, Acta. Philadelphia: JB Lippincott, 1983: 43–45.
214. Ryan SJ, Smith RE. Retinopathy associated with olivopentocerebellar degeneration. Am J Ophthalmol 1971; 71:839–843.
215. Anttinen A, Nikoskelainen E, Marttila RJ, et al. Familial olivopontocerebellar atrophy with macular degeneration: a separate entity among the olivopontocerebellar atrophies. Acta Neurol Scand 1986; 73:180–190.
216. Traboulsi EI, Maumenee IH, Green WR, et al. Olivopontocerebellar atrophy with retinal degeneration. A clinical and ocular histopathologic study. Arch Ophthalmol 1988; 106:801–806.
217. Marmor MF, Jacobson SG, Foerster MH, Kellner U, Weleber RG. Diagnostic clinical findings of a new syndrome with night blindness, maculopathy, and enhanced S cone sensitivity. Am J Ophthalmol 1990; 110:124–134.
218. Jacobson SG, Marmor MF, Kemp CM, Knighton RW. SWS (blue) cone hypersensitivity in a newly identified retinal degeneration. Invest Ophthalmol Vis Sci 1990; 31: 827–838.
219. To KW, Adamian M, Jakobiec FA, Berson EL. Clinical and histopathologic findings in clumped pigmentary retinal degeneration. Arch Ophthalmol 1996; 114:950–955.
220. Jacobson SG, Roman AJ, Roman MI, Gass JD, Parker JA. Relatively enhanced S cone function in the Goldmann-Favre syndrome. Am J Ophthalmol 1991; 111:446–453.
221. Haider NB, Jacobson SG, Cideciyan AV, Swiderski R, Streb LM, Searby C, Beck G, Hockey R, Hanna DB, Gorman S, Duhl D, Carmi R, Bennett J, Weleber RG, Fishman GA, Wright AF, Stone EM, Sheffield VC. Mutation of a nuclear receptor gene, NR2E3, causes enhanced S cone syndrome, a disorder of retinal cell fate. Nat Genet 2000; 24:127–131.
222. Sharon D, Sandberg MA, Caruso RC, Berson EL, Dryja TP. Shared mutations in NR2E3 in enhanced S-cone syndrome, Goldmann-Favre syndrome, and many cases of clumped pigmentary retinal degeneration. Arch Ophthalmol 2003; 121:1316–1323.
223. Dahl N, Pettersson U. Use of linked DNA probes for carrier detection and diagnosis of X-linked juvenile retinoschisis. Arch Ophthalmol 1988; 106:1414–1416.
224. Gardner EJ, Richards RC. Multiple cutaneous and subcutaneous lesions occurring simultaneously with hereditary polyposis and osteomatosis. Am J Hum Genet 1953; 5:139–148.

14

Inherited Diseases Involving the Choroid

INTRODUCTION

There are three inherited disorders that involve primarily the choroid or in which the choroid is presumed to be the primary site of the disease. Gyrate atrophy of the retina and choroid is an autosomal recessive disease, choroideremia is X-linked, and the inherited choroidal atrophies are usually autosomal dominant disorders. A characteristic clinical picture makes these diseases readily diagnosable in the more advanced stages. However, in the early stages, the differential diagnosis with disorders primarily affecting the neural retina or the retinal pigment epithelium (RPE), including retinitis pigmentosa, may be difficult. Recent advances in molecular genetics and cytogenetics make the first two disorders particularly interesting and provide hope for more efficient clinical approaches to therapy and prevention.

GYRATE ATROPHY

Gyrate atrophy, gyrate atrophy of the retina and choroid, hyperornithinemia with gyrate atrophy (HOGA), ornithinemia with gyrate atrophy of choroid and retina, ornithine-δ-aminotransferase deficiency, ornithine ketoacid aminotransferase (OKA) deficiency, and ornithine aminotransferase (OAT) deficiency, are some of the synonyms used for an autosomal recessive, progressive disease of the choroid and the retina, leading to legal blindness in middle age in most cases. For simplicity and clarity, I will use the term gyrate atrophy (GA).

Description and Clinical Findings

Gyrate atrophy affects the eye and several other tissues and organs of the body, such as the muscular system, brain, and hair. Blood chemistry results are abnormal with the characteristic very high plasma levels of ornithine. In spite of this widespread abnormality, which classifies GA as a systemic disease, the ocular symptoms are always predominant and usually the only ones.

The first symptom of GA is night blindness, which usually starts in the first decade of life. Later, visual acuity may decrease, preceded or followed by loss of side vision.

The reduction in visual acuity may be gradual because of the development of a cataract or more rapid because of the development of a maculopathy. In a study of 29 Finnish patients who were followed up for 2 to 31 years, Takki and Milton (1) reported considerable variability in the age of onset of symptoms and in the age of legal blindness. Visual acuity was between 6/60 and light perception in all patients over 60 years old, but some patients had poor visual acuity at age 30 or earlier. The visual fields became gradually more constricted and, at age 40, almost all patients had tunnel vision with less than 10° diameter of visual field in the center only. Myopia gradually developed. Finally, about 40% of patients had a myopia of 4–7 D about the same number had 8–12 D, and the rest had 13–20 D (1).

Characteristically, considerable variability exists for the age of onset of symptoms, age of legal blindness, age of loss of central vision, and age of occurrence of the tunnel vision. This variability can be seen as both an interfamilial and an intrafamilial phenomenon. It is possible, however, that the disease may have a different rate of progression in different populations. For instance, in Japanese patients, the disease is unexpectedly more severe than in Finnish patients (2). Japanese patients had visual acuity of 6/30 in the second or third decade of life, tunnel vision at 20 years of age and myopia of −10.0 D or more before age 20. The fundus changes are progressive. Round, separated, or partially fused areas of chorioretinal atrophy are seen initially around and anterior to the equator, but not reaching the ora serrata (Fig. 1), Later

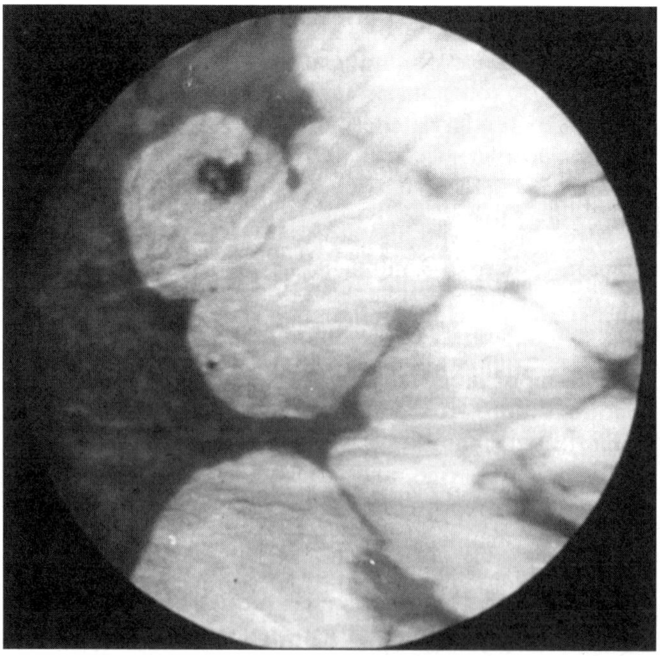

Figure 1 The fundus of a 4-year-old patient with gyrate atrophy: note the prominent areas of chorioretinal atrophy, characteristic of the disease. Pigmentation around and within the lesions can also be seen.

the lesions enlarge and become fused, followed in final stages by peripapillary atrophy and macular atrophy (3) (Fig. 2). Pigmentary changes increase with time, appearing as dark brown pigment clumps within the atrophic lesions and as a continuous dark area around the lesions, sometimes combined with colorless, elongated crystals over the pigmentations (3). The larger choroidal vessels can be seen through the lesion before pigmentation occurs.

Cataracts frequently develop in the second decade of life and are the major cause of visual loss in the third decade of life.

Night vision progressively worsens. The psychophysical dark adaptation test shows high thresholds, with a relative sparing of the cone threshold (3). The electro-oculogram (EOG) is normal and the electro-retinogram (ERG) is nonrecordable or very subnormal (4), even at an early age.

In all the variable clinical manifestations of GA, the progression of the disease is generally slow. Caruso and associates (5) assessed that the median half-life of each of three visual functions: visual acuity, visual fields, and electrophysiology exceeds ten years.

Patients show general wasting of practically all skeletal muscles, including in the face (6). Proximal musculature is more affected than distal. Patients are reported to be thinner than their nonaffected siblings (6).

Abnormal hair, which is sparse, fine, and straight, with intermittent dark cores in the medullary zone, was reported in all 10 patients in one series (7). Other tests, such as the electroencephalogram (7), the electrocardiogram, and the electromyogram (4), were reported to be abnormal in most patients examined, indicating malfunction of the brain, heart, and muscles. Amazingly, this is not related to any

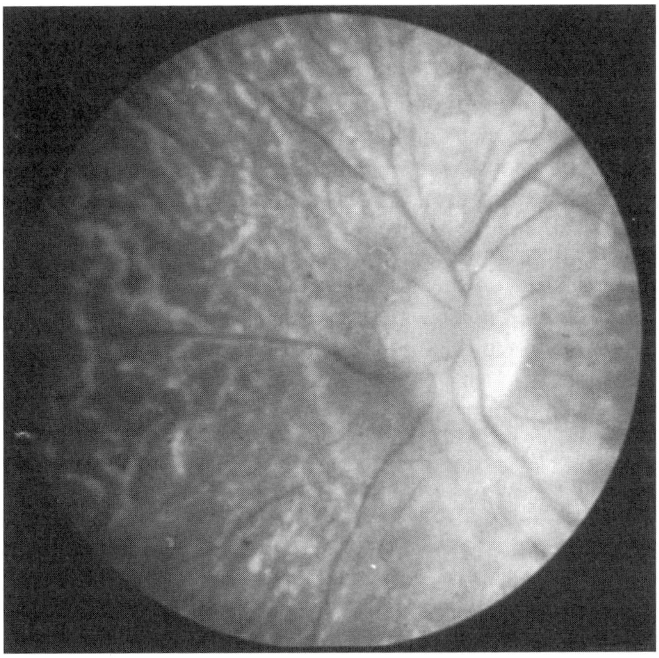

Figure 2 The posterior pole of the fundus of a 19-year-old girt with gyrate atrophy: note the extensive atrophy of the retinal pigment epithelium and the choriocapillaris.

functional clinical abnormality. Patients have no systemic complaints and no substantial muscle weakness.

In spite of the lack of CNS-associated symptoms, MRI revealed degenerative lesions in the brain of 50% of GA patients and premature atrophic changes in 70% of such patients with striking increase in the number of Virchow's spaces (8).

Vannas-Sulonen (9) followed up 21 patients with GA by fluorescein angiography. She noted the enlargement of pigment epithelial window defects into the typical patches of chorioretinal atrophy. Increased visibility of the larger choroidal vessels was noted, even in areas of ophthalmoscopically intact retina. The macula was affected in some patients, even when ophthalmoscopically it appeared normal. Six patients showed pigment epithelial window defects, two had typical patches of chorioretinal atrophy and one had cystoid macular edema. At the borders of the peripheral atrophic patches, blocked fluorescence was seen.

The Clinical and Genetic Types of Gyrate Atrophy

In 1982, it became clear (4,10–12) that some patients with GA respond to vitamin B (pyridoxine) treatment by significant reduction of the plasma ornithine level, whereas others do not show such a response. This characteristic seems to be patient- and family-specific, and the prevalence of the two responses varies in different populations. Therefore, in spite of similar clinical manifestations, two genetic types seem to exist. In addition, it is possible that a normo-ornithinemic GA may mimic hyper-orinthinemic GA.

Gyrate Atrophy, Pyridoxine Nonresponsive

Pyridoxine nonresponsive GA is the more common of the two types. It occurs in about two-thirds of the GA patients in the United States or Japan and in all patients in Finland (11), where the disease is common.

Gyrate Atrophy, Pyridoxine Responsive

Patients with this type of GA respond to diet supplementation by large doses [300 mg/day or more (10)] or by low doses [15–18 mg/day (4) for two weeks] by a reduction of their plasma ornithine level of more than 50%, and increase of their plasma lysine level to normal or near normal. Vitamin B_6 is the cofactor necessary for the normal metabolism of ornithine (Fig. 3), and the mode of action seems to be an increase in catabolism of ornithine. The characteristic of vitamin B_6 responsiveness can be detected also in vitro, in cultured skin fibroblasts of these patients (12). The two variants can be distinguished by the responsiveness of ornithine ketoacid transaminase (OKT) deficiency to pyridoxal phosphate stimulation (13).

Normo-Ornithinemic Gyrate Atrophy

It is not clear whether normo-ornithinemic GA of the choroid and retina actually exists as a separate nosologic entity, as was suggested (14). Punched-out lesions of chorioretinal atrophy in the midperiphery of the fundus often can be seen in isolated cases and have been described to occur in families (14). Ophthalmoscopically, they may mimic GA, but ornithine plasma levels are normal, the ERG is normal or only

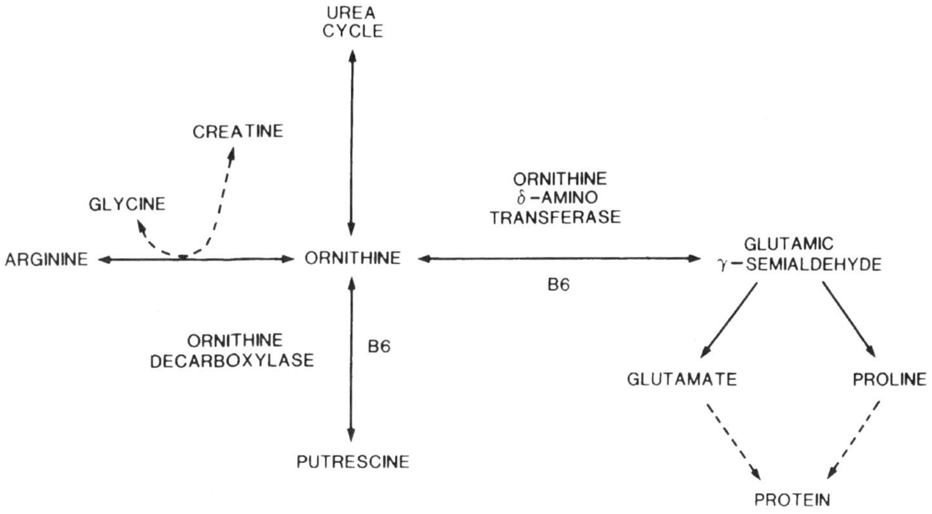

Figure 3 Simplified scheme of ornithine metabolism pathways.

mildly reduced, and the disease is mild. The cause of the atrophic patches is unknown.

Diagnosis and Laboratory Tests

The abnormally raised level of plasma ornithine in patients with GA was first reported in 1973 by Simell and Takki from Finland (15). The normal plasma ornithine level is in the range of 30–64 μmol/L, whereas GA patients display levels that are 10–20 times higher than normal. High levels of ornithine are found in all patients with GA, regardless of age. In fact, there is no relation among age, severity of disease, and level of plasma ornithine (16). High ornithine concentrations have also been detected in the cerebrospinal fluid and in the aqueous humor of the eye (3).

In 1977, three groups of investigators reported the finding of a marked deficiency in ornithine aminotransferase in cultured skin fibroblasts and in transformed lymphocytes of a patient with GA (17–19), whereas obligatory heterozygotes had values that were intermediate between normal controls and patients (20). Ornithine decarboxylase activity was normal. Figure 3 indicates the relevant main pathways of ornithine metabolism. Ornithine is produced from arginine of exogenous origin or from the urea cycle. However, the urea cycle does not add much to the body ornithine, as it is remetabolized within the cycle. Therefore, the major source for "new" ornithine is exogenous arginine from the diet. OAT is the enzyme necessary for catabolism of ornithine into glutamate and proline that, in turn, are incorporated into protein.

The plasma lysine level is low in patients with GA, reaching one-fourth to one-half of the normal concentration (16). The cause of the low lysine concentration in the plasma is not clear. It was suggested that it is a result of urinary loss of lysine, related to the constantly elevated filtered load of ornithine (16). In fact, GA patients have hyperlysinuria along with hyperornithiauria.

After an ornithine loading dose of 100 mg/kg, the plasma ornithine increases even further in all patients. Obligatory heterozygotes had an abnormally high ornithine plasma concentration at 30–120 min after oral ingestion of ornithine (21); however, another study (16) showed an overlap between some heterozygotes and normal controls.

Abnormally low plasma levels of glutamate, glutamine, and creatine, along with low lysine, have been reported in patients with GA (4).

Muscle biopsy detected structural abnormalities in all patients with GA who underwent biopsy. Characteristic findings were a preponderance of type 1 fibers and variable atrophy of type 2 fibers, subsarcolemmal inclusions, and, by electron microscopy, large dysmorphic mitochondria and mutliple areas of tubular aggregates (4,6). These changes were age-related and were more marked in older patients (6).

Ornithine aminotransferase is defined as an intramitochondrial, pyridoxal-dependent enzyme, and the structural changes of the muscle mitochondria may be related to an intramitochondrial accumulation of ornithine (4,6). The general muscle wasting of GA patients may also be related to the abnormally low concentration of creatine, which is needed for the metabolism of muscle fibers.

Pathology and Pathogenesis

A histopathologic study of three iridectomy specimens from Finnish patients with GA was reported by Vannas-Sulonen and colleagues (22). The dilator muscle showed changes similar to those described in skeletal muscles, such as generalized atrophy of fibers; and, by electron microscopy, abnormal mitochondria and tubular aggregates were evident. The pigmented epithelium of the iris was abnormal in having dilated, intercellular spaces, abnormal cellular matrix, and dropout of cellular organelles.

Localization of OAT in the rat showed widespread activity of this enzyme in many tissues of the body, especially cerebral neurons, hepatocytes, epithelial cells of renal tubuli, gut mucous membranes, and ocular tissues (23). In the eye, strong immunoreactivity detected OAT in the epithelial cells of the ciliary body, iris, and lens and in the RPE and Muller's cells (23,24). The choroid showed very little activity of OAT. This could simply be because the RPE is primarily affected and the choroid undergoes secondary atrophy (24).

In 1981, Kuwabara and coworkers (25) reached a similar conclusion that the RPE is the primary tissue affected in GA, by experimental methods. They used an animal model of GA by injecting L-ornithine intravitreally. Both rats and monkeys showed swelling of the RPE as the primary visible response to the increased ornithine. Later, underlying patches of atrophy and denuded areas mimicked the human ophthalmoscopic findings of GA. Secondary degeneration of photoreceptors occurred in areas overlying damaged RPE.

The pathogenetic mechanisms by which OAT deficiency causes the ocular defects of GA is not known, but these studies indicate the RPE as the probable primary site of the disease. Speculations that the cellular damage is caused by hyperornithinemia, by high intracellular ornithine, by the low lysine levels, by low glutamate and glutamic acid levels, or by the general abnormal function of the structurally abnormal mitochondria were not confirmed by any study.

Heinanen and associates proposed a different pathway of pathogenesis (26,27). They found that creatine and creatine phosphate are significantly reduced in GA patients. High ornithine concentration inhibits the activity of the enzyme arginine–glycine transaminidase, needed in creatine synthesis, and, in turn, results in the deficiency of creatine phosphate, a key intracellular energy source. They suggested that disturbed intracellular energy production might explain, completely or partially, the pathogenesis of GA (26,27).

The pathogenesis of GA was studied in a mouse model. Wang and coworkers (28,29) produced an OAT-deficient mouse by gene targeting. The oat −/− mouse exhibits hyperornithinema at rates 10- to 15-fold normal levels, similar to the rates found in human patients with GA. The initial site of insult was in the RPE cell. Degeneration of RPE cells was noted at two months of age, followed later by the degeneration of photoreceptors (28). The reduction of plasma ornithine by a long-term (12 months) arginine-restrictive diet prevented retinal degeneration (29).

Epidemiology and Genetics

About 160 cases of GA have been described in the literature, but the disease is undoubtedly more common. It has been found in several different populations, including in Finland, Western Europe, United States, and Israel.

Gyrate atrophy is transmitted as a regular autosomal recessive disease, but, as outlined earlier, two different genetic forms occur: B_6-nonresponsive in the majority and the B_6-responsive in the minority (11). These two forms are caused by allelic genes, as was suggested by experimental fusion of fibroblasts from B_6-responsive and B_6-nonresponsive patients (30). No complementation occurred. These studies also indicated that both the activity of OAT and the buildup of proteins was higher in B_6-responsive patients. Such a difference may also cause clinical variability in expression. Studies have demonstrated heterogeneity even within each of these two groups of patients (31).

Cytogenetic and molecular genetic research in the field of GA led to amazing successes in a mere three-year period. In 1985, the assignment of the GA locus to chromosome 10 was first reported by O'Donnell and.coworkers (32). Later, two loci for functional OAT genes in the human were located by Barrett and colleagues (33) and by Ramesh and colleagues (34) at 10q26 (10q23–10qter), near the distal end of the long arm of chromosome 10, and at Xp11.2 (Xp21–Xp11), near the proximal part of the short arm of chromosome X at the same location as the gene for X-linked retinitis pigmentosa. That the gene for functional OAT is located on the X chromosome does not bear any importance for GA, as the disease is autosomal recessive without any apparent sex influence. In fact, by using restriction fragment length polymorphisms (RLFPs), Ramesh and coworkers (35) determined that the OAT locus on chromosome 10 segregates concordantly with GA in one family with this disease. Another study by O'Donnell and coworkers (36) also assigned the structural gene for OAT to human chromosome 10, with no locus coding for OAT enzyme activity on chromosome X.

In 1986, the complementary DNA (cDNA) clone for the messenger RNA (mRNA) of human OAT was isolated and characterized by Inana and coworkers (37). This cDNA contained 2073 nucleotides with an open-reading frame from position 1 to 1371. The respective protein contains 439 amino acid residues, with a molecular mass of 48,534 Da. At position 55 the transitional initiation (the beginning of translation of codons, groups of three nucleotides or bases, into amino acids) was identified as a methionine codon (37,38).

This OAT cDNA, however, did not show any evidence of gene deletion or rearrangement in seven patients with GA, as the size and approximate amount of the mRNA formed by this cDNA was similar to the mRNA of normal OAT (39).

In another study (40), 13 of 14 patients with GA had an apparently normal OAT mRNA. The conclusion of these studies was that the defect in patients with GA must be caused by a subtle sequence alteration in the mRNA. This proved accurate when, in 1988, Mitchell and coworkers (41) found a single mutation in the genomic DNA of four patients with GA. The normal initiator codon for OAT is ATG (adenine-thymidine-guanine), which translates into the amino acid methionine. In patients with GA, a G→A takes place and the codon becomes ATA, which cannot be translated (41). The next methionine at which the enzyme can start is 138 amino acids downstream, and thus, the entire leader sequence will not be translated, and the enzyme will ineffective.

Mitchell and coworkers cloned the cDNA and analyzed the structure of the OAT gene (42). The gene was located on chromosome 10q; later it was mapped and refined to chromosome 10q26.13 (43). The gene contains 11 exons and spans 21 kb in length (42). The OAT gene encodes a nuclear-encoded mitochondria matrix enzyme that catalyzes conversion of ornithine and alpha-ketoglutarate to glutamate semialdehyde and glutamate (44). Brody and associates (44) identified 24 disease-bearing mutations. The majority of these mutations resulted in the inactivation of this function, but the amount and size of the enzyme remained normal. The mutations inactivate the enzyme and cause GA (44). In some reported mutations, however, nonsense mutations, as well as occasional missense mutations resulting in a truncated protein, were reported (45). Currently, about 60 mutations were identified (46).

About half of the currently reported 160 GA patients are Finnish (46). A strong founder effect is found (47). Peltola and colleagues (46) described the phenotype of the common Finnish founder mutation Leu402Pro. The first symptom is reduction in night vision or reduced day vision due to the rapidly growing myopia. However, the authors did not find a clear genotype/phenotype relationship, variability of expression was great, and no association between the genotype and plasma ornithine concentration was detected (46).

Comparison of B_6-responsive to B_6-nonresponsive GA patients demonstrated that the two respective cDNAs contained different single missense mutations (48). Ramesh and colleagues (48) demonstrated that both forms of GA result from different mutations in OAT as the structural-only gene. A study of cultured fibroblasts demonstrated a 50% decrease of both OAT mRNA and enzyme activity in obligate heterozygotes.

Management

Medical and Surgical

Once the biochemical abnormalities of GA became known, different approaches to treat the disease were attempted. Reduction of blood ornithine levels can best be achieved by a low arginine diet. Arginine is the dietary precursor of ornithine (see Fig. 3). The diet has to control arginine levels which are necessary to keep normal levels of ornithine in the plasma. Therefore, the diet is usually low in arginine and protein and supplemented by essential amino acids (10). All studies (4,10,49–51) reported an amazing decrease in plasma ornithine on such a diet, often reaching almost normal levels. However, except for one patient who seemed to show improvement in dark adaptation thresholds, enlargement of visual fields, and improvement in color vision (49,50), other patients did not benefit from this treatment (10). In fact, both the chorioretinal atrophy and the ERG changes progressed, even in young patients with excellent biochemical control for several years (51). Ornithine in the plasma can also be reduced by administration of α-aminoisobutyric acid, which increases urinary excretion of ornithine (4). I am not aware of any studies that have been done with patients by this method of ornithine reduction.

Later studies indicated that the arginine-restricted diet does have a beneficial effect, especially when used for a prolonged period. Kaiser-Kupfer and associates (52) treated six pairs of siblings by arginine-restricted diet and demonstrated a slow-down in the progression of the chorioretinal atrophy. Extended use of this diet for 16–17 years demonstrated a slower progression of the chorioretinal atrophy only if treatment started at an early age (53).

Using his mouse model of GA, Wang and coworkers encountered much better results. Arginine-restricted diet over a 12-month period substantially reduced plasma omithine levels and completely prevented retinal degeneration (29).

The poorer results in humans may be a result of poor compliance. The arginine-restrictive diet is unpleasant and 80% of patients could not follow it (29).

Supplementation of oral lysine caused increased levels of plasma lysine but seemed to have no effect on the ocular condition (16). The supplementation, however, was only administered for a short time. In another study, Elpeleg and Koman (54) used oral lysine as a food supplement in three patients with B6-nonresponsive GA patients. Within 1–2 days a reduction of plasma omithine by 21–31% was noted (54). This treatment was previously recommended by Peltola et al. (55).

Supplementation of creatine (1.5 g/day) for five years also had no effect on the ocular condition (56). The disease continued to progress, in spite of this treatment, especially in the younger individuals. However, creatine supplementation had a significant effect on the abnormalities in the skeletal muscles. In all patients who had these abnormalities before treatment, tubular aggregates and atrophy of type 2 muscle fibers disappeared (57). This would indicate a different pathogenesis of the ocular (not related to creatine) and muscular (creatine-related) abnormalities.

Heinanen and associates (27) gave oral supplementation with creatine or a creatine precursor (guanidinoacetate-methionine). Supplementation almost normalized low creatine (27).

Supplementation of pyridoxine (vitamin B_6), even in small amounts (15–18 mg/day), in the pyridoxine-responsive form of the disease, effectively reduced plasma ornithine and increased plasma lysine concentration to normal (4). However, no effect on the natural course of the disease was detected.

Mashima and colleagues (58) studied the increase of OAT activity with pyridoxine (B6) supplementation of daily amounts of 600–750 mg, in four patients with the Glu318Lys mutation. This is one of several mutations associated with the pyridoxine-responsive form, which include also Val332Met, Ala226Val, and Thr181Met missense mutations (58). Pyridoxine supplementation increased OAT activity, reduced ornithine by about 50%, and increased the level of lysine. Kaiser-Kupfer and associates (52) pointed out that pyridoxine supplementation results in partial correction of hyperornithinemia in less than 5% of GA patients, and that creatine supplementation appears not to have any effect (52).

Enzyme replacement by various methods or genetic engineering of the now-known abnormality of the gene may be the future approaches. In the meantime, these are only theoretical possibilities.

Genetic Counseling

Because GA is an autosomal recessive disease (Fig. 4), the chances for the sibling of a patient to be affected are 25%. Heterozygotes can be detected, by testing OAT activity in transformed lymphocytes or in cultured fibroblasts, as they show intermediate activity between normal individuals and patients (20). As mentioned earlier, at least two genetic forms are known: B_6-responsive and B_6-non-responsive. Metabolic or genetic studies can distinguish between the two.

Prenatal Diagnosis

Two methods of prenatal diagnosis were suggested by O'Donnell and colleagues (57). Amniotic fluid cells can be cultured in tissue culture and then direct measure of their OAT activity is performed using high-pressure liquid chromatography (HPLC). By the second method, the differential incorporation of [^{14}C]ornithine and [^{3}H]leu-cine into cell protein is measured. Cells from an embryo affected by GA show no, or very little, radioactive ornithine uptake, probably because it cannot be metabolized into proline (57).

Roschinger and associates (59) found deficient activity of the OAT enzyme in chorionic villus sampling and recommended this method for prenatal diagnosis.

In families with recognized mutations, a research for the mutation can be performed.

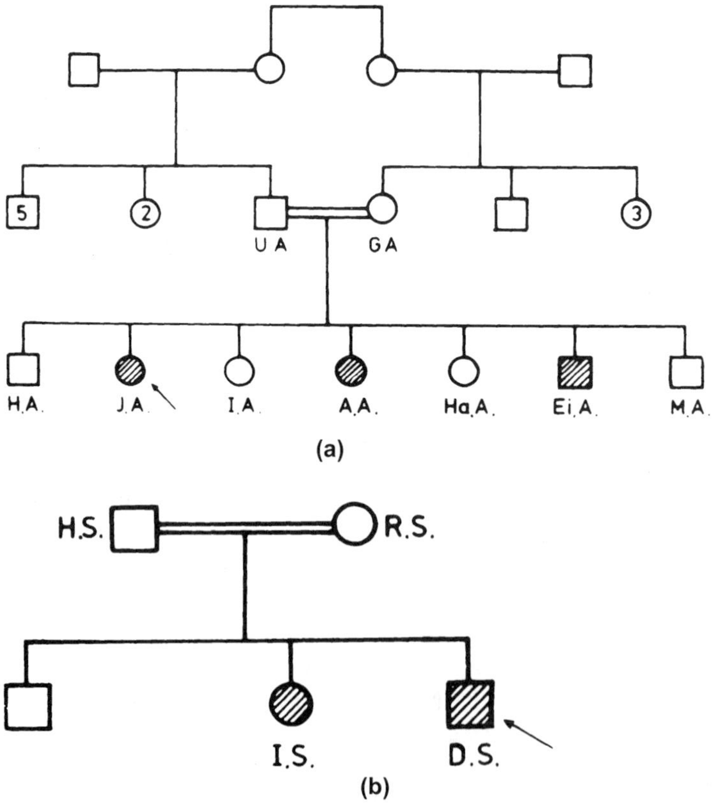

Figure 4 Two families, family A (a) and family S (b), with hyperornithinemia and gyrate atrophy of the retina and choroid, indicating an autosomal recessive transmission.

CHOROIDEREMIA

Several large families living in Canada, the United States, and Finland and suffering from choroideremia were the main sources for learning about the disease. The first classic large clinical study, done on 86 patients from one family, was performed in Canada by McCulloch and McCulloch (60). The family originated from an Irish farmer, who emigrated to Canada in the middle of the 19th century, bringing along his two sons and seven daughters. By the 1960s, there were 1600 descendants of the Irish farmer, who himself became blind from choroideremia in old age in Canada (61), and many of those descendants were affected. It is interesting that the McCullochs' report of 1948 (60) met with much opposition, both for the definition of the disease as choroideremia, rather than retinitis pigmentosa, and for its mode of inheritance (60, discussion). It was erroneously argued that if women carriers manifest some abnormalities this cannot be a sex-linked disorder.

Description and Clinical Findings

The term *choroideremia* defines an absence of choroid, which is characteristic of the late ("burned-out") stages of the disease. It is never a congenital absence, and it is rarely seen in childhood.

Choroideremia is a bilateral progressive dystrophy of the choroid and retina, which affects primarily men, but is also manifest in carrier women. Various other names have been given to the disease, such as diffuse total choroidal vascular atrophy of X-linked inheritance (62) or progressive tapetochoroidal dystrophy, used more in Europe. Choroideremia is probably the most frequently used term for the disease.

The onset of the disease is quite variable; the first symptoms appear as early as three years of age and as late as 40 years, with a peak occurrence between 10 and 30 (63). The visual fields become progressively constricted so that patients usually reach legal blindness by 25 years of age. Loss of central vision occurs, usually after 35 years of age (64).

The fundus changes are progressive, starting with fine pigmentary stippling, which continues with spots of depigmentation and increasing areas of loss of choriocapillaris (Fig. 5). Finally, loss of choriocapillaris and of the larger choroidal blood vessels bares the sclera. The disease starts in the midperiphery, but eventually all of the choroid becomes affected. A study of 84 patients with choroideremia from Finland confirmed the variable expressivity of the disease, with a very wide range of age of onset of symptoms and its progression (65). Fundus changes were identified in two boys aged 3 and eight months with choroideremia. Some patients were blind before aged 30 years, whereas others were subjectively symptom-free at age 50 or older (64).

Color vision, initially normal, turns into a tritanopia (63). Dark adaptation tests indicate an increasing rod threshold with age. The ERG is affected early. All 47 affected males in one series had an unrecordable ERG or showed the presence of some rod and cone function. Cone responses were normal or subnormal in amplitude, but delayed in implicit times (65).

Psychophysical tests and densitometric studies in two patients with choroideremia showed rod sensitivity much more impaired than cone sensitivity (66). Female carriers of the disease usually show abnormalities of the fundus in the form of pigment stippling with tiny patches of RPE depigmentation (Fig. 6). Brownish granular

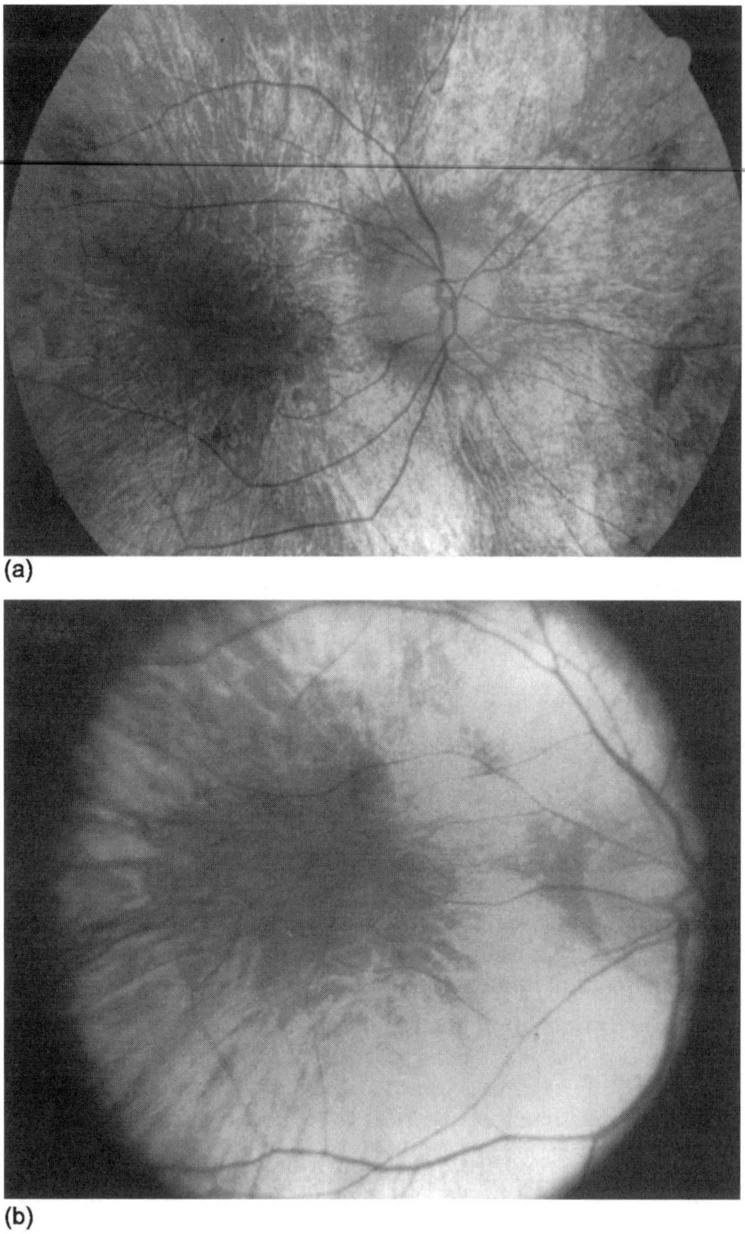

(a)

(b)

Figure 5 The fundus changes of choroideremia are progressive: initially, pigmentary stippling is replaced by mixed areas of pigment and atrophy of the choriocapillaris and RPE (a). In the final stages (b), most of the choriocapillaris disappears, with extensive atrophy of the RPE and loss of large choroidal vessels. (Courtesy of G.A. Fishman, MD)

pigmentation and peripapillary atrophy of the RPE and choroid may occur later (64). In contrast, visual acuity and dark adaptation thresholds are usually normal, except in rare cases of severe disease in a female carrier (65). The ERG is usually normal in carriers of choroideremia. In one series of 26 carriers, 22 had a normal ERG, but only 1 of the 26 had a normal fundus (65).

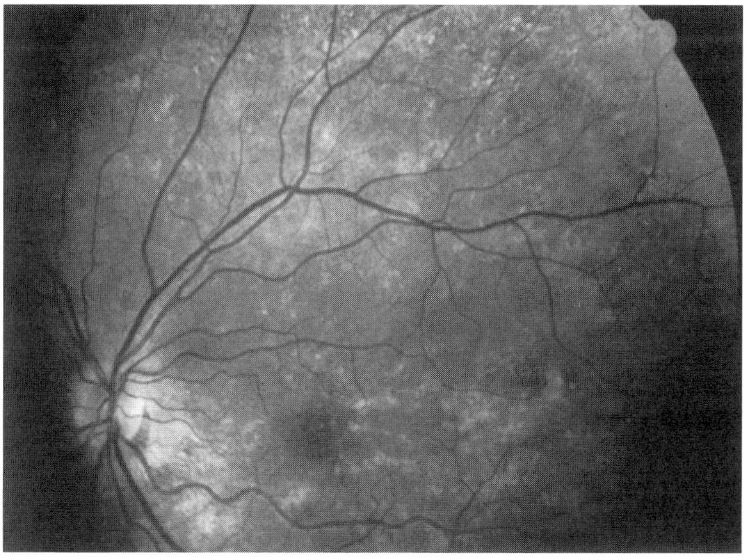

Figure 6 The fundus of a female carrier of choroideremia: note the pigmentary stippling and tiny areas of RPE and choroidal atrophy. Most female carriers of the disease have such abnormalities. (Courtesy of G.A. Fishman, MD)

In contrast to routine ERG, multifocal ERG (mfERG) may be a sensitive tool to measure functional abnormalities in carriers of choroideremia (67). Severely reduced amplitudes by mfERG were obtained in one eye of a carrier with an atrophic band across the macula.

Patients with choroideremia often complain of glare. This may be the result of intraocular light scatter associated with the severe reduction of the intraocular pigment (68).

Subretinal neovascularization in the macular area was reported in a 14-year-old boy with choroideremia (69), possibly a result of an abnormal RPE of the proximal long arm of the X chromosome caused choroideremia with severe mental retardation (70,71), or choroideremia with mental retardation and congenital deafness (72–74). In one patient, coarse facial features, microcephaly, and cleft lip and palate were also described (74). In all of these families, the mothers were carriers, showing the same deletions without the severe clinical manifestations. The disease can, therefore, be familial, with transmission of the chromosomal deletion of the X chromosome.

Other associations have been described. Ayazi (75) described a family in which three of four male subjects were affected by "choroideremia, obesity, and congenital deafness." It was transmitted as an X linked disorder. No chromosomal studies were performed. Judisch and coworkers (76) described a "chorioretinopathy and pituitary dysfunction" in five unrelated patients, four of whom were males. Patients had diffuse atrophy of the choroid and retina, with coarse pigmentation in the fundus, resembling choroideremia. There was growth retardation and sexual infantilism, with hypothyroidism in some. Sparse and fine scalp hair, along with abnormally long lashes (trichomegaly), was also present. Mental retardation was found in three males, but not in the female patient. Karyotypes were normal, except in one case which was unclear.

It is possible that the patients described by Ayazi (75) and Judisch et al. (76) had a deletion, or a submicroscopic deletion, of the X chromosome. It would then bring them into the same group of choroideremia associated with X chromosomal deletions and transmitted by nonmanifesting carriers.

The Clinical and Genetic Types

Isolated Choroideremia

Isolated choroideremia has been reported only as an X-linked disease, transmitted by regular mendelian X-linked recessive mode. Patients do not display any extra-ocular abnormality related to the disease. Its clinical description appears in the foregoing.

Associated Choroideremia

Choroideremia with mental retardation was described in several patients, who had a deletion of part of the long arm of the X chromosome, including the region of Xq21, which is supposed to harbor the gene for choroideremia. Such an interstitial deletion may result in isolated choroideremia or choroideremia with deafness, mental retardation cleft lip and palate, and other abnormalities (see below).

Diagnosis and Laboratory Tests

The diagnosis is based on the typical fundus abnormalities, the progressive course, and the combination of typical symptoms, with ERG abnormalities. The family history is helpful. When the diagnosis is in doubt, examination of obligatory heterozygotes, such as the mother, will reveal in almost all cases fundus abnormalities as described in carriers.

Nevertheless, I believe that many patients with choroideremia are misdiagnosed as having retinitis pigmentosa. In the early stages, both diseases may have very similar symptoms, and even the carrier state of both may be similar. Proper evaluation of the patient will distinguish between the two disorders.

As will be shown later, choroideremia-associated mutations result in the deficiency of Rab escort protein-1 (REP-1). No REP-1 has been detected in the circulating lymphocytes of male patients with choroideremia. MacDonald and colleagues (77) recommended using a simple immunoblot analysis with anti-REP-1 antibody to confirm the presence or absence of plasma Rep-1. This may confirm or exclude choroideremia.

Pathology and Pathophysiology

Cameron and colleagues (78) reviewed the pathologic reports of 12 eyes of 8 patients with choroideremia studied until 1987 and reported the findings in the eyes of a 66-year-old man with choroideremia. They found extensive atrophy of the retina and choroid, with a calcified Bruch's membrane. Muller's cells produced a basement membrane of various thickness on the choroidal (collagenous) side of Bruch's membrane. An epiretinal membrane was found, together with gliosis of the neural retina and loss of axons in the optic nerve in all studies on older patients. There was loss of choroidal structures, and the midperiphery was most affected. The macular area and the far periphery were preserved in most studies. In their study, Cameron et al. (78) found abnormalities of the vascular endothelial cells and pericytes, with hypoproduction of the normal basement membrane. These abnormalities were found throughout the uveal tract. The RPE cells were missing opposite the affected choroid, and dilator muscle fibers were missing, with flattening of the iris pigment epithelium in the affected iris. They concluded that this vascular hypoproduction of the basement membrance may be the primary abnormality in choroideremia.

Syed and associates studied the eye of an 88-year-old symptomatic female carrier of choroideremia (79). The mutation, a T-A substitution at nt1542 in exon 13 of REP-1 gene results in a stop codon and a severely truncated protein. They found a localization of REP-1 product in rods but not in cones and suggested that rods may be the primary sites of the disease. The choriocapillaris seemed well preserved except in areas that had lost all photoreceptors.

Flannery et al. (80) and MacDonald et al. (81) reached different conclusions from the histopathological study of eyes of choroideremia carriers. In the first study, islands of irregular pigmentation and depigmentation at the RPE level were present while photoreceptors were generally normal except in midperiphery-localized areas of short or absent outer segments (80). In the second study rather subtle changes were seen at the RPE level but scanning electron microscopy revealed striking changes of pleomorphic RPE cells of various shapes and sizes with loss of the usual polygonal structure and villi. Both groups concluded that the RPE is the primary site of the disease.

The youngest patient examined pathologically was a 19-year-old asymptomatic patient with choroideremia who died in an accident. Rodrigues and coworkers (82) found, even at this young age, absence of choriocapillaris and atrophy of the inner choroid and midchoroid. Marked degeneration of the outer retina and midretina, with loss of the RPE and Bruch's membrane, was also noted. Photoreceptor phagosomes were found in the remaining RPE cells, indicating normal phagocytic activity. No epiretinal membrane was found at this stage. Histochemical examinations of the same eye revealed a significantly lower-than-normal concentration of the interphotoreceptor retinol-binding protein (IRBP), a several-fold higher-than-normal cAMP level, and an almost normal cGMP concentration (82).

In their psychophysical and densitometric study, Fulton and Hansen found in dark-adapted choroideremia patients only a modest loss of rhodopsin, but abnormally slow kinetics of rhodopsin regeneration in some areas (66). This could be related to the decrease in IRBP.

Epidemiology and Genetics

The prevalence of the disease is not known, but it seems to vary in different populations.

The X chromosome-linked transmission of choroideremia is well known since the McCullochs' 1948 report (60). In 1985, the use of the RFLP technique enabled Nussbaum et al. (83) and Lewis and coworkers (84) to locate the gene for choroidseremia to the proximal part of the long arm of chromosome X at the Xql3–q21 location. In three families they found no recombinations between one polymorphic DNA probe, *DXYSI,* and the gene for choroideremia, with a significant lod (logarithm of odds) score of 5.78 that the two are linked. This very close linkage to *DXYSI* was confirmed in 15 families from Britain by Jay and coworkers (85), in 2 families from Germany by Gal and colleagues (86), in 12 families in the United States by Leske et al. (87), in 3 families from Canada by MacDonald and coworkers (88,89), and in 36 patients of 1 big Finnish family by Sankilla et al. (90). All of these studies indicate a very close linkage between the gene for choroideremia and the polymorphic probe *DXYSI* located at Xq13–q21. The distance between these two locations is 3 centimorgans (cM) or less (90).

The fact that identical results were achieved in different populations indicates that one and the same gene location is responsible for choroideremia.

Studies on families with choroideremia and visible deletions of the X chromosome were performed to achieve a more accurate localization. The locus *DXYSI* located at Xq13–Xq21 was detected, together with the *TCD* gene in all cases. The deletion did not include *DXS 17*, a DNA probe located at Xq22, which ruled out this location (91). The deleted segment was Xql3–21.3 in one report (91). Xq21.1–21.3 in the second report (51), Xq13–21 in the third (52), Xq21.1–21.31 in the fourth (72), Xq21 in the fifth (54), and Xq21.1–21.33 and Xq21.2–21.31 in the sixth (74). Bands Xq13 and Xq21.1 were apparently normal (69). The most likely location for the gene *TCD,* causing choroideremia is, therefore, the locus on Xq21.2. Xq21 also harbors genes for congenital deafness and mental retardation and nearby genes for X-linked cleft lip and palate and agenesis of corpus callosum.

Complicated molecular genetics methods let Nussbaum et al. (73) prove the presence of a microdeletion in one family. Cremers and coworkers (92), using a polymorphic DNA probe for locus *DXS 165,* suggested a microdeletion of the *DXS 165* locus in all the eight patients they examined. All of these patients had isolated choroideremia without any other abnormalities. The same group of investigators subdivided the Xq21 region into seven intervals and assigned the gene locus for choroideremia to interval 3 and the gene locus for X-linked deafness and mental retardation to interval 2 (93).

The same group of investigators partially cloned the cDNA of the gene at chromosome Xq21.2 using reverse genetics methods, 1 year later (94). Cremens et al. (94) found sequence alterations in eight choroideremia patients and in a female carrier of choroideremia due to a balanced translocation. Merry and coworkers partially cloned the gene (95). Van Bokhoven and colleagues (96) finally cloned and characterized the whole human gene. The gene responsible for choroideremia, initially named TCD (for tapetochoroidal dystrophy) was renamed CHM (for choroideremia). It consists of 15 exons, spans about 150 kb pairs, and encodes a protein of 653 amino acids. The gene has a large open reading frame, but also exceptionally large introns, with an average length of 10 kb each. The gene is expressed in many human tissues and is homologous to the gene of rats and mice (96). The encoded protein is Rab escort protein-1, so the gene is now frequently termed the REPl gene (97).

Many different mutations of the REPl gene are associated with choroideremia. All mutations, with possibly one exception, lead to the synthesis of a truncated, nonfunctional polypeptide (97). Among European choroideremia patients, 25% manifested large deletions or translocations that disrupt the CHM gene and 40% had point mutations or deletions causing premature stop codons (97). Similarly, nonsense, frameshift, splice-site mutations and deletions (all leading to a truncated Rep-1 protein) were identified in all studies (98–102). The studied population was from Sweden, Denmark, Canada, and Holland. A study of 57 Dutch families detected 42% transitions and transversions, 28% 1–5 bp deletions, 9% intragenic larger deletions, 4% complete deletion of the *gene* or deletion/insertion, and 13% splice site mutations (102). In all of these (96% of the examined), a total loss of the protein or a severe truncation of the protein was encountered (102). This renders the Rep-1 protein nonfunctional.

It seems that we lack a molecular genetics explanation for the considerable interfamilial and intrafamilial variability in the severity of the disease. In some patients the progressive constriction of the visual fields will lead to complete blindness in middle life (98). In other families, some members have a severe disease with extinguished ERG while other affected members will have a mild phenotype with only slight reduction of ERG (99). No clear genotype/phenotype correlation has been detected. We have no explanation for, sometimes seen, great assymetry between the two eyes of a manifest carrier of choroideremia.

The protein REP-1 is a component of intracellular traffic. It is essential in moving Rab to the cell membrane. Loss of REP-1 protein or its nonfunction results in defects in Rab protein prenylation (attachment of prenyl to the protein) and renders Rab inactive. This leads to the arrest of the intracellular traffic pathways (97), and is associated with the defects found in all cases of choroideremia.

Two additional genes, which have an association with the REP1 gene, were identified. A gene named Rep2 or CHML (for choroideremia-like) was located on chromosome 1q42–qter. It produces a protein that can compensate for the nonfunctioning REP1 gene, including the prenylation of Rab proteins, but only outside the eye. It shows little effect in the eye (97).

RAB27A is the gene on chromosome 15q15–q21.1 that produces the Rab protein which becomes nonfunctional due to lack of prenylation in choroideremia (103).

Management

Medical and Surgical

No treatment is available for choroideremia. We do not know if any external environmental factors, such as light, contribute to the progression of the disease, or if genetic factors alone are responsible for the great variability in the disease's expression. It is conceivable that an additional gene or genes may play a role in the phenotype variability of choroideremia. Possible genes with influence on choroideremia might be the CHML gene on chromosome 1 or the RAB27A gene on chromosome 15.

Optical aids such as those for correction of the refractive errors or low vision aids can help in patients with choroideremia.

Gene therapy will likely be the future treatment. It seems feasible since Anand and associates (104) succeeded, in vitro, in rescuing the affected lymphocytes and fibroblasts from choroideremia patients. They prepared a human cDNA that encodes REP-1 protein under the control of a cytomegalovirus promoter and used a recombinant adenovirus to deliver it in vitro to affected cells. Protein and enzyme assays proved the rescue of the defective cells (104).

Genetic Counseling

Choroideremia is transmitted by a regular mendelian gene. The risk for an affected male to have an affected brother or for a carrier mother to have an affected son is 50%. All daughters of an affected male will be carriers, and 50% of the daughters of a carrier mother will be carriers.

Prenatal Diagnosis

Sex determination alone can predict that a male embryo of a carrier mother has a 50% chance to be affected by choroideremia.

DNA analysis can reliably distinguish between an affected and nonaffected male embryo. Chorionic villus sampling was performed during the 12th week of pregnancy to find out whether the allele at risk had or had not been passed to the fetus (105).

INHERITED CHOROIDAL ATROPHIES

The choroidal atrophies are a group of disorders in which localized areas of choroidal atrophy are the predominant finding. The nomenclature is terribly confusing and several attempts have been made to reclassify these diseases. Krill and Archer (62), in 1971, classified the diseases according to the tissue affected—choriocapillaris only or all of the choroid—and according to the region affected—macular, paramacular, or peripapillary. Generalized atrophies were separately classified as total choroidal atrophy (choroideremia and GA) and diffuse choroidal sclerosis. The regional central areolar choroidal sclerosis was described as a sporadic autosomal dominant and autosomal recessive disease. The diffuse choriocapillaris atrophy was described as transmitted by the autosomal dominant mode (4). Carr and colleagues (106) tried to simplify this classification.

Most cases of regional choroidal atrophies, called "central" (meaning that they occur in the macular area) for peripapillary, are sporadic. However, a familial form of central areolar choroidal sclerosis, probably better named central areolar choroidal dystrophy, does occur. It has been reported to be transmitted more often by an autosomal dominant gene (62,106,107) or, less frequently, by an autosomal recessive gene (62,108,109).

The onset of visual loss may be as early as the late teens or beginning of the third decade (106), but usually, it is later in life. The disease often starts with nonspecific macular changes (106) and continues to form a sharply defined atrophic area (110) of the choriocapillaris and RPE. The large vessels of the choroid are seen through the atrophic choriocapillaris (Fig. 5). Fluorescein angiography confirms the absence of choriocapillaris. Color vision indicates a tritan defect. The EOG is reduced and may be flat (107). Dark adaptation shows a mild reduction in rod sensitivity and the scotopic ERG is subnormal (107). The affected area may enlarge to involve much of the fundus. A histopathologic study of an eye with regional choroidal dystrophy (central areolar choroidal dystrophy) was done by Weiter and Fine (111). In the affected region, the choriocapillaris, RPE, and photoreceptors were mostly missing. Choroidal veins were fewer than choroidal arteries. Müller cells produced a new "basement membrane," along the outer retinal surface on Bruch's membrane. Comparing different areas, Weiter and Fine indicate that the earliest sign of the disease is loss of endothelial fenestrae of the choriocapillaris. This is followed by a loss of the whole capillary bed in the affected region. Finally, atrophy of the venous drainage occurs. The conclusion is that central areolar choroidal dystrophy is primarily a vascular disorder, followed by secondary degeneration of the RPE and of photoreceptors.

No medical treatment is available for this disease, but low-vision aids may be helpful.

Helicoid peripapillary chorioretinal degeneration (HPCD) is a rare condition described by Sveinsson in Iceland (112). It carries clinical similarities to serpiginous choroidopathy, a nongenetic disease. HPCD is transmitted by the autosomal dominant mode. In childhood, the chorioretinal degeneration can be seen radiating from the disk, but later in life a progression of atrophic "fingers" may reach the macula and substantially reduce vision (112).

The fundus manifests serpiginous-like, sharply demarcated borders of "rays" of lesions, which radiate from the disk in all directions including the macula (113). In the affected area, atrophy of the RPE and the choriocapillaris is seen. The EOG was found subnormal in 15 of 17 patients while the ERG responses were normal in about a third, moderately reduced in another one-third, and severely reduced in the last third (114). Eysteinsson and the other authors (114) concluded that the RPE is the first to be affected by the disease.

The locus for HPCD was mapped to chromosome 11p15 (115).

The disease is known in Iceland and was described in one single family in Switzerland (113). It is not clear whether some of the sporadic serpiginous choroidopathy cases are also of the hereditary type.

A rare systemic metabolic disease, *long-chain 3-hydroxyacyl-CoA dehydrogenase deficiency*, is a severe disease affecting the heart, the CNS, and the liver. It is also associated with hypoketotic hypoglycemia, epilepsy, mental retardation, and other abnormalities. The eyes may be affected with a choroideremia-like disease (116). Granular RPE with or without pigment clumping in childhood progresses to the loss of RPE cells and choriocapillaris. All affected were found to carry a G–C transition at nt1528 in the for mitochondrial trifunctional protein, subunit A at chromosome 2p23 (117).

Central areolar choroidal dystrophy and *central areolar pigment epithelium* dystrophy are both discussed in Chapter 8 (Macula).

HLA-associated eye disorders and uveitis are discussed in Chapter 5 ("The Iris").

REFERENCES

1. Takki K, Milton RC. The natural history of gyrate atrophy of the choroid and retina. Ophthalmology 1981; 88:292–301.
2. Hayasaka S, Shiono T, Mizuno K, et al. Gyrate atrophy of the choroid and retina: 15 Japanese patients. Br J Ophthalmol 1986; 70:612–614.
3. Takki K. Gyrate atrophy of the choroid and retina associated with hyperornithinemia. Br J Ophthalmol 1974; 58:3–23.
4. Weleber RG, Kennaway NG, Buist NRM. Gyrate atrophy of the choroid retina Approaches to therapy. Int Ophthalmol 1981; 4:23–32.
5. Caruso RC, Nussenblatt RB, Csaky KG, Valle D, Kaiser-Kupfer MI. Assessment of visual function in patients with gyrate atrophy who are considered candidates for gene replacement. Arch Ophthalmol 2001; 119(5):667–669.
6. Shapira Y, Yatziv S, Merin S, et al. Myopathy in hyperornithimemic gyrate atrophy of choroid and retina. Isr J Med Sci 1981; 17:271–276.
7. Kaiser-Kupfer MI, Kuwabara T, Askanas V, et al. Systemic manifestations of gyrate atrophy of the choroid and retina. Ophthalmology 1981; 88:302–306.
8. Valtonen M, Nanto-Salonen K, Jaaskelainen S, Heinanen K, Alanen A, Heinonen OJ, Lundbom N, Erkintalo M, Simell O. Central nervous system involvement in gyrate atrophy of the choroid and retina with hyperornithinaemia. J Inherit Metab Dis 1999; 22(8):855–866.
9. Vannas-Sulonen K. Progression of gyrate atrophy of the choroid and retina. A long term follow-up by fluorescien angiography. Acta Ophthalmol 1987; 65:101–109.

10. Berson EL, Shih VE, Sullivan PL. Ocular findings in patients with gyrate atrophy on pyridoxine and low-protein tow-arginine diets. Ophthalmology 1981; 88:311–315.
11. Weleber RG, Kennaway NG. Clinical trial of vitamin B_6 for gyrate atrophy of the choroid and retina. Ophthalmology 1981; 88:316–324.
12. Hayasaka S, Saito T, Nakajima H, et al. Gyrate atrophy with hyperornithinemia: different responsiveness to vitamin B_6. Br J Ophthalmol 1981; 65:478-483.
13. Shih VE, Mandell R, Berson EL. Pyridoxine effects on ornithine ketoacid transaminase activity in fibroblasts from carriers of two forms of gyrate atrophy of the choroid and retina. Am J Hum Genet 1988; 43:929–933.
14. Bargum R. Differential diagnosis of normoornithinaemic gyrate atrophy of the choroids and retina. Acta Ophthalmol 1986; 64:369–373.
15. Simell O, Takki K. Raised plasma ornithine and gyrate atrophy of the choroid and retina. Lancet 1973; 1:1031–1033.
16. Yatziv S, Statter M, Merin S. Metabolic studies in two families with hyperornithinemia and gyrate atrophy of choroid and retina. J Lab Clin Med 1979; 93:749–757.
17. O'Donnell JJ, Sandman RP, Martin JR. Deficient L-ornithine:2-oxoacid aminotransferase activity in cultured fibroblasts from a patient with gyrate atrophy of the retina. Biochem Biophys Res Commun 1977; 79:396.
18. Kenneway NG, Weleber RG, Buist NRM. Gyrate atrophy of choroid and retina: deficient activity of ornithine keto acid aminotransferase in cultured skin fibroblasts. N Engl J Med 1977; 297:1180..
19. Valle O, Kaiser-Kupfer MJ, del Valle LA. Gyrate atrophy of the choroid and retina: deficiency of ornithine amino transferase in transformed lymphocytes. Proc Natl Acad Sci USA 1977; 74:5159.
20. Kaiser-Kupfer MI, Valle D, del Valle LA. A specific enzyme defect in gyrate atrophy. Am J Ophthalmol 1978; 85:200–204.
21. Takki K, Simell O. Genetic aspects in gyrate atrophy of the choroid and retina with hyperornithinemia. Br J Ophthaimol 1981; 58:907–916.
22. Vannas-Sulonen K, Vannas A, O'Donnell JJ, et al. Pathology of iridectomy specimens in gyrate atrophy of the retina and choroid. Acta Ophthalmol 1983; 61:9–19.
23. Kasahara M, Matsuzawa T, Kokubo M, et al. Immunohistochemical localization of ornithine aminotransferase in normal rat tissues by Fab′-horseradish peroxidase conjugates. J Histochem Cytochem 1986; 34:1385–1388.
24. Takahashi O, Ishiguro S, Mito T, et al. Immunocytochemical localization of ornithine aminotransferase in rat ocular tissues. Invest Ophthalmol Vis Sci 1987; 28:1617–1619.
25. Kuwabara T, Ishikawa Y, Kaiser-Kupfer MI. Experimental model of gyrate atrophy in animals. Ophthalmology 1981; 88:331–336.
26. Heinanen K, Nanto-Salonen K, Komu M, Erkintalo M, Heinonen OJ, Pulkki K, Valtonen M, Nikoskelainen E, Alanen A, Simell O. Muscle creatine phosphate in gyrate atrophy of the choroid and retina with hyperornithinaemia—clues to pathogenesis. Eur J Clin Invest 1999; 29(5):426–431.
27. Heinanen K, Nanto-Salonen K, Komu M, Erkintalo M, Alanen A, Heinonen OJ, Pulkki K, Nikoskelainen E, Sipila I, Simell O. Creatine corrects muscle 31P spectrum in gyrate atrophy with hyperornithinaemia. Eur J Clin Invest. 1999; 29(12):1060–1065.
28. Wang T, Milam AH, Steel G, Valle D. A mouse model of gyrate atrophy of the choroid and retina. Early retinal pigment epithelium damage and progressive retinal degeneration. J Clin Invest 1996; 97(12):2753–2762.
29. Wang T, Steel G, Milam AH, Valle D. Correction of ornithine accumulation prevents retinal degeneration in a mouse model of gyrate atrophy of the choroid and retina. Proc Nat Acad Sci USA. 2000; 97(3):1224–1229.
30. Wirtz MK, Kennaway NG, Weleber RG. Heterogeneity and complementation analysis of fibroblasts from vitamin B_6 responsive and non-responsive patients with gyrate atrophy of the choroid and retina. J Inherit Metab Dis 1985; 8:71–74.

31. Kennaway NG, Stankova L, Wirtz MK, Weleber RG. Gyrate atrophy of the choroids arid retina: Characterization of mutant ornithine aminotransferase and mechanism of response to vitamin B_6. Am J Hum Genet 1989; 44:344–352.
32. O'Donnell JJ, Vannas-Sulonen KM, Shows TB, Cox DR. Ornithine aminotransferase maps to human chromosome 10 and mouse chromosome 7 abstract. Cytogenet Cell Genet 1985; 40:716A.
33. Barrett DJ, Bateman JB, Sparkes RS, et al. Chromosomal localization of human ornithine aminotransferase gene sequences to 10q26 and Xp11.2. Invest Ophthalmol Vis Sci 1987; 28: 1037–1042.
34. Ramesh V, Eddy R, Bruns GA, et al. Localization of the ornithine aminotransferase gene and related sequences on two human chromosomes. Hum Genet 1987; 76:121–126.
35. Ramesh V, Benoit LA, Crawford P, et al. The ornithine aminotransferase (OAT) locus: analysis of RFLPs in gyrate atrophy. Am J Hum Genet 1988; 42:365–372.
36. O'Donnell JJ, Vannas-Sulonen KM, Shows TB, Cox DR. Gyrate atrophy of the choroids and retina: assignment of the ornithine aminotransferase structural gene to human chromosome 10 mouse chromosome 7. Am J Hum Genet 1988; 43:922–928.
37. Inana G, Totsuka S, Redmond M, et al. Molecular cloning of human ornithine amino transferase mRNA. Proc Natl Acad Sci USA 1986; 53:1203–1207.
38. Inana G, Totsuka S, Zintz C, et al. Molecular genetics of gyrate atrophy. Prog Clin Biol Res 1987; 247:163–172.
39. Ramesh V, Shaffer MM, Allaire JM, et al. Investigation of gyrate atrophy using a cDNA clone for human ornithine aminotransferase. DNA 1986; 5:493–501.
40. Inana G, Hotta Y, Zintz C, et al. Expression defect of ornithine aminotransferase gene in gyrate atrophy. Invest Ophthalmol Vis Sci 1988; 29:1001–1005.
41. Mitchell GA, Brody LC, Looney J, et al. An initiator codon mutation in ornithine-delta-aminotransferase causing gyrate atrophy of the choroid and retina. J Clin Invest 1988; 81:630–633.
42. Mitchell GA, Looney JE, Brody LC, Steel G, Suchanek M, Engelhardt JF, Willard HF, Valle D. Human ornithine-delta-aminotransferase. cDNA cloning and analysis of the structural gene. J Biol Chem. 1988; 263(28):14288–14295.
43. RetNet (retrieval system on the internet) Texas: The University of Texas Health Science Center C1996–2004 (cited 2004) URL: http://www.sph.uth.tmc.edu/retnet/.
44. Brody LC, Mitchell GA, Obie C, Michaud J, Steel G, Fontaine G, Robert MF, Sipila I, Kaiser-Kupfer M, Valle D. Ornithine delta-aminotransferase mutations in gyrate atrophy. Allelic heterogeneity and functional consequences. J Biol Chem. 1992; 267(5): 3302–3307.
45. Online Mendelian inheritance in Man, OMIM (TM). McKusick-Nathas Institute for Genetic Medicine, Johns Hopkins University, Baltimore MD, and National Center for Biotechnology Information, National Library of Medicine, Bethesda, MD, 2000 URL: http://www.ncbi.nlm.nih.gov/omim/.
46. Peltola KE, Nanto-Salonen K, Heinonen OJ, Jaaskelainen S, Heinanen K, Simell O, Nikoskelainen E. Ophthalmologic heterogeneity in subjects with gyrate atrophy of choroid and retina harboring the L402P mutation of ornithine aminotransferase. Ophthalmology 2001; 108(4):721–729.
47. Peltonen L, Jalanko A, Varilo T. Molecular genetics of the Finnish disease heritage. Hum Mol Genet. 1999; 8(10):1913–1923.
48. Ramesh V, McClatchey AI, Ramesh N, et al. Molecular basis of ornithine aminotransferase deficiency in B_6 responsive and non-responsive forms of gyrate atrophy. Proc Natl Acad Sci USA 1988; 85:3777–3780.
49. Kaiser-Kupfer MI, de Monasterio FM, Valle D, et al. Gyrate atrophy of the choroid and retina: improved visual function following reduction of plasma ornithine by diet. Science 1980; 210:1128–1131.

50. Kaiser-Kupfer MI, de Monasterio F, Valle O, et al. Visual results of a long-term trial of a low-arginine diet in gyrate atrophy of choroid and retina. Ophthalmology 1981; 88:307–310.
51. Vannas-Sulonen K, Simell O, Sipil AI. Gyrate atrophy of the choroid and retina. The ocular disease progresses in juvenile patients despite normal or near normal plasma ornithine concentration. Ophthalmology 1987; 94:1428–1433.
52. Kaiser-Kupfer MI, Caruso RC, Valle D. Gyrate atrophy of the choroid and retina. Long-term reduction of ornithine slows retinal degeneration. Arch Ophthalmol 1991; 109(11):1539–1548.
53. Kaiser-Kupfer MI, Caruso RC, Valle D. Gyrate atrophy of the choroid and retina: further experience with long-term reduction of ornithine levels in children. Arch Ophthalmol. 2002; 120(2):146–153.
54. Elpeleg N, Korman SH. Sustained oral lysine supplementation in ornithine delta-aminotransferase deficiency. J Inherit Metab Dis. 2001; 24(3):423–424.
55. Peltola K, Heinonen OJ, Nanto-Salonen K, Pulkki K, Simell O. Oral lysine feeding in gyrate atrophy with hyperornithinaemia—a pilot study. J Inherit Metab Dis. 2000; 23(4):305–307.
56. Vannas-Sulonen K, Sipila I, Vannas A et al. Gyrate atrophy of the choroid and retina: a five year follow up of creatine supplementation. Ophthalmology 1985; 92:1719–1727.
57. O'Donnell JJ, Sipila I, Vannas A et al. Gyrate atrophy of the retina and choroid: two methods for prenatal diagnosis. Int Ophthalmol 1981; 4:33–36.
58. Mashima YG, Weleber RG, Kennaway NG, Inana G. Genotype-phenotype correlation of a pyridoxine-responsive form of gyrate atrophy. Ophthalmic Genet 1999; 20(4): 219–224.
59. Roschinger W, Endres W, Shin YS. Characteristics of L-ornithine: 2-oxoacid amino-transferase and potential prenatal diagnosis of gyrate atrophy of the choroid and retina by first trimester chorionic villus sampling. Clin Chim Acta. 2000; 296(1–2):91–100.
60. McCulloch C, McCulloch RJP. A hereditary and clinical study of choroideremia. Trans Am Acad Ophthalmol Otolaryngol 1948; 52:160–196.
61. McCulloch C. Choroideremia: a clinical and pathologic review. Trans Am Ophthalmol Soc 1969; 67:142–195.
62. Krill AE, Archer D. Classification of the choroidal atrophies. Am J Ophthalmol 1971; 72:562–585.
63. Rubin ML, Fishman RS, McKay RA. Choroideremia: study of a family and literature review. Arch Ophthalmol 1966; 76:563–574.
64. Karna J. Choroideremia A clinical and genetic study of 84 Finnish patients and 126 female carriers. Acta Ophthalmol Suppl 1986; 176:1–68.
65. Sieving PA, Niffeneggere JH, Berson EL. Electroretinographic findings in selected pedigrees with choroideremia. Am J Ophthalmol 1986; 101:361–367.
66. Fulton AB, Hansen RM. The relation of rhodopsin and scotopic sensitivity in choroideremia. Am J Ophthalmol 1987; 104:524–532.
67. Cheung MC, Nune GC, Wang M, McTaggart KE, MacDonald IM, Duncan JL. Detection of localized retinal dysfunction in a choroideremia carrier.. Am J Ophthalmol 2004; 137(1):189–191.
68. Grover S, Alexander KR, Choi DM, Fishman GA. Intraocular light scatter in patients with choroideremia. Ophthalmology 1998; 105(9):1641–1645.
69. Robinson D, Tiedeman J. Choroideremia associated with a subretinal neovascular membrane. Case report. Retina 1987; 7:70–74.
70. Rosenberg T, Schwartz M, Niebuhr E et al. Choroideremia in interstitial deletion of the X chromosome. Ophthalmic Paediatr Genet 1986; 7:205–210.
71. Hodgson SV, Robertson ME, Fear CN et al. Prenatal diagnosis of X-Iinked choroideremia with mental retardation, associated with a cytologicaily detectable X-chromosome deletion. Hum Genet 1987; 75:286–290.

72. Rosenburg T, Niebuhr E, Yang HM, et al. Choroideremia, congenital deafness and mental retardation in a family with an X chromosomal deletion. Ophthalmic Paediatr Genet 1987; 8:139–143.
73. Nussbaum RL, Lesko JG, Lewis RA, et al. Isolation of anonymous DNA sequences from within a submicroscopic X chromosomal deletion in a patient with choroideremia, deafness, and mental retardation. Proc Natl Acad Sci USA 1987; 84:6521–6525.
74. Schwartz M, Yang HM, Niebuhr E, et al. Regional localization of polymorphic DNA loci on the proximal long arm of the X chromosome using deletions associated with choroideremia. Hum Genet 1988; 78:156–160.
75. Ayazi S. Choroideremia, obesity, and congenital deafness. Am J Ophthalmol 1981; 92:63–69.
76. Judisch GF, Lowry RB, Hanson JW, McGillivary BC. Chorioretinopathy and pituitary dysfunction. The CPD syndrome. Arch Ophthalmol 1981; 99:253–356.
77. MacDonald IM, Mah DY, Ho YK, Lewis RA, Seabra MC. A practical diagnostic test for choroideremia. Ophthalmology. 1998; 105(9):1637–1640.
78. Cameron JD, Fine BS, Shapiro I. Histopathologic observations in choroideremia with emphasis on vascular changes of the uveal tract. Ophthalmol 1981; 99:187–196.
79. Syed N, Smith JE, John SK, Seabra MC, Aguirre GD, Milam AH. Evaluation of retinal photoreceptors and pigment epithelium in a female carrier of choroideremia. Ophthalmology. 2001; 108(4):711–720.
80. Flannery JG, Bird AC, Farber DB, Weleber RG, Bok D. A histopathologic study of a choroideremia carrier. Invest Ophthalmol Vis 1990; 31(2):229–236.
81. MacDonald IM, Chen MH, Addison DJ, Mielke BW, Nesslinger NJ. Histopathology of the retinal pigment epithelium of a female carrier of choroideremia. Can J Ophthalmol 1997; 32(5):329–333.
82. Rodrigues MM, Ballantine EJ, Wiggert BB, et al. Choroideremia: clinical electron microscopic and biochemical report. Ophthalmology 1984; 91:873–883.
83. Nussbaum RL, Lewis RA, Lesko JG, Ferrel R. Choroideremia is linked to the restriction fragment length polymorphism *DXYSI* at Xq13-21. Am J Hum Genet 1985; 37:473–481.
84. Lewis RA, Nussbaum RL, Ferrell R. Mapping X-linked ophthalmic diseases: provisional assignment of the locus for choroideremia to Xq13-q24. Ophthalmology 1985; 92:800–806.
85. Jay M, Wright AF, Clayton JF, et al. A genetic linkage study of choroideremia. Ophthalmic Paediatr Genet 1986; 7:201–204.
86. Gal A, Brunsmann F, Hogenkamp D, et al. Choroideremia-locus maps between *DXS3* and *DXS11* on Xq. Hum Genet 1986; 73:123–126.
87. Lesko JG, Lewis RA, Nussbaum RL. Multipoint linkage analysis of loci in the proximal long arm of the human X chromosome: application to mapping the choroideremia locus. Am J Hum Genet 1987; 40:303–311.
88. MacDonald IM, Sandre RM, Hunter AG, Tenniswood MP. Gene mapping of X-linked choroideremia with restriction fragment-length polymorpisms. Can J Ophthalmol 1987; 22:310–315.
89. MacDonald IM, Sandre RM, Wong P, et al. Linkage relationships of X-linked choroideremia to *DXS1* and *DXS3*. Hum Genet 1987; 77:235–235.
90. Sankila EM, de la Chapelle A, Karna J, et al. Choroideremia: close linkage to *DXYS1* and *DXYS12* demonstrated by segregation analysis and historical-genealogical evidence. Clin Genet 1987; 31:315–322.
91. Schwartz M, Rosenberg T, Niebuhr E, et al. Choroideremia: further evidence for assignment of the locus to Xql3-Xq21. Hum Genet 1986; 74:449–452.
92. Cremers FP, Brunsmann F, van de Pol TJ, et al. Deletion of the *DSI65* locus in patients with classical choroideremia. Clin Genet 1987; 32:421–423.

93. Cremers FP, van de Pol DJ, Diergaarde PJ, et al. Physical fine mapping of the choroideremia locus using Xq21 deletions associated with complex syndromes. Genomics 1989; 4:41–46.
94. Cremers FP, van de Pol DJ, van Kerkhoff LP, Wieringa B, Ropers HH. Cloning of a gene that is rearranged in patients with choroideraemia. Nature 1990; 347(6294):674–677.
95. Merry DE, Janne PA, Landers JE, Lewis RA, Nussbaum RL. Isolation of a candidate gene for choroideremia. Proc Nat Acad Sci USA 1992; 89(6):2135–2139.
96. van Bokhoven H, van den Hurk JA, Bogerd L, Philippe C, Gilgenkrantz S, de Jong P, Ropers HH, Cremers FP. Cloning and characterization of the human choroideremia gene. Hum Mol Genet 1994; 3(7):1041–1046.
97. Seabra MC. New insights into the pathogenesis of choroideremia: a tale of two REPs. Ophthalmic Genet 1996; 17(2):43–6.
98. van den Hurk JA, Schwartz M, van Bokhoven H, van de Pol TJ, Bogerd L, Pinckers AJ, Bleeker-Wagermakers EM, Pawlowitzki IH, Ruther K, Ropers HH, Cremers FP. Molecular basis of choroideremia (CHM): mutations involving the Rab escort protein-1 (REP-1) gene. Hum Mutat 1997; 9(2):110–117.
99. Ponjavic V, Abrahamson M, Andreasson S, Van Bokhoven H, Cremers FP, Ehinger B, Fex G. Phenotype variations within a choroideremia family lacking the entire CHM gene. Ophthalmic Genet 1995; 16(4):143–150.
100. van Bokhoven H, Schwartz M, Andreasson S, van den Hurk JA, Bogerd L, Jay M, Ruther K, Jay B, Pawlowitzki IH, Sankila EM, et al. Mutation spectrum in the CHM gene of Danish and Swedish choroideremia patients. Hum Mol Genet 1994; 3(7):1047–1051.
101. Nesslinger N, Mitchell G, Strasberg P, MacDonald IM. Mutation analysis in Canadian families with choroideremia. Ophthalmic Genet 1996; 17(2):47–52.
102. McTaggart KE, Tran M, Mah DY, Lai SW, Nesslinger NJ, MacDonald IM. Mutational analysis of patients with the diagnosis of choroideremia. Hum Mutat 2002; 20(3):189–196.
103. Tolmachova T, Ramalho JS, Anant JS, Schultz RA, Huxley CM, Seabra MC. Cloning, mapping and characterization of the human RAB27A gene. Gene 1999; 239(1):109–116.
104. Anand V, Barral DC, Zheng Y, Brunsmann F, Maguire AM, Seabra MC, Bennett J. Gene therapy for choroideremia: in vitro rescue mediated by recombinant adenovirus. Vision Res 2003; 43(8):919–926.
105. van den Hurk JA, van Zandvoort PM, Brunsmann F, Pawlowitzki IH, Holzgreve W, Szabo P, Cremers FP, van Oost BA. Prenatal exclusion of choroideremia. Am J Med Genet 1992; 44(6):822–823.
106. Carr RE, Mittl RN, Noble KG. Choroidal abiotrophies. Trans Am Acad Ophthalmol Otolaryngol 1975; 79:796–816.
107. Hayasaka S, Shoji K, Kanno C, et al. Differential diagnosis of choroidal atrophies: Diffuse choriocapillary atrophy, choroideremia and gyrate atrophy of the choroid and retina. Retina 1985; 5:30–37.
108. Waardenburg PJ. Angio-sclerose familiale de la choroide. J Genet Hum 1952; 1:83–93.
109. Sorsby A, Crick RP. Central areolar choroidal sclerosis. Br J Ophthalmol 1953; 37:129–139.
110. Takki K. Differential diagnosis between the primary total choroidal vascular atrophies. Br J Ophthalmol 1974; 58:24–35.
111. Weiter J, Fine BS. A histologic study of regional choroidal dystrophy. Am J Ophthalmol 1977; 83:741–750.
112. Sveinsson K. Helicoidal peripapillary chorioretinal degeneration. Acta Ophthalmol 1979; 57(1):69–75.
113. Brazitikos PD, Safran AB. Helicoid peripapillary chorioretinal degeneration. Am J Ophthalmol 1990; 109(3):290–294.

114. Eysteinsson T, Jonasson F, Jonsson V, Bird AC. Helicoidal peripapillary chorioretinal degeneration: electrophysiology and psychophysics in 17 patients. Br J Ophthalmol 1998; 82(3):280–285.
115. Fossdal R, Magnusson L, Weber JL, Jensson O. Mapping the locus of atrophia areata, a helicoid periapillary chorioretinal degeneration with autosomal dominant inheritance, to chromosome 11p15. Hum Mol Genet 1995; 4(3):479–483.
116. Tyni T, Kivela T, Lappi M, Summanen P, Nikoskelainen E, Pihko H. Ophthalmologic findings in long-chain 3-hydroxyacyl-CoA dehydrogenase deficiency caused by the G1528C mutation: a new type of hereditary metabolic chorioretinopathy. Ophthalmol 1998; 105(5):810–824.
117. Ijlst L, Ruiter JP, Hoovers JM, Jakobs ME, Wanders RJ. Common missense mutation G1528C in long-chain 3-hydroxyacyl-CoA dehydrogenase deficiency. Characterization and expression of the mutant protein, mutation analysis on genomic DNA and chromosomal localization of the mitochondrial trifunctional protein alpha subunit gene. J Clin Invest 1996; 98(4):1028–1033.

15
Night Vision Disorders

INTRODUCTION

Decreased night vision, usually referred to as night blindness or nyctalopia, comprises conditions in which the rod vision mechanism is absent or subnormal. There is no parallel involvement of the cone vision mechanism. Nyctalopia is probably the preferred term, as many patients are not necessarily "night-blind," (although this Greek term means not seeing at night: *nycta*, night; *al*, no; *opia*, vision).

Nyctalopia generally stems from one of five groups of disorders. First, it may result from a nutritional factor, such as vitamin A deficiency (1) and acquired or inherited visceral and gastrointestinal diseases (2). Vitamin A deficiency leads to decreased amounts of rhodopsin, with subsequent deterioration of night vision and reduced electric activity of the retina (3). Second, nyctalopia can result from inherited retinal dystrophies that primarily affect the rod system. Some acquired conditions such as chloroquine retinopathy may mimic these conditions by affecting the rod visual system. Third, decreased night vision can be related to the physiologic process of aging (4). Fourth, other ocular disorders can reduce night vision by the selective involvement of the rod system, for example, myopia (5) and some cases of glaucoma with visual field loss. Fifth, congenitally inherited disorders of scotopic vision, which are discussed in this chapter, affect the largest group of patients living in developed countries without serious malnutrition problems. They suffer from severe reduction or total absence of night vision.

The inherited disorder of night vision has been known since 1830, when the Belgian ophthalmologist Cunier described night blindness that affected "Jean Nougaret, the butcher from Provence, and his family." Nyctalopia had been transmitted by an autosomal dominant mode, and the pedigree has been reported several times (6). Later, Donders (7) and Nettleship (8) demonstrated night blindness transmitted by the X-linked mode and linked to myopia.

Congenital stationary night blindness (CSNB) was the term used by Nettleship (9) and later by Carr (10) for one group of night vision disorders. The term stresses the two common characteristics of this group: the occurrence at birth and the stationary nature. This chapter will use the terms CSNB, congenital stationary night blindness and congenital nyctalopia synonymously.

Congenital nyctalopia consists of distinct genetic and clinical entities sharing a severe congenital and inherited reduction in night vision. These entities vary by clinical appearance, pathophysiology, and mode of inheritance. The heterogeneity of this disorder was confirmed in the 1990s with the identification of several mutated genes linked to CSNB.

The identification in the last decade of several genes which, when mutated, are associated with CSNB, confirmed the heterogeneity of this disorder.

In this chapter, CSNB will be classified into two large groups. CSNB with normal fundi (with or without high myopia) and CSNB with abnormal fundi. These groups will be subdivided by the mode of genetic transmission and then each distinct genetic and/or clinical entity will be described.

In all cases of CSNB, the scotopic function of the eye (night vision) is impaired. However, the distinct entities vary as to the degree of scotopic function loss, the involvement of the cones, and the pathophysiology of the dark adaptation and electroretinography.

Usually, it is easy to distinguish between CSNB and retinal dystrophies or acquired diseases. However, difficulties arise with the differential diagnosis of fundus albipunctatus between rare cases of vitamin A deficiency (11,12) and a progressive form of retinal dystrophy, retinitis punctata albescens (13). Also problematic may be the distinction between CSNB with normal fundi or CSNB with high myopia and certain cases of reduced night vision secondary to myopia.

CONGENITAL STATIONARY NIGHT BLINDNESS WITH NORMAL FUNDI

Description and Clinical Findings

Congenital nyctalopia with normal fundi can be detected in early childhood, through symptoms such as a child expressing fear when room lights are turned out at night. Not infrequently, an affected person will be unaware of the handicap until much later in life because modern life does not provide many opportunities for the use of scotopic vision. In many patients, the disorder is detected when they attempt to drive at night, serve in the army, or during summer camp activities. It is strictly a functional disorder. It predominantly affects night vision, although photopic vision may also exhibit other minor symptoms, such as disturbance in color vision. No physical abnormalities are related to this disorder, in sharp contrast with individuals with nyctalopia and high myopia or those with nyctalopia and abnormal fundi.

Because CSNB with normal fundi is often familial, apprehensive parents usually recognize the condition early in their offspring. Two modes of inheritance have been described, autosomal dominant and autosomal recessive.

Diagnosis and Laboratory Findings

Congenital nyctalopia with normal fundi is diagnosed by the results of laboratory tests, which also provide insight into the pathophysiology of night vision disorders.

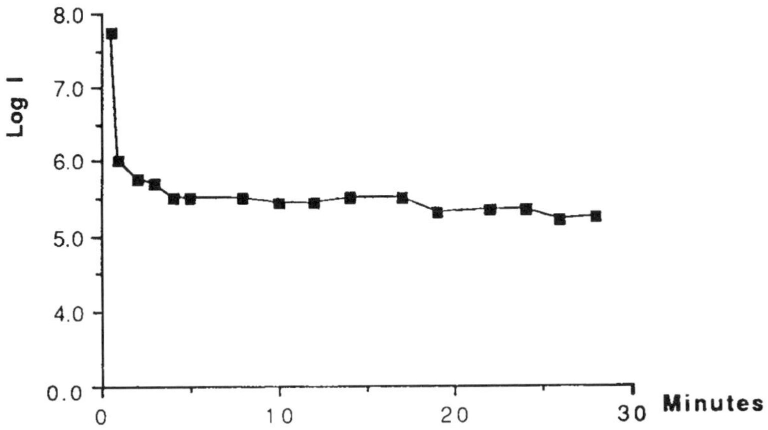

Figure 1 The dark adaptation curve of a patient with congenital nyctalopia and normal fundi: the monophasic curve has a cone level slightly higher than normal. There is no further decrease in threshold with time. No cone–rod transition is apparent. Log I indicates the light intensity in logarithmic units. The abscissa indicates the time in darkness.

Dark Adaptation Curves

The psychophysical test of dark adaptation reveals a monophasic curve (10) or a biphasic curve, with a delayed cone–rod transition and a highly raised rod threshold (14) (Fig. 1). Photopic visual mechanisms are also somewhat subnormal (14), manifested by slower-than-normal and elevated cone thresholds (15). The cone threshold curve was elevated in one patient with autosomal dominant CSNB 0.5 log unit over the normal cone threshold and 3 log units over the normal rod threshold (10). There is no change with prolonged adaptation time. Miyake and coworkers (16–18) have suggested a separation between complete types, in which the dark adaptation curve is monophasic and elevated above normal cone thresholds, and incomplete types, in which a cone–rod transition and some rod function can be documented.

Electroretinography

Auerbach and coworkers (14) identified two electroretinographic (ERG) responses in a large group of 95 patients with various types of congenital nyctalopia. The first response was originally described by Schubert and Bornschein (19); it consisted of a normal or almost normal a-wave and a small or absent b-wave (Fig. 2). The second response, originally described by Riggs (20), was a small negative and a small positive wave (Fig. 3). In most patients who exhibited the first response (43 of 59), the b-wave initially increased during dark adaptation, but later decreased owing to increased implicit time. In the others, the b-wave was small, increasing somewhat later in darkness, or was completely absent (10). The implicit times of both the a- and b-waves were slower than normal, and flicker fusion frequencies were decreased, indicating subnormal cone vision (15).

Ruether and associates (21) demonstrated that three different ERG responses exist in CSNB. The first, "complete Schubert–Bornschein," shows no rod b-wave, a negative ERG, and variable cone responses. The second, "incomplete Schubert–Bornschein," manifests an attenuated rod b-wave, a negative ERG and reduced cone

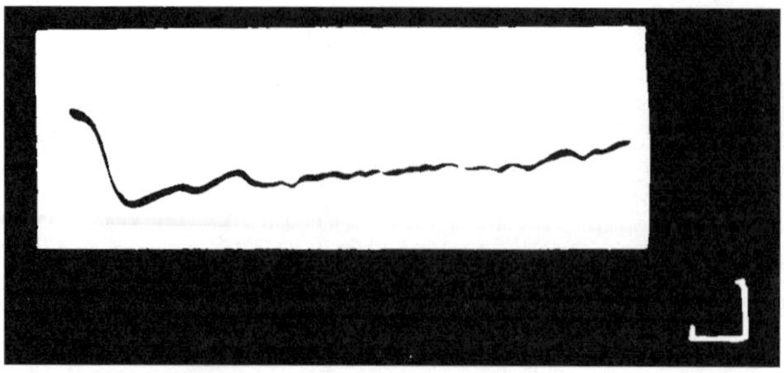

Figure 2 The Schubert–Bornschein-type ERG: Note the normal-sized a-wave and small b-wave. The patient was dark adapted for 30 min. The vertical line indicates 100 μV, the horizontal line 25 msec.

potentials. The third, Riggs type, demonstrates reduced cone and rod amplitudes. The reduced or absent a-wave of the Riggs-type ERG is evidence that the rod photoreceptors are defective, while the reduced or absent b-wave of the Schubert–Bomschein-type ERG is evidence that the synaptic connections of the bipolar cells are defective (22).

Electro-Oculography

The electro-oculogram (EOG), or the light peak/dark trough ratio of the standing potential may be normal or abnormal in CSNB with normal fundi. It was very subnormal in one autosomal dominant patient with a Riggs-type ERG, and normal in an autosomal recessive patient with a Schubert–Bornschein-type ERG (23). The EOG is unrelated to the complete loss of night vision; some patients with the complete and others with the incomplete forms had both normal and abnormal EOGs (16).

Spectral Sensitivity Curves

Spectral sensitivity curves performed on patients with congenital nyctalopia with normal fundi showed a maximal luminous efficiency in some cases during dark adaptation at 555–570 nm without a Purkinje shift (14,24). In other cases, a shift toward 500–510 nm was noted (10,14).

Reflectometry and Rhodopsin Regeneration

Reflectometry or densitometry is a laboratory test for rhodopsin regeneration not yet routinely used for patients with nyctalopia. It was introduced by Ripps and Weale

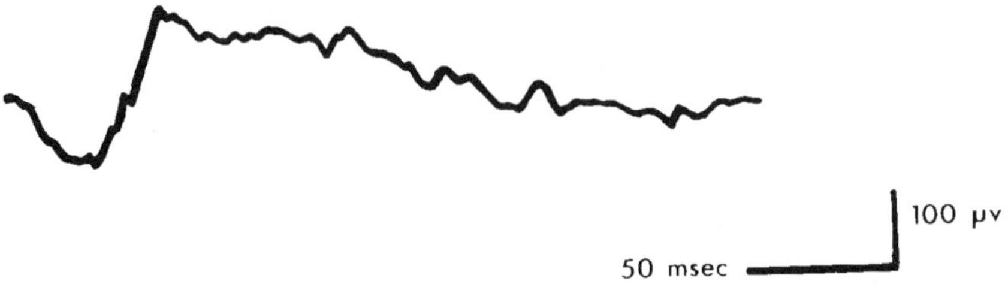

Figure 3 The Riggs–type ERG: Note a- and b-waves are small. The patient was dark adapted for 30 min.

(25) and then extensively studied by Ripps, Carr, and Siegel in patients with congenital nyctalopia. Light of different spectral wavelengths is emitted into the eye and measured on its exit. This light traverses the retina twice, and is partially absorbed by the pigment epithelium and visual pigments. A comparison of measurements after the visual pigment is bleached by a strong light with those of dark-adapted visual pigments indicate the amount of visual pigment present. The kinetics of visual pigment regeneration can also be established through proper timing of measurements (25). Such tests show that for cases of CSNB with normal fundi, rhodopsin has normal concentration, spectral position, and kinetics of regeneration (10) (Fig. 4).

Pathology and Pathogenesis

No abnormalities have been detected in two studies on eyes of patients with CSNB and normal fundi. Babel examined histologically the eye of a patient with autosomal dominant CSNB found a slightly weak staining of the outer segments of the photoreceptors, but summarized it as normal (26). Vaghefi and coworkers detected a normal proportion of rods and cones and a normal pattern of outer segments by light microscopic examination of an eye from a patient with multiple ocular disorders, including CSNB (27).

Our understanding of the pathogenesis improved enormously with the identification of several genes responsible for CSNB. This will be discussed with the distinct entities. However, some generalizations will be discussed here. Based on previous results of physiologic tests and reflectometry, some suggestions have been made to explain the two types of ERG responses. For the autosomal dominant type, with very attenuated or absent ERG a- and b-waves, Carr has proposed an abnormality at the level of the inner segments of the photoreceptor (10). Siegel and colleagues studied a patient with CSNB of the Schubert–Bornschein type transmitted as an autosomal recessive trait and concluded that the absence of rod–cone interaction, together

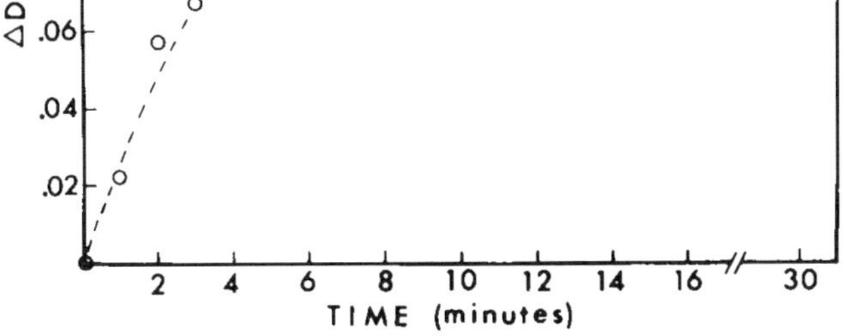

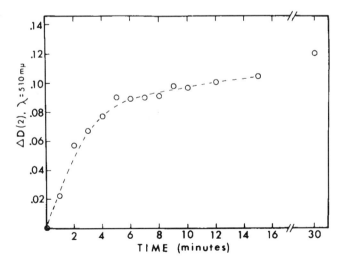

Figure 4 Results of reflectometry indicating normal regeneration of rhodopsin in a patient with congenital nyctalopia and normal fundi: The measured wavelength was 510 nm. Light traversed the retina twice (from Ref. 10).

with an absent scotopic b-wave, implies that the defect is in the midretinal layers and that the interplexiform cell may be involved in some manner (28). The presence of normal rhodopsin, with such a subnormal or absent ERG response, led Ripps to hypothesize that an inherited enzymatic defect may be causing an abnormal excitability of the photoreceptor, along with an inability to transfer the photic impulse into electrical energy (29). Ripps and associates (30) believe that patients with autosomal recessive CSNB and normal fundi have a condition similar to vincristine-induced night blindness, because the responses on ERG (normal a-wave, very subnormal b-wave) and the presence of normal rhodopsin occur in both. Vincristine interferes with the renewal system in the microtubules affecting the synaptic transmission at the proximal end of the photoreceptors (29,30). Thus, the mechanism for the first response is that of abnormal transduction and, in the second, abnormal transmission (29).

Animal Models

Very different animal models serve for human congenital nyctalopia with normal fundi. Under photopic conditions, the Appaloosa horse shows a normal a-wave and a reduced b-wave of longer than normal implicit time. Under scotopic conditions, the negative a-wave and normal c-wave are seen, but the b-wave is unrecordable (31). Histologically, no structural abnormality has been detected. The presence of a c-wave in the dark-adapted state also indicates normally functioning rods and a normal rod–retinal pigment epithelium relationship (29). Another animal model is the pearl mutant mouse, which has reduced sensitivity to light under dark-adapted conditions, a normal ERG a-wave, normal photoreceptors, and normal concentration of visual pigment (32). However, it also shows a hypopigmented retinal pigment epithelium and reduced ipsilateral retinofugal projections, as observed in albinos. The mouse may be a better model for CSNB with high myopia.

Other animal models for CSNB were also reported. The Briard dog suffers from an autosomal recessive congenital stationary night blindness with an ERG resembling Riggs type (33). Zhang and associates (34) reported a rat model with X-linked CSNB, a significantly reduced b-wave with a normal a-wave and reduced cone ERGs. Gregg et al. (35) identified the mutation (an 85 bp deletion) in the mouse nyx gene of a mutant mouse named nob (for no b-wave). Thus, the nob mouse is a model for human CSNB1 associated with a Schubert–Bornschein ERG (little or no b-wave) and NYX gene mutations.

Autosomal Dominant CSNB

Several distinct clinical and genetic entities comprise this subtype of CSNB with normal fundi. Table 1 summarizes the main clinical and genetic varieties of autosomal dominant (AD) CSNB.

In a large study, Auerbach and coworkers found no relationship between the type of ERG response and the mode of hereditary transmission (14). Some families with AD congenital nyctalopia had a Schubert–Bornschein-type ERG, whereas other families had a Riggs-type ERG. No family had both types of responses confirmed (14). Similarly, Miyake and associates have found no families displaying more than one form (complete or incomplete) (16).

Table 1 Clinical and Genetic Varieties of AD-CSNB

Clinical type	Gene	Chromosomal location	Mutation(s)	ERG	Dark adaptation
1 Nougaret	GNAT1	3p21.31	Gly38Asp	Riggs	Monophasic cones: normal or reduced
2 CSNB/Rambusch	PDE6B	4p16.3	His258Asn	Riggs	Monophasic cones: normal or reduced
3 CSNB-rhodopsin linked	RHO	3q21–q24	Gly90Asp, Ala292Glu, Thr94lle	Riggs	Rod sensitivity reduced by 2–3 log-units, cones normal

Note: AD—autosomal dominant; CNSB—congenital stationary night blindness. Other entities may exist.

The Nougaret Type of CSNB and the GNATl gene

The best known of the autosomal dominant type of CSNB with normal fundi is the Nougaret type. Affected patients are emmetropic and have normal visual acuity. The fewer affected vs. unaffected identified in this family (136/246) (6) may reflect that some members were not historically known to be affected, although, in fact, they were. The Riggs-type ERG has a small a-wave and photopic b-wave (36).

The dark adaptation curve is monophasic, and the EOG is normal (36). Another family, reported by Francois as not belonging to the Nougaret family, had similar findings, but larger Riggs-type ERG responses (37). The cone vision was far more affected than in the Nougaret type. It may be, but most likely is not, the same genetic entity in the two families. In the dominant cases described by Carr and coworkers, the ERG was the Riggs type, with very small a- and b-waves; the EOG was subnormal [130%]; rod vision was completely absent; and cone threshold was elevated (23,38,39).

The rod function is present in Nougaret-type CSNB but it is very subnormal and the cone function is also slightly impaired (40). Patients may have no rod a-wave response (41).

Dryja and associates (41) identified a missense mutation in the gene encoding the alpha subunit of rod transducin. The gene guanine nucleotide-binding protein, alpha-transducing activity polypeptide 1 (GNATl) was mapped to chromosome 3p21.31 (42). Only one disease-bearing mutation was identified. This was a Gly38Asp missense mutation, identified in descendants of Jean Nougaret (40,41). The alpha subunit of transducin is involved in the second step of the rod photoreceptor transduction cascade. It is a G-protein that couples rhodopsin with GDP to create GTP, with phosphodiesterase (PDE) as the catalyst (41,43). The mutant transducin fails to bind the inhibitory PDE-gamma subunit in order to activate the enzyme.

These findings confirm that the pathogenic defect of the Nougaret type of CSNB lies within the rod photoreceptor. However, the exact mechanism is not clear. Dryja (22) pointed out that being heterozygous, Nougaret-type patients should have about half of their alpha-type transducin functional. It is not clear, therefore, why about 99% of this transducin becomes nonfunctional.

CSNB Type 3 and the PDE6B Gene

In 1909 Sigurd Rambusch described a large Danish family with CSNB. Rosenberg and associates followed up this family in 1990 and reconstructed the family pedigree (44) (Fig. 5). This type became known as Rambusch type or CSNB type 3. The transmission is autosomal dominant, seemingly with full penetrance. However, in the family reported by Rosenberg et al. (44), the female patients had a typical CSNB in one eye and were practically normal in the other eye. Rod function was very abnormal and the ERG was of Riggs type, but rod responses could be seen.

In 1993, McLaughlin and coworkers reported the second human locus for autosomal recessive retinitis pigmentosa (ARRP) (45). They reported several different mutations in the gene encoding the beta subunit of rod CGMP PDE (45). In 1994 Gal and colleagues (46,47) identified a heterozygous missense mutation, His258Asn, linked to CSNB in the same gene. The gene PDE6B encodes a retinal rod photoreceptor-specific cGMP phosphodiesterase 6B and maps to the chromosome 4pl6.3 (46).

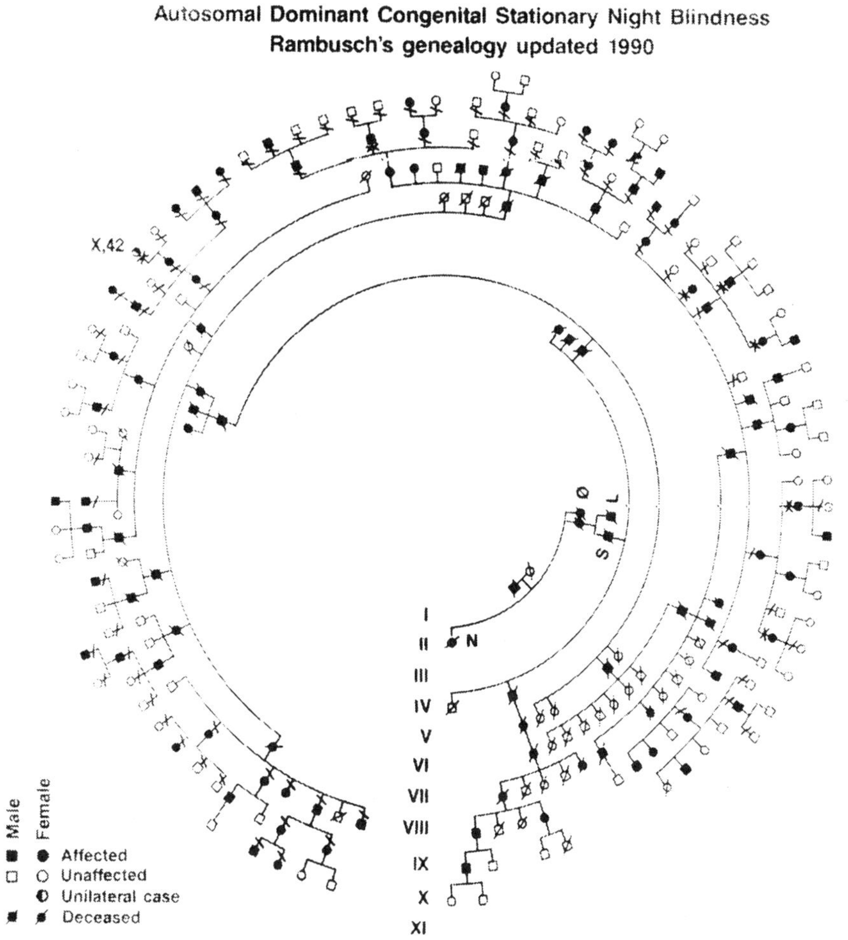

Figure 5 Congenital Stationary Night Blindness type 3: This large family was studied by Rambusch and reconstructed by Rosenberg et al. (by permission; from Rosenberg et al. Ref. 44).

It is not known how or why this mutation leading to 50% reduction in phosphodiesterase interferes with the phototransduction cascade to desensitize the rods and reduce their sensitivity by approximately 1000 times (3 log units) (22).

CSNB and the Rhodopsin Gene

In 1993, Dryja and associates (48) identified heterozygous missense mutations in the rhodopsin gene associated with AD-CSNB. The mutation Ala292Glu was found to cause complete loss of rod function. The ERG was of the Riggs type without a- or b-wave rod response (48). Additional mutations were identified later by other investigators. These included Gly90Asp (49,50) and Thr94Ile (51).

The associated night blindness does not worsen with age. Patients have normal visual acuity, full visual fields, and normal fundi (22). Their scotopic threshold is 2–3 log units above normal, rhodopsin density is normal, and so is cone function (50).

All investigators (22,48–51) speculated that the night blindness is associated with the abnormal continuous activation of transducin by the mutated opsin protein after it releases its chromophore.

Other AD-CSNB

It is not clear whether other entities of AD-CSNB really exist. Auerbach and coworkers (14) described AD nyctalopia with a Schubert–Bornschein-type of ERG. However, this has not been found in other families.

Autosomal Recessive CSNB

No genes responsible for autosomal recessive congenital stationary night blindness have yet been identified. However, there is no doubt that such entities exist.

Patients with autosomal recessive CSNB with normal fundi, usually have a Schubert–Bornschein ERG, as described by Armington and Schwab (24). The a-wave is normal, the b-wave is very subnormal, the EOG is normal, and the scotopic functions are present although reduced (23,38,39). A second autosomal recessive type, however, must exist, with a Riggs-type ERG response, as originally described in two sisters by Riggs (20), found in several families by Auerbach and associates (14), and described in an "incomplete type" by Miyake and associates (16). The adaptation curve is biphasic, with present, but severely reduced, scotopic vision.

Clinically, autosomal recessive CSNB with high myopia resembles X-linked CSNB with high myopia (52). Merin and associates reported two such families, as compared to 12 families with the X-linked form, in their series (52). (Fig. 6).

X-linked CSNB

Two Subtypes and High Myopia

Miyake and associates (16–18) and Miyake (53) established that there are two types of X-linked CSNB (XL-CSNB): the complete type in which no functional rod activity can be determined and the incomplete type in which rod activity exists to a varying degree. This classification proved to be correct with the identification of two genes on the X-chromosome, which, when mutated, are associated with these two separate entities, now referred to, respectively, as loci CSNB1 and CSNB2.

Most patients with XL-CSNB have myopia varying from moderate to high. CSNB with high myopia is a much more serious disorder than CSNB alone. It merits description. Families have typical X-linked recessive transmission (Fig. 7).

In 32 patients in 25 families, Merin and associates found congenital and stationary nyctalopia (52). Myopia varied from –4.00 to –14.50, was congenital, and usually bilaterally symmetric. Frequently, patients had strabismus (24 of 32), nystagmus (21 of 32), and astigmatism. Visual acuity was reduced in all, ranging from 6/12 to less than 6/60 in the worst eye. The fundus was abnormal in the majority, usually displaying myopic changes such as hypopigmented pigment epithelium, abnormal disc, absent foveal reflex, and pigmentary disturbance in the posterior pole (52). Tilted disks (54) or pale disks (55) have been noted frequently in persons with this syndrome.

The dark adaptation curve is essentially monophasic (52), but a small cone–rod break may be seen at 15 min (10). The initial adaptation to the final cone level is slower than normal, and the final threshold level is above normal (10,52).

The ERG is of the Schubert–Bornschein type, with a normal a-wave and a very reduced b-wave amplitude (10,32), The b-wave implicit time has been normal, in sharp contrast with those of patients with early autosomal recessive retinitis pigmentosa, thereby differentiating the two conditions (56). Under suprathreshold

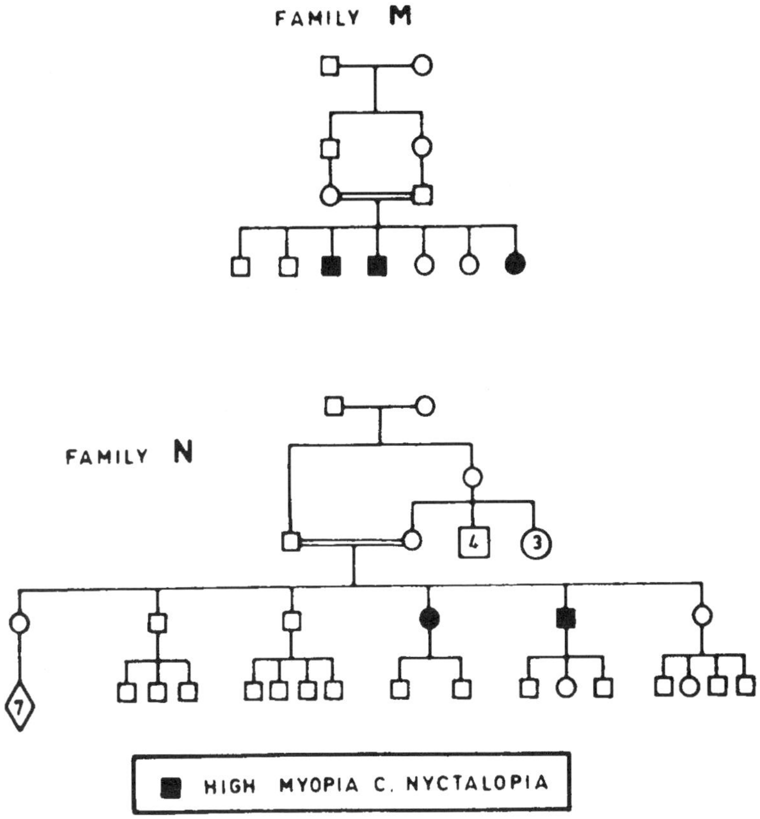

Figure 6 Pedigree of two families with autosomal recessive congenital nyctalopia and high myopia (from Ref. 52).

photopic conditions, the ERG displays decreased b-wave amplitude with preserved normal implicit time (57). The oscillatory potentials were conspicuously absent in all examined patients with CSNB and high myopia (55,57), in contrast with other congenital nyctalopia groups. The amplitudes of the oscillatory potentials were also statistically smaller than normal in one group of 12 female carriers of CSNB with high myopia (58), and in another group of nine female carriers (59). Normal vitreous fluorophotometric values in two patients with X-linked CSNB with myopia (60) indicate normally functioning outer (at the level of the retinal pigment epithelium) and inner (at the level of the retinal vessels) blood-retinal barriers.

The EOG is normal in these patients (10). Difference spectra and regeneration data from reflectometry indicate normal concentrations of rhodopsin, spectral position, and kinetics of regeneration.

Congenital nyctalopia with high myopia occurs in two genetic entities that are clinically very similar and carry a similar prognosis.

Most cases are transmitted by the X-linked recessive mode, a condition well-known since the reports by Donders (7) and the Eisdell pedigree by Nettleship (61). A few have an autosomal recessive inheritance (16,52,62).

All except three reported families with X-linked recessive CSNB also had associated myopia (63). It is possible that in these families the presence of one or more of "hyperopic genes" masks the effect of the myopia.

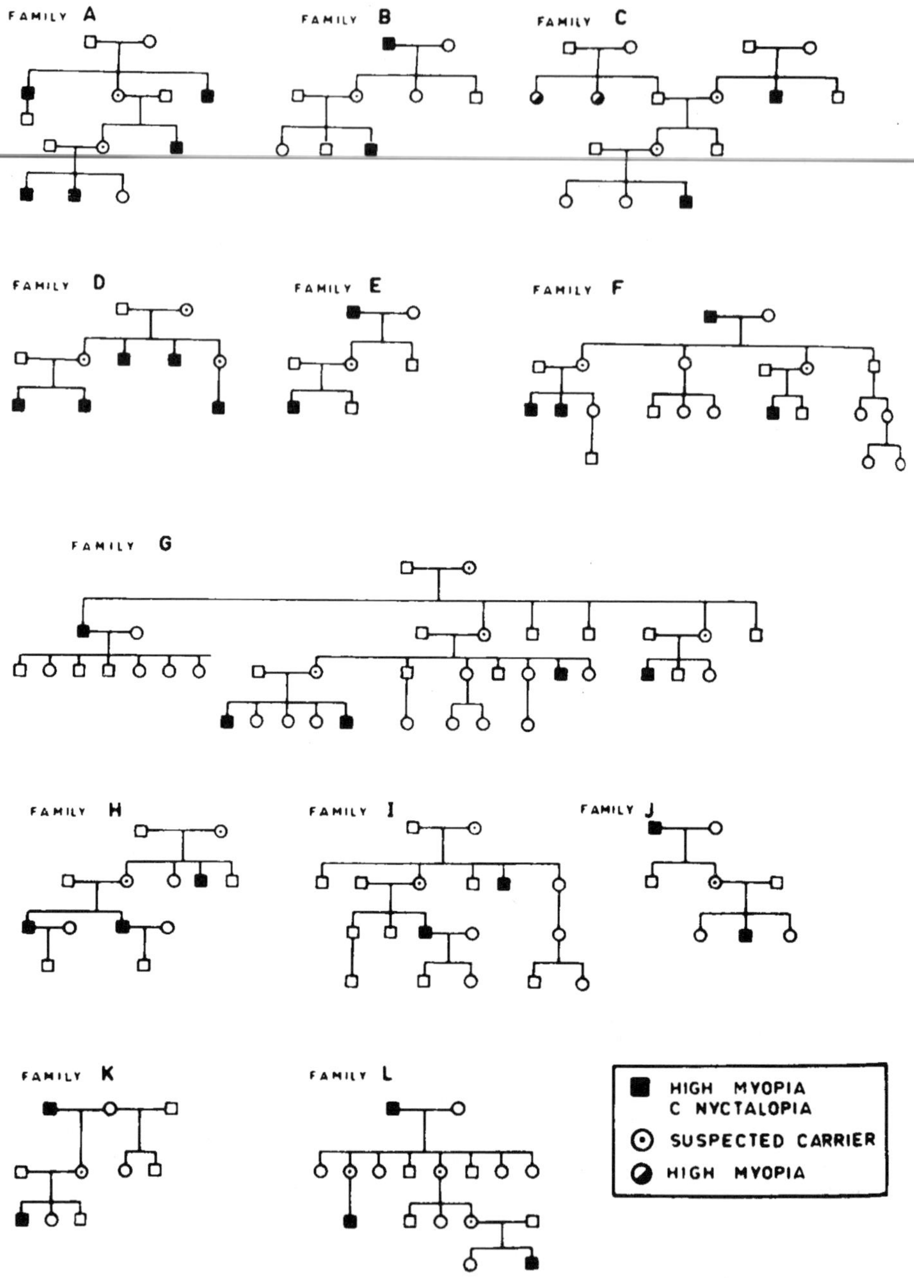

Figure 7 Pedigree of 12 families with X-linked congenital nyctalopia and high myopia (from Ref. 52).

Close linkage without recombination was found between the disease locus and the anonymous locus *DXS7,* mapped to Xp11.3, assigning the mutation to the proximal short arm of the X chromosome (64). Interestingly, this is the same area to which both XLRP and Norrie disease were assigned. This was the first mapping of an XL-CSNB.

CSNB1 and the NYX Gene

In 1989, Musarella and associates identified the linkage of complete XL-CSNB to chromosome Xp11.3 (65). In spite of the confusing intrafamilial variability in the expression of the disorder (66), it became clear that two separate loci for XL-CSNB exist (67). Boycott and coworkers examined 32 families and found 11 with the clinically complete form, now termed CSNB1 locus and mapped to chromosome Xp11.4–p11.3 (67). Nearby was the locus CSNB2 of the clinically incomplete form, with 21 of the 32 families (67). In the year 2000, two groups of investigators identified the gene responsible for the complete type of XL-CSNB as NYX, a new and unique member of the small leucine-rich proteoglycan family (68,69). NYX (for nyctalopin on X-chromosome) encodes a glycosylphosphatidyl-anchored protein called nyctalopin (68). Nyctalopin is expressed in many tissues including retina, brain, testis, and muscle. Many different disease-bearing mutations were identified in the NYX gene (68,69). Nyctalopin, a polypeptide of 481 amino acids, is assumed to disrupt the developing retinal interconnections involving the ON bipolar cells (68). Nyctalopin is an extracellular, membrane-bound protein and is functionally conserved in the mouse and in humans (70). Mapping of the NYX gene was later refined to chromosome Xp11.4 (71).

Clinically, the disease is a nonprogressive retinal disorder, manifesting impaired or absent night vision, myopia of variable degree, nystagmus in many cases, and reduced visual acuity (67). The ERG reveals a nonrecordable rod b-wave and the classic Schubert–Bornschein type. Cone responses are usually normal but some loss of cone function may be seen and tests demonstrate a defect of the ON pathway (68). The scotopic oscillatory potentials are absent (72). Studies of families from Germany, Holland, Sweden, Sardinia, and the United Kingdom demonstrated evidence of homogeneity in all families (71).

The female carriers of CSNB1 usually manifest very few abnormalities such as reduced oscillatory potentials in the ERG described above. Bech–Hansen and Pearce described a family in which three daughters demonstrated a disease indistinguishable from that of affected men (73). A study showed that they all were homozygous, carrying a mutated gene on each X-chromosome, both from their affected father and from their carrier mother.

Regarding pathogenesis, Carr suggested the existence of an abnormality in the neural transmission at the proximal end of the photoreceptors or in the bipolar cells (10). This theory was strengthened by its pathophysiologic similarities to vincristine-induced night blindness and to autosomal recessive congenital nyctalopia with normal fundi (29) and also to the paraneoplastic night blindness reported with malignant melanoma (74). It is not clearly known how mutated nyctalopin causes CSNB1 but it is likely associated with the neural transmission either at the bipolar cells–photoreceptors synapsis or along the bipolar cell.

No specific treatment is available. The high myopia is most probably congenital and stationary, like the night blindness. Parents are often more concerned with high myopia than with the night vision disturbance, although the myopia usually does not worsen. Attempts to improve visual acuity by antiamblyopia treatment commonly fail (52). Surgery for strabismus may be performed for cosmesis.

CSNB2 and the CACNA1F Gene

Heterogeneity of X-linked nyctalopia was confirmed by the existence of two clinical types as suggested by Miyake (53) and by the existence of two separate loci on the

Table 2 Clinical and Genetic Varieties of XL-CSNB

Clinical type	Gene	Chromosomal location	Mutation(s)	ERG[a]	Dark adaptation
1 CSNB1/complete	NYX	Xp11.4	Multiple; in most: truncated protein	Rod: undetected; cone: normal or near so; S–B	Monophasic curve
2 CSNB2/incomplete	CACNA1F	Xp11.23	Multiple; in most: truncated protein	Very subnormal rod; subnormal cone S–B	Scotopic threshold elevated 2–3 log units
3 AIED	RPGR(?)	Xp21	—	S–B	Elevated thresholds of rods and cones

[a]S–B Schubert–Bornschein-type of ERG. CSNB–Congenital Stationary Night Blindness. AIED–Åland Island Eye Disease. RPGR(?)–gene not yet identified.

X-chromosome (67). The terms complete and incomplete CSNB are used in regard to the ERG rod b-wave, which is nonrecordable in the complete type and recordable in the incomplete type. Other clinical differences also exist.

In contrast to the scotopic activity, the photopic function is generally more affected in the incomplete form (75). Visual acuity is often reduced and nystagmus and strabismus may be found (22). Scotopic oscillatory potentials were subnormal (they were absent in the complete form) and subnormal OFF responses were recorded (72). The ERG manifests reduced amplitudes in both the scotopic and the photopic functions (76).

Obligate carriers demonstrated few clinical abnormalities. However, a significant reduction in the sum of oscillatory potentials amplitudes was recorded (76).

The locus CSNB2 maps to chromosome Xp11.23 (42). Strom et al. (77) and Bech–Hansen et al. (78) identified CSNB2 associated mutations in a retina specific calcium channel alpha-1 subunit gene (CACNA1F) in the same region. The gene is large and it consists of 48 exons predicted to produce a 1977-amino acid protein (79). A large number of different mutations were identified. Most were predicted to cause premature termination and result in a truncated protein (75,77–79). Most detected mutations were private mutations, meaning that they affected only one single family. Wutz and colleagues (80) identified 30 different mutations in 36 families.

Nakamura and associates (81) described a Japanese family with CSNB type 2 and optic atrophy. The identified mutation was a 4 bp deletion between nucleotides 271 and 274 with an insertion of a 34 bp sequence in the CACNA1F gene.

Åland Island Eye Disease

Aland Island Eye disease (AIED), also named Forsius–Eriksson syndrome, is a congenital nyctalopia associated with high myopia. It has many clinical similarities to the incomplete CSNB form (82,83) except for the accentuation of a diffuse loss of intraocular pigment so that the disorder was sometimes classified with albinism.

The locus was mapped to chromosome Xp21 (82) and it is likely to be the same disorder and the same locus as Oregon eye disease found in Duchenne-type muscular dystrophy (84). The "novel X-linked CSNB" described by Bergen et al. (85) was also mapped to chromosome Xp21. The gene has not yet been identified. However, the location being the same as for RP3 (85) and the gene on this location being the retinitis pigmentosa GTPase regulator (RPGR) suggests that this is the prime candidate gene.

A clinically similar disease, named AIED-like disease was described by Carlson and associates (83). The disorder seems to be similar to AIED but presents somewhat different ERG responses and more cone abnormalities. Wutz and coworkers identified mutations in the CACNA1F gene in two patients with AIED-like disease but not in patients with AIED. This may explain why in some studies the locus for AIED was erroneously linked to chromosome Xp11 (86).

In summary, AIED disease seems to be a separate entity, with a locus at chromosome Xp21, while that disease classified as AIED-like is identical with CSNB2.

CONGENITAL NYCTALOPIA WITH ABNORMAL FUNDI

Fundus albipunctatus, Oguchi's disease, and other rare disorders compose this heterogenous group of CSNB. They have many similarities, especially improved rod visual function after prolonged dark adaptation, but their differences are enough to warrant separate discussions.

Fundus Albipunctatus

In 1910, Lauber accurately indicated that two distinct entities should be differentiated: (1) retinitis punctate albescens, a progressive disease leading to blindness, and (2) fundus albipunctatus cum hemeralopia, a congenital and stationary familial disorder manifesting as night blindness (13), without a progressive decrease of day vision. Lauber reviewed all 30 cases of both conditions reported in the literature and added an additional family with fundus albipunctatus of an autosomal recessive inheritance (13). Actually, a distinction between fundus albipunctatus and vitamin A deficiency (11,12) or oxalate retinopathy (87) should also be made.

Each of these conditions can be distinguished by ophthalmoscopy. In fundus albipunctatus, the multitude of spots start as a ring around the macula, leaving this area unaffected (Fig. 8), and spreading toward the equator. The dots are white, yellowish white, or greyish white, distinct and similarly sized. The fundus appears normal except for the dots. In retinitis punctata albescens, most of the dots are distinct, many are confluent, and they may invade the macular area. Above all, a distinct tapetal reflex, as occurs in the retinal dystrophies, is always present. In vitamin A deficiency, the dots are few and usually located in the retinal periphery. In generalized oxalosis, the spots are somewhat small, irregular, and extend into the posterior pole and macula (88). The dots of fundus albipunctatus are seen deep to the retinal vessels. Although their exact location cannot be determined by slit-lamp examination, they appear to be in the outer neural retina or on the pigment

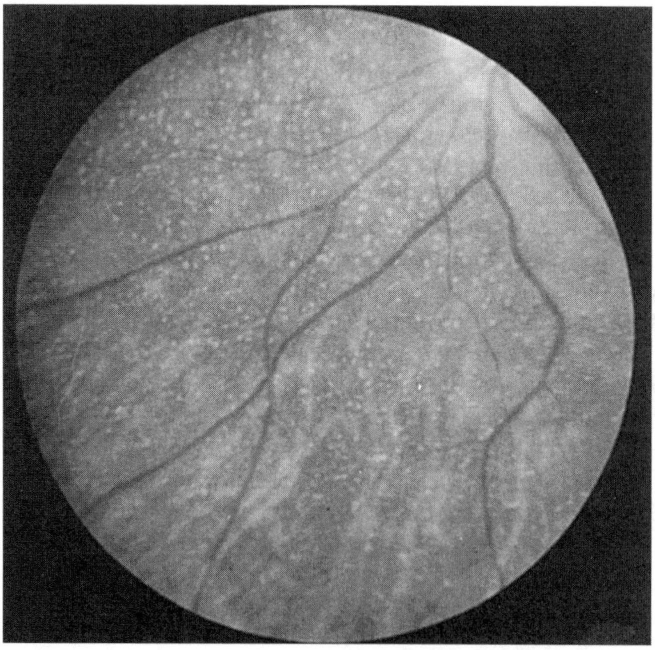

Figure 8 Patient with fundus albipunctatus demonstrates distinct gray-white spots: the macular area was unaffected.

epithelium. On fluorescein angiography, most of these dots are not seen or they block fluorescence (87,88). Surprisingly, multiple areas of retinal pigment epithelial atrophy, unrelated to the location of the albipunctate spots, can be found (87,89).

The general ophthalmoscopic picture of the fundus and the functional abnormality remain stationary. In one 59-year-old patient, it stayed essentially the same 49 years after the first examination (90), even though some albipunctate spots had changed (89). The dark adaptation curve (Fig. 9) characteristically remains at the cone level, with a threshold of 3–4 log units above the normal rod threshold for about 2.5 hr. Then, a cone–rod break occurs with a rapid increase of rod sensitivity to normal at about 3 hr (87). The ERG is very abnormal and of Riggs type. Both the a- and b-waves are very small, but return to normal after 3 hr of dark adaptation (10,61,87) (Fig. 10). The EOG is subnormal (about 130% light rise level), but normalizes after prolonged dark adaptation (10,89). It must be remembered, however, that in fundus albipunctatus there is a wide spectrum of fundoscopic abnormalities in both psychophysical and electrophysiological tests (91).

Normal blood levels of vitamin A, carotene, retinol-binding protein, amino acids, lipoproteins, and oxalates have been recorded (87,89).

Reflectometry shows abnormal kinetics of visual pigment regeneration, with 60 min half-time for rhodopsin regeneration (instead of the normal 3 min) and 20 min for cone pigment regeneration (instead of the normal 75 sec) (10) (Fig. 11). This abnormally slow regeneration of visual pigments in the photoreceptors could result from a malfunctioning retinal pigment epithelial cell, the abnormal transportation of products between this cell and the photoreceptor, or the anomalous utilization by the photoreceptor outer segment (10,27).

In 1999, two groups of investigators reported the identification of mutations in the RDH5 gene associated with fundus albipunctatus (92,93).

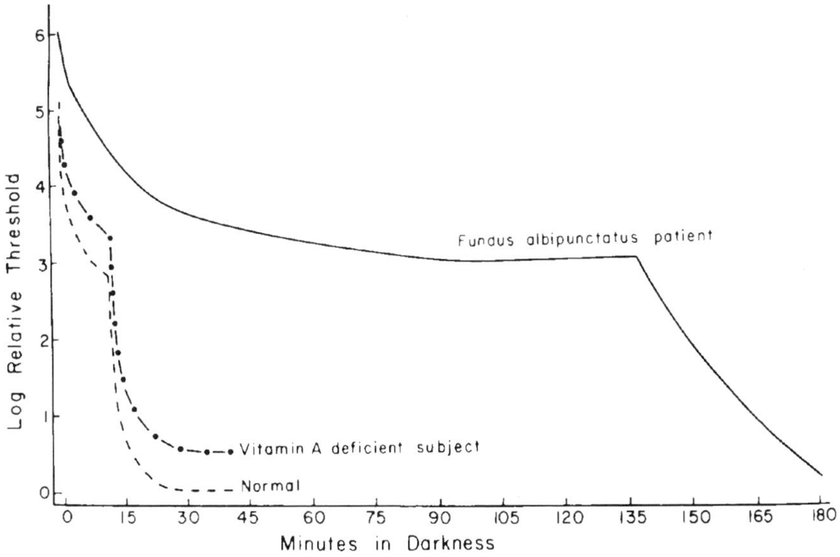

Figure 9 The dark adaption curve of a patient with fundus albipunctatus has slow cone recovery: the cone–rod break occurs at about 2.5 hr, and the final threshold is normal, compared with the dark adaptation curve of a normal and vitamin A-deficient subject (from Ref. 87).

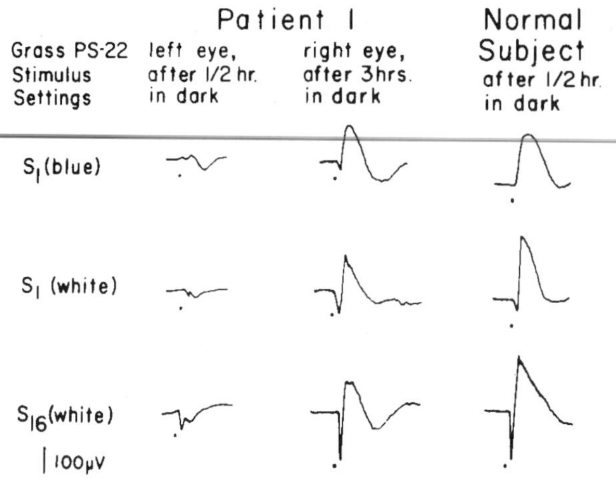

Figure 10 Electroretinographic responses to blue, white, and intense white light in a patient with fundus albipunctatus and a normal subject: The patient's response after 30 min is abnormal, then normalizes after 3 hr of dark adaption under all three conditions (from Ref. 87).

The gene RDH5 encoding 11-*cis*-retinol dehydrogenase was mapped to chromosome 12ql3–ql4 (94). It is expressed predominantly in the RPE (95). The enzyme 11-*cis* retinol dehydrogenase is a 32 kDa, membrane-bound enzyme consisting of 318 amino acids (96). It is a key enzyme necessary for the production in RPE cells of 11-*cis* retinal, which is then transported to the photoreceptors (22). The enzyme catalyzes the conversion of 11-cis retinol to 11-*cis* retinal.

Several missense mutations in the RDH5 were identified as causes of fundus albipunctatus. These included Gly238Trp, Ser73Phe, Vall77Gly, Arg280His, and Ala294Pro. Patients were homozygous or compound heterozygous in all cases (92–96).

In one 76-year-old patient, fundus albipunctatus was associated with an atrophic maculopathy and fading of the albipunctatus spots, associated with a Vall64Phe homozygous mutation (97). In some cases a progressive cone dystrophy is associated with fundus albipuncatus (95), possibly caused by a different mutation.

No treatment for fundus albipunctatus is available. An attempt has been made to treat the disorder with large amounts of vitamin A administered orally or parenterally (89). Dryja (22) suggested that the wearing of dark sunglasses may reduce the photoreceptors' need for 11-*cis* retinal and thus prevent or slow cone degeneration.

Oguchi Disease and the Two Causative Genes

Oguchi's disease, a relatively rare and interesting condition, was described in Japan at the turn of the century by Oguchi (98,99). Later, the disease was found in Europeans and blacks. In 1956, Francois and associates reviewed the literature and noted 72 Japanese and 22 non-Japanese case reports (100). The condition is congenital and stationary. Poor night vision is the major symptom. Ophthalmoscopy reveals an unusual ash-gray to yellow-white discoloration with strong fundus reflexes in whites and in Japanese and golden yellow with broad reddish-brown bands in blacks (101). After 2–3 hr of dark adaptation, the Mizuo phenomenon occurs: the

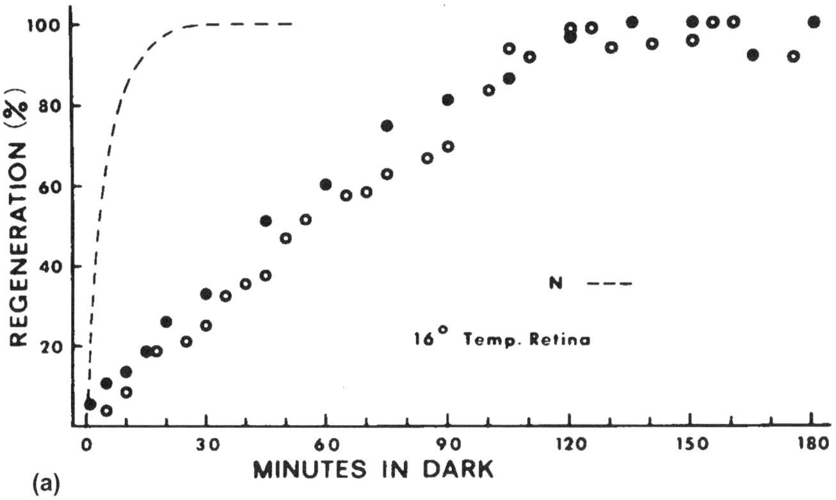

(a)

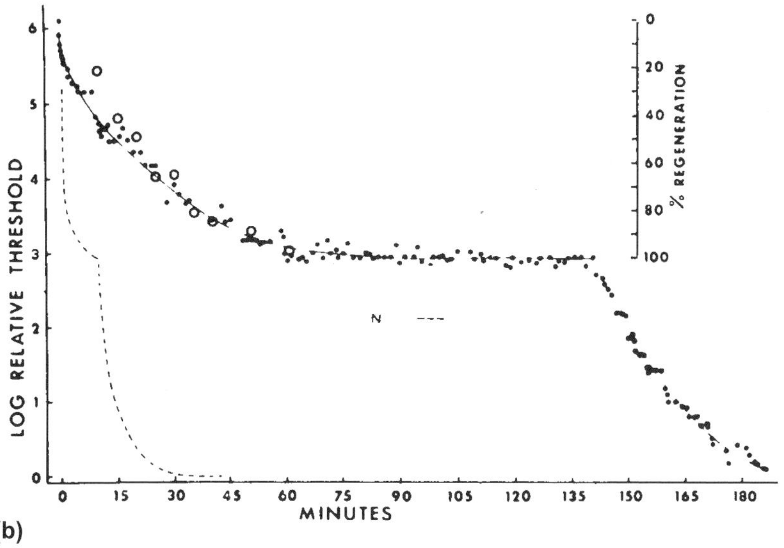

(b)

Figure 11 Rhodopsin regeneration in the dark (a) and the dark adaptation curve (b) of a patient with fundus albipunctatus: note the slow regeneration of both cone and rod pigments, which grossly parallels the cone and rod visual recovery in the dark adaptation curve (from Ref. 10).

fundus regains its normal color (102). The retinal vessels appear abnormal. Ophthalmoscopy under normal illumination cannot distinguish retinal arteries from retinal veins. After prolonged dark adaptation, the retinal vessels regain normal color (103).

Psychophysical dark adaptation curves show a normal, but very delayed, cone adaptation. Initially, rod function is completely absent; after about 2 hr of dark adaptation, the rod vision threshold decreases until it reaches a fully dark-adapted level at about 3 hr (10) (Fig. 11).

The ERG is essentially normal under photopic conditions. In the dark, small a- and b-waves (10,101), reminiscent of the Riggs type, are seen. Surprisingly, no change occurs after 2–3 hr (99) or even 24 hr (10) of dark adaptation. The EOG is

Table 3 Clinical and Genetic Varieties of CSNB with Abnormal Fundus

Clinical type	Gene	Chromosomal location	Mutation(s)	ERG	Dark adaptation (DA)
Fundus albipunctatus	RDH 5	12q13–q14	Gly238Trp and several other missense	Riggs type: normal after 2–3 hr of DA	Monophasic; normal after 2–3 hr of DA
Oguchi 1	SAG	2q37.1	1147delA	Cone: normal; rod: Riggs; no change with DA	Normal after 3 hr of adaptation
Oguchi 2	RHOK	13q34	Missense or deletions	As above	As above

normal, but the fluorescein angiogram shows areas of pigment epithelium atrophy (window defect) (101), not unlike those in fundus albipunctatus.

The rhodopsin regeneration kinetics are normal, as is the rhodopsin concentration (10). These findings imply that the abnormality is proximal to the outer segments or to the photoreceptors (10); however, the nature of any such abnormality may be more distal.

One histologic study by Yamanaka showed extensively damaged rods and cones (103). The parents of the patient, however, had retinitis pigmentosa, which confounded the diagnosis. Light and electron microscopic studies by Kuwabara and associates (104) disclosed an abnormal amorphic layer between the neural epithelium and the pigment epithelium, an accumulation of fuscin granules in the inner portion of the retinal pigment epithelial cells, and abnormal outer segments, which had microvascular and tubular internal structures instead of the ordinary lamellae.

These histologic findings suggest that the pathogenetic abnormality lies in the area of the pigment epithelium outer segments, possibly related to abnormal electric activity and severely prolonged adaptation.

The origin of the abnormal fundus in Oguchi disease is unknown. Usui et al. (105) studied the disorder by helium–neon laser ophthalmoscopy with a wavelength of 633 nm. It showed diffuse, fine white particles in the fundus, not found in normal subjects. The authors considered these particles the origin of the abnormal reflex.

In 1995 (106), Fuchs, Nakazawa et al. identified a mutation in the arrestin gene in Japanese patients with Oguchi disease.

Arrestin, an intrinsic rod photoreceptor protein, is implicated in the recovery phase of light transduction (106). The gene consists of 16 exons and encodes a protein of 405 amino acids. It was mapped to chromosome 2q37.1 (107). The protein is known by several names including arrestin, S-arrestin, or S-antigen (107). The gene is termed SAG for S-antigen.

Most Japanese patients with an identified mutation in the arrestin gene have a single mutation: a homozygous deletion of nucleotide 1147 [1147delA] (106,108,109). In some Japanese patients, probably 10–20%, this mutation is not found, which indicates the heterogeneity of this disorder.

In 1997, Yamamoto and associates (110) identified mutations in the rhodopsin kinase (RHOK) gene in non-Japanese patients with Oguchi disease. RHOK functions together with arrestin in shutting off rhodopsin after it has been activated by a photon of light (110). Various mutations in the gene were reported, such as a homozygous deletion of exon 5 or compound heterozygosity of one deletion and one missense mutation (110,111). No mutations were identified in association with retinitis pigmentosa (112). The locus was mapped to chromosome 13q34 (107). Lack of rhodopsin kinase has, probably, the same effect as lack of arrestin, prolongation of the lifetime of photoactivated rhodopsin. Photoactivated rhodopsin will remain active until it regains 11-*cis* retinal as chromophore. Even a small amount of photoactivated rhodopsin is sufficient to desensitize the photoreceptor. Rhodopsin regeneration in such a photoactivated rod is very slow and takes 2–4 hr (110).

Other Flecked Retinal Disorders

Three other conditions should be considered in relation to congenital nyctalopia with abnormal fundi.

Flecked Retina of Kandori

In this rare autosomal recessive condition, sharply defined, dirty yellow flecks are observed in the equatorial regions of the fundus. The flecks are deep in the retina and irregular in size, varying from tiny dots to flecks of 1.5-disk diameter (113).

Patients are asymptomatic or have only minimal disturbance in night vision. Psychophysical and electrophysiologic tests indicate a delay in the recovery of rod vision. The EOG is normal.

The pigment epithelium is disturbed with spots of hypertrophy and atrophy.

Benign Familial Fleck Retina

A condition that is ophthalmoscopically identical with fundus albipunctatus, but without night blindness, has been reported by Aish and Dajani (114). The mode of transmission is autosomal recessive. Because no psychophysical or electro-physiologic studies have been described, this condition may be the same as fundus albipunctatus.

Familial Fleck Retina with Night Blindness

In this retinal condition, multiple yellowish white flecks occur in the anterior part of the fundus, starting at the equator, sparing the posterior pole (115), Fluorescein angiography demonstrates, similar to other disorders of this group, retinal pigment epithelial atrophy unrelated to the flecks. The dark adaptation curve is monophasic; the cone level is 3–3.5 log units above the normal rod level. After prolonged dark adaptation (more than 2 hr) the rod visual threshold is at a normal level. The ERG in the dark initially displays a typical, large Schubert–Bornschein-type a-wave and a very small b-wave. These normalize after prolonged dark adaptation.

This condition, described by Miyake and Harada (62), shows many similarities to fundus albipunctatus, but enough differences to justify a separate classification. The inheritance seems to be autosomal recessive.

REFERENCES

1. Sommer A. Nutritional Blindness. New York: Oxford University Press, 1982:19–27.
2. Perlman I, Barzilai D, Haim T, Schramek A. Night vision in a case of vitamin A deficiency due to malabsorption. Br J Ophthalmol 1983; 67:37–42.
3. Dowling JE, Wald G. Vitamin A deficiency and nightblindness. Proc Natl Acad Sci USA 1958; 44:648–661.
4. Jayle GE, Ourgaud AG, Baisinger LF, Holmes WJ. Night Vision. Spring-field: Charles C Thomas, 1959:147–150.
5. Jayle GE, Ourgaud AG, Baisinger LF, Holmes WJ. Night Vision. Spring-field: Charles C Thomas, 1959:274–280.
6. Snyder C. Jean Nougaret, the butcher from Provence and his family. Arch Ophthalmol 1963; 69:676–678.
7. Donders FC. Torpeur de la retine congenitale héréditaire. Ann Ocul 1855; 34:270–272.
8. Nettleship E. On some hereditary diseases of the eye (Bowman lecture). Retinitis pigmentosa, night blindness with myopia, ocular albinism. Trans Ophthalmol Soc UK 1909; 29:57–148.
9. Nettleship E. A pedigree of congenital night blindness with myopia. Trans Ophthalmol Soc UK 1912; 32:21–45.

10. Carr RE. Congenital stationary night blindness. Trans Am Ophthalmol Soc 1977; 72:448–487.
11. Uyemura M. Ueber ein merkwurdige Augenhintergrundveränderung bei zwei Fällen von idiopatischer Hemeralopie. Klin Monatsbl Augenheilkd 1928; 81:471–473.
12. Levy NS, Toskes P. Fundus albipunctatus and vitamin A deficiency. Am J Ophthalmol 1974; 78:926–929.
13. Lauber H. Die sogenannte Retinitis Punctata Albescens. Klin Monatsbl Augenheilkd 1910; 48:133–148.
14. Auerbach E, Godel V, Rowe H. An electrophysiological and psychophysical study of two forms of congenital night blindness. Invest Ophthalmol 1969; 8:332–345.
15. Krill AE, Martin D. Photopic abnormalities in congenital stationary nightblindness. Invest Ophthalmol 1971; 10:625–636.
16. Miyake Y, Yagasaki K, Horiguchi M, et al. Congenital stationary night blindness with negative electroretinogram: a new classification. Arch Ophthalmol 1986; 104: 1013–1020.
17. Miyake Y, Yagasaki K, Horiguchi M. A rod-cone dysfunction syndrome with separate clinical entity: incomplete-type congenital stationary night blindness (Miyake). Prog Clin Biol Res 1987; 247:137–145.
18. Miyake Y, Horiguchi M, Ota I, Shiroyama N. Characteristic ERG-flicker anomaly in incomplete congenital stationary night blindness. Invest Ophthalmol Vis Sci 1987; 28:1816–1823.
19. Schubert G, Bornschein H. Beitrag zur Analyse des meuschlichen Elektroretinogramms. Ophthalmologica 1952; 123:396–413.
20. Riggs LA. Electroretinography in cases of night blindness. Am J Ophthalmol 1954; 38(pt II):70–78.
21. Ruether K, Apfelstedt-Sylla E, Zrenner E. Clinical findings in patients with congenital stationary night blindness of the Schubert-Bornschein type. Ger J Ophthalmol 1993; 2(6):429–435.
22. Dryja TP. Molecular genetics of Oguchi disease, fundus albipunctatus, and other forms of stationary night blindness: LVII Edward Jackson Memorial Lecture. Am J Ophthalmol 2000; 130(5):547–63.
23. Carr RE, Ripps H, Siegel IM, Weale RA. Rhodopsin and the electrical activity of the retina in congenital night blindness. Invest Ophthalmol 1966; 5:497–507.
24. Armington JC, Schwab GJ. Electroretinogram in nyctalopia. Arch Ophthalmol 1954; 52:725–733.
25. Ripps H, Weale RA. Rhodopsin regeneration in man. Nature 1969; 222:775–777.
26. Babel J. Constations histologiques dans l'amaurose infantile de Leber et dans diverses formes d'héméralopie. Ophthalmologica 1963; 145:399–402.
27. Vaghefi HA, Green WR, Kelley JS, et al. Correlation of clinicopathologic findings in a patient. Congenital night blindness, branch retinal vein occlusion, cilioretinal artery, drusen of the optic nerve head and intraretinal pigmented lesion. Arch Ophthalmol 1978; 96:2097–2104.
28. Siegel IM, Greenstein VV, Seiple WH, Carr RE. Cone function in congenital nyctalopia. Ophthalmology 1987; 65:307–318.
29. Ripps H. Night blindness revisited: from man to molecules. Invest Ophthalmol Vis Sci 1982; 23:588–609.
30. Ripps H, Carr RE, Siegel IM, Greenstein VC. Functional abnormalities in vincristine induced night blindness. Invest Ophthalmol Vis Sci 1984; 25:787–794.
31. Witzel DA, Smith EL, Wilson RD, Aguirre GD. Congenital stationary night blindness: An animal model. Invest Ophthaimol Vis Sci 1978; 17:788–795.
32. Balkema GW, Mangini NJ, Pinto LH. Discrete visual defects in pearl mutant mice. Science 1983; 4:1085–1087.
33. Narfstrom K, Wrigstad A, Nilsson SE. The Briard dog: a new animal model of congenital stationary night blindness. Br J Ophthalmol 1989; 739:750–756.

34. Zhang Z, Gu Y, Li L, Long T, Guo Q, Shi L. A potential spontaneous rat model of X-linked congenital stationary night blindness. Doc Ophthalmol 2003; 107(1):53–57.
35. Gregg RG, Mukhopadhyay S, Candille SI, Ball SL, Pardue MT, McCall MA, Peachey NS. Identification of the gene and the mutation responsible for the mouse nob phenotype. Invest Ophthalmol Vis Sci 2003; 44(1):378–384.
36. François J, Verriest G, De Rouck A, et al. Les fonctions visuelles dans l'héméralopie essentielle nougarienne. Ophthalmologica 1956; 132:244–257.
37. François J, Verriest G, De Rouck A. A new pedigree of idiopathic congenital night blindness: transmitted as a dominant hereditary trait. Am J Ophthalmol 1965; 59: 621–625.
38. Carr RE, Ripps H, Siegel IM. Rhodopsin and visual threshold in congenital nightblindness (abstract). J Physiol 1966; 186:103.
39. Carr RE, Ris H, Siegel IM, Weale RA. Visual functions in congenital night blindness. Invest Ophthalmol 1966; 5:508–514.
40. Sandberg MA, Pawlyk BS, Dan J, Arnaud B, Dryja TP, Berson EL. Rod and cone function in the Nougaret form of stationary night blindness. Arch Ophthalmol 1998; 116(7):867–872.
41. Dryja TP, Hahn LB, Reboul T, Arnaud B. Missense mutation in the gene encoding the alpha subunit of rod transducin in the Nougaret form of congenital stationary night blindness. Nat Genet 1996; 13(3):358–360.
42. RetNet (retrieval system on the Internet). Texas: The University of Texas Health Science Center. C1996–2004 (cited Jun 24, 2004). Available from: http ://www.sph.uth.tmc.edu/retnet/.
43. Muradov KG, Artemyev NO. Loss of the effector function in a transducin-alpha mutant associated with Nougaret night blindness. J Biol Chem 2000; 275(10):6969–6974.
44. Rosenberg T, Haim M, Piczenik Y, Simonsen SE. Autosomal dominant stationary night-blindness. A large family rediscovered. Acta Ophthalmol 1991; 69(6):694–702.
45. McLaughlin ME, Sandberg MA, Berson EL, Dryja TP. Recessive mutations in the gene encoding the beta-subunit of rod phosphodiesterase in patients with retinitis pigmentosa. Nat Genet 1993; 4(2):130–139.
46. Gal A, Xu S, Piczenik Y, Eiberg H, Duvigneau C, Schwinger E, Rosenberg T. Gene for autosomal dominant congenital stationary night blindness maps to the same region as the gene for the beta-subunit of the rod photoreceptor cGMP phosphodiesterase (PDEB) in chromosome 4pl6.3. Hum Mol Genet 1994; 3(2):323–325.
47. Gal A, Orth U, Baehr W, Schwinger E, Rosenberg T. Heterozygous missense mutation in the rod cGMP phosphodiesterase beta-subunit gene in autosomal dominant stationary night blindness. Nat Genet 1994; 7(1):64–68.
48. Dryja TP, Berson EL, Rao VR, Oprian DD. Heterozygous missense mutation in the rhodopsin gene as a cause of congenital stationary night blindness. Nat Genet 1993; 4(3):280–283.
49. Rao VR, Cohen GB, Oprian DD. Rhodopsin mutation G90D and a molecular mechanism for congenital night blindness. Nature 1994; 367(6464):639–642.
50. Sieving PA, Richards JE, Naarendorp F, Bingham EL, Scott K, Alpern M. Dark-light: model for nightblindness from the human rhodopsin Gly-90—>Asp mutation. Proc Natl Acad Sci USA 1995; 92(3):880–884.
51. al-Jandal N, Farrar GJ, Kiang AS, Humphries MM, Bannon N, Findlay JB, Humphries P, Kenna PF. A novel mutation within the rhodopsin gene (Thr-94-Ile) causing autosomal dominant congenital stationary night blindness. Hum Mutat 1999; 13(1):75–81.
52. Merin S, Rowe H, Auerbach E, Landau J. Syndrome of congenital high myopia with nyctalopia. Am J Ophthalmol 1970; 70:541–547.
53. Miyake Y. Establishment of the concept of new clinical entities—complete and incomplete form of congenital stationary night blindness. Nippon Ganka Gakkai Zasshi-Acta Soc Ophthalmol Jpn 2002; 106(12):737–755; discussion 756.

54. Hittner HM, Borda RP, Justice J Jr. X-linked recessive congenital stationary night blindness, myopia and tilted discs. J Pediatr Ophthalmol Strabismus 1981; 18:15–20.
55. Heckenlively JR, Martin DA, Rosenbaum AL. Loss of electroretinographic oscillatory potentials, optic atrophy and dysplasia in congenital stationary night blindness. Am J Ophthalmol 1983; 96:526–534.
56. Hill DH, Arbel KF, Berson EL. Cone electroretinograms in congenital nyctalopia with myopia. Am J Ophthalmol 1974; 78:127–136.
57. Lachapelle P, Little JM, Polomeno RC. The photopic electroretinogram in congenital stationary night blindness with myopia. Invest Ophthalmol Vis Sci 1983; 24:442–450.
58. Miyake Y, Kawase Y. Reduced amplitude of oscillatory potentials in female carriers of X-linked recessive congenital stationary night blindness. Am J Ophthalmol 1984; 98: 208–215.
59. Young RSL, Chaparro A, Price J, Walters J. Oscillatory potentials of X-linked carriers of congenital stationary night blindness. Invest Ophthalmol Vis Sci 1989; 30:806–812.
60. Miyake Y, Ando F, Ichikawa H. Vitreous fluorophotometry in congenital stationary nightblindness. Arch Ophthalmol 1983; 101:574–576.
61. Jay M. The Eisdell pedigree. Congenital stationary night-blindness with myopia. Trans Ophthalmot Soc UK 1983; 103:221–226.
62. der Kaloustian VM, Baghdassarian SA. The autosomal recessive variety of congenital stationary night blindness with myopia. J Med Genet 1972; 9:67–69.
63. Khouri G, Mets MB, Smith VC, et al. X-linked congenital stationary night blindness. Review and report of a family with hyperopia. Arch Ophthalmol 1988; 106:1417–1422.
64. Gal A, Schinzel A, Orth U, et al. Gene of X-chromosomal congenital stationary night blindness is closely linked to *DXS7* on Xp. Hum Genet 1989; 81:315–318.
65. Musarella MA, Weleber RG, Murphey WH, Young RS, Anson-Cartwright L, Mets M, Kraft SP, Polemeno R, Litt M, Worton RG. Assignment of the gene for complete X-linked congenital stationary night blindness (CSNB1) to Xp11.3. Gen 1989; 5(4):727–737.
66. Pearce WG, Reedyk M, Coupland SG. Variable expressivity in X-linked congenital stationary night blindness. Can J Ophthalmol 1990; 25(1):3–10.
67. Boycott KM, Pearce WG, Musarella MA, Weleber RG, Maybaum TA, Birch DG, Miyake Y, Young RS, Bech-Hansen NT. Evidence for genetic heterogeneity in X-linked congenital stationary night blindness. Am J Hum Gen 1998; 62(4):865–875.
68. Bech-Hansen NT, Naylor MJ, Maybaum TA, Sparkes RL, Koop B, Birch DG, Bergen AA, Prinsen CF, Polomeno RC, Gal A, Drack AV, Musarella MA, Jacobson SG, Young RS, Weleber RG. Mutations in NYX, encoding the leucine-rich proteoglycan nyctalopin, cause X-linked complete congenital stationary night blindness. Nat Genet 2000; 26(3):319–323.
69. Pusch CM, Zeitz C, Brandau O, Pesch K, Achatz H, Feil S, Scharfe C, Maurer J, Jacobi FK, Pinckers A, Andreasson S, Hardcastle A, Wissinger B, Berger W, Meindl A. The complete form of X-linked congenital stationary night blindness is caused by mutations in a gene encoding a leucine-rich repeat protein. Nat Genet 2000; 26(3):324–327.
70. Zeitz C, Scherthan H, Freier S, Feil S, Suckow V, Schweiger S, Berger W. NYX (nyctalopin on chromosome X), the gene mutated in congenital stationary night blindness, encodes a cell surface protein. Invest Ophthalmol Vis Sci 2003; 44(10):4184–4191.
71. Pusch CM, Maurer J, Ramser J, Tomiuk J, Achatz H, Pesch K, Lichtner P, Apfelstedt-Sylla E, Jacobi FK, Berger W, Meindl A, Wissinger B. Complete form of X-linked congenital stationary night blindness: refined mapping and evidence of genetic homogeneity. Int J Mol Med 2001; 7(2):155–161.
72. Allen LE, Zito I, Bradshaw K, Patel RJ, Bird AC, Fitzke F, Yates JR, Trump D, Hardcastle AJ, Moore AT. Genotype-phenotype correlation in British families with X-linked congenital stationary night blindness. Br J Ophthalmol 2003; 87(11):1413–1420.
73. Bech-Hansen NT, Pearce WG. Manifestations of X-linked congenital stationary night blindness in three daughters of an affected male: demonstration of homozygosity. Am J Hum Genet 1993; 52(1):71–77.

74. Berson EL, Lessell S. Paraneoplastic night blindness with malignant melanoma. Am J Ophthalmol 1988; 106:307–311.
75. Jacobi FK, Hamel CP, Arnaud B, Blin N, Broghammer M, Jacobi PC, Apfelstedt-Sylla E, Pusch CM. A novel CACNA1F mutation in a French family with the incomplete type of X-linked congenital stationary night blindness. Am J Ophthalmol 2003; 135(5): 733–736.
76. Rigaudiere F, Roux C, Lachapelle P, Rosolen SG, Bitoun P, Gay-Duval A, Le Gargasson JF. ERGs in female carriers of incomplete congenital stationary night blindness (I-CSNB). A family report. Doc Ophthalmol 2003; 107(2):203–212.
77. Strom TM, Nyakatura G, Apfelstedt-Sylla E, Hellebrand H, Lorenz B, Weber BH, Wutz K, Gutwillinger N, Ruther K, Drescher B, Sauer C, Zrenner E, Meitinger T, Rosenthal A, Meindl A. An L-type calcium-channel gene mutated in incomplete X-linked congenital stationary night blindness. Nat Genet 1998; 19(3):260–263.
78. Bech-Hansen NT, Naylor MJ, Maybaum TA, Pearce WG, Koop B, Fishman GA, Mets M, Musarella MA, Boycott KM. Loss-of-function mutations in a calcium-channel alpha1-subunit gene in Xp11.23 cause incomplete X-linked congenital stationary night blindness. Nat Genet 1998; 19(3):264–267.
79. Boycott KM, Maybaum TA, Naylor MJ, Weleber RG, Robitaille J, Miyake Y, Bergen AA, Pierpont ME, Pearce WG, Bech-Hansen NT. A summary of 20 CACNA1F mutations identified in 36 families with incomplete X-linked congenital stationary night blindness, and characterization of splice variants. Hum Genet 2001; 108(2):91–97.
80. Wutz K, Sauer C, Zrenner E, Lorenz B, Alitalo T, Broghammer M, Hergersberg M, de la Chapelle A, Weber BH, Wissinger B, Meindl A, Pusch CM. Thirty distinct CACNA1F mutations in 33 families with incomplete type of XLCSNB and Cacna1f expression profiling in mouse retina. Eur J Hum Genet 2002; 10(8):449–456.
81. Nakamura M, Ito S, Piao CH, Terasaki H, Miyake Y. Retinal and optic disc atrophy associated with a CACNA1F mutation in a Japanese family. Arch Ophthalmol 2003; 121(7):1028–1033.
82. Weleber RG, Pillers DA, Powell BR, Hanna CE, Magenis RE, Buist NR. Aland Island eye disease (Forsius-Eriksson syndrome) associated with contiguous deletion syndrome at Xp21. Similarity to incomplete congenital stationary night blindness. Arch Ophthalmol 1989; 107(8):1170–1179.
83. Carlson S, Vesti E, Raitta C, Donner M, Eriksson AW, Forsius H. Clinical electroretinographic comparison between Aland Island eye disease a newly found related disease with X-chromosomal inheritance. Acta Ophthalmol 1991; 69(6):703–710.
84. Pillers DA, Seltzer WK, Powell BR, Ray PN, Tremblay F, La Roche GR, Lewis RA, McCabe ER, Eriksson AW, Weleber RG. Negative-configuration electroretinogram in Oregon eye disease. Consistent phenotype in Xp21 deletion syndrome. Arch Ophthalmol 1993; 111(11):1558–1563.
85. Bergen AA, ten Brink JB, Riemslag F, Schuurman EJ, Tijmes N. Localization of a novel X-linked congenital stationary night blindness locus: close linkage to the RP3 type retinitis pigmentosa gene region. Hum Mol Genet 1995; 4(5):931–935.
86. Glass IA, Good P, Coleman MP, Fullwood P, Giles MG, Lindsay S, Nemeth AH, Davies KE, Willshaw HA, Fielder A, et al. Genetic mapping of a cone and rod dysfunction (Aland Island eye disease) to the proximal short arm of the human X chromosome. J Med Genet 1993; 30(12):1044–1050.
87. Carr RE, Margolis S, Siegel IM. Fluorescein angiography and vitamin A and oxalate levels in fundus albipunctatus. Am J Ophthalmol 1976; 82:549–558.
88. Bullock JD, Albert DM, Skinner CW, et al. Calcium oxalate retinopathy associated with generalized oxalosis. X-ray diffraction and electron microscopic studies of crystal deposits. Invest Ophthalmol 1974; 13:256–265.
89. Marmor MF. Fundus albipunctatus: a clinical study of the fundus lesions, the physiological deficit and vitamin A metabolism. Doc Ophthalmol 1977; 43:277–302.

90. Franceschetti A, Chome-Bercioux N. Fundus albipunctatus cum hemeralopia (cas stationnaire depuis 49 ans). Ophthalmologica 1951; 121:185–193.
91. Margolis S, Siegel IM, Ripps H. Variable expressivity in fundus albipunctatus. Ophthalmol 1987; 94:1416–1422.
92. Gonzalez-Fernandez F, Kurz D, Bao Y, Newman S, Conway BP, Young JE, Han DP, Khani SC. 11-cis retinol dehydrogenase mutations as a major cause of the congenital night-blindness disorder known as fundus albipunctatus. Mol Vis 1999; 5:41.
93. Yamamoto H, Simon A, Eriksson U, Harris E, Berson EL, Dryja TP. Mutations in the gene encoding 11-cis retinol dehydrogenase cause delayed dark adaptation and fundus albipunctatus. Nat Genet 1999; 22(2):188–191.
94. Wada Y, Abe T, Sato H, Tamai M. A novel Gly35Ser mutation in the RDH5 gene in a Japanese family with fundus albipunctatus associated with cone dystrophy. Arch Ophthalmol 2001; 119(7):1059–1063.
95. Nakamura M, Hotta Y, Tanikawa A, Terasaki H, Miyake Y. A high association with cone dystrophy in fundus albipunctatus caused by mutations of the RDH5 gene. Invest Ophthalmol Vis Sci 2000; 41(12):3925–3932.
96. Kuroiwa S, Kikuchi T, Yoshimura N. A novel compound heterozygous mutation in the RDH5 gene in a patient with fundus albipunctatus. Am J Ophthalmol 2000; 130(5): 672–675.
97. Yamamoto H, Yakushijin K, Kusuhara S, Escano MF, Nagai A, Negi A. A novel RDH5 gene mutation in a patient with fundus albipunctatus presenting with macular atrophy and fading white dots. Am J Ophthalmol 2003; 136(3):572–574.
98. Oguchi C. On a type of night-blindness. Acta Soc Ophthalmol Jpn 1907; 11:123–134.
99. Oguchi C. Ueber die eigenartige Hemeralopie mit diffuser Weissgraulicher Verfärbung des Augenhintergrundes. Albrecht von Graefes Arch Klin Exp Ophthalmol 1912; 81: 109–117.
100. François J, Verriest G, De Rouck A. La maladie d'Oguchi. Ophthalmologica 1956; 131:1–40.
101. Winn S, Tasman W, Spaeth G, et al. Oguchi's disease in Negroes. Arch Ophthalmol 1969; 81:501–507.
102. Mizuo G. A new discovery in dark adaptation in Oguchi's disease. Arch Soc Ophthalmol Jpn 1913; 17:1148–1150.
103. Yamanaka M. Histologic study of Oguchi's disease. Am J Ophthalmol 1969; 68:19–26.
104. Kuwabara Y, Ishihara K, Akiya S. Histopathological and electron microscopic studies of the retina of Oguchi's disease. Acta Soc Ophthalmol Jpn 1963; 67:1323–1351.
105. Usui T, Ichibe M, Ueki S, Takagi M, Hasegawa S, Abe H, Sekiya K, Nakazawa M. Mizuo phenomenon observed by scanning laser ophthalmoscope in a patient with Oguchi disease. Am J Ophthalmol 2000; 130(3):359–361.
106. Fuchs S, Nakazawa M, Maw M, Tamai M, Oguchi Y, Gal A. A homozygous 1-base pair deletion in the arrestin gene is a frequent cause of Oguchi disease in Japanese. Nat Genet 1995; 10(3):360–362.
107. Online Mendelian Inheritance in Man, OMIM (TM). McKusick-Nathans Institute for Genetic Medicine, Johns Hopkins University (Baltimore, MD) and National Center for Biotechnology Information, National Library of Medicine, Bethesda, MD, 2000. http ://www.ncbi.nim.nih. gov/omim/.
108. Wada Y, Nakazawa M, Abe T, et al. Clinical variability of patients associated with gene mutations of visual cycle protein, arrestin RPE 65 and RDH5 genes. Invest Ophthalmol Vis Sci 2000; 41:ARVO Abstract 617.
109. Nakamachi Y, Nakamura M, Fujii S, Yamamoto M, Okubo K. Oguchi disease with sectoral retinitis pigmentosa harboring adenine deletion at position 1147 in the arrestin gene. Am J Ophthalmol 1998; 125(2):249–251.
110. Yamamoto S, Sippel KC, Berson EL, Dryja TP. Defects in the rhodopsin kinase gene in the Oguchi form of stationary night blindness. Nat Genet 1997; 15(2):175–178.

111. Khani SC, Nielsen L, Vogt TM. Biochemical evidence for pathogenicity of rhodopsin kinase mutations correlated with the Oguchi form of congenital stationary night blindness. Proc Natl Acad Sci USA 1998; 95(6):2824–2827.
112. Yamamoto S, Khani SC, Berson EL, Dryja TP. Evaluation of the rhodopsin kinase gene in patients with retinitis pigmentosa. Exp Eye Res 1997; 65(2):249–253.
113. Kandori F, Tamai A, Kurimoto S, Fukunaga K. Fleck retina. Am J Ophthalmol 1972; 73:673–685.
114. Aish SFS, Dajani B. Benign familial fleck retina. Br J Ophthalmol 1980; 64:652–659.
115. Miyake Y, Harada K. Familial fleck retina with night blindness. Ann Ophthalmol 1982; 14:836–841.

16
Glaucoma

INTRODUCTION

Glaucoma is generally defined as an elevated intraocular pressure (IOP) that is sufficiently high to cause optic nerve demage. Formerly, it was assumed that any intraocular pressure above 21–24 mmHg characterized glaucoma.

Glaucoma was also thought to be hereditary and familial. Since the turn of the century, many descriptions of families with glaucoma have been published, indicating that glaucoma is transmitted by a single gene, usually autosomal recessive or autosomal dominant, with incomplete penetrance. However, most of these family studies were flawed, because they were based on one or more of three possibly erroneous assumptions. First, the diagnosis of glaucoma was occasionally wrong; affected patients with lower pressure were missed, and unaffected members of the family were included. Second, the age factor was often unaccounted for: In many pedigrees, family members were considered normal and unaffected because they had not reached the usual age at which the glaucoma became manifest. Third, gonioscopy was not performed routinely, resulting in an equivocal diagnosis.

Therefore, in spite of the general impression that glaucoma is indeed hereditary, the confusion related to the exact mode of inheritance remained. Some of this confusion cleared up when glaucoma was properly subdivided into separate clinical entities on the basis of different symptoms, clinical signs, clinical test results, and gonioscopic findings. These separate clinical entities were also noted to be individual genetic entities, each with its own form of inheritance. Although some points of controversy still exist, genetics may now be used to understand the underlying processes in glaucoma better and to manage the individual glaucoma patient more sucessfully.

The last decade witnessed the identification of several glaucoma-associated genes, and multiple disease-causative mutations. These included six primary open-angle glaucoma-associated genes, two congenital glaucoma-associated genes and two pigmentary glaucoma-associated genes, in addition to genes associated with secondary syndromic glaucoma, such as Rieger, aniridia and others. Blumenthal and Weinreb, in their review (1) and Wirtz and Samples in a subsequent review (2) pointed out that these developments in genetics may be valuable in advising patients concerning diagnoses such as in cases of suspicious discs; decisions about target IOP;

and decisions about treatment, such as preventive iridotomy. All these can be reflected from the diagnosed genetic entity and the specific clinical picture of affected family members.

The identification of the glaucoma genes greatly enhanced our understanding of pathogenic factors related to glaucoma. The discovery of the involved genes also led to some surprising findings. The first glaucoma-associated gene to be identified was TIGR (for: trabecular meshwork-inducible glucocorticoid response), a gene associated with the response to corticosteroid topical administration but also with both early-onset (juvenile) glaucoma and late-onset glaucoma. The glaucoma-causative mutation is heterozygous in effect, therefore transmitted by the autosomal dominant mode. However, no glaucoma results in people with the homozygous state of two mutated alleles (3).

The identified genes apply only to a proportion of patients with glaucoma. The mode of inheritance of the majority is not known, and is subject to speculation. A likely possibility is the transmission of hereditary glaucoma by more than one gene. This could be digenic (4), meaning that only when both genes are mutated, glaucoma occurs. It could also be polygenic (5), meaning that more than two genes are involved. In addition, environmental factors may play a role.

PRIMARY OPEN-ANGLE GLAUCOMA

Introduction

Chronic open-angle glaucoma (COAG), or primary open-angle glaucoma (POAG), is the most common primary glaucoma, which probably causes more blindness than all the other forms in most populations (but not in all). On the basis of older family reports, it has been suggested that the transmission is autosomal recessive or autosomal dominant, with incomplete penetrance, partial expressivity, and a high preponderance of sporadic cases. The study of POAG took a new and entirely different course in the 1960s, with the discovery of the effect of corticosteroids on the intraocular pressure (IOP) and its relation to glaucoma. The study took another new turn with the identification of several genes associated with POAG.

Corticosteroids and Glaucoma

Fifty years ago corticosteroids were shown to increase IOP in susceptible subjects (6). Becker and Mills (7) demonstrated an incerase in IOP in 30% of normal voluenteers who applied corticosteroid eye drops topically four times a day for two months. The same regimen caused large and highly significant increases in IOP in 44 glaucomatous patients and in 32 glaucoma suspects. These increases in IOP were reversible when the corticosteroids were stopped. On the basis of camparison of the volunteers and patients and their distribution in the population (8–10), Becker posulated the existence of three different genotypes with two alleles: n and g on one locus, the homozygote gg having glaucoma (Table 1). This, of course, assumed a monomeric inheritance of glaucoma, transmitted in the intermediate mode, with glaucoma being recessive.

The major problems with this theory were that not every high responder had glaucoma and that some POAG patients were not highly responsive to corticosteroid treatment. Armaly, therefore, suggsted a different theory, in which the pair of allelles $p^L p^H$ replaced the genes g and n of Becker (11). Armaly used the amount of IOP

Table 1 Inheritance of Corticosteroid Responsiveness and Glaucoma According to Becker

Group	Genotype	Final IOP[a]	Phenotype	Description
1	*nn*	<20 mmHg	Poor responder	Normal homozygote
2	*ng*	20–31 mmHg	Intermediate responder	Carrier
3	*gg*	>31 mmHg	High responder	Glaucoma homozygote

[a]After 6 weeks of topical dexamethasone treatment.

increase after corticosteroid administration as an end point for his three groups, instead of the final IOP (Table 2). The main difference between the two theories was, Armaly assumed, that the p^Lp^H gene were responsible for the corticosteroid response only. Although improtant for the development of open-angle glaucoma, they are not the only factor. According to Armaly's theory, open-angle glaucoma is a polygenic disease, of which p^Lp^H are just one of several genes (7). In family studies, Armaly found consistent results, indicating a monomeric transmission of corticosteroid responsiveness (Fig. 1).

The reproducibility of the corticosteroid test as was reasonably good at 73% (10) if one accounted for some noncompliance, disparate IOP measurements, diurnal changes in pressure, and other such factors.

Most studies were performed using topical dexamethasone, which elevates the IOP especially high, although other topical corticosteroids may also increase pressure. Fluoromethone, which reduces the risk of increasing the IOP compared with topical dexamethasone, also has a strong effect, sometimes comparable with dexamethasone (13).

High corticosteroid responsiveness is undoubtedly a factor in the development of glaucoma. A 10-year follow-up study indicated that IOP elevation is more likely to develop in corticosteroid-responsive indiviuals, and that they run a higher risk of developing glaucomatous field changes (14).

Some doubts were raised about the inheritance of corticosteroid responsiveness. After analyzing the available figures, Francois and Francois et al. (15,16) could not confirm the hereditary transmission of corticosteroid responsiveness by a single mendelian gene. However, they found an almost double prevalence of responsiveness to corticosteroids in families with glaucoma when compared with families without glaucoma (15). Akingbehin (17) claimed that corticosteroid responsiveness was related to POAG through a damaged trabeculum and not hereditary factors, pointing out that a high frequency of high responders occurs in various conditions associated with trabecular damage, such as trauma, goniodysgenesis, pigmentary glaucoma, and in patients after an acute attack of angle-closure glaucoma.

Table 2 Inheritance of Corticosteriod Responsiveness According to Armaly[a]

Group	Genotype[a]	Final IOP	Phenotype
1	p^Lp^L	<6 mmHg	Poor responder
2	p^Lp^H	6–15 mmHg	Intermediate responder
3	p^Lp^H	>15 mmHg	High responder

[a]p^Lp^H are one pair of genes (albeit the most important one) in a polygenic inheritance of chronic open-angle glaucoma.

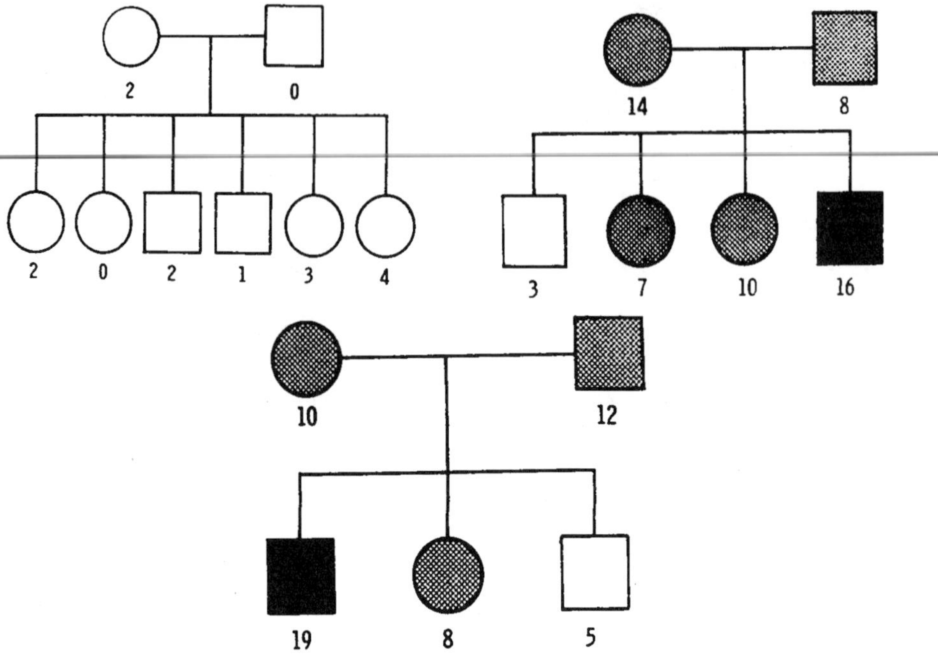

Figure 1 The pedigrees of three different families indicating a simple mendelian transmission of corticosteroid responsiveness. Open symbols indicate p^Lp^L, stippled symbols indicate p^Lp^H, solid symbols indicate $p^H\mathrm{p}^H$. Numbers indicate the increase in IOP after four-receiving weeks of topical 0.1% dexamethasone, three times a day (from Ref. 11).

The pathogenesis of corticosteroid-induced response and glaucoma is uncertain. Francois et al. (16,18) suggested that free mucopolysaccharides are found in the anterior chamber angle in the normal state. These may be polymerized, retain water, and cause narrowing of the trabecular apertures, or they may be depolymerized when no water is retained and the trabecular openings widen. This depolymerization occurs when catabolic enzymes are released from lysosomes in the goniocytes. Corticosteroids tend to strengthen the membrane of the lysosomes in sensitive goniocytes. Thus the release of catabolic enzymes is pervented, mucopolysaccharides remain polymerized, trabecular openings stay narrow, and the IOP increases. The different response to corticosteroids by the membrane of the lysosomes is genetically determined. This sequence of events has not, however, been confirmed by other studies.

The identification of the trabecular meshwork-(TIGR) gene (locus GLC1A) responsible (see below) both for the corticosteroid responsiveness and for POAG, did not solve the question of the exact pathogenic mechanism of increased pressure. Polansky et al. (19), conducting in vitro studies of the effect of prolonged use of glucocorticoids with a TIGR clone on human trabecular meshwork, concluded that TIGR is the candidate gene for outflow obstruction. They also concluded (20) that their data suggest the activation of stress/apoptotic pathways by environmental and genetic interaction in glaucoma pathogenesis. Nguyen et al. (21), having conducted similar in vitro studies, demonstrated that the gene product interacts with trabecular meshwork cells to form oligomeric complexes resulting in high levels of new extracellular protein/glycoproteins. These may obstruct the normal aqueous pathways.

Considering all the information, it seems to confirm that corticosteroid responsiveness is genetically determined. The only or possibly the most important gene is TIGR. However, other genes and even environmental factors may also play a role.

This theory is supported by findings in family studies (11), indicating a much higher-than-normal responsiveness in glaucoma families (15), a very high response (80%) in glaucoma patients (22), an increased tendency to develop glaucoma in corticosteroid-responsive subjects (14), and in population statistics on corticosteroid responsiveness. In addition, a predisposition to develop glaucoma after trauma to the eye was found in corticosteroid responders. Armaly (12) showed that a higher frequency of angle-recess glaucoma occurred when the fellow eye was a positive responder. Corticosteroid responsiveness is an inborn characteristic found in very young infants (23), which somewhat increases with age (24), possibly indicating a modifying influence of additional (such as local, anatomic) factors on the genetic predisposition.

Family Studies

Several studies to determine the prevalence of glaucoma among relatives of index patients were perfomed by taking histories and examining these relatives (25). Perkins (26) found that 5.25% of 190 first-degree relatives (siblings, parents, childern) of patients with POAG had glaucoma. If those under 40 were excluded, this figure rose to 7.62%. None of the 22 more-distant relatives had glaucoma. A 10-year follow-up of a group of subjects with a family history of open-angle glaucoma revealed that 3% develpoed frank glaucoma and an additional 6% were suspected of having glaucoma (27). Jay and Paterson (28) studied 135 first-degree relatives of patients with glaucoma and concluded that multifactorial inheritance was most likely, as was suggested by Armaly (29).

A study by Shin and associates (30) showed that 50% of patients with POAG had a positive family history for glaucoma. This prevalence was much higher on the maternal side, in spite of an even distribution of POAG in both sexes.

Schwartz et al. (31) evaluated corticosteroid responsiveness in 37 pairs of monozygotic (MZ) twins and in 26 pairs of dizygotic (DZ) twins. They found a low-to-top-midrange heritability index and concluded that (i) genetic factors alone cannot be reponsible for the corticosteroid responsiveness, and (ii) simple monogenic determination of this characteristic is unikely. In recent investigation perfomed as a part of the Finnish twin cohort sudy, Teikari et al. (32) assessed 103 pairs of twins with glaucoma. A significantly greater concordance was noted in the MZ group, compared with the DZ group, indicating an active role by genetic factors. However, the heritability index in these groups was low, indicating enviornmental influence. Analyzing these studies, one must consider poor patient compliance (33), which may reduce the rate of agreement.

Kalenak and Paydar examined the difference in IOP of pairs of twins (34). They found an intrapair difference of 1.2 mmHg in 61 pairs of MZ twins and of 2.3 mm in 32 pairs of DZ twins. This intrapair difference was statistically significantly smaller for MZ twins but the difference could also indicate that additional factors exist.

In a study of IOP in normal eyes of twins and their immediate families (159) subjects and of 658 normal subjects of 209 famalies, Armaly found a similar degree of correlation among three subgroups: offspring and father, offspring and mother, and between siblings (29). This pattern would be expected in multifactorial inheritance.

Wolfs et al. (35) found a prevalence of POAG in 10.4% of siblings of patients, (6.7% in controls) and 1.1% in offspring of patients (controls: 0%). The authors calculated the lifetime risks for first-degree relatives of patients as 42.5% for elevated IOP (6.7% in controls), 62.2% for enlarged C/D ratio (16.6% in controls), and 22% for POAG (2.3% in controls) (35).

Risk Factors

The identification of genes associated with POAG does not exclude the possibility of other factors playing a role in the pathogenesis of this disorder. Thus, an individual may carry the mutant gene but not exhibit glaucoma. Other factors must also exist.

In a multifactorial disease, various other diseases and findings may be associated. In POAG, the other findings are often referred to as "risk factors," some of which have been confirmed, whereas others have not. The following have been suggested as possible risk factors:

1. *A family history of glaucoma* may well be the most important risk factor (36). It increases up to ten times a person's chance of developing glaucoma or ocular hypertension over the general population (27,35).
2. *Diabetes mellitus*, Becker claimed in 1971 (37), that diabetes was often associated with open-angle glaucoma, ocular hypertension, corticosteroid responsiveness, and large cup/disc ratios. Moreover, it has been claimed that diabetes mellitus has been more common in glaucoma patients or in corticosteroid responders (37,38). This association, however, may be only of low (39–41) or even no (36) significance. Ocular hypertension was substantially increased in patients with type 2 diabetes mellitus (non-insulin-dependent diabetes mellitus) (40). The Rotterdam study found that diabetic patients had a threefold increased presence of high-tension glaucoma (42). Newly diagnosed diabetic patients also had a higher mean IOP. However, one study (43) did not find such an association.
3. *Myopia*, especially high myopia, has been associated with corticosteroid responsiveness (44) and open-angle glaucoma (41,44,45). No long-term studies have been available to confirm this association. The Blue Mountain Eye study and the Barbados study found a strong relationship between myopia and glaucoma (46,47). Myopic subjects had a two-fold to three-fold increased risk of glaucoma compared to nonmyopic subjects.
4. *Age* accounted for an increase in mean IOP of 1.2 mmHg (in men) and 2.2 mmHg (in women) between young (aged 20 years) and old (aged 70 years) subjects (34).
5. *No sexual predisposition* has been noted in the mean IOP of young men and women, but an increase in IOP with age is significantly greater in women.
6. *Systemic vascular disease*, characterized by elevated blood pressure, has been associated with high IOP (36,39,48). With an increase of 100 mmHg in the systemic pressure, there is an average increase of 2–4 mmHg in IOP.

The Rotterdam study also found that hypertension was associated with high-tension glaucoma (odds ratio 2.72) but not with normotensive glaucoma (49).

7. *Race* is an important risk factor, as reported in both the Baltimore Eye Survey (50) and the Barbados study (51). Age-adjusted prevalence rates for POAG were persistently higher in blacks when compared with whites. The prevalence rate for POAG, in the Baltimore study, in the age group above 80 was 2.16% for whites and 11.26% for blacks. A recent editorial again stressed race as risk factor for glaucoma (52).
8. *Optic disk abnormality* represented by a large cup, increases the risk for the development of glaucoma (53).
9. *Histocompatibility locus antigen (HLA) linkage*. It was claimed that HLA-B7 or HLA-B12 antigen, or both, have been found in high association (up to 88%) with POAG (54). In addition, the presence of HLA-A11 or HLA-BW35 protects white patients with ocular hypertension from developing visual field loss (55). However, these studies have not been confirmed, and the evidence for linkage of POAG with HLA antigens is not clear. Many studies have shown no association between POAG and HLA antigens (56–58). In one investigation, the only association was found in a group of familial POAG (59).
10. *Attempts to find other possible genetic markers* linked to the development of glaucoma seem inconclusive. An association between rhesus and Duffy blood group antigens and POAG (60); ABO blood groups (61); the secretion of ABO blood group antigens in saliva, or nontasting of phenylthiocarbamide and POAG (62); and the relation of plasma cortisol suppression by oral dexamethasone to the development of POAG (63), all have been suggested. These studies have not been confirmed, and subsequent studies have yielded contradictory results. A laboratory in vitro test was performed, based on the claim that an increased lymphocyte transformation sensitivity to corticosteroids exists in glaucoma patients (64). This hypothesis was not confirmed in subsequent studies (65).

One study indicated a possible association of ROAG with apolipoprotein E gene mutations (66) but another study did not confirm it (67). A possible association with a specific p53-gene haplotype has been suggested but not yet confirmed (68).

Epidemiology

Glaucoma is, in most populations, the second leading cause of blindness (69). Its impact is immense. In 1996, Quigley estimated that 6.7 million people, worldwide, suffer from glaucoma (69). He also estimated that in developed countries, one half of glaucoma patients are not aware of their disease. In developing countries even fewer know and treat their condition.

The carefully conducted Framingham Eye study found a prevalence of 1.2% of the population in the group aged 52–85 (70). This figure was much lower in studies that were not age-adjusted. In population studies in Sweden the prevalence was 0.5% (71) and in Wales it was 0.43% (72). However, the Swedish and Welsh groups were younger than those in Framingham and the definition of glaucoma varied between these studies.

Variable prevalence of POAG was reported in different populations. In North Italy 2.1% of the population over age 40 had ocular hypertension (OH), 1.4% had POAG, and 0.6% had angle-closure glaucoma (73). In Melbourne, Australia the prevalence was 0.1% in the fifth decade of life and 9.7% in the ninth decade (74). Prevalence of POAG in the United States population was estimated to be 1.86% (75). Black subjects were found to have, age-adjusted, a three-fold rate of that of white subjects. This higher rate of prevalence exists in blacks all over Africa without significant variation among the different African populations (76). In Japan and Mongolia the prevalence of POAG is low and the prevalence of angle closure glaucoma is high (77,78).

The Genetic and Clinical Types of POAG

The identification of several loci for glaucoma revolutionized our classification of this disease. The clinical expression of glaucoma may often depend upon the associated glaucoma-bearing gene and upon the specific mutation involved. We know still less about associated additional factors. The first gene to be identified, the MYOC/TIGR gene at locus GLC1A became the most studied and the most interesting. Table 3 summarizes the genetic types of POAG.

GLC1A Locus and the MYOC/TIGR Gene

In 1993, Sheffield et al. (79) mapped the first locus of a juvenile autosomal dominant glaucoma, GLC1A, to chromosome 1q21-q31. Twenty-two of 37 family members were affected by autosomal-dominant POAG with normal angles on gonioscopy. The age at diagnosis was 8–30, a mean of 18 years (80). Additional families were reported (81,82). The mean age at diagnosis was similar in another big family, ranged from 5 to 30; mean 18.5 years (82). Initial IOP was high, on average 38.5 mm Hg, and 83% needed surgical treatment (82); 87% had myopia. A large French Canadian family had glaucoma linked to the same location on chromosome 1, but phenotypically manifested either POAG of late onset (over 40 of age) or the juvenile form, or (83). A similar wide range of age of onset (11–51) was found in a second French Canadian family (84) and in a large American family (6–62 years) (85), thus confirming the wide age of onset of the POAG associated with GLC1A locus. The mapping of locus GLC1A was refined in 1997 (86) and 1998 (87) to chromosome 1q24.3-q25.2. The gene and three POAG associated mutations were identified in 1997 by Stone et al. (88) and they named the gene, associated with GLC1A locus, TIGR. Of the glaucoma population studied 3.9% had one of three mutations in the gene (88). The term TIGR was later changed to MYOC when it was discovered that its protein product is myocilin, a protein expressed in many human tissues including heart, muscles, and others.

GLC1A mutations were reported in families of German, English, Irish, Danish, French, and French Canadian origin (89), Other reports came from Italy (90), Australia (4,91), Japan (92,93), Britain and Turkey (94) and from the United States of a family of British descent (95). It seems that the GLCIA POAG-associated mutations have a worldwide distribution.

Many different mutations were reported. Most were missense mutations such as Gly357Val, Tyr430His (88), Thr377Met, Thr353Ile, Gly367Arg, Pro370Leu, Val426Phe, Tyr437His, Ile477Ser, Ile499Phe (91), Asp380Ala, Ser502Pro, Arg76Lys (94), Arg272Gly, Ile499Ser (93), Ile345Met, Val251Ala(3), Gly434Ser, Asn450Asp

Table 3 The Genetic Types of Autosomal Dominant POAG

Locus	Gene	Protein	Chromosomal location	Clinical characteristics	Remarks
GLC1A	MYOC/ TIGR	myocilin	1q24.3-q25.2	JOAG in most; late POAG in same families	Gln368STOP most common mutation; worldwide distribution
GLC1B	–	–	2cen-q13	NTG or POAG, severe	Several British families
GLC1C	–	–	3q21-q24	POAG, moderate to severe	One Oregon, USA and one Greek family
GLC1D	–	–	8q23	POAG	One family from the USA
FLC1E	OPTN	optineurin	10p15-p14	NTG; severe	One family
GLC1F	–	–	7q35-q36	POAG, high IOP	
Nail-patella syndrome	NPS	–	9q34	POAG, high IOP	Absent thumbnails, hypoplastic patella and other abnormalities

JOAG – juvenile onset open angle glaucoma.
POAG – primary poen angle glaucoma.
NTG – normotensive glaucoma.

and Ser393Asn (96). One reported mutation consisted of the deletion of two amino acids and replacement by another one amino acid (90). Another common mutation was the Gln368Stop mutation, which causes premature termination at codon 368 thus producing a truncated protein missing the final 135 amino acids of the myocilin protein (97).

A review of 1703 glaucoma patients in three races and five populations by Fingert et al. (98) revealed that 2–4% of glaucoma patients carry a GLC1A-associated mutation, and up to 5% in other studies. The phenotypes were variable. Most mutations resulted in juvenile open-angle glaucoma (JOAG) but adult-onset (late) POAG was described, often in other members of the same family. When only patients with juvenile OAG were selected, the rate of GLC1A-associated cases, increased to 8% in one study (99) while other studies showed a higher rate.

The most common mutation is undoubtedly the Gln368Stop mutation (4,97,100,101). Alward et al. (97) claimed that it is responsible for 1.6–2% of the whole population of glaucoma cases. Craig et al. (4) examined eight Australian families with this nonsense mutation and found in addition to juvenile OAG an increasing number of OHT and POAG. OHT or POAG were found in 72% of family members with this mutation and 82% at age of 65 (4). The adult-onset glaucoma seemed similar to the late POAG of patients without this mutation (101). Individuals were described that carried the mutation but did not have glaucoma (4,100).

Alward et al. determined (102) that GLC1A mutations are responsible for 4.6% of all POAG. The clinical variability is great, and the variable age of onset may be found associated with most missense mutations. Juvenile and late-onset glaucoma may be found in the same family (103). Mackey et al. (91) examined a family with a Thr377Met mutation and found a younger age of onset, higher peak of IOP, and a greater need for filtering surgery than with the GLC1A Glu368Stop mutation. Age of onset was 41.2 ± 11.5 and peak IOP was 31.7 ± 9.9 for the Thr377Met mutation, and a mean age of 52 with a mean IOP of 28 for the Glu368STOP mutation. Mabuchi et al. (92) showed that the same mutation caused POAG (high-tension glaucoma) in one individual, NTG (normal tension glaucoma) in a second individual and no glaucoma in a third. In a large survey of several different GLClA-associated mutations age of onset was 8–77 years and IOP peak ranged from 12 to 77 mmHg (102).

The gene on the GLC1A locus is MYOC (previously named TIGR). It consists of three exons and encodes a 504 amino acid protein known as myocilin (93,102). The gene has wide expression in the body but in the eye its function was isolated from cultured trabecular meshwork and from the connecting cilium of the photoreceptors (99). It is normally present in the cornea and in many extraocular tissues (104). The function of the normal protein myocilin is not known; nor do we know how myocilin is associated with glaucoma. Three theories were suggested (104). First, that excess extracellular myocilin increases outflow resistance by blocking channels; second, that the mutant myocilin is unable to fulfill the (unknown) function of normal myocilin in the a.c. angle; third, that interaction between normal and mutant myocilin is not possible, while two mutant forms of the same sort may interact normally (104). In this respect, it must be mentioned that in almost all autosomal dominant disease, a homozygous state leads to more severe disease, but not so in POAG. Morissette et al. (3) examined a large family with the Lys423Glu mutation and found that almost all heterozygotes (who had both normal and mutated myocilin) showed signs of glaucoma (90% over 40 years old) but four homozygotes (who had only mutated myocilin) did not show any signs of the disease. This is unique among autosomal dominant diseases.

In summary, GLC1A mutations are associated with glaucoma but the clinical expressivity is variable. The presence of a mutation may be associated with juvenile glaucoma, late-onset glaucoma, OH, or no glaucoma. No glaucoma was detected even in an individual that was hemizygous with this portion of chromosome 1q deleted, meaning that he had only 50% of GLC1A wild type (105). GLC1A mutations have a much higher association with JOAG than with late-onset POAG, but in most cases both forms of glaucoma may be found. The detection of juvenile glaucoma in a family with POAG increases the likelihood of a GLC1A mutation (93).

At least 50 different mutations were reported (93). The vast majority are missense mutations and some are nonsense mutations. The Glu368STOP mutation is the most common, providing about half of all GLC1A mutations.

GLC1B Locus

It became clear that in some families with autosomal-dominant glaucoma the disorder is not associated with the GLC1A locus (106). In 1996, Stoilova et al. identified a second locus GLC1B associated with POAG in several British families (107). GLC1B was localized near the centromere of chromosome 2 at chromosome 2cen-ql3. Clinically, affected individuals had low to moderate IOP, onset in the fifth decade of life and good response to medical therapy (107). The gene has not yet been identified.

GLC1C Locus

The third locus for AD-POAG was mapped by Wirtz et al. (108) at chromosome 3q21-q24 and designed GLC1C. In a large North American Caucasian family from Oregon, they found 12 of 44 members to be affected by a typical POAG. The range of IOP was 18–26 mmHg but the optic disk and visual fields were badly affected (108). A second family from Epirus, Greece, also showed linkage, associated with their glaucoma, to the long arm of chromosome 3 (109).

The gene is currently not identified but Wirtz et al. suggested that the candidate gene is MME-membrane endopeptidase, located in the same area (108).

GLC1D Locus

Trifan et al. mapped the fourth locus of autosomal-dominant glaucoma to chromosome 8q23 (110). GLC1D was detected in one North American family with glaucoma of late onset. In most affected persons, the IOP was in the low 20s. The gene has not yet been identified.

GLC1E Locus and the Optineurin Gene

Sarfarazi et al. described a large British family with classical normotensive glaucoma (NTG), transmitted by the autosomal dominant mode (111). They designated the locus as GLC1E and mapped it to chromosome 10pl5-pl4. The IOP was low or normal, ranging from 14 to 21 mm, but visual fields were very abnormal and optic disks excavated (0.8–0.9). Rezaie et al. (112,112a) identified mutations in the optineurin gene at the location of GLC1E in 16.7% of 54 families with hereditary glaucoma. They re-named the gene, which had already been cloned, OPTN, for optineurin. Two missense mutations and one nonsense mutation in the OPTN gene were identified in association with the severe NTG (112). However, two subsequent studies, one from the United States (52) and the other from Japan, where NTG is a common form of glaucoma (113), did not identify any glaucoma-bearing mutations in the OPTN gene in a large number of patients.

GLC1F Locus

A new locus for POAG was identified by Wirtz et al. (114) and designated GLC1F. It was mapped to chromosome 7q35-q36. The one family examined [which had 10 affected members with classic POAG of adult onset (range 28–70 years)], had high IOP that was easily controlled by medication (114,115).

The glaucoma-nail patella syndrome

Nail and bone abnormalities with open-angle glaucoma were transmitted by the autosomal-dominant mode in two families. Lichter et al. (116) mapped this condition to chromosome 9q34 in both families and designated the locus as NPS1 (for nail patella syndrome). Clinically, patients have skeletal abnormalities including hypoplastic patellae, thumbnails missing or abnormal and open-angle glaucoma with high IOP and variable age of onset (116).

Other genetic transmission of POAG

The assignment of the seven loci of POAG to specific chromosomal location does not change the fact that in the majority of POAG patients, the genetic background is not known. In addition, it is not known why one person with a known mutated glaucoma-associated gene develops glaucoma while another such person does not show any sign of the disease.

It is unlikely that many more loci for autosomal-dominant POAG will be identified. It is also unlikely that a large percentage of POAG patients will suddenly be found to have a single gene-associated autosomal-dominant inheritance.

Autosomal-recessive transmission as the only mode of inheritance is also highly unlikely. The fewer than expected affected members in families of patients, the lack of influence of consanguinity, and the lack of affected offspring when both parents have COAG preclude this mode of transmission.

It appears that the multifactorial mode is the most plausible inheritance for all, or for most, cases of POAG, and that single-gene inheritance is unlikely (117). Several support Armaly's theory of multifactorial inheritance of POAG (118).

1. The number of affected first-degree relatives was variously reported as being between 5 and 10%. The latter figure occurred in relatives over 40, when glaucoma becomes clinical. These figures are far too low for any monomeric transmission.
2. The number of affected second-degree relatives is only slightly more than in the general population. This is an expected feature in a multifactorial inheritance.
3. Twin studies indicated the influence of hereditary factors; the concordance between MZ twins was significantly higher than between DZ twins (119). However, the heritability index (HI) was rather low, indicating additional environmental factors.
4. Edward's law states that, in a multifactorial disease, the risk to first-degree relatives is the square root of the frequency of the disease in the general

population (120,121). A frequency of about 10% in first-degree relatives of patients with COAG over 40 years old fits well with the square root of 1.3 % prevalence in the general population recorded in the Framingham study.

5. Corticosteroid responsiveness is an important factor related to the development of POAG, but not the only one. Its inheritance is possibly by a pair of alleles on a single locus, but also may be multifactorial.
6. Several ocular characteristics that appear to be important in the development of glaucoma seem to be inherited separately, with possible some common genetic determinants (118), including IOP and outflow facility (118), horizontal cup/disk ratio (119), and corticosteroid responsiveness. It has been suggested that IOP, outflow facility, and disk abnormality are transmitted multifactorially (118).
7. Other related risk factors such as diabetes or glaucoma indicate additional genetic or environmental factors.
8. POAG in blacks represents a much more severe disease than in whites, because of existence of additional factors. Especially noted are a higher IOP, inborn pathologic disk changes, and younger age at onset (122).
9. Some affected families exhibit a much more severe disease than others. In general, POAG is more severe in familial than in sporadic cases.

Digenic or multigenic inheritance with additional environmental influence currently seems to be the most likely explanation for the mode of transmission in the majority of POAG patients. Autosomal-recessive genes associated with POAG maybe detected in the future. Digenic or polygenic inheritance may also explain an association between POAG and Alzheimer's disease and between POAG and Parkinson's disease (123). None of the above excludes additional environmental factors influencing onset of glaucoma.

Management of Chronic Open-Angle Glaucoma

Surgical and Medical Treatment

Details of the regimens to treat POAG are beyond the scope of this book. In most cases, the accepted approach is to treat POAG first medically. If such treatment fails, then laser trabeculoplasty or a modified filtering operation is suggested.

In familial cases, especially if the existence of a POAG-associated mutation is confirmed, extra attention should be taken. The disease that manifests itself earlier often takes a more severe course and leads more frequently to blindness, compared to non-familial cases. A more aggressive approach to treatment may be considered, including earlier surgery.

Higginbotham et al. recently reported results of the Ocular Hypertension Treatment Study that indicated that medical treatment is effective in preventing glaucoma of patients with OH and higher than average risk (124). African Americans with OH developed glaucoma with visual fields damage twice as often if not treated: 16.1% in the observation only group compared to 8.4% in the treatment group.

These results should, in my opinion, be applied to any other ocular hypertensive patient with additional risk, especially if such a patient carries a mutated POAG-associated gene.

Should a young family member, who carries such a mutation but currently shows no sign of glaucoma, receive treatment? At present, no study has been performed that unequivocally answers this question. Some mutation carriers will develop POAG, while others will not, and close supervision of any known mutation carrier should be lifelong.

Genetic Counseling

A member of a family with autosomal dominant form of POAG should be tested for glaucoma gene mutations. The risk for offspring will be, in any case, less than 50%, as some members will carry the gene but not show any signs of glaucoma all their life. Finding of a mutation that is POAG-associated helps in the diagnosis and management and may enable prenatal diagnosis if so desired.

In non-familial cases, the largest group of patients, genetic counseling should be given as for a multifactorial disease. The following applies:

1. In general, the risk for first-degree relatives (parents, offspring, siblings) to develop COAG after the age of 40 is about 10%.
2. Recurrence rates increase if more than one family member is affected.
3. Recurrence rates increase with the severity of the disease of the proband.
4. The disease tends to be more severe if more family members are affected.
5. Elevated IOP and decreased outflow facility occur in predisposed family members who show no visual field loss.
6. Prenatal diagnosis is not possible or likely for COAG.

PRIMARY ANGLE CLOSURE GLAUCOMA

Introduction

Primary angle closure glaucoma (PACG) predisposes the patient to an acute attack or to a chronic stage of slowly progressive irreversible angle changes. Numerous reports on the familial occurrence of the disease, on one hand, and an acute attack, often triggered by nonhereditary factors, on the other hand, have led to the assumption that hereditary and environmental factors are important in the development of this disease. Even opponents of a multifactorial pathogenesis for POAG would agree that angle closure glaucoma is require both (125,126).

Family Studies

In a study of 67 first-degree relatives of patients with PACG, Perkins found 5.97% to be affected. This number increased to 10.26% when only relatives over aged 40 were considered (26). None of 14 more distant relatives was affected. A relatively shallow anterior chamber was found in first- and second-degree relatives of patients (127). A study of 20 pairs of twins led Teikari (128) to conclude that the findings support multifactorial inheritance of chronic closed-angle glaucoma.

Risk Factors and Primary Angle Closure Glaucoma

For more than a century, the relation of this type of glaucoma to shallow anterior chambers has been known. Now, a series of additional risk factors have also been recognized.

1. *A shallow anterior chamber* is the most obvious predisposing factor to PACG (127). In Eskimos (129), no patient with an anterior chamber depth of at least

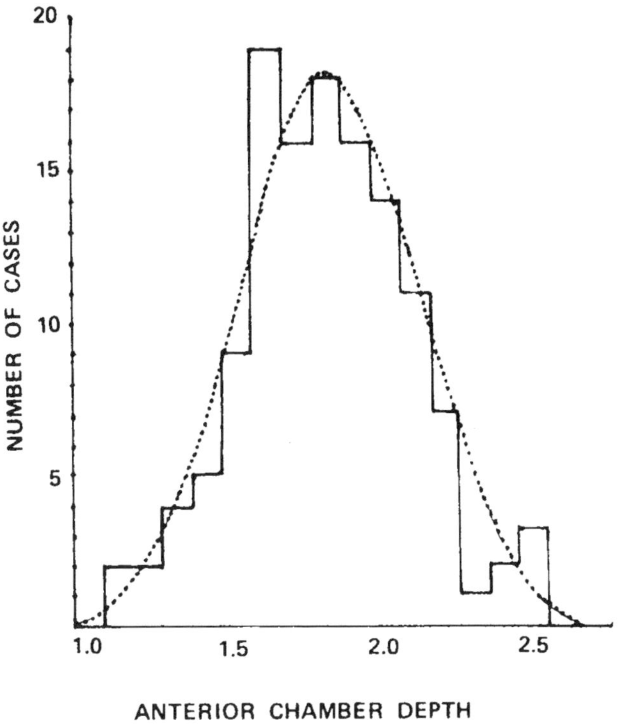

Figure 2 The distribution of anterior chamber depth (in mm) in 129 eyes with primary angle closure glaucoma. Note the normal population (Gaussian) curve. Compared with normal controls, it is skewed toward the shorter, depth measurements (from Ref. 129).

2.5 mm developed acute glaucoma. A depth of 2.0–2.5 mm, will trigger an acute attack in about 1%; a depth of 1.5–2.0 mm; will precipitate such an attack in about 20%. When the anterior chamber depth is shallower than 1.5 mm, about 85% will have acute closure (129). These predicted figures may be different in other populations. However, anterior chamber depth is not an "all-or-none" phenomenon. The distribution of the different measurements of anterior chamber depth in PACG patients is a Gaussian curve (Fig. 2), as in the normal population, except shifted to the shorter depth measurements (130).

The volume of the anterior chamber is another related factor; the risk of closure increases if the volume of the anterior chamber is <100 μL (131).

The major determining factors of anterior chamber depth are lens thickness, lens position, and height of the corneal dome (129), In patients with PACG, the mean lens thickness is greater, its mean position more anterior, and the corneal dome shallower than in normal controls. These variables seem to be genetically or "constitutionally" determined (132,133). A resemblance was noted between family members of patients with angle closure glaucoma when these measurements were compared with a normal control group (133).

Ultrasound biomicroscopy of patients diagnosed as PACG revealed a thicker, more anteriorly located lens, with a shorter ocular axial length, a shallower anterior chamber (a.c.) depth, a narrower a.c. angle, a shorter trabecular-ciliary process distance, a shorter iris-zonule distance, and a larger iris-lens contact (134).

One or more additional factors, as yet unknown, are needed to turn these risk factors into closed angle glaucoma. In one study, Wilensky et al. followed 129 patients diagnosed to be at risk by gonioscopy, refraction, pachymetry, ultrasound biometry, and provocative tests (135). Twenty-five of the 129 developed a closed angle, eight developed an acute attack, but none of the above tests showed high sensitivity or positive predictive accuracy (135).

2. *Other ocular dimensions*. The mean corneal dimensions are smaller in patients with PACG than in the general population, with a smaller anterior chamber diameter (131). The axial length of the eye also tends to be smaller, and there is increased frequency of hypermetropia in patients with PACG and in their relatives (134,136).

3. *Women* are more affected by angle closure glaucoma than men by a ratio of 3:1 (129). The mean difference in anterior chamber depth between white men and women is only 0.1 mm, which seems inadequate to explain the large difference in propensity for angle closure glaucoma in women (130). It is possible, however, that the decrease in anterior chamber depth with age is greater in women than in men, which could accentuate this difference.

4. The *mean depth of the anterior chamber lessens with increasing age* (130). This decrease is probably related to the increasing thickness of the aging lens.

5. Primary angle closure glaucoma has an uneven distribution among the *different populations and races*, probably reflecting the constitutional anatomic dimensions of the eye. PACG is very rare in American Indians, Australian Aborigines, and New Zealand Maoris. It is rare, in its acute form, in Africans. It is neither rare nor common in whites. It is more common than POAG in Chinese, Japanese, and Indonesians (130), and it has the highest known incidence in the Eskimos of Greenland (131), in whom it is 20–40 times more frequent than in whites (125).

Chinese ethnic origin and female sex were significant risk factors for development of acute angle closure glaucoma (138). A high prevalence of occludable angles was detected in Vietnamese (139). An angle of grade 2 or less was found in 29.5% of the Vietnamese, 47.8% in Vietnamese older than 55 years and 3.8% in whites older than 55 (139). An angle of 0–1 was found in 8.5% of Vietnamese and was rare in whites. A study of the a.c. angle in three populations revealed that iris insertion into the scleral wall was most anterior in Asians, most posterior in Caucasians and intermediate in Afro-Americans (140). Congdon et al. (141) found a smaller radius of corneal curvature in Chinese compared to white and black populations.

6. *Environmental factors*, such as mental factors, darkness, fatigue, or trauma (130), have been known to increase the risk of the acute attack.

7. Patients with angle closure glaucoma have had a significantly increased frequency of *familial type 2 diabetes mellitus* (noninsulin-dependent diabetes mellitus) (40). This tendency could indicate a common genetic background or secondary lens change in this type of diabetes.

8. Patients with *retinitis pigmentosa* have a much higher prevalence of angle closure glaucoma than the general population. This was reported for isolated retinitis pigmentosa, sector retinitis pigmentosa (142), and retinitis pigmentosa associated with nephropathy (143). Between approximately 2 and 12.5% of all patients with retinitis pigmentosa will have angle closure glaucoma. It may be caused by secondary lens changes in the form of lens thickening.

9. *Corticosteroid responsiveness* has no relationship to the development of PACG. The frequency of corticosteroid responsiveness among angle closure glaucoma patients is similar to that in the general population (144).

Epidemiology and Genetics

The prevalence of PACG varies in different populations. In whites, its frequency is between 0.1 and 0.5% (125) and about one third of the prevalence of chronic open-angle glaucoma. In Eskimos, who compose the population with the highest known prevalence, 2% of the population over 40 years old suffer from PACG, including 5.1% of women and 1.6% of men (129).

PACG comprises approximately 6% of all glaucoma patients and occurs in 0.1% of people older than 40, according to one study performed on a North American white population (139). Another study found in Italian whites over 40 years old, an incidence of 0.6% (73). This may reflect a genuine variation among white populations but it could likely reflect differences in diagnosing PACG.

Primary angle closure glaucoma was assumed by Lowe (132) to be transmitted as a multifactorial disease, characterized by a combination of hereditary and environmental factors.

The inherited factors include (i) dimensions of anterior chamber, (ii) size and position of lens, (iii) axial length of eye, and (iv) size of cornea.

The acquired factors include (i) aging changes in the lens and anterior chamber dimensions, and (ii) various mental and environmental trigger factors. The mode of action of the other factors mentioned, such as diabetes or retinitis pigmentosa, is not certain.

Management

Surgical and Medical

The usual approach to the treatment of angle closure glaucoma is surgical, by laser iridectomy or iridotomy or by surgical peripheral iridectomy. The argon, krypton, or YAG:Nd laser could be used. The YAG laser requires less total energy than the other two. A successful laser or surgical treatment results in elimination of the relative pupillary block, increased depth of the peripheral anterior chamber and an expanded anterior chamber volume (131).

Genetic Counseling

Francois (125) estimated the risk to first-degree relatives of patients with PACG to be 2–5%. However, multifactorial inheritance varies the risk among different families. The average risk to first-degree relatives is probably higher, about 6% in all, and about 10% over the age of 40 years (26). The modifying factors for a specific family are as follows: There is an increase if (i) more than one person of the family is affected, (ii) if the proband is male, (iii) if the proband has a more serious state of disease or rather shallow anterior chamber, and (iv) if a heavy genetic load exists, such as from a racial predisposition.

First-degree relatives, and a lower proportion of second-degree relatives, will have, on average, shallower anterior chambers than the general population.

In a review of all studies, Congdon et al. (145) summarized the risk for first-degree relatives as 1–12%, average four to five times of the general white population. They listed the list of risks as headed by family history and followed by age, sex, history of symptoms, and presence of hyperopia in this order (145).

PRIMARY INFANTILE GLAUCOMA

Introduction

Primary infantile glaucoma is an inborn type of glaucoma that may be present at birth or during the first year of life. It may be associated with the development of a big eye (buphthalmos), especially in the congenital form. Structural changes in the angle are present at birth, but often are not apparent. The term *primary* should be used to distinguish this disease from other inborn glaucomas associated with systemic diseases or occurring later in life. The term *infantile* is probably better than congenital, to distinguish it from a congenital glaucoma that appears later in life, such as juvenile glaucoma.

Family Studies

The number of familial cases of patients with primary infantile glaucoma is rather small. Of 63 families studied by Merin and Morin (146) (Fig. 3), only eight had another first-degree relative affected by the disease. Jay and Rice (147) found only seven familial cases among 163 patients with primary infantile glaucoma. The affected relative was a parent in three cases, a maternal uncle in two, and a sibling in two. Briard et al. (148) found that 13.6% of 221 cases had more than one affected family member. The parental prevalence ranged from 2.7 to 4.4%. Gencik et al. (149) found a high prevalence and a high risk of familial occurrence among gypsies of Slovakia. In 126 families, 205 affected members were identified.

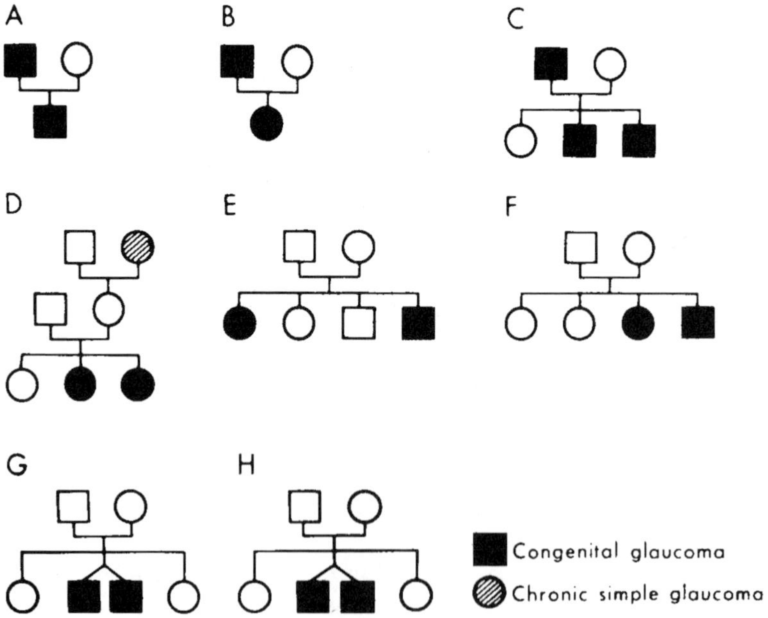

Figure 3 The pedigrees of eight of 63 families with primary infantile glaucoma. Families A–C have an affected father and child. Families C–F have two affected siblings, and families G and H have each a pair of affected monozygote twins. The remaining 55 families had only one affected member (the proband) (from Ref. 145).

Risk Factors

No specific risk factors or associations are known for primary infantile glaucoma. The associated anatomic abnormalities of the anterior segment of the eye, such as corneal changes, angle or size disorders, and associated myopia or optic disk changes, appear to be part of the same disease process (150). It is unlikely that the inborn angle changes will cause a primary open-angle glaucoma in the future, and the occurrence in the same families of such cases (Fig. 3) is most probably coincidental.

Some anatomic abnormalities stem from the high IOP. Seven of 10 eyes successfully operated for congenital glaucoma showed stability in the increase of the axial length and thereafter normal growth (151); three of 10 eyes showed reduction of their axial length; two eyes with failed surgeries continued to increase.

Corticosteroid responsiveness in patients with infantile glaucoma and their families is similar to that of the general population, unlike those with POAG (152).

Epidemiology

The incidence of primary infantile glaucoma is estimated to be 1:12,500 (146) to 1:22,000 (153) newborns. Familial cases occur in 4.3% (147) to 13.6% (148) of the total, with approximately one-half affecting a parent and child, and the other half affecting siblings. Males are affected more than females by a ratio of about 2:1 (71,72,77). In most patients, the disease is bilateral; about 30% are monocular and the second, unaffected eye in most of these instances shows angle changes indicating an arrested state of glaucoma.

Genetics and Molecular Genetics

The last decade witnessed the identification of two primary infantile glaucoma (PCG- for primary congenital glaucoma)-associated genes. These cover a variable proportion of PCG cases, according to the population.

GLC3A Locus and CYP1B1 Gene

The loci for congenital glaucoma were named GLC3. Sarfarazi et al. reported the assignment of the GLC3A locus to chromosome 2p21 (154), and in 1997 Stoilov et al. (155) identified three different truncating mutations on the CYP1B1 gene in five families with congenital glaucoma. The gene CYP1B1 encodes cytochrome P450, subfamily 1, polypeptide 1. It consists of three exons and two introns but coding starts from exon 2 (184), Its location was refined to the region of chromosome 2p21-p22 (156). A large number of various mutations in the CYP1B1 gene were reported. In one study 16 mutations were detected in 22 PCG families (157). The mutations included missense, nonsense, deletions, insertions, duplications, and one large deletion. In all families, segregation was consistent with autosomal recessive disease (157).

The gene belongs to a group of P450 superfamily multigenes. The encoded protein contains 543 amino acids and is expressed in many human tissues including the trabecular meshwork (158).

The CYP1B1 gene and the GLC3A locus are a major factor responsible for congenital glaucoma transmitted by the autosomal recessive mode. Reports from various countries demonstrated the importance of the GLC3A locus. In Japan primary congenital glaucoma is not common. About 20% of PCG is associated with the GLC3A locus (158,159). Two mutations were identified: a truncated protein due to a premature termination at codon 430 (158) and a missense mutation Arg444Gln (159). Three missense mutations were identified in Saudi Arabian PCG and these represent about 85% of all the PCG cases (160). In the Slovak Gypsies a single mutation Gly387Lys, was identified in all affected (161). The Slovak Gypsies suffer from an exceptionally high incidence of congenital glaucoma (161). This primary infantile glaucoma had been previously described in the Slovakian gypsies as an autosomal recessive disease with full penetrance (149,162). The disease was differentiated from other PCG by being bilateral in all cases, manifest at birth, severe and showing no sexual predilection. The prevalence in the affected population was extremely high: 1:1250 people. The gene frequency was calculated as 2.8% (162). The disease in this group differed from a clinically similar disease in the rest of the Slovakian population (153).

In all described cases of primary infantile glaucoma the disease-associated mutations in the CYPlBl gene were homozygous or compound heterozygous.

GLC3B Locus and PCG

The second locus for primary congenital glaucoma has been mapped by Akarsu and coworkers to chromosome 1p36 (163). The authors screened 17 Turkish PCG families who had at least two affected offspring. Host had parental consanguinity. Eight families were not linked to GLC3A locus and half of these were identified as associated with locus GLC3B (163). The gene and its mutations were not yet identified. The transmission of the GLC3B locus-associated disorder is autosomal recessive.

Other Genetic Transmission of PCG

In isolated populations with a high rate of consanguinity, as in Saudi Arabia, Turkey or the Slovak Gypsies, GLC3A locus is responsible for most cases of PCG. In most other populations this is certainly not the case, and hereditary transmission of primary infantile glaucoma remains unknown and controversial. Only few families with three affected generations have been reported and therefore autosomal dominant inheritance is unlikely. Autosomal recessive inheritance with reduced penetrance has been suggested. It was confirmed in the Saudi Arabian population for the GLC3A locus (160) but it is not likely to be widespread, as it cannot be linked to the equal number of affected parents and siblings (164).

Multifactorial inheritance, with multiple genes acting together with an environmental influence, has been hypothesized (146,148,164–166). In support of this theory are the following: (i) The number of affected sibs parallels the number of affected parents in familial cases, indicating a genetic similarity between child and parent and between siblings. (ii) Inheritance is indicated by a high concordance in reported MZ twins. The unusual appearance of a discordance of MZ twins (165,167) can be explained by additional factors modifying the genetic process. (iii) The unequal distribution among sexes, with a propensity for boys, may indicate additional genetic or nongenetic factors consistent with the multifactorial history. (iv) Sib incidence fits fairly well with the expected square root of the population incidence (146), as suggested by Edwards, for multifactorial inheritance (120). (v) Additional factors, that may be genetic or not are responsible for many unilateral cases (almost one third of all) (168), variously called "arrested," "incomplete," or "abortive" congenital glaucoma (169), which occur in the "unaffected" eye of the monocular patients or in unaffected siblings of the patients. (vi) The frequency of affected family members substantially decreases in second-degree relatives.

Several authors have suggested a genetic heterogeneity for primary infantile glaucoma. Jay and Rice (147) described some cases as autosomal recessive and the rest as nongenetic. Others (117,170) have proposed a combination of various genetic backgrounds, including autosomal recessive, autosomal dominant, and muitifactorial.

A clinically similar disease to primary infantile glaucoma, which was unilateral in some and bilateral in others, was described in association with a pericentric inversion of chromosome 11 (171). A rare chromosomal abnormality, it was not previously reported in association with clinical anomalies (172). Infantile glaucoma was reported in selected cases of chromosomal anomalies that affected the eye (117).

Nishimura et al. (173) described congenital glaucoma in a person with a balanced translocation involving 6p25 and 13q22. In a second person with congenital glaucoma a deletion in the short arm of chromosome 6 was found. This hinted at 6p25 as a suspected locus for congenital glaucoma (174).

Management

Medical and Surgical

Primary infantile glaucoma is usually treated surgically. Goniotomy, trabeculotomy, and trabeculoplasty are the customary approaches, usually in that order of preference.

Failure of these procedures occurs. Other options include seton implants, such as Molteno, Baerveldt or Ahmed valves, but these procedures carry a high rate of complications (174). A regular filtering operation carries a high rate of failure and the use of MMC (mitomycin C) is justified (174). Combined trabeculotomy and trabeculectomy as an initial procedure using MMC renders a high rate of success according to one study (175), but MMC-associated complications may occur (176).

Genetic Counseling

In most patients, genetic counseling should be based on a model of multifactorial transmission. A monomeric theory of inheritance will likely overestimate the risks for additional offspring, and a non-genetic viewpoint will underestimate such risks.

The following facts should be kept in mind: (i) The risk of recurrence in offspring is about 5% (147), (ii) the risk to siblings is greater if more than one member of the family is affected, (iii) the risk is greater if the proband is of the less-affected sex (female), (iv) cases of abortive primary infantile glaucoma can sometimes be found among relatives, in whom some or all of the genes for the disease are present, but they do not manifest the fullblown disease.

Prenatal diagnosis is not possible. Hopefully, future methods will be developed to measure the size of the eye in utero.

HEREDITARY JUVENILE GLAUCOMA

Hereditary juvenile glaucoma is an uncommon, but not rare, specific clinical entity, which was named by Berg (177) to describe the autosomal dominant transmission of glaucoma in the young. Jerndal extended the pedigree described by Berg and showed that the transmission was autosomal dominant, with complete penetrance, that the iridocorneal angle was similar to that observed in primary infantile glaucoma, and that rarely did the affected patients have a high IOP in the neonatal period (178). By 1974, about 100 pedigrees had been published (179), many covering several generations (146,179,180) (Fig. 4). In all, the transmission was by a single autosomal dominant gene with full penetrance. There were suggestions that the disease was a late manifestation of congenital glaucoma or an early manifestation of chronic open-angle glaucoma. Shaffer termed this type of glaucoma "late developing infantile type" (181). Jerndal proposed the term "dysgenic glaucoma," reflecting the inborn angle changes and objections to the classification by age of onset (182).

Stegman et al. (183) studied the a.c. angle of eyes with juvenile OAG (JOAG) and reported that the trabecular meshwork is small compared to non-glaucomatous eyes.

The single determined JOAG-associated gene is MYOC and, as described above, GLC1A is the common locus for both JOAG and POAG. At least, 10% of all JOAG cases are associated with MYOC mutations. About 50 different mutations in the MYOC gene have been reported and every one of them is responsible for both JOAG and POAG, often found in the same family.

The hereditary transmission of the majority of patients with JOAG is unknown. Varied modes of transmission may occur, including autosomal recessive, autosomal dominant not associated with GLC1A and MYOC or multifactorial. Vincent et al. (184) studied 60 individuals with JOAG, which they termed "early onset glaucoma" as age of onset ranged from 5 to 40 years. They found MYOC gene mutations in 13.3% and CYP1B1 mutations in 5%. A variable phenotype was seen. In one family with a clear autosomal dominant transmission an early-onset JOAG segregated with both MYOC and CYP1B1 mutations, indicating digenic inheritance. The CYP1B1 mutation was Arg368His and the authors suggested that the heterozygous state could be the cause of a mild phenotype or may modify the expression of MYOC (182).

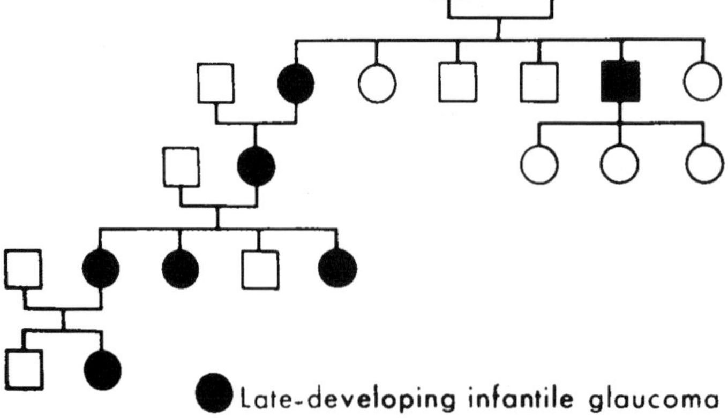

Figure 4 A family with hereditary juvenile glaucoma. Note the autosomal dominant transmission, with full penetrance. All patients manifested the disease after age 5 years (from Ref. 145).

Treatment of JOAG is medical, by topical anti-glaucoma medications, or surgical. In some cases, JOAG is treated like congenital glaucoma by goniotomy (146) or as POAG by filtering operations (185), now often using mitomycin C(MMC).

Genetic counseling is for an autosomal dominant inheritance with full penetrance. If the pedigree so indicates, MYOC gene mutations may be sought.

PIGMENTARY GLAUCOMA

Pigmentary glaucoma, as one sign of pigmentary dispersion syndrome, appears to be a distinct entity, separate from chronic open-angle glaucoma. As suggested by both clinical and electron microscopic studies (186,187), pigmentary dispersion results from the liberation of pigment when the iris pigment epithelium rubs against the zonules. It was thought that this occurred in individuals with a specific, genetically determined, configuration of the iris (186).

When a large amount of pigment accumulates, it tends to block the filtering angle, causing glaucoma. This occurrence is more common in males, by a ratio from 2:1 (188) to 3:1 (189,190) is rarely found in blacks, but has been reported in a black albino who had enough pigment dispersal to cause glaucoma (190).

The pigmentary dispersion syndrome is rare before age 10, is usually diagnosed between ages 20 and 40 years, and may go into remission, with an actual reduction in amount of pigment. The clinical features of the syndrome include increased pigmentation in the anterior chamber, on the corneal endothelium, and on the filtering angle, and the presence of Kurkenberg's spindle. Careful slit-lamp examination will often detect iris defects. There is an increased incidence of moderate to high myopia and of pigmentary glaucoma. Midperipheral iris transillumination defects and a heavily pigmented trabecular meshwork are the hallmarks of pigmentary glaucoma. The presumed pathogenesis is the rubbing away of the iris pigment epithelium, possibly by an inherent abnormality of the iris PE, and the accumulation of the pigment granules blocking the trabecular meshwork (191).

Approximately 50% of patients with the pigment dispersion syndrome (PDS) will develop glaucoma (191). The risk factors to develop PDS are young adult age (typical 20–30), white race, male gender and myopia (191). A more posterior insertion of the iris into the ciliary body is also a risk factor for PDS, because it increases the likelihood for iridozonular contact and pigment dispersion (192). An additional risk factor is a midperipheral iris concavity that increases with accommodation (193). The posterior iris bowing is reversible on inhibition of blinking and is restored by blinking (194). High-resolution ultrasound biomicroscopy confirms all these findings. Mid-peripheral iris concavity was found in 56% of PDS patients, irido-zonular contact in 25% and iridociliary process contact in 75% (195).

Two risk factors that predict that a patient with PDS will develop pigmentary glaucoma are higher myopia (190,195) and male gender. PDS affects men and women similarly but glaucoma is more common in men by threefold (194,196). Ritch considered the existence of three "hits" or stages in the progression of PDS to pigmentary glaucoma. First, enough pigment deposit to decrease trabecular function; second, a meshwork susceptible to develop high IOP; third, the susceptibility of the disk to damage (192).

Siddiqui et al. (197), on examining patients with pigmentary glaucoma in Minnesota in the US, concluded that only 10% of PDS patients would develop glaucoma in five years. The most important sign of developing glaucoma was intraocular pressure of 21 mmHg or more (197).

The prevalence of PDS was established by Ritch et al. as 2.45% in a white population they screened (198).

The epidemiology and genetics of the pigmentary dispersion syndrome were studied by Mandelcorn et al. (197) in four families. Three families had two affected generations, and one had one affected generation. In all, 10 of 23 family members had pigmentary dispersion syndrome, probably with autosomal dominant inheritance. The study of an additional family (200) gave the same results; the transmission of the syndrome was independent of other factors such as sex, iris color, or refractive error. However, the results of the large number of published pedigrees of *pigmentary glaucoma* cast some doubts on this claim, chiefly because of the smaller number of affected individuals than expected, the preponderance of males, and the increased prevalence of myopia. The possible modes of transmission, therefore, could be (i) autosomal dominant, with complete penetrance, but varying expressivity; (ii) autosomal dominant, with incomplete penetrance and varying expressivity; (iii) autosomal dominant inheritance of the pigmentary dispersion syndrome, in which additional genetic or environmental factors, including myopia, male bias, and others, determine the presence or absence of heavy pigmentation and glaucoma; or (iv) multifactorial inheritance.

Andersen et al. (201) mapped a locus for PDS at the telomeric end of the long arm of chromosome 7. The assigned locus was named GPDS1 for glaucoma related pigment dispersion syndrome (202). Four families with 28 affected members had the PDS association to the GPDS1 locus at chromosome 7q35-q36 (201).

A second locus for PDS and pigmentary glaucoma may also exist. Andersen et al. reported linkage of the second locus to chromosome 18qll-q21 (203).

The treatment of pigmentary glaucoma should be attempted initially as in POAG. Anti-glaucoma medications are usually the first line of management followed by laser iridotomy (189,204–206). Laser iridotomy reduces or abolishes any future elevation of IOP (205) and significantly decreases iridolenticular contact (206).

Until the inheritance is completely clarified, genetic counseling should probably be as for an autosomal dominant disease, incomplete penetrance, and varying expressivity, with glaucoma determined by the presence or absence of additional factors.

SECONDARY DEVELOPMENTAL GLAUCOMAS

Glaucoma may develop as a secondary phenomenon in a series of ocular and systemic genetic diseases. Increased IOP may manifest in infancy, childhood, or young adulthood. It may be caused by an anterior chamber cleavage syndrome (goniodysgenesis) (Table 4), other filtration angle anomalies (Table 5), lens subluxation (Table 6), or other causes, such as tumors or blood vessels in the angle (Table 7). Developmental glaucoma is much more common in peripheral dysgenesis of the iris if anterior chamber cleavage syndromes are divided into three groups, namely, peripheral, central, and mixed (207). Secondary glaucomas are not rare in childhood.

In one series, they composed about 30% of all cases of infantile glaucoma; the rest were primary glaucomas (168). They may also be caused by nongenetic factors, such as infectious embryopathies (208). These different diseases are discussed in other chapters and listed here only in tables. Most of these rather uncommon

Table 4 The Anterior Chamber Cleavage Syndromes

Syndromes	Inheritance
Axenfeld–Rieger anomaly	AD
Rieger syndrome type 1, type 2, type 3	AD
Peters anomaly	AR
Congenital microcoria with goniodysgenesis (207)	AD
Iridogoniodysgenesis syndrome (210)	AD

AD, autosomal dominant; AR, autosomal recessive.

Table 5 Infantile Glaucoma Caused by Developmental Anomaly or Gradual Closure of the Anterior Chamber Angle

Disorder	Inheritance
Aniridia	AD
Neurofibromatosis	AD
Microcornea	AD
Nanophthalmos	AD
Oculodentodigital syndrome (211)	AD
Marfan syndrome	AD
Klippel-Trenaunay-Weber syndrome	AD
Von Hippel-Lindau syndrome	AD
Lowe syndrome	XL

AD, autosomal dominant; XL, sex-linked recessive.

Table 6 Infantile Glaucoma Caused by Lens Subluxation

Lens disorder	Inheritance
Ectopia lentis et pupillae	AR
Weill–Marchesani syndrome	AR
Marfan syndrome	AR
Homocystinuria	AR
Ehlers–Danlos syndrome	AR

AR, autosomal recessive.

Table 7 Other Angle Anomalies Causing Glaucoma

Anomaly	Inheritance
Neurofibromatosis	AD
Von Hippel-Lindau disease	AD
Retinoblastoma	AD
Sturge–Weber syndrome	
Congenital rubella	

AD, autosomal dominant.

disorders have loci mapped and many have genes cloned and mutations known. These can be found in the appropriate chapters.

REFERENCES

1. Blumenthal EZ, Weinreb RN. Molecular genetics in the clinical practice. Ophthalmol Clin N Am 2000; 13(3):489–500.
2. Wirtz MK, Samples JR. The genetic loci of open-angle glaucoma. Ophthalmol Clin N Am 2003; 16(4):505–514.
3. Morissette J, Clepet C, Moisan S, Dubois S, Winstall E, Vermeeren D, Nguyen TD, Polansky JR, Cote G, Anctil JL, Amyot M, Plante M, Falardeau P, Raymond V. Homozygotes carrying an autosomal dominant TIGR mutation do not manifest glaucoma. Nat Genet 1998; 19(4):319–321.
4. Craig JE, Baird PN, Healey DL, McNaught AI, McCartney PJ, Rait JL, Dickinson JL, Roe L, Fingert JH, Stone EM, Mackey DA. Evidence for genetic heterogeneity within eight glaucoma families, with the GLC1A Gln368STOP mutation being an important phenotypic modifier. Ophthalmology 2001; 108(9):1607–1620.
5. Samples JR. Discussion of the article by Graig JE et al. Ophthalmology 2001; 108:1620.
6. François J. Cortisone et tension oculaire. Ann Ocul 1954; 187:805–816.
7. Becker B, Mills DW. Corticosteroids and intraocular pressure. Arch Ophthalmol 1963; 70:500–507.
8. Becker B, Hahn KA. Topical corticosteroids and heredity in primary open-angle glaucoma. Am J Opthalmol 1964; 57:543–551.
9. Becker B. Intraocular pressure response to topical corticosteroids. Invest Ophthalmol 1965; 4:198–205.
10. Palmberg PF, Mandell A, Wilensky JT et al. The reproducibility of the intraocular pressure response to dexamethasone. Am J Ophthalmol 1975; 80:844–856.
11. Armaly MF. The heritable nature of dexamethasone induced ocular hypertension. Arch Ophthalmol 1966; 75:32–35.
12. Armaly MF. Inheritance of dexamethasone hypertension and glaucoma. Arch Ophthalmol 1967; 77:747–751.
13. Morrison E, Archer DB. Effect of fluorometholone (FML) on the intraocular pressure of corticosteroid responders. Br J Ophthalmol 1984; 68:581–584.
14. Kitazawa Y, Horie T. The prognosis of corticosteroid responsive individual. Arch Ophthalmol 1981; 99:819–823.
15. Francois J, Heintz-De Bree G, Tripathi RC. The cortisone test and the heredity of primary open angle glaucoma. Am J Ophthalmol 1966; 62:844–852.
16. Francois J. Corticosteroid glaucoma. Ann Ophthalmol 1977; 9:1075–1080.
17. Akingbehin T. Corticosteroid provocative tests. Trans Ophthalmol Soc UK 1982; 102:253–256.
18. Francois J, Victoria Troncoso V. Mucopolysaccharides at hypertension oculaire (pathogenie du glaucome cortisonique). Ann Ocul 1974; 207:625–641.
19. Polansky JR, Fauss DJ, Chen P, Chen H, Lutjen-Drecoll E, Johnson D, Kurtz RM Ma ZD, Bloom E, Nguyen TD. Cellular pharmacology and molecular biology of the trabecular meshwork inducible glucocorticoid response gene product. Ophthalmologica 1997; 211(3):126–139.
20. Polansky JR, Fauss DJ, Zimmerman CC. Regulation of TIGR/MYOC gene expression in human trabecular meshwork cells. Eye 2000; 14:503–514.
21. Nguyen TD, Chen P, Huang WD, Chen H, Johnson D, Polansky JR. Gene structure and properties of TIGR, an olfactomedin-related glycoprotein cloned from glucocorticoid-induced trabecular meshwork cells. J Biol Chem 1998; 273(11):6341–6350.

22. Nordmann J, Lobstein A, Gerhard JP et al. La test a la cortisone dans le glaucome simple a champ visual normal. Ophthalmologica 1965; 150:46–50.
23. Kass MA, Kolker AE, Becker B. Chronic topical corticosteroid use simulating congenital glaucoma. J Pediatr 1972; 81:1175–1177.
24. Armaly MF. Effect of corticosteroids on intraocular pressure and fluid dynamics. I. The effect of dexamethasone in the normal eye. Arch Ophthalmol 1963; 70:482–491.
25. Leighton DA. Survey of the first degree relatives of glaucoma patients. Trans Ophthalmol Soc UK 1976; 96:28–32.
26. Perkins ES. Family studies in glaucoma. Br J Ophthalmol 1974; 58:529–535.
27. Rosenthal AR, Perkins ES. Family studies in glaucoma. Br J Ophthalmol 1985; 69: 664–667.
28. Jay B, Paterson G. The genetics of simple glaucoma. Trans Ophthalmol Soc UK 1970; 90:161–171.
29. Armaly MF. The genetic determination of ocular pressure in the normal eye. Arch Ophthalmol 1967; 78:187–192.
30. Shin DH, Becker B, Kolker AE. Family history in primary open-angle glaucoma. Arch Ophthalmol 1977; 95:598–600.
31. Schwartz JT, Reuling FH, Feinleib M et al. Twin study on ocular pressure following topically applied dexamethasone. II. Inheritance of variation in pressure response. Arch Ophthalmol 1973; 90:281–286.
32. Teikari JM, Kaprio J, Koskenvuo M et al. Heredity of chronic open angle glaucoma. a twin study [Abstract]. Invest Opthalmol Vis Sci 1985; 26(suppl):109.
33. Apt L, Henrick A, Silverman LM. Patient compliance with use of topical ophthalmic corticosteroid suspensions. Am J Ophthalmol 1979; 87:210–214.
34. Kalenak JW, Paydar F. Correlation of intraocular pressures in pairs of monozygotic and dizygotic twins. Ophthalmology 1995; 102(10):1559–1564.
35. Wolfs RC, Klaver CC, Ramrattan RS, van Duijn CM, Hofman A, de Jong PT. Genetic risk of primary open-angle glaucoma. Population-based familial aggregation study. Arch Ophthalmol 1998; 116(12):1640–1645.
36. Seddon JM, Schwartz B, Flowerdew G. Case-control study of ocular hypertension. Arch Ophthalmol 1983; 101:891–894.
37. Becker B. Diabetes mellitus and primary open-angle glaucoma. The 27th Edward Jackson Memorial Lecture. Am J Ophthalmol 1971; 71:1–16.
38. Krupin T, Schoch LH, Cooper D, Becker B. Lack of correlation between ocular hypertensive response to topical corticosteroids and progression of retinopathy in insulin-dependent diabetes mellitus. Am J Ophthalmol 1983; 96:52–56.
39. Leske MC, Podgor MJ. Intraocular pressure, cardiovascular risk variables and visual field defects. Am J Epidemiol 1983; 118:280–287.
40. Clark CV, Mapstone R. The prevalence of diabetes mellitus in the family history of patients with primary glaucoma. Doc Ophthalmol 1986; 62:161–163.
41. Vacharat N. Risk factors in glaucoma. Int Ophthalmol Clin 1979; 19:157–197.
42. Dielemans I, de Jong PT, Stolk R, Vingerling JR, Grobbee DE, Hofman A. Primary open-angle glaucoma, intraocular pressure, and diabetes mellitus in the general elderly population. The Rotterdam Study. Ophthalmology 1996; 103(8):1271–1275.
43. Ellis JD, Evans JM, Ruta DA, Baines PS, Leese G, MacDonald TM, Morris AD. Glaucoma incidence in an unselected cohort of diabetic patients: is diabetes mellitus a risk factor for glaucoma? Br J Ophthalmol 2000; 84(11):1218–1224.
44. Podos SM, Becker B, Morton WR. High myopia and primary open-angle glaucoma. Am J Ophthalmol 1966; 62:1038–1043.
45. Linner E. The association of ocular hypertension with the exfoliation syndrome, the pigmentary dispersion syndrome and myopia. Surv Ophthalmol 1980; 25:145–147.
46. Mitchell P, Hourihan F, Sandbach J, Wang JJ. The relationship between glaucoma and myopia: the Blue Mountains Eye Study. Ophthalmology 1999; 106(10):2010–2015.

47. Wu SY, Nemesure B, Leske MC. Glaucoma and myopia. Ophthalmology 2000; 107(6):1026–1027.
48. Ganley JP. Epidemiological aspects of ocular hypertension. Surv Ophthalmol 1980; 25:130–135.
49. Dielemans I, Vingerling JR, Algra D, Hofman A, Grobbee DE, de Jong PT. Primary open-angle glaucoma, intraocular pressure, and systemic blood pressure in the general elderly population. The Rotterdam Study. Ophthalmology 1995; 102(1):54–60.
50. Tielsch JM, Sommer A, Katz J, Royall RM, Quigley HA, Javitt J. Racial variations in the prevalence of primary open-angle glaucoma. The Baltimore Eye Survey. JAMA 1991; 266(3):369–374.
51. Leske MC, Connell AM, Wu SY, Hyman LG, Schachat AP. Risk factors for open-angle glaucoma. The Barbados Eye Study. Arch Ophthalmol 1995; 113(7):918–924.
52. Miller E. Race and the risk of glaucoma. Arch Ophthalmol 2004; 122(6):909–910.
53. Kass MA. When to treat ocular hypertension. Surv Ophthalmol 1983; 28(suppl):229–34.
54. Shin DH, Becker B, Waltman SR et al. The prevalence of HLA-B12 and HLA-B7 antigens in primary open-angle glaucoma. Arch Ophthalmol 1977; 95:224–225.
55. Shin DH, Becker B. HLA-A11 and HLA-Bw35 and resistance to glaucoma in white patients with ocular hypertension. Arch Ophthalmol 1977; 95:423–424.
56. Gieser DK, Wilensky JT. HLA antigens and acute angle-closure glaucoma. Am J Ophthalmol 1979; 88:232–235.
57. Ticho U, Cohen T, Brautbar C. Absense of association between HLA antigens and primary open angle glaucoma in Israel. Isr J Med Sci 1979; 15:124.
58. Sears ML. Clinical and scientific basis for the management of open glaucoma. Arch Ophthalmol 1986; 104:191–195.
59. Rosenthal AR, Payne R. Association of HLA antigens and primary open-angle glaucoma. Am J Ophthalmol 1979; 88:479–182.
60. David R, Jenkins T. Genetic markers in glaucoma. Br J Ophthalmol 1980; 64:227–231.
61. Brooks AM, Gillies WE. Blood groups as genetic markers in glaucoma. Am J Ophthalmol 1988; 72:270–273.
62. Genetic associations of glaucoma [Editorial]. Br J Ophthalmol 1980; 64:225–226.
63. Becker B, Podos SM, Asseff CF, Cooper DG. Plasma cortisol suppression in glaucoma. Am J Ophthalmol 1973; 75:73–76.
64. Bigger JF, Palmberg PF, Becker B. Increased cellular sensitivity to glucocorticoids in primary open-angle glaucoma. Invest Ophthalmol 1972; 11:832–837.
65. Ben-Ezra D, Ticho U, Sacks U. Lymphocyte sensitivity to glucocorticoids. Am J Ophthalmol 1976; 82:866–870.
66. Vickers JC, Craig JE, Stankovich J, McCormack GH, West AK, Dickinson JL, McCartney PJ, Coote MA, Healey DL, Mackey DA. The apolipoprotein epsilon4 gene is associated with elevated risk of normal tension glaucoma. Mol Vis 2002; 8:389–393.
67. Ressiniotis T, Griffiths PG, Birch M, Keers S, Chinnery PF. The role of apolipoprotein E gene polymorphisms in primary open-angle glaucoma. Arch Ophthalmol 2004; 122(2):258–261.
68. Ressiniotis T. Griffiths PG, Birch M, Keers S, Chinnery PF. Primary open angle glaucoma is associated with a specific p53 gene haplotype. J Med Genet 2004; 41(4):296–298.
69. Quigely HA. Number of people with glaucoma worldwide. Br J Ophthalmol 1996; 80(5):389–393.
70. Kahn HA, Milton RC. Revised Framingham eye study prevalence of glaucoma and diabetic retinopathy. Am J Epidemiol 1980; 111:769–776.
71. Stromberg U. Ocular hypertension. Acta Ophthalmol 1962; Suppl 69:1-75.
72. Hollows FC, Graham PA. Intraocular pressure, glaucoma and glaucoma suspects in a defined population. Br J Ophthalmol 1966; 50:570–586.
73. Bonomi L, Marchini G, Marraffa M, Bernardi P, De Franco I, Perfetti S, Varotto A, Tenna V. Prevalence of glaucoma and intraocular pressure distribution in a defined population. The Egna-Neumarkt Study. Ophthalmology 1998; 105(2):209–215.

74. Wensor MD, McCarty CA, Stanislavsky YL, Livingston PM, Taylor HR. The prevalence of glaucoma in the Melbourne Visual Impairment Project. Ophthalmology 1998; 105(4):733–739.
75. Friedman DS, Wolfs RC, O'Colmain BJ, Klein BE, Taylor HR, West S, Leske MC, Mitchell P, Congdon N, Kempen J. Eye Diseases Prevalence Research Group. Prevalence of open-angle glaucoma among adults in the United States. Arch Ophthalmol 2004; 122(4):532–538.
76. Rotchford AP, Johnson GJ. Glaucoma in Zulus: a population-based cross-sectional survey in a rural district in South Africa. Arch Ophthalmol 2002; 120(4):471–478.
77. Shiose Y, Kitazawa Y, Tsukahara S, Akamatsu T, Mizokami K, Futa R, Katsushima H, Kosaki H. Epidemiology of glaucoma in Japan – a nationwide glaucoma survey. Jpn J Ophthalmol 1991; 35(2):133–155.
78. Foster PJ, Baasanhu J, Alsbirk PH, Munkhbayar D, Uranchimeg D, Johnson GJ. Glaucoma in Mongolia. A population-based survey in Hovsgol province, northern Mongolia. Arch Ophthalmol 1996; 114(10):1235–1241.
79. Sheffield VC, Stone EM, Alward WL, Drack AV, Johnson AT, Streb LM, Nichols BE. Genetic linkage of familial open angle glaucoma to chromosome 1q21-q31. Nat Genet 1993; 4(1):47–50.
80. Johnson AT, Drack AV, Kwitek AE, Cannon RL, Stone EM, Alward WL. Clinical features and linkage analysis of a family with autosomal dominant juvenile glaucoma. Ophthalmology 1993; 100(4):524–529.
81. Wiggs JL, Haines JL, Paglinauan C, Fine A, Sporn C, Lou D. Genetic linkage of autosomal dominant juvenile glaucoma to 1q21-q31 in three affected pedigrees. Genomics 1994; 21(2):299–303.
82. Wiggs JL, Del Bono EA, Schuman JS, Hutchinson BT, Walton DS. Clinical features of five pedigrees genetically linked to the juvenile glaucoma locus on chromosome 1q21-q31. Ophthalmology 1995; 102(12):1782–1789.
83. Morissette J, Cote G, Anctil JL, Plante M, Amyot M, Heon E, Trope GE, Weissenbach J, Raymond V. A common gene for juvenile and adult-onset primary open-angle glaucomas confined on chromosome lq. Am J Hum Genet 1995; 56(6):1431–1442.
84. Meyer A, Bechetoille A, Valtot F, Dupont de Dinechin S, Adam MF, Belmouden A, Brezin AP, Gomez L, Bach JF, Garchon HJ. Age-dependent penetrance and mapping of the locus for juvenile and early-onset open-angle glaucoma on chromosome lq (GLC1A) in a French family. Hum Genet 1996; 98(5):567–571.
85. Johnson AT, Richards JE, Boehnke M, Stringham HM, Herman SB, Wong DJ, Lichter PR. Clinical phenotype of juvenile-onset primary open-angle glaucoma linked to chromosome lq. Ophthalmology 1996; 103(5):808–814.
86. Belmouden A, Adam MF, Dupont de Dinechin S, Brezin AP, Rigault P, Chumakov I, Bach JF, Garchon HJ. Recombinational and physical mapping of the locus for primary open-angle glaucoma (GLC1A) on chromosome 1q23-q25. Genomics 1997; 39(3): 348–358.
87. Michels-Rautenstrauss KG, Mardin CY, Budde WM, Liehr T, Polansky J, Nguyen T, Timmerrnan V, Van Broeckhoven C, Naumann GO, Pfeiffer RA, Rautenstrauss BW. Juvenile open angle glaucoma: fine mapping of the TIGR gene to 1q24.3-q25.2 and mutation analysis. Hum Genet 1998; 102(1):103–106.
88. Stone EM, Fingert JH, Alward WL, Nguyen TD, Polansky JR, Sunden SL, Nishimura D, Clark AF, Nystuen A, Nichols BE, Mackey DA, Ritch R, Kalenak JW, Craven ER, Sheffield VC. Identification of a gene that causes primary open angle glaucoma. Science 1997; 275(5300):668–670.
89. Lichter PR, Richards JE, Boehnke M, Othman M, Cameron BD, Stringham HM, Downs CA, Lewis SB, Boyd BF. Juvenile glaucoma linked to the GLClA gene on chromosome 1q in a Panamanian family. Am J Ophthalmol 1997; 123(3):413–416.

90. Angius A, De Gioia E, Loi A, Fossarello M, Sole G, Orzalesi N, Grignolo F, Cao A, Pirastu M. A novel mutation in the GLC1A gene causes juvenile open-angle glaucoma in 4 families from the Italian region of Puglia. Arch Ophthalmol 1998; 116(6):793–797.
91. Mackey DA, Healey DL, Fingert JH, Coote MA, Wong TL, Wilkinson CH, McCartney PJ, Rait JL, de Graaf AP, Stone EM, Craig JE. Glaucoma phenotype in pedigrees with the myocilin Thr377Met mutation. Arch Ophthalmol 2003; 121(8):1172–1180.
92. Mabuchi F, Yamagata Z, Kashiwagi K, Tang S, Iijima H, Tsukahara S. Analysis of myocilin gene mutations in Japanese patients with normal tension glaucoma and primary open-angle glaucoma. Clin Genet 2001; 59(4):263–268.
93. Shimizu S, Lichter PR, Johnson AT, Zhou Z, Higashi M, Gottfredsdottir M, Othman M, Moroi SE, Rozsa FW, Schertzer RM, Clarke MS, Schwartz AL, Downs CA, Vollrath D, Richards JE. Age-dependent prevalence of mutations at the GLClA locus in primary open-angle glaucoma. Am J Ophthalmol 2000; 130(2):165–177.
94. Stoilova D, Child A, Brice G, Desai T, Barsoum-Homsy M, Ozdemir N, Chevrette L, Adam MF, Garchon HJ, Pitts Crick R, Sarfarazi M. Novel TIGR/MYOC mutations in families with juvenile onset primary open angle glaucoma. J Med Genet 1998; 35(12):989–992.
95. Richards JE, Ritch R, Lichter PR, Rozsa FW, Stringham HM, Caronia RM, Johnson D, Abundo GP, Willcockson J, Downs CA, Thompson DA, Musarella MA, Gupta N, Othman MI, Torrez DM, Herman SB, Wong DJ, Higashi M, Boehnke M. Novel trabecular meshwork inducible glucocorticoid response mutation in an eight-generation juvenile-onset primary open-angle glaucoma pedigree. Ophthalmology 1998; 105(9): 1698–1707.
96. Michels-Rautenstrauss K, Mardin C, Wakili N, Junemann AM, Villalobos L, Mejia C, Soley GC, Azofeifa J, Ozbey S, Naumann GO, Reis A, Rautenstrauss B. Novel mutations in the MYOC/GLC1A gene in a large group of glaucoma patients. Hum Mutat 2002; 20(6):479–480.
97. Alward WL, Kwon YH, Khanna CL, Johnson AT, Hayreh SS, Zimmerman MB, Narkiewicz J, Andorf JL, Moore PA, Fingert JH, Sheffield VC, Stone EM. Variations in the myocilin gene in patients with open-angle glaucoma. Arch Ophthalmol 2002; 120(9):1189–1197.
98. Fingert JH, Heon E, Liebmann JM, Yamamoto T, Craig JE, Rait J, Kawase K, Hoh ST, Buys YM, Dickinson J, Hockey RR, Williams-Lyn D, Trope G, Kitazawa Y, Ritch R, Mackey OA, Alward WL, Sheffield VC, Stone EN. Analysis of myocillin mutation's in 1703 glaucoma patients from five different populations. Hum Mol Genet. 1998; 8(5):899–905.
99. Wiggs JL, Allingham RR, Vollrath D, Jones KH, De La Paz M, Kern J, Patterson K, Babb VL, Del Bono EA, Broomer BW, Pericak-Vance MA, Haines JL. Prevalence of mutations in TIGR/myocilin in patients with adult and juvenile primary open-angle glaucoma. Am J Hum Genet 1998; 63(5):1549–1552.
100. Angius A, Spinelli P, Ghilotti G, Casu G, Sole G, Loi A, Totaro A, Zelante L, Gasparini P, Orzalesi N, Pirastu M, Bonomi L. Myocilin Gln368stop mutation and advanced age as risk factors for late-onset primary open-angle glaucoma. Arch Ophthalmol 2000; 118(5):674–679.
101. Graul TA, Kwon YH, Zimmerman MB, Kim CS, Sheffield VC, Stone EM, Alward WL. A case–control comparison of the clinical characteristics of glaucoma and ocular hypertensive patients with and without the myocilin Gln368Stop mutation. Am J Ophthalmol 2002; 134(6):884–890.
102. Alward WL, Fingert JH, Coote MA, Johnson AT, Lerner SF, Junqua D, Durcan FJ, McCartney PJ, Mackey DA, Sheffield VC, Stone EM. Clinical features associated with mutations in the chromosome 1 open-angle glaucoma gene (GLC1A). New Engl J Med 1998; 338(15):1022–1027.
103. Bruttini M, Longo I, Frezzotti P, Ciappetta R, Randazzo A, Orzalesi N, Fumagalli E, Caporossi A, Frezzotti R, Renieri A. Mutations in the myocilin gene in families with

primary open-angle glaucoma and juvenile open-angle glaucoma. Arch Ophthalmol 2003; 121(7):1034–1038.
104. Johnson DH, Myocilin. Myocilin and glaucoma: a TIGR by the tail? Arch Ophthalmol 2000; 118(7):974–978.
105. Wiggs JL, Vollrath D. Molecular and clinical evaluation of a patient hemizygous for TIGR/MYOC. Arch Ophthalmol 2001; 119(11):1674–1678.
106. Richards JE, Lichter PR, Herman S, Hauser ER, Hou YC, Johnson AT, Boehnke M. Probable exclusion of GLC1A as a candidate glaucoma gene in a family with middle-age-onset primary open-angle glaucoma. Ophthalmology 1996; 103(7):1035–1040.
107. Stoilova D, Child A, Trifan OC, Crick RP, Coakes RL, Sarfarazi M. Localization of a locus (GLCIB) for adult-onset primary open angle glaucoma to the 2cen-q13 region. Genomics 1996; 36(1):142–150.
108. Wirtz MK, Samples JR, Kramer PL, Rust K, Topinka JR, Yount J, Koler RD, Acott TS. Mapping a gene for adult-onset primary open-angle glaucoma to chromosome 3q. Am J Hum Genet 1997; 60(2):296–304.
109. Kitsos G, Eiberg H, Economou-Petersen E, Wirtz MK, Kramer PL, Aspiotis M, Tommerup N, Petersen MB, Psilas K. Genetic linkage of autosomal dominant primary open angle glaucoma to chromosome 3q in a Greek pedigree. Eur J Hum Genet 2001; 9(6):452–457.
110. Trifan OC, Traboulsi El, StoilovaD, Alozie I, Nguyen R, Raja S, Sarfarazi M. A third locus (GLCID) for adult-onset primary open-angle glaucoma maps to the 8q23 region. Am J Ophthalmol 1998; 126(1):17–28.
111. Sarfarazi M, Child A, Stoilova D, Brice G, Desai T, Trifan OC, Poinoosawmy D, Crick RP. Localization of the fourth locus (GLC1E) for adult-onset primary open-angle glaucoma to the 10pl5-pl4 region. Am J Hum Genet 1998; 62(3):641–652.
112. Rezaie T, Child A, Hitchings R, Brice G, Miller L, Coca-Prados M, Heon E, Krupin T, Ritch R, Kreutzer D, Crick RP, Sarfarazi M. Adult-onset primary open-angle glaucoma caused by mutations in optineurin. Science 2002; 295(5557):1077–1079.
112a. Wiggs JL, Auguste J, Allingham RR, Flor JD, Pericak-Vance MA, Rogers K, LaRocque KR, Graham FL, Broomer B, Del Bono E, Haines JL, Hauser M. Lack of association of mutations in optineurin with disease in patients with adult-onset primary open-angle glaucoma. Arch Ophthalmol 2003; 121(8):1181–1183.
113. Tang S, Toda Y, Kashiwagi K, Mabuchi F, Iijima H, Tsukahara S, Yamagata Z. The association between Japanese primary open-angle glaucoma and normal tension glaucoma patients and the optineurin gene. Hum Genet 2003; 113(3):276–279.
114. Wirtz MK, Samples JR, Kramer PL et al. Identification of a new adult-onset primary open angle glaucoma locus- GLC1F. Invest Ophthalmol Vis Sci 1998; 39:(ARVO Abstract 512).
115. Wirtz MK, Samples JR, Rust K, Lie J, Nordling L, Schilling K, Acott TS, Kramer PL. GLCIF, a new primary open-angle glaucoma locus, maps to 7q35-q36. Arch Ophthalmol 1999; 117(2):237–241.
116. Lichter PR, Richards JE, Downs CA, Stringham HM, Boehnke M, Farley FA. Cosegregation of open-angle glaucoma and the nail-patella syndrome. Am J Ophthalmol 1997; 124(4):506–515.
117. Heckenlively J, Isenberg S. Glaucoma and buphthalmus. In: Emery AEH, Rimoin DL, eds. Principle and Practice of Medical Genetics. Edinburgh: Churchill-Livingstone, 1983:488–496.
118. Armaly MF, Monstavicius BF, Sayegh RE. Ocular pressure and aqueous outflow facility in siblings. Arch Ophthalmol 1968; 80:354–360.
119. Schwartz JT, Reuling FH, Feinleib M. Size of the physiologic cup of the optic nerve head. hereditary and environmental factors. Arch Ophthalmol 1975; 93:776–780.
120. Edwards JH. The simulation of mendelism. Acta Genet 1960; 10:63–70.
121. Armaly MF. Applanation pressure in husbands-wife pairs. Am J Ophthalmol 1966; 62:635– 639.

122. Coulehan JL, Helzlsouer KJ, Rogers KD, Brown SI. Racial difference in intraocular tension and glaucoma surgery. Am J Epidemiol 1980; 111:759–768.
123. Bayer AU, Keller ON, Ferrari F, Maag KP. Association of glaucoma with neurodegenerative diseases with apoptotic cell death: Alzheimer's disease and Parkinson's disease. Am J Ophthalmol 2002; 133(1):135–137.
124. Higginbotham EJ, Gordon MO, Beiser JA, Drake MV, Bennett GR, Wilson MR, Kass MA. Ocular Hypertension Treatment Study Group The Ocular Hypertension Treatment Study: topical medication delays or prevents primary open-angle glaucoma in African American individuals. Arch Ophthalmol 2004; 122(6):813–820.
125. Francois J. Genetic predisposition to glaucoma. Dev Ophthalmol 1981; 3:1–45.
126. Francois J. Multifactorial or polygenic inheritance in ophthalmology. Dev Ophthalmol 1985; 10:1–39.
127. Tornquist R. Shallow anterior chamber in acute glaucoma: a clinical and genetic study. Acta Opthalmol 1953; 31(suppl 39):1–74.
128. Teikari JM. Closed-angle glaucoma in 20 pairs of twins. Can J Ophthalmol 1988; 23: 14–16.
129. Alsbirk PH. Primary angle-closure glaucoma. Oculometry, epidemiology and genetics in a high risk population. Acta Ophthalmol 1976; 127(suppl):5–31.
130. Lowe RF. Primary angle closure glaucoma. Inheritance and environment. Br J Ophthalmol 1972; 56:13–20.
131. Lee DA, Brubaker RF, Ilstrup DM. Anterior chamber dimensions in patients with narrow angles and angle closure glaucoma. Arch Ophthalmol 1984; 102:46–50.
132. Lowe RF. Aetiology of the anatomical basis for primary angle-closure glaucoma. Bio-metrical comparisons between normal eyes and eyes-with primary angle-closure glaucoma. Br J Ophthalmol 1970; 54:161–169.
133. Tomlinson A, Leighton DA. Ocular dimensions in the heredity of angle-closure glaucoma. Br J Ophthalmol 1973; 57:475–486.
134. Marchini G, Pagliarusco A, Toscano A, Tosi R, Brunelli C, Bonomi L. Ultrasound biomicroscopic and conventional ultrasonographic study of ocular dimensions in primary angle-closure glaucoma. Ophthalmology 1998; 105(11):2091–2098.
135. Wilensky JT, Kaufman PL, Frohlichstein D, Gieser DK, Kass MA, Ritch R, Anderson R. Follow-up of angle-closure glaucoma suspects. Am J Ophthalmol 1993; 115(3): 338–346.
136. Lowe RF. Causes of shallow anterior chamber in primary angle-closure glaucoma. Am J Ophthalmol 1969; 67:87–93.
137. Alsbirk PH. Anterior chamber of the eye. A genetic and anthropological study in Greenland Eskimos. Hum Hered 1975; 25:418–427.
138. Seah SK, Foster PJ, Chew PT, Jap A, Oen F, Fam HB, Lim AS. Incidence of acute primary angle-closure glaucoma in Singapore. An island-wide survey. Arch Ophthalmol 1997; 115(11):1436–1440.
139. Nguyen N, Mora JS, Gaffney MM, Ma AS, Wong PC, Iwach AG, Tran H, Dickens CJ. A high prevalence of occludable angles in a Vietnamese population. Ophthalmology 1996; 103(9):1426–1431.
140. Oh YG, Minelli S, Spaeth GL, Steinman WC. The anterior chamber angle is different in different racial groups: a gonioscopic study. Eye 1994; 8(pt 1):104–108.
141. Congdon NG, Youlin Q, Quigley H, Hung PT, Wang TH, Ho TC, Tielsch JM. Biometry and primary angle-closure glaucoma among Chinese, white, and black populations. Ophthalmology 1997; 104(9):1489–1495.
142. Omphroy CA. Sector retinitis pigmentosa and chronic angle-closure glaucoma: a new association. Ophthalmologica 1984; 189(Pt 1):12–20.
143. Fiore C, Santoni G, Reggiani FM et al. Familial nephropathy with retinitis pigmentosa and closed-angle glaucoma. Ophthalmic Paediatr Genet 1985; 6:39–49.
144. Kitazawa Y. Primary angle-closure glaucoma: corticosteroid responsiveness. Arch. Oph thalmol 1970; 84:724–727.

145. Congdon N, Wang F, Tielsch IM. Issues in the epidemiology and population-based screening of primary angle-closure glaucoma. Surv Ophthalmol 1992; 36(6):411–423.
146. Merin S, Morin D. Heredity of congenital glaucoma. Br J Ophthalmol 1972; 56:414–417.
147. Jay MR, Rice NSC. Genetic implications of congenital glaucoma. Metab Ophthalmol 1978; 2:257–258.
148. Briard ML, Feingold J, Kaplan J et al. Genetique du glaucome congenital un etude sur 231 cas. J Genet Hum 1976; 24(suppl):107–123.
149. Gencik A, Gencikova A, Gerinec A. Genetic heterogeneity of congenital glaucoma. Clin. Genet 1980; 17:241–248.
150. Morin JD, Merin S, Sheppard RW. Primary congenital glaucoma—a survey. Can J Ophthalmol 1974; 9:17–28.
151. Law SK, Bui D, Caprioli J. Serial axial length measurements in congenital glaucoma. Am J Ophthalmol 2001; 132(6):926–928.
152. Leighton DA, Phillips CI. Infantile glaucoma. Steroid testing in parents of affected children. Br J Ophthalmol 1970; 54:27–30.
153. Gencik A, Kadasi L, Gencikova A, Gerinec A. Notes on the genetics of congenital glaucoma. Ophthalmologica 1979; 179:209–213.
154. Sarfarazi M, Akarsu AN, Hossain A, Turacli ME, Aktan SG, Barsoum-Homsy M, Chevrette L, Sayli BS. Assignment of a locus (GLC3A) for primary congenital glaucoma (buphthalmos) to 2p21 and evidence for genetic heterogeneity. Genomics 1995; 30(2):171–177.
155. Stoilov I, Akarsu AN, Sarfarazi M. Identification of three different truncating mutations in cytochrome P4501B1 (CYP1B1) as the principal cause of primary congenital glaucoma (buphthalmos) in families linked to the GLC3A locus on chromosome 2p21. Hum Mol Genet 1997; 6(4):641–647.
156. Tang YM, Wo YY, Stewart J, Hawkins AL, Griffin CA, Sutter TR, Greenlee WF. Isolation and characterization of the human cytochrome P450 CYP1B1 gene. J Biol Chem 1996; 271(45):28324–28330.
157. Stoilov I, Akarsu AN, Alozie I, Child A, Barsoum-Homsy M, Turacli ME, Or M, Lewis RA, Ozdemir N, Brice G, Aktan SG, Chevrette L, Coca-Prados M, Sarfarazi M. Sequence analysis and homology modeling suggest that primary congenital glaucoma on 2p21 results from mutations disrupting either the hinge region or the conserved core structures of cytochrome P4501B1. Am J Hum Genet 1998; 62(3):573–584.
158. Kakiuchi T, Isashiki Y, Nakao K, Sonoda S, Kimura K, Ohba N. A novel truncating mutation of cytochrome P4501B1 (CYP1B1) gene in primary infantile glaucoma. Am J Ophthalmol 1999; 128(3):370–372.
159. Kakiuchi-Matsumoto T, Isashiki Y, Ohba N, Kimura K, Sonoda S, Unoki K. Cytochrome P450 1B1 gene mutations in Japanese patients with primary congenital glaucoma(l). Am J Ophthalmol 2001; 131(3):345–350.
160. Bejjani BA, Lewis RA, Tomey KF, Anderson KL, Dueker DK, Jabak M, Astle WF, Otterud B, Leppert M, Lupski JR. Mutations in CYP1B1, the gene for cytochrome P4501B1, are the predominant cause of primary congenital glaucoma in Saudi Arabia. Am J Hum Genet 1998; 62(2):325–333.
161. Plasilova M, Stoilov I, Sarfarazi M, Kadasi L, Ferakova E, Ferak V. Identification of a single ancestral CYP1B1 mutation in Slovak Gypsies (Roma) affected with primary congenital glaucoma. J Med Genet 1999; 36(4):290–294.
162. Gencikova A, Gencik A. Congenital glaucoma in gypsies from Slovakia. Hum Hered 1982; 32:270–273.
163. Akarsu AN, Turacli ME, Aktan SG, Barsoum-Homsy M, Chevrette L, Sayli BS, Sarfarazi M. A second locus (GLC3B) for primary congenital glaucoma (buphthalmos) maps to the Ip36 region. Hum Mol Genet 1996; 5(8):1199–1203.
164. Demenais F. Further analysis of familial transmission of congenital glaucoma. Am J Hum Genet 1983; 35:1156–60.

165. Fried K, Sachs R, Krakowsky D. Congenital glaucoma in only one of identical twins. Ophthalmologeca 1977; 174:185–187.
166. Bardelli AM, Hadjistilianou T, Frezzotii R. Etiology of congenital glaucoma. Genetic and extragenetic factors. Ophthalmic Paediatr Genet 1985; 6:265–270.
167. Zhang K, Jampel HD. Discordance of primary infantile glaucoma in monozygotic twins. Am J Ophthalmol 1999; 128(1):97–98.
168. Azuma I. Ein bericht zum kongenitalen glaucoma. Klin Monatsbl Augenheilkd 1984; 184:287–289.
169. Pollack A, Oliver M. Congenital glaucoma and incomplete congenital glaucoma in two siblings. Acta Ophthalmol 1984; 62:359–363.
170. Demenais F, Bonaiti C, Briard ML et al. Congenital glaucoma: genetic models. Hum Genet 1979; 46:305–317.
171. Broughton WL, Rosenbaum KN, Beauchamp GR. Congenital glaucoma and other ocular abnormalities associated with pericentric inversion of chromosome 11. Arch Ophthalmol 1983; 101:594–597.
172. Wahrman J, Atidia J, Goitein R et al. Pericentric inversions of chromosome 9 in two families. Cytogenet Cell Genet 1972; 11:132–144.
173. Nismimura DY, Patil S, Alward WLM, et al. Fine mapping of the chromosomal breakpoints in an individual with congenital glaucoma and a 6:13 translocation. Invest Ophthalmol Vis Sci 1995; 36:(ARVO Abstract 554).
174. Mandal AK, Walton DS, John T, Jayagandan A. Mitomycin C-augmented trabeculectomy in refractory congenital glaucoma. Ophthalmology 1997; 104:996–1001; discussion 1002–1003.
175. Mullaney PB, Selleck C, Al-Awad A, Al-Mesfer S, Zwaan J. Combined trabeculotomy and trabeculectomy as an initial procedure in uncomplicated congenital glaucoma. Arch Ophthalmol 1999; 117(4):457–460.
176. Sidoti PA, Belmonte SJ, Liebmann JM, Ritch R. Trabeculectomy with mitomycin-C in the treatment of pediatric glaucomas. Ophthalmology 2000; 107(3):422–429.
177. Berg I. Erbliches jugendliches Glaukom. Acta Ophthalmol 1932; 10:568–587.
178. Jerndal T. Goniodysgenesis and hereditary juvenile glaucoma. A clinical study of a Swedish pedigree. Acta Ophthalmol 1970; (suppl 107).
179. Martin JP, Zorab EC. Familial glaucoma in nine generations of a South Hampshire family. Br J Ophthalmol 1974; 58:536–542.
180. Lee DA, Brubaker RF, Hruska L. Hereditary glaucoma: a report of two pedigrees. Ann Ophthalmol 1985; 17:739–741.
181. Shaffer RN. Genetics and the congenital glaucomas. Am J Ophthalmol 1965; 60: 981–994.
182. Jerndal T. Congenital glaucoma due to dominant goniodysgenesis. A new concept of the heredity of glaucoma. Am J Hum Genet 1983; 35:654–651.
183. Stegman Z, Sokol J, Liebmann JM, Cohen H, Tello C, Ritch R. Reduced trabecular meshwork height in juvenile primary open-angle glaucoma. Arch Ophthalmol 1996; 114(6):660–663.
184. Vincent AL, Billingsley G, Buys Y, Levin AV, Priston M, Trope G, Williams-Lyn D, Heon E. Digenic inheritance of early-onset glaucoma: CYP1B1, a potential modifier gene. Am J Hum Genet 2002; 70(2):448–460.
185. Wyatt HT, Pearce WG, Boyd TA, Ombres RS, Salter AB. Autosomal dominant iridogoniodysgenesis: glaucoma management. Can J Ophthalmol 1983; 18:11–14.
186. Campbell DG. Pigmentary dispersion and glaucoma: a new theory. Arch Ophthalmol 1979; 97:1667–1672.
187. Kamplik A, Green WR, Quigley HA, et al. Scanning and transmission electron microscopic studies of two cases of pigment dispersion syndrome. Am J Ophthalmol 1981; 91:573–587.
188. Speakman JS. Pigmentary dispersion. Br J Ophthalmol 1981; 65:249–251.
189. Sugar HS. Pigmentary glaucoma: a 25-year review. Am J Ophthalmol 1966; 62:499–507.

190. Weber PA, Dingle JB. Pigmentary glaucoma in a black albino. Ann Ophthalmol 1983; 15:454–455.
191. Farrar SM, Shields MB. Current concepts in pigmentary glaucoma. Surv Ophthalmol 1993; 37(4):233–252.
192. Sokol J, Stegman Z, Liebmann JM, Ritch R. Location of the iris insertion in pigment dispersion syndrome. Ophthalmology 1996; 103(2):289–293.
193. Ritch R, A unification hypothesis of pigment dispersion syndrome. Trans Am Ophthalmol Soc 1996; 94:381–405; discussion 405–409.
194. Ritch R. Going forward to work backward. Arch Ophthalmol 1997; 115(3):404–406.
195. Potash SD, Tello C, Liebmann J, Ritch R. Ultrasound biomicroscopy in pigment dispersion syndrome. Ophthalmology 1994; 101(2):332–339.
196. Farrar SM, Shields MB, Miller KN, Stoup CM. Risk factors for the development and severity of glaucoma in the pigment dispersion syndrome. Am J Ophthalmol 1989; 108(3):223–229.
197. Siddiqui Y, Ten Hulzen RD, Cameron JD, Hodge DO, Johnson DH. What is the risk of developing pigmentary glaucoma from pigment dispersion syndrome? Am J Ophthalmol 2003; 135(6):794–799.
198. Ritch R, Steinberger D, Liebmann JM. Prevalence of pigment dispersion syndrome in a population undergoing glaucoma screening. Am J Ophthalmol 1993; 115(6):707–710.
199. Mandelkorn RM, Hoffman ME, Olander KW, et al. Inheritance and the pigmentary dispersion syndrome. Ann Ophthalmol 1983; 15:577–582.
200. Mandelkorn RM, Hoffman ME, Olander KW, et al. Inheritance and the pigmentary dispersion syndrome. Ophthalmic Paediatr Genet 1985; 6:325–331.
201. Andersen JS, Pralea AM, DelBono EA, Haines JL, Gorin MB, Schuman JS, Mattox CG, Wiggs JL. A gene responsible for the pigment dispersion syndrome maps to chromosome 7q35-q36. Arch Ophthalmol 1997; 115(3):384–388.
202. Online Mendelian Inheritance in Man, OMIM (TM). Mckusick-Nathans Institute for Genetic Medicine, Johns Hopkins University, Baltimore, MD and National Center for Biotechnology Information. National Library of Medicine, Bethesda, MD, 2000. URL: http://www.ncbi.nlm.nih.gov/omim/.
203. Andersen JS, Parrish R, Greenfield D, et al. A second locus for pigment dispersion syndrome and pigmentary glaucoma maps to 18qll-q21. Am J Hum Genet 1998; 63: A279.
204. Karickhoff JR. Pigmentary dispersion syndrome and pigmentary glaucoma: a new mechanism concept, a new treatment, and a new technique. Ophthal Surg 1992; 23(4):269–277.
205. Gandolfi SA, Vecchi M. Effect of a YAG laser iridotomy on intraocular pressure in pigment dispersion syndrome. Ophthalmology 1996; 103(10):1693–1695.
206. Breingan PJ, Esaki K, Ishikawa H, Liebmann JM, Greenfield DS, Ritch R. Iridolenticular contact decreases following laser iridotomy for pigment dispersion syndrome. Arch Ophthalmol 1999; 117(3):325–328.
207. Waring GO, Rodrigues MM, Laibson PR. Anterior chamber cleavage syndrome: a stepladder classification. Surv Ophthalmol 1975; 20:3–27.
208. Crandall AS. Developmental ocular abnormalities and glaucoma. Int Ophthalmol Clin 1984; 24:73–86.
209. Tawara A, Inomata H. Familial cases of congenital microcoria associated with late onset congenital glaucoma and goniodysgenesis. Jpn J Ophthalmol 1983; 27:63–72.
210. Chisholm IA, Chudley AE. Autosomal dominant iridogoniodysgenesis with associated somatic anomalies: four-generation family with Rieger's syndrome. Br J Ophthalmol 1983; 67:529–534.
211. Novotny L, Sterbova S. Meyer-Schwickerath syndrome with microphthalmia. Klin Monatsbl Augenheilkd 1984; 185:282–285.

17

Inherited Diseases of the Optic Nerve

INTRODUCTION

The possibility that an atrophy of the optic nerve may be inherited became widely known to ophthalmologists in the classic report by Leber in 1871 (1). It is interesting that Leber considered it "congenitally induced" (1), although it usually appeared much later in life, and that it was considered a sex-linked disorder until very recently, when its nonmendelian transmission was documented. Leber's disease remained the classic inherited optic atrophy. However, other inherited optic atrophies were described and do not seem to be uncommon. These diseases were placed in various different classifications, but it seems to me that the natural and logical classification should be based on the mode of transmission of the disease, with subdivision into the different entities. Table 1 provides such a basic classification of the inherited optic atrophies.

Other diseases of the optic nerve were shown to be inherited. These include drusen of the optic nerve, various congenital malformations, and inherited tumors.

AUTOSOMAL DOMINANT OPTIC ATROPHY

Clinical Classification

The identification of a gene responsible for the vast majority of cases of autosomal dominant optic atrophy (DOA), the OPA1 gene (mapped to chromosome 3q28–q29), fundamentally changed the clinical classification of DOA. Older attempts at classification distinguished between an infantile form and a more serious congenital form associated with nystagmus (2) or between a congenital form and a juvenile form with onset between 6 and 12 years of age (3). However, classification according to age of onset seems inappropriate. Age of onset of symptoms varies even within the same family.

Genetic investigations of OPAl-associated optic atrophy demonstrated homogeneity and lack of genetic heterogeneity (4,5). However, a great variability was noted in age of onset, severity of loss of visual acuity and visual fields, and rate of loss (5). The variability was much more pronounced by intrafamilial comparison, possibly indicating heterogeneity at the allelic level. Intrafamilial variability might indicate environmental influence or a function of additional modifying genes (5).

Table 1 Inherited Atrophies of the Optic Nerve

Classification	McKusick catalog No.	Locus	Chromosome location
Dominant optic atrophies (DOA)			
a. Severe form	165500	OPA1	3q28–q29
b. Mild form (Kjer and Caldwell)	165500		
c. Variant form	—	OPA4	18q12.2–q12.3
d. DOA with hearing loss	125250		
e. DOA with hearing loss and ophthalmoplegia	165490		
f. DOA with hearing loss and peripheral neuropathy	165199		
Recessive optic atrophies (ROA)			
a. Behr syndrome	210000		
b. Wolfram (DIDMOAD) syndrome	222300	WFS1 WFS2	4q16.1 4q22–q24
c. GAPO syndrome	230740		
d. Opticocochleodentate syndrome	258700		
e. Rosenberg and Chutorian syndrome	311070		
f. Infantile optic atrophy (Went)	311050	OPA2	Xp11.4–p11.21
g. Opticoacoustic atrophy with dementia (Jensen)	311150		Xq22
Leber optic atrophy (LOA, LHON)	535000		Mitochondrial

The following is therefore a strictly clinical classification, although the different DOA forms may possibly be shown as associated with different allelic mutations on the OPA1 gene.

DOA, Severe Form

In the severe clinical form, visual acuity is already low (6/60 or less) in the first decade of life and is sometimes accompanied by nystagmus. Visual acuity tends to remain stationary; at levels within the definition of blindness. This form is the less common of the two forms of DOA, and it tends to occur earlier in life. Roggeveen and colleagues found that among seven families with DOA living in the Leiden district of the Netherlands (6), one family had the severe form. Figure 1 compares the visual acuities of patients with this form of DOA vs. those with the mild form. The two forms are one genetic entity, as was considered by some investigators in the past (7,8). However, they might be associated with different mutations.

DOA, Mild Form

The mild form of DOA was extensively described by Kjer in 19 affected families in Denmark (9). Visual acuity decreases progressively and slowly, but some patients are asymptomatic. In some families, patients are only mildly affected (3).

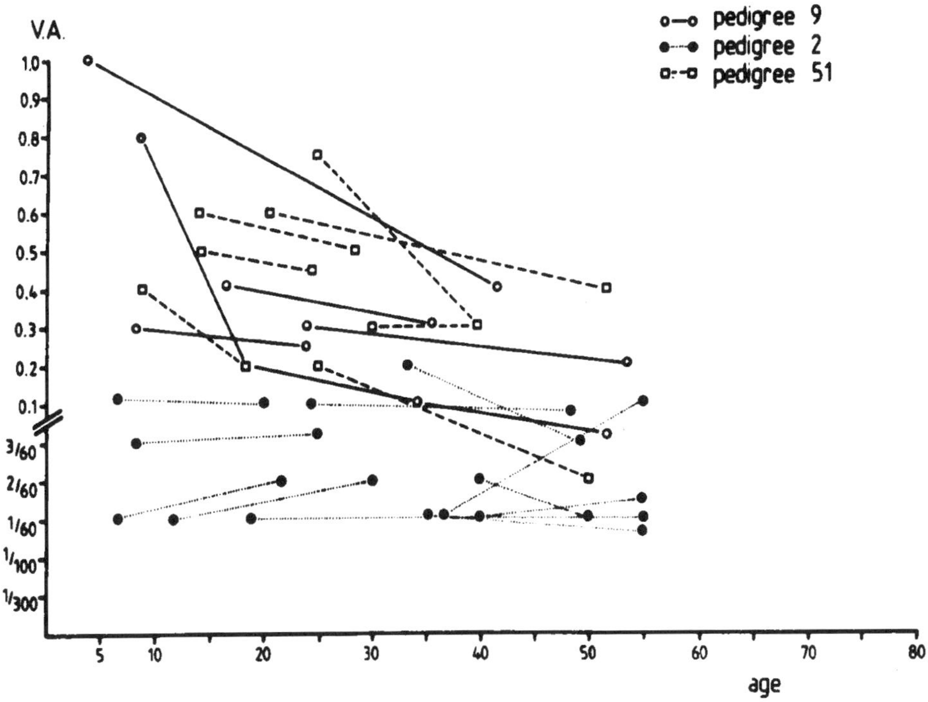

Figure 1 Visual acuity and age of patients with DOA stemming from three different families, indicated by filled circles (first family), open circles, and open squares. Note that the first family suffers from DOA, severe form, with visual acuity less than 6/60 in the first decade of life, with little change thereafter. The other two families suffer from the mild form of DOA, with visual acuities ranging from 6/6 to 3/60 and averaging 6/12–6/18 (from Ref. 6).

DOA with Hearing Loss

In this entity, autosomal dominant optic atrophy is associated with hearing loss (10,11). The loss of visual acuity is similar to that found in DOA, mild form, and is progressive. The hearing loss may be congenital or may occur later in life (11). At least seven families have been described (11) since the first description in 1968 (12).

DOA with Hearing Loss and Ophthalmoplegia

This combination of findings together with ptosis, dystaxia, and a nonspecific myopathy was described in 23 members of one family by Treft and associates (13). The family described by Meire et al. (14) might have the same genetic entity. Like the loss of visual function, the other clinical signs and symptoms become progressively worse during life.

Dominant Atrophy with Hearing Loss and Peripheral Neuropathy

Hagemoser and colleagues (15) described this phenotype in two families with DOA and surveyed the published literature.

Clinical Findings in DOA

Loss of visual acuity in the mild form of DOA is insidious. Visual loss usually starts in early childhood, becomes manifest at school age, but never leads to blindness; however, visual acuity may become as poor as 6/60 in the fifth decade of life (9). The average patient will have a visual acuity of 6/15 at age 25 years and 6/30 to 6/60 at age 45 (16). Considerable variability among patients is found in both the rate of progression of functional loss and the final visual outcome. Some patients remain asymptomatic or show very little loss of function throughout their life (3,9,17).

The rate of progression of visual loss was studied by Eliott et al. (18) and Vortuba et al. (19). In both studies 65% of DOA patients retained stable visual acuity and visual fields. In the rest, the progression was slow. In the first study, the range of the visual acuity was measured as 20/20–20/400. However, the median visual acuity was 20/60 and during follow-up of five to ten years it was only reduced to 20/80 (18).

Visual fields usually manifest a full periphery with a central or centrocecal scotoma occurring later in life (9,16,20). However, peripheral loss with a preferential loss of the upper temporal field was also reported (19).

Color vision is initially normal. Later, when visual acuity decreases, to 20/40 or less, a blue-yellow (tritan) defect is usually found (16,19,21). Further loss of visual acuity may be associated with both blue-yellow and red-green defects (mixed deficits) (19) (Fig. 2).

The anterior segments are normal. Ophthalmoscopy reveals an optic atrophy that may be mild or greater up to total optic atrophy. Vortuga and colleagues (19) found temporal pallor in 55% and total disk pallor in 44% of DOA patients.

Strabismus was detected in 10% of DOA patients (19).

The severe form of DOA is rare. Severe optic atrophy may be seen clinically in the first years of life and, if so, it is associated with gross loss of vision, achromatopsia, and sometimes nystagmus (20). Visual acuity, as pointed out, is less than 6/60 before the end of the first decade of life and remains so or slowly deteriorates.

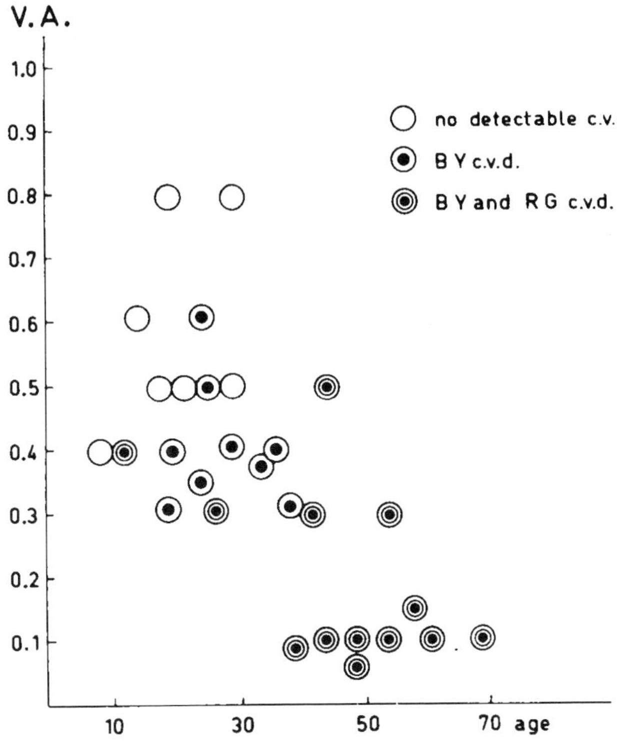

Figure 2 Color vision and visual acuity in 29 patients with DOA, mild form V.A., visual acuity; c.v.d., color vision defect; BY, blue-yellow; RG, red-green (from Ref. 16).

Among the seven described families with DOA with hearing loss, there was great interfamilial and intrafamilial variation in onset and severity of both visual and hearing losses (11). In general, visual functions were similar to those described for DOA in the mild form. The deafness was sometimes congenital, but, usually, occurred later, up to the second decade of life. The hearing loss was moderate to severe, with a total loss of 50–100 dB.

Dominant optic atrophy with hearing loss and ophthalmoplegia also shows the same characteristic of insidious loss of visual function that occurs in the mild form of DOA. Loss of muscular function is also slowly progressive, with paralysis causing ptosis and ophthalmoplegia (13).

Dominant infantile optic atrophy (DIOA) (22) is very likely a variant of DOA associated with the same OPA1 gene.

Diagnosis, Laboratory Tests, and Pathology

The diagnosis of dominant optic atrophy is based on the ophthalmoscopic findings, the reduced visual acuity, the central or centrocecal scotoma, and the family history. Color vision tests will reveal the defects in color vision parallel to the loss of visual acuity. In early cases, when visual acuity is normal, perception of desaturated colors may be reduced, and contrast sensitivity to low spatial frequencies is also reduced (23). The electroretinogram (ERG), electro-oculogram (EOG), and pattern ERG (p-ERG) are all normal in early cases (24). In advanced cases the p-ERG becomes abnormal (24), the p–ERG N 95 component and the PVEP become reduced and delayed (19).

The differential diagnosis with normotensive glaucoma (NTG) may present a problem. Fournier and associates (25) pointed out that contrary to NTG, in DOA onset is earlier, visual fields manifest preferential loss of central vision, with sparing of peripheral visual fields, with pallor of the remaining rim of the optic nerve and family history of the specific disorder (25).

The mild form of DOA should be distinguished from congenital tritanopia. In both conditions, some functional loss with mild pallor of the optic disk can be found, and a loss of blue color vision can be detected. The distinction can be made by blue cone ERGs, as they are unrecordable in patients with congenital tritanopia and are normal in patients with DOA (26). Jaeger (27) recently advised use of the blue vision defects as a screening test for preschool children (27).

A pathologic specimen from a 56-year-old patient with DOA, mild form, who died of a subdural hemorrhage, indicated a marked reduction in the number of ganglion cells in the macular area, normal outer segments, a nerve fiber layer reduced in thickness, and loss of myelin from axons of the optic nerve (28) (Figs. 3 and 4). Abnormal structures were also found more posteriorly, with a massive loss of ganglion cells in the lateral geniculate body, but the calcarine cortex was normal (29).

These pathologic studies led to the conclusion that DOA is a primary degeneration of the ganglion cell layer, followed by ascending optic atrophy (28,29). However, this statement was disputed by other authors on electrophysiological grounds (24).

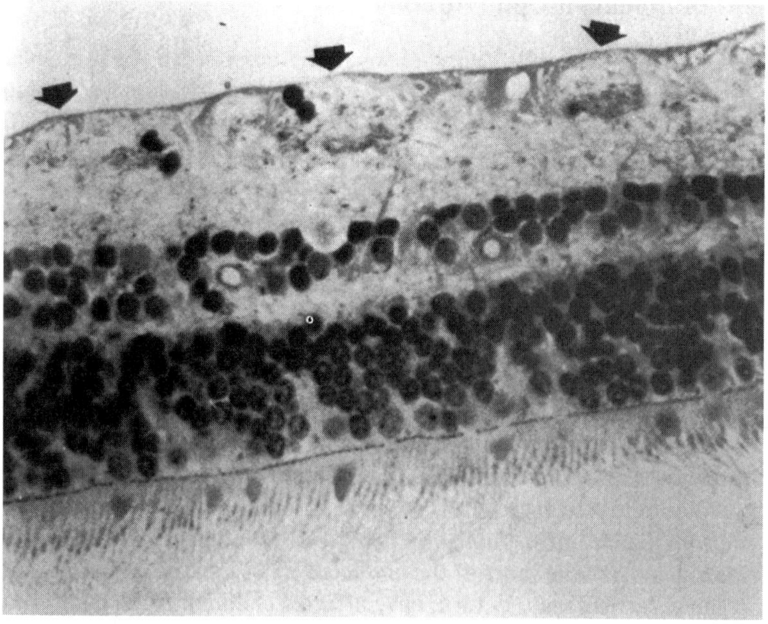

Figure 3 Histopathologic appearance of the eye of an 86-year-old patient with DOA, mild form. Note the degenerated ganglion cells in the posterior retina (arrows) and the few normal-looking ganglion cells (from Ref. 29).

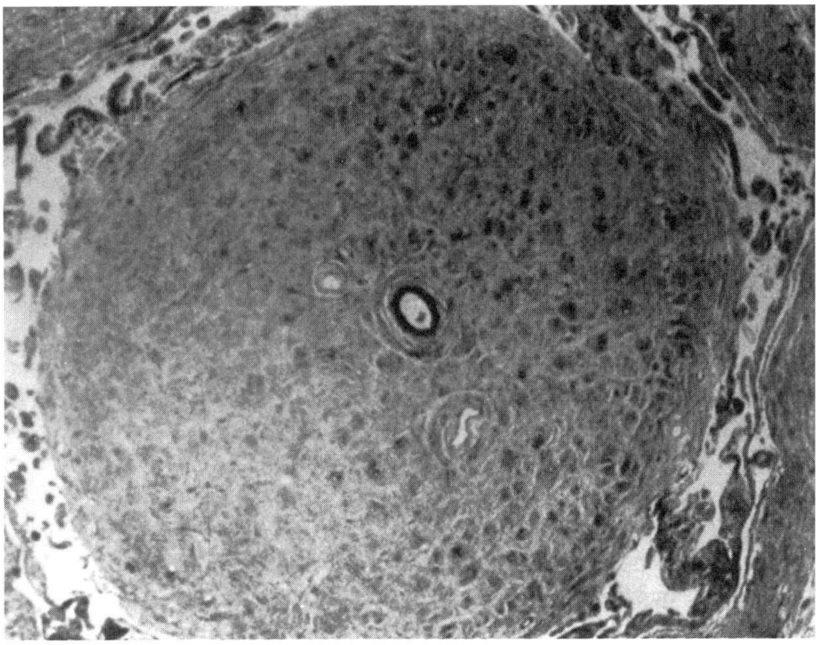

Figure 4 Histopathologic appearance of the same eye as that shown in Figure 3. Note the atrophy of the temporal half of the nerve (from Ref. 29).

Epidemiology and Genetics

The incidence of DOA is not known but was reported within the wide range of 1:10,000–1:50,000 newborns (21). The incidence probably varies among different ethnic populations. OPA1 associated DOA was reported from the United Kingdom, France, Cuba, and the United States (21). In Denmark, Kjer found the mild form of DOA considerably more common than Leber hereditary optic atrophy (9). In Jamaica six children blind from DOA were found among 108 blind children (30). This may indicate a high incidence of DOA (as children with DOA are only very rarely blind), or reflect a peculiar susceptibility of the Jamaicans, as reflected in the well-known Jamaican neuropathy.

The OPA1 Locus and Gene

Former speculations (based on linkage studies and on chromosomal abnormalities) that the gene causing DOA mild form is located on chromosome 2 (31,32) were not confirmed.

In 1994, Eiberg and associates mapped the locus OPA1 (for optic atrophy 1) at the telomere of the long arm of chromosome 3 in three Danish families with Kjer type of DOA (157). Lunkes et al. (34) refined the location to chromosome 3q28–q29 (34). This location was confirmed for patients from Cuba (34), France (35), Denmark, the United Kingdom, and the United States. The location and the homogeneity for all DOA patients studied were confirmed for British and Danish families (36–38). It was also confirmed for patients with the severe form of DOA (39).

Two groups of investigators, Alexander and associates (40) and Delettre and associates (41), identified the gene responsible for OPA1. The OPA1 gene encodes a dynamin-related protein targeted or localized to mitochondria (40,41). The gene contains 30 exons (42). Various mutations were identified including missense, nonsense, deletions, and insertions (40,41). Sixty-five percent of the mutations were of premature termination in one of the exons 8–28 and produced a truncated protein. In the other cases, missense mutations in the GTPase domain (exons 8–15) were identified (42). By 2001, 25 mutations had been reported (43) and by 2002, 54 mutations were known (44).

The pathophysiology is only speculative. Olichon et al. (45) demonstrated that OPA1 gene encodes a large GTPase related to dynamins anchored to the mitochondrial cristae inner membrane facing the intermembrane space. Therefore, OPA1 seems to be a major organizer of the mitochondrial inner membrane. A defective protein may start the apoptosis pathway (45).

Mutations in the OPA1 gene were found in 47% of DOA patients (44).

It is likely that specific clinical subtypes are associated with specific mutations. Amati–Bonneau and associates (46) reported that a missense mutation Arg445His was associated with DOA and hearing loss.

The OPA4 Locus

Kerrison and associates demonstrated genetic heterogeneity of DOA after identifying a second locus associated with autosomal dominant optic atrophy, Kjer type (49). The locus, later designated as OPA4, maps to chromosome 18q12.2–q12.3. The gene is currently not identified. Clinically, the affected family members have a mild type of DOA; however, great variability exists (47).

Management of DOA

Medical and Surgical

No specific medical treatment is available for DOA. Low-vision aids may be successfully used in a patient with a low visual acuity and a central scotoma.

In one study, 12 patients with DOA had a craniotomy performed and opto-chiasmatic arachnoiditis was found (48). The thickened arachnoid was incised or excised, and good results, in the form of arrest of the progressive functional loss and even improvement, were claimed (48). These results were not confirmed by any other source, and this approach is not recommended.

Genetic Counseling

The diseases of this group are transmitted by an autosomal dominant single gene (Fig. 5), and genetic counseling should be given accordingly. However, one should remember the considerable interfamilial and even intrafamilial variabilities in severity of expression of the disease (16,17). The disease in the next generation may be milder or more severe. One should also take into account that some carriers of the gene are completely asymptomatic. In most published pedigrees of families with DOA, the number of affected members falls short of the predicted 50%, indicating asymptomatic carriers. These carriers may, in turn, have affected children. Autosomal dominance with reduced penetrance is probably the rule, rather than the exception, in

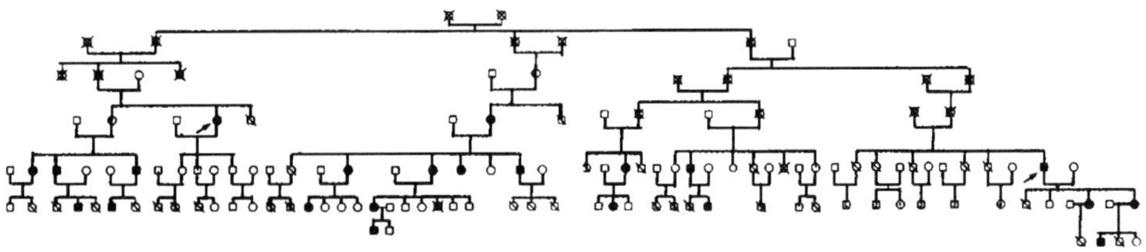

Figure 5 A large Dutch family with DOA, mild form: filled circles and squares indicate affected members; half-filled symbols, obligatory carriers; a diagonal line, an examined uninvolved member; and two diagonal lines, a deceased member (from Ref. 6).

families with DOA. The claim that DOA may be more severe in males (sex-influenced severity) (49) was not substantiated by any other study.

The mutations of the OPA1 gene may be sought and the results used for better counseling and for prenatal diagnosis.

RECESSIVE OPTIC ATROPHIES

In sharp contrast with dominant optic atrophies, in which the optic atrophy is usually an isolated event, the recessive optic atrophies (ROA) are multisystem diseases. The central nervous system (CNS) is affected along with the optic atrophy and other organs. This involves both the autosomal recessive and the sex-linked recessive diseases of this group. Table 2 lists the entities of autosomal recessive and X-linked recessive inherited optic atrophies.

The Clinical and Genetic Types of Recessive Optic Atrophy

Behr Syndrome

Behr, in 1909, described a syndrome in which optic atrophy with neurologic abnormalities occurred in infancy and was transmitted by the autosomal recessive mode (50,51). The optic atrophy is not complete. Visual acuity may remain stable or progressively decrease. Nystagmus may be present. The neurologic signs include pyramidal and extrapyramidal signs such as Babinsky, increased tendon reflexes, spastic gait, and ataxia. Mental deficiency may be present.

It has been suggested that Behr syndrome is a heterogenous group of disorders (52). The name was undoubtedly applied to different diseases in various published reports. The term should, in my opinion, be reserved for a disease in which autosomal ROA is coupled with neurologic signs of the nature and severity described by Behr (50). The differential diagnosis with other ROAs, which also involve the nervous system, should be considered for each patient.

Copeliovitch and associates (53) reported a high prevalence of Behr syndrome in the Iraqi–Jewish population in Israel. Seventeen patients suffered from optic atrophy diagnosed in the first decade of life and from nystagmus noted in the first year of life. Most suffered from ataxia and spasticity, and 70% had severe lower limb contractures, which progressively worsened (53).

An autopsy of a patient with Behr syndrome revealed atrophy of the optic nerves with loss of neurons, gliosis, and loss of the normal laminar structure of the lateral geniculate body. Similar cell loss and gliosis were found in other thalamic

Table 2 The Recessive Optic Atrophies

Name of syndrome	Other names	Heredity	Main ocular findings	Main other findings
Behr	Optic atrophy with neurologic signs	AR	Optic atrophy in infancy stationary or progressive	Pyramidal and extrapyramidal signs
ROA, nonsyndromic	Optic atrophy, AR	AR	Optic atrophy	None
Wolfram	DIDMOAD WFS1 WFS2	AR	Optic atrophy in second decade of life, progressive, cataract, DR, nystagmus	Diabetes mellitus, diabetes insipitus, deafness, peripheral neuropathy
Costeff	3-Methylglutaconic aciduria, III, OPA3	AR	Partial optic atrophy	Spastic paraparesis
GAPO		AR	Optic atrophy in first decade of life	Alopecia, lack of teeth, small stature
Nyssen–van Bogaert	Opticocochleodentate degeneration	AR	Severe optic atrophy and blindness in first decade	Progressive condition of spastic quadriplegia, hearing loss, mental deficiency, early death
McDermot	(Syndrome not established)	AR	Optic atrophy	Motor and sensory neuropathy with mental deficiency
Chalmers	(Syndrome not established)	AR	Progressive optic atrophy starting in first decade	Progressive hearing loss, distal form of spinal muscular atrophy
Rosenberg and Chutorian	Familial opticoacoustic nerve degeneration	XR	Progressive optic atrophy	Progressive hearing loss, distal muscular atrophy
Went	OPA2	XR	Optic atrophy in infantile period	Mental retardation, pyramidal and extrapyramidal signs
Jensen	Opticoacoustic TIMM8A-associated	XR	Progressive optic atrophy in first and second decades	Progressive hearing loss, dementia in second decade

Note: AR—autosomal recessive; XR—X-linked recessive.

nuclei and less in the pallida (52). This study seems to indicate that, in contrast with DOA, in Behr syndrome the optic atrophy is a descending phenomenon starting in the brain.

ROA, Nonsyndromic

Autosomal recessive optic atrophy not associated with a syndrome or CNS involvement is rare. Barbet and colleagues described this disorder in a large French family (54). This homozygous disease was localized to chromosome 8q21–q22, so that it was not associated with DOA and not with syndromic ROA (54).

Wolfram (DIDMOAD) Syndrome

An autosomal recessive syndrome in which optic atrophy is coupled with diabetes mellitus, with an onset in childhood was described by Wolfram and Wagener in 1938 (55). Later, some patients with this syndrome were found to have diabetes insipidus and hearing loss. The acronym of DIDMOAD (Diabetes Insipidus, Diabetes Mellitus, Optic Atrophy, Deafness) was therefore given to this syndrome and often used. Both optic atrophy and juvenile diabetes mellitus, the hallmarks of the syndrome, show in the first or second decade of life. Ataxia, nystagmus, mental retardation, and seizures may also occur (56).

Wolfram syndrome is uncommon, with an estimated prevalence of 1:100,000 population (57).

Of 11 patients reported by Mtanda and coworkers (58), all 11 had optic atrophy and diabetes mellitus, 5 had diabetes insipidus, 4 were deaf, and 5 had anosmia. The diabetes mellitus preceded optic atrophy and visual loss by an average of five years. Two patients had nystagmus. Other findings were probably secondary to the diabetes and included peripheral neuropathy in three patients, cataract in six, and diabetic retinopathy in three.

In electrophysiologic studies the ERG and the EOG are normal, whereas the visual-evoked potentials are of very low amplitude (58). Color vision, initially normal, becomes a red-green defect and may become progressively worse, up to total color blindness. MRI may show a diffuse neurodegenerative disease (56).

A curious phenomenon was described by Swift (59) in that heterozygous carriers, otherwise asymptomatic, have an increased tendency to psychiatric disease and suicide.

Pathologic studies showed gliosis and loss of myelin in the optic nerves, chiasm, and optic tracts; atrophy of the lateral geniculate body; and brain stem hypoplasia and thinning (60). As with Behr syndrome, these studies indicate a primary brain disease, with secondary descending atrophy of the optic nerves.

Some studies implied a relationship between Wolfram syndrome and HLA-DR2 (61,62), whereas others indicated no relationship (63).

The locus for Wolfram syndrome, WFS1, was mapped to chromosome 4pl6.1 (64). The gene encodes a transmembrane protein that appears to function in various tissues including neurons and the pancreas (65). El–Shanti and associates localized a second locus for Wolfram disease, WFS2 locus, to chromosome 4q22–q24 (66). In contrast to WFS1, patients with a WFS2 mutation do not suffer from diabetes insipidus (66).

The OPA3 Locus and Gene

Costeff and associates (67) described a familial syndrome of infantile onset optic atrophy with spastic paraparesis (the Costeff syndrome). All 19 affected were offspring of Iraqi–Jewish immigrants to Israel and 17 of the 19 affected were females (67). The metabolic associated disorder is 3-methylglutaconic aciduria, type III, and 40 patients were reported by Aniksler et al. (68).

The locus OP A3 was localized to chromosome 19ql3.2–ql3.3 and the gene was identified (68). The gene consists of two exons and encodes a peptide of 179 amino acids, expressed in the kidney and in skeletal muscle (68).

GAPO Syndrome

The acronym GAPO is used for an autosomal recessive syndrome consisting of *g*rowth retardation, *a*lopecia, *p*seudoanodontia, and *o*ptic atrophy. The syndrome is very rare, with only about 20 reported cases. The striking appearance of the lack of hair, apparent lack of teeth, the small stature, and sometimes other craniofacial abnormalities should make the diagnosis apparent early in life (69). Optic atrophy is slowly progressive. It starts with blurring of the disk margins. Computed tomographic (CT) scan indicates thickened optic nerves (70).

Other Autosomal Recessive Optic Atrophies

Rare causes of autosomal recessive optic atrophies include the opticocochleodentate syndrome, described in 1965 (71). Optic atrophy is found together with severe neurologic abnormalities, such as progressive spastic quadriparesis. Mental deficiency and hearing loss are present, and both become increasingly worse. Visual loss leads to blindness. The disease is fatal, with death occurring before ten years of age. About 10 cases have been described.

An isolated case of inherited optic atrophy, with motor and sensory neuropathy with mental retardation and pyramidal signs (72), and of an opticoacoustic atrophy with weakness and wasting of small muscles (73) have also been described.

Optic atrophy associated with hereditary motor and sensory neuropathy plays an essential part in the diagnosis of Charcot–Marie–Tooth syndrome subtype 6, now known as HMSN type VI (74). The locus CMT6 was found not be associated with OPA1 gene (74).

Sex-Linked Recessive Optic Atrophies

This group probably includes several distinct and very rare syndromes. The first was described by Rosenberg and Chutorian (75) in two brothers and a maternal nephew who suffered from visual loss owing to optic atrophy, hearing loss owing to degeneration of the acoustic nerve, and progressive polyneuropathy. Distal muscular atrophy resembled Charcot-Marie-Tooth disease.

Went and coauthors (76) described an X-linked disorder, in which optic atrophy in early childhood coexists with neurologic abnormalities and mental deficiency in some members. Assiuk et al. (77) studied the same family and assigned the locus, named OP A2, to chromosome Xp 11.4–p 11.21. A follow-up of many years indicated a very early onset of the disease but no or slow progression (77).

More recently, Jensen (78,79) described a sex-linked recessive condition of a progressive optic atrophy together with progressive hearing loss and dementia. The disorder presents in the second or third decade of life. Demyelination and calcifications are found spread in the central nervous system.

Later Tranebjaerg and associates identified a stop mutation in the DDP gene associated with Jensen syndrome (80). The gene DDP1 (for deafness-dystonia peptide 1) or TIMM8A (for translocase of inner mitochondrial membrane) was mapped to chromosome Xq22 (64).

This syndrome accentuates the fact that many genes responsible for hereditary optic atrophy are associated with mitochondrial function, thus forming a pathogenic link between the different modes of inheritance including mitochondrial (Leber), autosomal dominant (DOA), and different recessive modes.

Diagnosis and Management

In all ROAs, the systemic problems involved in the diseases usually outweigh the ocular problems. The main role of the ophthalmologist in this group of rare diseases is to assist with the proper diagnosis. Table 2 tabulates the basic findings in each of these complex syndromes. The differential diagnosis with secondary optic atrophy resulting from primary diseases of the central nervous system should always be considered.

No particular management is available.

LEBER OPTIC ATROPHY

Description and Clinical Findings

This disorder is known under several different names, such as Leber's optic atrophy (used for many years), Leber optic atrophy (or LOA), Leber's hereditary neuroretinopathy (or Leber hereditary optic neuroretinopathy or LHON). All of these synonyms can be still found used in books and in articles. I will also use them synonymously.

The occurrence of optic atrophy with its accompanying visual loss in LOA is an acute and dramatic event. The patient, usually male, is unaware of any health problems when visual disturbances begin in one eye and rapidly progress to profound loss of vision. In one case, two affected brothers (Fig. 6) had no family history of visual problems, when the vision of the older brother's left eye decreased to 1m finger counting (fc) in 1 week. Six weeks later a similar event occurred in the right eye. The boy was 16 when he became blind. His younger brother had good vision up to age 21, when his right eye became blind (visual acuity of 10cm fc), followed 1 month later by the left eye (final visual acuity of 5 m fc).

The onset of the disease may be at any age between 8 and 60 years, but 16–23 is the most frequent age of onset. Visual acuity, which is rapidly reduced in the acute stage of the disease, may improve somewhat in the chronic stage. Visual fields always show a large central or centrocecal scotoma. This starts as a relative scotoma, rapidly becomes a large absolute scotoma, and later "breaks" into the periphery, upward or inward (81).

Once LOA was considered to be a primary optic atrophy, but Nikoskelainen and several collaborators have shown that ophthalmoscopically the disease starts as a disease of the peripapillary neural retina and the peripapillary and epipapillary vasculature (81–85).

Four stages of the development of LOA can be distinguished (Table 3; Figs. 7 and 8). In the presymptomatic phase, peripapillary teleangiectatic microangiopathy is seen, together with nonedematous swelling and some atrophy of the

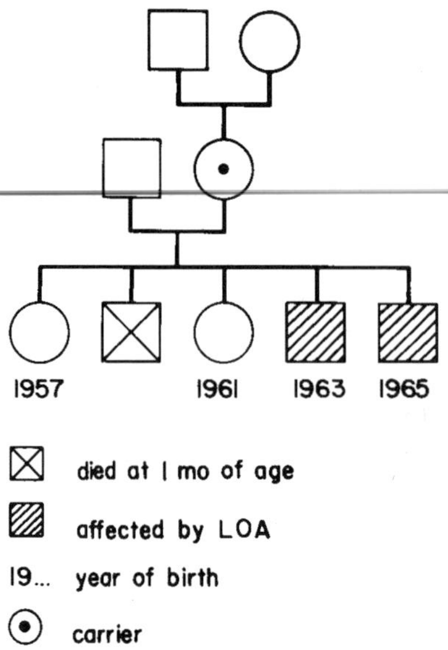

Figure 6 Pedigree of family with LOA.

peripapillary retinal nerve fibers (81). In fact, these findings do not always continue into the acute stage and may only serve to prove the existence of the genetic background of the disease (86,87). Later, microangiopathy grows and, during the acute stage, the small peripapillary retinal vessels become dilated, tortuous, and teleangiectatic, with possibly evident retinal hemorrhages (83). Nikoskelainen, therefore, suggested the term of Leber's hereditary neuroretinopathy instead of LOA (84).

Table 3 Development of Fundus Findings in LHON

Phase	Clinical findings	Fluorescein angiography	Remarks
Presymptomatic	Peripapillary microangiopathy; swelling and atrophy of peripapillary nerve fibers	No staining or leakage	In some patients, may remain without progression to the next stage
Acute	Peripapillary microangiopathy increases; dilated peripapillary retinal vessels, retinal hemorrhages	Dilated shunt vessels	
Atrophic, early	Narrowing of peripapillary vessels, involution of microangiopathy; atrophy of nerve fibers	Occluded capillaries and vessels; small areas of capillary nonperfusion	
Atrophic, late	Optic atrophy	Decreased staining	Amount of optic atrophy varies from moderate to severe in different patients

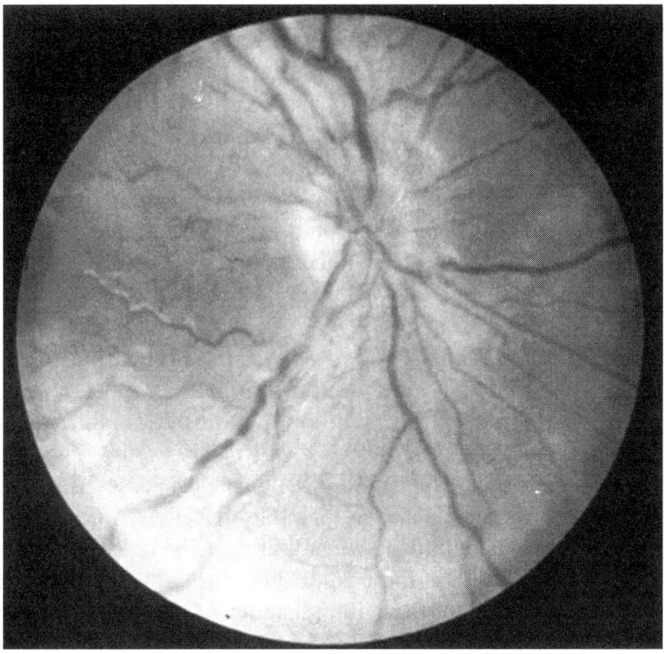

Figure 7 Fundus of patient with Leber optic atrophy in the acute phase (elder brother in Fig. 8). Note mild peripapillary microangiopathy.

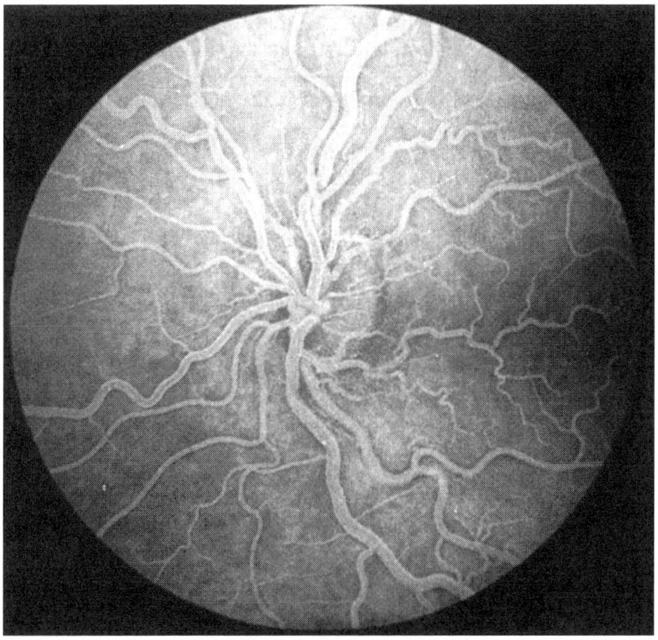

Figure 8 Fluorescein angiogram of a patient with Leber optic atrophy in the acute phase (younger brother in Fig. 7). Note absence of leakage or staining and presence of peripapillary microangiopathy.

Toward the end of the acute phase, reduced filling of the papillomacular capillaries can be seen (82). Finally, all vessels become narrow and the nerve becomes pale.

The outcome in most patients is severe optic atrophy with profound loss of vision. A few have a partial optic atrophy, with some preserved vision.

Color vision tests indicate a red-green defect in the beginning of the acute stage (81) and total achromatopsia in the late stages.

Additional studies showed that Leber hereditary neuroretinopathy is a heterogenous disorder caused by a series of mutations of the mitochondrial DNA.

Diagnosis and Laboratory Tests

No single test (except molecular genetics techniques) is pathognomonic of LHON. The diagnosis is based on the typical family history, the suggestive clinical course, and the characteristic progression of fundus changes as outlined in Table 3 .

The ERG and EOG are normal. The visual-evoked potential (VEP) is extinct in severe cases and is reduced in size and delayed in less severe cases (88).

The electrocardiogram (ECG) is abnormal in a high percentage of patients and asymptomatic members of families with LOA of the descending female line (87). It includes abnormalities of cardiac excitation and conduction in the form of Wolff-Parkinson-White (WPW) or Lown–Ganong–Levine (LGL) syndromes. In WPW syndrome, the duration of QRS complex is longer than 0.10 sec, and an additional delta wave is found. In LGL syndrome, the PR interval is less than 0.12 sec, while the QRS interval is normal. These abnormalities were found in all 10 Finnish families with LHON that were investigated (87).

Biochemically no abnormality was found in the serum of patients with LHON. Muscle biopsy showed by histochemistry focally increased activity of many type 1 fibers in the form of red-staining material. These areas were shown by electron microscopy to be aggregates of enlarged mitochondria in the subsarcolemmal regions of the fibers (89). In addition, myofilaments were disrupted. This study indicated the existence of mild myopathic changes in LHON in spite of clinical absence of muscle weakness or overt atrophy (89).

Wilson in 1965 was probably the first to call attention to the possibility that a defect in cyanide metabolism may be the basis of LHON (90). Cyanide is so powerfully toxic that it cannot be tolerated, even in small amounts, in the human body. Normally, it is rapidly detoxified by the enzyme rhodanese (thiosulfate sulfurtransferase) into an inactive compound, thiocyanate. The activity of rhodanese was significantly reduced in patients with LHON in both the liver (91) and the rectal mucosa (92).

In another study of muscle biopsies of 13 patients with LHON, 8 had abnormally large mitochondria (93). The activity of rhodanese in the muscle was normal (93). In one study low glutathione levels were found in erythrocytes (94).

Epidemiology and Genetics

The unusual epidemiology and incomprehensible genetic transmission of LHON captured the imagination of physicians for decades. Initially, the fact that mainly men are affected, whereas women are usually asymptomatic carriers and transmitters of the disease, classified LHON as yet another sex-linked recessive disease. However, many facts did not fit such transmission. The descendants of an affected man were never affected and were never carriers, almost all daughters of a carrier mother were carriers themselves, and the number of affected daughters was higher than expected. Therefore, it was suggested that LOA may possibly be autosomal recessive in females and autosomal dominant in males (95), with reduced viability of the trait-carrying spermatozoa (96). Another suggestion was that the inheritance is X-linked, but, in a female trait-carrying gamete, there is no further development after fertilization (96). It was later shown that all women born in the female lines of descent in affected families are carriers (96,97). Carrier females transmit the disease to about half of their sons and to all of their daughters (93). In a very large study on the entire Dutch population, van Senus (98) found 352 affected persons in 27 kindreds. He was the first to show that all sisters of patients or carriers are carriers themselves (98). Many unaffected sons of carrier mothers show the typical triad of peripapillary microangiopathy, pseudoedema of the peripapillary retina, and absence of staining by fluorescein angiography, a triad that seems to be the genetic marker of LHON (86). If these signs are included, then all sons and daughters of a female carrier inherit the trait.

These findings do not fit any known trait of hereditary mendelian transmission, whatever the "additional" explanations will be. As early as 1956, Imai and Moriwaki (99) suggested cytoplasmic inheritance as a possible mechanism of transmittance of LHON. This theory was revived, when mitochondrial inheritance was suggested to be responsible for some human disease (100). Suggested diseases transmitted by this mode were blood dyscrasias related to drug sensitivity. Mitochondria carry less than 1% of DNA, but this DNA is distinct from the nuclear and carries different genetic characteristics.

Human mitochondrial DNA in both males and females is inherited only from the mother. In the cow, the ovum contains 10^6 mitochondria, whereas the spermatid contains only 70 mitochondria (100). It is likely that all cytoplasm derived from the spermatozoon is destroyed upon fertilization. LHON, if transmitted by mitochondrial DNA through cytoplasmic inheritance, would be transmitted by females only. Affected men would not be able to transmit the disease.

Studies by Wallace and others confirmed that a mitochondrial DNA mutation is the cause of LHON (101). This mutation converted a highly conserved arginine to a histidine at codon 340 (102,103). Hotta and associates (104) also demonstrated a point mutation at nucleotide position 11778 in the mitochondrial DNA of three siblings, two affected brothers and a carrier sister, with LHON.

Now, molecular genetics techniques, using the appropriate probes, offer a rapid method of confirmation of the diagnosis of LHON on a small blood sample of the patient.

The reason for the strong male bias of LHON is not clear. It has been suggested that an interaction between an X-linked gene and the mitochondrial gene causes the male preponderance, but linkage analysis has almost excluded X-linked involvement (105).

The Genetic and Clinical Types of LOA

Introduction

By 1994, 16 mitochondrial DNA (mtDNA) missense mutations were known to be associated with LHON, and Brown and Wallace (106) confirmed its extensive genetic heterogeneity. All mutations were in mitochondrial DNA and by 2004, the number of known mutations associated with LHON had increased to approximately 20.

Brown and Wallace classified the mutations into two groups: primary mutations that are specific to LHON patients, and secondary mutations that are expressed as LHON only when they occur in certain combinations with other mutations (106). Approximately 90% of LHON is caused by one of the three primary mutations at nucleotides 3460, 11778, or 14484 (107). These mutations are preferentially associated with mtDNA haplogroup J. A haplogroup or haplotype of a population is the specific combination of alleles and polymorphisms related to the mtDNA. Haplogroup J is one of nine western Eurasian mtDNA linkages (107). The secondary mutations delineate the 15 or so other mutations each reported in a limited number of families. Secondary mutations cause LHON only if they occur in combination with one or more other, mildly deleterious mtDNA mutations (106,108). The worldwide division of LHON-associated primary mutation was summarized by Nikoskelainen et al. (108) as 50–76% for np (nucleotide pair) 11778, 17–30% for np 3460 and 10–31% for np 14484.

The onset of the disease ranges from 6 to 62 years of age in all types (108,109). With all mutations the disease is bilateral in almost all cases and appears simultaneously in 22% and sequentially with a median interval of eight weeks in 78% (109). A younger onset in childhood gives a better visual prognosis (108,109). In all types, the disorder is mostly or exclusively homoplasmic with a minority manifesting heteroplasmy (some cells carry the mutant mtDNA while others carry normal mtDNA).

Table 4 lists the three primary LHON-associated mtDNA mutations.

The np11778 Mutation

This is the most common LHON-associated mtDNA mutation. Sadun and associates (112–114) performed an extensive investigation of the clinical aspects of LHON in a very large Brazilian family with a homoplasmic 11778 mutation and of haplogroup J. The penetrance rate of the affection decreased with consecutive generations from 71% in the first generation through 60%, 34%,15% to 9% in the fifth generation (112). Percentage of affected males went up from 60% to 100% (112). Risk factors that increased risk of LHON in individuals carrying the 11778 mutations were smoking, alcohol consumption, and toxic exposure (pesticides and others). Affected members smoked much more than carriers (70% vs. 16%), consumed more alcohol (50% vs. 14.5%), and had greater exposure to toxins (40% vs. 7%) (112,113). Smokers also had poorer visual acuity (114). Warner and Lee also concluded that cigarette smoking, alcohol consumption and use of ephedrine alkaloids may be precipitating factors for LHON (115). However, Kerrison and colleagues did not find any significant association with these factors (116).

The np 11778 mutation is associated with a more severe disease than other mutations (108). Final visual acuity was 20/200 or less in 86% of affected according to one study (117) and 98.2% according to another study (118). Recovery is extremely rare, as retinal ganglion cells very likely die through an apoptotic process (119). In some studies, no evidence of recovery was seen (114).

The np 11778 is generally considered homoplasmic for the primary mutation but in reality, various tissues are differentially affected. Homoplasmy occurs 100% in the retina, sclera, and skeletal muscles, 95% in extraocular and heart muscle, 95% in the optic nerve, and 33% in circulating leukocytes (120).

Sadun and associates (121) studied the pathology of the optic nerve in two female patients, one harboring the 11778 mutation and the other the 3460 mutation.

Table 4 The Primary LHON-Associated mtDNA Mutations

Nucleotide	Complex 1 gene	Worldwide % LHON	Homoplasmy/heteroplasmy	Maternal relatives affected (%)	Males affected (%)	Vision recovery (%)
11778	ND4	50–76	Homoplasmy in most; heteroplasmy in some families	33–60	80	4
3460	ND1	17–30	15% heteroplasmic; rest homoplasmic	14–40	33–67	22
14484	ND6	10–31	Homoplasmy	27–80	68	37

Note: Figures from Refs. 64, 108, 110, 111; ND is the gene for NADH-ubiquinone oxidoreductase (NADH dehydrogenase); the numbers 4, 1, 6 refer to the subunits of the seven known subunits of the mitochondrial respiratory complex 1.

They found a 95–99% depletion of axons, a preferential loss of the smaller axons and spared fibers limited to periphery. The pathological abnormalities were similar in both mutations and, in fact, were similar to the pathology described in toxic and nutritional optic neuropathies (121).

MRI is usually normal in LHON but enlargement of the optic nerves and chiasm can be sometimes seen (122).

The np 3460 Mutation

Huoponen and coworkers identified this mutation and reported it in 1991 (123). Various phenotypes were displayed, ranging from normal fundi to complete optic atrophy (123). Johns et al. (110) compared the clinical characteristics of the np 3460 mutation to those of the 11778 mutation. The np 3460 mutation manifested a higher incidence of visual recovery (20% vs. 4%), a higher percentage of pedigrees with more than one affected member (78% vs. 43%), and a greater frequency of tobacco and alcohol abuse (110). The phenotype severity was less than that with np 11778 (108).

The np 14484 Mutation

The clinical characteristics of the np 14484 mutation are similar to those of the other mutations but the visual recovery rate is the highest; more than one third (37%) (111). Recovery is higher when onset is earlier (109,111). Mackey (124) also found in Australia that the np 14484 mutation was associated with a high (the most frequent in Australia) recovery rate, unlike in the np 11778 or the np 3460 mutation.

Kerrison and coworkers found in a 14484 mutation associated optic nerve histopathological specimen, calcifications in the mitochondria (125), but Sadun and Sadun (126) did not find any calcifications in a 11778 mutation-associated optic nerve specimen.

Howell and associates demonstrated that many Dutch families and French Canadian families had the same 14484 mutations associated with LHON and calculated that all share a common founder ancestor who lived 900–1800 years ago (127).

Secondary LHON Associated Mutations

The np 8993 mutation results in a variable phenotype ranging from mild to Leigh syndrome, the severity depending on load of heteroplasmy (128). Usually a retinal dystrophy is seen but sometimes an optic atrophy as in LHON occurs (128). LHON was associated with mutations at np 9101 (129), np 13730 (130), np 14495 (131), and np 15257 (132). Other reported mutations (64) included nucleotides 3394, 4136, 4160, 4171, 4216, 4640, 5244, 4917,10663 (with haplogroup J only), 13708, 13730, 14453 (causing MELAS), 14459, 14495, and 14596.

These "secondary" mutations are associated with additional mitochondrial mutations and it is the combination of two or more that cause the clinical phenomenon of LHON. All of these secondary mutations are uncommon. It may also be difficult to distinguish between a disease-bearing mutation and a non-disease associated polymorphism, as mutations are 10 times more frequent in mtDNA than in nuclear DNA(133).

Management of LHON

Medical and Surgical

No medical treatment has been effective in LHON, even if administered in the acute phase of the disease. However, some physicians have given systemic corticosteroids for two to three weeks, in doses similar to those used in optic neuritis, when the patient is seen in the acute phase. Others have given vitamin B_{12} injections (hydroxocobalamin) in amounts of 1000 μg (a single-dose ampule) three times a week for two to three weeks. I have seen definite improvement in patients who received this treatment, but such improvement, as mentioned before, could have been spontaneous and unrelated to the medication. The effect of any medication in the acute phase of LHON is, therefore, uncertain. No medication should be used in the atrophic phase.

Idebenone therapy administered during the acute phase was reported as resulting in visual recovery in several patients with LHON (111,134).

One group of investigators (135) used 4–8 g/day of oral cystine with 1000 μg of intramuscular hydroxocobalamin three times a week. This treatment resulted in a increase in thiocyanate production, indicating an increase in cyanide detoxification. The authors claimed that up to 35% of their patients recovered if treated within 1 year of onset (135). In another study, the investigators used a three-day thiosulfate infusion and showed an increase in urinary thiocyanate, again indicating improvement in cyanide detoxification (91).

Genetic Counseling

Genetic counseling is based on the assumption that LHON is inherited by the cytoplasmic (nonmendelian) mode of inheritance. Mitochondrial DNA, and not nuclear DNA, contains the abnormal gene. Only carrier women can transmit the gene. Affected men or asymptomatic carrier men cannot transmit the disease to any of their descendants. All female children of a female carrier will be carriers themselves (136). If a woman carrier is not affected, then 49% of her sons and 8–15% of her daughters will be affected. If a woman carrier is affected, then 52% of her sons and 24–32% of her daughters will be affected (137).

Harding and associates (138) studied 85 families with LHON and listed the recurrence risks as 30% for brothers, 8% for sisters, 46% for maternal nephews, 10% for maternal nieces, 31% for maternal male cousins, and 6% for maternal female cousins.

Prenatal Diagnosis

Leber's optic atrophy presents a unique situation, in which the presence or absence of a gene in an unborn child can be accurately predicted by genetic considerations and counseling, as all descendants of a female carrier are carriers. However, no method of prenatal diagnosis can distinguish between a future affected and a future unaffected carrier.

Drusen of the Optic Nerve

Drusen of the optic disk are probably better termed drusen of the optic nerve, since in many cases they are found deeper in the nerve and more posterior than the disk. They usually occur in older persons as sporadic, nonfamilial phenomena. However, their familial occurrence is not rare and, possibly, is much more common than generally assumed.

Drusen of the optic nerve were first defined as a clinical entity in 1891 (139). Lauber, in 1907 (140), first described inherited drusen, and Braun, in 1935 (141), demonstrated their autosomal dominant inheritance. Lorentzen, in a large study on 70 patients in Denmark, confirmed the autosomal dominant nature of inheritance (142).

Inherited drusen of the optic nerve are probably much more common among children than among adults. The prevalence of drusen of the optic nerve in children is less than 0.5% with 3.4:1000 population in the Danish study (142) and 4.0:1000 in a Finnish study (143). However, the true prevalence is not known, and must be much higher. Autopsy figures indicate 20 cases per 1000 (144). Ultrasound of the optic nerve often shows the existence of deep drusen not seen ophthalmoscopically.

Computerized tomography, magnetic resonance imaging (MRI), fluorescein angiography and B-mode ultrascan are all used for diagnosis of drusen of optic nervehead (145). The best results are obtained with B-mode ultrasound (145,146).

Nischal et al. reported finding an extremely high incidence of optic nerve drusen in Alagille syndrome (147). Alagille syndrome is a liver disease, one of several forms of intrahepatic cholestasis, transmitted by the autosomal dominant mode. Nischal et al. (147) examined 20 children with Alagille syndrome and found unilateral optic nerve drusen in 95% and bilateral in 80%. The reason for this phenomenon is not clear but one could speculate that optic nerve drusen could be a secondary phenomenon to vascular anomalies that are common in Alagille syndrome (148) that cause secondary drusen (146).

Clinically, drusen of the optic nerve may be asymptomatic. In the symptomatic minority, transient loss of vision, lowered visual acuity, visual fields defects of various and sometimes bizarre forms all can be found (142–150). Ophthalmoscopically, the optic disk may have blurred margins all around, show some irregularities at the margins or show frank pseudopapilledema. Retinal and subretinal hemorrhages may be seen. Subretinal neovascularization in the macular area is seen frequently in children with drusen of optic nerve (Fig. 9). It is my impression that familial cases of optic nerve drusen tend to be more severe and occur earlier than sporadic cases, hence their higher frequency in children. However, no study has been done to confirm this impression.

Genetically, patients should be advised of the autosomal dominant transmission of the disease in familial cases.

The expressivity of the gene may vary, with some affected persons being asymptomatic and having a normal optic disk.

Congenital Abnormalities of the Optic Nerve Head

Most congenital abnormalities of the optic disk are sporadic; their cause is unknown, but they result from an abnormal development of the eye or the brain in the embryo. Some abnormalities may be inherited, such as drusen, tumors, and colobomata. Table 5 classifies the congenital optic nerve anomalies with reference to their inherited or nonfamilial nature.

Autosomal dominant deep colobomatous excavations of the optic nerve head may be associated with normal or abnormal vision. Most patients have profound loss of vision (Fig. 10). Variable expression was described between the two eyes and among the affected members of the same family (154). The spectrum of morphologic variants

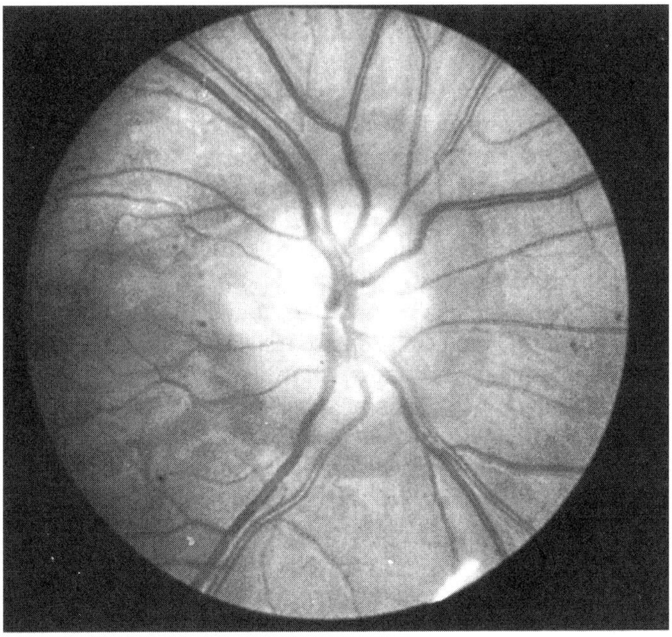

(a)

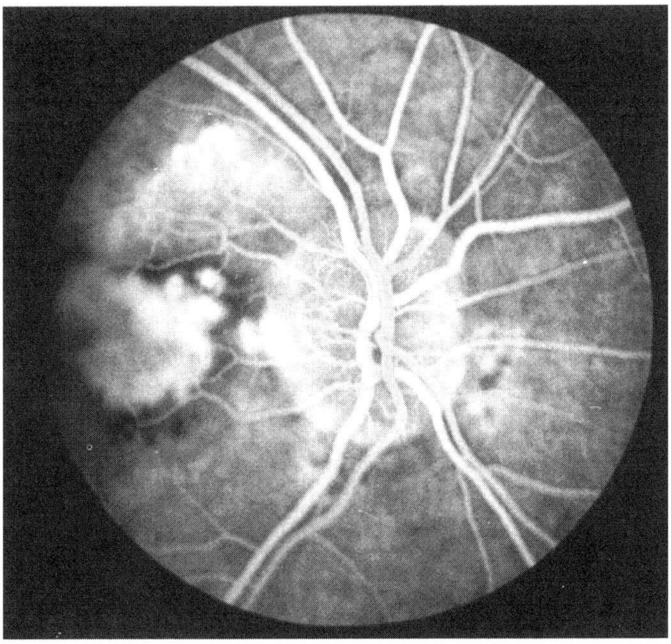

(b)

Figure 9 The fundus (a) and fluorescein angiogram (b) of a nine-year-old girl with drusen of the optic nerve. Her mother also had drusen of the optic disk, but was asymptomatic. The girl had subretinal neovascularization at the age of eight years in the left eye and at nine years in right eye, reducing her vision to finger counting.

Table 5 Congential Anomalies of the Optic Nerve (ON)

Group anomaly	Disease of ON or syndrome	Inheritance[a]
Dimension or volume	Megalopapilla	NG
	Hypoplasia	NG
	Hypoplasia and absent septum pellucidum (De Morsier syndrome)	NG
	Hypoplasia absent septum pellucidum and pituitary dysfunction (Hoyt syndrome)	NG
	Aplasia	NG
	Congenital excavation	NG
	Papilledema or pseudopapilledema	Rarely familial
Shape	Oval malformation	NG
	Tilted disk	NG
Colobomatous	Pit	NG or AD
	Coloboma	NG or AD
	Morning glory syndrome	NG
	Congential cresent	NG
Numerical	Duplication	NG
Tumors or other space-occupying lesions	Drusen	NG or AD
	Angioma	NG or AD
	Gilioma	NG or AD
	Astrocytoma	NG or AD
	Melanocytoma	NG

[a]NG, nongenetic; AD, autosomal dominant inheritance with variable expressivity.
Source: Adapted from Refs. 151–153

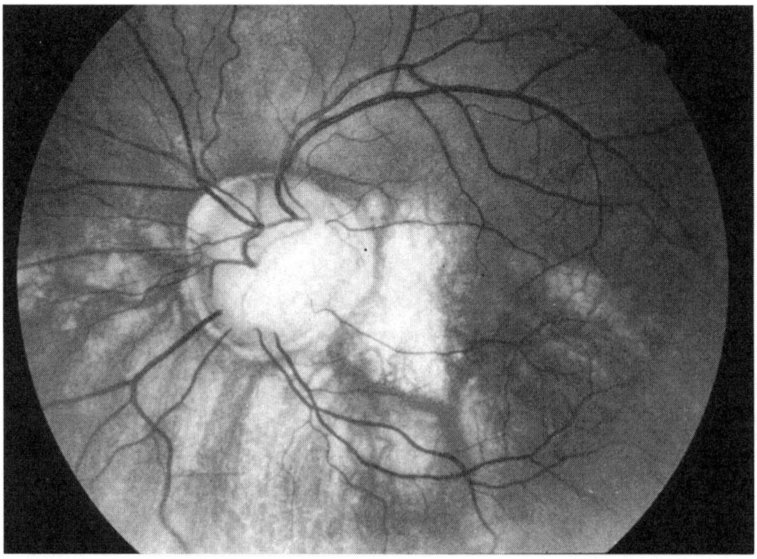

Figure 10 Autosomal dominant transmission of colobomatous excavation of the optic nerve head in two siblings: the brother (in the figure) displayed diffuse peripapillary atrophy of the RPE. The sister (not shown) had reduced vision owing to a shallow nonrhegmatogenous retinal detachment in the posterior pole.

ranged in one large family from small optic nerve pits to large colobomatous excavations (155).

Pits of the optic nerve were reported in one family with three generations affected (156). Optic nerve colobomas were described in a boy with congenital renal hypoplasia (157). The authors considered it a variant of the renal-coloboma syndrome and identified a mutation in the PAXL gene.

REFERENCES

1. Leber TH. Ueber hereditäre und congenital anglelegte Sehnervenleiden. Arch Ophthalmol 1871; 17:249–291.
2. Lodberg CV, Lund A. Hereditary optic atrophy with dominant transmission. Three Danish families. Acta Ophthalmol 1950; 28:437–468.
3. Caldwell JBH, Howard RO, Riggs LA. Dominant juvenile optic atrophy. A study of two families and review of hereditary disease in childhood. Arch Ophthalmol 1971; 85: 133–147.
4. Johnston RL, Burdon MA, Spalton DJ, Bryant SP, Behnam JT, Seller MJ. Dominant optic atrophy, Kjer type. Linkage analysis and clinical features in a large British pedigree. Arch Ophthalmol 1997; 115(1):100–103.
5. Wiggs JL. Genomic mapping of Kjer Dominant Optic Atrophy. Arch Ophthalmol 1997; 115(1):115–116.
6. Roggeveen HC, de Winter AP, Went LN. Studies in dominant optic atrophy. Ophthalmic Paediatr Genet 1985; 5:103–109.
7. Hoyt CS. Autosomal dominant optic atrophy. A spectrum of disability. Ophthalmology 1980; 87:245–250.
8. Pearce WG. Variable severity in autosomal dominant optic atrophy. Ophthalmic Paediatr Genet 1985; 5:99–102.
9. Kjer P. Infantile optic atrophy with dominant mode of inheritance. Acta Ophthalmol Suppl 1959; 54:1–146.
10. Kollaritis CR, Pinheiro ML, Swann WR, et al. The autosomal dominant syndrome of progressive optic atrophy and congenital deafness. Am J Ophthalmol 1979; 87:789–792.
11. Mets MB, Mhoon E. Probable autosomal dominant optic atrophy with hearing loss. Ophthalmic Paediatr Genet 1985; 5:85–89.
12. Szmigielski M, Ptasinska-Urbanska M, Mitkiewicz-Bochener M. Atrophie optique heredo-familiale dominante associee a la surdi-mutite. Ann Oculist 1968; 201:431–435.
13. Treft RL, Sanborn BE, Carey J, et al. Dominant optic atrophy, deafness, ptosis, ophthalmoplegia, dystaxia, and myopathy. A new syndrome. Ophthalmology 1984; 91:908–915.
14. Meire F, de Laey JJ, de Bie S, et al. Dominant optic nerve atrophy with progressive hearing loss and chronic progressive external ophthalmoplegia (CPEO). Ophthalmic Paediatr Genet 1985; 5:91–97.
15. Hagemoser K, Weinstein J, Bresnick G, Nellis R, Kirkpatrick S, Pauli RM. Optic atrophy, hearing loss, and peripheral neuropathy. Am J Med Genet 1989; 33(l):61–65.
16. Volker-Dieben HJ, van Lith GHM, Oosterhuis JA, Swart-van den Berg M. Examination methods and their significance for the analysis of hereditary optic atrophies. Doc Ophthalmol Proc Ser 1978; 17:117–125.
17. Went LN. Optic atrophy. In: Emery AEG, Rimoin DL, eds. Principle and Practice of Medical Genetics. Edinburgh: Churchill-Livingstone, 1983:482–487.
18. Eliott D, Traboulsi EI, Maumenee IH. Visual prognosis in autosomal dominant optic atrophy (Kjer type). Am J Ophthalmol 1993; 115(3):360–367.

19. Votruba M, Fitzke FW, Holder GE, Carter A, Bhattacharya SS, Moore AT. Clinical features in affected individuals from 21 pedigrees with dominant optic atrophy. Arch Ophthalmol 1998; 116(3):351–358.
20. Neetens A, Rubbens MC. Dominant juvenile optic atrophy. Ophthalmic Paediatr Genet 1985; 5:79–83.
21. Johnston RL, Seller MJ, Behnam JT, Burdon MA, Spalton DJ. Dominant opticatrophy. Refining the clinical diagnostic criteria in light of genetic linkage studies. Ophthalmology 1999; 106(1):123–128.
22. Berninger TA, Jaeger W, Krastel H. Electrophysiology and colour perimetry in dominant infantile optic atrophy. Br J Ophthalmol 1991; 75(l):49–52.
23. Wildberger H. Acquired disorders of contrast sensitivity and color vision in mild optic neuropathies. Klin Monatsbl Augenheilkd 1985; 186:194–199.
24. Papst N, Bopp M, Wundrack EM. Autosomal dominant infantile optic atrophy: ascending or descending degeneration? Klin Monatsbl Augenheilkd 1985; 187:101–104.
25. Fournier AV, Damji KF, Epstein DL, Pollock SC. Disc excavation in dominant optic atrophy: differentiation from normal tension glaucoma. Ophthalmology 2001; 108(9): 1595–1602.
26. Miyake Y, Yagasaki K, Ichikawa H. Differential diagnosis of congenital tritanopia and dominantly inherited juvenile optic atrophy. Arch Ophthalmol 1985; 103:1496–1501.
27. Jaeger W. Diagnosis of dominant infantile optic atrophy in early childhood. Ophthalmic Paediatr Genet 1988; 9:7–11.
28. Johnston PB, Gaster RN, Smith VC, Tripathi RC. A clinicopathologic study of autosomal dominant optic atrophy. Am J Ophthalmol 1979; 88:868–875.
29. Kjer P, Jensen OA, Klinken L. Histopathology of eye, optic nerve and brain in a case of dominant optic atrophy. Acta Ophthalmol 1983; 61:300–312.
30. Moriarty BJ. Childhood blindness in Jamaica. Br J Ophthalmol 1988; 72:65–67.
31. Kivlin JD, Lovrien EW, Bishop DT, Maumenee IH. Linkage analysis in dominant optic atrophy. Am J Hum Genet 1983; 35:1190–1195.
32. Meyer E, Navon D, Aloni U, et al. Bilateral optic atrophy associated with abnormality of chromosome No. 2. Metab Pediatr Syst Ophthalmol 1983; 7:207–210.
33. Eiberg H, Kjer B, Kjer P, Rosenberg T. Dominant optic atrophy (OPA1) mapped to chromosome 3q region. I. Linkage analysis. Hum Mol Genet 1994; 3(6):977–980.
34. Lunkes A, Hartung U, Magarino C, Rodriguez M, Palmero A, Rodriguez L, Heredero L, Weissenbach J, Weber J, Auburger G. Refinement of the OPA1 gene locus on chromosome 3q28-q29 to a region of 2–8 cM, in one Cuban pedigree with autosomal dominant optic atrophy type Kjer. Am J Hum Genet 1995; 57(4):968–970.
35. Bonneau D, Souied E, Gerber S, Rozet JM, D'Haens E, Journel H, Plessis G, Weissenbach J, Munnich A, Kaplan J. No evidence of genetic heterogeneity in dominant optic atrophy. J Med Genet 1995; 32(12):951–953.
36. Kjer B, Eiberg H, Kjer P, Rosenberg T. Dominant optic atrophy mapped to chromosome 3q region. H Clinical and epidemiological aspects. Ada Ophthalmol Scand 1996; 74(1):3–7.
37. Jonasdottir A, Eiberg H, Kjer B, Kjer P, Rosenberg T. Refinement of the dominant optic atrophy locus (OPA1) to a 1.4-cM interval on chromosome 3q28-3q29, within a 3-Mb YAC contig. Hum Genet 1997; 99(1):115–120.
38. Votruba M, Moore AT, Bhattacharya SS. Genetic refinement of dominant optic atrophy (OPA1) locus to within a 2 cM interval of chromosome 3q. J Med Genet 1997; 34(2):117–121.
39. Brown J Jr, Fingert JH, Taylor CM, Lake M, Sheffield VC, Stone EM. Clinical and genetic analysis of a family affected with dominant optic atrophy (OPA1). Arch Ophthalmol 1997; 115(l):95–99.
40. Alexander C, Votruba M, Pesch UE, Thiselton DL, Mayer S, Moore A, Rodriguez M, Kellner U, Leo-Kottler B, Auburger G, Bhattacharya SS, Wissinger B. OPA1, encoding

a dynamin-related GTPase, is mutated in autosomal dominant optic atrophy linked to chromosome 3q28. Nat Genet 2000; 26(2):211–215.
41. Delettre C, Lenaers G, Griffoin JM, Gigarel N, Lorenzo C, Belenguer P, Pelloquin L, Grosgeorge J, Turc-Carel C, Perret E, Astarie-Dequeker C, Lasquellec L, Arnaud B, Ducommun B, Kaplan J, Hamel CP. Nuclear gene OPA1, encoding a mitochondrial dynamin-related protein, is mutated in dominant optic atrophy. Nat Genet 2000; 26(2):207–210.
42. Delettre C, Griffoin JM, Kaplan J, Dollfus H, Lorenz B, Faivre L, Lenaers G, Belenguer P, Hamel CP. Mutation spectrum and splicing variants in the OPA1 gene. Hum Genet 2001; 109(6):584–591.
43. Toomes C, Marchbank NJ, Mackey DA, Craig JE, Newbury-Ecob RA, Bennett CP, Vize CJ, Desai SP, Black GC, Patel N, Teimory M, Markham AF, Inglehearn CF, Churchill AJ. Spectrum, frequency and penetrance of OPA1 mutations in dominant optic atrophy. Hum Mol Genet 2001; 10(13):1369–1378.
44. Thiselton DL, Alexander C, Taanman JW, Brooks S, Rosenberg T, Eiberg H, Andreasson S, Van Regemorter N, Munier FL, Moore AT, Bhattacharya SS, Votruba M. A comprehensive survey of mutations in the OPA1 gene in patients with autosomal dominant optic atrophy. Invest Ophthalmol Vis Sci 2002; 43(6):1715–1724.
45. Olichon A, Baricault L, Gas N, Guillou E, Valette A, Belenguer P, Lenaers G. Loss of OPA1 perturbates the mitochondrial inner membrane structure and integrity, leading to cytochrome c release and apoptosis. J Biol Chem 2003; 278(10):7743–7746.
46. Amati-Bonneau P, Odent S, Derrien C, Pasquier L, Malthiery Y, Reynier P, Bonneau D. The association of autosomal dominant optic atrophy and moderate deafness may be due to the R445H mutation in the OPA1 gene. Am J Ophthalmol 2003; 136(6): 1170–1171.
47. Kerrison JB, Amould VJ, Ferraz Sallum JM, Vagefi MR, Barmada MM, Li Y, Zhu D, Maumenee IH. Genetic heterogeneity of dominant optic atrophy Kjer type: Identification of a second locus on chromosome 18ql2.2-12.3. Arch Ophthalmol 1999; 117(6): 805–810.
48. Imachi J, Mimura O. Infantile dominant optic atrophy. Doc Ophthalmol Proc Ser 1978; 17:127–137.
49. Gorgone G, Volti S, Cavallaro N, et al. Familial optic atrophy with sex-influenced severity. A new variety of autosomal-dominant optic atrophy? Ophthalmologica 1986; 192:28–33.
50. Behr C. Die komplizierte, hereditar-familiare optikusatrophie des Kindesalters: ein bisher nicht beschriebener Symptomenlcomplex. Klin Monatsbl Augenheilkd 1909; 47:138–160.
51. Franceschetti A. L'atrophie optique infantile compliquee (maladie de Behr). J Genet Hum 1966; 15:322–331.
52. Horoupian DS, Zucker DK, Moshe S, Peterson HD. Behr syndrome: a clinicopathologic report. Neurology 1979; 29:323–327.
53. Copeliovitch L, Katz K, Arbel N, Harrie N, Bar-On E, Soudry M. Musculoskeletal deformities in Behr syndrome. J Pediatr Orthop 2001; 21(4):512–514.
54. Barbet F, Gerber S, Hakiki S, Perrault I, Hanein S, Ducroq D, Tanguy G, Dufier JL, Munnich A, Rozet JM, Kaplan J. A first locus for isolated autosomal recessive optic atrophy (ROA1) maps to chromosome 8q. Eur J Hum Genet 2003; 11(12):966–971.
55. Wolfram DJ, Wagener HP. Diabetes mellitus and simple optic atrophy among siblings: report of four cases. Proc Staff Meet Mayo Clin 1938; 13:715–718.
56. Rando TA, Horton JC, Layzer RB. Wolfram syndrome: evidence of a diffuse neurodegenerative disease by magnetic resonance imaging. Neurology 1992; 42(6):1220–1224.
57. Fraser FC, Gunn T. Diabetes mellitus, diabetes insipidus and optic atrophy. An autosomal recessive syndrome? J Med Genet 1977; 14:190–193.
58. Mtanda AT, Cruysberg JR, Pinckers AJ. Optic atrophy in Wolfram syndrome. Ophthalmic Paediatr Genet 1986; 7:159–165.

59. Swift RG, Polymeropoulos MH, Torres R, Swift M. Predisposition of Wolfram syndrome heterozygotes to psychiatric illness. Mol Psychiatry 1998; 3(1):86–91.
60. Khardori R, Stephens JW, Page OC, Dow RS. Diabetes mellitus and optic atrophy in two siblings. a report on a new association and a review of the literature. Diabetes Care 1983; 6:67–70.
61. Monson JP, Boucher BJ. HLA type and islet cell antibody status in family with (diabetes insipidus and mellitus, optic atrophy, and deafness) DIDMOAD syndrome. Lancet 1983; 4:1286–1287.
62. Deschamps I, Lestradet H, Schrnid M, Hors J. HLA-DR2 and DIDMOAD syndrome. Lancet 1983; 2:109.
63. Bertrams J, Wendel U, Koletzko S. HLA and Wolfram (DIDMOAD) syndrome. Lancet 1983; 2:573.
64. Online Mendelian Inheritance in Man, OMIM (TM). McKusick-Nathans Institute for Genetic Medicine, Johns Hopkins University (Baltimore, MD) and National Center for Biotechnology Information, National Library of Medicine (Bethesda, MD), 2000. http://www.ncbi.nlm.nih.gov/omim/.
65. Inoue H, Tanizawa Y, Wasson J, Behn P, Kalidas K, Bernal-Mizrachi E, Mueckler M, Marshall H, Donis-Keller H, Crock P, Rogers D, Mikuni M, Kumashiro H, Higashi K, Sobue G, Oka Y, Permutt MA. A gene encoding a transmembrane protein is mutated in patients with diabetes mellitus and optic atrophy (Wolfram syndrome). Nat Genet 1998; 20(2):143–148.
66. El-Shanti H, Lidral AC, Jarrah N, Druhan L, Ajlouni K. Homozygosity mapping identifies an additional locus for Wolfram syndrome on chromosome 4q. Am J Hum Genet 2000; 66(4):1229–1236.
67. Costeff H, Gadoth N, Apter N, Prialnic M, Savir H. A familial syndrome of infantile optic atrophy, movement disorder, and spastic paraplegia. Neurology 1989; 39(4): 595–597.
68. Anikster Y, Kleta R, Shaag A, Gahl WA, Elpeleg O. TypeIII 3-methylglutaconic aciduria (optic atrophy plus syndrome, or Costeff optic atrophy syndrome): identification of the OPA3 gene and its founder mutation in Iraqi Jews. Am J Hum Genet 2001; 69(6): 1218–1224.
69. Tipton RE, Gorlin RJ. Growth retardation, alopecia, pseudo-anodontia, and optic atrophy—the GAPO syndrome. report of a patient and review of the literature. Am J Med Genet 1984; 19:209–216.
70. Gagliardi AR, Gonzales CH, Pratesi R. GAPO syndrome: report of three affected brothers. Am J Med Genet 1984; 19:217–223.
71. Muller J, Zeman W. Degenerescence systematisee optico-cochleo-dentate. Acta Neuropathol 1965; 5:26–39.
72. MacDermot KD, Walker RW. Autosomal recessive hereditary motor and sensory neuropathy with mental retardation, optic atrophy and pyramidal signs. J Neurol Neurosurg Psychiatry 1987; 50:1342–1347.
73. Chalmers N, Mitchell JD. Optico-acoustic atrophy in distal spinal muscular atrophy. J Neurol Neurosurg Psychiatry 1987; 50:238–239.
74. Voo I, Allf BE, Udar N, Silva-Garcia R, Vance J, Small KW. Hereditary motor and sensory neuropathy type VI with optic atrophy. Am J Ophthalmol 2003; 136(4):670–677.
75. Rosenberg RN, Chutorian A. Familial opticoacoustic nerve degeneration and polyneuropathy. Neurology 1967; 17:827–832.
76. Went LN, de Vries-de Mol EC, Völker-Dieben HJ. A family with apparently sex linked optic atrophy. J Med Genet 1975; 12:94–98.
77. Assink JJ, Tijmes NT, ten Brink JB, Oostra RI, Riemslag FC, de Jong PT, Bergen AA. A gene for X-linked optic atrophy is closely linked to the Xp l 1.4-Xp l 1.2 region of the X chromosome. Am J Hum Genet 1997; 61(4):934–939.
78. Jensen PKA. Nerve deafness, optic atrophy and dementia: A new X-linked recessive syndrome? Am J Med Genet 1981; 9:55–60.

79. Jensen PKA, Reske-Nielsen E, Hein-Sorensen O, Warburg M. The syndrome of opticoacoustic nerve atrophy with dementia. Am J Med Genet 1987; 28:517–518.
80. Tranebjaerg L, Van Ghelue M, Nilssen O, et al. Jensen syndrome is allelic to Mohr-Tranebjaerg syndrome and both are caused by stop mutations in the DDP gene. Am J Hum Genet 1997; 61(Suppl):A349.
81. Nikoskelainen E, Sogg RL, Rosenthal AR, et al. The early phase in Leber hereditary optic atrophy. Arch Ophthalmol 1977; 95:969–978.
82. Nikoskelainen E, Hyot WF, Nuinmelin K, Schatz H. Fundus findings in Leber's hereditary optic neuroretinopathy. III. Fluorescein angiographic studies. Arch Ophthalmol 1984; 102:981–989.
83. Nikoskelainen E, Hoyt WF, Nummelin K. Ophthalmoscopic findings in Leber's hereditary optic neuropathy. II. The fundus findings in the affected family members. Arch Ophthalmol 1983; 101:1059–1968.
84. Nikoskelainen E, Hoyt WF, Nummelin K. Fundus findings in Leber's hereditary optic neuroretinopathy. Ophthalmic Paediatr Genet 1985; 5:125–130.
85. Nikoskelainen E. The clinical findings in Leber's hereditary optic neuroretinopathy. Leber's disease. Trans Ophthalmol Soc UK 1985; 104:845–852.
86. Lopez PF, Smith JL. Leber's optic neuropathy. New observations. J Clin Neurol Ophthalmol 1986; 6:144–152.
87. Nikoskelainen EK, Savontaus ML, Wanne OP, et al. Leber's hereditary optic neuroretino-pathy, a maternally inherited disease. A genealogic study in four pedigrees. Arch Ophthalmol 1987; 105:665–671.
88. Carroll WM, Mastaglia FL. Leber's optic neuropathy. a clinical and visual evoked potential study of affected and asymptomatic members of a six generation family. Brain 1979; 102:559–580.
89. Uemura A, Osame M, Nakagawa M, et al. Leber's hereditary optic neuropathy: mitochondrial and biochemical studies on muscle biopsies. Br J Ophthalmol 1987; 71: 531–536.
90. Wilson J. Leber's hereditary optic atrophy: a possible defect of cyanide metabolism. Clin Sci Mol Med 1965; 29:505–515.
91. Cagianut B, Schnebli HP, Rhyner K, Furrer J. Decreased thiosulfate sulfur transferase (rhodanese) in Leber's hereditary optic atrophy. Klin Wochenschr 1984; 62:850–854.
92. Poole CJ, Kind PR. Deficiency of thiosuiphate sulphurtransferase (rhodanese) in Leber's hereditary optic neuropathy. Br Med J 1986; 292:1229–1230.
93. Nikoskelainen E, Hassinen IE, Paljärvi L, et al. Leber's hereditary optic neuroretinopathy, a mitochondrial disease? Lancet 1984; 2:1474.
94. Cotticelli L, Rinaldi E, D'Alessandro L. Red cell glutathione in Leber's optic atrophy. Metab Ophthalmol 1985; 8:31–34.
95. Walsh FB. Clinical Neuro-Ophthalmology. Baltimore: Williams & Wilkins, 1957:605–611.
96. Seedorff T. Leber's disease. Acta Ophthalmol 1968; 46:4–25.
97. Seedorff T. The inheritance of Leber's disease. A genealogical follow-up study. Acta Ophthalmol 1985; 63:135–145.
98. van Senus AHC. Leber's disease in the Netherlands. Doc Ophthalmol 1963; 17:1–162.
99. Imai Y, Moriwaki D. A probable case of cytoplasmic inheritance in man; a critique of Leber's disease. J Genet 1936; 33:163–167.
100. Fine PEM. Mitochondrial inheritance and disease. Lancet 1978; 2:659–661.
101. Merz B. Eye disease linked to mitochondrial gene defect. J Am Med Assoc 1988; 260:894.
102. Wallace DC, Singh G, Lott MT, et al. Mitochondrial DNA mutation associated with Leber's hereditary optic neuropathy. Science 1988; 242:1427–1430.
103. Singh G, Lott MT, Wallace DC. A mitochondrial DNA mutation as a cause of Leber's hereditary optic neuropathy. N Engl J Med 1989; 320:1300–1305.
104. Hotta Y, Hayakawa M, Saito K et al. Diagnosis of Leber's optic neuropathy by means of polymerase chain reaction amplification. Am J Ophthalmol 1989; 108:601–602.

105. Chen J, Cox I, Denton MJ. Preliminary exclusion of an X-linked gene in Leber optic atrophy by linkage analysis. Hum Genet 1989; 82:203–207.
106. Brown MD, Wallace DC. Spectrum of mitochondrial DNA mutations in Leber's hereditary optic neuropathy. Clin Neurosci 1994; 2:138–145.
107. Brown MD, Starikovskaya E, Derbeneva O, Hosseini S, Allen JC, Mikhailovskaya IE, Sukernik RI, Wallace DC. The role of mtDNA background in disease expression: a new primary LHON mutation associated with Western Eurasian haplogroup J. Hum Genet 2002; 110(2):130–138.
108. Nikoskelainen EK, Huoponen K, Juvonen V, Lamminen T, Nummelin K, Savontaus ML. Ophthalmologic findings in Leber hereditary optic neuropathy, with special reference to mtDNA mutations. Ophthalmology 1996; 103(3):504–514.
109. Riordan-Eva P, Sanders MD, Govan GG, Sweeney MG, Da Costa L, Harding AE. The clinical features of Leber's hereditary optic neuropathy defined by the presence of a pathogenic mitochondrial DNA mutation. Brain 1995; 118(Pt 2):319–337.
110. Johns DR, Smith KH, Miller NR. Leber's hereditary optic neuropathy. Clinical manifestations of the 3460 mutation. Arch Ophthalmol 1992; 110(11):1577–1581.
111. Johns DR, Heher KL, Miller NR, Smith KH. Leber's hereditary optic neuropathy. Clinical manifestations of the 14484 mutation. Arch Ophthalmol 1993; 111(4):495–498.
112. Sadun AA, Carelli V, Salomao SR, Berezovsky A, Quiros P, Sadun F, DeNegri AM, Andrade R, Schein S, Belfort R. A very large Brazilian pedigree with 11778 Leber's hereditary optic neuropathy. Trans Am Ophthalmol Soc 2002; 100:169–178; discussion 178–179.
113. Sadun AA, Carelli V, Salomao SR, Berezovsky A, Quiros PA, Sadun F, DeNegri AM, Andrade R, Moraes M, Passos A, Kjaer P, Pereira J, Valentino ML, Schein S, Belfort R. Extensive investigation of a large Brazilian pedigree of 11778/haplogroup J Leber hereditary optic neuropathy. Am J Ophthalmol 2003; 136(2):231–238.
114. Sadun F, De Negri AM, Carelli V, Salomao SR, Berezovsky A, Andrade R, Moraes M, Passos A, Belfort R, da Rosa AB, Quiros P, Sadun AA. Ophthalmologic findings in a large pedigree of 11778/Haplogroup J Leber hereditary optic neuropathy. Am J Ophthalmol 2004; 137(2):271–277.
115. Warner RB, Lee AG. Leber hereditary optic neuropathy associated with use of ephedra alkaloids. Am J Ophthalmol 2002; 134(6):918–920.
116. Kerrison JB, Miller NR, Hsu F, Beaty TH, Maumenee IH, Smith KH, Savino PJ, Stone EM, Newman NJ. A case-control study of tobacco and alcohol consumption in Leber hereditary optic neuropathy. Am J Ophthalmol 2000; 130(6):803–812.
117. Hotta Y, Fujiki K, Hayakawa M, Nakajima A, Kanai A, Mashima Y, Hilda Y, Shinoda K, Yamada K, Oguchi Y, et al. Clinical features of Japanese Leber's hereditary optic neuropathy with 11778 mutation of mitochondrial DNA. Jpn J Ophthalmol 1995; 39(1):96–108.
118. Newman NJ, Lott MT, Wallace DC. The clinical characteristics of pedigrees of Leber's hereditary optic neuropathy with the 11778 mutation. Am J Ophthalmol 1991; 111(6):750–762.
119. Howell N. Leber hereditary optic neuropathy: mitochondrial mutations and degeneration of the optic nerve. Vis Res 1997; 37(24):3495–3507.
120. Howell N, Xu M, Halvorson S, Bodis-Wollner L, Sherman J. A heteroplasmic LHON family: tissue distribution and transmission of the 11778 mutation. Am J Hum Genet 1994; 55(l):203–206.
121. Sadun AA, Win PH, Ross-Cisneros FN, Walker SO, Carelli V. Leber's hereditary optic neuropathy differentially affects smaller axons in the optic nerve. Trans Am Ophthalmol Soc 2000; 98:223–232; discussion 232–235.
122. Phillips PH, Vaphiades M, Glasier CM, Gray LG, Lee AG. Chiasmal enlargement and optic nerve enhancement on magnetic resonance imaging in leber hereditary optic neuropathy. Arch Ophthalmol 2003; 121(4):577–579.

123. Huoponen K, Vilkki J, Aula P, Nikoskelainen EK, Savontaus ML. A new mtDNA mutation associated with Leber hereditary optic neuroretinopathy. Am J Hum Genet 1991; 48(6):1147–1153.
124. Mackey DA. Three subgroups of patients from the United Kingdom with Leber hereditary optic neuropathy. Eye 1994; 8(Pt 4):431–436.
125. Kerrison JB, Howell N, Miller NR, Hirst L, Green WR. Leber hereditary optic neuropathy. Electron microscopy and molecular genetic analysis of a case. Ophthalmology 1995; 102(10):1509–1516.
126. Sadun AA, Sadun F. Leber hereditary optic neuropathy. Ophthalmology 1996; 103(2):201–202.
127. Howell N, Oostra RJ, Bolhuis PA, Spruijt L, Clarke LA, Mackey DA, Preston G, Herrnstadt C. Sequence analysis of the mitochondrial genomes from Dutch pedigrees with Leber hereditary optic neuropathy. Am J Hum Genet 2003; 72(6):1460–1469.
128. Carelli V, Sadun AA. Optic neuropathy in Lhon and Leigh syndrome. Ophthalmology 2001; 108(7):1172–1173.
129. Lamminen T, Majander A, Juvonen V, Wikstrom M, Aula P, Nikoskelainen E, Savontous ML. A mitochondrial mutation at nt 9101 in the ATP synthase 6 gene associated with deficient oxidative phosphorylation in a family with Leber hereditary optic neuroretinopathy. Am J Hum Genet 1995; 56(5):1238–1240.
130. Howell N, Halvorson S, Burns J, McCullough DA, Paulton J. When does bilateral optic atrophy become Leber hereditary optic neuropathy? Am J Hum Genet 1993; 53(4): 959–963.
131. Chinnery PF, Brown DT, Andrews RM, Singh-Kler R, Riordan-Eva P, Lindley J, Applegarth DA, Turnbull DM, Howell N. The mitochondrial ND6 gene is a hot spot for mutations that cause Leber's hereditary optic neuropathy. Brain 2001; 124(Pt 1): 209–218.
132. Johns DR, Smith KH, Savino PJ, Miller NR. Leber's hereditary optic neuropathy. Clinical manifestations of the 15257 mutation. Ophthalmology 1993; 1000:981–986.
133. Johns DR. Seminars in medicine of the Beth Israel Hospital, Boston. Mitochondrial DNA and disease. N Engl J Med 1995; 333(10):638–644.
134. Carelli V, Ghelli A, Cevoli S, Cortelli P, Lugaresi E, Baruzzi A, Leuzzi V, Degli Esposti M, Barboni P, Montagna P. Idebenone therapy in Leber's hereditary optic neuropathy: report of six cases. Neurology 1998; 50(suppl 4):A4.
135. Syme IG, Bronte-Stewart J, Foulds WS, et al. Clinical and biochemical findings in Leber's hereditary optic atrophy. Trans Ophthalmol Soc UK 1983; 103:556–559.
136. Seedorf T. Leber's disease. Acta Ophthalmol 1970; 48:187–213.
137. Nikoskelainen E. New aspects of the genetic, etiologic, and clinical puzzle of Leber's disease. Neurology 1984; 34:1482–1484.
138. Harding AE, Sweeney MG, Govan GG, Riordan-Eva P. Pedigree analysis in Leber hereditary optic neuropathy families with a pathogenic mtDNA mutation. Am J Hum Genet 1995; 57(1):77–86.
139. Hirschberg J, Cirincione G. Über Drusen im Sehnervenkopf. Zentralbl Prakt Augenheilkd 1891; 15:166–168, 198–211.
140. Lauber H. Drusen im Sehnervenkopf. Zentralbl Augenheilkd 1907; 17:391–392.
141. Braun W. Über familiares Vorkommen von Drusen der Papille. Klin Monatol Augenheilkd 1935; 94:734–738.
142. Lorentzen SE. Drusen of the optic disk: a clinical and genetic study. Acta Ophthaimol Suppl 1966; 90:1–180.
143. Erkkiia H. Optic disc drusen in children. Acta Ophthalmol Suppl 1977; 129:1–44.
144. Friedman AH, Gartner S, Modi SS. Drusen of the optic disc. Br J Ophthalmol 1975; 59:413–421.
145. Kheterpal S, Good PA, Beale DJ, Kritzinger EE. Imaging of optic disc drusen: a comparative study. Eye 1995; 9(Pt 1):67–69.

146. Antcliff RJ, Spalton DJ. Are optic disc drusen inherited? Ophthalmology 1999; 106(7): 1278–1281.
147. Nischal KK, Hingorani M, Bentley CR, Vivian AJ, Bird AC, Baker AJ, Mowat AP, Mieli-Vergani G, Aclimandos WA. Ocular ultrasound in Alagille syndrome: a new sign. Ophthalmology 1997; 104(1):79–85.
148. Kamath BM, Spinner NB, Emerick KM, Chudley AE, Booth C, Piccoli DA, Krantz ID. Vascular anomalies in Alagille syndrome: a significant cause of morbidity and mortality. Circulation 2004; 109(11):1354–1358.
149. Friedman AH, Beckerman B, Gold DH, et al. Drusen of the optic disc. Surv Ophthalmol 1977; 21:375–390.
150. Levinson JB. Pseudopapilledema secondary to optic nerve drusen: ophthalmoscopic differentiation. J Am Optom Assoc 1986; 57:373–375.
151. Acers TE. Congenital Abnormalities of the Optic Nerve and Related Forebrain. Philadelphia: Lea & Feblger, 1983.
152. Magli A, Cennamo G, Corvino C, Mele A. Genetic and ultrasound study of abnormalities of the optic nerve head. Ophthalmic Paediatr Genet 1985; 5:71–78.
153. Taylor DS. The genetic implications of optic disc anomalies. Trans Ophthalmol Soc UK 1985; 104:853–856.
154. Yamashita T, Kawano K, Ohba N. Autosomal dominantly inherited optic nerve coloboma. Ophthalmic Paediatr Genet 1988; 9:17–24.
155. Slusher MM, Weaver RG, Greven CM, et al. The spectrum of cavitary optic disc anomalies in a family. Ophthalmol 1989; 96:342–347.
156. Stefko ST, Campochiaro P, Wang P, Li Y, Zhu D, Traboulsi EI. Dominant inheritance of optic pits. Am J Ophthalmol 1997; 124(1):112–113.
157. Chung GW, Edwards AO, Schimmenti LA, Manligas GS, Zhang YH, Ritter R 3rd. Renal-coloboma syndrome: report of a novel PAX2 gene mutation. Am J Ophthalmol 2001; 132(6):910–914.

18
Strabismus

INTRODUCTION

Hippocrates has been credited with being the first (almost 2500 years ago) to note that strabismus tends to be inherited, remarking that "children of parents having distorted eyes squint also for the most part" (1,2). Because strabismus is easily noticed very early in life, parent–offspring comparisons may be readily made, strengthening the impression of an inherited entity.

The mode of inheritance has not been always clear-cut. In most families, strabismus is single and sporadic. Some of the previous confusion about inheritance stems from a poor understanding of the genetic concept of multifactorial heredity and an unclear definition of the subject. For example, does esophoria in a sibling occur as an expression of the same gene that causes esotropia in another sibling? A number of studies have dealt differently with this question.

We classify strabismus into two subgroups: isolated concomitant strabismus and associated strabismus. Associated strabismus occurs as part of a systemic syndrome or an orbital disease, incomitant strabismus, and ophthalmoplegias.

ISOLATED CONCOMITANT (NONSTRABISMIC) STRABISMUS

Concomitant strabismus, heterotropia, or squint, is a misalignment of the eyes that does not change in magnitude in any horizontal gaze of view. Isolated concomitant strabismus occurs as an isolated phenomenon. It may manifest itself as an esotropia or exotropia, with or without the A, X, or V syndrome; it may be a large-angle squint or a raicrostrabismus; and it may be permanent, intermittent (irregularly appearing and disappearing), or cyclic (regularly appearing and disappearing).

Studies on Heredity of Strabismus

Studies of families, twins, and general populations have been performed. Some have dealt with specific subtypes of concomitant strabismus as well.

Family Studies

Siblings of strabismic patients have a significantly higher prevalence of strabismus than the general population, as demonstrated by a large study of children's diseases in families (3) and from many investigations of individual pedigrees.

A positive family history has been found in 65% of 254 consecutive patients with concomitant strabismus in Vancouver, Canada (4), in 65% of 195 such patients in France (5), and in 43% of 345 patients in Greece (6). Earlier studies of families with strabismus have suggested an autosomal recessive inheritance by one or two genes (7). Many later investigators have accepted Waardenburg's view (8) of an irregular autosomal dominant transmission (autosomal dominant with incomplete penetrance) (5,9). His theory was based on a large number of affected siblings and affected parent–offspring pairs. The genes causing esotropia had been assumed to be separate and different from those causing exotropia (6,8,9). Maumenee and colleagues (10) analyzed the pedigrees of 173 families with congenital esotropia and concluded that the results are compatible with a mendelian codominant model, with homozygotes who carry a relatively common allele having a high probability of being affected. However, the data have not been analyzed for multifactorial inheritance.

In the Vancouver study (4), congenital concomitant squint had a higher rate of positive family history (76%) than that which occurred after the first year of life (59%). When studied, a high rate of refractive disorders, mainly hypermetropia with esotropia, and sensory anomalies, such as amblyopia and defective binocular function, were noted in other family members (4,6,9,11).

In 1967, after studying 697 strabismic children and their 3123 relatives in Berlin, Richter concluded that strabismus is multifactorially transmitted (11). She found a high incidence of ametropias in family members; also sensory anomalies, such as low fusional amplitudes, anomalous retinal correspondence, or amblyopia; and motor anomalies, such as heterophorias. The risk for the siblings of a patient was 30–50% if one or both parents were also affected and 20–30% if the parents were unaffected (11).

Studies of large families showed wide variation in the incidence of affected family members (12) and affected/unaffected ratios that could not support the hypothesis of a single mutant gene (13), but could uphold multifactorial inheritance.

Aurell and Norrsell (14) followed up children who had at least one parent who had suffered from strabismus. Of these children 17.6% developed strabismus, a figure that is more than four times the general population. All children who developed esotropia were hyperopic.

Pedgor and colleagues (15) also found a significant familial component in their family studies. Odds for esotropia in a sibling more than doubled if another sibling was affected. A strong association of exotropia with multiple births was also found (15).

Studies of Twins

After studying II monozygotic (MZ) twins, 58 similar cases in the literature and 51 dizygotic (DZ) twins (8), Waardenburg reported a very high concordance for MZ twins (81%; 14% for DZ twins). He suggested that discordance could be explained by one gene that "can manifest itself in different phenotypes of squint, with and without amblyopia." Richter (11) detected a concordance of 92% in 12 pairs of MZ twins and 26% in 27 pairs of DZ twins. Rubin and colleagues (16) collected information on twins and strabismus from 50 ophthalmologists in 20 different countries. On the basis of numerous twins for each trait, they concluded that the heritability factors are high for exotropia, hyperopia, and myopia, and moderate for esotropia eccentric fixation, and astigmatism. Hereditary factors were also observed in a study of 17 pairs of MZ twins, of which at least one was affected by squint (17) In each of two sets of monozygotic female twins, one was esotropic and one was orthophoric; in each case the esotropic twin had the higher hyperopia, which supports a multifactorial mode of inheritance (18).

Population Studies

Population studies on the prevalence of strabismus have been varied in their results ranging from 1.3% to 4.6% in whites. A screening of 38,000 young children in welfare clinics in Israel showed 1.3% to have strabismus, 0.5% strabismic amblyopia, and 0.3% nonstrabismic amblyopia (19). Similar findings were obtained in other studies in Israel. In Germany, Molnar recorded a strabismus rate of 2.93% and 3.37% in the general population (20). Several surveys in England showed a frequency of 4.3% (21). The highest figure, 4.6%, was reported in Finnish schoolchildren (22).

The frequency of all types of squints varies among different populations. A much lower rate of esotropia occurs in blacks than in whites, especially for accommodative esotropia (12). In Hawaii, esotropia is more common in whites, and exotropia more usual in Asians, whereas both were equally observed in a racially mixed population (23).

Chew and associates (24) reported the results of a multicenter study performed on about 40,000 children. Esotropia was more frequent in whites compared to blacks (3.9% vs 2.2%) and exophoria was similar in both whites and blacks (1.2%). They reported associations with various factors that increase the risk of strabismus. Low birth weight and maternal cigarette smoking were significant risk factors for both esotropia and exotropia. Increased maternal age was a significant risk factor for esotropia (24). Mohney and associates studied the risk factors for congenital strabismus in one county in Minnesota (25). The strabismus odds ratio (OR) was 11.5 for prematurity; 4.6 for birth weight of less than 2,500 grams; 4.3 if APGAR was low at 1 min, 6.3 if it remained low at 5 min; and 3.5 if there was a family history of strabismus (25).

A group of investigators from Iowa (26), conducted a large study on three populations of patients and their families. These included 118 families of patients with esotropia, 27 families with exotropia, and 163 families without squint. They noted a higher frequency of esophoria in families with esotropic patients and of exophoria in families with exotropic probands than in the general population (27). They also recorded a moderate heritability factor for accommodation convergence/accommodation (AC/A) ratio (0.38 ± 0.09) and for the cover test (heterophoria) results (0.42 ± 0.12) With the amblyoscope, heritability estimates were greater for convergence than for divergence and for recovery than for break points (28). Interestingly, the difference in refractive power between strabismic and nonstrabismic populations was not due to a difference in corneal power, although this characteristic had a high heritability of 0.89 ± 0.05. This finding indicates that the difference in refraction between strabismic and nonstrabismic populations depends on axial length (29,30).

Scott and colleagues studied the familial occurrence of primary monofixation syndrome after excluding families with overt strabismus (31). They found primary monofixation syndrome in 9% of families and 6% of parents, significantly higher than the 1% of this syndrome in the general population. The authors concluded that monofixation might be a mild, subthreshold effect of one or more genes that cause congenital strabismus (31).

Numerous studies have shown that more women than men suffer from strabismus (7,32). Also, heterophoria found in family members of patients with strabismus reflects the mother's state significantly more often than that of the father (27). Waardenburg has suggested that this sexual predisposition may result from some difference in orbital anatomy or in the innervation of the extraocular muscles (8).

Microtropia and Cyclic Strabismus

Both subtypes of concomitant esotropia have demonstrated a high familial tendency toward strabismus.

Microtropia, microstrabismus, or monofixational syndrome is a unilateral strabismus of less than 5°, usually with harmonious anomalous correspondence, that occurs in about 1% of the population (33). Cantolino and von Noorden compared the parents and siblings of 20 patients with microtropia with normal control families (34). They noted that 8.1 % of the parents and 7.2% of the siblings of the probands had strabismus, as expected in multifactorial inheritance. If the patient had microstrabismus, a significantly higher incidence of family members had sensory, motor, and refractive anomalies, including heterotropia, diminished fusional amplitude, eccentric fixation, anomalous retinal correspondence, deficient stereopsis, large-angle strabismus, microtropia, anisometropia, and hypermetropia (34). In another family study, both microtropia and large-angle strabismus frequently occurred in the same family (35).

Cyclic strabismus is a condition in which orthophoria and esotropia alternate in cycles, usually of 24 hr each (36). All other biologic functions are normal in patients with this condition, but a high incidence of manifest strabismus has been found in their families (36).

The Inheritance of Strabismus and Genetic Counseling

Conclusions from Studies

Studies of twins indicate a high heritability factor for strabismus. The concordance rate is approximately four times as large for MZ twins as for DZ twins, making a genetic background indisputable (2,8,11,16). Nevertheless, the frequency and variability of clinical strabismus in families do not fit any known single-gene modes of mendelian inheritance. Investigators formerly overcame this problem by postulating a mechanism of two recessive genes or of an accessory gene for an autosomal dominant main gene (8). In 1961, Francois assumed that an irregular dominant gene transmitted heterophoria and environmental factors and refractive disorders caused manifest heterotropia (9). Later, most investigators and reviewers of the subject accepted Richter's theory (11) of a multifactorial inheritance for strabismus (2,7,37–39). Actually, the earlier approach (of more than one gene, such as two recessive or an accessory gene and environmental influence) would be interpreted today as a multifactorial inheritance. Miller and Folk have suggested that both multifactorial

Table 1 Factors Involved in Strabismus

Sensory anomalies
Eccentric fixation
Anomalous retinal correspondence
Reduced stereopsis
Amblyopia
Motor anomalies
Diminished fusional amplitudes
Heterophoria
Microtopia
Refractive anomalies
Hypermetropia
Myopia
Astigmatism
Anisometropia

inheritance and complex Mendelian models can explain the inheritance of strabismus (12). Although the latter is possible, the multifactorial theory is most tenable.

Considering the reviewed studies, multifactorial inheritance implies the following: (1) a polygenic and environmental influence with a threshold effect; 2) different genetic backgrounds for esotropias and exotropias; and 3) the same genetic background for large-angle manifest strabismus, microstrabismus, and cyclic strabismus.

Table 1 lists the various etiologic factors of strabismus. Most are genetically influenced, although the environmental impact is also present. The more factors at hand, or the stronger these factors are, the more likely an individual will reach the "threshold" and exhibit manifest strabismus. The additive effect of the different genes may take any of various combinations. The etiologic factors are different for esotropia and exotropia; thus, hypermetropia is important in the development of esotropia, and myopia is important in exotropia.

It is likely, therefore, that many or most cases of nonsyndromic strabismus are determined by two or more mutated genes with the additional influence of environmental factors. This certainly does not mean that in some cases a different mode of inheritance occurs. Paul and Hardage in a review of the heritability of strabismus (40) implied that isolated strabismus that clusters in families might be transmitted by the autosomal dominant, multifactorial, mitochondrial or sporadic mode.

In addition to the unequivocal hereditary background of strabismus, environmental factors may play a role. Some of these factors are known, such as low birth weight unrelated to a specific cause, advanced maternal age, or others that are not known.

More recently, one strabismus susceptibility locus was detected on the short arm of chromosome 7, Parikh and coworkers (41) performed a linkage analysis in one large multiplex family with strabismus and identified a presumptive strabismus locus at chromosome 7p22.1. Six other multiplex families did not show such a linkage (41). No gene responsible for isolated strabismus has yet been identified. Unfortunately, even the name of a possible strabismus gene (STRAB) will not be available for use in ophthalmic genetics. STB1 and STB2 for strabismus 1 and 2 were named for *Drosophila* strabismus and *Xenopus* strabismus (42). The human homologs are tumor suppressor genes, unrelated to ophthalmology (43).

Genetic Counseling

First-degree relatives of probands with strabismus have a 16–50% risk of having strabismus (6,11,18,44). This risk, however, varies from family to family and depends on the number of factors present.

When a child is born with strabismus, the risk to an additional sib is 20–30% if the parents are unaffected and increases to 30–50% if one or both parents have strabismus (11). This risk is higher if the mother, rather than the father, is affected (20); the reason for this is not clearly understood. The risk increases if a parents' familial history is positive, even if the parents are healthy (44). The risk also is enhanced if more factors (see Table 1) are found in first-degree relatives of the proband.

The risk to second-degree relatives is dramatically reduced, as expected in a multifactorial inheritance. For example, the figure of 8.1% was cited for grandparents (20).

When a second case of strabismus appears in a family, it tends to be of the same type and manifests at approximately the same age as the first (6).

Families with a heavy genetic background of strabismus should be advised about early examinations to detect and treat the various possible manifestations of a similar disorder in their offspring, such as large-angle heterotropia, microtropia, or amblyopia. If they are detected too late, useful treatment is precluded.

ASSOCIATED AND SYNDROMIC STRABISMUS

Strabismus, when it occurs as an essential part of a syndrome, is usually transmitted by a single mutated gene. This group includes multisystem disorders in which strabismus is an essential part of the syndrome and local disorders in which strabismus is associated with a congenital nerve abnormality. In most cases an incomitant strabismus occurs. Most are transmitted by autosomal dominant mutations. Often several genes are responsible for the rather uncommon disorders. Currently, there are three known loci associated with each of the following disorders, Duane syndrome, Moebius and congenital fibrosis of extraocular muscles (45). Table 2 lists the main genetic types of associated syndromic strabismus.

Duane Retraction Syndrome

In 1905, Duane described (46) a case of decreased abduction and adduction, retraction into the orbit on adduction, oblique elevation or depression, with narrowing of the palpebral fissure on adduction, and deficient convergence. The syndrome is now classified into one of three subtypes and is considered a congenital abnormal innervation of the extraocular muscles. Most cases of Duane syndrome are sporadic, but 5–10% are familial (47–49). It has been described in three generations of one family (37), as discordant in a pair of DZ twins (one bilaterally affected and one unaffected) (38), as concordant with mirror imaging in a pair of MZ twins (49), and as concordant, with one esotropic and one orthotropic, in another pair of MZ twins (50). In this last family, the mother and one twin had Duane syndrome in the right eye, whereas the other twin had an affected left eye. Smith and Cibis reported a fourth case of MZ twins, discordant for Duane syndrome. They suggested that the intrauterine environment (which is different for each of the twins) might have resulted in the syndrome in one of them (51).

Table 2 The Main Genetic Types of Associated Strabismus

	Name	Locus	Gene	Chromosomal location	Inheritance	Remarks
1	Duane syndrome Duane retraction s. DRS, type 1	DURS1	—	8q13	AD	Variable phenotypes, genetic typing unrelated to clinical types
2	Duane, type 2	DURS2	—	2q31	AD	—
3	Duane radial ray syndrome	DRRS	SALL4	20q13	AD	Duane syndrome associated with radial bone anomalies
4	Congenital superior oblique palsy		ARIX	11q13.3–q13.4	AD	
5	CFEOM type 1	FEOM1	KIF21A	12q12	AD	Characteristic phenotype
6	CFEOM type 2	FEOM2	ARIX	11q13.3–q13.4	AR	Exotropic strabismus fixus
7	CFEOM type 3	FEOM3	—	16q24.2–q24.3	AD	Rare

Duane syndrome is usually unilateral, the left eye affected about twice as often as the right (52). It was reported as unilateral in 80% (40). Both esotropia and exotropia may appear in different members of the same affected family (40). As in concomitant strabismus, there is a propensity for females (53). Chung et al. studying a large family with Duane syndrome (54) reported a variable severity of manifestations. Amblyopia was found in almost half of the 25 affected members. The disorder was associated with some other abnormalities including third or fourth cranial nerve palsies, nystagmus, seizures, and deafness (54).

Other associated anomalies have included innervation anomalies, such as facial palsy, facial hypoplasia, crocodile tears, Klippel–Feil syndrome, and Goldenhar–Wilderwanck syndrome with perceptive deafness (47,49). When familial, Duane syndrome shows an autosomal dominant inheritance.

Duane syndrome is a heterogenous disease with a variety of phenotypes. Variability of manifestations can be found even within the same family. The first locus DURS1 (for Duane retraction syndrome 1) has been mapped to chromosome 8ql3 (55). The second locus DURS2 has been mapped by Appukuttan and associates (56) to chromosome 2q31. Neither gene is yet identified. A third locus is DRRS for Duane radial ray syndrome (Okihiro syndrome) in which abnormalities in the radial bone or hand occur with Duane. Al-Baradie and associates mapped the DRRS locus to chromosome 20ql3 and identified three different truncating mutations in the SALL4 gene in this area (57).

It is likely that other genes are also associated with Duane syndrome, as some families could not be linked to the reported locations. One location could be chromosome 4q27–q31 as reported by Chew et al. (58) in a boy with bilateral Duane syndrome and deletion of this chromosomal segment. Another possibility is on chromosome 22 (56,59).

Brown's Syndrome (Superior Oblique Tendon Sheath Syndrome)

Brown's syndrome is an incomitant strabismus, with limitation in supraduction and adduction. It is usually isolated and sporadic, but may be familial (60). In one family, two siblings, in another two siblings, their mother and aunt were affected (53). In two pairs of MZ twins, a mirrorlike manifestation of Brown's syndrome occurred (61,62), presenting the well-known occurrence of mirrorlike congenital characteristics in MZ twins. The mode of inheritance of familial Brown's syndrome is unclear.

Congenital Superior Oblique Palsy

While most cases are sporadic, families with several affected members were reported by Wallace and von Noorden (63), Botelho and Giangiacomo (64) and Bhola et al. (65). In all reports the inheritance seems to be autosomal dominant. Jiang and associates found a mutation in the ARIX gene, segregating with congenital superior oblique palsy in one family (66). The ARIX gene (for Aristaless homeobox, homolog of *Drosophila*), a gene of three exons, is located at chromosome 11ql3.3–ql3.4 (55).

Congenital Fibrosis of the Extraocular Muscles

This congenital condition was originally described as a fibrosis of the extraocular muscles and Tenon's capsule, with adhesions among these muscles, Tenon's capsule, and the globe. Muscle movements are absent or very restricted and associated with blepharoptosis, little oronhorizontal movement, absence of elevation or depression of the eyes, eyes fixed below the horizontal line, and a chin-up head posture (67). The condition is transmitted by a single autosomal dominant gene, with regular penetrance (67,51). Although complicated, repeated operations can improve the condition and are advised (51,67,68). Pathologically, muscle tissue is replaced by collagen and dense fibrous tissue (51).

Paul and Hardage (40) described the characteristics of a patient with congenital fibrosis of extraocular muscles (CFEOM). CFEOM is always congenital. Fibrosis of EOMs and Tenon's capsule, and adhesions between muscles and the globe render the eyes fixed. No elevation or depression of either eye exists, with little or no horizontal movements and eyes fixed in downgaze of 20°–30°. Bilateral ptosis, chin elevation, and fragility with no elasticity of the conjunctiva also occur (40).

Computerized tomography (CT) may be a valuable tool in order to demonstrate the atrophy of extraocular muscle (69). The clinical spectrum of CFEOM is diverse, especially as to additional abnormalities (70,71).

CFEOM is generally heterogenous. Several loci have been mapped. Engle (72) suggests that all CFEOMs result from a primary defect in cranial nerves or in their nuclei.

CFEOM1 is probably the most common or listopathologuc. Engle et al. performed a histopathologic study and demonstrated the absence of the superior division of the third cranial nerve and the corresponding alpha motor neurons (73). The study also revealed abnormalities in the levator palpebrae superioris and the superior rectus. An increased number of internal nuclei and of central mitochondrial clumping were found in other muscles (73). Engle and colleagues (74) mapped the locus of CFEOM1 to the pericentromeric region of chromosome 12. A study of seven families refined the location to chromosome 12pl1.2–ql2 (75), and finally to

12q12 (55). CFEOM1 is an autosomal dominant disease with full penetrance and typical clinical characteristics as outlined above. Yamada and associates identified six different heterozygous mutations in 44 out of 45 probands with CFEOM type 1 disorder. The KIF21A for Kinesin family member 21A gene encodes a kinesis motor protein (76).

CFEOM2 is the locus for an autosomal recessive disease. Engle (72) claims that in CFEOM2 the fourth and sixth cranial nerves are also undeveloped, in addition to the congenital absence of the ophthalmic branch of the third nerve. Bilateral ptosis with extreme exotropia and little or no deviation are the hallmarks of this disorder. Wang and associates mapped the locus for this recessive type to chromosome 11ql3 (77). Nakano and associates (78) identified three different homozygous mutations in the ARIX gene, in four patients with autosomal recessive CFEOM2. Yazdani et al. (79) identified a novel nonsense mutation in two members of an Iranian family with autosomal recessive CFEOM2. The ARIX gene, for Aristaless homeobox, homolog of Drosophila, seems to play a critical role in the development of midbrain nuclei (78). In the mouse and in the zebrafish ARIX encodes a homeodomain transcription factor protein required for development of cranial nerves (78). The mutated gene results in CFEOM2.

CFEOM3 is an autosomal dominant disorder. Clinical characteristics are similar to type 1, but manifest more diversity in findings (80). Ptosis may be variable. External ophthalmoplegia is restrictive and in primary gaze the eyes are fixed in hypo- and exotropic position. However, expressivity varies and mild or moderate cases have much less involvement. Doherty and associates, by linkage studies, located CFEOM type 3 to chromosome 16q24.2–q24.3 (89).

Traboulsi and colleagues found heterogeneity among the autosomal recessive CFEOM, as in one Yemenite family they excluded the FEOM2 and FEOM3 locus (81).

Surgical management of all CFEOM cases is difficult and necessitates repeated surgeries (82).

Another congenital fibrosis syndrome caused by deficient innervation to extraocular muscles involves cranial nerves three to six (83). It is different from the above-mentioned three types of CFEOMs. It combines the clinical manifestation of simultaneous abduction with intorsion and depression of the eye with a jaw winking elevation of the ptotic eyelid.

Progressive Dystrophy of Extraocular Muscles

This autosomal dominant condition is also termed ocular myopathy or oculopharyngeal muscular dystrophy and is similar pathologically to other types of progressive muscular dystrophies. The onset may occur at any age, but is usually in the first two decades of life. The dystrophy affects the levator palpebrae, extraocular muscles, and muscles of mastication (84).

Progressive Ophthalmoplegia and Retinitis Pigmentosa

Retinitis pigmentosa (retinal dystrophy) demonstrates a progressive paresis of the extraocular muscles in several inherited syndromes. External ophthalmoplegia with, retinitis pigmentosa and heart block (Kearns–Sayre syndrome), is now known as one of the mitochondrial diseases characterized by ragged-red fibers. Clinically observed findings are external progressive ophthalmoplegia, cardiac conductive defects, acousticovestibular abnormalities, abnormal electroencephalogram, high levels of cerebrospinal fluid protein, retinitis pigmentosa, myopathy, neuropathy, cerebellar signs, and others (85). Four affected generations have been described (86). Progressive ophthalmoplegia may occur in Refsum's syndrome, in which retinitis pigmentosa is associated with progressive peripheral polyneuropathy, ataxia, and deafness. This disease is transmitted by the autosomal recessive mode.

Surgery by resection of muscles rather than recession may be more effective in mitochondrial associated strabismus (87).

Congenital Ophthalmoplegia, Recessive X-Unked

A congenital condition that includes partial or complete ophthalmoplegia, with bilateral ptosis, myopia, and progressive chorioretinal degeneration, has been described by Ortiz de Zarate (88). The condition is transmitted by the X-linked recessive mode affecting males.

Machado–Joseph Disease

People of Portuguese ancestry may demonstrate ataxia, dysarthria, spasticity, and external ophthalmoparesis. The condition is transmitted by the autosomal dominant mode (89). It seems to be the same disease as spinocerebellar ataxia type 3. It was mapped to chromosome 14q24.3–q31. Mutations were identified in the ATX3, the ataxin-3 gene (55).

Ataxia-Teleangiectasia

AT1 or Louis–Bar syndrome is a severe disease that involves various abnormalities in both the homozygote and the heterozygote state. In the homozygote form, ocular abnormalities are common with strabismus in 38% of patients, nystagmus 29%, apraxia of horizontal gaze 30% and poor accommodation (90). The gene for AT1 was mapped to chromosome 11q22.3 (91). Mutations in the ATM gene were identified in patients with AT1 (92). However, heterogeneity is established.

Williams Syndrome

A rare autosomal dominant condition, in which a congenital heart disease, elfin facies, and strabismus (93), are transmitted by autosomal dominant mode.

Bencze Syndrome

A rare syndrome, Bencze syndrome, consists of facial asymmetry in the form of congenital hemifacial hyperplasia with congenital esotropia. It is transmitted by the autosomal dominant mode (94,95).

Strabismus with Other Disorders

Without being an essential or recognized part of a syndrome, strabismus still occurs frequently in groups of diseases and congenital hereditary syndromes. In the craniofacial dysostoses, strabismus is frequently observed in Apert's syndrome (acrocephalo-syndactyly) of irregular autosomal dominant or autosomal recessive inheritance; the autosomal dominant Crouzon's disease or Scheuthauer–Marie–Sauton syndrome (7,12,13,32), and in Goltz syndrome, a rare ectodermal and mesodermal syndrome that has numerous abnormalities and a females predisposition. Strabismus is also common in many chromosomal aberrations. It has been described in partial chromosomal deficiencies such as 4p– (Wolf–Hirschhorn syndrome), 4r, 5p–, 13r, 18p–, 18q–, 18r, 21r, 21p– r q–, and 45 XO, and in partial duplications, balanced translocations, and trisomies (96).

Strabismus also appears commonly as a secondary phenomenon in most retinal or optic nerve diseases if they are congenital or early (infantile)-onset conditions.

REFERENCES

1. Adams F. The Genuine Works of Hippocrates vol. 1. New York: Wood, 1886:171.
2. Yazawa K, Grützner P, Spivey BE. II. Concepts of heredity of strabismus. Surv Ophthalmol 1970; 14:450–456.
3. Simpson NE, Alleslev JL. Association of children's diseases in families from record linkage data. Can J Genet Cytol 1972; 14:789–800.
4. Pratt-Johnson JA, Lunn CT. Early case finding and the hereditary factor in strabismus. Can J Ophthalmol 1967; 2:50–53.
5. Duffier JL, Briard ML, Bonaiti C, et al. Inheritance in the etiology of convergent squint. Ophthalmologica 1979; 179:225–234.
6. Chimonidou E, Palimeris G, Koliopoulas J, Velissaropolous P. Family distribution of concomitant squint in Greece. Br J Ophthalmol 1977; 61:27–29.
7. Isenberg S. Genetic aspects of strabismus. In: Emery AEH, Rimoin DL, eds. Principles and Practice of Medical Genetics. Edinburgh: Churchill-Livingstone, 1983:555–561.
8. Waardenburg PJ. Squint and heredity. Doc Ophthalmol 1954; 7:422–494.
9. Francois J. Heredity in Ophthalmology. St Louis: CV Mosby Co, 1961:239–269.
10. Maumenee IH, Alston A, Mets MB, et. al. : Inheritance of congenital esotropial. Trans Am Ophthalmol Soc 1986; 84:85–93.
11. Richter S. Untersuchungen über die Heredität des Strabismus Concomitants. VEB Leipzig: Georg Thieme, 1967.
12. Miller MT, Folk ER. Strabismus. In: Renie WA, ed. Goldberg's Genetic and Metabolic Eye Disease. 2nd ed. Boston: Little Brown & Co, 1986:257–273.
13. Cross HE. The heritability of strabismus. Am Orthopt J 1975; 25:11–17.
14. Aurell E, Norrsell K. A longitudinal study of children with a family history of strabismus: factors determining the incidence of strabismus. Br J Ophthalmol 1975; 74(10):589–594.
15. Podgor MJ, Remaley NA, Chew E. Associations between siblings for esotropia and exotropia. Arch Ophthalmol 1996; 114(6):739–744.
16. Rubin W, Helm C, McCormack MK. Ocular motor anomalies in monozygotic and dizygotic twins. In: Reinecke R, ed. Strabismus. New York: Grune & Stratton, 1978:89–95.
17. De Vries B, Houtman WA. Squint in monozygotic twins. Doc Ophthalmol 1979; 46: 305–308.
18. Bucci FA Jr, Catalano RA, Simon JW. Discordance of accommodative esotropia in monozygotic twins. Am J Ophthalmol 1989; 107:84–85.
19. Friedman Z, Newmann E, Peleg B. Screening for strabismus and amblyopia in child welfare clinics. Metab Ophthalmol 1978; 2:109.
20. Molnar L. Hereditary features of strabismus. Klin Monatsbl. Augenheilkd 1967; 150:557–668.
21. Adelstein AM, Scully J. Epidemiological aspects of squint. Br Med J 1967; 3:334–338.
22. Laatikainen L, Erkkila H. Refractive errors and other ocular findings in school children. Acta Ophthalmol 1980; 58:129–136.
23. Ing MR, Pang SWC. The racial distribution of strabismus. In: Reinecke ED, ed. Strabismus. New York: Grune & Stratton, 1978:107–109.
24. Chew E, Remaley NA, Tamboli A, Zhao J, Podgor MJ, Klebanoff M. Risk factors for esotropia and exotropia. Arch Ophthalmol 1994; 112(10):149–155.

25. Mohney BG, Erie JC, Hodge DO, Jacobsen SJ. Congenital esotropia in Olmsted County, Minnesota. Ophthalmology 1998; 105(5):846–850.
26. Mash AJ, Spivey BE. Genetic aspects of strabismus. Doc Ophthalmol 1973; 34:285–291.
27. Mash AJ, Hegmann JP, Spivey BE. Genetic analysis of cover test measures and AC/A ratio in human populations with varying indices of strabismus. Br J Ophthalmol 1975; 59:380–384.
28. Mash AJ, Hegmann JP, Spivey BE. Genetic analysis of vergence measures in populations with varying incidences of strabismus. Am J Ophthalmol 1975; 79:978–984.
29. Hegmann JP, Mash AJ, Spivey BE. Genetic analysis of human visual parameters in populations with varying incidences of strabismus. Am J Hum Genet 1974; 26:549–562.
30. Mash AJ, Hegmann JP, Spivey BE. Genetic analysis of indices of corneal power and corneal astigmatism in human populations with varying incidences of strabismus. Invest Ophthalmol 1975; 14:826–832.
31. Scott MH, Noble AG, Raymond WR 4th, Parks MM. Prevalence of primary monofixation syndrome in parents of children with congenital esotropia. J Pediatr Ophthalmol Strabismus 1994; 31(5):298–301; discussion 302.
32. Mash AJ, Grutzner P, Hegmann JP, Spivey BE. In: Goldberg MF, ed. Genetic and Meta bolic Eye Disease. Boston: Little Brown & Co, 1974:261–277.
33. Lang J. Microtropia. Int Ophthalmol 1983; 6:33–36.
34. Cantolino SJ, von Noorden GK. Heredity in microtropia. Arch Ophthalmol 1969; 81:753–757.
35. Oggel K, Rochels R. Ueber die heredität des Mikrostabismus und die Prëdisposition zum grossen Schielwinkel. Klin Monatsbl Augenheilkd 1979; 175:697–703.
36. Friendly DS, Manson RA, Albert DG. Cyclic strabismus. A case study. Doc Ophthalmol 1973; 34:189–202.
37. Keith CG. Genetics and counselling in ophthalmology. Aust J Ophthalmol 1981; 9: 74–76.
38. Francois J. Multifactorial or polygenic inheritance in ophthalmology. Dev Ophthalmol 1985; 10:1–39.
39. Grützner P, Yazawa K, Spivey BE. Heredity and strabismus-I. Surv Ophthalmol 1970; 14:441–450.
40. Paul TO, Hardage LK. The heritability of strabismus. Ophthalmic Genet 1994; 15(1): 1–18.
41. Parikh V, Shugart YY, Doheny KF Zhang J, Li L, Williams J, Hayden D, Craig B, Capo H, Chamblee D, Chen C, Collins M, Dankner S, Fiergang D, Guyton D, Hunter D, Hutcheon M, Keys M, Morrison N, Munoz M, Parks M, Plotsky D, Protzko E, Repka MX, Sarubbi M, Schnall B, Siatkowski RM, Traboulsi E, Waeltermann J, Nathans J. A strabismus susceptibility locus on chromosome 7p. Proc Natl Acad Sci USA 2003; 100(21):12283–12288.
42. Katoh M. Strabismus (STB)/Vang-like (VANGL) gene family. Int J Mol Med 2002; 10(1):11–15.
43. Katoh M. Structure and expression of Strabismus 1 gene on human chromosome 1q21-q23. Int J Oncol. 2002; 20(6):1197–1203.
44. Spivey BE. Strabismus: Factors in anticipating its occurrence. Aust J Ophthalmol 1980; 8:5–9.
45. Lorenz B. Genetics of isolated and syndromic strabismus: facts and perspectives. Strabismus 2002; 10(2):147–156.
46. Duane A. Congenital deficiency of abduction, associated with impairment of adduction, retraction movements, contraction movements, contraction of the palpebral fissure and oblique movements of the eye. Arch Ophthalmol 1905; 34:133–159.
47. Okihiro MM, Tasaki T, Nakano KK, Bennett BK. Duane syndrome and congenital upper-limb anomalies: a familial occurrence. Arch Neurol 1977; 34:174–179.
48. Rosenbaum AL, Weiss SJ. Monozygotic twins discordant for Duane's retraction syndrome. J Pediatr Ophthalmol Strabismus 1978; 15:359–361.

49. Mehdorn E, Kommerell G. Inherited Duane's syndrome. Mirror-like localization of oculomotor disturbances in monozygotic twins. J Pediatr Ophthalmol Strabismus 1979; 16:152–155.
50. Hoffman RJ. Monozygotic twins concordant for bilateral Duane's retraction syndrome. Am J Ophthalmol 1985; 99:563–566.
51. Harley RD, Rodrigues MM, Crawford JS. Congenital fibrosis of the extraocular muscles. Trans Am Ophthalmol Soc 1978; 76:197–226.
52. Isenberg S, Urist MJ. Clinical observations in 101 consecutive patients with Duane's retraction syndrome. Am J Ophthalmol 1977; 84:419–425.
53. Gowan M, Levy J. Heredity in the superior oblique tendon sheath syndrome. Br Orthop J 1968; 25:91–93.
54. Chung M, Stout JT, Borchert MS. Clinical diversity of hereditary Duane's retraction syndrome. Ophthalmology 2000; 107(3):500–503.
55. Online Mendelian Inheritance in Man, OMIM (TM). McKusick-Nathans Institute for Genetic Medicine, Johns Hopkins University (Baltimore, MD) and National Center for Biotechnology Information, National Library of Medicine (Bethesda, MD), 2000. http://www.ncbi.nlm.nih.gov/omim/.
56. Appukuttan B, Gillanders E, Juo SH, Freas-Lutz D, Ott S, Sood R, Van Auken A, Bailey-Wilson J, Wang X, Patel RJ, Robbins CM, Chung M, Annett G, Weinberg K, Borchert MS, Trent JM, Brownstein MJ, Stout JT. Localization of a gene for Duane retraction syndrome to chromosome 2q31. Am J Hum Genet. 1999; 65(6):1639–1646.
57. Al-Baradie R, Yamada K, St Hilaire C, Chan WM, Andrews C, Mclntosh N, Nakano M, Martonyi EJ, Raymond WR, Okumura S, Okihiro MM, Engle EC. Duane radial ray syndrome (Okihiro syndrome) maps to 20ql3 and results from mutations in SALL4, a new member of the SAL family. Am J Hum Genet 2002; 71(5):1195–1199.
58. Chew CK, Foster P, Hurst JA, Salmon JF. Duane's retraction syndrome associated with chromosome 4q27–31 segment deletion. Am J Ophthalmol 1995; 119(6):807–809.
59. Ott S, Borchert M, Chung M, Appukuttan B, Wang X, Weinberg K, Stout JT. Exclusion of candidate genetic loci for Duane retraction syndrome. Am J Ophthalmol. 1999; 127(3):358–360.
60. Moore AT, Walker J, Taylor D. Familial Brown's syndrome. J Pediatr Ophthalmol Strabismus 1988; 25:202–204.
61. Katz NNK, Whitmore PV, Beauchamp GR. Brown's syndrome in twins. J Pediatr Ophthalmol Strabismus 1981; 18:32–34.
62. Wortham EV, Crawford JS. Brown's syndrome in twins. Am J Ophthalmol 1988; 105:562–563.
63. Wallace DK, von Noorden GK. Clinical characteristics and surgical management of congenital absence of the superior oblique tendon. Am J Ophthalmol 1994; 118(1): 63–69.
64. Botelho PJ, Giangiacomo JG. Autosomal-dominant inheritance of congenital superior oblique palsy. Ophthalmology 1996; 103(9):1508–1511.
65. Bhola RM, Horne GV, Squirrell DM, Chan TK, Kumar D. Autosomal dominant congenital superior oblique palsy. Eye 2001; 15(Pt 4):479–484.
66. Jiang Y, Matsuo T, Fujiwara H, Hasebe S, Ohtsuki H, Yasuda T. ARDC gene polymorphisms in patients with congenital superior oblique muscle palsy. Br J Ophthalmol 2004; 88(2):263–267.
67. Laughlin RC. Congenital fibrosis of the extraocular muscles. A report of six cases. Am J Ophthalmol 1956; 41:432–438.
68. Apt L, Axelrod RN. Generalized fibrosis of the extraocular muscles. Am J Ophthalmol 1978; 85:822–829.
69. Hupp SL, Williams JP, Curran JE. Computerized tomography in the diagnosis of the congenital fibrosis syndrome. J Clin Neuro-Ophthalmol 1990; 10(2):135–139.

70. Traboulsi EL, Jaafar MD, Kattan HM, Parks MM. Congenital fibrosis of the extraocular muscles: report of 24 cases illustrating the clinical spectrum and surgical management. Am Orthop J 1993; 43:45–53.
71. Sener EC, Lee BA, Turgut B, Akarsu AN, Engle EC. A clinically variant fibrosis syndrome in a Turkish family maps to the CFEOM1 locus on chromosome 12. Arch Ophthalmol 2000; 118(8):1090–1097.
72. Engle EC. Applications of molecular genetics to the understanding of congenital ocular motility disorders. Ann NY Acad Sci 2002; 956:55–63.
73. Engle EC, Goumnerov BC, McKeown CA, Schatz M, Johns DR, Porter JD, Beggs AH. Oculomotor nerve and muscle abnormalities in congenital fibrosis of the extraocular muscles. Ann Neurol 1997; 41(3):314–325.
74. Engle EC, Kunkel LM, Specht LA, Beggs AH. Mapping a gene for congenital fibrosis of the extraocular muscles to the centromeric region of chromosome 12. Nat Genet 1994; 7(1):69–73.
75. Engle EC, Marondel I, Houtman WA, de Vries B, Loewenstein A, Lazar M, Ward DC, Kucherlapati R, Beggs AH. Congenital fibrosis of the extraocular muscles (autosomal dominant congenital external ophthalmoplegia): genetic homogeneity, Linkage refinement, and physical mapping on chromosome 12. Am J Hum Genet 1995; 57(5): 1086–1094.
76. Yamada K, Andrews C, Chan WM, McKeown CA, Magli A, de Berardinis T, Loewenstein A, Lazar M, O'Keefe M, Letson R, London A, Ruttum M, Matsumoto N, Saito N, Morris L, Del Monte M, Johnson RH, Uyama E, Houtman WA, de Vries B, Carlow TJ, Hart BL, Krawiecki N, Shoffmer J, Vogel MC, Katowitz J, Goldstein SM, Levin AV, Sener EC, Ozturk BT, Akarsu AN, Brodsky MC, Hanisch F, Cruse RP, Zubcov AA, Robb RM, Roggenkaemper P, Gottlob I, Kowal L, Battu R, Traboulsi EL, Franceschini P, Newlin A, Demer XL, Engle EC. Heterozygous mutations of the kinesin KEF21A in congenital fibrosis of the extraocular muscles type 1 (CFEOM1). Nat Genet 2003; 35(4):318–321.
77. Wang SM, Zwaan J, Mullaney PB, Jabak MH, Al-Awad A, Beggs AH, Engle EC. Congenital fibrosis of the extraocular muscles type 2, an inherited exotropic strabismus fixus, maps to distal 1lql3. Am J Hum Genet 1998; 63(2):517–525.
78. Nakano M, Yamada K, Fain J, Sener EC, Selleck CJ, Awad AH, Zwaan J, Mullaney PB, Bosley TM, Engle EC. Homozygous mutations in ARIX(PHOX2A) result in congenital fibrosis of the extraocular muscles type 2. Nat Genet 2001; 29(3):315–320.
79. Yazdani A, Chung DC, Abbaszadegan MR, Al-Khayer K, Chan WM, Yazdani M, Ghodsi K, Engle EC, Traboulsi EL. A novel PHOX2A/ARIX mutation in an Iranian family with congenital fibrosis of extraocular muscles type 2 (CFEOM2). Am J Ophthalmol 2003; 136(5):861–865.
80. Doherty EJ, Macy ME, Wang SM, Dykeman CP, Melanson MX, Engle EC. CFEOM3: a new extraocular congenital fibrosis syndrome that maps to 16q24.2–q24.3. Invest Ophthalmol Vis Sci 1999; 40(8):1687–1694.
81. Traboulsi EL, Lee BA, Mousawi A, Khamis AR, Engle EC. Evidence of genetic heterogeneity in autosomal recessive congenital fibrosis of the extraocular muscles. Am J Ophthalmol 2000; 129(5):658–662.
82. Yazdani A, Traboulsi EL. Classification and surgical management of patients with familial and sporadic forms of congenital fibrosis of the extraocular muscles. Ophthalmology 2004; lll(5):1035–1042.
83. Brodsky MC. Hereditary external ophthalmoplegia synergistic divergence, jaw winking, and oculocutaneous hypopigmentation: a congenital fibrosis syndrome caused by deficient innervation to extraocular muscles. Ophthalmology 1998; 105(4):717–725.
84. Kiloh LG, Nevin S. Progressive dystrophy of the external ocular muscles (ocular myopathy). Brain 1951; 74:115–143.
85. Drachrnann DA. Ophthalmoplegia plus; the neurodegenerative disorders associated with progressive external ophthalmoplegia. Arch Neurol 1968; 18:654–674.

86. Iannacconne ST, Griggs RC, Markesbery WR, Joynt RJ. Familial progressive external ophthalmoplegia and ragged-red fibers. Neurology 1974; 24:1033–1038.
87. Sorkin JA, Shoffner JM, Grossniklaus HE, Drack AV, Lambert SR. Strabismus and mitochondrial defects in chronic progressive external ophthalmoplegia. Am J Ophthalmol 1997; 123(2):235–242.
88. Ortiz de Zarate JC. Recessive sex-linked inheritance of congenital external ophthalmoplegia and myopia coincident with other dysplasias. Br J Ophthalmol 1966; 50:606–607.
89. Dawson DM, Feudo P, Zubick HH, et al. Electro-oculographic findings in Machado-Joseph disease. Neurology 1982; 32:1272–1276.
90. Farr AK, Shalev B, Crawford TO, Lederman HM, Winkelstein JA, Repka MX. Ocular manifestations of ataxia-telangiectasia. Am J Ophthalmol 2002; 134(6):891–896.
91. Gatti RA, Berkel I, Boder E, Braedt G, Channley P, Concannon P, Ersoy F, Foroud T, Jaspers NG, Lange K, et al. Localization of an ataxia-telangiectasia gene to chromosome llq22–23. Nature 1988; 336(6199):577–580.
92. Savitsky K, Sfez S, Tagle DA, Ziv Y, Sartiel A, Collins FS, Shiloh Y, Rotman G. The complete sequence of the coding region of the ATM gene reveals similarity to cell cycle regulators in different species. Hum Mol Genet 1995; 4(11):2025–2032.
93. Kapp ME, von Noorden GK, Jenkins R. Strabismus in Williams syndrome. Am J Ophthalmol 1995; 119(3):355–360.
94. Bencze J, Schnitzler A, Walawska J. Dominant inheritance of hemifacial hyperplasia associated with strabismus. Oral Surg 1973; 35:489–500.
95. Kurnit D, Hall JG, Shurtleff DB, Cohen MM Jr. An autosomal domiantly inherited syndrome of facial assymetry, esotropia, amblyopia and submucous left palate (Bencze syndrome). Clin Genet 1979; 16:301–304.
96. Jay M. The Eye in Chromosome Duplications and Deficiencies. New York: Marcel Dekker, 1977.

19

Ametropia

INTRODUCTION

Myopia, or nearsightedness, has been known since ancient times. It is thought that Emperor Nero of Rome used a modified concave lens to correct his myopia. Not until the early 17th century did the work of the Czech physicist Kepler establish the geometric basis for ametropia. Kepler was the first to point out that good vision depended on a clear retinal image, which was determined by incoming light being focused on the retina.

Research on ametropia started about 120 years ago with a monumental study by Donders (1). Since then it has flourished; literally hundreds of studies have been performed, and thousands of articles, reviews, and books have been published. Among the findings of this research are certain characteristics: (i) very little of the work has dealt with astigmatism, hypermetropia, or presbyopia; (ii) studies have been concerned mainly with the cause of myopia; and (iii) the relative effect of hereditary predisposition and environment on the cause of myopia is still a controversial issue.

Genetics and environment in the etiology of myopia have been a central area of research since Donders claimed that it was caused by close work (1). Results of the studies were equivocal; they could be variably interpreted, supporting opposite position. The "environmentalists" considered that refutation of their views seriously damaged efforts to prevent and eradicate myopia (2). On the other hand, the "geneticists" believed environmental factors to be unworthy of mention (3).

Studies in the last decade did not change the picture of the combination of both genetic load and near work that is responsible for myopia. In this decade several genes associated with pathologic myopia were identified. However, these are associated with familial cases that do not represent the bulk of myopia (4). The "debate of nature versus nurture," as Mutti et al. (5) expressed it, goes on. Saw et al. (6), after reviewing the literature on this subject, concluded that the two strongest risk factors to develop myopia are both family history of myopia and the occupational hazard of close-up work.

STUDIES ON ETIOLOGY OF MYOPIA

Studies concerning the cause of myopia can be subdivided into the following: the biologic components of refraction, family and twin studies, general and specific populations, myopia in animals, and the effect of myopia on ocular structures.

Results of Studies

The Biologic Components of Refraction

In 1913, Steiger (7) showed that the refractive power of an eye depends on a series of different genetically determined components, the free association of which decide the final refraction. About the same time, Straub (8) pointed out that the eye tries to overcome ametropia by a process called emmetropization, which he assumed results from changes in the refractive power of the lens. The different components of refraction and the emmetropization effect were further delineated by Tron (9), Stenström (10), and Sorsby (11). The various components of refraction included the radius or refractive power of the cornea, depth of the anterior chamber, refractive power of the lens, and axial length. The distribution in the population of each value matched the expected population curve (Gaussian curve) (3) (Fig. 1). This type of curve was indicative of a multifactorial inheritance (3,12), similar to characteristics such as height, weight, and intelligence. However, the distribution of the total spherical refractive error differed from the expected population curve by two variations: an excess of persons in the emmetropic range (the emmetropization effect) and an increase of high myopia outside the curve (Fig. 2).

The emmetropization effect appeared so powerful that Francois (12) thought it surprising how few ametropias exist, considering the total refractive power of the eye is about 60 D and a change of only 1% could cause ametropia. Although the phenomenon of emmetropization was not in dispute, little is known about its mechanism. It was suggested to be a vision–dependent phenomenon that is seriously disturbed by subnormal vision in infancy; therefore, infants with ocular diseases will develop myopia because emmetropization is absent (13). It may also be related to the resting point of accommodation (the intermediate position assumed by the lens when an appropriate stimulus for distance or near is absent), which was lowest in corrected myopes, intermediate in emmetropes, and highest in corrected hypermetropes (14).

This was later confirmed when a study showed that myopic children have insufficient accommodative response to blur (15). Gwiazda and associates claimed that the emmetropization effect is strongest in preschool children with a reduction to a much smaller effect at six years of age (16). Disruption of emmetropization occurs in certain children such as premature-born or children with Down syndrome (17). The failure in emmetropization results in more myopia or hyperopia in these children.

Family Studies

A large number of studies concerning pedigrees of families with myopia have been reported, especially in the first half of this century. Summarizing these studies, Francois (18) concluded that myopia is a heterogeneous condition. Simple benign myopia was transmitted by several autosomal dominant genes, with incomplete penetration, whereas high myopia was transmitted by autosomal recessive or autosomal dominant genes (18). Little attention was paid to findings indicating that

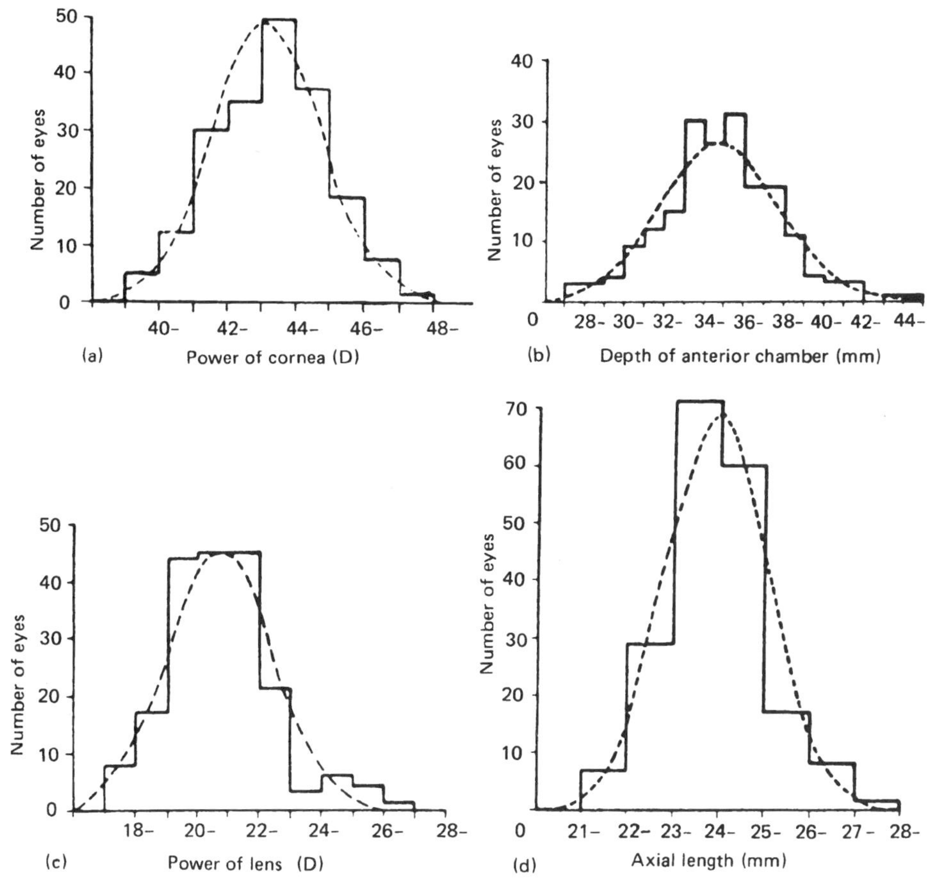

Figure 1 Distribution of various components of refraction: note that the curves of distribution of corneal refractive power, depth of anterior chamber, refractive power of lens, and axial length fit normal population curves (from Ref. 3).

mothers with high myopia had more myopic children (19), and that, in families with myopia, 35% of the siblings were affected when the parents were not, and 49% of the siblings were myopic if one or both parents were affected (20). These results obviously did not fit any known monogenic inheritance. Also, if close work played a role in the etiology of myopia, then it is possible that intrafamilial similarities in education and near work could increasingly resemble refraction and exaggerate genetic factors (21). More recent studies on intrafamilial resemblance such as sibling–sibling or offspring–parent correlation concluded that myopia is not a monogenic, but a polygenic trait, with gene dosage effect (22) and that environmental factors were important (23). Some family analyses even concluded that most variation is nongenetic in origin (24).

Pacella and associates (25) reported a 24-year longitudinal study of 43 pedigrees with juvenile-onset myopia. Children with two myopic parents were 6.42 times more likely to become myopic as children with one or no affected parents (25). Lee et al. (26), reporting on the Beaver Dam study showed a sibling correlation odds ratio (OR) of 4.18 for myopia and 2.87 for hyperopia. However, the Framingham offspring Eye Study Group discovered a large increase in the prevalence of

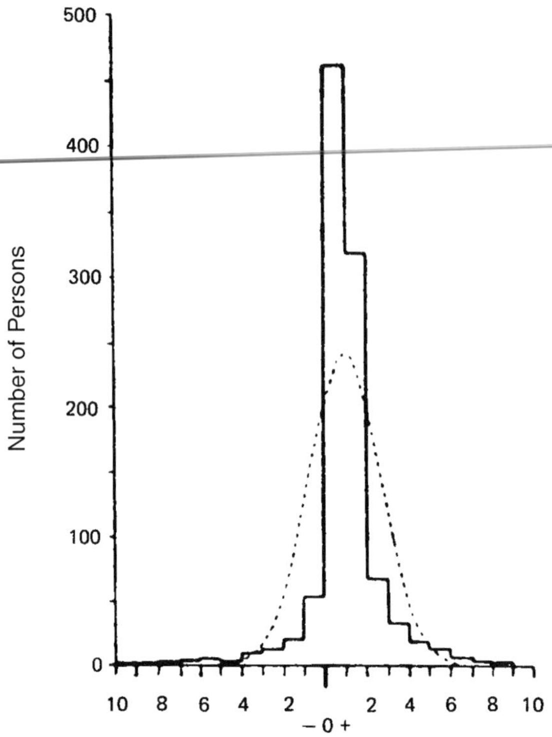

Figure 2 The emmetropization effect and the excess of high myopia. The distribution curve for the total refractive power of the eye shows an increase in its center over the expected calculation from the normal population, and shows more high myopes (from Ref. 3).

myopia in more recent-birth cohorts ranging from 60% myopia at the age of 23 to 20% myopia at the age of 65, and decrease in strength of between-siblings association for myopia (27). The results of the Framingham study demonstrate an important and increasing role for monitoring environmental factors.

An unusual incident occurred with the study of ambient light, the dim light which parents leave at night near the bed of their offspring. Quinn et al. (28) studied 479 children aged 2–16 years and found a strong association between the use of night-time ambient light and myopia. Nine percent of children sleeping in darkness, 31% of children sleeping with ambient light and 48% of children sleeping with room light, had myopia (28). However, Gwiazda et al. (29) did not find a difference in the prevalence of myopia between the groups in their study, Zadnik et al. (30) found an association between parents being myopic and the use of ambient light in children under the age of two years. This would confirm the view that myopic parents tend to use more night-light and a higher prevalence of myopia in their offspring is related to their genetic predisposition to myopia (30).

Twin Studies

The results of reported twin studies consistently proved a hereditary background in the etiology of ametropia. The concordance rate for monozygotic (M2) twins was far higher than for dizygotic (DZ) twins. After studying 78 MZ twins, 40 DZ twins, and

48 unrelated subjects, Sorsby (31) concluded that refraction, emmetropia, the various ametropias, and the separate components of refraction, such as axial length and refractive power of the cornea, were genetically determined individually.

In a study that was based on 742 pairs of Norwegian twins, Nance et al. (32) found a heritability factor of 0.92 for myopia, 0.82 for hyperopia, and 0.62 for astigmatism. In the same study, the segregation rates for half-sibs, however, were substantially lower than the expected minimum of half for full-sibs, supporting the theory of multifactorial inheritance. A similar investigation of a large group of Chinese twins detected both a significant genetic influence and environmental impact of studying and reading (33). Results were similar when the methods of twin research were changed, that is, using only MZ twins as a study group, but comparing those who lived apart with those who lived together (34).

Teikari et al. (35) studied 109 same-sex age 30–31 years, 54 MZ and 55 DZ twins. The mean difference in refraction between MZ twins was 1.17 and 2.4 D between DZ twins (35). Hammond et al. (36) found a heritability of 84–86% both for myopia and hyperopia. These and other studies stressed the important role of heritability of myopia and hyperopia. However, astigmatism showed a persistently lower heritability ratio (36–38).

General Population Studies

Statistics on general populations were the preferred methods of investigation, according to a number of published studies. Performed in many countries in the world on diverse populations such as schoolchildren, whole villages and settlements, and total areas or conscripts, the studies attempted to test the influence of ethnic background, occupation, sex, working habits, and many other features on the frequency of myopia.

As early as 1883, Tscherning (39) studied the refraction of conscripts in Denmark, and found a frequency of 8.33% of myopia over–2.00 D. About 100 years later, Goldschmidt (40) evaluated a similar population of Danish conscripts and demonstrated an amazingly similar 9.2% for myopia of over –1.50 D. Tscherning also found large differences in myopia according to education and occupation. The highest figures occurred in scholars and university graduates (more than 32%), which was about 10 times as high as in unskilled workers. He concluded that three types of myopia exist: (i) incidental, or mild myopia in a normal eye; (ii) functional, resulting from close work; and (iii) pathologic or high myopia, similar in frequency in all populations and not influenced by close work. Goldschmidt (40) confirmed these studies as well. He found a similar difference in frequency of myopia between educated and less-educated schoolchildren and agreed with the importance of environmental influence, in addition to decisive genetic factors. Goldschmidt also postulated three types of myopia: (i) low myopia, which is genetically determined and polymeric In transmission; (ii) high myopia, a heterogeneous group with monomeric or polymeric transmission, a possible environmental influence, and a propensity for females; and (iii) late myopia (spatmyopie), which is environmental in nature and has an onset in late teens and later.

Guggenheim et al. (41) re-analyzed the data of Goldschmidt (40), and found compelling evidence that both environmental and genetic factors are involved in the etiology of myopia. However, they stressed the differences between mild and moderate myopia with lower heritability rates and high myopia with higher heritability rates. Prevalence of myopia in Europe and the United States is usually estimated as 10–25% and that of high myopia, as 0.5–2.5%. For high myopia, monogenic inheritance is not uncommon; in the study, nine of 36 high myopia families had evidence of autosomal dominant transmission (41).

In Finland, all schoolchildren are routinely screened. The frequency of myopia of 0.50 D or more was 22–23% at the age of 15, and the frequency of hyperopia of 2.0 D or more was 3.6% (42,43). Far more girls than boys were myopic at schoolage (44), but this probably represented the earlier development of girls compared with boys (Fig. 3). During the school years, there was a shift toward myopia in the whole curve of refractive powers (Fig. 4).

In west Greenland, Alsbirk examined Eskimos and found both genetic and environmental factors important in the development of myopia. The heritability

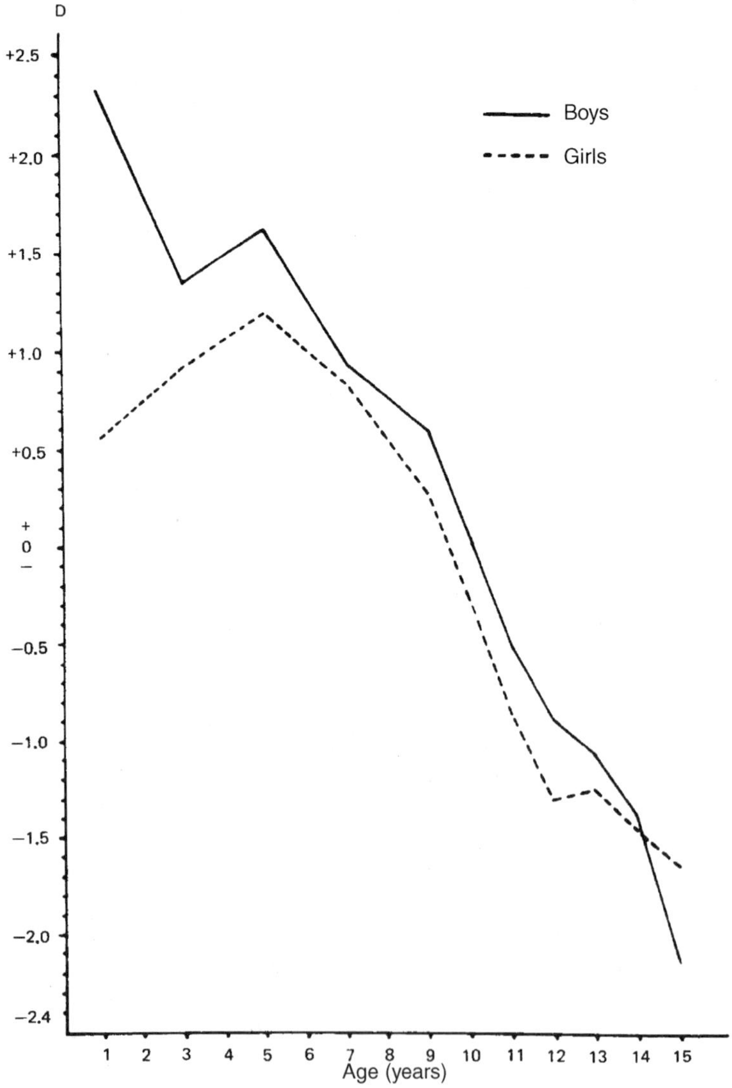

Figure 3 The increase in onset of myopia in boys and girls: at age 15 years, the mean refraction equalizes (from Ref. 44).

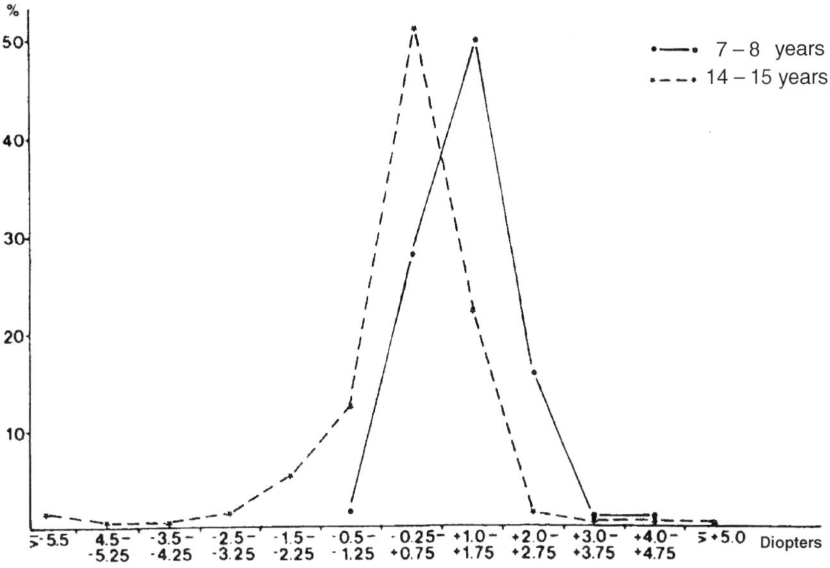

Figure 4 The spherical equivalents of the refractive power in two groups of schoolchildren. With advancing age, the population curve shifts to the left (toward myopia) and an additional "tail" (extension toward high myopia) appears (from Ref. 42).

factor was high for axial length, corneal curvature, and anterior chamber depth, and low for total refractive error (45,46). This result suggested that the emmetropization effect depends on environmental factors.

Richler and Bear found much less myopia in the older uneducated population in Newfoundland (47,48) (Fig. 5), similar to results from four other studies done in Alaska, Ontario, United States, and Greenland (48) (Fig. 6). The authors concluded that close work in childhood contributes to the incidence of clinical myopia.

In Iceland, low and moderate myopia increased between 1935 and 1975 from 3.6% to 20.5% in the 10–25 year aged group (49). There was no similar increase in hypermetropia in the same period.

In the United States, the incidence of myopia was 26.3% in whites and 13.0% in blacks (50). It was lower in the 52–85-year age group (17.7%; Framingham study; 51), and higher in the 12–17-year aged group, with 25% in blacks and 32.7% in whites (52). All of these findings implied that more education increased the frequency of myopia. A study of prevalence and risk factors of myopia, hyperopia, astigmatism and anisometropia in a mixed population in the inner city of Baltimore, came to similar conclusions. Myopia has become more prevalent over the years. Its incidence parallels increasing years of personal education (53).

In Israel, the incidence was 18.4% for myopia, 57.1 % for emmetropia, and 24.5% for hypermetropia in subjects 40 years or older living in settlements of the Jezreel Valley (54). All subjects were literate, Jewish, and on average read a lot, facts that question the accuracy of the theory that Jews have an exceptionally high incidence of myopia (55).

A high prevalence of myopia was found in Japanese, Chinese, and Egyptian populations; it involved more than half the total population (54,55). A low incidence was noted in Africans (56) and in Australian aborigines (57) (Fig. 7). Melanesian

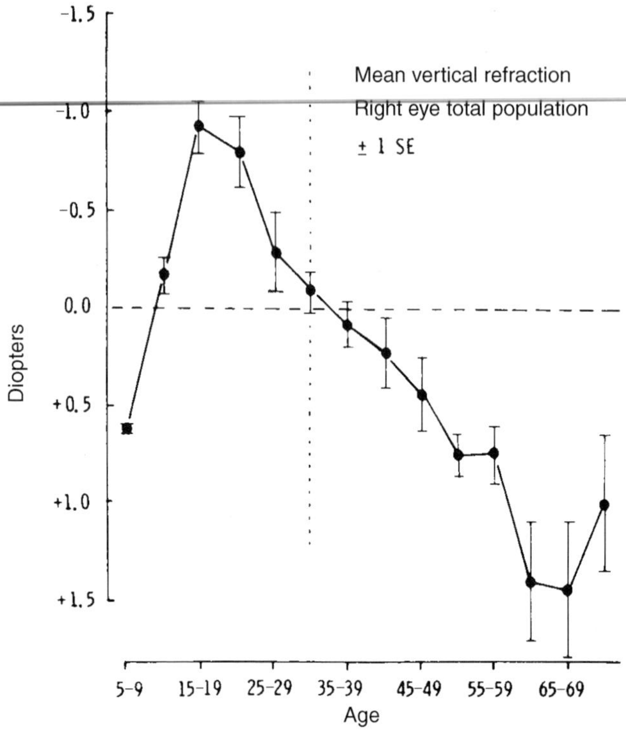

Figure 5 Refraction (mean and standard error) for different aged groups of the total population studied in western Newfoundland: myopia was more common and higher in the younger who were more educated (from Ref. 48).

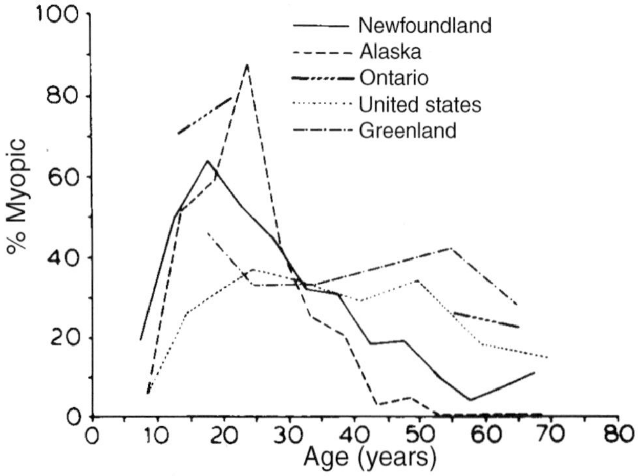

Figure 6 Percentage of myopic persons in different age groups, compiled from five studies: Note the difference in the incidence of myopia between old and young, especially in Alaska. (from Ref. 48).

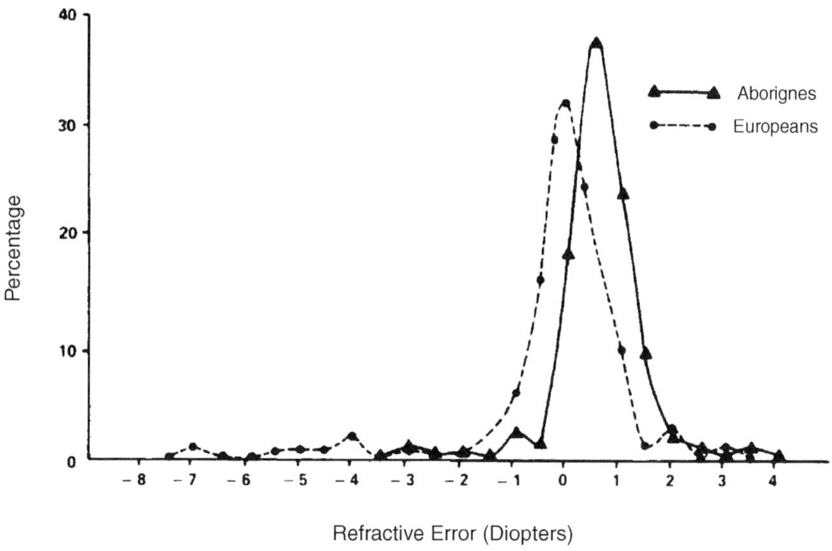

Figure 7 The spherical refractive error of Australian Aborigines and Europeans, presented as percentages. The Aborigines have less myopia, no high myopia, more emmetropization effect and more hypermetropia (from Ref. 57).

children had a very low prevalence of myopia in spite of normal educational features (58), indicating the importance of genetic factors.

In many population studies, myopia was related to other variables. Its prevalence was higher in females than in males, in whites than in blacks, and in families on the higher ends of the income, social status, and advanced education ladders (50,52,55). On the average, myopic children were taller and heavier, had a somewhat higher IQ, and better mean school ability than nonmyopic children (40,44,55,59,60). Although these facts have not been earnestly disputed, their interpretation has been. Both a genetic background and environmental influences can be argued.

Specific Population Studies

Several studies performed on specific populations have shown increased myopia during the follow–up period. Joffe (61) studied a group of textile workers and found that the incidence of myopia increased from 17.9% after four years to 37.6% after nine years, to 68.1% thereafter. Dunphy et al. (62) noted a continuously increasing incidence of myopia among students at Harvard Business School and Harvard Law School, sometimes as much as –0.75 D/year. The smallest annual increase in myopia occurred in the third decade of life in pilots (0.05 D/year) (63); the highest recorded increase of 80% was found among Jewish theological students in Jerusalem who devote almost all of their time to reading (64).

A study of the influence of near work on development of myopia among Norwegian engineering students (65) demonstrated a significant relationship between refractive change toward increasing myopia and time spend in reading or in practical near work or time spend in lectures. No relationship was found with watching TV or watching video–displays (65). There was no obvious trend of worsening of "academic myopia" among Danish medical students in whom rate of myopia remained stable at 50% during their studies (66). In contrast, in Taiwan, Singapore and Hong Kong, myopia among medical students significantly increased in the last decade both by rate and by degree of myopia (66),(67). Myopia prevalence rate at admission reached a surprising high of 92.8%, and continued to increase, to 95.8% after five years of medical studies (67). These results reflect the results of other university students in Singapore (68).

Animal Models and Their Human Counterparts

Many animals have natural myopia. Domestic animals, such as horses, have a high prevalence of myopia, that, however has not advanced our knowledge of human myopia. A serious search for an experimental model of myopia in animals started in the early 1960s. Impressed by the effect of close work on the production of myopia in children, Young tried to produce a similar effect in young monkeys. The monkeys were confined in a space, so that their distance vision was restricted to < 20 in. and they were forced to use their near vision (69). These animals developed myopia, however, it was highly variable; myopia of −0.50 D or more (mean, −1.75 D) developed in 86%. The rest had no myopia. More females than male monkeys developed myopia (69).

Young chickens, tree shrews, and kittens have also been as models for experimental myopia. Normally developing chicks showed a progressive decrease in the variability of refractive power and a decline in hypermetropia during the first eight weeks of life (70), reminiscent of human emmetropization (Fig. 8). Monocular or binocular lid closure in the neonatal chick produced myopia by increasing the axial length of the eye (71).

The results of lid suture experiments in cats were conflicting. Some experiments resulted in increased axial length and myopia, but only a small degree of myopia or no effect was achieved in others (72). *Experimental anisometropia* was produced by using negative lenses of −10.0 or more diopters before one eye of a developing kitten to cause blurred vision. The eye with the negative lens developed axial myopia by 12 weeks of life (73). Lid suture myopia produced in tree shrews was prevented by daily administration of atropine (74).

The most consistent and reliable model of experimental myopia was developed by Wiesel and Raviola (75–79). Since 1977, the investigators showed in repeated experiments that lid suturing in monkeys for a limited period during the first year of life causes axial myopia (76). It was produced in both *Macaca mulatto* (rhesus monkey) and in *M. arctoides* (stump–tailed monkey), but could not be repeated in mature monkeys. The myopia was unilateral when one eye was sutured, bilateral when both eyes were sutured, and occurred in every case (76). The myopia was always axial, showing enlargement of the whole posterior segment of the occluded eye (Fig. 9). Myopia did not develop if the monkeys were reared in darkness, suggesting that visual stimulation in the form of blurred vision through translucent lids was necessary for the development of experimental myopia (77). Visual blur caused by an experimentally cloudy cornea produced a similar myopia (78). Raviola and Wiesel (79) used this latter model to assess the pathogenetic factors producing myopia. After they removed the striate and substriate cortex, they found that the myopia continued to develop, even without the visual cortex. Also, the removal of the superior cervical ganglion or a section of the trigeminal nerve had no effect on the experimental myopia.

Surprisingly, some experiments had a different effect in each of the two monkey species. In stump-tailed monkeys, the myopia could be prevented by

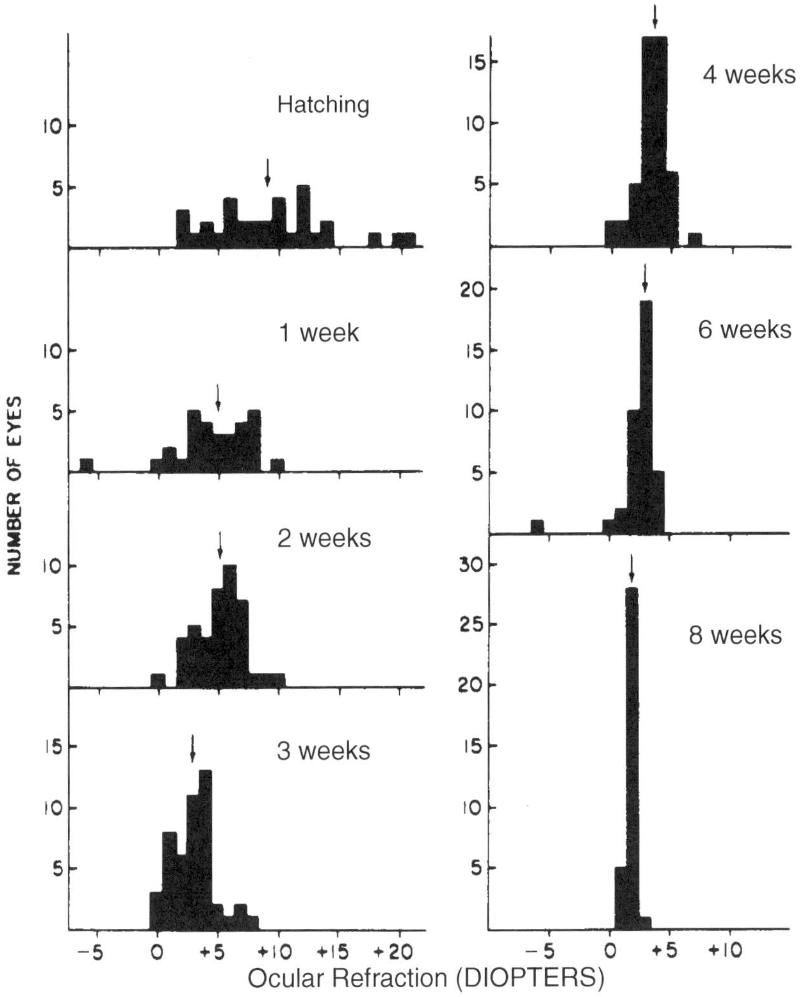

Figure 8 The refractive error in chickens in the first 8 weeks of life: arrows indicate medians. Note emmetropization effect (from Ref. 70).

sectioning the optic nerve at the chiasm or by preventing accommodation with atropine eyedrops or by removing the ciliary ganglion. In rhesus monkeys, sectioning the optic nerve, using atropine, or removing the ciliary ganglion had no effect on the experimental myopia (79).

Similar myopia-producing eyelid closure and visual deprivation was documented in humans. Large hemangiomas involving the eyelids caused myopia (of 7.0 D or more) and high astigmatism on the affected side (80). Also, eyelid closure by unilateral or bilateral ptosis increased myopia in affected eyes by an average of –2.75 D (81). Other causes of prolonged eyelid occlusion such as third nerve palsy, plexiform neuroma, or birth trauma, also caused unilateral myopia of –4.25 to –7.00 D (82). As in experimental lid suture myopia, this myopia was of axial origin, not affecting keratometric measurements (82). Axial myopia also occurred in infants with visual deprivation from diverse conditions such as retrolental fibroplasia, persistent pupillary membrane, cloudy vitreous, cataract, trauma (13), and monocular cataract in one of

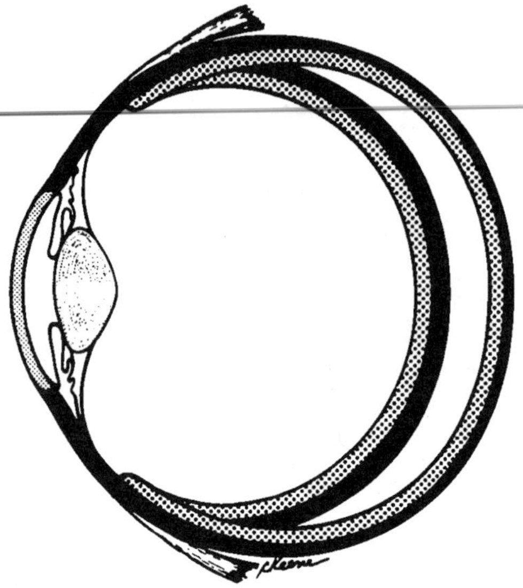

Figure 9 The effect of lid fusion on one eye of *Macaca mulatto* monkey. The myopic eye is superimposed on the open eye. Note the enlargement of the posterior segment in experimental myopia (from Ref. 79).

four eyes of two monozygotic twins (83). Although the other three eyes had a similar refraction of +0.50, the one deprived eye had myopic astigmatism and was longer by 2 mm (83). Focus-induced changes, such as those associated with a blur, cause changes in ocular growth and refraction, similar to those of other forms of deprivation (84).

Visual deprivation is an environmental influence that may contribute to myopia. However, this does not rule out genetic participation as an additional factor. Several studies have been performed on animals with experimental myopia. The studies detected the expression in the retina of genes and proteins that may be mediators in the process of myopia formation. McKenzie et al. (85) demonstrated that deprivation of form vision by the fitting of translucent occluders suppressed the diurnal cycling of enkephalinergic amacrine cells in the chicken. Fischer et al. (86) showed two genes that may be associated with developing myopia. Experimenting with chickens deprived of good vision by plus or minus lenses, they detected a gene ZENG (Zif 268, Egr-1) in glucagon-containing amacrine cells that synthesizes a protein that suppresses ocular elongation.

The synthesis of the protein is suppressed under conditions that enhance ocular elongation, such as minus defocus or form deprivation. Its synthesis is increased by plus defocus or by termination of form deprivation. Synthesis of another protein associated with ocular elongation, Fos, was also enhanced by termination of form deprivation. These authors concluded that glucagon-containing amacrine cells may mediate lens-induced changes in ocular growth and refraction (86). Morgan et al. (87) found that levels of alphaB-crystallin mRNA in the retina of form-deprived chicken eyes were increased compared to controls and were reduced to below normal after removal of the diffusers.

Attempts to prevent experimental myopia by medications were performed. Chronic administration of the muscarinic antagonist, atropine, prevents experimental form-deprivation-induced myopia in the chicken, by a nonaccommodative mechanisms (88).

Myopia and Other Ocular Changes

The vast majority of patients with myopia can have good visual acuity by correction with negative lenses. Vision is rarely decreased in young children from macular disease or retinal detachment. In high myopia, vision is usually well preserved until after 50–60 years, when posterior pole changes may cause decreased visual acuity (89). A significant correlation of myopic fund us changes, such as peripapillary crescent formation, chorioretinal atrophy, and posterior staphyloma with increased axial length of the eye, suggests a biomechanical, not a genetic effect (90). On the contrary, peripheral retinal degenerative changes may be genetically determined. In a study of unilateral high myopic patients, Zauberman and Merin (91) found a significantly high prevalence of peripheral retinal "myopic" degenerative changes in the nonmyopic or less myopic eye.

Loci and Genes for Isolated (Nonsyndromic) Myopia. Several loci associated with myopia have been detected in the recent years. Most were autosomal dominant and in all cases they were associated with high or pathologic myopia. Table 1 lists the currently known loci for isolated familial high myopia.

Schwartz, et al. (92) described in 1988 and in 1990 a family with X-linked high myopia, which became known as Bornholm Eye Disease (BED). The clinical phenotype was of males affected by high myopia (median of –8.50 D and range of 0–11.50), mild astigmatism, RPE atrophy, hypoplasia of optic disc in some, subnormal ERG and deuteranopia. The study indicated a location on chromosome Xq28 (92). The locus was later named MYP1. Young et al. (93) described in 1994 a second family with BED. The family, from Minnesota (United States.), showed similar clinical findings to the family from Bomholm (Denmark), including high myopia, optic nerve hypoplasia and reduced ERG flicker. However, instead of deuteranopia, the affected males suffered from protanopia and the astigmatism rate was higher.

In 1998, Young et al. (94) reported the first locus for autosomal dominant high myopia, which was later named MYP2. Seven of eight families manifested linkage of the myopia to the locus on chromosome 18pl1.31. The average myopia was –9.48.

Table 1 Loci for High Myopia

Locus	Synonyms	Genetic transmission	Chromosomal location	Remarks
MYP1	Bornholm eye disease	XL	Xq28	Myopia: mean–8.50; mild cone deficiency, deuteranopia or protanopia
MYP2	High myopia	AD	18p11.31	Mean myopia: –9.48; (seven families)
MYP3	High myopia	AD	12q21-q23	Mean myopia: –9.47; (one family)
MYP4	High myopia	AD	7q36	French families
MYP5	High myopia	AD	17q21-q23	One English-Canadian family

XL, X-chromosome linked; AD-automsomal dominant

In the same year, Young et al. (95) described the second locus for AD-high myopia, MYP3, and mapped it to chromosome 12q21–q23. Mean myopia was –9.47 and range was –6.25 to –15.00. The eyes were large with an axial length of 30.06 ± 0.54 (95).

Naiglin et al. (96) studied 23 French and Algerian families with bilateral nonsyndromic high myopia. They reported in 2002 that in one family the transmission was by the autosomal recessive mode, and in the rest by autosomal dominant mode. They mapped a novel locus for familial autosomal dominant myopia to chromosome 7q36 (96).

In 2003, Paluru et al. (97) reported a novel locus for AD severe high myopia located at chromosome 17q, in one English-Canadian family.

None of the genes have yet been identified. Young et al. recommended laminin gene as the candidate gene for MYP2 (94) and decorin gene or lumican gene as the candidate gene for MYP3 (95).

Conclusions From Studies

An analysis of the studies related to the etiology of myopia indicates evidence for both a genetic background and environmental influence.

The evidence for genetic factors appears to be (i) high heritability factor detected in twin studies; (ii) high–heritability factor detected in familial studies comparing similarities of each parent–offspring midparent–offspring, and sib–sib; and (iii) ethnic differences with extreme variations in prevalence of myopia.

The evidence for environmental influence is as follows: (i) much higher prevalence of myopia among educated than uneducated workers; (ii) increased prevalence of myopia in the same population with better education and more close work; (iii) an increasing incidence of myopia, even after age 20 years, in specific groups performing much close work; and (iv) the rapid increase in rate of myopia in Singapore and Taiwan in the last two decades. This increase involves people of Chinese, Malay, and Indian origin, but Malays and Indians have a much higher rate of myopia in Singapore than in other countries (98).

The emmetropization effect is the main factor in reducing the genetically determined myopia, and environmental factors may be able to reduce this effect.

The emmetropization effect may have a genetic component in the process of its modification of the refraction. Animal experiments imply that putable proteins expressed in the retinal amacrine cells may have both enhancing and arresting influence on the axial length of the eyeglobe. This "homeostasis effect" seems to be controlled by the same factors that increase or slow down the normal increase of the eyeglobe.

If myopia is both genetically and environmentally influenced, then it is logical that the etiology of myopia and other ametropias is multifactorial, at least in most cases. This theory is based on the following:

1. Each component of refraction in the population fits a typical Gauss curve, as would be expected in multifactorial transmission.
2. The incidence of refractive errors fits a Gauss curve, except for the emmetropization effect, and "the tail" on the high myopic side. The first aspect may indicate additional unknown and probably environmental factors. The latter suggests additional, nonmultifactorial types of high myopia, probably monomeric.

3. Mothers with higher degrees of myopia have more high myopic children.
4. Intrafamilial coefficients of correlation indicate polygenic inheritance of emmetropia and low and moderate ametropias (99).
5. Segregation rates for half–sibs, when compared with full–sibs, fit a multifactorial inheritance (32).

Multifactorial transmission means polygenic inheritance, with several genes of additive action for each component of refraction and environmental impact, in the form of near work or visual deprivation at a young age.

Exceptions to the polygenic and multifactorial inheritance exist. Monogenic inheritance of myopia was described only for high myopia, transmitted in families with the autosomal dominant or with the X-linked mode of transmission. In addition, some pedigrees of families with high myopia or high hyperopia point to a possible autosomal recessive (96,99) or autosomal dominant (12,41,99) trait. Several loci for autosomal dominant high myopia and one locus for X-linked high myopia are known (see Table 1). Common juvenile myopia is likely not associated with these genes (4).

It is not clear whether "late myopia," a condition occurring between late teens and the third decade of life as a result of close work (40,100) actually exists as a separate entity. There appears to be much evidence to the contrary.

The genetic or environmental mechanisms by which myopia is produced are not clear. The main factors in the pathogenesis of myopia have been suggested as increased intraocular pressure, increased accommodation, excessive convergence with pressure of the extraocular muscles on the eye, abnormal control of the autonomic nervous system, and central or peripheral visual stimulation (101). It is possible, as explained above, that a homeostasis mechanism, becomes defective in ametropias.

Animal models have advanced our knowledge of these mechanisms, but they deal with only one type of myopia, axial myopia. Different mechanisms cause this type of myopia in two species of monkeys (79). Two separate mechanisms might indicate different genetic backgrounds that respond to the same external stimulus by producing myopia. Possibly, each represents a loss of the emmetropization abilities of a normal eye.

MYOPIA IN SYNDROMES AND OTHER OCULAR DISEASES

Associated myopia refers to myopia in association with a syndrome or another ocular disease, such as is found in several monogenic diseases (Table 2). In all cases the myopia is high. The associated disease can be classified as one of three: connective tissue disease such as Ehlers-Danles syndrome, multisystem diseases such as myopia, intellectual impairment and deafness and associated ocular disaease such as achromatop or blidness. Table 2 lists associated myopia. Some cases have been reported in only one or a few families, but others such as Stickler disease, or congenital nyctalopia with high myopia are not uncommon.

Myopia may result from a disorder affecting the crystalline lens, as in Alport syndrome or in ectopia Lentis (see Chapter. 7), or secondary to eye globe distension, as in congenital glaucoma. Myopia frequently occurs in chromosomal disorders, such as trisomy 17, 21, and 22, and in Turner's (XO) syndrome (118). In some connective tissue diseases, myopia may be lens-induced or a true myopia caused by

Table 2 Associated Myopia

No.	Eponym	Myopia	Ref	Inheritance
1.	Ehlers-Danlos syndrome	High	102	AD
2.	Stickler disease (hereditary progressive arthroophthalmopathy)	High	103	AD
3.	Dysplasia spondyloepiphysaria congenita	High and progressive	104	AD
4.	Myopia, multiple epiphyseal dysplasia and deafness	High	105	AD
5.	Myopia, intellectual impairment and deafness	High	106	AR
6.	Myopia, epiphyseal dysplasia and deafness	High	107	AR
7.	Microcornea and myopia	High	108, 109	AD
8.	Congenital external ophthalmoplegia and myopia	High	110	XL
9.	Congenital nyctalopia with high myopia, sex-linked	High	111, 112	XL
10.	Congenital nyctalopia with high myopia, autosomal recessive	High	112, 113	AR
11.	Congenital X-linked achromatopsia with myopia	High	114, 115	XL
12.	Congenital achromatopsia with myopia (Pingelapese disease)	High	116	AR
13.	Infantile myopia with hypoplasia of optic nerve head	Variable	117	XL

AD, autosomal dominant; AR, autosomal recessive; XL, X-linked recessive.

increased axial length, including Marfan syndrome and homocystinuria. A higher incidence of myopia in open-angle glaucoma has been described (119), but not confirmed. It was suggested that high myopes, white but not black, have low serum concentrations and low urinary excretion of copper (120), but these studies also have not been confirmed.

High myopia was also described in Marfan syndrome, in Stickler syndrome of type I and type II, in other vitreoretinopathies and in Åland Island disease. These disorders and the others listed in Table 2 are discussed in detail in their proper chapters.

MANAGEMENT AND GENETIC COUNSELING

Attempts, other than corrective lenses, to prevent and treat myopia started in the 19th century, when a "proper ocular hygiene" was advised for children to prevent increases in myopia. This regimen included restricted reading time, proper close work distance, and good light. No long-term study was ever conducted to evaluate this approach.

The major techniques used to prevent, treat, or check the degree of myopia in the 20th century, besides prescribing glasses, have included surgery for reinforcement of the sclera, short-acting and long-acting cycloplegics to reduce accommodation effort, and the use of hard contact lenses (118). Short-acting cycloplegics have been ineffective (118), and the effectiveness of cycloplegics alone (121) or in use with bifocals (122) has not been confirmed in long-term prospective studies. Similarly, no long-term evaluations have confirmed the efficacy of contact lenses or consistent undercorrection with glasses. However, clinical trials continue with both the use of cycloplegics and corrective glasses. Atropine has been used with possible effective slowdown of the growth of myopia (123). However, atropine has many side effects and more selective muscarinic antagonists, such as pirenzepine, are being investigated (123).

A randomized trial of rigid gas permeable contact lenses was performed for two years in 428 Singaporean children (124). The children were 6–12 years old and had myopia of –1.0 to –4.0 D with a small astigmatism. After two years, 78% remained in follow up. The contact lenses did not slow down the rate of myopia progression (124).

Some investigators believe that the studies point to no clear advantage of any treatment to reliably slow down or prevent myopia development (125). However, two large recent studies, on the use of progressive lenses in children 9–12 years old in Hong Kong (126) and 6–11 years old in the United States (127), indicated a slowdown of the progression of myopia after a period of two years.

The risk of myopia or ametropia should never prevent the birth of any child. The ophthalmologist, however, is confronted with frequent questions about the inheritance of ametropias. For most, the family's history and ethnic and educational background should be studied. In rare cases, monomeric inheritance will be found, mainly the autosomal recessive or autosomal dominant transmission of high ametropias. In others, associated myopia may be detected.

In the majority, however the transmission is multifactorial, polygenic, and environmental. Risks are different in different families. Such facts as the presence or absence of myopia in the parents, their degree of ametropia, and mentioned environmental features are important. The risk of myopia is greater when both parents have high degrees of myopia than if one parent is myopic and the other is hypermetropic.

REFERENCES

1. Donders FC. On the Anomalies of Accomodation and Refraction of the Eye. London: New Sydeuham Society, 1864.
2. Cohn H. Lehrbuch der Hygiene des Auges. Wien und Leipzig, 1892. English translation. In: Turnbull WP, ed. The Hygiene of the Eye in Schools. London: Simpkin Marshall, 1886.
3. Sorsby A. Epidemiology of refraction. In: Safir A, ed. Refraction. International Ophthalmology Clinics. Vol .II. Boston: Little, Brown & Co., 1971:1–18.
4. Mutti DO, Semina E, Marazita M, Cooper M, Murray JC, Zadnik K. Genetic loci for pathological myopia are not associated with juvenile myopia. Am J Med Genet 2002; 112(4):355–360.
5. Mutti DO, Zadnik K, Adams AJ. Myopia. The nature versus nurture debate goes on. Invest Ophthalmol Vis Sci 1996; 37(6):952–957.
6. Saw SM, Katz J, Schein OD, Chew SJ, Chan TK. Epidemiology of myopia. Epidemiologic Reviews 1996; 18(2):175–87.
7. Steiger A. Die entstehung des sphärischen refraktionen des mensehlichen Auges. Berlin: S Karger, 1913.

8. Straub M. Ueber die Aetiologie der Brechungsanomalien des Auges und der Ursprung der Emmetropie. Albrecht Von Graefes Arch Ophthalmol 1909; 70:130–199.
9. Tron E. Ueber die optischen Grundlagen der Ametropie. Albrecht Von Graefes Arch Ophthalmol 1934; 132:182–223.
10. Stenström S. Untersuchungen ueber die variation und Ko-variation der optischen Elemente des mensehlichen Auges. Acta Ophthalmol 1946; Suppl 26.
11. Sorsby A, Benjamin D, Davey JB, et al. Emmetropia and its Aberrations. Spec Rep Ser Med Res Counc No 293. London: HMSO, 1957.
12. Francois J. Multifactorial or polygenic inheritance in ophthalmology. Dev Ophthalmol 1985; 10:1–39.
13. Rabin J, Van Sluyters RC, Maiach R. Emmetropization: a vision–dependent phenomenon. Invest Ophthalmol Vis Sci 1981; 20:561–569.
14. Maddock RJ, Miilodot M, Leat S, Johnson CA. Accommodation responses and refractive error. Invest Ophthal Vis Sci 1981; 20:387–391.
15. Gwiazda J, Bauer J, Thorn F, Held R. Myopic children show insufficient accommodative response to blur. Invest Opthalmol Vis Sci 1993; 34(3):690–694.
16. Gwiazda J, Bauer J, Thorn F, Held R. A dynamic relationship between myopia and blur-driven accomodation in school-aged children. Vision Res 1995; 35(9):1299–1304.
17. Gwiazda J, Thorn F. Development of refraction and strabismus. Current Opinion in Ophthalmology 1999; 10(5):293–299.
18. Francois J. L'heredite de la myopie. Ann Ocul, 1973; 206:477–485.
19. Paul L. Untersuchungen über die erbliche Entstehung der Kurzsichtigkeit. Albrecht Von Graefes Arch Ophthalmol 1938; 139:378–402.
20. Wold KC. Hereditary myopia. Arch Ophthalmol, 1949; 42:225–237.
21. Bear JC, Richler A. Environmental influences on ocular refraction [Letter]. Am J Epidemiol 1982; 115:138–139.
22. Basu SK, Jindal A. Genetic aspects of myopia among the Shia Muslim Dawoodi Bohras of Udaipur Rajasthan. Hum Hered 1983; 33:163–169.
23. Bear JC, Richler A, Burke G. Near–work familial resemblances in ocular refraction: a population study in Newfoundland. Clin Genet 1981; 19:462–472.
24. Ashton GC. Segregation analysis of ocular refraction and myopia. Hum Hered 1985; 35:232–239.
25. Pacella R, McLellan J, Grice K, Del Bono EA, Wiggs JL, Gwiazda JE. Role of genetic factors in the etiology of juvenile-onset myopia based on a longitudinal study of refractive error. Optometry & Vis Sci 1999; 76(6):381–386.
26. Lee KE, Klein BE, Klein R, Fine JP. Aggregation of refractive error and 5-year changes in refractive error among families in the Beaver Dam Eye Study. Arch Ophthalmol 2001; 119(11):1679–1685.
27. Anonymous. Familial aggregation and prevalence of myopia in the Framingham Offspring Eye Study. The Framingham Offspring Eye Study Group. Archives of Ophthalmology. 1996; 114(3):326–332.
28. Quinn GE, Shin CH, Maguire MG, Stone RA. Myopia and ambient lighting at night. Nature 1999; 399(6732):113–114.
29. Gwiazda J, Ong E, Held R, Thron F. Myopia and ambient night-time lighting. Nature 2000; 404(6774):144.
30. Zadnik K, Jones LA, Irvin BC, Kleinstein RN, Manny RE, Shin JA, Mutti DO. Myopia and ambient night–time lighting. CLEERE Study Group. Collaborative Longitudinal Evaluation of Ethnicity and Refractive Error. Nature 2000; 404(6774):143–144.
31. Sorsby A, Leary GA, Fraser GR. Family studies on ocular refraction and its components. J Med Genet 1966; 3:269–273.
32. Nance WE, Corey LA, Boughman JA, et al. Distribution of common eye disease in the families of Norwegian twins. Birth Defects 1982; 18:669–678.
33. Chen CJ, Cohen BH, Diamond EL. Genetic and environmental effects on the development of myopia in Chinese twin children. Ophthalmic Paediatr Genet 1985; 6:353–359.

34. Gedda L, Brenci G. Twins living apart test: progress report. Acta Genet Med Gemellol (Roma) 1983; 32:17–22.
35. Teikari JM, O'Donnell J, Kaprio J, Koskenvuo M. Impact of heredity in myopia. Hum Hered 1991; 41(3):151–156.
36. Hammond CJ, Snieder H, Gilbert CE, Spector TD. Genes and environment in refractive error: the twin eye study. Invest Ophthalmol Vis Sci 2001; 42(6):1232–1236.
37. Valluri S, Minkovitz JB, Budak K, Essary LR, Walker RS, Chansue E, Cabrera GM, Koch DD, Pepose JS. Comparative corneal topography and refractive variables in monozygotic and dizygotic twins. Am J Ophthalmol 1999; 127(2):158–163.
38. Teikari JM, O'Donnell JJ. Astigmatism in 72 twin pairs. Cornea 1989; 8(4):263–268.
39. Tscherning M. Studien ueber die Aetiologie der Myopie. Aibrecht von Graefes Arch Ophhalmol 1883; 29:201–272.
40. Goldschmidt E. On the etiology of myopia. An etiological study. Acta Ophthalmol 1968; Suppl 98.
41. Guggenheim JA, Kirov G, Hodson SA. The heritability of high myopia: a reanalysis of Goldschmidt's data. J Med Genet 2000; 37(3):227–231.
42. Laatikainen L, Erkkiia H. Refractive errors and other ocular findings in school children. Acta Ophthalmol 1980; 58:129–136.
43. Mantyjarvi M. Incidence of myopia in a population of Finnish school children. Acta Ophthalmol 1983; 61:417–423.
44. Krause U, Krause K, Rantakallio P. Sex differences in refraction errors up to the age of 15 . Acta Ophthalmol 1982; 60:917–926.
45. Alsbirk PH. Variation and heritability of ocular dimensions. A population study among adult Greenland Eskimos. Acta Ophthalmol 1977; 55:443–456.
46. Alsbirk PH. Refraction in adult West Greenland Eskimos. A population study of spherical refractive errors, including oculometric and familial correlations. Acta Ophthalmol 1979; 57:84–95.
47. Richler A, Bear JC. Refraction, near–work and education: a population study in Newfoundland. Acta Ophthalmol 1980; 58:468–478.
48. Richler A, Bear JC. The distribution of refraction in three isolated communities in western Newfoundland. Am J Optom Physiol Opt 1980; 57:861–871.
49. Sveinsson KJ. The refraction of Icelanders. Acta Ophthalmol 1982; 60:779–787.
50. Sperduto RD, Seigel D, Roberts J, Rowland M. Prevalence of myopia in the U.S. Arch Ophthalmol 1983; 101:405–407.
51. Leibowitz KM, Krueger DE, Maunder LR, et al. The Framingham Eye Study Monograph. VIII. Visual acuity. Surv Ophthalmol, 1980; 24(suppl):472–479.
52. Angle J, Wissman DA. The epidemiology of myopia. Am J Epidemiol 1980; 111:220–227.
53. Katz J, Tielsch JM, Sommer A. Prevalence and risk factors for refractive errors in an adult inner city population. Invest Ophthalmol Visl Sci. 1997; 38(2):334–340.
54. Hyams SW, Pokotilo E, Shkurko G. Prevalence of refractive errors in adults over 40: a survey of 8102 eyes. Br J Ophthalmol 1977; 61:428–432.
55. Baldwin WR. A review of statistical studies of relations between myopia and ethnic, behavioral and physiological characteristics. Am J Optom Physiol Opt 1981; 58: 516–527.
56. Av–Shalom A, Berson D, Blumenthal M, et al. Prevalence of myopia in Africans. Am J Ophthalmol 1967; 63:1728–1731.
57. Taylor HR. Racial variations in vision. Am J Epidemiol 1981; 113:62–80.
58. Garner LF, Kinnear RF, Klinger JD, McKellar MJ. Prevalence of myopia in school children in Vanuatu. Acta Ophthalmol 1985; 63:323–326.
59. Rosner M, Belkin M. Intelligence education myopia in males. Arch Ophthalmol 1987; 105:1508–1511.
60. Teikari JM. Myopia and stature. Acta Ophthalmol 1987; 65:673.
61. Joffe CM. Vest Oftal 1949; 28:18. (Cited by Goldschmidt E. On the etiology of myopia, an etiological study. Acta Ophthalmol Suppl, 1968:98).

62. Dunphy EB, Stoll MR, King SH. Myopia among American male graduate students. Am J Ophthalmol 1968; 65:518–521.
63. Diamond S. Acquired myopia in airline pilots. J Aviation Med 1957; 28:559–568.
64. Berson D, Jedwab E, Stollman EB. Incidence of myopia among theological and high school students in Jerusalem. Harefuah 1982; 102:16–17 [in Hebrew].
65. Kinge B, Midelfart A, Jacobsen G, Rystad J. The influence of near-work on development of myopia among university students. A three-year longitudinal study among engineering students in Norway. Acta Ophthalmol Scand 2000; 78(1):26–29.
66. Fledelius HC. Myopia profile in Copenhagen medical students 1996–98. Refractive stability over a century is suggested. Acta Ophthalmol Scand 2000; 78(5):501–505.
67. Lin LL, Shih YP, Lee YC, Hung PT, Hou PK. Changes in ocular refraction and its components among medical students—a 5-year longitudinal study. Opt Vis Sci 1996; 73(7):495–498.
68. Au Eong KG, Tay TH, Lim MK. Education and myopia in 110,236 young Singaporean males. Singapore Med J 1993; 34(6):489–492.
69. Young FA. The effect of restricted visual space on the refractive error of the young monkey eye. Invest Ophthalmol 1963; 2:571–577.
70. Wallman J, Adams JI, Trachtman JN. The eyes of young chickens grow towards emmetropia. Invest Ophthalmol Vis Sci 1981; 20:557–561.
71. Yinon U, Rose L, Shapiro A. Myopia in the eye of developing chicks following monocular and binocular lid closure. Vision Res 1980; 20:137–141.
72. Kirby AW, Sutton L, Weiss H. Elongation of cat eyes following neonatal lid suture. Invest Ophthalmol Vis Sci 1982; 22:274–277.
73. Smith EL III, Maguire GW, Watson JT. Axial lengths and refractive errors in kittens reared with an optically induced anisometropia. Invest Ophthalmol Vis Sci 1980; 19:1250–1255.
74. McKanna JA, Casagrande VA. Atropine affects lid-suture myopia development: Experimental studies of chronic atropinization in tree shrews. Doc Ophthalmol Proc Ser 1981; 28:187–192.
75. Kolata G. What causes nearsightedness [News]? Science 1985; 229:1249–1250.
76. Wiesel TN, Raviola E. Myopia and eye enlargement after neonatal lid fusion in monkeys. Nature 1977; 266:66–68.
77. Raviola E, Wiesel TN. Effect of dark-rearing on experimental myopia in monkeys. Invest Ophthalmol Vis Sci 1978; 37:485–488.
78. Wiesel TN, Raviola E. Increase in axial length of the macaque monkey eye after corneal opacification. Invest Ophthalmol Vis Sci 1979; 38:1232–1236.
79. Raviola E, Wiesel TN. An animal model of myopia. N Engl J Med 1985; 312:1609–1635.
80. Robb RM. Refractive errors associated with hemangiomas of the eyelids and orbit in infancy. Am J Ophthalmol 1977; 83:52–58.
81. O'Leary DJ, Millodot M. Eyelid closure causes myopia in humans. Experientia 1979; 35:1478–1479.
82. Hoyt CS, Stone RD, Fromer C, Billson FA. Monocular axial myopia associated with neonatal eyelid closure in human infants. Am J Ophthalmol 1981; 91:197–200.
83. Johnson CA, Post RB, Chalupa LM, Lee TJ. Monocular deprivation in humans: a study of identical twins. Invest Ophthalmol Vis Sci 1982; 23:135–135.
84. Naxasimhan K. Signaling myopia. Nat Neurosci 1999; 2(8):691.
85. McKenzie C, Megaw P, Morgan I, Boelen MK. Deprivation of form vision suppresses diurnal cycling of retinal levels of leu-enkephalin. Austral N Zeal J Ophthalmol 1997; 25(suppl 1):S79–S81.
86. Fischer AJ, McGuire JJ, Schaeffel F, Stell WK. Light-and focus-dependent expression of the transcription factor ZENK in the chick retina. Nat Neurosci 1999; 2(8):706–712.
87. Morgan I, Kucharski R, Krongkaew N, Firth SI, Megaw P, Maleszka R. Screening for differential gene expression during the development of form-deprivation myopia in the chicken. Opt Vis Sci 2004; 81(2):148–155.

88. McBrien NA, Moghaddam HO, Reeder AP. Atropine reduces experimental myopia and eye enlargement via a nonaccommodative mechanism. Invest Ophthalmol Vis Sci 1993; 34(1):205–215.
89. Weigelin E, Neumann G. Statistische Untersuchungen zum Verlauf der Hochgradigen Myopie. Ophthalmologica 1959; 137:1–14.
90. Curtin BJ, Karlin DB. Axial length measurements and fundus changes of the myopic eye. Am J Ophthalmol 1971; 71:42–53.
91. Zauberman H, Merin S. Unilateral myopia associated with bilateral degenerative changes in fundus. Am J Opthalmol 1969; 67:756–759.
92. Schwartz M, Haim M, Skarsholm D. X-linked myopia: Bornholm eye disease. Linkage to DNA markers on the distal part of Xq. Clin Genet 1990; 38(4):281–286.
93. Young TL, Deeb SS, Ronan SM, Dewan AT, Alvear AB, Scavello GS, Paluru PC, Brott MS, Hayashi T, Holleschau AM, Benegas N, Schwartz M, Atwood LD, Oetting WS, Rosenberg T, Motulsky AG, King RA. X-linked high myopia associated with cone dysfunction. Arch Ophthalmol 2004; 122(6):897–908.
94. Young TL, Ronan SM, Drahozal LA, Wildenberg SC, Alvear AB, Oetting WS, Atwood LD, Wilkin DJ, King RA. Evidence that a locus for familial high myopia maps to chromosome 18p. Am J Hum Genet 1998; 63(1):109–119.
95. Young TL, Ronan SM, Alvear AB, Wildenberg SC, Oetting WS, Atwood LD, Wilkin DJ, King RA. A second locus for familial high myopia maps to chromosome 12q. Am J Hum Genet 1998; 63(5):1419–1424.
96. Naiglin L, Gazagne C, Dallongeville F, Thalamas C, Idder A, Rascol O, Malecaze F, Calvas P. A genome wide scan for familial high myopia suggests a novel locus on chromosome 7q36. J Medi Genet 2002; 39(2):118–124.
97. Paluru P, Ronan SM, Heon E, Devoto M, Wildenberg SC, Scavello G, Holleschau A, Makitie O, Cole WG, King RA, Young TL. New locus for autosomal dominant high myopia maps to the long arm of chromosome 17. Invest Ophthalmol Vis Sci 2003; 44(5):1830–1836.
98. Morgan I, Megaw P. Using natural STOP growth signals to prevent excessive axial elongation and the development of myopia. Ann Acad Med Singapore 2004; 33(1):16–20.
99. Sorsby A, Benjamin B. Modes of inheritance of errors of refraction. J Med Genet 1973; 10:161–164.
100. Letocha CC. Myopia [letter]. Arch Ophthalmol 1983; 101:1301.
101. McBrien NA, Barnes DA. A review and evaluation of theories of refractive error development. Ophthalmic Physiol Opt 1984; 4:201–213.
102. Pemberton JW, Freeman HM, Schepens CL. Familial retinal development and the Ehlers-Danlos syndrome. Arch Ophthalmol 1966; 76:817–824.
103. Stickler GB, Belau PG, Farrell FJ, et al. Hereditary progressive arthro-ophthalmopathy. Mayo Clin Proc 1965; 40:433–455.
104. Fraser GR, Friedmann AI, Maroteaux P, et al. Dysplasia spondyloepiphysaria congenita and related generalized skeletal dysplasias among children with severe visual handicaps. Arch Dis Child 1969; 44:490–498.
105. Beighton P, Goldberg L, Op't Hof J. Dominant inheritance of multiple epiphyseal dysplasia, myopia and deafness. Clin Genet 1978; 14:173–177.
106. Eldridge R, Berlin CI, Money JW, McKusick VA. Cochlear deafness, myopia and intellectual impairment in an Amish family. A new syndrome of hereditary deafness. Arch Otolaryngol 1968; 88:49–84.
107. Pfeiffer RA, Junemann G, Polster J, Bauer H. Epiphyseal dysplasia of the femoral head, severe myopia and perceptive hearing loss in three brothers. Clin Genet 1973; 4: 141–144.
108. Mollica F, Li Volti S, Tomarchio S, et al. Autosomal dominant cataract and microcornea associated with myopia in a Sicilian family. Clin Genet 1985; 28:42–46.
109. Batra DV, Paul SD. Microcornea with myopia. Br J Ophthalmol 1967; 51:57–60.

110. Ortiz de Zarate JC. Recessive sex-linked inheritance of congenital external ophthalmolplegia and myopia coincident with other dysplasias. Br J Ophthalmol 1966; 50:606–607.
111. Jay M. The Eisdell pedigree. Congenital stationary night-blindness myopia. Trans Ophthalmol Soc UK 1983; 103:221–226.
112. Merin S, Rowe H, Auerbach E, Landau J. Syndrome of congenital high myopia with nyctalopia. Am J Ophthalmol 1970; 70:541 547.
113. der Kaloustian VM, Baghdassarian SA. The autosomal recessive variety of congenital stationary night blindness with myopia. J Med Genet 1972; 9:67–69.
114. Spivey BE, Pearlman JT, Burian HM. Electroretinographic findings (including flicker) in carriers of congenital X-linked achromatopsia. Doc Ophthalmol 1964; 18:367–375.
115. Francois J, Verriest G, Matton-Van Leuven MT, et al. Atypical achromatopsia of sex-linked recessive inheritance. Am J Ophthalmol 1966; 61:1101–1108.
116. Brody JA, Hussels I, Brink E, Torres J. Hereditary blindness among Pingelapese people of eastern Caroline Islands. Lancet 1970; (7659):1253–1257.
117. Haim M, Fledelius HC, Skarshol M. X-linked myopia in Danish family. Acta Ophthalmol 1988; 66:450–456.
118. Curtin BJ. Myopia: a review of its etiology pathogenesis treatment. Surv Ophthalmol 1970; 15:1–17.
119. Podos SM, Becker B, Morton WR. High myopia primary open-angle glaucoma. Am J Ophthalmol 1966; 62:1038–1043.
120. Silverstone BZ, Berson D, Seelenfreund M, Mendelsohn D. Copper metabolism study in high myopia in the African. Metab Pediatr Syst Ophthalmol 1983; 7:173–176.
121. Bedrossian RH. The effect of atropine on myopia. Ann Ophthalmol 1971; 3:891–897.
122. Brodstein RS, Brodstein DE, Olson RJ, et al. The treatment of myopia with atropine and bifocals: a long–term prospective study. Ophthalmology 1984; 91:1373–1378.
123. Saw SM, Gazzard G, Au Eong KG, Tan DT. Myopia: attempts to arrest progression. Br J Ophthalmol 2002; 86(11):306–311.
124. Katz J, Schein OD, Levy B, Cruiscullo T, Saw SM, Rajan U, Chan TK, Yew Khoo C, Chew SJ. A randomized trial of rigid gas permeable contact lenses to reduce progression of children's myopia. Am J Ophthalmol 2003; 136(1):82–90.
125. Wildsoet CF, Norton TT. Toward controlling myopia progression. Optom Vis Sci 1999; 76(6):341–342.
126. Leung JT, Brown B. Progression of myopia in Hong Kong Chinese schoolchildren is slowed by wearing progressive lenses. Optom Vis Sci 1999; 76(6):346–354.
127. Gwiazda JE, Hyman L, Norton TT, Hussein ME, Marsh-Tootle W, Manny R, Wang Y, Everett D. Accommodation and related risk factors associated with myopia progression and their interaction with treatment in COMET children. Invest Ophthamol Vis Sci 2004; 45(7):2143–2151.

20

Inherited Tumors of the Eye

INTRODUCTION

Although the inherited nature of some malignant and benign ocular tumors has been known for several generations, it has been viewed by many physicians as just another curiosity of their profession. Only since the second half of the 20th century has increased knowledge and understanding of the genetic background of these tumors evolved into practical tools in the clinical management of affected patients. Hereditary retinoblastoma has been known for many decades to be transmitted by a single autosomal dominant gene, but it has also been believed that only a small percentage of retinoblastomas are genetically transmitted. In the last decades, new studies into the nature of retinoblastoma have greatly improved genetic counseling, diagnosis, and even treatment of these patients. In addition, new cytogenetic studies performed in the United States, Canada, Japan, and some European countries have brought the subject of retinoblastoma into the forefront of all human cancer research.

An inherited tendency to develop malignant melanoma of the eye and of the skin will be described separately in this chapter, as will xeroderma pigmentosum, an inherited disease predisposing to several different malignant tumors.

RETINOBLASTOMA AND RETINOMA

General Description

Retinoblastoma is by far the most common malignant intraocular tumor of childhood and one of the more common hereditary malignant tumors of humans. Some reports have suggested that its incidence is increasing (1,2). Retinoblastoma is a tumor of early childhood, about 90% of all cases are diagnosed before the age of three years (mean age, 18 months) (3). Nevertheless, the age of onset encompasses an extremely wide range from newborn to 62 years old (3). A review of the literature indicates that, although only 6–8% of affected patients have a family history of retinoblastoma, about 40% of all cases are hereditary (4,5).

The tumor arises from retinal cells related to the differentiation of the photoreceptors. Verhoeff has named these cells retinoblasts (6). It was suggested that these same cells may develop into a benign variant of a tumor termed retinoma (5), retinocytoma (7), or retinoblastoma grade 0 (8). Since James Wardrop advised excision of the eye as the first useful treatment for retinoblastoma in 1809 (9), treatment in developed societies has become so efficient that the survival rate for retinoblastoma is now among the highest of all malignant tumors. The long-term survival rate is reported to be 80–90% (10–12), with one study from the United States citing 76% for three years survival (13).

Retinoblastoma may be unilateral, bilateral, or "trilateral" It also may be hereditary, transmitted by an autosomal dominant gene from a parent, or due to a new mutation. It may be nonhereditary or due to a new chromosomal aberration. The hereditary tumor differs, in many aspects, from the nonhereditary form. One of the best known differences is that bilateral tumors are virtually always hereditary, whereas most unilateral tumors are sporadic and nonhereditary.

Clinical Findings

Age of Onset

The vast majority of patients initially show symptoms of the disease before the age of three years. However, the age of onset between hereditary and nonhereditary cases clearly differs. Bilateral cases, considered generally to be hereditary, have a mean age of onset and diagnosis between 10 and 15 months of age, whereas unilateral cases have a mean age of onset between 24 and 35 months (14–17). The onset of symptoms occurs before age one in 78–79% of bilateral cases and 15–36% of unilateral cases (6,18), and before age two in 96% of bilateral cases and 22% of unilateral cases (18).

Figure 1 shows graphically the age at diagnosis in 95 patients with sporadic retinoblastoma studied in New Zealand by Fitzgerald et al. (15). When the tumor is bilateral, both eyes are found to be affected concurrently or the second tumor is detected shortly after the first. However, Carlson et al. (14) found five of 27 bilateral cases to have a delayed onset of the tumor in the fellow eye, ranging from one year to more than 11 years.

Several assumptions can be made from these figures. First, the earlier the onset of symptoms, the more likely the patient will have bilateral disease (19). This was also shown in a study of 50 patients by Aherne and Roberts (18) (Table 1). Second, the likelihood of bilaterality sharply decreases (4–6%) if the first symptoms do not appear by age two. Third, it is conceivable that early onset characterizes hereditary cases; consequently, age of onset may assist the differentiation of hereditary sporadic unilateral cases from nonhereditary sporadic unilateral cases.

Rarely does retinoblastoma appear after childhood. Only 11 cases of retinoblastoma have been reported after the age of 20 years. It is possible that in these patients embryonal retinal cells persisted for some unknown reason and were subject to late malignant transformation (20).

Presenting Signs and Symptoms

The most common presenting sign of retinoblastoma is an abnormal, greenish, white, or grayish reflex from the pupil (Fig. 2), variously referred to as leukocoria (in North America) and as "amaurotic cat's eye" (in Europe). This is the first sign in more than half of all patients (54–56%), followed by strabismus (18–20%), and signs of inflammation, with or without glaucoma (7–15%] (2,3,21). The rest present with less common first symptoms and signs, such as loss of vision (in older children)

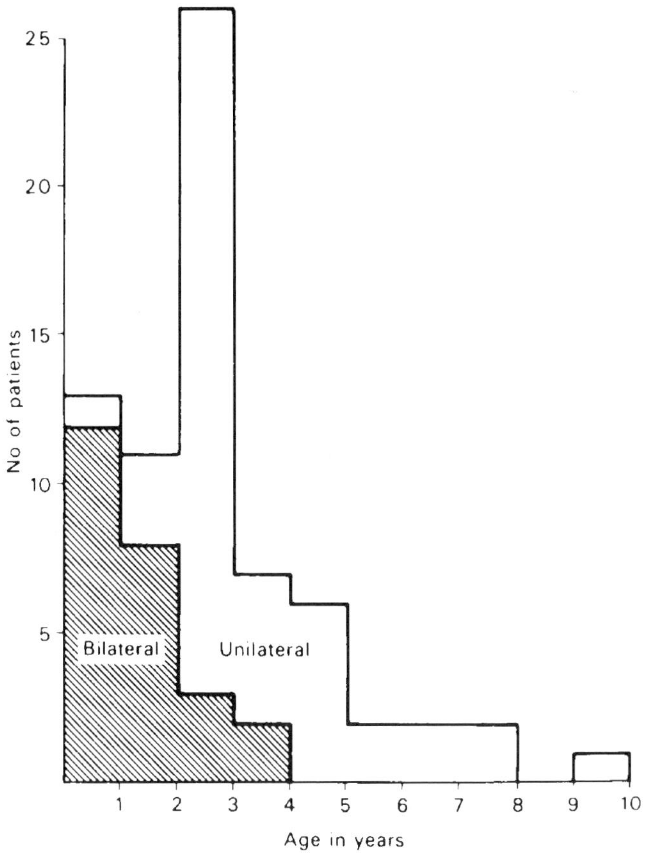

Figure 1 Age of diagnosis in 95 patients with sporadic retinoblastoma, studied in New Zealand by Fitzgerald et al. Note that most bilateral cases were diagnosed before the age of 2 years, whereas most unilateral cases were diagnosed later (from Ref. 15).

unilateral mydriasis, and hyphema, or indications of infiltration into the anterior chamber, such as hypopyon or white spots on the iris. Sometimes orbital involvement or a routine examination leads to the diagnosis.

Clinical Examination and Natural History

In most cases, the tumor can be seen ophthalmoscopically (Fig. 3). The indirect ophthalmoscope should always be used for the examination. In young children,

Table 1 Probability of Bilaterality According to Age of Onset

Age at onset of first tumor (months)	Probability that tumor will be bilateral (%)
0–5	85
6–11	82
12–17	44
18–23	44
24 and over	6

Source: From Ref. (19)

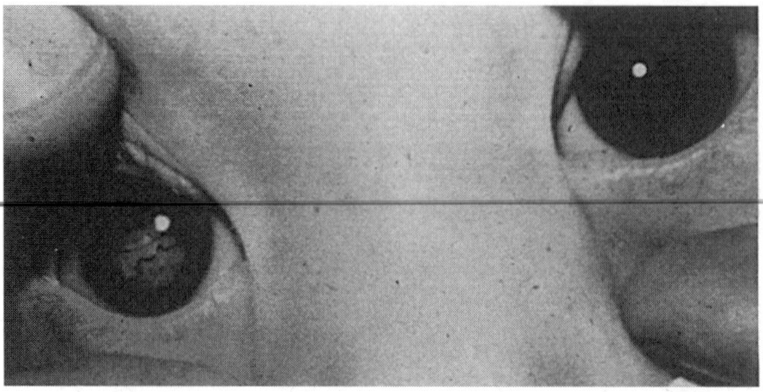

Figure 2 Leukocoria: the clinical appearance varies from a faint gray or green reflex in the pupil to a well-distinguished massive growth with a retinal detachment as in this patient.

general anesthesia is preferable to obtain a reliable view of the fundus. The tumor may be solitary or multiple. In advanced cases, vitreous hemorrhage, cataract, and other anterior segment changes may obscure the view of the fundus. It is customary to divide the patients into clinical groups, as suggested by Ellsworth (21). Such a classification (Table 2) is helpful in defining the patient's clinical status and prognosis and in making decisions about treatment.

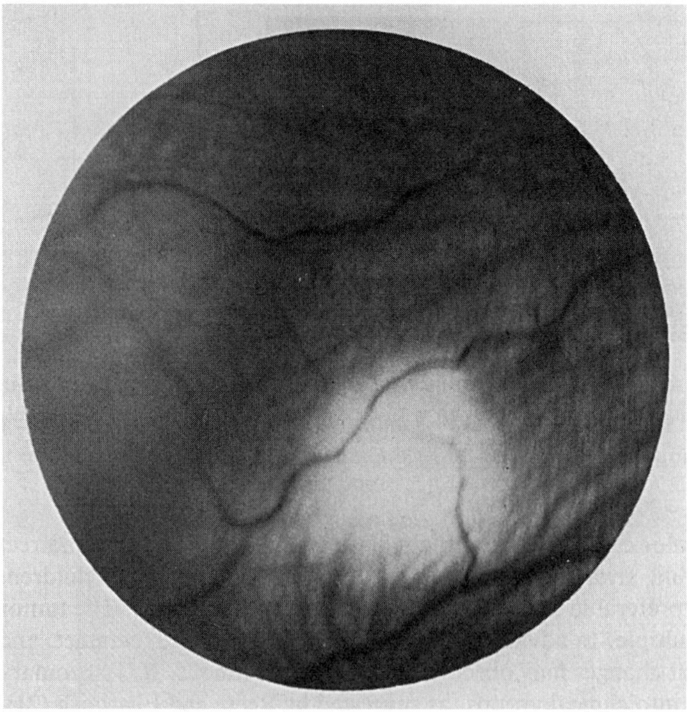

(a)

Figure 3 Retinoblastoma: typical ophthalmoscopic appearance of a tumor of group 1 (a), group 2 (b), and groups 3 and 4 (c).

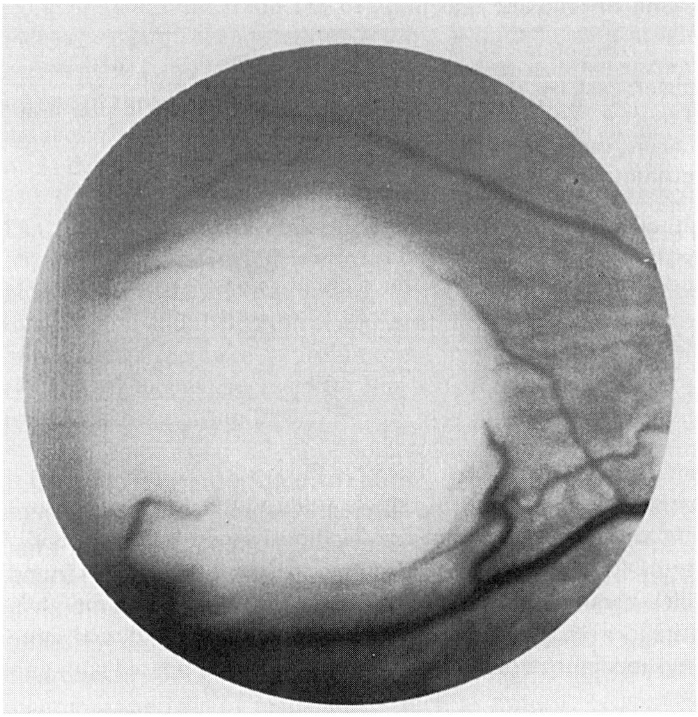

(b)

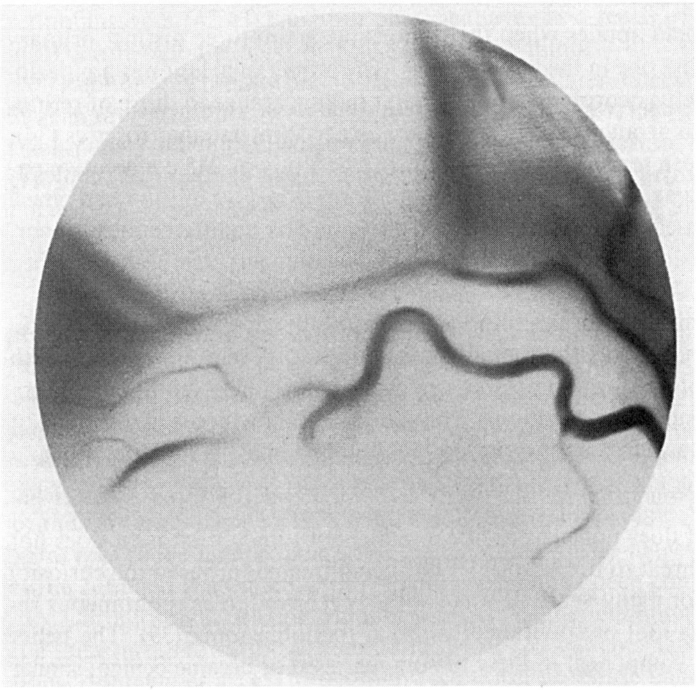

(c)

Figure 3 *(Continued)*

Table 2 The Reese-Elsworth Division into Groups

Group	Type	Description
1	Tumor only	One or more tumors, each <4 DD in size, at or posterior to equator
2	Tumor and subretinal fluid	One or more, each 4–10 DD in size, including subretinal fluid
3	Tumor with focal seeds	3a—subretinal seeds, 3b—vitreous seeds
4	Tumor with diffuse seeds	4a—subretinal seeds, 4b—vitreous seeds
5	Massive tumors	Neovascular glaucoma, invasive retinoblastoma, massive tumor filling the eye

DD, disc diameter.
Source: Modified from Refs. 21 and 210.

Untreated, the tumor invariably grows. The growth is called exophytic when it expands mainly under the retina and toward the choroid, and endophytic when it expands inward toward the vitreous. The spread of the tumor occurs most frequently through direct invasion of the optic nerve toward the chiasm. Less frequently, the tumor perforates Bruch's membrane and extends into the choroid, sending early metastases mainly to the liver. Least frequently, the tumor infiltrates directly into the anterior segment or subconjunctival and orbital spaces.

The Clinical and Genetic Types of Retinoblastoma

Relatively few patients with retinoblastoma have a positive family history. Various studies have reported this as 5% (22), 5.1% (23), 10.5% (24), and 11% (2). However, the percentage of patients with hereditary retinoblastoma is much higher than this, reaching about 40%, for many sporadic cases without a familial history carry a germinal mutation. We will discuss the different types as they are clinically characterized.

Bilateral Retinoblastoma

In patients with a positive family history, the pedigree shows autosomal dominant inheritance with reduced penetrance, which is cited in most reports as being 90% (25). Usually, the disease is transmitted to the patient by an affected parent. However, sporadic bilateral cases are assumed to be hereditary, as it is very unlikely that a patient without such germinal mutation will have two (or more) different primary foci of retinoblastoma in the two eyes. About one of three patients has bilateral retinoblastoma (24,26). In review of the literature, Francois (27) showed that between 1930 and 1965, the percentage of bilateral cases increased from 19% to 36%. It seems that this percentage has continued to increase after 1965 (25). Of all new germinal mutations, about two-thirds have bilateral involvement and one-third are unilateral (27). This is about the same ratio as in all inherited cases (25). The fraction of bilateral cases differs among families (25), possibly indicating a difference in expressivity of the gene. This proportion is not influenced by the sex of the carrier parent (28). However, the mean age of both parents was higher in patients with bilateral tumors when compared with those demonstrating unilateral tumors (14), possibly caused by a higher number of new germinal mutations in bilateral cases.

It was claimed that bilateral retinoblastoma patients afflicted with blindness, have an IQ higher by about 10 points than controls (29,30), but these studies are inconclusive and not confirmed. However, a more recent study also found an association between bilateral retinoblastoma and superior cognitive capacities (31). As such an association was not found with unilateral retinoblastoma, it might indicate a link between the RBI gene and intelligence.

Unilateral Retinoblastoma

About two of three patients with retinoblastoma have unilateral involvement. Of these sporadic (nonfamilial) cases, about 10–15% are assumed to be germinal mutations (25,27), as found in the follow-up of such patients. The ophthalmologist faces a difficult decision in determining whether or not a particular unilateral case is hereditary, as the management of the patient (examinations of the fellow eye, frequency of follow-up, and sometimes treatment) may be different. Certainly, the genetic counseling is different. Several epidemiologic findings may indirectly assist in the diagnosis. After studying 66 patients with unilateral retinoblastoma, Abramson et al.(32) found that in hereditary familial cases the age at diagnosis was lower (25 vs. 27 months), the average number of tumors per affected eye was greater (2.4 vs. 1.2), and more patients had multiple intraocular tumors (42 vs. 12%), when compared with unilateral nonfamilial cases.

Patients with unilateral retinoblastoma must be followed up, as 10–20% of such individuals will develop a tumor in the other eye.

"Trilateral" Retinoblastoma

Trilateral retinoblastoma applies when the tumor appears in three distinct primary foci, one in each eye and one in the brain (33–35). The intracranial lesion is a pinealo-blastoma, which contains neuroblastic cells similar in appearance to those of retinoblastoma, including an arrangement resembling Flexner–Wintersteiner rosettes (35). About 40 cases had been reported by 1989 (36). In one study of 245 patients with retinoblastoma, seven (3%) had the trilateral form (36). Five of the seven had pineal body tumors, one a suprasellar neuroblastoma, and one an undifferentiated parasellar tumor. A unilateral retinoblastoma with a pineal body malignancy has also been described (37,38).

Kivela (39) reviewed 103 reported children with trilateral retinoblastoma. The median age at diagnosis was five months, with a range of 0–29 months. The second and third generations of families with hereditary retinoblastoma were much more affected than the first generation. The five-year survival was 27% (39).

In spite of its rarity, trilateral retinoblastoma is very intriguing because it indicates the powerful tendency of these malignant tumors to develop in patients with the inherited gene. Interestingly, in lower vertebrates, the pineal body has photoreceptors as well as endocrine functions. This could explain why the association of bilateral tumors with a pineal body primary "retinoblastoma" is not fortuitous.

Retinoma or Benign Retinoblastoma

A retinoblastoma that does not behave like a malignant tumor, that is, it does not grow or constitute a threat to life without treatment, aroused the curiosity of ophthalmologists for many years. It was variously referred to as spontaneous regressed retinoblastoma (40) or spontaneous-healed retinoblastoma (41). The belief was that the malignant component in these tumors regressed or became benign, similar to the neuroblastoma, another malignant tumor with a high rate of regression (42).

Compared with the frequency of occurrence of retinoblastoma, there are few documented cases of benign retinoblastoma. Khodadoust et al. (40) described 50 cases, between 1911 and 1975. The authors suggested that this phenomenon may be caused by one of three possibilities: (i) the tumor outgrows its blood supply and the necrosis induces "healing"; (ii) the deposited calcium serves as an inhibitor of tumor growth; or (iii) development of immunity stops the growth.

Gallie et al. (43) have suggested that spontaneous-regressed retinoblastoma is, in fact, the benign manifestation of the retinoblastoma gene *(RB)* and proposed the term retinoma for it. This view is supported by the facts that retinomas show a blood supply (they do not outgrow their vasculature); they never change, even after many years; and their clinical appearance is typical. This view is similar to the opinion that regressed neuroblastoma is a neuroblastoma remaining in situ (42). Other names suggested for this benign tumor have been retinocytoma (44) and retinoblastoma group 0 (8).

Retinomas may be more common than previously assumed. Gallie et al. (5) studied 1400 documented carriers of the *RB* gene and found 32 (2%) to have a retinoma. Retinoma presents a typical clinical appearance (Fig. 4), described by the same group of authors as a "homogeneous, translucent gray elevated mass," often with white nodules of calcium like "cottage cheese" and migration and proliferation of the pigment epithelium (43). Histologically, the tumor is composed of benign-appearing cells, with calcific foci and a well-vascularized ground substance. Typically, fleurettes are present (Fig. 4). A histologic study by Aaby et al. (8), showed no sign characteristic of malignancy, such as mitosis, cellular plemorphism, signs of tumor necrosis, or regression. In fact, there may be two kinds of untreated, nonma-lignant retinoblastomas: the benign variant, spontaneously arrested retinoblastoma (retinoblastoma in situ, retinoma, or retinocytoma); and the spontaneously regressed retinoblastoma (44,45) found in phthisical eyes as a result of a vascular occlusion, insufficient blood supply, and necrosis of the tumor.

Retinoma is usually unilateral (46,47), but bilateral occurrence has been found in as many as 10–20% of all affected patients (40,43). This figure is far higher than the expected 2% of the benign variant of all *RB* gene carriers. In some families, "regression" seems to be familial, with several members affected by the benign tumor (40,48). These two facts may indicate that, in addition to the inherited *RB* gene, some individuals may have an inherited tendency to the benign version of the tumor, which is of genetic importance.

Balmer et al. (49) also found that about 10% of retinoblastoma patients developed a retinoma (11 of 103 patients). Average age at diagnosis was 23 years. About half were unilateral and half were bilateral. Seven of 11 retinoma patients had a history of familial retinoblastoma. Genetically, similarities with hereditary retinoblastoma were noticed. Twelve of 16 offspring of retinoma patients had retinoblastoma that was almost all bilateral. One child with retinoma, who had the other eye enucleated at two years of age, developed an osteosarcoma at the age of nine years (49).

Lommatzsch et al. (50) found an incidence of retinoma of 3.2% among retinoblastoma patients. They stressed that this incidence of an associated benign tumor is 1000-fold more than in other malignancies (50).

Singh et al. (51) studied 17 patients, who had features compatible with retinocytoma (retinoma). Age at diagnosis ranged from 4 to 45, with a median of 15 years. The clinical manifestation was a translucent retinal mass (88%), calcification (63%) and RPE alterations (54%). One of 17 had a malignant transformation (51).

Lueder et al. (52) reported two patients with retinoma and vitreous seeding. They were followed up for 8 and 33 years without any treatment and without any other sign of malignant transformation (52).

Chromosomal-Deletion Retinoblastoma

Approximately 5% of all retinoblastoma patients have a detectable deletion of band 14 on the long arm of chromosome 13 (del13q14). In 1976, Knudson et al. (53) examined the karyotype of one patient with retinoblastoma and mental retardation and reviewed 12 previous reports of similar chromosomal aberrations with retinoblastoma. They reported that 11 of these patients had 13q14 deletions. Confirmation of their findings came in 1978 from Yunis and Ramsey (54), after they analyzed two karyotypes in the late prophase and prometaphase. The suggestion (55) that 13q14.2 is the subband associated with retinoblastoma has been confirmed.

Chromosomal deletion retinoblastoma is neither common nor rare. In reviewing the literature, Howard (56) found that 14 of 259 patients had chromosomal aberrations. Johnson et al. (57) used high-resolution prophase banding techniques to

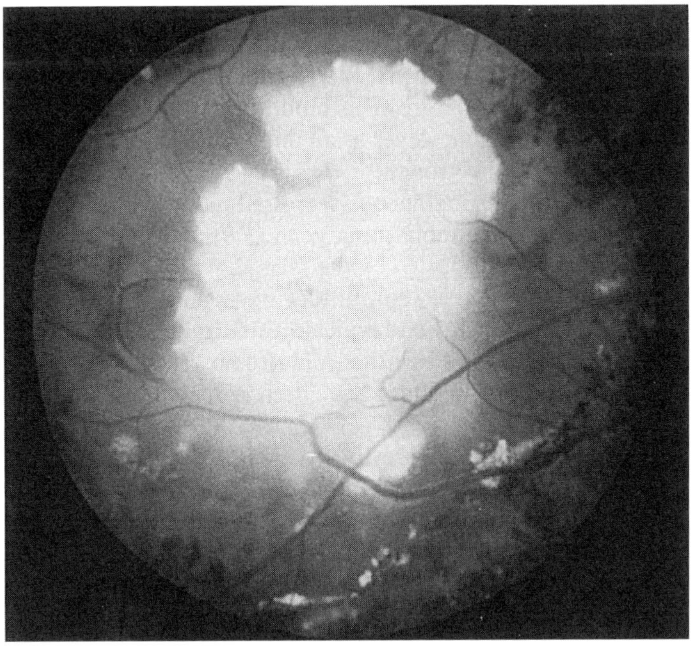

(a)

Figure 4 Retinoma: (a) Ophthalmoscopically, the lesion is large, gray, and elevated, with scattered white nodules of calcium; (b) a family with five of six siblings affected by retinoblastoma; (c) a large retinoma was found in the fundus of the right eye of their father.

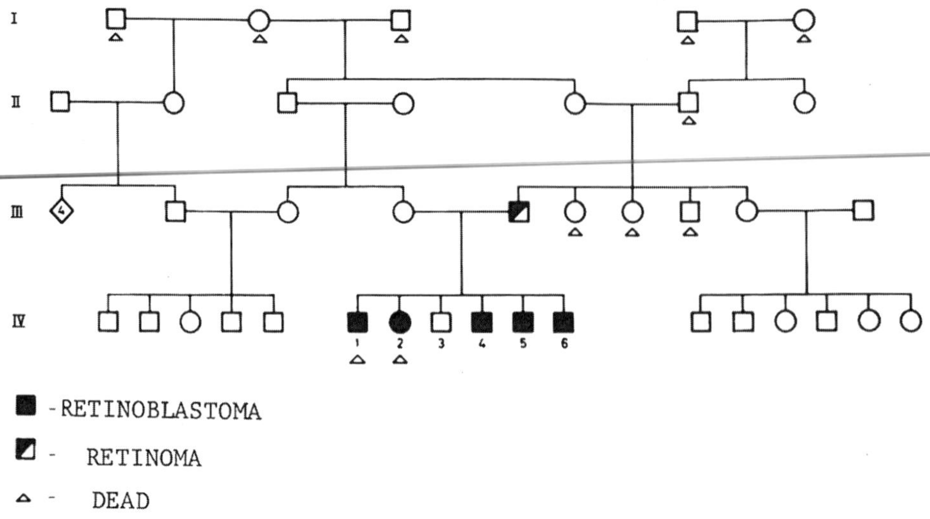

(b)

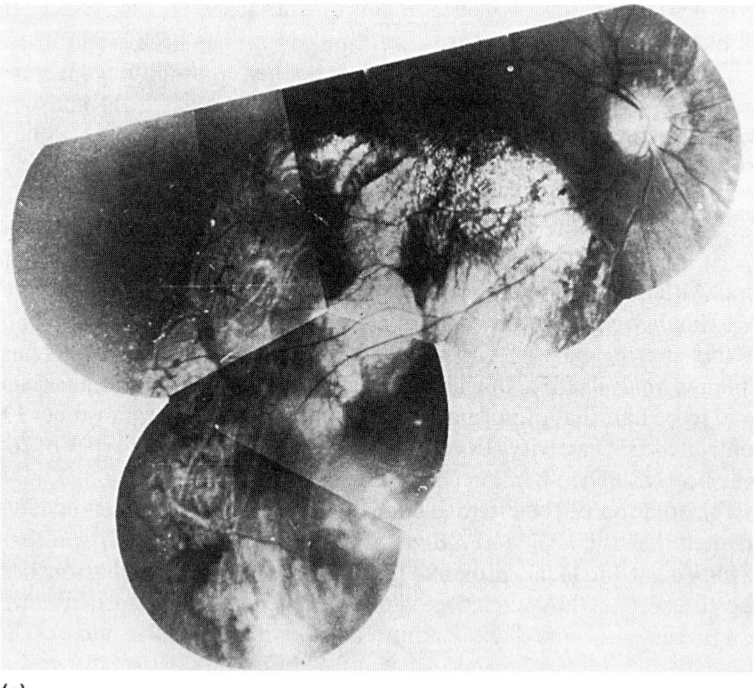

(c)

Figure 4 *(Continued).*

examine 12 patients with retinoblastoma and found three with an interstitial deletion of band ql4 on one chromosome 13. Of 51 patients with a deletion involving band 14 on chromosome 13, 50 had retinoblastoma (58).

Table 3 describes the clinical findings in patients with a deletion of band 14 on one long arm of chromosome 13. Retinoblastoma, mild or severe mental and developmental retardation, and facial anomalies occur in practically every one. Other

Table 3 Clinical Findings in Patients with Deletion of 13q14

Findings	Remarks
Retinoblastoma	50/51 cases
Mental retardation	50% mild, 50% severe
Developmental retardation	
Microcephaly	
Microphthalmus or coloboma	
Skeletal abnormalities	
Facial abnormalities	
Low-set ears	
Micrognathia	
Prominent eyebrows	
Broad nasal bridge	
Bulbous tip of nose	
High-arched palate	
Thin upper lip and long philtrum	
Large mouth	
Genitourinary anomalies	
Muscle defects	
Polydactyly and clinodactyly	

Source: From Refs. 53, 56, 57, 59.

reported malformations are less frequent, depending on the length and the points of beginning and end of the deleted segment. Figure 5 shows a schematic drawing of chromosome 13 and the deleted parts in three patients. In most described cases of 13q with retinoblastoma, the deleted segment affects different portions of the long arm of chromosome 13, somewhere between band 13 and band 22, but always includes the proximal or middle part of band 14. There are indications (55) that mental retardation is related to deletion of portions distal to locus ql4, whereas facial abnormalities are related to the deletion of portions proximal to ql4.

It is not surprising that chromosomal deletion retinoblastoma has the same bilateral/unilateral case ratio as hereditary retinoblastoma. Approximately two of every three reported cases are bilateral, a similarity that has theoretical genetic importance.

Studies using deletion technique mapping were performed to detect nearby loci on chromosome 13. The most important result was the discovery of a locus on 13ql4, which controls activity of esterase D (ESD), an enzyme of unknown function that is found in most human tissues (55). It was suggested that the locus for the ESD activity and the locus for retinoblastoma is one and the same (56,58), but this seems unlikely (60,61). Rather, the two loci are close together, but distinct from each other. In one family, a mother and her daughter had a small deletion within chromosomal region 13ql4, and 50% of normal ESD levels but no retinoblastoma (62). On the basis of studies of patients with constitutional deletion of 13ql4, it is now assumed that the *ESD* gene lies proximally to the *RB* gene within region 13q14 (63). The fact that two allelic forms of this enzyme exist and can be differentiated by electrophoresis has been used for linkage analysis (61). In chromosomal deletion retinoblastoma, ESD activity was found to be half that of normal, as only one of the two chromosomes 13 had the gene-controlled ESD activity. In contrast, ESD activity in other types of retinoblastoma was normal (64).

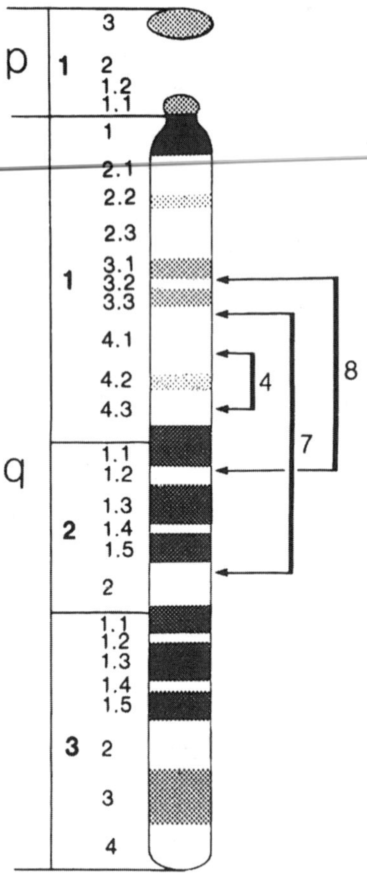

Figure 5 Schematic drawing of chromosome 13, with the deleted segments of three patients marked. Note that band q14.2 is deleted in all three. The other deleted parts influence associated anomalies, in addition to the retinoblastoma (from Ref. 57).

The successful isolation of the esterase D cDNA clone was established in 1986 (65,66). It confirmed that the *ESD* and *RB* genes are two separate genes, and that the *ESD* gene is located at 13ql4.11, proximal to the *RB* gene. Young et al. (67) reported the complete cDNA sequence of the *ESD* gene. A long open-reading frame encodes a predicted protein of 282 amino acids, with molecular mass of 30 kDa.

It was also suggested that another locus on 13ql4 is related to increased sensitivity of fibroblasts to x-ray irradiation (68), but this finding has not been confirmed.

A fluorescent marker on the short arm of chromosome 13 was of no value for genetic linkage studies (69).

Second Malignant Tumor in Retinoblastoma

Survivors of bilateral retinoblastoma have been particularly susceptible to development of a second malignant tumor, especially osteogenic sarcoma (70,71). This was assumed to result from therapy by irradiation, but in a national epidemiologic study in the United States, Jensen and Miller (10) pointed out that approximately half the patients with a second malignant tumor either had the neoplasm in a nonirradiated area or never received any irradiation. This high susceptibility for various malignant tumors also has been found in family members not manifesting retinoblastoma, but possibly carrying the *RB* gene (70,71); retinoblastoma survivors who carry the germinal mutations and not the sporadic unilateral type are at risk (72). In a large study of 2300 cases of retinoblastoma, Abramson et al. (73) found 84 nonocular malignant tumors in 80 patients, of which 97.5% had bilateral retinoblastoma. In patients who received irradiation to the eye and survived, about one in four had the second tumor outside the field of irradiation (74).

It seems, therefore, that the gene *RB* increases the susceptibility to develop a second malignant neoplasm. The development of such a malignancy may, in turn, be further stimulated by irradiation. Patients irradiated for retinoblastoma have a tremendous increase in the number of certain neoplasms in the irradiated field, even after receiving relatively low amounts of irradiation; this is in addition to second malignancies unrelated to the irradiation.

Of all retinoblastoma patients who did not survive, 15% died of another malignant tumor and not of the retinoblastoma (10). A second malignancy developed in 14% of survivors of bilateral retinoblastoma who did not receive irradiation (75), and in 22.8% of survivors who received two courses or more of irradiation (74). These latter patients show a high mortality from a nonocular malignancy (Fig. 6).

The incidence of second malignancies increases with time. Of 215 patients with bilateral retinoblastoma, 4.4% developed a second tumor in course of the first ten years, 18.3% after 20 years, and 26.1% after 30 years (76). The incidence of such tumors was more than four times higher in patients who received irradiation treatment compared with nonirradiated patients (35.1 vs. 8.1%).

Several investigators assumed that such figures, as reported by Abramson and others, are greatly overestimated because of lack of properly controlled studies (77–79), and that the cumulative incidence of a second malignancy in retinoblastoma survivors is "only" 19% at 35 years, or 14 times that of the general population (79).

The most common second malignancy is an osteogenic sarcoma of the orbit or of the femur. This occurs in patients with retinoblastoma at least 500 times more

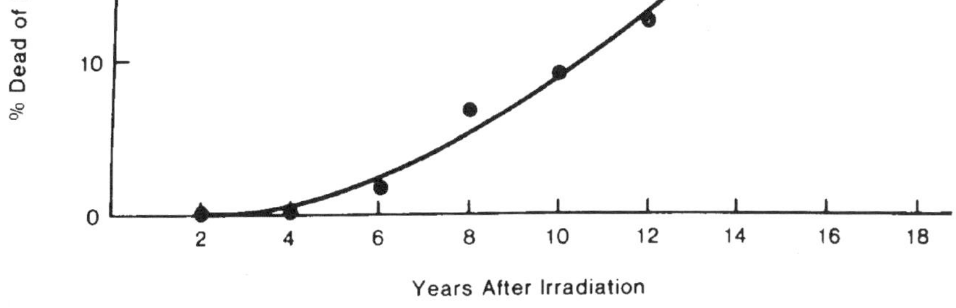

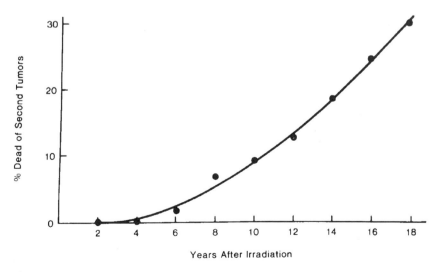

Figure 6 Mortality from a nonocular malignancy in retinoblastoma survivors: the risk for death was calculated from life-table curves (from Ref. 74).

Table 4 Second Malignant Tumors Reported in Retinoblastoma Survivors

Osteogenic sarcoma
Rhabdomyosarcoma (74)
Anaplastic tumor of orbit
Testicular tumor
Ewing's sarcoma
Cutaneous melanoma (75,80)
Leiomyosarcoma (81,82)
Renal cell adenocarcinoma (81)
Epidermoid carcinoma of tongue (83)
Carcinoma of lung (6,84)
Carcinoma of bladder (6)
Breast tumor (85)
Hodgkin lymphoma (85)
Brain tumors (86)

frequently than in the general population (73). Other sites of secondary tumors are listed in Table 4. It has been suggested that survivors of bilateral retinoblastoma should undergo an annual bone scan for the detection of such tumors (87). A scan carries little risk because the amount of radiation is low.

Evidence is accumulating that a second malignancy in retinoblastoma survivors may result from a genetic abnormality subsequent to the development of homozygosity at one or more loci on the long arm of chromosome 13 (88), including a defective or missing *RB* gene with development of homozygosity at this locus (84).

The consensus about the genetic background of second malignancies with RBI mutations is unequivocal and no longer disputed. However, other influencing factors remained disputable. Kony et al. concluded that both genetic factors and exposure to radiation have independent effects on the risk of second malignant neoplasms (89). Eng et al. (85) claimed that their study of 1458 retinoblastoma cases implicates germinal mutations within the RB1 gene in second cancer mortality, but that radiotherapy enhances the inborn susceptibility to develop such second malignancies. Abramson and Frank found no increased risk for second malignant tumors out of the field of radiation in patients who underwent external beam radiation (90) after the age of 12 months. The risk was high if the treatment was given in the first year of life. Abramson et al. (91) detected only 46 children diagnosed with retinoblastoma in the first month of life. The incidence of second nonocular cancer was at a mean age of 23.7 years, 54% for patients who received radiation therapy and 0% for patients who did not receive such treatment.

On the other hand, some studies demonstrated that second malignancies developed equally (92) or mostly (93) outside the field of irradiation. This included patients who were irradiated in the course of their first year of life. These studies assumed that it was not the irradiation per se that was implicated with the growth of the second tumor (92). Wong et al. pointed out that subsequent cancers were evident only in the group of hereditary retinoblastoma. At 50 years after the diagnosis, 51% of hereditary retinoblastoma developed a secondary malignancy compared to 5% for sporadic RB (94).

More than one second tumor may occur. Abramson et al. (95) followed 1506 retinoblastoma patients and found 211 with second tumors, 28 with third malignancies, six had a fourth tumor and two had a fifth tumor. The majority of these more than two-tumor patients had received radiation therapy in the past (95).

Other factors may also play a role in causing second tumors. Germline RB1 mutations carry an increased risk of lung cancer (96). Kleinerman et al. found five cases of lung neoplasm among 964 patients with hereditary retinoblastoma and none in the nonhereditary group. They concluded that possibly RB1 carriers may be more susceptible to complications due to cigarette smoking (96).

A second malignancy is a serious problem that interferes with the management of retinoblastoma patients. Doctors must be aware of this problem. In the United States in the last decade, 95% or more of all children with retinoblastoma survived the disease. Approximately 1% of the survivors go on to have a second nonocular tumor every year, and half of them will die from the second malignancy (97). In a study of 1458 patients, Eng et al. (85) detected 305 cases of death as follows: 167 from retinoblastoma, 96 from second malignancy, 21 from other known causes and 21 from unknown causes.

Tumor suppressor genes, such as retinoblastoma or p53 are an important cause of brain tumor formation (86). The incidence of osteosarcoma is increased 500-fold in patients with mutated RB1 gene. Thomas et al. studied osteogenesis and found that loss of the Rb protein blocks late osteoblast differentiation and this increases susceptibility to osteogenic sarcoma (98).

Laboratory Tests and Additional Examinations

The single most important examination for the diagnosis of retinoblastoma is ophthalmoloscopy. However, advanced cases require a differential diagnosis with other causes of leukocoria, and early and atypical cases may result in an uncertain diagnosis.

Radiologic Examination

Almost all eyes excised for retinoblastoma demonstrated histologic evidence of calcifications (99,100). Klintworth (100) showed that such eyes have typical radiographic densities that are multiple, discrete, relatively uniform, and small. Unfortunately, only about 20% of patients with retinoblastoma show signs of calcification on routine skull roentgenograms. This percentage can be increased by using hypocycloidal tomography or computed tomography (CT) (Fig. 7). Evidence of calcification is seen in 83% of tumors by CT scan (101). However, other cases of leukocoria also may show calcifications.

Ultrasonography

Like radiology, ultrasonography is not a definitive test for retinoblastoma. A B-scan may show a solid intraocular echo with numerous dense focal echoes persisting at lower sensitivities, indicating calcifications within the mass (102). Occasionally, extremely high reflectivity varies with areas of strong sound attenuation, indicating the nature of the tumor, in which areas of rosette arrangements are replaced by large vessels and sections of necrosis (103). These ultrasonographic changes are highly indicative, but are not specific, and may yield both false-positive and false-negative results.

Ultrasonography is used for evaluation of treatment such as globe-conserving radiotherapy or chemotherapy (104). It permits monitoring of the response to

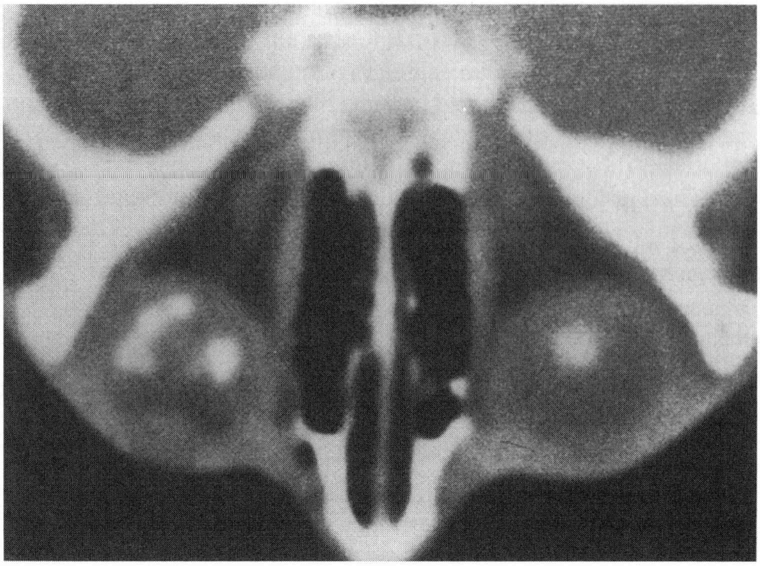

Figure 7 A CT scan of orbits of a patient with retinoblastoma: Note the prominent bilateral calcifications. (Courtesy of M. Maffee, MD.).

treatment and detects tumor growth or failure to respond (104). High frequency ultrasound can be used to evaluate extension into the anterior segment (105).

Fluorescein Angiography

Fluorescein angiography may detect tiny tumors because all tumors leak. According to Shields et al. (106), angiography may differentiate between a tumor within the retina (well-circumscribed staining) and a tumor with seeding into vitreous (ill-defined staining). This technique also may be helpful in evaluating results of conservative treatment. After successful destruction of the tumor, no leakage occurs, except accumulation of dye in the sclera (107). It has no value in detecting exophytic tumors, however.

Magnetic Resonance Imaging

Magnetic resonance imaging (MRI) is a useful examination in the evaluation of a patient with retinoblastoma (108,109). In children with an intraocular mass, MRI reliably distinguished between retinoblastoma and Coats' disease, toxocariasis, or persistent hyperplastic primary vitreous (PHPV), if the lesion was 4 mm or larger (109).

A newer high-resolution MRI carries a superb resolution of intraocular and orbital structures and can be successfully used to define the structure of the intraocular and orbital malignancy (110). Choroidal infiltration sometimes can be visualized but MRI is of limited value in visualization of prelaminar or postlaminar infiltration of the optic nerve (111).

Enzyme Assays

Dias et al. (112), suggested that lactic dehydrogenase (LDH) activity in the aqueous can be used as a test for retinoblastoma. Although the control subjects with various nonmalignant ocular diseases had aqueous levels of < 350 units/100 mL, four retinoblastoma patients had levels of 1800–3250 units/100 mL. However, following this discovery, the test was more frequently used, and cases of retinoblastoma were found with a low enough level of aqueous LDH activity to fall within the normal range. To increase the reliability of the test, it was suggested that the LDH aqueous level be compared with the serum ratio (113) and that the LDH aqueous isoenzyme pattern be measured (114). Total aqueous LDH level seem to be the most accurate index for the presence of retinoblastoma. Only about 10% of all patients will have false-negative findings (levels within normal values). To increase reliability, the sample used for the test must be fresh, not frozen, and free of blood (115).

High aqueous LDH levels may precede the appearance of a visible tumor by several months (116). This feature gives the best quantitative as well as qualitative value. Dias claims (117) that aqueous LDH increases in direct proportion to the duration of the tumor, the amount of undifferentiated cells and tumor necrosis, and the occurrence of retinal arterial occlusions.

Increased levels of both the γ- and α-subunits, with reduced levels of the β-subunit of the enzyme enolase were demonstrated by enzyme immunoassay of the aqueous (118). This could be useful in diagnosis of retinoblastoma.

Cytologic Examinations

If the diagnosis of retinoblastoma continues to be equivocal after all other examinations have been performed, then selected cases may undergo cytologic examination of aqueous and vitreous (119). Aqueous is aspirated, and vitreous is obtained by biopsy with a 19-gauge needle. The specimens undergo centrifugation and the sediment is stained and examined microscopically according to the Papanicolau technique. Again, false-negative results may occur.

Chromosomal Studies

Every retinoblastoma patient who shows mental retardation or any other systemic abnormality possibly related to chromosomal deletion retinoblastoma should undergo studies of the karyotype. The banding technique should be used in these studies.

Genetic Tests

With the advance in our understanding of the molecular genetics of retinoblastoma (see below), tests were developed to be used for diagnosis.

Polymerase chain reaction (PCR) has the potential to amplify minute amounts of DNA and to enable precise analysis of the mutation. Its use was implemented in the 1990s to analyze the RB1 gene and the loss of heterozygosity (120). Improvement in techniques and equipment continue.

Richter et al. (121) advised a combined, relatively rapid, sensitive and efficient method that was composed of three laboratory tests. First, an improved PCR, named quantitative multiplex PCR (QM-PCR) was performed. Second, mutations were sought by double-exon sequencing of the gene. Third, the promoter region, which may also harbour mutations, was searched by promoter-targeted methylation sensitive PCR. The turnaround time was three weeks, and the method detected 89% of the mutations (121). A less sensitive but more rapid method is the PTT-protein truncation testing. Tsai et al. (122) suggested this technique based on synthesis of protein from amplified RNA in vitro. The detection of a truncated protein signals the presence of a germline truncating mutation and yields 70% sensitive results and no false positives (122).

Esterase D Activity

Esterase D, an enzyme of unknown function that is found in most tissues of the body, can be tested in the peripheral blood by measuring its activity in erythrocytes. Normal red blood cells have an ESD activity of 68.9 ± 6.7 units. A low activity that is 50% of normal indicates a deletion of 13q14, which rarely is submicroscopic (123). There are two electrophoretic types of ESD: type I and type II. Some families have both alleles, and the intrafamilial segregation of these types may be helpful with genetic counseling (61).

Other Tests

There is probably no correlation between the occurrence of any retinoblastoma types and HLA antigens (124), although one study claimed a significantly increased frequency of HLA-w5 in retinoblastoma patients in Germany (125). There is no correlation with ABO blood types (126).

It has been suggested that fibroblasts obtained by skin or conjuctival biopsy from patients with hereditary retinoblastoma, and grown in tissue cultures, appear to be more sensitive to the lethal effect of irradiation (127). This method can be used to differentiate hereditary from the sporadic type. It was also claimed (128) that fibroblasts from patients with the hereditary type, grown in low concentrations of fetal calf serum, show significantly better growth than fibroblasts from patients with the sporadic type. However, these studies are controversial and are not used clinically (128,129). Wide-field specular microscopy displayed irregular oval dark structures on the endothelium in one patient (130). These were shown to be clusters of retinoblastoma cells.

Uric acid was elevated in the aqueous of patients with retinoblastoma, Coats' disease, and choroidal melanoma (131).

Pathology

The histologic features of retinoblastoma and retinoma are characteristic (Fig. 8). Tso et al. (131) recognized photoreceptor elements in retinoblastoma cells. Their neuronal nature is indicated by both the Flexner–Wintersteiner rosettes and the even more highly differentiated fleurettes (132). The type of cell population may classify the tumor into three groups: (i) differentiated tumors, with rosettes and fleurettes; (ii) intermediate or partially differentiated tumors, with trabeculoid patterns; and (iii) undifferentiated tumors, without any pattern of cells, found in the most malignant forms, mainly in extraocular tumors (133). In bilateral cases, the tumor may show dissimilar differentiation in. the two eyes (11,132). This may even occur in the same eye, indicating different primary foci. The initial deposit of calcium is surprisingly intramitchondrial, with plasmalemma disruption in tumor cells (134). Later, calcium aggregates in microbodies around a central calcified cone. The prognosis depends on the extent of invasion into surrounding tissues. Choroidal invasion, without scleral, iris, and optic nerve involvement results in 100% survival, as does optic nerve invasion that does not require resection (135).

Several lines of retinoblastoma cells are available in tissue cultures for studies (4). The study of the Y-79 human retinoblastoma cell line indicated that retinoblastoma

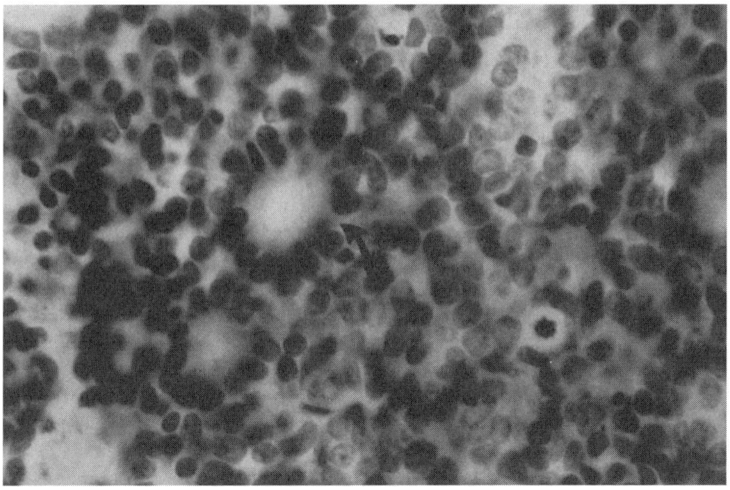

(a)

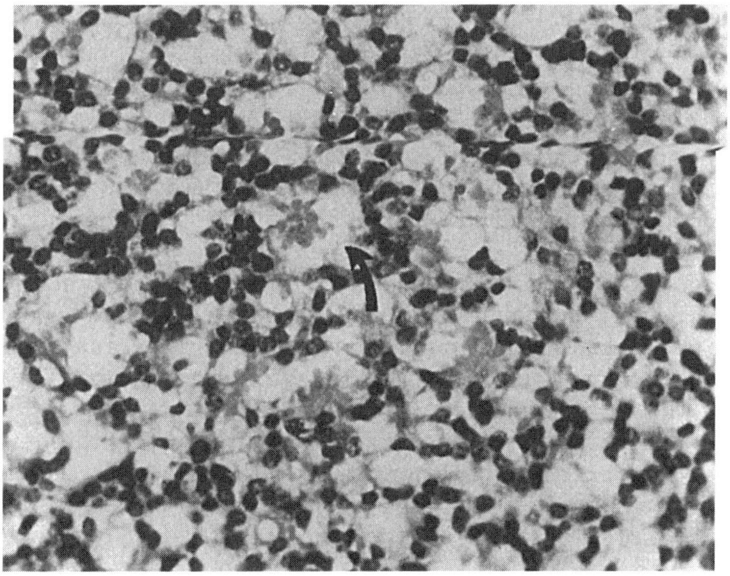

(b)

Figure 8 Histology of retinoblastoma: note the typical small cells with hyperchromatic nuclei. A well-differentiated malignant tumor (a) shows the Flexner–Wintersfeiner rosettes (arrows). A retinoma (b) shows the typical formation of fleurettes (arrow) (Courtesy of M. Tso, MD).

cells originate from a primitive retinal cell with multipotential characteristics and capability to differentiate into pigment epithelial, neuronal, or glial cells (136,137). However, the tumor cells have a predominantly neuronal nature with significant photoreceptor-like differentiation (138).

Immunocytochemical techniques, by which numerous retinal proteins were tested, confirmed that differentiated retinoblastoma cells most likely originate from the rod photoreceptor and possibly, from Muller cells (139).

Studies of a transgenic mouse model of retinoblastoma also confirmed the outer retinal origin of the tumor. Oncogenes were linked to retinal genes to produce both undifferentiated and well-differentiated retinoblastomas (140).

Electron microscopic studies indicate that, as a result of tumor necrosis and cell death, DNA precipitation occurs in the anterior segment of the affected eye (141), and that this phenomenon may be more common than suspected from routine histopathologic studies.

Retinoma, the benign form of the tumor, is composed of a thick mass of compact, well-differentiated neural elements, split by strands of Muller fibers and astrocytes (7,142) and fleurettes.

Karotype examinations of the tumor cells have yielded conflicting results. Report of different chromosomal anomalies have included 13q–, 14q–, 1q– or 6p anomalies, and many others (128,143,144). It seems that none of these changes is pathognomonic of retinoblastoma, except the loss of the segment 13ql4, as described in the following section.

Epidemiology and Genetics of Retinoblastoma

Incidence

The incidence of retinoblastoma is usually expressed as frequency per live births. Table 5 lists this frequency in different countries. The incidence of retinoblastoma seems to be fairly similar in most European countries (26). Extremes of 1:12,300 and 1:34,000 have been reported (3,18,150), but not confirmed. It appears that the range of frequencies is much narrower, around 1:16,000 to 1:20,000. A higher incidence of retinoblastoma has been reported in African blacks, American Navajo Indians, Haitians (see Table 5), and Hawaiians (13). The death rate from retinoblastoma is many times higher among American blacks than among American whites (146), but this is probably a result of delayed diagnosis and treatment, not a true difference of incidence (13,146,152). People of Maori and Polynesian origin in New Zealand have a incidence similar to that of the general population (22).

The general impression is that the frequency of retinoblastoma is increasing. In Finland, between 1912 and 1964, the frequency per live births increased in a stepwise

Table 5 Frequency of Retinoblastoma as Related to Live Births in Different Countries

Country	Year of publication (Ref.)	Ratio
Japan	1976 (16)	1:22,326
Ireland	1971 (145)	1:20,500
France	1974 (24)	1:20,000
United States	1975 (146)	1:18,000
Sweden	1979 (26)	1:18,000
New Zealand	1982 (22)	1:17,500
England	1975 (18)	1:16,000
South Africa (blacks)	1976 (147)	1:10,000
Malawi (Africans, blacks)	1976 (148)	1:10,000
American Navajo Indians	1983 (149)	1:6550
Haiti	1974 (150)	1:3300
Sweden, Finland[a]	2004 (151)	1:16,642

[a]Small changes in incidence during 40 years.

manner from 1:82,000 to 1:16,000 (2). Francois (27) estimated that the incidence apparently doubled between 1930 and 1965. Increases also have been noted in African blacks (153). Moreover, the incidence of bilateral blindness is increasing (27); conceivably, the rise in incidence may be mostly or wholly due to a greater number of hereditary cases.

A recent study of the incidence of retinoblastoma based on a national registry and cohort analysis was performed in Sweden and Finland. The incidence of retinoblastoma essentially remained stable, except for an insignificant increase during 40 years, and remained as 1:16,642 (151).

New Mutation Rates

The mutation rate of new cases of retinoblastoma is high. It has been calculated to be as high as 2.3×10^{-5} per generation (11,24). In Japan (16) the germinal mutation per generation was 8×10^{-6} and $9.3–10.9 \times 10^{-6}$ in New Zealand (15).

The Genetics of Retinoblastoma

Most retinoblastoma cases are sporadic, unilateral, and not inherited from parents. Such patients obviously cannot transmit the disease to their children. However, a large minority (about 40%) are hereditary cases. These patients carry the autosomal dominant *RB* gene and will transmit the disease to somewhat fewer than half of their children because of the incomplete penetrance of the gene. About 6–8% of all retinoblastomas (or 15–20% of all hereditary cases) are familial. In the rest, the distinction between hereditary and nonhereditary retinoblastoma may be difficult, unless the patient has bilateral retinoblastoma, indicating a carrier of the retinoblastoma *RB* gene.

These figures indicate that many heritable cases of retinoblastoma are due to new mutations. About 40% of retinoblastoma cases are of a germ-line mutation (154). About one-third of all new cases (after excluding familial cases) will be heritable (5). About 5% of all cases result from a chromosome 13 deletion (1).

The penetrance of the *RB* autosomal dominant gene is not complete, meaning that some carriers of the gene will not develop the disease. This penetrance is usually estimated at 80–90%. Merin et al. (41) suggested that the incomplete penetrance may, in part, be due to the occurrence of unrecognized spontaneously regressed tumors. Matsunaga (155) showed that penetrance of the gene varies among families. The proportion of gene carriers who manifest the disease (or gene penetrance) depends on the parent transmitting the gene. According to Matsunaga (155), the figures are 0.624 ± 0.0056 if the parent is an unaffected carrier, 0.836 ± 0.1 if the parent is unilaterally affected, and 0.984 ± 0.092 if the parent is bilaterally affected. Vogel (25) gave higher estimates of penetrance ranging from 0.927 ± 0.015 (when two children are affected and both parents are not) to 0.984 ± 0.007 (one unilaterally affected parent), and 0.996 ± 0.003 (one bilaterally affected parent).

Table 6 lists the manifestations of the *RB* gene. Familial occurrence, bilaterality, and a tumor of benign manifestation (retinoma) are extremely unlikely in nonhereditary cases and, for all practical purposes, confirm the inherited nature of the disease. Decreased ESD activity in the red blood cells is found in patients with 13ql4 deletions. It was described in one patient who had a submicroscopic deletion of 13ql4 (156), but not in other inherited cases. Most patients with inherited retinoblastoma have multiple primary tumors. Two or more tumors, proved histologically to be of different primary foci, confirm the diagnosis of inherited retinoblastoma.

Table 6 Manifestations of the *RB* Gene

Findings that confirm the presence of *RB* gene or 13q– in retinoblastoma patients
Familial occurrence
Retinoma
Two primary foci
Chromosomal aberrations
Decreased esterase D activity
Findings that increase the likelihood of an *RB* gene
Multiple tumors
Low age of onset
Second malignant tumor
Findings of questionable or unconfirmed value
Sensitivity of fibroblasts to x-ray
Growth rate of fibroblasts

However, a clinical distinction between multiple tumors from one primary focus and those from two primary foci may be very difficult. The mere existence of multiple tumors increases the chances of an inherited tumor.

It must be remembered that 5% of RB carriers show no tumor and 15% have only one tumor (129). The occurrence of a second malignant tumor is likely to be related to the *RB* gene (74,84,88).

Most patients with hereditary retinoblastomas demonstrate symptoms before age 1 year and rarely after age 2, a feature useful for differential diagnosis.

Different biologic characteristics of fibroblasts between patients with hereditary and nonhereditary retinoblastomas are still being investigated.

Molecular Background

How is this genetic entity translated into the phenotype of retinoblastoma? How could the *RB* gene form one or several primary foci of malignant tumors? Knudson (157) tried to answer this question in 1971 with his two-hit theory. According to Knudson, the formation of a retinoblastoma is a two-mutational event; the first event is germinal (and inherited), and the second is somatic (occurs directly in the affected retinal cells). In nonhereditary forms both mutations are at the somatic level. If an individual with a germinal mutation has an average of three primary tumors, statistical analysis can also explain the phenomena of a single tumor in one eye only and an RB carrier having no tumor at all. Knudson et al. elaborated further to include chromosomal deletion retinoblastoma and more quantitative analysis (53,158). If this theory is true, then retinoblastoma is a recessive disease at the cellular level and a double dose of the gene is required for the induction of the disease (53). The chances of a RB carrier developing retinoblastoma are extremely high because the "second event" needs to occur only once in any of many millions of predisposed cells. The chances of a non-RB carrier (general population) to develop retinoblastoma are extremely small because rarely do two separate events hit the same cell in the developing retina.

Cavenee et al. (159) and Dryja et al. (160) showed that homozygosity of large portions of chromosome 13 is common in the tumor cells, and that the recessive nature of the tumor at the cellular level is frequently manifested by chromosomal mechanisms. These included mitotic nondisjunction, with loss of wild-type (hemizygous chromosome); mitotic nondisjunction, with reduplication of the mutant type (homozygous chromosomes); and mitotic recombination between *RB* locus and centromere (partially homozygous chromosomes). Such chromosomal anomalies were found in both inherited and sporadic possibly noninherited cases, as would be expected if Knudson's theory is correct.

The phenomenon of a benign tumor occurring in retinoblastoma was explained by Knudson's theory as being a result of only one event, the germinal hit. In these patients cells proliferate until delayed maturation occurs, resulting in benign hyperplasia. Knudson extended his two-hit theory to include all other tumors with a benign counterpart: neuroblastoma vs. neuroblastoma IV-S or ganglioneuroma; neurofibrosarcoma vs. hereditary neurofibroma; medullary carcinoma of thyroid vs. C-cell hyperplasia; and pheochromocytoma vs. adrenal medullary hyperplasia (161).

Other studies support Knudson's theory in principle. Studies involving ESD activity and chromosomal deletion technique showed that a second event does occur at the tumor cellular level. Some studies of the karyotype of tumor cells have suggested that the second hit involves other chromosomes, such as 1 and 6 (128). However, this seems unlikely. Recent studies involving ESD activity (a distinct gene located very close to the *RB* gene), indicated the close involvement of this area on chromosome 13 in both the first and second hit (162). Benedict et al. (155), studying the tumor karyotype of a patient with submicroscopic deletion of one 13ql4, concluded that, in tumor cells of their patient, the parallel area on the normal chromosome 13 was lost. The two hits resulting in the development of retinoblastoma are one and the same: loss of a gene at 13ql4 (156). When this happens, the tumor may develop because of a similar defect on both chromosomes of the same cell. This would be evidence that, at the cellular level, retinoblastoma is a recessive disease.

Malignant transformation of a retinal cell occurs when both homologous copies of the *RB* gene have a loss-of-function mutation (141). Therefore, the *RB* gene is an antioncogene. One copy of the normal *RB* gene is sufficient to prevent malignant transformation of the primitive retinal cell. Its loss by deletion or other loss-of-function mutation will induce the formation of retinoblastoma (163). A group of human cancers in addition to retinoblastoma, are now suspected to be caused by the loss of a "cancer suppression gene." These include osteosarcoma, Wilms' tumor, hepatoblastoma, rhabdomyosarcoma, uveal melanoma, bladder cell carcinoma, acoustic neuroma, and meningioma (164).

Some objections were raised to Knudson's theory. Gallie et al. (43) suggested that retinoma also results from a two-mutational event, but that the second hit occurs in mature or relatively mature retinoblasts. Retinoblastoma develops when the second hit occurs in immature retinoblasts. Carlson et al. (14) introduced terms, such as mutational mosaicism and cryptic mosaics, which could account for these inconsistencies. Mutational mosaicism explains cases of unilateral involvement with transmission of bilateral retinoblastoma. A mutation occurs early in embryogenesis, and mutant cells enter both the embryonic gonad and one of the two developing optic cups. The term *cryptic mosaics* explains families with more than one affected sibling and normal parents. Here, according to Carlson et al. (14), a new mutation occurs in early embryogenesis in the inferior region of the embryo, affecting the primordial germ cells. These suggestions are at variance with Knudson's theory, which postulates that such events are simply a result of normal statistical distribution.

Knudson's theory assumes that the second hit occurs randomly, in accordance with statistical laws, and, therefore, does not explain phenomena such as the familial occurrence of retinomas (40,48), similar age of onset of the disease in both eyes (17), and the different number of affected children according to the phenotype of the affected parent (155). Matsunaga suggests that factors involving inherited host resistance determine the age of onset and expressivity (bilateral, unilateral, or no tumor) (17,155).

In summary, it is assumed that Knudson's two-hit theory is basically correct. The second hit is, at the cellular level, similar to the first hit, which is the loss or inactivation of a gene. However, the second hit is not completely random, but is somewhat influenced by other factors. These factors are likely to be inherited, to render the gene or chromosome more vulnerable to the second hit, but they could be environmental, or a combination of the two.

Knudson calculated that the average number of primary retinoblastoma tumors in a heritable case would be three. This calculation was based on the number of retinal cells and the likelihood of a "second hit" (154). To form a malignant tumor the second mutation must occur before the final differentiation of the cell occurs.

The location of the retinoblastoma gene was studied initially by chromosomal deletions and translocations, and later by cDNA probes. It was mapped to chromosome 13ql4.1-ql4.2 (165). The cloning of the gene, named *RB1*, was achieved in 1986 (166) and its structure was confirmed, identified and sequenced in 1987 (167,168). The gene *RB1* is a large gene. It contains 27 exons, spans 180–200 kb pairs, and is grouped in three domains separated by two large introns (120,169). It encodes a protein, pRb, which is a nuclear phosphoprotein expressed in all human cells. It consists of 928 amino acids (169,170). The protein plays a role in the regulation of the cell division cycle and cell apoptosis (169,170). Possibly, pRb protein is the master regulator of the balance between cell cycle, differentiation and apoptosis. Loss of its function leads to severe disturbance of differentiation and either death through apoptosis or unlimited multiplication. Therefore, pRb is a tumor suppressor protein. In some cases it cooperates with p53 protein, another tumor-suppressor protein (170).

In retinoblastoma tumors, early studies demonstrated a high frequency of mutations, deletions or breakpoints (171–173). Translocation breakpoints with intragenic deletions were also detected. The gene *RB1* was also found to have binding activity to both cellular DNA (174) and adenovirus polypeptides (142).

A large number of retinoblastoma-associated mutations were identified in the *RB1* gene. Mutations were identified in all 27 exons and in the promoters (169). No hot spot of mutation was detected but there was a preference for more mutations on exons 3, 8, 18, 19 (169), 13, 17 (175) and 23 (176). Exons 25–27 are less affected or not affected (177); most identified mutations were small (1-bp or 2-bp) deletions, leading to premature termination (175). Harbour (176) listed 192 patients with identifiable mutations. Seventy-eight percent had nonsense or frameshift mutations; only 6% had missense mutations, and the rest were introns mutations, in-frame deletions and promoter mutations (176). Lohmann et al. (177) found 42% of base substitutions. They also found no correlation between the location of frameshift or nonsense mutation and the phenotypic features including age at diagnosis, number of tumors or manifestation of second malignancy (177).

In summary of the mutations, missense mutations and inframe deletions are rare while premature terminations leading to a truncated protein are the rule (178).

Mutations of the "second hit" are different. They include intragenic mutations, whole gene deletion, and chromosomal loss by nondisjunction and somatic recombinations (154). Hogg et al. (179) found independent mutations in the two alleles in four of 12 retinoblastoma cases. In the rest, only one mutation was identified, consistent with the loss of heterozygosity (LOH) theory. Some mutations probably tend to cause a specific phenotype, Low-penetrance retinoblastoma may be caused by a specific location or by missense mutation (180,181). Harbour (182) claimed that nine different mutations are associated with low penetrance retinoblastoma (182). This occurs in one of two ways. One, when the mutation alone reduces the level of expression of the normal pRb. These are rare and occur when the mutation is in the promoter region or in a splice-site. Two, when the mutation produces a partially inactivated pRb. This happens with some missense point mutations (182).

The mutation in a case of an ectopic intracranial retinoblastoma has been identified as a nonsense mutation in exon 17, codon 556 (183).

The inactivation of the retinoblastoma susceptibility gene is the crucial step in the formation of retinoblastoma or osteosarcoma. This hypothesis was proven by gene transfer. A cloned *RB* gene that was introduced into retinoblastoma and osteosarcoma cells suppressed the neoplastic phenotype (184), thereby confirming the hypothesis.

The Management of Retinobiastoma

Faced with a possible case of retinoblastoma, the ophthalmologist should (i) verify the diagnosis by ophthalmoscopy and other examinations; (ii) decide if the patient has a hereditary, a chromosome-deletion, or a nonhereditary retinoblastoma; (iii) estimate where the patient belongs in the Reese-Ellsworth classification; (iv) decide on a treatment for the patient; (v) examine other family members if hereditary retinoblastoma is suspected; and (vi) provide genetic counseling to the family, including advice about prenatal diagnosis, if needed.

Surgical and Medical Treatment

Only a brief description of the approaches to treatment of retinoblastoma will be covered here. The subject is detailed thoroughly in standard textbooks on tumors of the eye (185–188) and in the referred articles.

The treatment of retinoblastoma (9) has greatly changed since the beginning of the 19th century when some patients with retinoblastoma survived the disease after undergoing simple excision of the eye. In 1977, the survival rate approached 90% of all retinoblastoma patients (12). More than pure numbers, the change of the objectives expresses the progress in the treatment of retinoblastoma. The goal of preservation of life has shifted to preservation of vision; from preservation of vision in one eye in bilateral cases, to preservation of vision in the one affected eye in unilateral cases.

There is a definite trend away from enucleation as the primary treatment of retinoblastoma. By 1988, 25% of unilaterally affected eyes and 25% of both bilaterally affected eyes were salvaged (189). Anterior chamber involvement is, however, an indication for enucleation without delay (190). Maximal optic nerve length should be obtained in this surgery since leaving any portion of an infiltrated nerve in the orbit means that the patient's life will not be saved. Abramson (191) advised the nasal approach for enucleation to obtain a longer optic nerve cut off.

Photocoagulation or cryotherapy can be used as the only treatment, resulting in a successful eradication of a retinoblastoma in groups 1 and 2 of the Reese-Ellsworth classification (192,193). Xenon arc photocoagulation is used for posterior pole tumors. Cryotherapy is applied to tumors located anterior to the equator, except when located at the vitreous base, for which such treatment failed (193). Cryotherapy may be repeated to increase its effectiveness, and it may be used following radiation therapy when dosage becomes critical and the tumor is not completely eradicated (133), The triple freeze-thaw technique is efficient in most of the treated tumors of these groups (194).

Larger tumors may be treated by external beam irradiation (192), with use of 3500 rad in favorable cases and 4500 rad in advanced cases (113). External high-energy radiotherapy by linear accelerators with 5 to 7-mV photon capacity is an effective treatment for most cases belonging to Reese-Ellsworth groups 1–4 (195,196). Complications of the treatment include cataract and vitreous hemorrhage, which can be reduced by proper alignment of the beam. Recurrences should be treated by photocoagulation, cryotherapy, or cobalt applicators, rather than by a second course of beam irradiation (82,192). Chemotherapy can be an adjunct in selected cases of group 4 tumors, and used to treat unrecognized micrometastases and metastatic disease, residual tumors after enucleation, or brain tumor in trilateral retinoblastoma (114,192,197–199).

External beam radiotherapy (EBR) became a concern because of the possible effect on second malignancies, both in the field of radiation and outside this field, in addition to other complications and side effects. The EBR whole eye technique was used as a primary treatment for retinoblastoma in 175 eyes with retinoblastoma of groups I–V. Fifty-seven percent of eyes were preserved, a figure that rose to 65% with additional salvage therapy (200). The lens sparing technique of EBR was used in 67 eyes of groups I–III with an overall of 72% success, a figure that turned into 93% with salvage therapy (201). The results of EBR, used in various modified techniques, seem to be good in most cases (202). Hall et al. (203) treated 74 children with bilateral retinoblastoma. by EBR. Sixty-two percent had one eye removed. Of the rest, 58% remained with vision of 20/20 to 20/40, 31% with vision of 20/50 to 20/400 and 9% with <9% (203). Blach et al. (204) compared the two modified techniques of EBR and concluded that the modified lateral beam technique was superior to the lens sparing technique for tumors in groups I–III.

The last decade marked a trend to a different approach and avoidance of external radiation because of the concern of secondary tumors, in spite of the fact that an association between EBR and such tumors is debatable (205). Chemotherapy or chemoreduction therapy is based on the use of carboplatin and etoposide (206) and to this vincristine sulfate is usually added (207,208). This combined treatment, named VEC for vincristine, etoposide and carboplatin, is given in six cycles (209,210). New tumors may develop in spite of chemotherapy (211), especially in eyes with vitreous or subretinal seeding. Lee et al. (212) found 1.1 new tumors per eye after carboplatin systemic treatment and more if the child was <six months old at the treatment.

Adjuvant therapy by cryo or laser or thermoapplications or brachytherapy or EBR increases the success rate (209,213). Other possible adjuvant therapies included 532-nm or 1064-nm laser, cryotherapy (214), and brachytherapy by iridium-192 plaque (215) or by subconjunctival delivery of carboplatin (216,217) and EBR (218). Histology of eyes enucleated after chemoreduction indicated that in some cases the tumor regression was not complete (219). Shields et al. (220) reported that the recurrence rate after a mean interval of five months was 9% in patients with sporadic retinoblastoma and 80% (1) in patients with familial retinoblastoma. This may indicate that some of these are new tumors and not recurrences of insufficiently treated tumors. Comparison of EBR with chemotherapy showed that chemoreduction yields earlier tumor reduction than EBR (221).

Enucleation is now usually used for patients of group IV or V if prior treatment by chemoreduction or EBR or both failed (192,222). EBR and adjuvant treatment may be successful in advanced cases (223).

For suitable cases, especially with small tumors, brachytherapy can be used. Cobalt plaques of different sizes are sometimes used as primary treatment (12,224,225) or as adjuvant treatment (226). Other scleral plaques, such as iodine-125, iridium-192, and ruthenium-162 have also been used for local irradiation (227,228).

Small tumors were also treated by thermotherapy as the only treatment. Of 188 retinoblastomas, with a mean base size of 3 mm and thickness of 2 mm complete regression occurred in 161 (85.6%) (229). In patients with massive orbital involvement, as often seen in developing countries, aggressive treatment that includes radical surgery, chemotherapy and EBR can be helpful (230).

Genetic Counseling

Table 7 lists the risk of siblings and children for developing retinoblastoma in different families. For proper counseling all facts related to the carrier state of the *RB* gene and its penetrance and expressivity in a particular family should be known. Risk figures are based on genetic calculations, penetrance figures, and empiric data (18,25).

In selected families, linkage studies can be done to improve counseling. As ESD activity is closely linked to the *RB* gene (61,123,162), families carrying two types of ESD enzyme may be suitable for such studies (231). Molecular genetic methods using restriction fragment length polymorphisms (RFLPS) and isozymic alleles of different loci at 13ql4, including the *ESD* gene may be helpful in the genetic evaluation of the family (232,233).

Since the *RB1* gene was identified and encoded, the cloned retinoblastoma gene can be used to detect the mutation predisposing to hereditary retinoblastoma. In two studies involving familial retinoblastoma, these DNA markers identified the genetic

Table 7 Risk for Siblings and Children to Develop Retinoblastoma[a]

Patient	Family history	Risk for being a carrier	Risk for children	Risk for siblings
Affected[b]	Parent affected	100	42–49	42–49
Bilateral	Negative	100	42–49	6[c,e]
Normal	One parent, one sib affected	9	4	42–49
Unilateral				
One tumor unilateral	Negative	10–12	5–6	1–1.5[e]
Two or more tumors[d]	Negative	100	42–49	

[a]Figures are in percent and are approximate.
[b]Including those affected by retinoma only.
[c]The risk to siblings exists because in some cases an unaffected parent may be a carrier of the gene.
[d]Confirmed to be separate primary foci.
[e]This figure may be lower in older fathers, as the patient has a higher chance for a new mutation (14).

risk with a confidence level of 90–99% (234,235). This high rate of accurate prediction is achieved only in families with two or more affected members, who share a common DNA marker.

Wiggs and Dryja (236) summarized the possibility of molecular genetics to predict occurrence of hereditary retinoblastoma in families with only one affected member.

First, high-resolution chromosome-banding technique can detect deletions of more than 2 million base pairs of DNA. As the *RB* gene is approximately 200,000 base pairs of DNA in size, this method can be used only in deletion retinoblastoma.

Second, the Southern blotting technique can detect mutations of the genomic DNA. An analysis of 20 families showed such mutations in 3 (15%).

Third, analysis of tumor DNA can sometimes allow the identification of the chromosome carrying the tumor-predisposing mutation because, in most cases (50–70%), it is the chromosome carrying the normal gene that becomes lost in the tumor cells. If the abnormal chromosome and its origin are identified, it can be used as a marker to detect the genetic risk of developing retinoblastoma.

Currently, more accurate and rapid methods of molecular genetics investigation have been developed and are being used (see "Laboratory Tests and Additional Examinations.").

The initial mutation in nonhereditary retinoblastoma occurred equally in genes of paternal or maternal origin. However, in new germline mutations of an inherited tumor, the initial mutation involved the paternal gene in all of eight patients examined (237). This is consistent with the view that new germline mutations arise primarily during spermatogenesis. Preferential inheritance of *RB1* among children of male carriers was also documented in another study (238).

Prenatal Diagnosis

Prenatal diagnosis was initially given only in cases of increased risk for chromosomal-deletion retinoblastoma, by examining cells of the amniotic fluid for their karyotype or for their ESD activity. A decreased ESD activity of approximately 50% indicated that the fetus would manifest chromosomal-deletion retinoblastoma (98,239). Five percent of patients with retinoblastoma carry such a detectable constitutional deletion of 13q (233). Later, polymorphic probes were used for prenatal counseling, based on the results of amniocentesis (234,235) or on chorionic villus sampling (240).

Since the 1990s RB1 gene mutations have been identified in some cases. Onadim et al. (241) used intragenic DNA probes based on RFLPs. Prenatal diagnosis was performed on chorionic villus sampling obtained in four embryos or by cord blood samples or by neonatal venipuncture. In one case, a mutated RB1 gene accurately predicted the development of retinoblastoma. In six others the results were negative and follow up showed them to be disease-free (241).

The end of the 1990s and the beginning of the 21st century marked the development of in-vitro fertilization (IVF) with pre-implantation genetic diagnosis (PGD) as a better alternative to prenatal diagnosis (242,243). PGD has been developed for prevention of pregnancies with severe inherited diseases of chromosomal aberration or single-gene defects. One or two blastomeres were biopsied from human embryos at the 8–10 cells stage, after IVF. The cells are DNA-tested to detect RB1 mutation. On day 5, after an initial negative response, the cells are transferred to the uterus for continuing pregnancy (242–245).

MALIGNANT MELANOMA

Malignant melanoma of the uvea is a relatively rare and usually sporadic disease that is unrelated to cutaneous malignant melanoma. The hereditary occurrence of a malignant melanoma is well known in different species of fish (246). In humans, a rare, inherited, autosomal dominant disease causes both uveal and cutaneous melanomas, as well as other malignant tumors. This rare inherited disease was variously referred to as "B–K mole syndrome" (247); FAMMM—Familial Atypical Multiple Mole-Melanoma Syndrome (248); and "dysplastic nevus syndrome" (249). We will use the term FAMMM because it appears more commonly in the literature.

The Clinical Manifestations of Familial Atypical Multiple Mole-Melanoma Syndrome

Skin Lesions

The most common lesions of FAMMM syndrome occur on the skin. Carriers of the gene have tan, brown, or pink large (more than 5 mm) moles (247). The number of moles ranges from 10 to 100, and they appear mostly on the upper trunk and extremities (247). They vary in size, shape, and color, and continue to grow during life (250). The moles have a high tendency for malignant transformation into cutaneous malignant melanoma, which is often multicentric.

Ocular Lesions

Uveal malignant melanomas, indistinguishable from the sporadic tumor, were described in a much higher incidence than expected in families with FAMMM syndrome (251–254). In one familial case, bilateral uveal malignant melanomas occurred (253).

Other Lesions

Several other malignancies occur in a high frequency in FAMMM syndrome, including carcinomas of lung, pancreas, and breast (254). One patient from a family with this syndrome had eight different tumors in her body, two of them malignant (250).

Pathology and Pathogenesis

The skin lesion shows histologically atypical melanocytic hyperplasia, lymphocytic infiltration, fibroplasia, and the growth of new blood vessels within a compound nevus (247). The transformation of two such moles into malignant melanomas was documented photographically by Clark et al. (247).

The hereditary intraocular melanoma is histologically similar to the sporadic melanoma. It usually affects the choroid, but melanomas of the iris and ciliary body have also been described (251).

Cytogenic studies found frequent structural aberrations and anomalies of chromosome 6 and, to a lesser extent, of chromosome 1 in tumor cells of malignant melanoma (255).

Epidemiology and Genetics

Malignant melanoma of the uvea has an incidence of about 1:160,000 in the general population, whereas cutaneous malignant melanoma occurs more frequently with a 1:25,000 incidence (252,256). Six new cases per million occur annually in the United States (257). The possibility of a random occurrence of both tumors in the same patient is possible (258), but extremely rare. The hereditary nature of some uveal melanomas is indicated by both the occurrence of uveal melanoma in families with FAMMM syndrome and by the occurrence of both cutaneous and uveal melanoma in the same family. In two families, each with two members affected by uveal melanoma, no genetic markers were detected (259).

The FAMMM syndrome is transmitted as an autosomal dominant disease with a high but unknown penetrance and a variable expressivity. A carrier of the gene may demonstrate a mole, a cutaneous melanoma, an uveal melanoma, or other cancers. However, some obligate carriers have shown no sign (249), indicating incomplete penetrance of the gene.

A retrospective study of 4600 patients with primary uveal melanoma revealed eight patients with a biopsy-proven FAMMM syndrome. Three of the eight had a positive family history of melanoma, two cutaneous and one uveal (260).

Families with three generations affected by malignant melanoma of the uvea have been reported (261). Some patients and their siblings have had additional malignant tumors documented, which stresses the pleiotropic effect of the autosomal dominant gene. Familial intraocular melanoma occurs about 20 years earlier than nonfamilial melanoma (251), a phenomenon also observed in other hereditary tumors.

Singh and Donoso (262) reviewed 14 families with familial uveal melanoma. Phenotypically they were similar to sporadic cases except for earlier onset. Young et al. (263) reviewed 15 reported families and added 11 additional families with two or more members affected. Singh et al. studied 4500 uveal melanoma patients and found 17 kindreds of probands with additional first degree relative (264) and 27 families with first or second degree relative (265). They conclude that familial occurrence of uveal melanoma is not coincidental. Singh et al. (265) described a father and son occurrence of choroidal melanoma and estimated the likelihood of familial uveal melanoma as 0.6% of all melanomas.

Both hereditary conditions, such as neurofibromatosis (267), and nonhereditary ones, such as nevus of Ota (268), may predispose the patient to the development of uveal melanoma.

Uveal malignant melanoma is known to be very rare in blacks. Miller et al. (269) estimated that the whites/blacks ratio for uveal malignant melanoma is 80:1. Why this tumor is so rare in blacks is unknown, but a similar difference in the incidence of cutaneous melanoma is well known. It has been suggested that HLA-DR4 is present in higher frequency in patients than in controls (270), but this has not been confirmed.

Cutaneous malignant melanoma and uveal malignant melanoma are generally independent and occur as separate diseases, except in the familial syndromes. A study of the family history of 400 patients with uveal melanoma revealed that at least 14 patients showed a family history of cutaneous melanoma and at least two had a family history of uveal melanoma (271). How this link is caused is unknown, but one study using immunohistochemical techniques has demonstrated antigens shared by both uveal and cutaneous melanomas (272).

Bilateral uveal melanoma may also be an indication for a hereditary tendency. Singh et al. (273) found eight such cases among 4500 uveal melanoma patients instead of a statistical prediction of one such case. In the world literature, 44 well-documented cases have been reported (273).

Association between familial uveal malignant melanoma and various gene mutations is reported for several families. Jay and McCartney (274) reported a four-generation family with uveal melanoma with a likely mutation of the p53 gene. Mouriaux et al. (275) reported that tumor cells of uveal melanoma carried mutations of p21 and p27, two proteins (out of three) of the cyclin-dependent kinase inhibitory proteins. These proteins play a critical role in the regulation of cell cycle. The third protein, p16, did not show any mutations in uveal melanoma (276). Foster et al. (277) demonstrated that mutations of the NFl (neurofibromatosis) gene may play a role in uveal melanoma.

Clinical Management

The treatment methods of familial uveal melanoma should be similar to the accepted methods of treatment of sporadic malignant melanoma. Genetic counseling for affected families should begin, after the family pedigree and the particular manifestation of the disease in the family are studied, keeping in mind the pleiotropic effect of the gene.

All potentially affected family members should undergo ophthalmologic and dermatologic examinations to rule out silent tumors.

XERODERMA PIGMENTOSUM

Most hereditary tumors develop from an interaction between the genetic predisposition of the patient and environmental factors that determine the formation of the malignancy (278). The best example of such interaction is seen in cases of xeroderma pigmentosum (XP), an autosomal recessive disease in which the injurious external factor is now well known.

Clinical Manifestations

The skin and the eye are affected most by xeroderma pigmentosum. Sometimes neurologic changes occur.

Skin Lesions

The earliest changes of xeroderma pigmentosum occur during the first two years of life, with increased skin sensitivity to sunlight and the appearance of erythema in exposed areas. Later, hyperpigmentation of the skin develops, mainly expressed as myriads of freckles. When areas of atrophy and telangiectasis are added, the skin appears to have "salt and pepper" spots. Still later, at a variable time during life, hyperkeratosis and malignant changes occur. The lesions may develop anywhere in exposed areas, but the face—around the mouth and the eyes—seems to be especially affected. Different malignant and benign tumors have been described in XP (Table 8), the most frequent being basal cell and squamous cell carcinomas (279).

Table 8 Frequent Benign and Malignant Skin Tumors in XP

Fibroma
Angioma
Keratoacanthoma
Basal cell carcinoma
Squamous cell carcinoma
Malignant melanoma
Sarcoma

Ocular Lesions

Stenson (279) has described two patients with XP and reviewed the literature on reported ocular changes in the disease.

The earliest ocular changes in XP are probably related to photophobia and eyelid disorders. Later, the conjunctiva shows xerosis, edema, keratinization, hyperpigmentation, and atrophy (279). There is an increased tendency for conjunctival infections and scarring. Tumors develop, starting with the common benign and large pinguecula, pterygia, and pseudopterygia, up to malignant tumors, such as squamous cell carcinomas. The cornea frequently opacifies or clouds and tends to develop infective ulcers and perforates. Keratomalacia, with dissolution of the whole cornea, has also been observed.

It has been suggested (280,281) that XP in blacks is clinically different from that in whites by being mild in the skin and severe in the eyes. In blacks the cornea may become opaque by age two years from invasive blood vessels (281).

Pathology and Pathogenesis

Histologic features of XP in the skin are nonspecific, but the combination of atrophy, hyperkeratosis, proliferation, accumulation of melanin, and inflammation may be suggestive of XP (282). In the later stage, basal cell carcinomas and (less frequently) squamous cell carcinomas or other tumors are found.

In 1968, Cleaver (283) showed that cells from XP patients are defective in repair of their DNA structure after damage from ultraviolet (UV) light. The damage by UV to cells of XP patients is like that of normal cells, except that normal cells can repair the damaged pyrimidine dimers of their DNA, but XP cells cannot or have a very reduced ability to do so (284).

In addition (284), cells from XP patients are deficient in repairing DNA damage from chemical mutagens or carcinogens. The XP cells also show an increased number of UV-induced sister chromatid exchanges. Because of these changes in the DNA, UV radiation induces mutations at the somatic cellular level. Robbins (284) reviewed these mutations as follows:

1. Freckles occur because UV-induced mutation causes a single melanin-producing cell to form a clone of melanocytes.
2. Hypopigmented areas are created because UV-induced mutation causes melanocytes to lose their ability to produce melanin.
3. Precancerous and cancerous lesions are demonstrated because the UV-induced mutation in the DNA forms a clone of such cells. The frequency of mutations per unit dose of UV and of UV-induced neoplastic transformation is higher in XP than in controls (285).

Epidemiology and Genetics

The incidence of XP is low, approximately 1:1million to 4:1million births (284). The disease is found throughout the world and in all races. Xeroderma pigmentosum is an autosomal recessive disease, but in the last years, at least eight genetic variants have been discovered (286). Of these eight, seven complementation groups (A–G) of patients with defective excision of pyrimidine dimers have been identified. Normal repair of DNA in fibroblasts occurs if two different complementation groups have their cells fused together. The last group has a defect in postreplicative repair (variant form). The genes were cloned and the mapping completed for the seven-

Table 9 The Genetic Variants of XP

	Complementation group	Symbol	Gene	Chromosomal location	Reference	Remarks
1	XPA correcting XP, group A XP type I	XPA	XP1	9q22.3	287	Fusion of cells with other groups, not mixing, can repair the DNA
2	XPB XP, group B XP type II	XPB	ERCC3	2q21	288	ERCC3 for: excision-repair, complementing defective, in Chinese hamster, 3
3	XPC XP, group C XP type III	XPC	XP3	3p25.1	289	XP3 gene repairs the defective DNA by selective repair of cyclobutane pyrimidine dimers.
4	XPD XP, group D XP type VIII	XPD	ERCC2	19q13.2	290	Clinically: trichothiodystrophy sulfur-deficient brittle hair with sun sensitivity. CNS abnormalities
5	XPE XP group E XP type V	XPE	DDB2	11p11-p12	233	DDB2 for DNA damage-binding protein 2
6	XPF XP group F XP type VI	XPF	ERCC4	16p13.3	291	Rare
7	XPG XP group G	XPG	ERCC5	13q32-q33	292	
8	XP variant	XPV	—	—	291	Uncloned; could be more than one gene

complementation groups. Mutations associated with XP were identified in each. XP-variant gene is currently not yet known (Table 9).

Groups A and C are the most common (286); group A is most frequent in Japan, and group C is most usual in Europe and the United States (284).

Clinical Management

The clinical management of a patient with XP should include treatment of lesions that already have formed and preventive measures, whereby exposure to UV is reduced. For ocular lesions, the use of topical antibiotics is necessary for infections and corneal inflammations. Surgical excision of tumors of the eyelid, conjunctiva, and limbus is frequently needed. Perforating keratoplasty may be performed to exchange a cloudy cornea or one on the verge of perforation or a scarred cornea causing high astigmatism. There is a high incidence of graft rejection and the use of immunosuppressive drugs has been suggested (281) to reduce this risk in blacks. As the risk of graft rejection is high in whites as well, immunosuppressives should be considered in all patients with XP.

Genetic counseling is based on the understanding that XP is an autosomal recessive disease with different genetic subgroups. Only if both parents carry the gene for the same complementation group will 25% of the children be affected. For the same reason, both parents may be homozygotes and affected, but if their complementation groups are different, no children will be affected. The frequency of the different complementation groups, however, depends on location; certain populations may have the same complementation group of XP.

Prenatal diagnosis can be made (293). Cells taken by amniocentesis have been found to have deficient DNA repair in an affected fetus. Postreplication repair can also be measured in amniotic cells to discover the variant form of XP.

REFERENCES

1. Roberts DF, Aherne GES. Retinoblastoma. In: Emery AEH, Rimoin DL, eds. Principles and Practice of Medical Genetics. Edinburgh: Churchill-Livingstone, 1983: 539–554.
2. Tarkkanen A, Tuovinen E. Retinoblastoma in Finland 1912–64. Acta Ophthalmol 1971; 49:293–300.
3. Zakka KA, Yee RD, Foos RY. Retinoblastoma in a 12-year old girl. Ann Ophthalmol 1983; 15:88–91.
4. McFall RC, Sery TW, Makadon M. Characterization of a new continuous cell line derived from a human retinoblastoma. Cancer Res 1977; 37:1003–1010.
5. Gallie BL, Phillips RA, Ellsworth RM, Abramson DM. Significance of retinoma and phthisis bulbi for retinoblastoma. Ophthalmology 1982; 89:1393–1399.
6. Smith JLS, Bedford MA. Retinoblastomas. In: Marsden HB, Stewart JK, eds. Tumors in Children. 2nd ed. Berlin: Springer-Verlag, 1976:245–281.
7. Margo C, Hidayat A, Kopelman J, Zimmerman LE. Retinocytoma: a benign variant of retinoblastoma. Arch Ophthalmol 1983; 101:1519–1531.
8. Aaby AA, Price RL, Zakov ZN. Spontaneously regressing retinoblastomas, retinoma or retinoblastoma group 0. Am J Ophthalmol 1983; 96:315–320.
9. Gailloud G. Retinoblastoma—introduction. Mod Probl Ophthalmol 1977; 18:92–93.
10. Jensen RD, Miller RW. Retinoblastoma: epidemiological characteristics. N Engl J Med 1971; 285:307–311.

11. Sang DN, Albert DM. Recent advances in the study of retinoblastoma. In: Peyman GA, Apple DJ, Sanders DR, eds. Intraocular Tumors. New York: Appleton-Century-Crofts, 1977:285–329.
12. Bedford MA. Management of retinoblastoma. Mod Probl Ophthalmol 1977; 18: 101–105.
13. Pendergrass TW, Davis S. Incidence of retinoblastoma in the United States. Arch Ophthalmol 1980; 98:1204–1210.
14. Carlson EA, Letson RD, Ramsay NKC, Desnick RJ. Factors for improved genetic counseling for retinoblastoma based on a survey of 55 families. Am J Ophthalmol 1979; 87:449–459.
15. Fitzgerald PH, Stewart J, Suckling RD. Retinoblastoma mutation rate in New Zealand and support for the two-hit model. Hum Genet 1983; 64:128–330.
16. Matsunaga E, Oggu H. Retinoblastoma in Japan: follow-up survey of sporadic cases. Jpn J Opthalmol 1976; 20:266–282.
17. Matsunaga E. Hereditary retinoblastoma: host resistance and age at onset. J Natl Cancer Inst 1979; 63:933–939.
18. Aherne GES, Roberts DF. Retinoblastoma: a clinical survey and its genetic implications. Clin Genet 1975; 8:275–290.
19. Rubenfeld M, Abramson DH, Ellsworth RM, Kitchin FD. Unilateral vs bilateral retinoblastoma: correlation between age and stage of ocular disease. Ophthalmology 1986; 93:1016–1019.
20. Takahashi T, Tamura S, Inoue M, et al. Retinoblastoma in a 26-year-old adult. Ophthalmology 1983; 90:179–183.
21. Ellsworth RM. The practical management of retinoblastoma. Trans Am Ophthalmol Soc 1969; 67:462–534.
22. Suckling RD, Fitzgerald PH, Stewart J, Wells E. The incidence and epidemiology of retinoblastoma in New Zealand: a 30-year survey. Br J Cancer 1982; 46:729–736.
23. Francois J, Matton MT, Debie S, et al. Genesis and genetics of retinoblastoma. Ophthalmologica 1975; 170:405–525.
24. Briard-Guillemot ML, Bonaiti-Pellie C, Feingold J, Frezal J. Etude genetique du retinoblastome. Humangenetik 1974; 24:271–284.
25. Vogel F. Genetics of retinoblastoma. Hum Genet 1979; 52:1–54.
26. Kock E, Naeser P. Retinoblastoma in Sweden 1958–71: a clinical and histopathological-study. Acta Ophthalmol 1979; 57:344–350.
27. Francois J. Genetics of retinoblastoma. Mod Probl Ophthalmol 1977; 18:165–172.
28. Matsunaga E. Hereditary retinoblastoma: lack of maternal effect. Hum Genet 1982; 62:124–128.
29. Levitt EA, Rosenbaum AL, Willerman L, Levitt M. Intelligence of retinoblastoma patients and their siblings. Child Dev 1972; 43:939–948.
30. Eldridge R, O'Meara K, Kitchin D. Superior intelligence in sighted retinoblastoma patients and their families. J Med Genet 1972; 9:331–335.
31. Ek U, Seregard S, Jacobson L, Oskar K, Af Trampe E, Kock E. A prospective study of children treated for retinoblastoma: cognitive and visual outcomes in relation to treatment. Acta Ophthalmol Scand 2002; 80(3):294–299.
32. Abramson DH, Marks RF, Ellsworth RM, et al. Management of unilateral retinoblastoma without primary enucleation. Arch Ophthalmol 1982; 100:1249–1252.
33. Bader JL, Miller RW, Meadows AT, et al. Trilateral retinoblastoma. Lancet 1980; 2:582–583.
34. Judisch GF, Patil SR. Concurrent heritable retinoblastoma, pinealoma and trisomy X. Arch Ophthalmol 1981; 99:1767–1769.
35. Zimmerman LE, Burns RP, Wankum G, et al. Trilateral retinoblastoma: ectopic intracranial retinoblastoma associated with bilateral retinoblastoma. Pediatr Ophthalmol Strabismus 1982; 19:320–325.

36. Pesin SR, Shields JA. Seven cases of trilateral retinoblastoma. Am J Ophthalmol 1989; 107:121–126.
37. Stannard C, Knight BK, Sealy R. Pineal malignant neoplasm in association with hereditary retinoblastoma. Br J Ophthalmol 1985; 69:749–753.
38. Whittle IR, McClellan K, Martin FJ, Johnston IH. Concurrent pineoblastoma and unilateral retinoblastoma. A forme fruste of trilateral retinoblastoma? Neurosurgery 1985; 17:500–505.
39. Kivela T. Trilateral retinoblastoma: a meta-analysis of hereditary retinoblastoma associated with primary ectopic intracranial retinoblastoma. J Clin Oncol 1999; 17(6): 1829–1837.
40. Khodadoust AA, Roozitalab HM, Smith RE, Green WR. Spontaneous regression of retinoblastoma. Surv Ophthalmol 1977; 21:467–478.
41. Merin S, Robinson E, Landau J. Spontaneous healed retinoblastoma as a factor in dominant heredity. J Pediatr Ophthalmol 1965; 2:43–46.
42. Marsden HB, Stewart JK. Tumors in Children. 2nd ed. Berlin: Springer-Verlag, 1976:231.
43. Gallie BL, Ellsworth RM, Abramson DH, Philips RA. Retinoma: spontaneous regression of retinoblastoma or benign manifestation of the mutation. Br J Cancer 1982; 45:513–521.
44. Abramson DH. Retinoma, retinocytoma and the retinoblastoma gene [Editorial]. Arch Ophthalmol 1983; 101:1517–1518.
45. Sanborn GE, Augsburger JJ, Shields JA. Spontaneous regression of bilateral retinoblastoma. Br J Ophthalmol 1982; 66:685–690.
46. Sabbah R, Berry FD, Schimmelpfennig W. An unusual family with retinoblastoma. Ann Ophthalmol 1981; 13:595–596.
47. Gangwar DN, Jain IS, Gupta A, Sharma PC. Bilateral spontaneous regression of retinoblastoma with dominant transmission. Ann Ophthalmol 1982; 14:479–480.
48. Migdal C. Spontaneous regression of retinoblastoma in identical twins. Br J Ophthalmol 1982; 66:691–694.
49. Balmer A, Munier F, Gailloud C, Retinoma. Case studies. Ophthalmic Paediatr Genet 1991; 12(3):131–137.
50. Lommatzsch PK, Zimmermann W, Lommatzsch R. Spontaneous growth inhibition in retinoblastoma. Klinische Monatsblatter fur Augenheilkunde. 1993; 202(3):218–223.
51. Singh AD, Santos CM, Shields CL, Shields JA, Eagle RC Jr. Observations on 17 patients with retinocytoma. Arch Ophthalmol 2000; 118(2):199–205.
52. Lueder GT, Heon E, Gallie BL. Retinoma associated with vitreous seeding. Am J Ophthalmol 1995; 119(4):522–523.
53. Knudson AG, Meadows AT, Nichols WW, Hill R. Chromosomal deletion and retinoblastoma. N Engl J Med 1976; 295:1120–3123.
54. Yunis JJ, Ramsey N. Retinoblastoma and subband deletion of chromosome 13. Am J Dis Child 1978; 132:161–163.
55. Sparkes RS, Sparkes MC, Wilson MG, et al. Regional assignment of genes for human esterase D and retinoblastoma to chromosome band 13ql4. Science 1980; 208: 1042–1044.
56. Howard RO. Chromosome errors in retinoblastoma. Birth Defects 1982; 18:703–727.
57. Johnson MP, Ramsay N, Cervenka J, Wang N. Retinoblastoma and its association with a deletion in chromosome 13: a survey using high-resolution chromosome techniques. Cancer Genet Cytogenet 1982; 6:29–37.
58. Howard RO. Origin of retinoblastoma [Letter to the Editor]. Lancet 1982; 2:490–491.
59. Motegi T, Kaga M, Yanagawa T, et al. A recognizable pattern of the midface of retinoblastoma patients with interstitial deletion of 13q. Hum Genet 1983; 64:160–162.
60. Mueller RF. Retinoblastoma and esterase D. Lancet 1982; 2:823.
61. Sparkes RD, Murphree AL, et al. Gene for hereditary retinoblastoma assigned to human chromosome 13 by linkage to esterase D. Science 1983; 219:971–973.

62. Cowell JK, Rutland P, Hungerford J, Jay M. Deletion of chromosome region 13ql4 is transmissible and does not always predispose to retinoblastoma. Hum Genet 1988; 80:43–45.
63. Mitchell CD, Cowell JK. Molecular evidence that the esterase D gene lies proximal to the retinoblastoma susceptibility locus in chromosome region 13ql4. Hum Genet 1988; 81:57–60.
64. Dryja TP, Bruns GAP, Gallie B, et al. Low incidence of deletion of the esterase D locus in retinoblastoma patients. Hum Genet 1983; 64:151–155.
65. Lee EY, Lee WH. Molecular cloning of the human esterase D gene, a genetic marker of retinoblastoma. Proc Natl Acad Sci USA 1986; 83:6337–6341.
66. Squire J, Dryja TP, Dunn J, et al. Cloning of the esterase D gene: a polymorphic gene probe closely linked to the retinoblastoma locus on chromosome 13. Proc Natl Acad Sci USA 1986; 86:6573–6577.
67. Young LJ, Lee EY, To HA, et al. Human esterase D gene: complete cDNA sequence, genomic structure, and application in the genetic diagnosis of human retinoblastoma. Hum Genet 1988; 79:137–141.
68. Nove J, Little JB, Weichselbaum RR, et al. Retinoblastoma, chromosome 13, and in vitro cellular radiosensitivity. Cytogenet Cell Genet 1979; 24:176–184.
69. Palmer RW, Hulten MA. Chiasma derived genetic maps and recombination fractions: Chromosome 13 with reference to the proposed 13ql4 retinoblastoma locus. J Med Genet 1982; 19:125–129.
70. Aherne G. Retinoblastoma associated with other primary malignant tumors. Trans Ophthalmol Soc UK 1974; 94:938–944.
71. Francois J. Retinoblastoma and osteogenic sarcoma. Ophthalmotogica 1977; 175: 185–191.
72. Kitchin FD, Ellsworth RM. Pleiotropic effects of the gene for retinoblastoma. J Med Genet 1974; 11:244–246.
73. Abramson DH, Ellsworth RM, Zimmerman LE. Nonocular cancer in retinoblastoma survivors. Trans Am Acad Ophthalmol Otolaryngol 1976; 81:454–457.
74. Abramson DH, Ellsworth RM, Rosenblatt M, et al. Retreatment of retinoblastoma with external beam irradiation. Arch Ophthalmol 1982; 100:1257–1260.
75. Abramson DH, Ronner HJ, Ellsworth RM. Second tumors in irradiated bilateral retinoblastoma. Am J Ophthalmol 1979; 87:624–627.
76. Roarty JD, McLean IW, Zimmerman LE. Incidence of second neoplasms in patients with bilateral retinoblastoma. Ophthalmology 1988; 95:1583–1587.
77. Lueder GT, Judisch GF, O'Gorman TW. Second nonocular tumors in survivors of heritable retinoblastoma. Arch Ophthalmol 1986; 104:372–373.
78. Mitchell C. Second malignant neoplasm in retinoblastoma. Fact and fiction. Ophthalmol Paediatr Genet 1988; 9:161–165.
79. der Kinderen DJ, Koten JW, Nagelkerke NJ, et al. Non-ocular cancer in patients with hereditary retinoblastoma and their relatives. Int J Cancer 1988; 43:499–504.
80. Traboulsi El, Zimmerman LE, Manz HJ. Cutaneous malignant melanoma in survivors. Arch Ophthalmol 1988; 106:1059–1061.
81. Font RL, Jurco S, Brechner RJ. Postradiation leiomyosarcoma of the orbit complicating bilateral retinoblastoma. Arch Ophthalmol 1983; 101:1557–1561.
82. Folberg R, Cleasby G, Flanagan JA, et al. Orbital leiomyosarcoma after medication therapy for bilateral retinoblastoma. Arch Ophthalmol 1983; 101:1562–1565.
83. Nuutinen J, Karja J, Sainio P. Epithelial second malignant tumors in retinoblastoma survivors. A review and report of a case. Acta Ophthalmol 1982; 60(1):133–140.
84. Harbour JW, Lai SL, Whang-Peng J, et al. Abnormalities in structure and expression of the human retinoblastoma gene in SCLC. Science 1988; 241:353–357.
85. Eng C, Li FP, Abramson DH, Ellsworth RM, Wong FL, Goldman MB, Seddon J, Tarbell N, Boice JD Jr. Mortality from second tumors among long-term survivors of retinoblastoma. J Nat Cancer Inst 1993; 85(14):1121–1128.

86. Liang XQ, Avraham HK, Jiang S, Avraham S. Genetic alterations of the NRP/B gene are associated with human brain tumors. Oncogene 2004; 23(35):5890–5900.
87. Romano P, Gross S, Quisling RG. Retinoblastoma [Letter to the Editor]. Arch Ophthalmol 1983; 101:487.
88. Dryja TP, Rapaport JM, Epstein J, et al. Chromosome 13 homozygosity in osteosarcoma without retinoblastoma. Am J Hum Genet 1986; 38:59–66.
89. Kony SL, de Vathaire F, Chompret A, Shamsaldim A, Grimaud E, Raquin MA, Oberlin O, Brugieres L, Feunteun J, Eschwege F, Chavaudra J, Lemerle J, Bonaiti-Pellie C. Radiation and genetic factors in the risk of second malignant neoplasms after a first cancer in childhood. Lancet 1997; 350(9071):91–95.
90. Abramson DH, Frank CM. Second nonocular tumors in survivors of bilateral retinoblastoma: a possible age effect on radiation-related risk. Ophthalmology 1998; 105(4):573–579; discussion 579–580.
91. Abramson DH, Du TT, Beaverson KL. (Neonatal) retinoblastoma in the first month of life. Arch Ophthalmol 2002; 120(6):738–742.
92. Moll AC, Imhof SM, Schouten-Van Meeteren AY, Kuik DJ, Hofinan P, Boers M. Second primary tumors in hereditary retinoblastoma: a register-based study, 1945–1997: is there an age effect on radiation-related risk? Ophthalmology 2001; 108(6): 1109–1114
93. Mohney BG, Robertson DM, Schomberg PJ, Hodge DO. Second nonocular tumors in survivors of heritable retinoblastoma and prior radiation therapy. Am J Ophthalmol 1998; 126(2):269–277.
94. Wong FL, Boice JD Jr. Abramson DH, Tarone RE, Kleinerman RA, Stovall M, Goldman MB, Seddon JM, Tarbell N, Fraumeni JF Jr, Li FP. Cancer incidence after retinoblastoma. Radiation dose and sarcoma risk. J Am Med Assoc 1997; 278(15): 1262–1267.
95. Abramson DH, Melson MR, Dunkel IJ, Frank CM. Third (fourth and fifth) nonocular tumors in survivors of retinoblastoma. Ophthalmology 2001; 108(10):1868–1876.
96. Kleinerman RA, Tarone RE, Abramson DH, Seddon JM, Li FP, Tucker MA. Hereditary retinoblastoma and risk of lung cancer. J Nat Cancer Inst 2000; 92(24):2037–2039.
97. Abramson DH. Second nonocular cancers in retinoblastoma: a unified hypothesis. The Franceschetti Lecture. Ophthalmic Genet 1999; 20(3):193–204.
98. Thomas DM, Carty SA, Piscopo DM, Lee JS, Wang WF, Forrester WC, Hinds PW. The retinoblastoma protein acts as a transcriptional coactivator required for osteogenic differentiation. Mol Cell 2001; 8(2):303–316.
99. Bullock JD, Campbell RJ, Waller RR. Calcification in retinoblastoma. Invest Ophthalmol Vis Sci 1977; 16:252–255.
100. Klintworth GK. Radiographic abnormalities in eyes with retinoblastoma and other disorders. Br J Ophthalmol 1978; 62:365–372.
101. Arrigg PG, Hedges TR, Char DH. Computed tomography in the diagnosis of retinoblastoma. Br J Ophthalmol 1983; 67:588–591.
102. Shields JA, Leonard BC, Michelson JB, Sarin LK. B-scan ultrasonography in the diagnosis of atypical retinoblastomas. Can J Ophthalmol 1976; 11:42–51.
103. Diamond JG, Ossoining KC. Contact A-scan and B-scan ultrasonography in the diagnosis of intraocular lesions. In: Peyman GA, Apple DJ, Sanders DR, eds. Intraocular Tumors. New York: Appleton-Century-Crofts, 1977:35–49.
104. Roth DB, Scott IU, Murray TG, Kaiser PK, Feuer WJ, Hughes JR, Rosa RH Jr. Echography of retinoblastoma: histopathologic correlation and serial evaluation after globe-conserving radiotherapy or chemotherapy. J Pediatr Ophthalmol Strabismus 2001; 38(3):136–143.
105. Finger PT, Meskin SW, Wisnicki HJ, Albekioni Z, Schneider S. High-frequency ultrasound of anterior segment retinoblastoma. Am J Ophthalmol 2004; 137(5):944–946.
106. Shields JA, Sanborn GE, Augsburger JJ, et al. Fluorescein angiography of retinoblastoma. Trans Am Ophthalmol Soc 1982; 80:98–112.

107. Ohnishi Y, Yamana Y, Minei M, Ibayashi H. Applications of fluorescein angiography in retinoblastoma. Am J Ophthalmol 1982; 93:578–588.
108. Schulman JA, Peyman GA, Mafee MF, et al. The use of magnetic resonance imaging in the evaluation of retinoblastoma. J Pediatr Ophthalmol Strabismus 1986; 23:144–147.
109. Mafee MF, Goldberg MF, Cohen SB, et al. Magnetic resonance imaging versus computed tomography of leukocoric eyes and use of in vitro proton magnetic resonance spectroscopy of retinoblastoma. Ophthalmology 1989; 96:965–976.
110. McCaffery S, Simon EM, Fischbein NJ, Rowley HA, Shimikawa A, Lin S, O'Brien JM. Three-dimensional high-resolution magnetic resonance imaging of ocular and orbital malignancies. Arch Ophthalmol 2002; 120(6):747–754.
111. Schueler AO, Hosten N, Bechrakis NE, Lemke AJ, Foerster P, Felix R, Foerster MH, Bornfeld N. High resolution magnetic resonance imaging of retinoblastoma. Br J Ophthalmol 2003; 87(3):330–335.
112. Dias PLR, Shanmuganathan SS, Rajaratanam M. Lactic dehydrogenase activity of aqueous humor in retinoblastoma. Br J Ophthalmol 1971; 55:130–132.
113. Swartz M, Herbst RW, Goldberg MF. Aqueous humor lactic acid dehydrogenase in retinoblastoma. Am J Ophthalmol 1974; 78:612–617.
114. Ellsworth RM. Retinoblastoma. Mod Probl Opthalmol 1977; 18:94–100.
115. Abramson DH, Piro PA, Ellsworth RM, et al. Lactate dehydrogenase levels and isozyme patterns: measurements in the aqueous humour and serum of retinoblastoma patients. Arch Ophthalmol 1979; 97:870–871.
116. Dias PLR. Prognostic significance of aqueous humour lactic dehydrogenase activity. Br J Ophthalmol 1979; 63:571–573.
117. Dias PLR. Correlation of aqueous humour lactic acid dehydrogenase activity with intraocular pathology. Br J Ophthalmol 1979; 63:574–577.
118. Nakajima T, Kato K, Kaneko A, et al. High concentrations of enolase, alpha- and gamma subunits, in the aqueous humor in cases of retinoblastoma. Am J Ophthalmol 1986; 101:102–106.
119. Rodriguez A. Diagnosis of retinoblastoma by cytologic examination of the aqueous and the vitreous. Mod Probl Ophthalmol 1977; 18:142–148.
120. Mastrangelo D, Squitieri N, Bruni S, Hadjistilianou T, Frezzotti R. The polymerase chain reaction (PCR) in the routine genetic characterization of retinoblastoma: a tool for the clinical laboratory. Surv Ophthalmol 1997; 41(4):331–340.
121. Richter S, Vandezande K, Chen N, Zhang K, Sutherland J, Anderson J, Han L, Panton R, Branco P, Gallie B. Sensitive and efficient detection of RB1 gene mutations enhances care for families with retinoblastoma. Am J Hum Genet 2003; 72(2):253–269.
122. Tsai T, Fulton L, Smith BJ, Mueller RL, Gonzalez GA, Uusitalo MS, O'Brien JM. Rapid identification of germline mutations in retinoblastoma by protein truncation testing. Arch Ophthalmol 2004; 122(2):239–248.
123. Murphree AL, Gomer CJ, Doiron R, Benedict WF. Recent developments in the genetics and treatment of retinoblastoma. Birth Defects 1982; 18:681–687.
124. Gallie B, Wong JJY, Ellsworth RM, et al. Immunological mechanisms in spontaneous-regression of retinoblastoma. In: Silverstein AM, O'Connor GR, eds. Immunology and Immunopathology of the Eye. New York: Masson, 1979:190.
125. Betrams J, Schildberg P, Hopping, et al. HLA antigens in retinoblastoma. Tissue Antigens 1973; 3:78–87.
126. Matsunaga E, Minoda K. Retinoblastoma and ABO blood groups. Hum Genet 1983; 63:87.
127. Weichselbaum RR, Nove J, Little JB. X-ray sensitivity of diploid fibroblasts from patients with hereditary or sporadic retinoblastoma. Proc Natl Acad Sci 1978; 75: 3962–3964.
128. Gallie BL, Phillips RA. Multiple manifestations of the retinoblastoma gene. Birth Defects 1982; 18:689–701.
129. Gallie BL. Gene carrier detection in retinoblastoma. Ophthalmology 1980; 87:591–594.

130. Roberts CW, Iwamoto M, Haik BC. Ultrastructural correlation of specular microscopy in retinoblastoma. Am J Ophthalmol 1986; 102:182–187.
131. Mendelsohn ME, Abramson DH, Senft S, Servodidio CA, Gamache PH. Uric acid in the aqueous humor and tears of retinoblastoma patients. J AAPOS: Am Assoc Pediatr Ophthalmol Strabismus 1998; 2(6):369–371.
132. Tso MOM, Zimmerman LE, Fine BS. The nature of retinoblastoma. Am J Ophthalmol 1970; 69:339–359.
133. Naves AE, Gaisiner PD. Different cell populations in retinoblastoma. Ann Ophthalmol 1981; 13:1073–1076.
134. Lin CCL, Tso MOM. An electron microscopic study of calcification of retinoblastoma. Am J Ophthalmol 1983; 96:765–774.
135. Stannard C, Lipper S, Sealy R, Sevel D. Retinoblastoma: correlation of invasion of the optic nerve and choroid with prognosis and metastases. Br J Ophthalmol 1979; 63: 560–570.
136. Kyritsis AP, Tsokos M, Triche TJ, Chader GJ. Retinoblastoma: a primitive tumor with multipotential characteristics. Invest Ophthalmol Vis Sci 1986; 27:1760–1764.
137. Tsokos M, Kyritsis AP, Chader GJ, Triche TJ. Differentiation of human retinoblastoma in vitro into cell types with characteristics observed in embryonal or mature retina. Am J Pathol 1986; 123:542–552.
138. Rodriguez MM, Wilson ME, Wiggert B, et al. Retinoblastoma: a clinical immunohistochemical and electron microscopic case report. Ophthalmology 1986; 93:1010–1015.
139. Nork TM, Schwartz TL, Doshi HM, Millecchia LL. Retinoblastoma. Cell of origin. Arch Ophthalmol 1995; 113(6):791–802.
140. Albert DM, Griep AE, Lambert PF, Howes KA, Windle JJ, Lasudry JG. Transgenic models of retinoblastoma: what they tell us about its cause and treatment. Trans Am Ophthalmol Soc 1994; 92:385–400.
141. Loeffler KU, McMenamin PG. An ultrastructural study of DNA precipitation in the anterior segment of eyes with retinoblastoma. Ophthalmology 1987; 94:1160–1168.
142. Smith JL. Histology and spontaneous regression of retinoblastoma. Trans Ophthalmol Soc UK 1974; 94:953–967.
143. Hashem N, Khalifa S. Retinoblastoma: a model of hereditary fragile chromosomal regions. Hum Hered 1975; 25:35–49.
144. Hossfeld DK. Chromosome 14q+ in a retinoblastoma. Int J Cancer 1978; 21:720–723.
145. Barry G, Mullaney J. Retinoblastoma in the Republic of Ireland. Trans Ophthalmol Soc UK 1971; 91:839–855.
146. Devesa MHS. The incidence of retinoblastoma. Am J Ophthalmol 1975; 80:263–265.
147. Freedman J, Goldberg L. Incidence of retinoblastoma in the Bantu of South Africa. Br J Ophthalmol 1976; 60:655–656.
148. Ben Ezra D, Chirambo MC. Incidence of retinoblastoma in Malawi. J Pediatr Ophthalmol 1976; 13:340–343.
149. Berkow RL, Fleshman JK. Retinoblastoma in Navajo Indian children. Am J Dis Child 1983; 137:137–138.
150. Albert DM, Lahav M, Lesser R, Craft J. Recent observations regarding retinoblastoma: I. Ultrastructure, tissue culture growth, incidence and animal models. Trans Ophthalmol Soc UK 1974; 94:909–928.
151. Seregard S, Lundell G, Svedberg H, Kivela T. Incidence of retinoblastoma from 1958 to 1998 in Northern Europe: advantages of birth cohort analysis. Ophthalmology 2004; 111(6):1228–1232.
152. Newell GR, Roberts JD, Baranovsky A. Retinoblastoma: presentation and survival in Negro children compared with whites. J Natl Cancer Inst 1972; 49:989–992.
153. Goldberg L. The rising incidence of retinoblastoma in blacks. S Afr Med J 1977; 51:368.
154. Knudson AG. Two genetic hits (more or less) to cancer. Nat Rev Cancer 2001; 1(2): 157–162.

155. Matsunaga E. On estimating penetrance of the retinoblastoma gene. Hum Genet 1980; 56:127–128.
156. Benedict WF, Murphee AL, Banerjee A, et al. Patient with 13 chromosome deletion: evidence that the retinoblastoma gene is a recessive cancer gene. Science 1983; 219: 973–975.
157. Knudson AG. Mutation and cancer: statistical study of retinoblastoma. Proc Natl Acad Sci USA 1971; 68:820–823.
158. Hethcote HW, Knudson AG. Model for the incidence of embryonal cancers: application to retinoblastoma. Proc Natl Acad Sci USA 1978; 75:2453–2457.
159. Cavenee WK, Dryja TP, Phillips RA, et al. Expression of recessive alleles by chromosomal mechanisms in retinoblastoma. Nature 1983; 305:779–784.
160. Dryja TP, Cavenee WK, White R, et al. Homozygosity of chromosome 13 in retinoblastoma. N Engl J Med 1984; 310:550–553.
161. Knudson AG, Meadows AT. Regression of neuroblastoma [V-S. N Engl J Med 1980; 302:1254–1256.
162. Goodbout R, Dryja TP, Squire J, et al. Somatic inactivation of genes on chromosome 13 is a common event in retinoblastoma. Nature 1983; 304:451–453.
163. Dryja TP, Rapaport JM, Joyce JM, Petersen RA. Molecular detection of deletions involving band q14 of chromosome 13 in retinoblastoma. Proc Natl Acad Sci USA 1986; 83:7391–7394.
164. Albert DM, Dryja TP. Recent studies of the retinoblastoma gene. What it means to the ophthalmologist. Arch Ophthalmol 1988; 106:181–182.
165. Online Mendelian Inheritance in Man, OMIM (TM). McKusick-Nathans Institute for Genetic Medicine, Johns Hopkins University (Baltimore, MD) and National Center for Biotechnology Information, National Library of Medicine (Bethesda, MD), 2000. http://www.ncbi.nlm.nih.gov/omim/.
166. Friend SH, Bernards R, Rogel JS, et al. A human DNA segment with properties of the gene that predisposes to retinoblastoma and osteosarcoma. Nature 1984; 323:643–646.
167. Lee WH, Bookstein R, Hong F, et al. Human retinoblastoma susceptibility gene: cloning, identification and sequence. Science 1987; 235:1394–1399.
168. Fung YK(T), Murphree AL, T'Ang A, et al. Structural evidence for the authenticity of the human retinoblastoma gene. Science 1987; 236:1657–1661.
169. Blanquet V, Turleau C, Gross-Morand MS, Senamaud-Beaufort C, Doz F, Besmond C. Spectrum of germline mutations in the RB1 gene: a study of 232 patients with hereditary and nonhereditary retinoblastoma. Hum Mol Genet 1995; 4(3):383–388.
170. Herwig S, Strauss M. The retinoblastoma protein: a master regulator of cell cycle, differentiation and apoptosis. Eur J Biochem 1997; 246(3):581–601.
171. Dunn JM, Phillips RA, Becker AJ, Gallie BL. Identification of germline and somatic mutations affecting the retinoblastoma gene. Science 1988; 241:1797–1800.
172. Bookstein R, Lee EY, To H, et al. Human retinoblastoma susceptibility gene: genomic organization and analysis of heterozygous intragenic deletion mutants. Proc Natl Acad Sci USA 1988; 85:2210–2214.
173. Goddard AD, Balakier H, Canton M, et al. Infrequent genomic rearrangement and normal expression of the putative *RB1* gene in retinoblastoma tumors. Mol Cell Biol 1988; 8:2082–2088.
174. Lee WH, Bookstein R, Lee EY. Studies on the human retinoblastoma susceptibility gene. J Cell Biochem 1988; 38:213–227.
175. Onadim Z, Hogg A, Cowell JK. Mechanisms of oncogenesis in patients with familial retinoblastoma. Br J Cancer 1993; 68(5):958–964.
176. Harbour JW. Overview of RB gene mutations in patients with retinoblastoma. Implications for clinical genetic screening. Ophthalmology 1998; 105(8):1442–1447.
177. Lohmann DR, Brandt B, Hopping W, Passarge E, Horsthemke B. The spectrum of RB1 germ-line mutations in hereditary retinoblastoma. Am J Hum Genet 1996; 58(5): 940–949.

178. Lohmann DR. RB1 gene mutations in retinoblastoma. Hum Mut 1999; 14(4):283–288.
179. Hogg A, Bia B, Onadim Z, Cowell JK. Molecular mechanisms of oncogenic mutations in tumors from patients with bilateral and unilateral retinoblastoma. Proc Nat Acad Sci USA 1993; 90(15):7351–7355.
180. Dryja TP, Rapaport J, McGee TL, Nork TM, Schwartz TL. Molecular etiology of low-penetrance retinoblastoma in two pedigrees. Am J Hum Genet 1993; 52(6):1122–1128.
181. Lohmann DR, Brandt B, Hopping W, Passarge E, Horsthemke B. Distinct RB1gene mutations with low penetrance in hereditary retinoblastoma. Hum Genet 1994; 94(4): 349–354.
182. Harbour JW. Molecular basis of low-penetrance retinoblastoma. Arch Ophthalmol 2001; 119(11):1699–1704.
183. Onadim Z, Woolford AJ, Kingston JE, Hungerford JL. The RB1 gene mutation in a child with ectopic intracranial retinoblastoma. Br J Cancer 1997; 76(11):1405–1409.
184. Huang HJ, Yee JK, Shew JY, et al. Suppression of the neoplastic phenotype by replacement of the *RB* gene in human cancer cells. Science 1988; 242:1563–1566.
185. Char DH. Clinical Ocular Oncology. New York: Churchill-Livingstone, 1989.
186. Shields JA. Diagnosis and Management of Intraocular Tumors. St Louis, MO: CV Mosby, 1983:480–492.
187. Shields JA, Shields CL. Intraocular Tumors: a Text and Atlas. Philapelphia: Saunders, 1992.
188. Albert DM, Polans A. Ocular Oncology. New York: Marcel Dekker, 2003.
189. Shields JA, Shields CL, Sivalingam V. Decreasing frequency of enucleation in patients with retinoblastoma. Am J Ophthalmol 1989; 108:185–188.
190. Haik BG, Dunleavy SA, Cooke C, et al. Retinoblastoma with anterior chamber extension. Ophthalmology 1987; 94:367–370.
191. Abramson DH. Two concerns about obtaining maximal optic nerve length during enucleation. Arch Ophthalmol 2001; 119(1):143–144.
192. Balmer A, Gailloud C. Retinoblastoma: diagnosis and treatment. Dev Ophthalmol 1983; 7:36–100.
193. Abramson DH, Ellsworth RM, Rozakis GW. Cryotherapy for retinoblastoma. Arch Ophthalmol 1982; 100:1253–1256.
194. Shields JA, Parson H, Shields CL, Giblin ME. The role of cryotherapy in the management of retinoblastoma. Am J Ophthalmol 1989; 108:260–264.
195. Monge OR, Flage T, Hatlevoll R, Vermund H. Sightsaving therapy in retinoblastoma. Experience with external magavoltage radiotherapy. Acta Ophthalmol 1986; 64: 414–420.
196. Harnett AN, Hungerford JL, Lambert GD, et al. Improved external beam radiotherapy for the treatment of retinoblastoma. Br J Radiol 1987; 60:753–760.
197. Malik RK, Friedman HS, Djang WT, et al. Treatment of trilateral retinoblastoma with vincristine and cyclophosphamide. Am J Ophthalmol 1986; 102:650–656.
198. Kingston JE, Hungerford JL, Plowman PN. Chemotherapy in metastatic retinoblastoma. Ophthalmic Paediatr Genet 1987; 8:69–72.
199. Zelter M, Gonzalez G, Schwartz L, et al. Treatment of retinoblastoma. Results obtained from a prospective study of 51 patients. Cancer 1988; 61:153–160.
200. Hungerford JL, Toma NM, Plowman PN, Kingston JE. External beam radiotherapy for retinoblastoma: I. Whole eye technique. Br J Ophthalmol 1995; 79(2):109–111.
201. Toma NM, Hungerford JL, Plowman PN, Kingston JE, Doughty D. External beam radiotherapy for retinoblastoma: II. Lens sparing technique. Br J Ophthalmol 1995; 79(2):112–117.
202. Scott IU, Murray TG, Feuer WJ, Van Quill K, Markoe AM, Ling S, Roth DB, O'Brien JM. External beam radiotherapy in retinoblastoma: tumor control and comparison of 2 techniques. Arch Ophthalmol 1999; 117(6):766–770.
203. Hall LS, Ceisler E, Abramson DH. Visual outcomes in children with bilateral retinoblastoma. J AAPOS: Am Assoc Pediatr Ophthalmol Strabismus 1999; 3(3):138–142.

204. Blach LE, McCormick B, Abramson DH. External beam radiation therapy and retinoblastoma: long-term results in the comparison of two techniques. Int J Radiat Oncol Biol Phys 1996; 35(1):45–51.
205. O'Brien JM. Alternative treatment in retinoblastoma. Ophthalmology 1998; 105(4): 571–572.
206. Greenwald MJ, Strauss LC. Treatment of intraocular retinoblastoma with carboplatin and etoposide chemotherapy. Ophthalmology 1996; 103(12):1989–1997.
207. Shields CL, De Potter P, Himelstein BP, Shields JA, Meadows AT, Maris JM. Chemoreduction in the initial management of intraocular retinoblastoma. Arch Ophthalmol 1996; 114(11):1330–1338.
208. Murphree AL, Villablanca JG, Deegan WF 3rd, Sato JK, Malogolowkin M, Fisher A, Parker R, Reed E, Gomer CJ. Chemotherapy plus local treatment in the management of intraocular retinoblastoma. Arch Ophthalmol 1996; 114(11):1348–1356.
209. Shields CL, Shields JA, Needle M, de Potter P, Kheterpal S, Hamada A, Meadows AT. Combined chemoreduction and adjuvant treatment for intraocular retinoblastoma. Ophthalmology 1997; 104(12):2101–2111.
210. Shields CL, Mashayekhi A, Demirci H, Meadows AT, Shields JA. Practical approach to management of retinoblastoma. Arch Ophthalmol 2004; 122(5):729–735.
211. Scott IU, Murray TG, Toledano S, O'Brien JM. New retinoblastoma tumors in children undergoing systemic chemotherapy. Arch Ophthalmol 1998; 116(12):1685–1686.
212. Lee TC, Hayashi NI, Dunkel IJ, Beaverson K, Novetsky D, Abramson DH. New retinoblastoma tumor formation in children initially treated with systemic carboplatin. Ophthalmology 2003; 110(10):1989–1994; discussion 1994–1995.
213. Ferris FL 3rd, Chew EY. A new era for the treatment of retinoblastoma. Arch Ophthalmol 1996; 114(11):1412.
214. Gallie BL, Budning A, DeBoer G, Thiessen JJ, Koren G, Verjee Z, Ling V, Chan HS. Chemotherapy with focal therapy can cure intraocular retinoblastoma without radiotherapy. Arch Ophthalmol 1996; 114(11):1321–1328.
215. Madreperla SA, Hungerford JL, Doughty D, Plowman PN, Kingston JE, Singh AD. Treatment of retinoblastoma vitreous base seeding. Ophthalmology 1998; 105(1): 120–124.
216. Murray TG, Cicciarelli N, O'Brien JM, Hernandez E, Mueller RL, Smith BJ, Feuer W. Subconjunctival carboplatin therapy and cryotherapy in the treatment of transgenic murine retinoblastoma. Arch Ophthalmol 1997; 115(10):1286–1290.
217. Mendelsohn ME, Abramson DH, Madden T, Tong W, Tran HT, Dunkel IJ. Intraocular concentrations of chemotherapeutic agents after systemic or local administration. Arch Ophthalmol 1998; 116(9):1209–1212.
218. Gunduz K, Shields CL, Shields JA, Meadows AT, Gross N, Cater J, Needle M. The outcome of chemoreduction treatment in patients with Reese-Ellsworth group V retinoblastoma. Arch Ophthalmol 1998; 116(12):1613–1617.
219. Bechrakis NE, Bornfeld N, Schueler A, Coupland SE, Henze G, Foerster MH. Clinicopathologic features of retinoblastoma after primary chemoreduction. Arch Ophthalmol 1998; 116(7):887–893.
220. Shields CL, Shelil A, Cater J, Meadows AT, Shields JA. Development of new retinoblastomas after 6 cycles of chemoreduction for retinoblastoma in 162 eyes of 106 consecutive patients. Arch Ophthalmol 2003; 121(11):1571–1576.
221. Sussman DA, Escalona-Benz E, Benz MS, Hayden BC, Feuer W, Cicciarelli N, Toledano S, Markoe A, Murray TG. Comparison of retinoblastoma reduction for chemotherapy vs external beam radiotherapy. Arch Ophthalmol 2003; 121(7):979–984.
222. Abramson DH, Ellsworth RM, Tretter P, et al. Simultaneous bilateral radiation for advanced bilateral retinoblastoma. Arch Ophthalmol 1981; 99:1763–1766.
223. Abramson DH, Ellsworth RM, Tretter P, et al. Treatment of bilateral groups I through III retinoblastoma with bilateral radiation. Arch Ophthalmol 1982; 99:1761–1762.

224. Buys RJ, Abramson DH, Ellsworth RM, Haik B. Radiation regression patterns after cobalt plaque insertion for retinoblastoma. Arch Ophthalmol 1983; 101:1206–1208.
225. Kock E, Rosengren B, Tengroth B, Trampe E. Retinoblastoma treated with a 60Co applicator. Radiother Oncol 1986; 7:19–25.
226. Abramson DH, Ellsworth RM, Haik B. Cobalt plaques in advanced retinoblastoma. Retina 1983; 3:12–15.
227. Standard C, Sealy R, Shackleton D, et al. The use of iodine-125 plaques in the treatment of retinoblastoma. Ophthalmic Paediatr Genet 1987; 8:89–93.
228. Amendola BE, Markoe AM, Augsburger JJ, et al. Analysis of treatment results in 36 children with retinoblastoma treated by scleral plaque irradiation. J Radiat Oncol Biol Phys 1989; 17:63–70.
229. Shields CL, Santos MC, Diniz W, Gunduz K, Mercado G, Cater JR, Shields JA. Thermotherapy for retinoblastoma. Arch Ophthalmol 1999; 117(7):885–893.
230. Kiratli H, Bilgic S, Ozerdem U. Management of massive orbital involvement of intraocular retinoblastoma. Ophthalmology 1998; 105(2):322–326.
231. Connolly MJ, Payne RH, Johnson G, et al. Familial, ESD-linked, retinoblastoma with reduced penetrance and variable expressivity. Hum Genet 1983; 65:122–124.
232. Cavenee WK, Murphree AL, Shull MM, et al. Prediction of familial predisposition to retinoblastoma. N Engl J Med 1986; 314:1201–1207.
233. Cowell JK, Thompson E, Rutland P. The need to screen submicroscopic patients for esterase D activity: detection of submicroscopic chromosome deletions. Arch Dis Child 1987; 62:8–ll.
234. Wiggs JL, Nordenskjold M, Yandell D, et al. Prediction of the risk of hereditary retinoblastoma, using DNA polymorphisms within the retinoblastoma gene. N Engl J Med 1988; 318:151–157.
235. Greger V, Kerst S, Messmer E, et al. Application of linkage analysis to genetic counseling in families with hereditary retinoblastoma. J Med Genet 1988; 25:217–221.
236. Wiggs JL, Dryja TP. Predicting the risk of hereditary retinoblastoma. Am J Ophthalmol 1988; 106:346–351.
237. Dryja TP, Mukai S, Petersen R, et al. Parental origin of mutation of the retinoblastoma gene. Nature 1989; 339:556–558.
238. Munier F, Spence MA, Pescia G, Balmer A, Gailloud C, Thonney F, van Melle G, Rutz HP. Paternal selection favoring mutant alleles of the retinoblastoma susceptibility gene. Hum Genet 1992; 89(5):508–512.
239. Junten C, Despoisse S, Turleau C, et al. Retinoblastoma, deletion 13ql4 and esterase D. application of gene dosage effect to prenatal diagnosis. Cancer Genet Cytogenet 1982; 6:281–287.
240. Mitchell C, Nicolaides K, Kingston J, et al. Prenatal exclusion of hereditary retinoblastoma [Letter]. Lancet 1988; 1:826.
241. Onadim Z, Hungerford J, Cowell JK. Follow-up of retinoblastoma patients having prenatal and perinatal predictions for mutant gene carrier status using intragenic polymorphic probes from the RB1 gene. Br J Cancer 1992; 65(5):711–716.
242. Sutterlin M, Sleiman PA, Onadim Z, Delhanty J. Single cell detection of inherited retinoblastoma predisposition. Prenat Diagn 1999; 19(13):1231–1236.
243. Xu K, Rosenwaks Z, Beaverson K, Cholst I, Veeck L, Abramson DH. Preimplantation genetic diagnosis for retinoblastoma: the first reported liveborn. Am J Ophthalmol 2004; 137(1):18–23.
244. Munne S, Wells D. Preimplantation genetic diagnosis. Curr Opin Obstetr Gynecol 2002; 14(3):239–244.
245. Girardet A, Hamamah S, Anahory T, Dechaud H, Sarda P, Hedon B, Demaille J, Claustres M. First preimplantation genetic diagnosis of hereditary retinoblastoma using informative microsatellite markers. Mol Hum Reprod 2003; 9(2):111–116.

246. Gordon M. Effect of 5 primary genes on the site of melanoma in fish and influence of 2 color genes on their pigmentations. In: Gordon M (ed): The Biology of Melanoma. New York: New York Health Science, 1948:216.
247. Clark WH, Reimer RR, Greene M, et al. Origin of familial malignant melanomas from heritable melanocytic lesions: "The B–K mole syndrome". Arch Dermatol 1978; 114:732–738.
248. Lynch HT, Fujaro RM, Pester J, Lynch JF. Naming the melanoma-prone syndrome [Letter to the Editor]. Lancet 1981; 2:817.
249. Greene MH, Sanders RJ, Chu FC, et al. The familial occurrence of cutaneous melanoma, intraocular melanoma and the dysplastic nevus syndrome. Am J Ophthalmol 1983; 96:238–245.
250. Abramson DH, Rodriguez-Sains RS, Rubman R. B–K mole syndrome, cutaneous and ocular malignant melanoma. Arch Ophthalmol 1980; 98:1397–1399.
251. Lynch HT, Anderson DE, Krush AJ. Heredity and intraocular malignant melanoma: study of two families and review of 45 cases. Cancer 1968; 21:119–125.
252. Bellet RE, Shields JA, Soll DB, Bernardino EA. Primary choroidal and cutaneous melanomas occurring in a patient with the B-K mole syndrome phenotype. Am J Ophthalmol 1980; 89:567–570.
253. Lynch HT, Fusaro RM, Pester J, et al. Tumor spectrum in the FAMMM syndrome. Br J Cancer 1981; 44:553–560.
254. Lynch HT, Fusaro RM, Danes BS, et al. A review of hereditary malignant melanoma including biomarkers in familial atypical multiple mole melanoma syndrome. Cancer Genet Cytogenet 1983; 8:325–358.
255. Becher R, Gibas Z, Sandberg AA. Chromosome 6 in malignant melanoma. Cancer Genet Cytogenet 1983; 9:173–175.
256. Oosterhuis JA, Went LN, Lynch HT. Primary choroidal and cutaneous melanomas, bilateral choroidal melanomas and familial occurrence of melanomas. Br J Ophthalmol 1982; 66:230–233.
257. Egan KM, Seddon JM, Glynn RJ, et al. Epidemiologic aspects of uveal melanoma. Surv Ophthalmol 1988; 32:239–251.
258. Augsburger JJ, Shields JA, Mastrangelo MJ, Frank PE. Diffuse primary malignant melanoma after prior primary cutaneous malignant melanoma. Arch Ophthalmol 1980; 98:1261–1264.
259. Canning CR, Hungerford J. Familial uveal melanoma. Br J Ophthalmol 1988; 72: 241–243.
260. Singh AD, Shields CL, Shields JA, Eagle RC, De Potter P. Uveal melanoma and familial atypical mole and melanoma (FAM-M) syndrome. Ophthalmic Genet 1995; 16(2): 53–61.
261. Walker JP, Weiter JJ, Albert DM, et al. Uveal malignant melanoma in three generations of the same family. Am J Ophthalmol 1979; 88:723–726.
262. Singh AD, Donoso LA. Genetic aspects of uveal melanoma. Int Ophthalmol Clin 1993; 33(3):47–52.
263. Young LH, Egan KM, Walsh SM, Gragoudas ES. Familial uveal melanoma. Am J Ophthalmol 1994; 117(4):516–520.
264. Singh AD, Wang MX, Donoso LA, Shields CL, Potter PD, Shields JA, Elston RC, Fijal B. Familial uveal melanoma, III Is the occurrence of familial uveal melanoma coincidental? Arch Ophthalmol 1996; 114(9):1101–1104.
265. Singh AD, Shields CL, De Potter P, Shields JA, Trock B, Cater J, Pastore D. Familial uveal melanoma. Clinical observations on 56 patients. Arch Ophthalmol 1996; 114(4): 392–399.
266. Singh AD, Shields CL, De Potter P, Shields JA, Trock B, Cater J, Pastore D. Familial uveal melanoma. Clinical observations on 56 patients. Arch Ophthalmol 1996; 114(4): 392–399.

267. Yanoff M, Zimmerman LE. Histogenesis of malignant melanomas of the uvea: III. The relationship of congenital ocular melanocytosis and neurofibromatosis to uveal melanomas. Arch Ophthalmol 1967; 77:331–336.
268. Nik NA, Giew WB, Zimmerman LE. Malignant melanoma of the choroid in the nevus of Ota of a black patient. Arch Ophthalmol 1982; 100:1641–1643.
269. Miller B, Abrahams C, Cole GC, Proctor NSF. Ocular malignant melanoma in South African blacks. Br J Ophthalmol 1981; 65:720–722.
270. Merz B. Melanoma linked with chromosome 6 genes. Arch Intern Med 1983; 143:1105.
271. Turner BJ, Siatkowski RM, Augsburger JJ, et al. Other cancers in uveal melanoma patients and their families. Am J Ophthalmol 1989; 107:601–608.
272. Folberg R, Donoso LA, Herlyn MF, Kopronski H. Antigens in ocular and cutaneous melanomas. Am J Ophthalmol 1983; 96:394–395.
273. Singh AD, Shields CL, Shields JA, De Potter P. Bilateral primary uveal melanoma. Bad luck or bad genes? Ophthalmology 1996; 103(2):256–262
274. Jay M, McCartney AC. Familial malignant melanoma of the uvea and p53: a Victorian detective story. Surv Ophthalmol 1993; 37(6):457–462.
275. Mouriaux F, Maurage CA, Labalette P, Sablonniere B, Malecaze F, Darbon JM. Cyclin-dependent kinase inhibitory protein expression in human choroidal melanoma tumors. Invest Ophthalmol Vis Sci 2000; 41(10):2837–2843.
276. Singh AD, Croce CM, Wary KK, Shields JA, Donoso LA, Shields CL, Huebner K Ohta M. Familial uveal melanoma: absence of germline mutations involving the cyclin-dependent kinase-4 inhibitor gene (p16). Ophthalmic Genet 1996; 17(1):39–40.
277. Foster WJ, Fuller CE, Perry A, Harbour JW. Status of the NF1 tumor suppressor locus in uveal melanoma. Arch Ophthalmol 2003; 121(9):1311–1315.
278. Purtilo DT, Paquin L, Gindhart T. Genetics of neoplasia: impact of ecogenetics on oncogenesis. Am J Pathol 1978; 91:609–688.
279. Stenson S. Ocular findings in xeroderma pigmentosum: report of two cases. Ann Ophthalmol 1982; 14:580–585.
280. Bellows RA, Lahav M, Lepreau FJ, Albert DM. Ocular manifestations of xeroderma pigmentosum in a black family. Arch Ophthalmol 1979; 92:113–117.
281. Freedman J. Corneal transplantation with associated histopathologic description in xeroderma pigmentosum occurring in a black family. Ann Ophthalmol 1979; 11:445–448.
282. Campbell RJ. Tumors of the eyelids, conjunctiva and cornea. In: Garner A, Klintworth GK, eds. Pathobiology of Ocular Disease, A Dynamic Approach. New York: Marcel Dekker, 1982:608–609.
283. Cleaver JE. Defective repair replication of DNA in xeroderma pigmentosum. Nature 1968; 218:652–656.
284. Robbins JH. Significance of repair of human DNA: evidence from studies of xeroderma pigmentation. J Natl Cancer Inst 1978; 61:645–655.
285. Maher VM, Ronan LA, Silinskas KC et al: Frequency of UV-induced neoplastic transformation of diploid human fibroblasts is higher in xeroderma pigmentosum cells than in normal cells. Proc Natl Acad Sci USA 1982; 79:2613–2617.
286. McKusick VA. Mendelian Inheritance in Man. 6th ed. Baltimore: Johns Hopkins University Press, 1983:976–977.
287. Satokata I, Uchiyama M, Tanaka K. Two novel splicing mutations in the XPA gene in patients with group A xeroderma pigmentosum. Hum Mol Genet 1995; 4(10): 1993–1994.
288. Weeda G, van Ham RC, Vermeulen W, Bootsma D, van der Eb AJ, Hoeijmakers JH. A presumed DNA helicase encoded by ERCC-3 is involved in the human repair disorders xeroderma pigmentosum and Cockayne's syndrome. Cell 1990; 62(4):777–791.
289. Legerski R, Peterson C. Expression cloning of a human DNA repair gene involved in xeroderma pigmentosum group C. Nature 1992; 359(6390):70–73.
290. Arrand JE, Bone NM, Johnson RT. Molecular cloning and characterization of a mammalian excision repair gene that partially restores UV resistance to xeroderma

pigmentosum complementation group D cells. Proc Nat Acad Sci US Am 1989; 86(18): 6997–7001.
291. Cleaver JE, Thompson LH, Richardson AS, States JC. A summary of mutations in the UV-sensitive disorders: xeroderma pigmentosum, Cockayne syndrome, and trichothiodystrophy. Hum Mut 1999; 14(1):9–22.
292. Nouspikel T, Clarkson SG. Mutations that disable the DNA repair gene XPG in a xeroderma pigmentosum group G patient. Hum Mol Genet 1994; 3(6):963–967.
293. Halley DJJ, Keijzer W, Jaspers NGJ et al. Prenatal diagnosis of xeroderma pigmentosum (group C) using assays of unscheduled DNA synthesis and postreplication repair. Clin Genet 1979; 16:137–146.

21
The Phakomatoses

INTRODUCTION

It is appropriate that following the chapter on ocular tumors is one devoted to the phakomatoses, a group of distinct clinical and genetic entities, with the common pathologic finding of hamartomas and/or tumors in various organs and tissues. This discussion on the phakomatoses will be limited to those in which the eye is also affected, including the four phakomatoses originally delineated by van der Hoeve in 1937 (1) and the others added since then.

A *hamartoma* is defined as a nodule composed of an aggregation of various cells that are normal in cellular structure and that normally occur in the affected tissue or organ. However, the cells are of abnormal density, abnormal organization, and occur in an abnormal ratio. A hamartoma can be congenital or appear later in life. It usually remains unchanged, but may grow during periods of normal growth of the body and may evolve into a benign tumor. More uncommonly, a hamartoma may become a malignant tumor.

Hamartomas are the most typical finding in the group of diseases termed phakomatoses. Since its introduction in a series of papers and lectures in the 1920s and 1930s by van der Hoeve (2), the term phakomatoses has evoked a controversy that continues into the present. The name was derived from the Greek word *phakos* for circumscribed spot, because the ophthalmologist van der Hoeve observed spots in the eye and in other organs in patients affected with the phakomatoses. He first used *phakoma* to describe the retinal lesion found in a patient with tuberous sclerosis. There is no doubt today that each of the diseases called by this term is a distinct genetic and clinical entity, so it is conceivable to object to using the same term for all of them (3). On the other hand, for the ophthalmologist, the similarities of the findings in the different diseases composing the phakomatoses are obvious. They are all multisystem diseases that affect mainly three organs: the eye, the skin, and the central nervous system (CNS). There is a great variability in expression of the same disease in different patients, including different affected members of the same family. Similar findings in the eye or skin can be found in more than one disease of the group. It seems to me that there is no reason to ridicule van der Hoeve's approach (4), but for the sake of certain classifications, mainly for clinical use, each distinct genetically unrelated disease may be grouped under the common term *phakomatoses*. It is also possible that their pathogenesis is similar.

A series of published case reports describe patients with more than one phakomatosis (5). It is beyond the scope of this text to describe all of the possible combinations, but it may be said that, in some, the combination is spurious, whereas in others, one disease causes changes usually found in another phakomatosis. The best-known example of this phenomenon is the finding of café au lait spots, the typical and often pathognomonic sign of neurofibromatosis, in patients with tuberous sclerosis.

The tendency to develop tumors that may affect the eye or other tissues is the hallmark of all phakomatoses. These tumors may be benign or malignant, as they are typically seen in the classical neurofibromatosis. The idea that cells derived from the embryonal neural crest may migrate and transform into another target cell in various tissues, is well established. The concept of neurocristopathies (diseases derived from abnormal neural crest tissue) as promoted by Bolande (6) and by the monograph of Kissel et al. (7) was verified by the identification in the last decade of disease-associated genes (8,9). Neurofibromatosis (NF) came to be known as the typical example of neurocristopathy, with the co–existence of three tumors of neural crest origin: neurofibroma, meningioma and malignant melanoma (10). It occurs in the more common NF type 1 (NF-1) and the less common NF type 2 (NF-2).

NEUROFIBROMATOSIS TYPE 1

Neurofibromatosis, or von Recklinghausen's disease, was described by von Recklinghausen in 1882. It is one of the most common autosomal dominant diseases in humans, and it is of special interest for the ophthalmologist because of its variety of manifestations in the visual system. NF may appear as one of three forms. The classic form of NF is the most common (it occurs in 1:3500 individuals) and is the only one with common ophthalmic manifestations. Two rare forms, a central form manifested by bilateral acoustic neurinomas (it occurs in 1:50,000 individual) and a segmented form have also been described. A 1988 conference statement (11) established the term NF-1 for the classic or peripheral form and the term NF-2 for the central form.

The Clinical Manifestations of Neurofibromatosis Type 1

A multitude of clinical findings in different organs of the body are typical of NF-1. Of the three mainly affected organs, the skin, the eye, and the CNS, each shows several different manifestations. The disease tends to be progressive (12). The number of skin and hamartomatous lesions increases with age. Hamartomas may start to grow and behave like benign tumors, and then malignant tumors may develop.

Skin Lesions

The most common findings in NF-1 are skin lesions, which consist of pigmentary changes and neurofibromas (12) (Fig. 1)

Pigmentary changes of the skin. Three different types of anomalies of skin hyperpigmentation can be seen (12). Café au lait spots are flat areas of

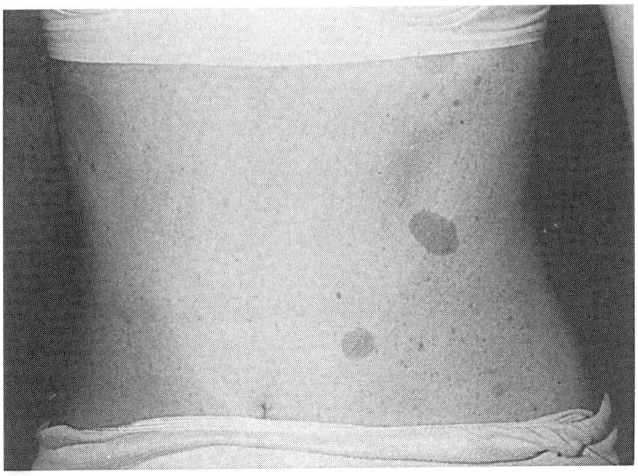

(a)

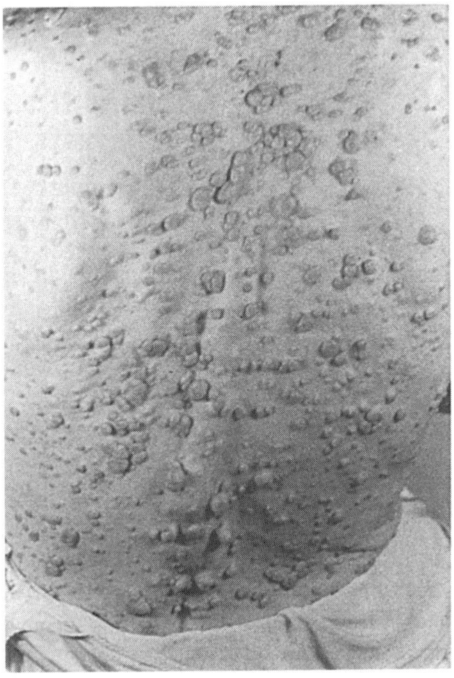

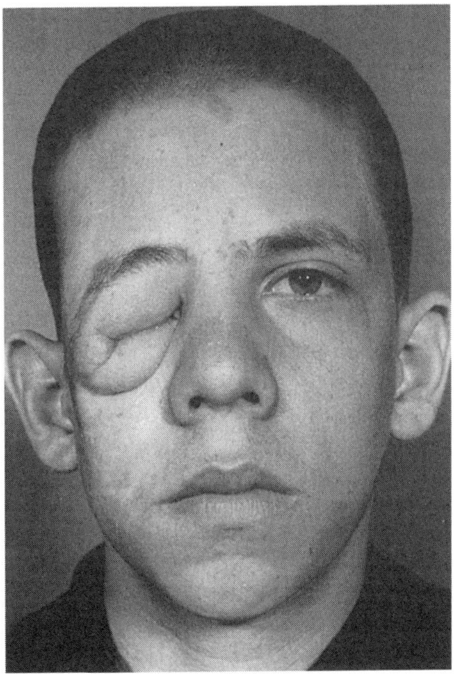

(b) (c)

Figure 1 Skin lesions in three patients with neurofibromatosis: (a) Typical café au lait spots, these are usually dark brown and may be of different sizes and numbers. (b) Multiple neurofibromas on the trunk; there are an unusually large number in this patient. (c) Neurofibroma of the eyelids; this is not an uncommon finding in NF.

hyperpigmentation, that range in size from 1–2 mm to more than 15 cm. Café au lait spots are found in practically all patients (99%) with NF-1 (12), and can be seen anywhere on the body, with a propensity for the trunk. Hyperpigmentation in the form of freckles or nevi also is found in NF patients in a much higher frequency than in controls. Finally, hyperpigmented patches can occur over elevated neurofibromas. The number of these pigmentary skin lesions varies considerably from patient to patient, ranging from a few spots to a very large number, but the number usually increases with age.

Skin hamartomas and tumors. Neurofibromas are the typical lesions of NF and consist of a combination of cellular elements normally found in the skin, such as fibroblasts, vascular elements, neurons, Schwann cells, and mast and pigmented cells. The lesions often increase at puberty and during pregnancy (13). Not uncommonly the upper eyelid is affected, causing ptosis and swelling of the eyelid. The ptosis is typically irregular, in that one part of the eyelid is lower than the other. Sometimes a plexiform neurofibroma produces a localized hypertrophy and severe cosmetic complications.

Ocular Manifestations

Ocular lesions are the second most common finding in NF after pigmented skin lesions.

Iris hamartomas. Lisch nodules were named after the ophthalmologist who described them as an important finding in NF. These typical NF lesions represent melanocytic hamartomas in the iris (14). They are discrete, often slightly elevated, and translucent to dark-brown. Sometimes, they can be seen in the depth of the iris tissue. Because they are small, the largest reaching about 1–2 mm, most can be seen only with the use of the slit lamp (Fig. 2). Lisch nodules should be distinguished from freckles, which are commonly found in the normal iris.

The number of Lisch nodules increases with age (15,16). In a study of 77 patients with NF, Lewis and Riccardi (17) found Lisch nodules to be rare before the age of six years; thereafter, 92% of patients had them. The number of Lisch nodules in their series varied from 1 to 190 and was partially related to age, even after age 6 (Fig. 3). There probably is a hormonal influence on the appearance and number of Lisch nodules, as evidenced by their increase with puberty (18) and pregnancy (3). In most postpubertal patients the finding is bilateral, but about one-third to one-fourth of all patients have only one affected iris.

Lisch nodules may often be difficult to diagnose. The iris changes of NF-1 are versatile and much more diverse than in the classic descriptions of Lisch nodules (19).

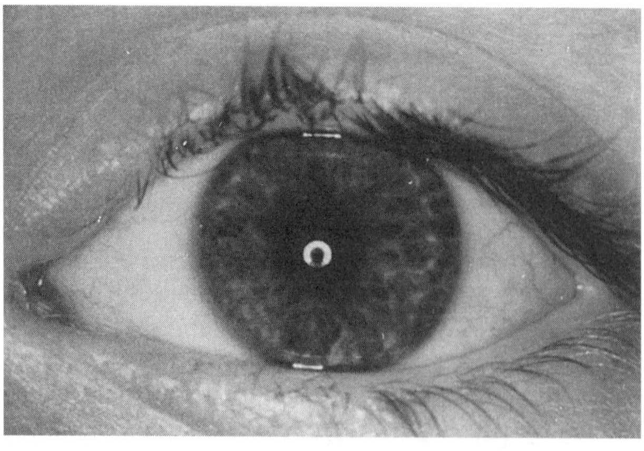

Figure 2 Iris nodules (Lisch nodules) in a middle–aged patient with neurofibromatosis.

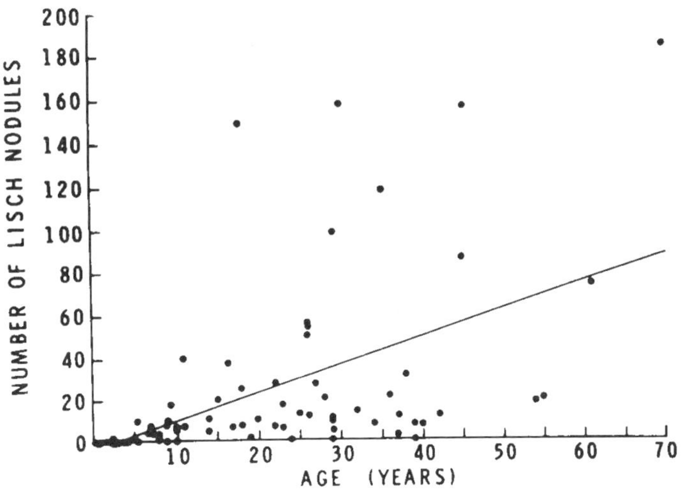

Figure 3 Number of Lisch nodules compared with age in 77 patients with neurofibromatosis. A least–squares linear regression is drawn through the data. Note that the youngest patient to have Lisch nodules is 6 years old, that most of the patients older than 9 years old had nodules, and that some patients did not have nodules up to age 39 (from Ref. 17).

Beauchamp (19) found poor interobserver reliability in diagnosis of 151 suspected patients. Generally of pale brown color and slightly elevated, their appearance varies according to the underlying color of the iris (20). They should be distinguished from iris nodular nevi and freckles (21). Ragge et al. (20) found Lisch nodules in 50% of their 5-year-old patients, 75% of their 15-year-old patients and close to 100% in patients over 30 years old.

Lisch nodules appear to be unrelated to other clinical features of NF-1, such as skin lesions, tumors, or brain findings. Their importance is mainly diagnostic. Rarely does a neurofibroma affect the iris (22).

Other ocular lesions. Not infrequently, a neurofibroma causes ptosis and disfigurement of the eyelid. Sometimes an uncommon conjunctival neurofibroma may be detected.

In about 25% of patients with NF-1, slit-lamp examination detects visibly thickened corneal nerves (17). In one case studied histologically, corneal nerves did not contain the usual increase in Schwann cells, but rather, a secondary hyperregeneration (23). This may have been an exception. Prominent nerves may be also found in conjunctiva. Thickened ciliary nerves are sometimes seen. Not uncommonly an anterior subcapsular cataract is detected (24).

An unknown percentage of patients with NF have congenital or infantile type glaucoma owing to an anomaly of the anterior chamber angle (25). Hamartomas also may appear in the choroid, but they are difficult to recognize. They occur as soft, flat, and ill-defined yellow-white to brown lesions (Fig. 4). Drusen of the optic disc may stem from the hamartomata of NF, and hyperplastic patches of the pigment epithelium may stem be the hyperpigmentation found in this disease. An intraocular neurilemoma (schwannoma) was detected in a 31–year–old patient with known NF–I and found to originate from the long posterior ciliary nerve (26).

The proportion of patients with NF-1 who develop a glioma of the optic nerve has not been firmly established. In various studies, 10–50% of all gliomas of the optic

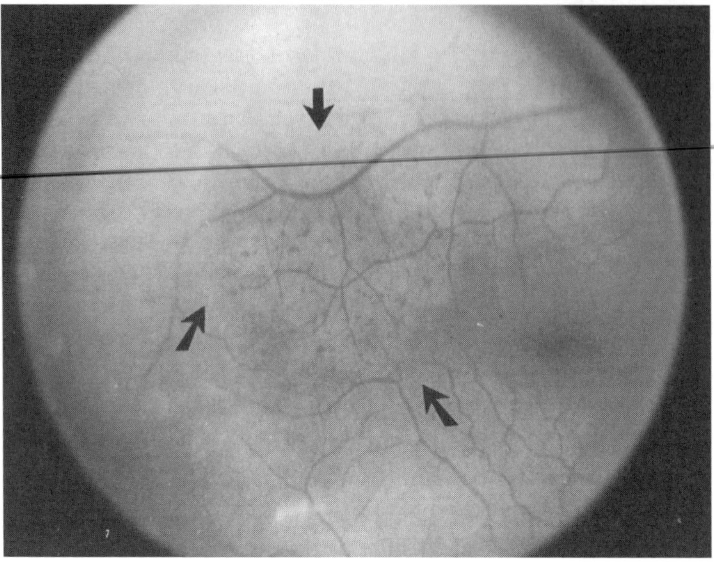

Figure 4 Choroidal hamartoma in a patient with NF. The borders of the faint, flat lesion are marked by arrows.

nerve were related to NF. However, this proportion was closer to the 50% figure in some studies (25) and to the 15% figure in other studies (27–29). The mean age of diagnosis was 5.2 years in one study (30) and 7.1 years in another (29). Stem et al. (31) found that the glioma occurs at a younger age in NF patients (mean 4.9 years), than in patients without NF (mean 12 years). Seventy-five percent of the affected patients were symptomatic before age 10, and 90% were symptomatic before age 20 (27). The tumor may be progressive or stable (29). Progression occurs usually soon after detection of the tumor. Twenty-two of 54 patients progressed within 1 year and six additional patients progressed after 1 year (30). Severe loss of vision to less than 20/200 occurs in about a third (30).

Optic nerve ganglioglioma, a rare tumor composed of both neural and glial tissue is rarely found (32). It is not malignant but tends to grow rapidly.

Bilateral primary gliomas in the two optic nerves are the hallmark of NF-1. They have never been were never reported in patients without NF1.

The clinical manifestation of these tumors are visual loss, optic nerve pallor, visual field change (in older children), proptosis, and, rarely, papilledema. It is important to distinguish between gliomas originating in the anterior part of the optic nerve, which have a favorable prognosis, and gliomas originating from the optic chiasm, which have a disastrous visual outcome and increased risk to life. Two pairs of monozygotic twins were described with optic nerve gliomas at an identical location (33). One pair of siblings with NF had both a similar pulsating left exophthalmos caused by an orbital tumor (34).

Central Nervous System Involvement

The CNS is affected in NF-1 in association with various tumors. The more common of these are optic nerve glioma, astrocytoma, acoustic neuroma or schwannoma, meningioma (often multiple), neurilemoma, and neurofibroma (12,25). The occurrence of tumors was estimated to be 5–10% of all patients with NF-1 (12), whereas the occurrence of NF-1 was 4.5% among 318 children with primary tumors of the CNS and a history of seizures (35).

Gliomas associated with NF-1 usually affected the anterior optic pathways including the optic nerve as far as the chiasm. Liu et al. (36) recently described seven patients with gliomas affecting the posterior optic pathways, such as the optic radiation.

Second brain tumors in patients, diagnosed as NF-1-associated glioma of optic nerve, are not uncommon. They may involve about half of all cases and it was, therefore, recommended to perform yearly follow-up examinations and include MRI (29).

In a small proportion of cases, CNS involvement may cause mental retardation, seizures, or an endocrine disorder, including reduced height. Pituitary-hypothalamic malfunction is not uncommon with chiasmal gliomas.

Malignant Tumors

As many as one of four patients with NF is estimated to develop a cancerous lesion during life (37). In addition, the mean age of diagnosis of the tumor at 38 years (38) is much lower than that for malignancies in the general population. Although reliable estimates are lacking for the frequency of malignancies in NF-1, it is safe to say that any patient with NF is much more likely to suffer from a malignant tumor than normal controls. These tumors may be of neural crest origin, such as neuroblastoma, pheochromocytoma, thyroid carcinoma, and melanoma; of CNS origin, such as glioblastoma multiforme or astroblastoma; or others, including childhood leukemia, rhabdomyosarcoma, Wilms' tumor, and stomach cancer. When malignancies occurred in more than one affected member of a family with NF, concordance of histologic tumor types was seen (39).

Several cases of choroidal malignant melanomas have been reported in patients with NF (40–42). As choroidal nevi seem to be a very common finding in NF (40), malignant melanoma possibly occurs more frequently than in the general population because choroidal nevi could be a source for malignant transformation. A choroidal melanoma has been described in a patient with NF and nevus of Ota, two conditions predisposing to this tumor (43). Malignant peripheral nerve sheath tumors (MPNST) occur in 2% of all NF-1 patients (44).

Other Findings

The skeletal system of patients with NF can be affected by kyphoscoliosis and pseudoarthrosis. Peripheral nerves of NF patients may demonstrate a variety of manifestations. It is beyond the scope of this text to describe all possible findings in NF. Almost any organ can be affected. These less common features are seen in fewer than 5% of all NF patients.

Diagnosis

There is no single laboratory test to confirm the diagnosis of NF. Therefore, the diagnosis must be based on the clinical manifestations of the disease. An accepted criterion for the diagnosis of NF is the finding of six or more café au lait spots, each larger than 1.5 cm in diameter (12). The Lisch nodule may be assumed as pathognomonic, if positively distinguished from iris freckles. The finding of Lisch nodules may confirm or exclude the diagnosis of NF if the patient is beyond puberty.

Slit-lamp examination of the iris is also an excellent method of screening relatives of a patient to find all affected persons.

The consensus accepted for the diagnosis of NF-1 is the finding of two or more of the following clinical presentations of the disease: (i) six or more café au lait spots; (ii) two or more neurofibromas or one plexiform neurofibroma; (iii) freckles in the axillary, inguinal, or other intertriginous regions; (iv) optic glioma, unilateral or bilateral; (v) two or more iris Lisch spots; (vi) an osseous lesion or thinning of the long bone cortices; and (vii) a first-degree relative in whom NF-1 has been diagnosed (45).

The size of the café au lait spots is important. Spots are considered for counting if the size of the largest diameter is 5 mm in prepubertal children and 15 mm in post-pubertal patients (24). In spite of the identification of the NF–1 causative gene, the diagnosis of NF-1 remains clinical. The identification of the causative mutation is time-consuming, expensive and complicated (46) because of the large size of the gene and the extremely high number of mutations. Currently, it makes sense to send for a DNA study only after the clinical diagnosis is established.

Any patient suspected to have NF should undergo extensive multisystem examinations, including dermatologic and ocular evaluations. Computed tomography (CT) scanning of the head and orbits and magnetic resonance imaging (MRI) are helpful for the evaluation of each patient (27,47).

Pathology and Pathogenesis

The pathology of an iris nodule was studied electron microscopically, by Perry and Font (14), in an iridectomy specimen removed for cataract extraction in a patient with NF. They found a hamartoma made of melanocytic cells, rich in cellular processes, and containing large immature melanosomes. In one patient with a large iris tumor, Wolter (22) found Schwann cells, and diagnosed a neurofibroma of the iris, the only report of its kind to date. The ovoid bodies in the choroid are a frequent histologic finding in patients with NF. Ultrastructural studies showed ovoid bodies to contain proliferated Schwann cells (48).

A study of the histology of Lisch nodules revealed condensations of spindle cells on the anterior iris surface (49). In contrast, pigmented nodules also have an underlying stromal nerve.

A pigmented iridocorneal tumor surgically removed in a 32-year-old woman with NF-1 was actually two tumors. Histology revealed a malignant melanoma of the iris and a separate malignant melanoma of the cornea (50).

In one clinical study (51), gliomas of the optic nerve were considered non-neoplastic hamartomas. However, after studying a chiasmal glioma histologically, Parker et al. (52) concluded that optic nerve gliomas are not hamartomas, but are "benign" tumors of a local invasive nature. They claimed that the astrocytes composing the glioma are not normal astrocytes (as required for the definition of hamartoma), but are morphologically abnormal and immature and contain microcystic changes and Rosenthal fibers: Stern et al. (31) suggested that the histologic features of optic nerve glioma in patients with NF are different from those in patients without NF. In patients with NF the optic nerve glioma is a tumor capable of invasion into surrounding tissues. The authors found that the tumor had a "circumferential-perineural pattern." It contained astrocytes, reactive meningoendothelial cells, fibroblasts, and collagen fibers, which were capable of invading the arachnoid and proliferating in the subarachnoid space around the optic nerve. In contrast, a glioma of a non-NF patient was intraneural, inside the optic nerve, and noninvasive. A recent clinicopathologic study of 30 cases of optic nerve and chiasmal gliomas, seems to confirm that leptomeningeal hyperplasia is more common in gliomas associated with NF, an association that is prognostically unfavorable (53).

A review of pathologic reports indicates that the tumor is a juvenile pilocytic astrocytoma, so called because the astrocytes are bipolar cells with greater elongated processes, reminiscent of hair (54). There is no histologic difference between optic nerve and chiasmal gliomas.

How can one disease, caused by a single gene, result in so many different manifestations in a multitude of tissues and organs? The basic pathogenesis is unknown, but Bolande has suggested a unifying concept to explain why certain cells are involved in the disease process and introduced the term *neurocristopathies* to describe all diseases that involve cells derived from the neural crest (6). At a certain period of embryonic development, the neural crest, a transient structure of ectoblastic origin, "sends out" cells that migrate to various parts of the body. These include many different cells, such as melanoblasts, Schwann cells, leptomeningeal cells, sympathetic cells, and others (7). An abnormality in the formation or migration of the cells may cause pathologic responses such as malformations, hamartomas, dysplasias, and tumors (7).

Epidemiology, Genetics and Molecular Genetics

The incidence of NF has been estimated as 1:3000 live births or approximately 1000 new cases each year in the United States alone (55), the ratio of 1:3500 was also cited in another study (24). Garty et al. (56) surveyed 17-year-old Jewish recruits in Israel and found 390 NF1 cases among 374,440 individuals. This gave a prevalence rate of 1.04/1000, the highest reported in any large population study. Gender-wise it was unevenly distributed with prevalence rates of 0.94:1000 in males and 1.19:1000 in females (56). About half are familial cases, and the rest are sporadic (13).

The new mutation rate was estimated as approximately 10^{-4}, probably the highest known in humans. New mutations were estimated to be responsible for about 50% of all new cases of NF-1 and about 39% of all cases of NF-1 (57,24). The mean paternal age in the new mutation cases was reported to be high: 36.7 years (57).

The disease is inherited by autosomal dominant transmission, with almost complete penetrance, but variable expressivity. There is nothing to substantiate the possibility that multiple alleles on one locus are the cause for the different phenotypes. Actually, the variable expression of the disease in different members of the same family seems to preclude this possibility, as far as "classic" NF (NF-1) is concerned. The extremely variable expressivity precludes a proper estimate of penetrance. For descendants of an affected patient with NF-1, a penetrance rate of 97% (57) or "close to 100%" (58) can be shown if minor changes, such as Lisch nodules are taken into account.

Linkage analyses of many families with NF led investigators in 1987 to believe that the gene for NF-1 is located in the pericentric region of chromosome 17 (59,60). There was no evidence for heterogeneity. A plethora of articles confirmed this assumption. The use of molecular probes for linkage analysis (61,62) and investigation of balanced translocations (63) pointed to the locus 17q11.2 as the most likely point for localization of the NF-1 gene. The joint data of a multipoint linkage analysis performed on 142 families by eight teams of investigators (64) confirmed that the locus for the gene of NF-1 is on the proximal part of the long arm of chromosome 17, flanked proximally by marker pHHH202 and distally by marker EW206.

Marchuk et al. (65) cloned the complete coding region of the NFl transcript after three other reports of partial coding. The gene is very large and extends 300–350 kb on chromosome 17. It has an open-reading frame that encodes a protein of 2818 amino acids (65). The genomic DNA is organized in 59 exons (66) or 60 exons (67). Three small genes were detected on one of the introns, reading in the opposite direction. The function of their products is unknown (24). The NF-1 gene has been, as mentioned, mapped to chromosome 17q11.2 (67).

The product of NF-1 is a protein named neurofibromin. One part of neurofibromin forms GAP, a GTPase-activating protein, which may act as a growth cell cycle regulator (24) and when defective be associated with oncogenesis.

NF-1 is a tumor suppressor gene. If the heterozygous state becomes coupled with the loss of function or physical loss of the second allele, benign or malignant tumors may occur, according to Knudson's two-hit theory (68). Legius et al. (69) examined neurofibrosarcoma tumor cells from a patient with NF-1 and demonstrated loss of heterozygosity (LOH) for all chromosome 17 polymorphisms tested. This was the first example of an NF-1-associated homozygous inactivation of the gene at the molecular level (69). Colman et al. (70) demonstrated somatic deletions involving NF-1 and confirmed LOH in benign neurofibromas associated with NF-1 mutations. Thus, Knudson's two-hit theory applies to the NF-1 gene for both malignant and benign tumor formation.

A multitude of mutations of the NF-1 gene have been reported. In most cases these are specific, family associated, private mutations. Heim et al. (71) identified 70 mutations among 78 individuals. These included 14 large (more than 25 bp) deletions, 18 small (<25 bp) deletions, eight small insertions, six nonsense, 14 missense and seven intronic mutations (71). This means that at least in 80% of these mutations the gene will encode a truncated, usually nonfunctional, protein. Similar truncating protein mutations were also found by others (72,73). Additionally, splice-site errors were responsible for exon skipping (72). Presence of pseudogenes of unknown function is another curious phenomenon (73).

The range of clinical expressivity of the mutated NF-1 gene is very large. This includes the large variety of different benign and malignant tumors that may occur. Why such large differences occur is not known, but some speculations can be proposed. First, it could be related to variable defective functions with different mutations of this long gene. Second, it could reflect a variable expression of the gene in different cells. Third, the variable phenotype could be associated with the expression of additional, modifying, genes.

Neurofibromin acts as a membrane-associated molecular switch that regulates cell–cell and cell–matrix signals. It inhibits cell proliferation by modulating mitogenic pathway signaling through inactivation of a protein named p21-ras (74). Neurofibromin also functions as a regulator of melanogenesis, a process specific to the melanocytes derived from the neural crest (75). This could be the background for both the benign and malignant tumors associated with NF-l. Hoffmeyer et al. (66) demonstrated unequal allelic expression of the NF-1 gene in various tissues. Low amount of allelic messages was obtained from fibroblasts, keratinocytes and melanocytes of normal tissue and high amount of such messages was obtained from café au-lait spots (66).

Some NF-l-associated malignant tumors may be age-specific. In young patients with NF-1 the risk of malignant myeloid disorder of the blood is 200–500 times the norm (67). In animals with NF1 mutations, the tendency to develop one of several tumors is great (76). Table 1 lists all the tumor-suppressor genes linked to the phakomatoses.

Lazaro et al. identified a novel mutation: a 12-kb deletion of the NF-1 gene. Later, another sibling developed neurofibromatosis in spite of the parents being normal. They identified that 10% of the father's spermatozoa carried this mutation (77). The authors stressed that most germ-line mutations occur in precursors of gametes. This report seems in agreement with the known fact that most of the new mutations in NF-1 gene are of paternal origin (24).

NF-1 Variants

NF-2, a neurofibromatosis of different genetic origins and different clinical phenotypes than NF-1 will be discussed as a separate entity. In the past it was combined with NF-1 because of some similarities in the clinical appearance such as café au lait spots and others.

The rare occurrence of both NF-1 and NF-2 in the same individual is most likely an incidental finding (78).

It has not yet been confirmed that NF-3 (a condition in which acoustic neuromas and intracranial tumors are common), exists as a separate genetic and clinical entity. Phenotypically it manifests combined findings of NF-1 and NF-2 (67).

Segmental neurofibromatosis is a condition in which the skin lesions of NF-1 occur in only one part of the body, while other parts are normal. Tinschert et al. (79) found mutations in the NF-1 gene derived from cells in the affected region, such as fibroblasts in the café au lait spot. No mutations were detected in fibroblasts derived from normal skin. The authors concluded that these findings prove that *segmental neurofibromatosis* is caused by somatic mutations (79). However, Oguzkan et al. (80) reported a familial occurrence of segmental neurofibromatosis. It seems feasible, therefore, that in the majority of cases sporadic mutations occur while in rare cases a germline mutation is associated with a segmental distribution of NF-1.

Management

The most important step in the clinical management of NF is the diagnosis, which then enables a rational approach to advise and treat the patient. Many patients who have a milder form of the external manifestation of the disease may be undiagnosed. This includes patients with optic nerve glioma who have no diagnosis for the underlying NF-1. I found that a most important step to diagnose NF-1 is by confirming the existence of Lisch nodules on the iris. The technique of using several consecutive methods to detect the truncation of the neurofibromin, as suggested by Messiaen et al. (73), seems a practical method to examine this difficult gene.

Medical and Surgical Management

Growths that cause disfigurement, such as tumors of the eyelids, should be surgically removed. Ptosis also may be surgically corrected. Lisch nodules are harmless and do not cause glaucoma. If glaucoma occurs, it should be treated according to the angle changes found.

Table 1 Phakomatosis-Associated Tumor-Suppressor Genes

	Disease	Synonyms	Gene/symbol	Protein	Chromosomal location	Remarks
1	Neurofibromatosis type I	von Recklinghausen disease NF-1	NF-1	Neurofibromin	17q11.2	Multitude of various germ-line and somatic mutation. Segmental NF1 may occur.
2	Neurofibromatosis type II	NF-2	NF-2	Merlin/ schwannomin	22q12.2	Severe and mild subtypes, probably associated with different mutations
3	Tuberous sclerosis type 1	TS-1	TSC1	Hamartin	9q34	Mosaicism may be common
4	Tuberous sclerosis type 2	TS-2	TSC2	Tuberin	16p13.3	Hamartin and tuberin interact for growth suppression
5	Von Hippel–Lindau disease	VHL disease	VHL	pVHL 30 KDa pVHL19 KDa	3p25-p26	Few new mutations. Several specific to family phenotypes
6	Neuro-oculocutaneous cavernous angiomatosis	Cavernoma multiplex CCM1	KRIT1	—	7q11.2-q21	Retinal and cerebral lesions may be asymptomatic
7	MEN 2B	Multiple endocrine neoplasia type 2B	RET	—	10q11.2	93% of MEN2B carry the Met918Thr mutation on exon 16
8	Basal cell nevus syndrome	Fifth phacomatosis	PTCH	—	9q22.3	

The treatment of optic nerve gliomas is still a subject of great controversy. Hoyt and Baghdassarian (51) claim that treatment is usually not necessary, as the tumor is self-limiting, vision does not change appreciably after diagnosis, and life expectancy is normal. On the other hand, some optic nerve gliomas do change after diagnosis; they may increase in size, infiltrate surrounding tissue, and reduce vision further. This may be especially true for optic nerve gliomas associated with NF.

Chiasmal gliomas also may be life threatening. One report describes a progressive chiasmal glioma treated with 4680 rad. Radiation seems to have stopped further growth and may prove to be palliative treatment (52). In one study, radiation therapy effectively controlled the disease in seven of nine patients (81). These authors favor biopsy-radiotherapy as the treatment of choice for chiasmal tumors and recommend a course of 4500–5000 rad over a 4.5- to 5-week period. They also claim that surgery can be successful if a clear margin is maintained between the tumor and the chiasm, and the tumor is completely excised (81).

More studies are needed to evaluate differences between gliomas of NF and those not related to NF. A course of surgery, irradiation, or just observation should be individually adjusted according to the clinical findings and the patient's progress.

The consensus of a 1988 National Institutes of Health (NIH) conference on the management of neurofibromatosis was that the best methods to detect optic nerve gliomas are CT scans and MRI, and the best therapeutic approach is usually conservative (11). Surgery, radiation, or chemotherapy can be used, but should be reserved for exceptionally large or dangerous tumors.

Genetic Counseling

Because NF is an autosomal dominant disease with a penetrance of close to 100%, statistically, chances are that 50% of children of an affected person will have the disease, whether the case is familial or a new mutation. The expressivity of the disease varies considerably, and about 25% of all affected persons are estimated to have the moderate or severe form of the disease, the rest will show only mild signs (3). Slit-lamp examination for Lisch bodies of the patient's immediate family members may disclose the familial occurrence of the disease and its severity. However, it is not possible to predict the severity of the disease in descendants from these findings. The use of molecular genetics methods for prenatal diagnosis or presymptomatic diagnosis will, undoubtedly, become available in the near future, but is not now accurate enough (64).

NEUROFIBROMATOSIS TYPE 2

Neurofibromatosis type 2 affects all three main organs that are affected in the other phakomatoses: the eye, the brain and the skin. Other organs may also be affected. The hallmarks of the disorder are bilateral eighth cranial nerve (vestibular branch) tumors. The eyes are more often affected than not.

The Clinical Manifestations of NF Type 2

Parry et al. (82) studied the clinical characteristics of their 63 patients with NF-2 disorder. They found that the clinical manifestations and course of progression were similar within the family but differed among families. They proposed to designate each family into a severe type or a mild type. The initial symptoms that marked the onset of the disease were from vestibular tumors (schwannomas) in 44% of the patients, from other tumors (22%), from skin abnormalities (13%), and from ocular signs in 13% (82).

Skin Lesions

Café–au–lait spots, counted like in NF-1, when more than 0.5 cm in the prepubertal period and more than 1.5 cm in the postpubertal period, were found in 47% of patients. Skin tumors were found in 68% of patients. Fifteen percent had more than 10 skin tumors (82).

CNS Tumors

Tumors affecting the CNS included bilateral vestibular schwannoma (92%), meningiomas (49%), spinal tumors (67%), and other brain tumors (5%). Schwannomas affected all cranial nerves, except the first, the second and the sixth (82). However, a menigioma of the optic nerve was detected in almost half of the cases (82).

Ocular Abnormalities

Ocular abnormalities were common. Cataracts usually of the posterior subcapsular type (PSC) were commonly found (81% of patients). In five, cataracts were seen at the age of 10. Retinal hamartomas were found in eight cases (82). Combined hamartomas of the retina and the RPE were found in five of 63 patients in one study (82), in four patients of the same family with NF2 (83), and in one of 15 patients in a third study (84). Epiretinal membranes in the macular region were reported in 12 of 15 patients (84) and in seven of nine patients in another study (85).

Retinal hamartomas are not uncommon and affect from 10% (85) to 22% of patients (86). Extraocular motor nerve involvement may lead to strabismus (86). Multiple astrocytomas may lead to retinal detachment (85).

In the severe type, various complications may occur. Increased intracranial pressure from tumors such as meningioma or schwannoma may cause chronic papilledema, optic atrophy and blindness (87). In an exceptionally severe case of NF-2, the patients suffered from blindness, deafness and quadriparesis (88).

Diagnosis

In spite of the identification of the gene, the diagnosis of NF-2 remains based on clinical findings, because of the difficulty of the search for mutations (46).

As mentioned above, the ocular abnormalities are very common in NF-2 patients and almost universally present. However, in only 13% were the initial symptoms related to the eye (82), or even less, with 10% only (24). The main initial symptoms, hearing loss, imbalance or tinnitus occur in 44–89%, according to different studies (89). NF-2 is usually not diagnosed until the late teen years or early adulthood. The mean age of diagnosis ranges in different studies, from 20 to 26 years (89). Ocular examination can confirm the diagnosis and reduce the time between first symptoms and diagnosis, estimated to be eight years. Laboratory tests are not very helpful but an inner retinal dysfunction was determined by ganzfeld ERG in one patient with NF-2 and congenital cataract (89). All NF-2 patients must be followed up by MRI.

The diagnostic criterion for NF-2 is one of the following: (i) bilateral tumors of the eighth nerve; (ii) a-first degree relative with NF-2 and a unilateral eighth nerve tumor or two neurofibromas, meningiomas or schwannomas, or a characteristic posterior cortical lens opacity of adolescent onset (45); (iii) two of the following: neurofibroma, meningioma, glioma, schwannoma, juvenile PSC cataract.

Epidemiology, Genetics and Molecular Genetics

The incidence of NF-2 is about one-tenth of the incidence of NF-1, ranging from 1 in 33,000 to 1 in 40,000, according to various studies (24). The genetic transmission is by the autosomal dominant mode with full penetrance but great intrafamiliar variance in expressivity, and to a much lesser degree intrafamilial variability. Intrafamilial similarity was reported as to the type of severity, mild or severe. Baser et al. (90) studied three pairs of monozygotic twins with NF-2. All had bilateral vestibular schwannomas. Each MZ pair was concordant as to the general type (mild or severe) and usually as to affected organ. They were discordant as to presence and type of associated cranial tumors.

The locus of the gene NF-2 was mapped to the proximal long arm of chromosome 22, between 22ql1.1 and 22ql3.1 (91,92). This is interesting, considering the reported loss of genes on chromosome 22 in pathologic specimens of meningiomas and acoustic neuromas (91). NF-2 was therefore suspected to be one of the tumor-suppressor genes, even before the gene was known.

The mapping of the gene was later refined to chromosome 22ql2.2 (67). The gene NF-2 was cloned in parts in 1993 (93,94) and in whole in 2002 (95). It consists of 17 exons (95) and encodes a 587 amino acid protein named merlin (94) or schwannomin (93). Sainz et al. (96) identified the protein as consisting of 595 amino acids and belonging to a new family of proteins with similarity to moesin, radixin and ezrin, whose function is to link the cell membrane and the cell cytoskeleton. Multiple mutations were identified (93,96–98). Most led to a truncated protein-product. Parry et al. (98) pointed out that patients with nonsense mutations or frameshifts leading to premature termination with earlier onset and earlier diagnosis, suffered from the severe type of NF-2. The diagnosis was usually established before the age of 20 and they developed many other CNS tumors, in addition to the bilateral schwannomas. Patients with splice-site mutations had milder disease of later onset. In addition to the bilateral Schwannoma they had few benign tumors (98).

NF-2 is a tumor suppressor gene as evident from several studies and from LOH detected in the tumors (8). Gutmann et al. demonstrated that the tumor suppressor protein merlin (or schwannomin) functions together with HRS (hepatocyte growth factor-regulated tyrosine kinase substrate) as cell regulators of Schwann cells. They suppress cell growth and motility (99).

Management

The most important first step in the management of NF-2 is its diagnosis, which frequently is made too late. It is based on the clinical findings and on the diagnostic criteria as outlined above. Once diagnosis is established, the patient must be thoroughly investigated in various disciplines, which should at least include a neurologist, dermatologist and an ophthalmologist. Imaging should be performed, using CT scan and MRI. Annual follow up by MRI will determine progression of the disease.

Genetic Counseling

Counseling is based on autosomal dominant transmission, full penetrance and variable expressivity. The high rate of mutations de novo should be considered. At least 50% of all cases are new mutations (24,100). The mutation of the NF-2 may be identified in spite of the difficulty. However, a certain proportion of sporadic cases and a larger proportion of mosaicism (100) must be accounted for. In the sporadic cases no disease-bearing mutations will be detected in the NF-2 gene in the circulating leukocytes.

Mutations and LOH will be detected in the tumors, likely to be a result of somatic mutations. In mosaicism, some leukocytes will carry mutations while others not. This seems to be a common finding in NF-2 (100).

Prenatal Diagnosis

When both the gene and the mutation are known, direct analysis of the DNA of the embryo and of other affected members can be performed (101). Pulst concluded from his studies of families that most want to have a prenatal diagnosis, in spite of the fact that two-thirds of the families would continue the pregnancy regardless of the results (101). Pre-implantation Genetic Diagnosis (PGD) has been successfully used (102,103). Standard in-vitro fertilization (IVF) techniques are used. A mutation-free oocyte is selected and introduced into the uterus (103).

TUBEROUS SCLEROSIS

Tuberous sclerosis (TS) or Bourneville's disease is, like NF, an autosomal dominant disease of high penetrance, variable expressivity, with a high rate of new mutations. Also like NF it affects many organs, mostly the skin, the eye, and the CNS.

The Clinical Manifestations of Tuberous Sclerosis

The largest group of patients with TS examined in a single study comprised 160 patients. This study from the Mayo Clinic (104) has been an invaluable source of information on the clinical manifestations of this disease.

Skin Lesions

The most common finding of TS in the skin are facial angiofibromas, formerly considered to be adenoma sebaceum, found in 70% of patients (104). Typically, the lesions are multiple red to pink papules with a smooth glistening surface (Fig. 5). They occur in a bilateral and symmetric arrangement over the cheeks, centrofacial area, and chin (105). Their number increases at puberty (105). The second most common skin lesions, hypomelanotic macular ash leaf spots, can be easily missed unless examined under a Wood's light. They were so named because they resemble the contours of the leaves of the European mountain ash tree. The spots can be easily detected under the 360-nm wavelength of the Wood's light (Fig. 5). These spots can occasionally be seen in normal babies.

Other skin lesions occur less frequently in TS. Table 2 lists the different skin lesions found in 160 patients at the Mayo Clinic (104).

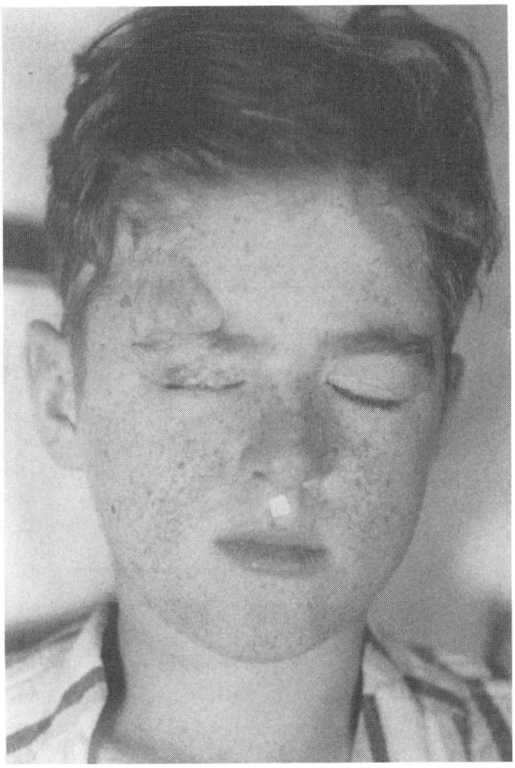

Figure 5 Adenoma sebaceum (multiple facial angiofibromata) in a patient with tuberous sclerosis: note the characteristic multiple papules diffusely and symmetrically distributed over cheeks, chin, and nose. These are red or pink in color. Note also a large angiofibroma over right eyelid and right forehead.

Ocular Lesions in Tuberous Sclerosis

Retinal hamartomas. The most common ocular lesion of TS is the retinal hamartoma. In some studies, retinal hamartomas were found in all patients with TS (106). In a study of 139 patients described by Robertson (107), retinal hamartomas occurred in approximately half of all patients. In a follow-up of his patients, Robertson (108) confirmed that about half of all TS patients manifested hamartomas of the retina or of the optic

Table 2 Skin Lesions in Tuberous Sclerosis

Lesion	Percentage[a]
Adenoma sebaceum (facial angiofibromas)	70
Hypomelanotic maculas (ash-leaf spots)	57
Shagreen patches	36
Fibromas at the nailbed	18
Café au lait spots	18
Cutaneous nodules	14

[a]The percentage of patients with tuberous sclerosis manifesting the lesion.
Source: Gomez MR (ed.) Tuberous Sclerosis. New York: Ravan Press, 1979.

nerve; in about half of these, the hamartomas were bilateral. In another study of 100 patients, Rowley et al. (109) detected 44 with retinal hamartomas.

The lesions (Fig. 6), manifest in one of three forms (107). One type of retinal lesion is flat, smooth-surfaced, nearly transparent, and circular or oval. It may be tiny, the size of a retinal exudate, or larger. This lesion may be unilateral or bilateral and may appear singly or in multiples. A second form occurs as larger, more elevated, glistening nodules, that are calcified, multinodular, or cystic. These have been variously referred to as "salmon-eggs," "tapioca," and "mulberries." A third type is a transitional form that combines features of the other two types of retinal lesions.

Rowley et al. (109) found that the most common hamartoma was the flat translucent lesion (31 of 44); the mulberry type (24 of 44) was less common and the transition type was uncommon (four of 44). The same eye may manifest more than one type of retinal hamartoma.

There is significant indication that most hamartomas can be ophthalmoscopically detected early in life. Shami et al. (110) diagnosed bilateral astrocytic hamartomas of the retina in a 7-day-old infant. Published reports indicated that TS-associated hamartomas had been found in 1-month and 3.5-month-old children (110). Zimmer-Galler and Robertson followed 16 patients with 37 TS–associated astrocytic hamartomas for a mean of 16 years (range 6–34). In this period only three tumors showed progression and one new hamartoma occurred (111). On the other hand, in one case, spontaneous regression of a documented hamartoma of the retina occurred (112).

The same eye may contain more than one type of retinal hamartoma. Most of these lesions remain unchanged, but at least one photographically documented report exists of a flat lesion that evolved into a calcified nodular tumor (113).

Abnormalities of fundus pigmentation. Abnormalities of fundus pigmentation may occur as pigment clumping, "black drusen" (107), or as areas of depigmentation. Depigmentation may appear as a "punched-out" spot anywhere in the fundus or as a depigmented line along the long posterior ciliary nerve (109,114).

Vascular changes in fundus. Retinal vascular changes may be found in conjunction with retinal hamartomas and may include sheathed vessels, dilated vessels, and a double vascular supply around the tumor (107).

Iris hypopigmentation. Rarely, a spot of iris depigmentation (115) or a depigmented iris sector (114) is found in patients with TS. The iris hypopigmentation illustrates the decreased melanin in the melanosomes, similar to that found in typical hypopigmented skin maculae (115).

Other ocular lesions. Rarely, a hamartoma may cause papilledema because of an optic nerve involvement, resulting in optic atrophy (107). Also rare are vitreous hemorrhages and retinal exudates (107). A rare case of persistent hyperplastic primary vitreous was also described (116). This patient also had a retinal tumor and detachment in the other eye. Hamartomas of the iris are uncommon (117).

Central Nervous System Lesions

Seizures or epilepsy and mental retardation were recognized as a common finding in TS, both by Vogt in 1908 and by van der Hoeve in 1921 (113). Seizures occurred in 88% of the Mayo Clinic patients, and mental retardation was found in 60% (104). Every patient with mental retardation had seizures. A study of monozygotic twins (118) suggested that mental retardation is related to the early onset of seizures.

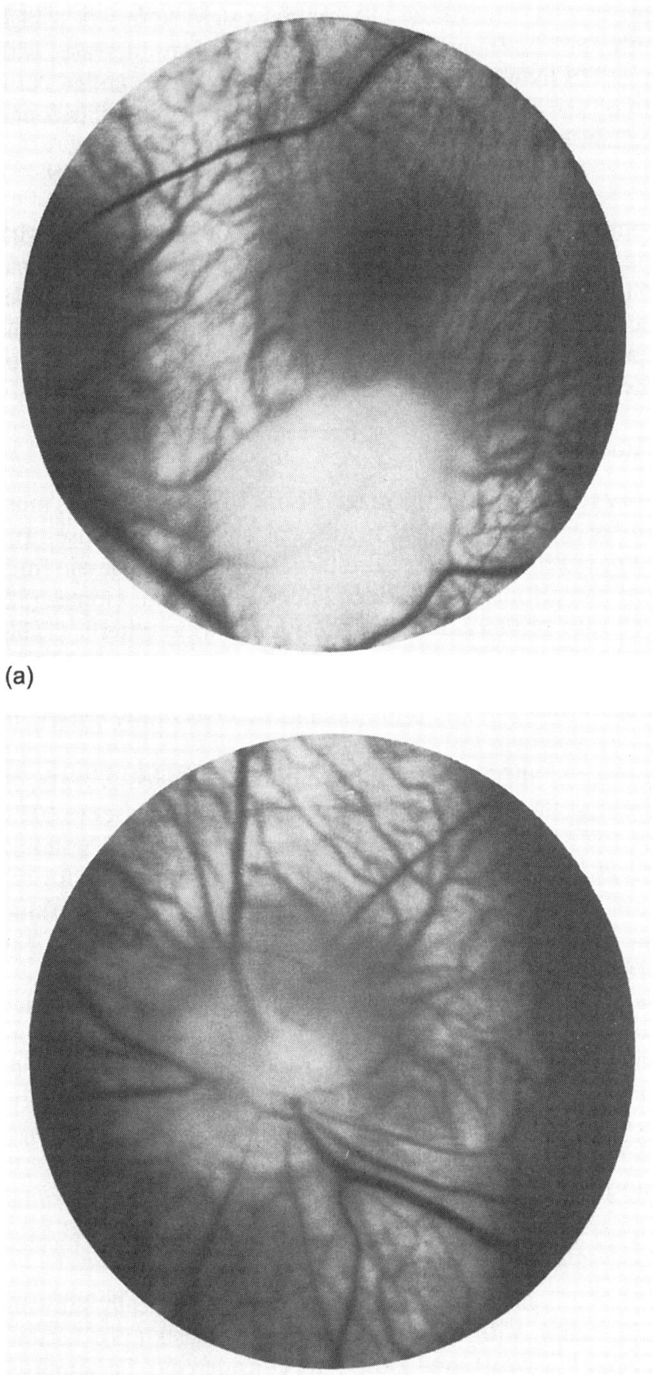

(a)

(b)

Figure 6 Retinal hamartoma in a patient with TS: one lesion was near the macula (a); the other partially surrounded the optic disk (b). Both lesions were almost transparent, elevated and glistening, and seemed to be transitional between the smooth-surfaced small lesion and the "tapioca" lesion.

Skull roentgenograms or CT scans show intracranial calcifications in a high percentage of patients with TS. The frequency of such calcifications increases with time. Two types of brain lesions may be detected (119): subependymal nodules, commonly <1 mm in size, and mineralized and cortical tubers, tiny bodies found in the cerebrum or cerebellum representing benign calcifying astrocytomas.

Single or multiple rhabdomyomas of the heart were found in 30% of patients with TS (120). A common association exists between TS and a heart conduction syndrome named Wolff-Parkinson-White (WPW), which may be the expression of the cardiac rhabdomyoma or result from supraventricular tachycardia (121).

Angiomyolipoma of the kidney is rather common. In one study of 38 patients with TS, angiomyolipoma was discovered in 23 (60%) (122). It is best detected by abdominal CT scans. Cysts may be found in the bones and kidneys. Colonic hamartomas or adenomatous polyps or both are also found in a high percentage of patients with TS (123). The lungs may also be affected.

The Diagnosis of Tuberous Sclerosis

There is no single laboratory test to confirm the diagnosis of TS. The diagnosis must be made by the physician based on the clinical manifestations of the disease. The triad of adenoma sebaceum, epilepsy, and mental retardation are the classic findings of the disease. Retinal hamartomas were added later to this triad. Gomez (104) divided the findings of TS into primary and secondary diagnostic criteria (Table 3) and suggested that the presence of three primary diagnostic criteria or two primary and any two secondary criteria make the diagnosis of TS. Later Osborne (124) considered the presence of one primary criterion and two secondary criteria as diagnostic of TS.

The diagnosis of TS may be difficult in young children. At age two years, as few as 25% of patients show manifestations of the disease; at age ten years, this increases to 60%, at 20 years 82% manifest the disease. All persons suspected of

Table 3 Primary and Secondary Diagnostic Criteria in Tuberous Sclerosis

Primary diagnostic criteria
Cortical tubers of subependymal hamartoraas
Retinal hamartomas
Adenoma sebaceum (facial angiofibroma)
Periungual fibroma
Renal angiomyolipomata
Secondary diagnoslic criteria
Infantile spasm; myotonic, tonic, or atonic seizures
Ash-leaf skin spots
Single retinal hamartoma
Brain calcifications
Bilateral polycystic kidneys
Cardiac rhabdomyoma
Pitting defects in tooth enamel
Radiographic "honeycomb" lungs
Fibrous plaque on forehead
Giant cell astrocytoma
First-degree relative with tuberous sclerosis

Source: After Refs. 104, 124

having TS should undergo a thorough dermatologic examination, using Wood's light to seek for the hypomelanotic maculae; a thorough ocular examination; and a neurologic workup, including roentgenograms and CT scans. Moreover, first-degree relatives of the patient should also undergo similar examinations.

An important differential diagnosis of the retinal lesion is retinoblastoma, which may look like the hamartoma of TS (106,107). It was suggested that when no definite diagnosis can be established, observation with weekly reexaminations is preferred. If the tumor grows, it is probably retinoblastoma, as hamartomas of TS usually remain unchanged.

Pathology and Pathogenesis

The ocular hamartomas were histologically found to be glial astrocytomas located in the retina or at the optic nerve head (107).

The facial skin changes represent a facial angiofibroma, histologically showing dermal fibrosis and vasodilatation with occasional large fibroblasts (105). Lesions occurring in the brain, retina, skin, heart, and kidney are considered to be hamartomas.

Electron microscopy can distinguish between hypomelanotic skin macules representing white ash-leaf skin spots of TS and simple white vitilligo spots. In the first, melanocyte density is normal, but melanization is suppressed, whereas, in the second, a decrease in number of melanocytes is found (125).

The pathogenesis of TS is unknown. Like other phakomatoses, TS probably should be classified as a neurocristopathy.

Epidemiology and Genetics

Estimates on the prevalence of TS in the general population vary from 1:23,000 to 1:170,000 (126). Newer estimates express a much higher prevalence, such as 1:10,000 of the general population (124,127). Some epidemiological studies cited the figure even higher, at 1:6,000 (128). A complete ascertainment of the population of west Scotland revealed a minimum prevalence of 1:12,000 in children (129). Most epidemiologic studies have been performed in institutions for the mentally retarded and, undoubtedly, indicate minimal figures only. The mutation rate is relatively high, with 6–14.6 mutants per million genes per generation (126), and may even be higher. The mutation rate in Scotland was calculated to be 25 mutations per million genes per generation (129).

The proportion of familial cases to sporadic ones is not known. The estimates vary from 20% to 44% of all TS patients having a family history of this disease (130). With proper examination of the immediate family, including the use of a Wood's lamp and CT scans, approximately one-third to one-half of all cases may reveal a positive family history.

Linkage analysis, by use of 26 polymorphic DNA markers in 19 families with TS, supported the assignment of the TS gene to the distal long arm of chromosome 9, near the locus for the ABO blood group (131). The exact location is probably at 9q34 (132,133).

It is now known that tuberous sclerosis is a group of diseases similar in their clinical appearance and caused by several different mutated genes. The group was given the symbol of tuberous sclerosis complex (TSC). Haines et al. reported in 1991 a study of 22 families with TS that strongly supported the heterogeneity of TS. One locus, later named TSC1 was linked to chromosome 9q32-34 and was detected in approximately a third of all families (134). The TSC1 locus was later mapped to chromosome 9q34 and considered to be responsible for about one half of all cases of TS (135,136). The gene has a transcript of 8.6 kb. It encodes a protein of 130 kDa, named hamartin, that consists of 1164 amino acids (137). Its function is unknown. Many studies demonstrated loss of alleles with LOH, thus confirming that TSC1 is a tumor-suppressor gene (116,137–139). Young et al. (140) screened the entire coding region of TSC1 in 79 tuberous sclerosis patients. They identified 26 mutations, all predicted to cause premature truncation of the protein and one splice-site mutation. Similarly van Slegtenhorst et al. (137) identified 32 distinct mutations and 30 of them were protein truncating.

Mosaicism can occur and may pose a serious problem for detection of the mutated allele. In most cases of mosaicism mild TS was reported; but Kwiatkowska et al. (141) described a young girl with a severe TS that included fits and mental retardation. Study of peripheral leukocytes revealed that only about one-third had the mutated allele.

TSC2 Locus

In 1993, the second locus for tuberous sclerosis has been identified. This locus has been previously mapped to a location on chromosome 16pl3 where a linkage with polycystic kidney disease exists (142). The European chromosome 16 tuberous sclerosis consortium reported the identification of TSC2 on chromosome 16p13.3 (143). Its protein product tubulin is a predicted 198 kDa protein (135). The gene contains 41 small exons spanning 45 kb of genomic DNA and encodes a 5.5 kb mRNA (144). TSC2 mutations, like TSC1 mutations, are responsible for approximately 50% of familial TS (144). TSC2 is also a tumor suppressor gene as demonstrated by loss of alleles and LOH (127,139). New mutations may occur in one-third to two-third of all cases of TS2 (127).

The two proteins, tuberin and hamartin interact for mediation of growth suppression (145). Their critical functions are likely to be closely linked. Binding of tuberin and hamartin is necessary, but not sufficient, for mediation of growth suppression (145).

TSC3 Locus

Fahsold et al. (146) reported the mapping of a third locus for tuberous sclerosis on chromosome 12q22-q24.1, close to or within the region of the gene of phenylalanine hydroxylase. It is not yet known if such a locus exists and is rarely associated with TS, or that it does not exist.

Clinical Management

The ocular lesions usually do not increase in size and do not affect vision. In rare cases, laser photocoagulation may be indicated. The lesions in the brain and in other organs must be evaluated individually for the best method of treatment.

Genetic counseling should be based on the fact that TS is an autosomal dominant gene with an unknown, but high (70–100%) penetrance and variable expressivity. Approximately 35–50% of children of an affected person will develop the disease. The number of sporadic cases owing to new mutations is high, forming the majority of TS cases, at least 60% of all such patients. In addition, many patients are mentally retarded, institutionalized, and never marry, thus further reducing the number of familial cases.

The successful use of fetal echocardiography for prenatal diagnosis of TS has been reported (147). Prenatal diagnosis using molecular genetic methods for detection of TSC genes and their mutations may soon be practical.

VON HIPPEL–LINDAU DISEASE

The hamartomatous lesion of von Hippel–Lindau disease (VHL) is a vascular angioma, described in the retina, brain, spinal cord, face, adrenal glands, lungs, liver, and other tissues. As with the other phakomatoses, VHL is an autosomal dominant trait, with variable expressivity, and a high mutation rate. Like the others, it is a progressive disease, and many times its characteristic manifestations are not evident before the third decade of life. The angioma of VHL affects a multitude of organs and tissues and may be benign or may undergo a malignant transformation.

The Clinical Manifestations of von Hippel–Lindau Disease

More than 20 years passed from the time the ophthalmologist von Hippel described the retinal angioma as a very rare disease in 1904 (148) until the neurologist Lindau reported on the second manifestation of VHL after pathologic studies of the brain (149). These two manifestations are the hallmark of VHL Other organs are less frequently affected, but Lindau (149) also described cysts in the pancreas, kidneys, adrenal glands, and liver. Different terms were used for this disease, including retinal angiomatosis, angiomatosis retinae, von Hippel's disease, and oculoneurovisceral syndrome of von Hippel and Lindau. The term VHL is the most accepted, however, and will be used here.

Ocular Lesions

Retinal angiomas. Angioma of the retina is the typical ocular lesion of VHL. In a review of the subject, Augsburger et al. (150) classified hereditary retinal angiomas into capillary and cavernous hemangiomatoses. Only capillary hemangiomatosis is related to VHL.

The classic picture of the angioma is a reddish or a yellow-red mass in the peripheral retina, fed by one or more dilated, tortuous, and congested arteries and veins. The lesion usually is clinically evident around the third decade of life (151). Salazar and Lamiell (152), who studied a large kindred with VHL in Hawaii, found three types of retinal lesions, which probably represent the development of the angiomas over time. The early lesions look like microaneurysms and do not stain with fluorescein. The intermediate group are pale gray tumors that stain with fluorescein, but have no abnormal feeder vessels. The advanced group is the classic angioma. Sometimes, the earliest findings in the retina may be tiny abnormalities in the vessels or microaneurysms, which hyperfluoresce (151). The "adult" tumor is a reddish or pink vascular lesion ranging in size from 0.5 to 10 mm or more (Fig. 7). It may grow anywhere on the retina, toward the vitreous (endophytic growth) or toward the choroid (exophytic growth), and appear singly or in multiples. About one of three patients have more than one tumor, and about 50% of all patients are affected bilaterally (151).

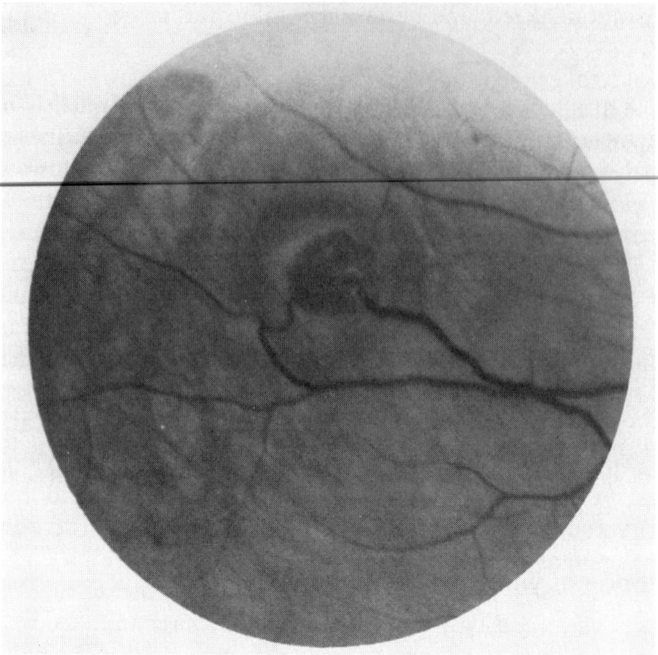

(a)

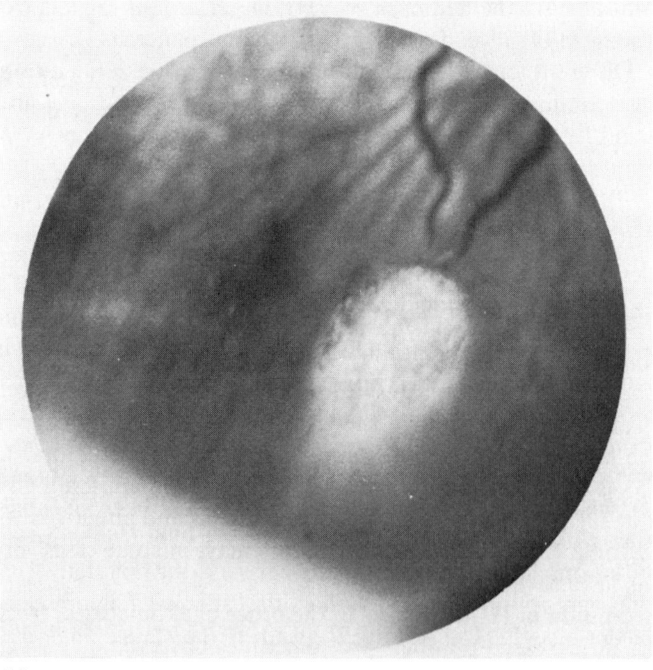

(b)

Figure 7 Retinal angioma of advanced VHL: The tumor varies in size and appearance and changes with time, (a) A small tumor, pink-red in appearance, with one congested arteriole supplying blood and one congested vein draining it; (b) an intermediate sized, gray elevated tumor with multiple vessels on it; (c) a large tumor, partially gray-white from fibrovascular tissue, with a heavy fibrotic component; and (d) a large tumor predominantly fibrotic.

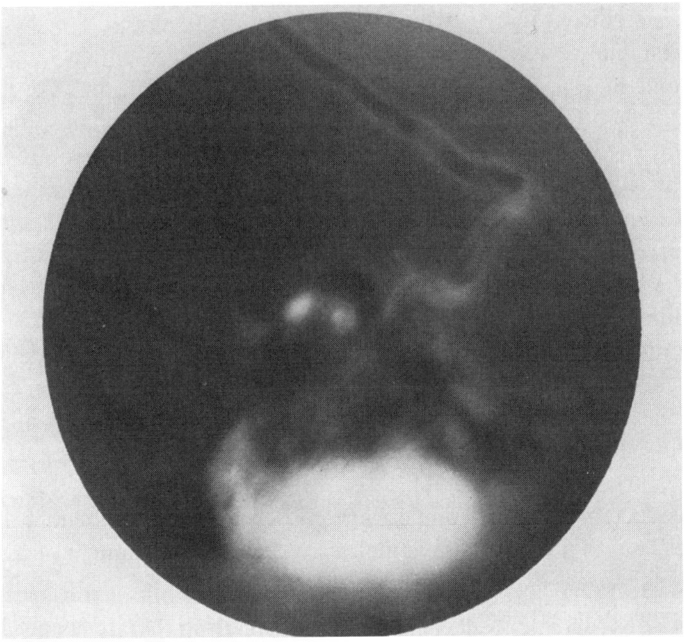

(c)

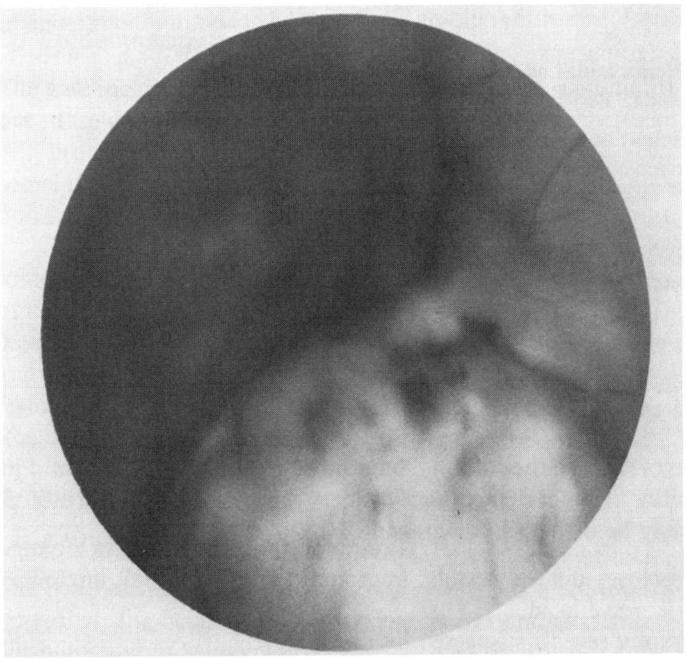

(d)

Figure 7 (*Continued*)

Maher et al. (153) studied 152 eyes with VHL. Mean age of onset of disease was 26.3 years. Retinal angioma was the first manifestation in 43% of patients, cerebellar hemangioblastoma in 39% and renal carcinoma in 10%. With time 59% developed a retinal angioma, 59% a CNS angioma, 28% renal cell carcinoma, 13% a spinal hemangioblastoma and 7% a pheochrornocytoma (153). Maher and Moore (154) consider the retinal tumors, usually referred to as angiomas, as hemangioblastomas. They are composed of endothelial-lined channels separated by masses of vacuolated foam cells. Shields et al. (155) reported 103 patients (113 eyes) with vascular retinal tumors that were not VHL angiomas. They used terms such as vasoproliferative retinal tumors or acquired retinal angiomas. They should be distinguished from primary genetic or sporadic angiomas. Schmidt and Neumann (156) displayed their findings of retinal vascular hamartomas in VHL patients that occur in addition to the typical hemangiomas They are located superficially near a retinal vein, and appear small and moss fiber-like. Ophthalmoscopically they are flat vascular lesions (156).

Secondary changes occur typically from leakage in the vascular endothelium of the tumor (157). These changes result in intraretinal edema, serous detachment of the retina, intraretinal and subretinal exudates, a star-shaped figure around the macula, and subretinal or vitreous hemorrhage (Fig. 8). In the final stages, the secondary changes progress to total retinal detachment, ġlaucoma, phthisis bulbi, and complete loss of vision. It is also possible, however, that some angiomas never change.

Optic disk angiomas: Optic disk angiomas are relatively uncommon and may be found in patients with retinal angiomas or may be an isolated finding. There are three types of optic disk angiomas (150). One is an ophthalmoscopically visible endophytic papillary hemangioma that grows on the optic nerve head. Surrounding the

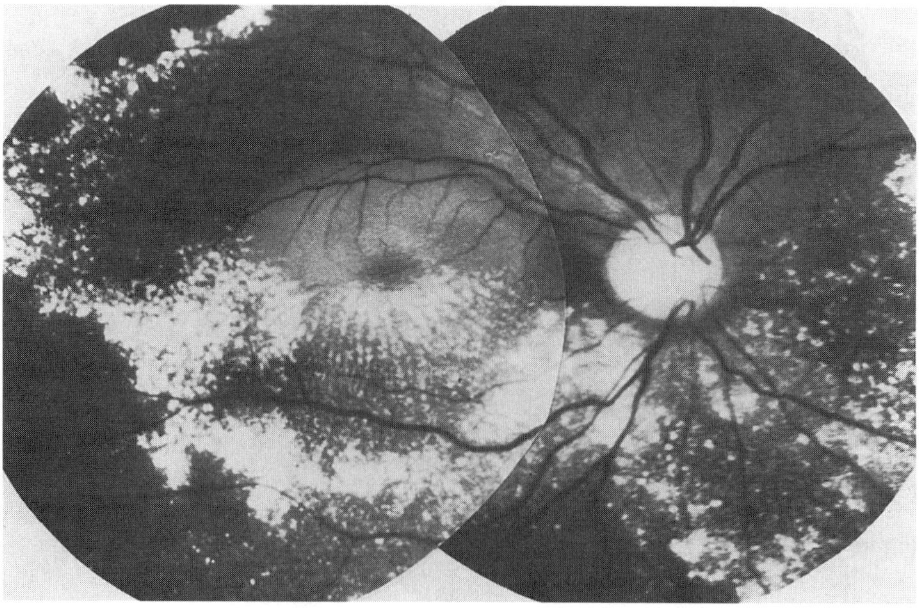

Figure 8 Heavy intraretinal and subretinal exudation in a patient with a peripheral large retinal angioma (Fig. 7d). Note the extensive involvement of the posterior pole including the macular star.

disk is a ring of exudates. The second type is a sessile hemangioma manifested by a thickening of the optic nerve head. The lesion should be suspected when a ring of exudates is seen. The third type is an exophytic hemangioma that grows as a nodular, yellow orange tumor into the subretinal space.

Central Nervous System Lesions

About 25% of patients with retinal or optic nerve disease develop clinical manifestations of CNS involvement, usually in the form of a cerebellar hemangioma or hemangioblastoma, but other parts of the CNS, such as the spinal cord, medulla, or the fourth ventricle may be affected. A screening of 47 patients with hemangioblastoma of the brain found 23% to have VHL (158). Eighty-three percent of these tumors were located in the cerebellum. The hemangioma may be solid or cystic. The frequency of CNS lesions is probably higher than estimations, because some are not manifested clinically and are found incidentally in autopsy specimens.

Other Lesions

Cysts, benign tumors, and malignant neoplasms in various locations are not uncommon findings in VHL Table 4 lists some of the growths reported in this disease, including nonprogressive hamartomas, benign tumors, and malignant tumors. Of all patients with VHL, 55% develop retinal angiomas, at least 60% manifest a CNS hemangioblastoma, about 33% will have renal or pancreatic cysts and about 7% will develop a pheochromocytoma (159–161). Abdominal tumors may, in some cases, precede symptomatic ocular lesions (162).

Later studies indicate an increase in the diagnosis of pheochromocytomas in patients with VHL. In one study, 64 of 246 individuals with VHL had pheochromocytoma (163). Thirty-five percent of pheochromocytoma patients were asymptomatic. In another study, 19 of 82 unselected patients with pheochromocytoma (23%) were found to be carriers of a familial disorder, VHL (19%) and MEN 4% (164).

A benign tumor of the epididymis, cystadenoma was detected in 54% of male patients with VHL and confirmed by ultrasound (165). Pancreatic tumors may include cysts, microcystic adenomas and malignant pancreatic neuroendocrine tumors. Libutti et al. (166) reported that 12% of VHL patients manifested neuroendocrine tumors in the pancreas, some already metastasized into the liver.

Skin lesions are uncommon in VHL, but, as in the other phakomatoses, freckles and café au lait spots in increased numbers are sometimes observed.

Table 4 Reported Hamartomas and Tumors in von-Hippel–Lindau Disease

Angioma (hemangioblastoma) of cerebellum
Hemangioblastoma of spinal cord or medulla
Cysts of pancreas
Microcystic adenoma of pancreas
Cysts of kidney
Cysts of liver
Cystadenomas of epididymis
Renal cell carcinoma
Pheochromocytoma
Carcinoma of pancreas
Neuroendocrine tumors of pancreas

The Diagnosis of von Hippel–Lindau Disease

No specific laboratory test exists to confirm or rule out the diagnosis of VHL. Most often, the diagnosis is made by an ophthalmologist who observes the typical picture of a retinal capillary angioma in a patient with visual complaints or during a routine eye examination. The diagnosis may be unsuspected, however, and difficult to confirm in early stages (before the "adult" angioma is seen in the retina) and in late stages when a "milky" retinal detachment distorts the classic picture. The following examinations may be of help in diagnosing HLD:

1. Ophthalmoscopy discloses dilated vessels, microaneurysms, or small angiomas in the retina or optic nerve head.
2. Fluorescein angiography reveals suspected lesions.
3. Eye examinations of first-degree relatives demonstrate the genetic factor.
4. CT scans of the brain show the neurologic elements.
5. Intravenous pyelogram or CT scan of the abdomen discloses other organ involvement.

A high incidence of presence of twin vessels, defined as a paired retinal arteriole and venule, separated by less than the diameter of one venule, and extending for a distance of more than 1-disk diameter, was found in patients with VHL (161). These vessels were found as early as six months of age and, therefore, may serve as a marker for the disease before the characteristic findings develop.

It is imperative to distinguish between a retinal angioma associated with genetic VHL and a sporadic, single, non-genetic angioma. Several factors can help make this distinction.

Patients with VHL-associated angioma have, as outlined above, a significant risk of extraocular tumors such as cerebellar hemangioblastoma, renal cell carcinoma, pheochromocytoma and others (167). Tumor susceptibility indicates a hereditary retinal angioma. Two or more primary retinal angiomas, separated in one eye or one (or more) in each eye, always indicate hereditary VHL. However, in many VHL cases the angioma is solitary. The mean number of retinal angiomas in VHL is 1.85, with a range of 0–15 (168). The appearance of a sporadic, solitary angioma is identical to that of the hereditary type and they cannot be thus distinguished (169). Singh et al. (170) claimed that onset is earlier in hereditary angiomas with a mean of 17.6 years vs. sporadic angiomas with onset at 36.1. years. Fifty-five percent of VHL patients had more than one tumor, 13% developed a new tumor growing within the follow-up period of ten years. The diagnosis was made on the basis of family history (plus one angioma) in 28%, systemic findings in 4% and multiple tumors in 14% (170). A new solitary retinal angioma detected in mid-life has a risk of 46% of being of hereditary origin. After age of 60 the risk is reduced to <1% (171).

McCabe et al. (172) compared genetic VHL-associated juxtapapillary hemangioblastomas to sporadic angiomas. In VHL (one-third of all patients) the visual acuities were poorer both initially and finally. The eye manifestations appeared earlier and were often bilateral and/or additional peripheral tumors were seen (172).

The evaluation of a patient suspected to have VHL must include screening for both brain and abdominal tumors. Because of the progressive nature of the disease, repeated examination should be performed. CT scanning and MRI of the head, spine, and abdomen are useful in both the diagnosis and the follow-up of VHL (173). However, in sporadic, non-genetic angioma the only necessary treatment and follow-up is ophthalmic. Maher et al. (174) and Webster et al. (169) suggested the following protocol for patients with VHL and for first-degree relatives with a retinal angioblastoma. Annually, a general physical, an ophthalmic examination, a renal ultrasound and a 24-hr urine collection for metanephrines and catecholamines should be performed. Every three years a MRI of the skull, spine and abdomen should be added. After the age of 50, these last tests can be done every five years (169,174).

Pathology and Pathogenesis

The earliest pathologic phenomenon of retinal angiomatosis is probably a nodule of endothelial hyperplasia, connected to both arterial and venous retinal systems (151). In the "adult phase" the retinal tumor shows a proliferation of endothelial cells, capillaries, and small blood vessels. The capillaries of the tumor, unlike normal retinal capillaries, are fenestrated and have few pericytes. Also, the basement membrane of the capillary wall is thickened and reduplicated (175). In addition, lipid-laden foam cells and glial cells that proliferate to induce fibrosis can be seen. Mottow-Lippa et al. (175) postulate that the foam cells do not derive from glia or macrophages, but that both the endothelial cells of the hamartoma and the interstitial foam cells originate from a pluripotential vasoformative skin cell.

Epidemiology, Genetics and Molecular Genetics

The incidence of VHL has been variably reported as 1:36,000 (176), 3:100,000 (177), or 1:35,000 to 1:40,000 (178). However, it is possibly more common. VHL is an autosomal dominant disease, with a high penetrance and variable expressivity. The new mutation rate is very low, probably <5%, because of the small size of the gene (179).

Three of 10 female patients with VHL, examined by high-resolution chromosome banding of lymphocytes, showed chromosomal mosaicism, with predominance of the normal cell line (180). The assignment of the VHL gene to the short arm of chromosome 3, at locus 3p25, was reported in 1988 (181). Tumor cells of both sporadic and VHL-related renal cell carcinomas were found to be associated with the loss of regions on chromosome 3p (181,182). This may indicate that the VHL gene acts through loss of function or absence of a "tumor suppressor" gene.

Latif et al. (183) reported the identification and positional cloning of the VHL gene. It encodes a transcript of approximately 6–6.5 kb, and in VHL disease many different mutations were identified, either deletions or single spot mutations (183). The gene contains three exons with an open-reading frame of 852 nucleotides, predicted to encode a protein of 284 amino acids (184), later considered to be 213 ammo acids. The locus VHL has been mapped to chromosome 3p25–p26 (177,179,183). A very large number of different mutations were identified in the VHL gene in a short time. About 500 were known in 1998 (167). Many of them were private and were detected only in one family. The mutations could be classified into two groups, protein truncating mutations and missense point mutations (167,168,177).

Several studies confirmed than VHL is a tumor suppressor gene by confirming loss of heterozygosity, "the second hit" according to Knudson's theory (185–188). Hypermethylation of the VHL gene has been detected in some cells without LOH. Hypermethylation is one cause of tumor-suppressor-gene inactivation (186). LOH was detected in vacuolated "stromal" cells of tumors but not in vascular cells or glial cells, considered to be reactive cells (187).

Most somatic mutations are deletions, insertions, frameshifts and nonsense, while most germline mutations are missense (189). Although not specific, missense point mutations in the VHL gene were associated much more with pheochromocytoma and renal cell carcinoma (190,191). Frequency of pheochromocytoma was 40% or 59% (age 30 and 50, respectively) with missense mutations and 6–9% with truncated protein. This frequency increased to 53% and 82%, respectively, when the missense mutations involved codon 167 (190). Benign hemangioblastoma of the retina and/or brain has a similar distribution with both types of mutation. One missense mutation at codon 98, Tyr98His, was reported as a benign mutation without malignant tumors (192). Chen et al. (193) classified VHL patients with truncated proteins as VHL type 1 without pheochromocytoma and VHL type 2 with 96% missense mutations. The family phenotype may be farther subdivided, as reviewed and summarized by Lonser et al. (194). Type 1 have low risk of pheochromocytoma but develop other tumors with the usual frequency. Type 2 have pheochromocytoma with high frequency and are classified into one of three familial subtypes. Type 2A have a low risk for renal cell carcinoma, type 2B have a high risk and type 2C have only pheochromocytomas (194).

It is believed that the VHL Protein inhibits the transcription elongation process (179), and that it is associated with two regulatory subunits of the transcription elongation factor (189). However, the exact mode of action is yet unknown. Newer methodology for detection of VHL mutations enables detection of close to 100% of the mutations (195,196). However, mosaicism exists and may be the cause for false-negative tests (197).

Clinical Management

Medical and Surgical Management

The progressive nature of the lesions of VHL is a constant threat to the patient. If untreated, the ocular lesion often results in blindness, and the brain lesion may be disabling and life-threatening. The surgical treatment of these lesions is easier and yields better results when performed in the early stage. Argon laser or xenon arc photocoagulation is probably the best management for small and medium-sized tumors (198,199). Goldberg (199) found that either of these modalities can be used successfully. Direct photocoagulation of the angioma is usually better than treatment of the feeder vessels, and the patient may benefit from a reduction in the size of the tumor, even if the tumor cannot be destroyed completely. Small tumors (up to 1/2-disk diameter) commonly respond well to a single session of treatment. Cryotherapy may be more suitable for anteriorly located and large tumors. The freeze-thaw technique, used twice, with temperatures of −70 to −80°C (75) or −60°C (151) has been advocated.

A combination of these two methods can be employed. If the response is insufficient, treatment may be repeated after a few weeks or months. This is often necessary in medium-sized tumors ($\frac{1}{2}$ to 1 $\frac{1}{2}$ -disk diameters). In patients with retinal detachment, surgery with a buckling procedure must be considered. In some cases cryoapplications apparently resulted in increased exudation and formation of a preretinal macular fibrosis (150).

Other forms of treatment have been suggested. Nicholson (200) uses photocoagulation over the afferent artery of the tumor during induced elevated intraocular pressure (by suction ophthalmodynamometry). Peyman et al. (201) have successfully removed two large angiomas in two patients using the eye wall resection method. Considering that large angiomas respond poorly to treatment with photocoagulation or cryotherapy, and that they carry a poor prognosis if left to their natural course, this surgical approach may be considered in selected cases.

Peripapillary or disk hemangioblastomas are especially difficult to treat. Treatment is important, as patients tend to develop retinal detachments. Garcia-Arumi et al. (202) treated successfully four patients with either argon laser or transpupillary thermotherapy (TTT) (202).

In large hemangioblastomas, external beam radiotherapy (EBRT) was used. Raja et al. treated six eyes of patients by EBRT. It resulted in reduction of tumor size by 40% and a mean improvement of visual acuity from 20/70 to 20/45 (203).

Aiello et al. (204) treated one patient with an optic nerve head hemangioblastoma by systemic administration of an experimental VEGF receptor inhibitor SU5416. Follow-up showed stability in size of the tumor and some improvement of visual acuity.

Extraocular benign and malignant tumors should be referred to the appropriate specialist.

Genetic Counseling

First-degree relatives should be examined before genetic counseling is given. It must be remembered that some persons may not show manifestations of the disease until later in life.

The gene penetrance is close to 100% but it varies with age, reaching close to full penetrance at age 60. The expressivity is variable, but certain family phenotypes have been delineated and they are useful for counseling. Identification of the mutation in the VHL gene will assist subclassification and proper counseling.

Prenatal diagnosis can be done with one of the accepted methods once the mutation has been identified.

STURGE-WEBER SYNDROME

This "phakomatosis" is included here only for completeness, as it most probably has no hereditary background (205). Single descriptions of two affected members in one family may have been coincidental.

The triad of choroidal hemangioma, ipsilateral nevus flammeus of the face, and angioma of the meninges is the hallmark of the disease. The facial hemangioma that occurs along the distribution of the trigeminal nerve is histologically a cavernous hemangioma. The brain angioma, which characteristically appears in the occipital region, may cause typical calcifications seen by roentogenography, and seizures with mental retardation.

In the eye, a broad spectrum of potential findings (206) include congested and tortuous epibulbar conjunctival or episcleral blood vessels, congenital or developmental glaucoma, diffuse choroidal hemangioma, retinal vascular changes in the form of peripheral arteriovenous anastomoses, and heterochromia iridis.

NEURO-OCULOCUTANEOUS CAVERNOUS HEMANGIOMATOSIS

Cavernous hemangiomas of the retina are uncommon, and only a few have been reported. In 1971, Gass (207) described three patients with a cavernous hemangioma of the retina. He suggested that in some cases this lesion is part of a syndrome that similarly affects the skin and the brain. Since that report, several more individuals and families have been described, confirming the existence of a distinct hereditary entity, neurooculocutaneous cavernous hemangiomatosis. The disease is transmitted as an autosomal dominant condition and includes the existence of vascular hamartomas in the same three structures as the other phakomatoses.

The Clinical Manifestations of Neurooculocutaneous Cavernous Hemangiomatosis

Ocular Lesions

The ophthalmoscopic appearance is characteristic (Fig. 9). It consists of one or more clusters of thin-walled vascular aneurysms, variously described as dark red grapelike structures or red globules. They are fed by venous blood, which often fills only part

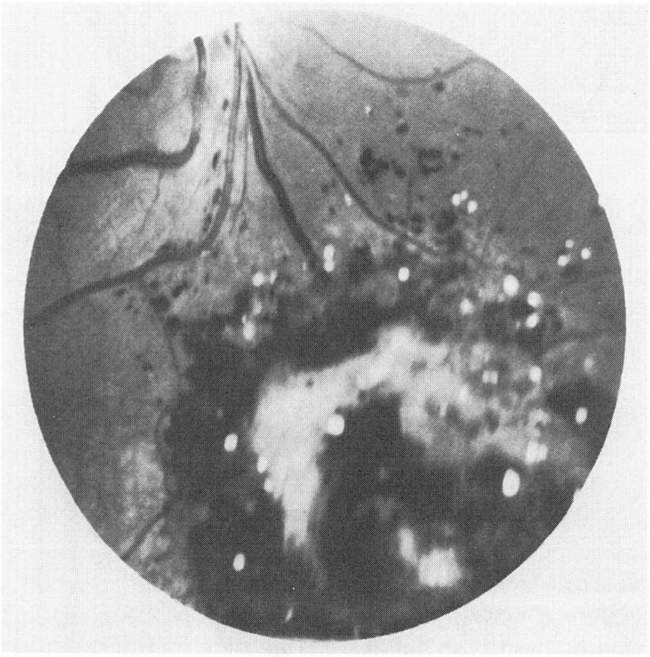

(a)

Figure 9 Neurooculocutaneous cavernous hemangiomatosis: (a) The patient was 27 years old when this picture of the fundus was taken. The tumor consisted of multiple dark red aneurysms of different sizes, from the size of a microaneurysm up to about $\frac{1}{3}$ -disk diameter. In the center of the tumor, the individual angiomas could not be separated from each other because of the thickness of the tumor. The whitish band is glial tissue covering part of the tumor. (b) Same tumor eight years later: note that very little change has occurred, except that in the periphery some new angiomas appeared (arrows), (c) Fluorescein angiography of same tumor, 20 sec after injection. Note the slow filling of the tumor by fluorescein. (d) Fluorescein angiography of same tumor 120 sec after injection. Some medium-sized angiomas show the separation of fluorescein-stained plasma above and dark erythrocytes below. Two such angiomas are outlined by arrows. (e) Fluorescein angiography of same tumor 309 sec after injection. Most angiomas show the typical separation and the fluorescein-blood level The patient had a single skin angioma, but no evidence of intracranial involvement (Courtesy of MF Goldberg, MD).

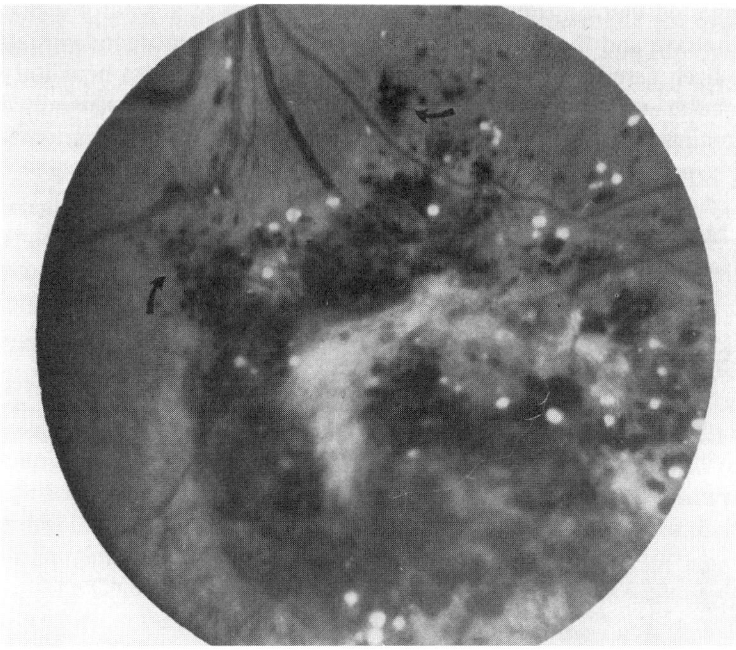

(b)

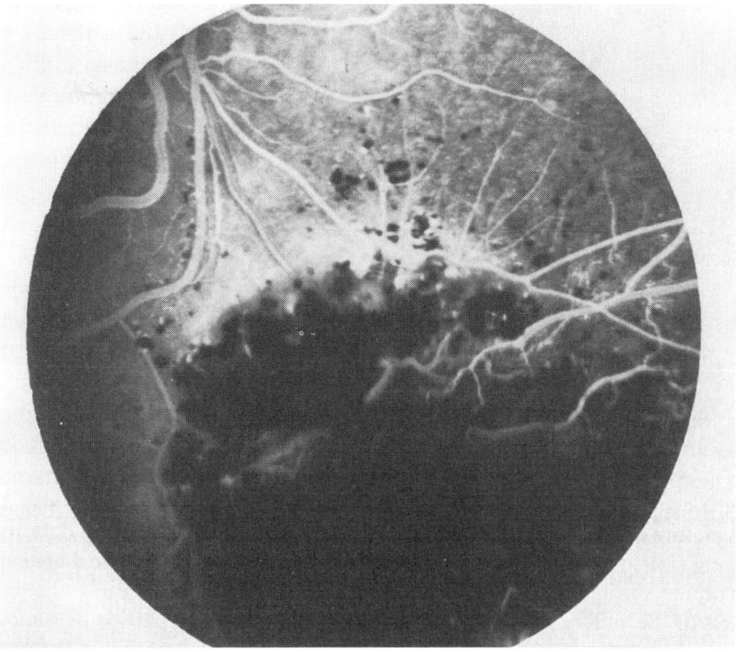

(c)

Figure 9 (*Continued*)

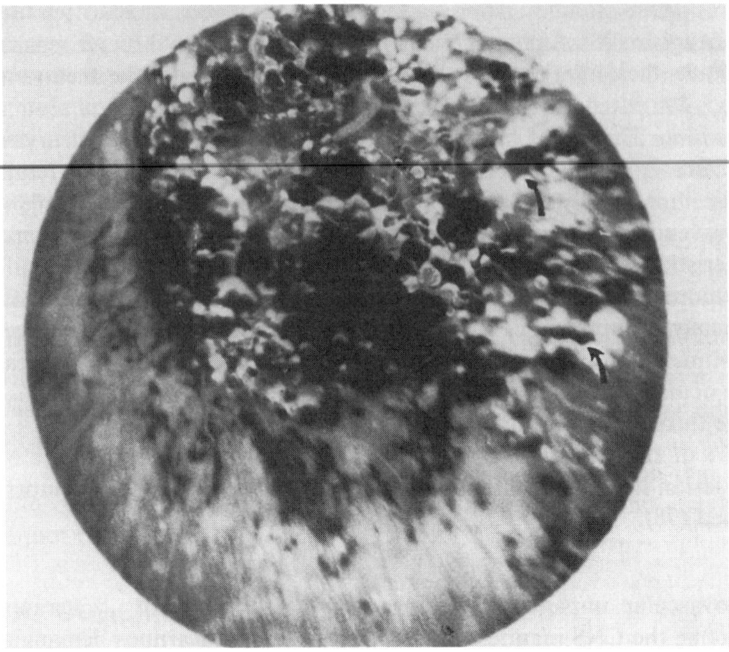

(d)

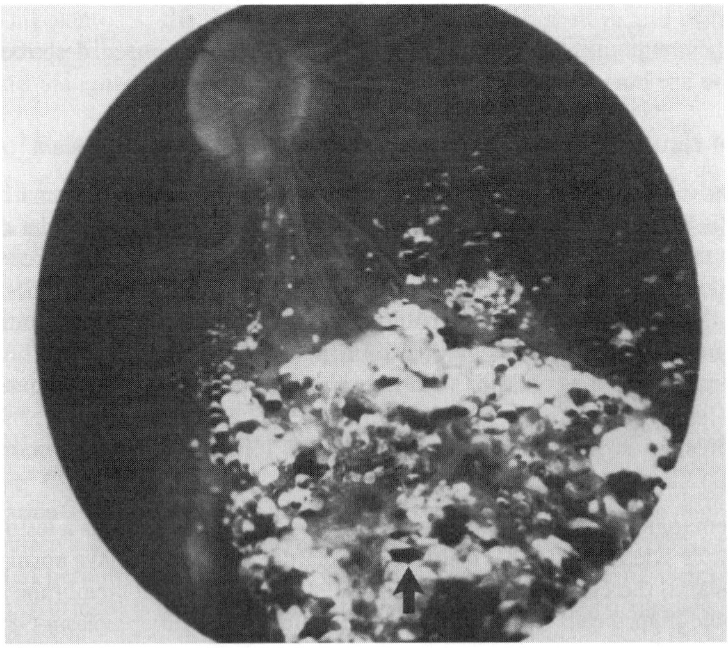

(e)

Figure 9 (*Continued*)

of the aneurysm (208). A characteristic finding is plasma-erythrocyte separation within the globule; the darker erythrocytes gravitate inferiorly inside the aneurysm. No unusual dilated, congested, or tortuous vessels feed the lesion. Exudate around the lesion is uncommon. The size of each aneurysm varies from a tiny microaneurysm to 1-disk diameter (150). The hemangioma may occur anywhere in the retina or on the optic disk. It is usually unilateral, but may be bilateral. Fluorescein angiography shows slow venous drainage without vascular permeability and without leakage (209). Characteristically, in the late phase of angiography, the aneurysms fill differentially, with fluorescein above, blood below, and an interface in the middle (206). The lesions are usually asymptomatic, but may bleed into the retina, subretinal space, or vitreous. Sometimes white-gray glial tissue covers the lesion (Fig. 9). Great variability of the ocular findings has been reported. A follow-up of patients suggested progressive thrombosis and organization of the angioma (210).

In about 10% of the patients, visual acuity may become reduced because of extension of the lesion into the macular area, and in about 15%, vitreous hemorrhage was described (210).

Brain Lesions

Seizures, cerebrovascular impairment, intracranial hemorrhage, or intracranial calcifications can all be the CNS manifestations of intracranial cavernous hemangiomas (150,211). Cranial nerve palsies are rare (212).

Cutaneous Lesions

Skin cavernous hemangiomas in different parts of the body have been described (207,209,212). These are hamartomas and usually do not change.

Diagnosis of Neuro-Oculocutaneous Cavernous Hemangiomatosis

Diagnosis is based on the clinical findings of a typical cavernous hemangioma in the retina or optic disk, and the presence of cutaneous cavernous hemangioma or seizures or other neurologic signs. Often the intracranial lesions are silent. CT scanning is the best and most reliable method to detect cavernous hemangiomas of the brain, but even this technique may not disclose the tiny lesions, which often are found only at autopsy (212,213).

The retinal lesions may be confused with Leber's miliary aneurysms and Coats' disease.

Pathology

The cavernous hemangioma is an endothelium-lined venous aneurysm. It is a lesion totally on the venous side of the retinal or brain vasculature. The vessels have normal anatomic features and, therefore, no leakage occurs (210). The preretinal membrane is composed of spindle-shaped cells with numerous glial filaments in their cytoplasm (210).

Epidemiology and Genetics

The disease is rare. The familial cases seem to be transmitted as an autosomal dominant trait, with unknown penetrance and quite variable expressivity. Only a proportion of patients with retinal cavernous hemangiomas have a positive familial history. In addition, most reported cases of cavernous hemangioma affect only one of three structures: retina (208,209), brain (211), or skin (212). Until 1975, only 24 cases of retinal cavernous hemangiomas had been reported; 14 affected the retina and one or two other structures (209). An unresolved question is whether or not some of these pure retinal cases have "hidden" and silent hemangiomas in the brain. By 1983, 70 cases were known and reported, most of them sporadic (214). By 1987, 17 families with 54 affected members were described (215).

Sarraf et al. described the familial occurrence of cavernous hemangiomas in several members of a three-generation family (216). The transmission was, as in all phakomatoses, autosomal dominant. Hemangiomas were found through a screening search in the brain, on the skin, in the retina and choroid. The authors also suggested the localization of the gene to chromosome 7q11–q22 (216).

Mutations in the KRIT1 gene were associated with cerebral and retinal cavernous angiomatosis (217). The KRITl gene is associated with locus cerebral cavernous malformation 1 (CCM1), a gene of unknown function that encodes a micro tubule-associated protein (218). The cerebral cavernous angiomas may be symptomatic and even cause cerebral hemorrhage, but in about 50% of all cases they are "silent" by age of 50 (219). Thus, a brain scan seems in order for each patient with retinal cavernous angioma.

Management

Usually, the retinal cavernous hemangioma is asymptomatic and does not change with time. No treatment is necessary. In several reported cases photocoagulation was performed when a hemorrhage occurred. Such treatment may cause bleeding because of the thin venous walls of the aneurysms.

Genetic counseling should be based on the assumption that the disease is an autosomal dominant trait, with unknown penetrance. The severity of the disease cannot be predicted.

OTHER MULTISYSTEM SYNDROMES

Two other multisystem diseases involving structures derived from the neural crest and of interest to the ophthalmologist should be mentioned here. As in the other phakomatoses, the skin and the CNS, along with the eye and other tissues, are affected. Also similar is the main clinical manifestation of hamartomas and benign and malignant tumors.

Multiple Endocrine Neoplasia Syndromes

Clinically, three syndromes were delineated in this group of diseases with predominantly endocrine system tumors. In multiple endocrine neoplasia (MEN) type I adenomas of the parathyroid, pituitary, thyroid, and adrenal cortex are found. In MEN type II (or IIa) the tumors are medullary carcinoma of the thyroid and pheochromocytoma. In MEN type III or (IIb) the facies have a characteristic appearance and the body structure is "marfanoid." Neuromas of the mucous membranes are found in all three types. In type III the conjunctiva is especially commonly affected. Café au-lait spots and the frequent neuromas resemble clinically other phakomatoses, and MEN can be erroneously diagnosed as neurofibromatosis.

Ocular findings are common in MEN type III syndrome (220). All affected patients have prominent corneal nerves (221). Most also have neuromas of the conjunctiva or the eyelids. Dryness of the eyes (keratoconjunctivitis sicca) and associated perilimbal congestion of blood vessels may be the first sign of the disease and may bring the patient to the ophthalmologist as the first physician.

The diagnosis of MEN type IIb (or MEN III) may be suspected with the typical findings of marfanoid habitus, thickened eyelids, thickened corneal nerves and subconjunctival neuromas. In each case medullary thyroid carcinoma and pheochromocytoma should be ruled out (222). Prominent corneal nerves are found in 100% of patients, conjunctival and eyelid neuromas are found in 80–87%, conjunctivitis sicca in 67%, and perilimbal prominent vessels in 40% (223).

A histologic study of four eyes with this syndrome showed that the basic anomaly of the thickened corneal nerves are numerous closely packed axons and Schwann cells (224). The authors stress that these thickened corneal nerves may be the first sign enabling the diagnosis of this potentially lethal disease. An early diagnosis may enable successful treatment of the malignancies that occur later.

All three types of MEN are autosomal dominant traits. Pasini et al. (225) cloned the entire genomic sequence of the RET proto-oncogene responsible for MEN types II and III. Therefore, the terms MEN2A and MEN2B may be the more proper terminology. The gene Rearranged during Transfection, (RET) so named for the way it was first identified, contains 20 exons, and encodes a transmembrane tyrosinase receptor. Fink et al. (226) described a point mutation, Met918Thr, in a patient with the classic ophthalmologic findings. The gene was mapped to chromosome 10q11.2. Other missense mutations of the same gene may cause other diseases. Familial medullary thyroid carcinoma is also associated, in most cases, with the Met918Thr mutation (227). In fact, this single mutation is associated with 93% of MEN2B disease (227). Probably about 50% of cases are sporadic.

Basal Cell Nevus Syndrome

Another relatively rare multisystem disease, which affects predominantly the skin, CNS, and skeleton, and occasionally the eye and other tissues is basal cell nevus syndrome. Multiple skin tumors in form of nodules of different shapes and sizes become apparent, usually in late childhood. These are basal cell carcinomas. Commonly and characteristically, a mandibular cyst occurs with associated dental problems. The skeletal changes include kyphoscoliosis, costal malformations, and shortened metacarpals. The CNS may be involved by the occurrence of medulloblastomas, calcification of dura, or partial agenesis of the corpus callosum.

The eye is affected in about 30% of all patients (228). Commonly, the eyelids have one or more typical basal cell carcinomas. The orbit may be invaded by the tumor, and strabismus may occur (228). A possibly associated tumor is a malignant melanoma of the iris, reported in one case (229). The disease is inherited by the autosomal dominant mode.

The disease results from mutations in the PTCH gene (for patched, *Drosophilia*, homolog), which has been mapped to chromosome 9q22.3 (67). Several studies provide evidence of LOH in tumor cells (67), thus confirming the tumor-suppressor nature of the gene.

Cerebroretinal Vasculopathy

A new hereditary syndrome involving the retina and the brain was reported in 1988 (230). In the described family, at least 10 members were affected. In the retina, small areas of capillary nonperfusion, dilated and tortuous capillaries, especially in the perifoveal zone, were described. In the brain, pseudotumors were found.

Histopathologic studies of the brain showed fibrinoid necrosis of blood vessels and necrosis of the white matter, whereas histopathologic studies of the eyes showed microinfarctions, with focal areas of loss of inner retina, combined with an intact photoreceptor layer (230).

The disease shows autosomal dominant transmission, variable expressivity, and progressive manifestations (230).

Gutmann et al. (231) described the combination of progressive visual loss and leukoencephalopathy in a family with this syndrome. Ophoff et al. (232) demonstrated that in three families, retinopathy (microaneurysms, microangiopathy and teleangiectatic capillaries) was associated with cerebral pathology (vascular anomalies, migraine, stroke) and nephropathy. They mapped the locus to chromosome 3p21.1–p21.3 (232). The gene has not yet been identified. Siveke and Schmid (233) supplied more evidence for systemic involvement with additional abnormalities in one patient with this syndrome: cerebroretinal vasculopathy, liver cirrhosis, and bilateral osteonecrosis of the femur.

REFERENCES

1. van der Hoeve J. Fourth type of phakomatosis. Arch Ophthalmol 1937; 18:679–682.
2. van der Hoeve J. Eye symptoms of phakomatoses [The Doyne Memorial Lecture]. Trans Ophthalmol Soc UK 1932; 52:330–401.
3. Riccardi VM. The phakomatoses. In: Emery AEH, Rimoin DL, eds. Principle and Practice of Medical Genetics. Edinburgh: Churchill–Livingstone, 1983:313–320.
4. Critchley M. Foreword. In: Gomez MR, ed. Tuberous Sclerosis. New York: Raven Press, 1979:VII–IX.
5. Riley FC, Campbell RJ. Double phakomatosis. Arch Ophthalmol 1979; 97:518–520.
6. Bolande RP. The neurocristopathies. a unifying concept of disease arising in neural crest maldevelopment. Hum Pathol 1974; 5:409–429.
7. Kissel P, Andre JM, Jackquier A. The Neurocristopathies. New York: Masson, 1981.
8. Nakamura T. Genetic markers and animal models of neurocristopathy. Histol Histopathol 1995; 10(3):747–759.
9. MacDonald M, Bech-Hansen NT, Britton WA Jr, Green J 2nd, Paterson M, Stone J. The phakomatoses: recent advances in genetics. Can J Ophthalmol 1997; 32(1):4–11.
10. Warwar RE, Bullock JD, Shields JA, Eagle RC Jr. Coexistence of 3 tumors of neural crest origin: neurofibroma, meningioma, and uveal malignant melanoma. Arch Ophthalmol 1998; 116(9):1241–1243.
11. National Institutes of Health Consensus Development Conference. Neurofibromatosis. Conference statement. Arch Neurol 1988; 45:575–578.
12. Riccardi VM. von Recklinghausen neurofibromatosis. N Engl J Med 1981; 305: 1617–1627.
13. Riccardi VM. Neurofibromatosis: an overview and new directions in clinical investigations. In: Riccardi VM, Mulvihill JJ, eds. Advances in Neurology. Vol. 29. New York: Raven Press, 1981:1–9.

14. Perry HD, Font RL. Iris nodules in von Recklinghausen's neurofibromatosis: electron-microscopic confirmation of their melanocytic origin. Arch Ophthalmol 1982; 100: 1635–1640.
15. Zehavi C, Romano A, Goodman RM. Iris (Lisch) nodules in neurofibromatosis. Clin Genet 1986; 29:51–55.
16. Toonstra J, Dandriew MR, Ippel PF, et al. Are Lisch nodules an ocular marker of the neurofibromatosis gene in otherwise unaffected family members? Dermatologica 1987; 174:232–235.
17. Lewis RA, Riccardi VM. Von Recklinghausen neurofibromatosis. Incidence of iris hamartomata. Ophthalmology 1981; 88:348–354.
18. Rubenstein AE, Mindel JS, Korczyn AD, Perla CS. Iris nevi in neurofibromatosis: evidence for a specific effect of puberty [Abstract]. Neurology 1981; 31(2)(suppl):64.
19. Beauchamp GR. Neurofibromatosis type 1 in children. Trans Am Ophthalmol Soc 1995; 93:445–472.
20. Ragge NK, Falk RE, Cohen WE, Murphree AL. Images of Lisch nodules across the spectrum. Eye 1993; 7(Pt l):95–101.
21. Ticho BH, Rosner M, Mets MB, Tso MO. Bilateral diffuse iris nodular nevi. Clinical and histopathologic characterization. Ophthalmology 1995; 102(3):419–425.
22. Wolter JR. Solitary neurofibroma of the iris: report of a case. J Pediatr Ophthalmol Strabismus 1969; 6:84–87.
23. Wolter JR. Corneal involvement in choroidal neurofibromatosis. J Pediatr Ophthalmol 1966; 3(2):19–24.
24. Ragge NK. Clinical and genetic patterns of neurofibromatosis 1 and 2. Br J Ophthalmol 1993; 77(10):662–672.
25. Grant WM, Walton DS. Distinctive gonioscopic findings in glaucoma due to neurofibromatosis. Arch Ophthalmol 1968; 79:127–134.
26. Freedman SF, Elner VM, Donev I, et al. Intraocular neurilemoma arising from the posterior ciliary nerve in neurofibromatosis. Pathologic findings. Ophthalmology 1988; 95:1559–1564.
27. Lewis RA, Gerson LP, Axelson KA, el al. von Recklinhausen neurofibromatosis. II. Incidence of optic gliomata. Ophthalmology 1984; 91:929–935.
28. Listernick R, Charrow J, Greenwald M, Esterly NB. Optic gliomas in children with neurofibromatosis type I. J Pediatr 1989; 114:788–792.
29. Kuenzle C, Weissert M, Roulet E, Bode H, Schefer S, Huisman T, Landau K, Boltshauser E. Follow-up of optic pathway gliomas in children with neurofibromatosis type 1. Neuropediatrics 1994; 25(6):295–300.
30. Thiagalingam S, Flaherty M, Billson F, North K. Neurofibromatosis type 1 and optic pathway gliomas: follow-up of 54 patients. Ophthalmology 2004; 111(3):568–577.
31. Stern J, Jakobiec FA, Housepian EM. The architecture of optic nerve gliomas with and without neurofibromatosis. Arch Ophthalmol 1980; 98:505–511.
32. Sadun F, Hinton DR, Sadun AA. Rapid growth of an optic nerve ganglioglioma in a patient with neurofibromatosis 1. Ophthalmology 1996; 103(5):794–799.
33. Crawford MJ, Buckler JMH. Optic gliomata affecting twins with neurofibromatosis. Dev Med Child Neurol 1983; 25:370–373.
34. Kennedy RE. Pulsating exophthalmos: orbital tumors in siblings. Trans Am Ophthalmol Soc 1982; 80:205–217.
35. Baptiste M, Nasca P, Metzger B, et al. Neurofibromatosis and other disorders among children with CNS tumors and their families. Neurology 1989; 39:487–492.
36. Liu GT, Brodsky MC, Phillips PC, Belasco J, Janss A, Golden JC, Bilaniuk LL, Burson GT, Duhaime AC, Sutton LN. Optic radiation involvement in optic pathway gliomas in neurofibromatosis. Am J Ophthalmol 2004; 137(3):407–414.
37. Rubenstein AE, Mytiluneoau C, Yahr MD, Revoltella RP. Neurological aspects of neurofibromatosis. In: Riccardi VM, Mulvihill JJ, eds. Advances in Neurology. New York: Raven Press, 1981:11–21.

38. Hope DG, Mulvihill JJ. Malignancy in neurofibromatosis. In: Riccardi VM, Mulvihill JJ, eds. Advances in Neurology. Vol. 29. New York: Raven Press, 1981:33–56.
39. Schneider M, Obringer AC, Zackai E, Meadows AT. Childhood neurofibromatosis: risk factors for malignant disease. Cancer Genet Cytogenet 1986; 21:347–354.
40. Noroman J, Brini A. von Recklinghansen's disease and melanoma of the uvea. Br J Ophthalmol 1970; 54:641–648.
41. Wiznia RA, Freedman JK, Mancini AD, Shields JA. Malignant melanoma of the choroid in neurofibromatosis. Am J Ophthalmol 1978; 86:684–687.
42. Friedman SM, Margo CE. Choroidal melanoma and neurofibromatosis type 1. Arch Ophthalmol 1998; 116(5):694–695.
43. Croxatto JO, Charles DE, Malbran ES. Neurofibromatosis associated with nevus of Ota and choroidal melanoma. Am J Ophthalmol 1981; 92:578–580.
44. King AA, Debaun MR, Riccardi VM, Gutmann DH. Malignant peripheral nerve sheath tumors in neurofibromatosis 1. Am J Med Genet 2000; 93(5):388–392.
45. Lewis RA, Riccardi VM. Neurofibromatosis classification clarified [correspondence]. Ophthalmology 1989; 96:1123.
46. Gutmann DH, Aylsworth A, Carey JC, Korf B, Marks J, Pyeritz RE, Rubenstein A, Viskochil D. The diagnostic evaluation and multidisciplinary management of neurofibromatosis 1 and neurofibromatosis 2. J Am Med Assoc 1997; 278(1):51–57.
47. Gray J, Swaiman KF. Brain tumors in children with neurofibromatosis: computed tomography and magnetic resonance imaging. Pediatr Neurol 1987; 3(6):335–341.
48. Kurosawa A, Kurosawa H. Ovoid bodies in choroidal neurofibromatosis. Arch Ophthalmol 1982; 100:1939–1941.
49. Williamson TH, Garner A, Moore AT. Structure of Lisch nodules in neurofibromatosis type 1. Ophthalmic Paediatr Genet 1991; 12(1):11–17.
50. Rehany U, Rumelt S. Iridocorneal melanoma associated with type 1 neurofibromatosis: a clinicopathologic study. Ophthalmology 1999; 106(3):614–618.
51. Hoyt WF, Baghdassarian SA. Optic glioma of childhood: natural history and rationale for conservative management. Br J Ophthalmol 1969; 53:193–798.
52. Parker JL, Smith JL, Reyes P, Vuksanovic MM. Chiasmal optic glioma after radiation therapy: neuroophthalmologic/pathologic correlation. J Clin Neuroophthalmol 1981; 1:31–43.
53. Borit A, Richardson EP. The biological and clinical behavior of pilocytic astrocytomas of the optic pathways. Brain 1982; 105:161–187.
54. Garner A, Klinworth GK. Tumors of the orbit, optic nerve and lacrimal sac. In: Garner A, Klintworth GK, eds. Pathobiology of Ocular Disease. A Dynamic Approach. New York: Marcel Dekker, 1982:741–821.
55. Riccardi VM. Neurofibromatosis: an overview and new directions in clinical investigations. In: Riccardi VM, Mulvihill JJ, eds. Neurofibromatosis (von Reckfinghansen Disease): Genetics, Cell Biology and Biochemistry. Adv Neurol 1981; 29:1–7.
56. Garty BZ, Laor A, Danon YL. Neurofibromatosis type 1 in Israel: survey of young adults. J Med Genet 1994; 31(11):853–857.
57. Toutain A, Kaplan J, Briard ML, Frezal J. Genetic counseling in neurofibromatosis. Apropos of a study of 53 families. J Genet Hum 1998; 36:163–171.
58. Riccardi VM, Lewis RA. Penetrance of von Recklinghausen neurofibromatosis. a distinction between predecessors and descendants. Am J Genet 1988; 42:284–289.
59. Barker D, Wright E, Nguyen K, et al. Gene for von Recklinghausen neurofibromatosis in the pericentromeric region of chromosome 17. Science 1987; 236:1100–1102.
60. Skolnick MH, Ponder B, Seizinger B. Linkage of NF 1 to 12 chromosome 17 markers: a summary of eight concurrent reports. Genomics 1987; 1:382–383.
61. Fountain JW, Wallace MR, Brereton AM, et al. Physical mapping of the von Recklinghausen neurofibromatosis region on chromosome 17. Am J Hum Genet 1989; 44: 58–67.

62. Fain PR, Wright E, Willard HF, et al. The order of loci in the pericentric region of chromosome 17, based on evidence from physical and genetic breakpoints. Am J Hum Genet 1989; 44:68–72.
63. Ledbetter DH, Rich DC, O'Connell P, et al. Precise localization of NF 1 to 17q11.2 by balanced translocation. Am J Hum Genet 1989; 44:20–24.
64. Goldgar DE, Green P, Parry DM, Mulvihill JJ. Multipoint linkage analysis in neurofibromatosis type I. an international collaboration. Am J Hum Genet 1989; 44:6–12.
65. Marchuk DA, Saulino AM, Tavakkol R, Swaroop M, Wallace MR, Andersen LB, Mitchell AL, Gutmann DH, Boguski M, Collins FS. cDNA cloning of the type 1 neurofibromatosis gene: complete sequence of the NF1 gene product. Genomics 1991; 11(4): 931–940.
66. Hoffmieyer S, Assum G, Griesser J, Kaufmann D, Nurnberg P, Krone W. On unequal allelic expression of the neurofibromin gene in neurofibromatosis type 1. Hum Mol Genet 1995; 4(8):1267–1272.
67. Online Mendelian Inheritance in Man, OMIM (TM). McKusick–Nathans Institute for Genetic Medicine, Johns Hopkins University (Baltimore, MD) and National Center for Biotechnology Information, National Library of Medicine (Bethesda, MD), 2000. World Wide Web URL: http ://www.ncbi.nlm.nih.gov/oniim/.
68. Knudson AG. Hereditary cancer: two hits revisited. J Cancer Res Clin Oncol 1996; 122(3):135–140.
69. Legius E, Marchuk DA, Collins FS, Glover TW. Somatic deletion of the neurofibromatosis type 1 gene in a neurofibrosarcoma supports a tumour suppressor gene hypothesis. Nat Genet 1993; 3(2):122–126.
70. Colman SD, Williams CA, Wallace MR. Benign neurofibromas in type 1 neurofibromatosis (NF1) show somatic deletions of the NFl gene. Nat Genet 1995; 11(l):90–92.
71. Heim RA, Silverman LM, Farber RA, Kam-Morgan LN, Luce MC. Screening for truncated NF1 proteins. Nat Genet 1994; 8(3):218–219.
72. Purandare SM, Lanyon WG, Connor JM. Characterisation of inherited and sporadic mutations in neurofibromatosis type-1. Hum Mol Genet 1994; 3(7):1109–1115.
73. Messiaen LM, Callens T, Mortier G, Beysen D, Vandenbroucke I, Van Roy N, Speleman F, Paepe AD. Exhaustive mutation analysis of the NF1 gene allows identification of 95% of mutations and reveals a high frequency of unusual splicing defects. Hum Mutat 2000; 15(6):541–555.
74. Gutmann DH. The neurofibromatoses: when less is more. Hum Mol Genet 2001; 10(7):747–755.
75. Suzuki H, Takahashi K, Yasumoto K, Shibahara S. Activation of the tyrosinase gene promoter by neurofibromin. Biochem Biophys Res Commun 1994; 205(3):1984–1991.
76. Jacks T, Shih TS, Schmitt EM, Bronson RT, Bernards A, Weinberg RA. Tumour predisposition in mice heterozygous for a targeted mutation in NF1. Nat Genet 1994; 7(3):353–361.
77. Lazaro C, Ravella A, Gaona A, Volpini V, Estivill X. Neurofibromatosis type 1 due to germ–line mosaicism in a clinically normal father. N Engl J Med 1994; 331(21):1403–1407.
78. Sadeh M, Martinovits G, Goldhammer Y. Occurrence of both neurofibromatoses 1 and 2 in the same individual with a rapidly progressive course. Neurology 1989; 39: 262–283.
79. Tinschert S, Naumann I, Stegmann E, Buske A, Kaufmann D, Thiel G, Jenne DE. Segmental neurofibromatosis is caused by somatic mutation of the neurofibromatosis type 1 (NF1) gene. Eur J Hum Genet 2000; 8(6):455–459.
80. Oguzkan S, Cinbis M, Ayter S, Anlar B, Aysun S. Familial segmental neurofibromatosis. J Child Neurol 2004; 19(5):392–394.
81. Dosoretz DE, Blitzer PH, Wang CC, Linggood RM. Management of glioma of the optic nerve and/or chiasm: an analysis of 20 cases. Cancer 1980; 45:1467–1471.

82. Parry DM, Eldridge R, Kaiser-Kupfer MI, Bouzas EA, Pikus A, Patronas N. Neurofibromatosis 2 (NF2): clinical characteristics of 63 affected individuals and clinical evidence for heterogeneity. Am J Med Genet 1994; 52(4):450–461.
83. Bouzas EA, Parry DM, Eldridge R, Kaiser-Kupfer MI. Familial occurrence of combined pigment epithelial and retinal hamartomas associated with neurofibromatosis 2. Retina 1992; 12(2):103–107.
84. Meyers SM, Gutman FA, Kaye LD, Rothner AD. Retinal changes associated with neurofibromatosis 2. Trans Am Ophthalmol Soc 93:245–252; discussion 1995; 252–257.
85. Kaye LD, Rothner AD, Beauchamp GR, Meyers SM, Estes ML. Ocular findings associated with neurofibromatosis type II. Ophthalmology 1992; 99(9):1424–1429.
86. Ragge NK, Baser ME, Klein J, Nechiporuk A, Sainz J, Pulst SM, Riccardi VM. Ocular abnormalities in neurofibromatosis 2. Am J Ophthalmol 1995; 120(5):634–641.
87. Thomas DA, Trobe JD, Cornblath WT. Visual loss secondary to increased intracranial pressure in neurofibromatosis type 2. Arch Ophthalmol 1999; 117(12):1650–1653.
88. Rettele GA, Brodsky MC, Merin LM, Teo C, Glasier CM. Blindness, deafness, quadriparesis, and a retinal malformation: the ravages of neurofibromatosis 2. Surv Ophthalmol 1996; 41(2):135–141.
89. Tong JT, Bateman JB. Selective b-wave reduction with congenital cataract in neurofibromatosis-2. Ophthalmology 1999; 106(9):1681–1683.
90. Baser ME, Ragge NK, Riccardi VM, Janus T, Gantz B, Pulst SM. Phenotypic variability in monozygotic twins with neurofibromatosis 2. Am J Med Genet 1996; 64(4):563–567.
91. Rouleau GA, Wertelecki W, Haines JL, et al. Genetic linkage of bilateral acoustic neurofibromatosis to a DNA marker on chromosome 22. Nature 1987; 329:246–248.
92. Wertelecki W, Rouleau GA, Superneau DW, et al. Neurofibromatosis 2: clinical and DNA linkage studies of a large kindred. N Engl J Med 1988; 319:278–283.
93. Rouleau GA, Merel P, Lutchman M, Sanson M, Zucman J, Marineau C, Hoang-Xuan K, Demczuk S, Desmaze C, Plougastel B, et al. Alteration in a new gene encoding a putative membrane–organizing protein causes neuro–fibromatosis type 2. Nature 1993; 363(6429):515–521.
94. Trofatter JA, MacCollin MM, Rutter JL, Murrell JR, Duyao MP, Parry DM, Eldridge R, Kley N, Menon AG, Pulaski K, et al. A novel moesin-, ezrin-, radixin-like gene is a candidate for the neurofibromatosis 2 tumor suppressor. Cell 1993; 72(5):791–800.
95. Chang LS, Akhmametyeva EM, Wu Y, Zhu L, Welling DB. Multiple transcription initiation sites, alternative splicing, and differential polyadenylation contribute to the complexity of human neurofibromatosis 2 transcripts. Genomics 2002; 79(1):63–76.
96. Sainz J, Huynh DP, Figueroa K, Ragge NK, Baser ME, Pulst SM. Mutations of the neurofibromatosis type 2 gene and lack of the gene product in vestibular schwannomas. Hum Mol Genet 1994; 3(6):885–891.
97. Twist EC, Ruttledge MH, Rousseau M, Sanson M, Papi L, Merel P, Delattre O, Thomas G, Rouleau GA. The neurofibromatosis type 2 gene is inactivated in schwannomas. Hum Mol Genet 1994; 3(1):147–151.
98. Parry DM, MacCollin MM, Kaiser-Kupfer MI, Pulaski K, Nicholson HS, Bolesta M, Eldridge R, Gusella JF. Germ–line mutations in the neurofibromatosis 2 gene: correlations with disease severity and retinal abnormalities. Am J Hum Genet 1996; 59(3): 529–539.
99. Gutmann DH, Haipek CA, Burke SP, Sun CX, Scoles DR, Pulst SM. The NF2 interactor, hepatocyte growth factor-regulated tyrosine kinase substrate (HRS), associates with merlin in the "open" conformation and suppresses cell growth and motility. Hum Mol Genet 2001; 10(8):825–834.
100. Kluwe L, Mautner VF. Mosaicism in sporadic neurofibromatosis 2 patients. Hum Mol Genet 1998; 7(13):2051–2055.
101. Pulst SM. Prenatal diagnosis of the neurofibromatoses. Clin Perinatol 1990; 17(4): 829–844.

102. Abou-Sleiman PM, Apessos A, Harper JC, Serhal P, Winston RM, Delhanty JD. First application of preimplantation genetic diagnosis to neurofibromatosis type 2 (NF2). Prenat Diagn 2002; 22(6):519–524.
103. Verlinsky Y, Rechitsky S, Verlinsky O, Chistokhina A, Sharapova T, Masciangelo C, Levy M, Kaplan B, Lederer K, Kuliev A. Preimplantation diagnosis for neurofibromatosis. Reprod Biomed Online 2002; 4(3):218–222.
104. Gomez MR. Clinical experience at Mayo Clinic. In: Gomez MR, ed. Tuberous Sclerosis. New York: Raven Press, 1979.
105. Rogers RS. Dermatologic manifestations. In: Gomez M, ed. Tuberous Sclerosis. New York: Raven Press, 1979:95–119.
106. Shelton RW. The incidence of ocular lesions in tuberous sclerosis. Ann Ophthalmol 1975; 7:771–773.
107. Robertson DM. Ophthalmic findings. In: Gomez MR, ed. Tuberous Sclerosis. New York: Raven Press, 1979:121–142.
108. Robertson DM. Ophthalmic manifestations of tuberous sclerosis. Ann NY Acad Sci 1991; 615:17–25.
109. Rowley SA, O'Callaghan FJ, Osborne JP. Ophthalmic manifestations of tuberous sclerosis: a population based study. Br J Ophthalmol 2001; 85(4):420–423.
110. Shami MJ, Benedict WL, Myers M. Early manifestation of retinal hamartomas in tuberous sclerosis. Am J Ophthalmol 1993; 115(4):539–540.
111. Zimmer-Galler IE, Robertson DM. Long-term observation of retinal lesions in tuberous sclerosis. Am J Ophthalmol 1995; 119(3):318–324.
112. Kiratli H, Bilgic S. Spontaneous regression of retinal astrocytic hamartoma in a patient with tuberous sclerosis. Am J Ophthalmol 2002; 133(5):715–716.
113. Nyboer JH, Robertson DM, Gomez MR. Retinal lesions in tuberous sclerosis. Arch Ophthalmol 1976; 94:1277–1280.
114. Lucchese NJ, Goldberg MF. Iris and Fundus pigmentary changes in tuberous sclerosis. J Pediatr Ophthalmol Strabismus 1981; 18(6):45–46.
115. Gutman I, Dunn D, Behrens M, Gold AP, Odel J, Olarte MR. Hypopigmented iris spot: an early sign of tuberous sclerosis. Ophthalmology 1982; 89:1155–1159.
116. Milot J, Michaud J, Lemieux N, Allaire G, Gagnon MM. Persistent hyperplastic primary vitreous with retinal tumor in tuberous sclerosis: report of a case including tumoral immunohistochemistry and cytogenetic analyses. Ophthalmology. 1999; 106(3):630–634.
117. Eagle RC Jr, Shields JA, Shields CL, Wood MG. Hamartomas of the iris and ciliary epithelium in tuberous sclerosis complex. Arch Ophthalmol 2000; 118(5):711–715.
118. Gomez MR, Kuntz NL, Westmoreland BF. Tuberous sclerosis, early onset of seizures and mental subnormality: study of discordant homozygous twins. Neurology 1982; 32:604–611.
119. Houser OW, McLeod RA. Roentgenographic experience at the Mayo Clinic. In: Gomez M, ed. Tuberous Sclerosis. New York: Raven Press, 1979:27–53.
120. Mair DD. Cardiac manifestations. In: Gomez M, ed. Tuberous Sclerosis. New York: Raven Press, 1979:155–169.
121. O'Callaghan FJ, Clarke AC, Joffe H, Keeton B, Martin R, Salmon A, Thomas RD, Osborne JP. Tuberous sclerosis complex and Wolff–Parkinson–White syndrome. Arch Dis Child 1998; 78(2):159–162.
122. van Baal JG, Fleury P, Brummelkamp WH. Tuberous sclerosis and the relation with renal angiomyolipoma. A genetic study on the clinical aspects. Clin Genet 1989; 35:167–173.
123. Devroede G, Lemieux B, Mass S, et al. Colonic hamartomas in tuberous sclerosis. Gastroenterology 1988; 94:182–188.
124. Osborne JP. Diagnosis of tuberous sclerosis. Arch Dis Child 1988; 63:1423–1425.

125. Hausser I, Anton-Lamprecht I. Electron microscopy as a means for carrier detection and genetic counseling in families at risk of tuberous sclerosis. Hum Genet 1987; 76:73–80.
126. Kuntz NL, Gomez MR. Genetics, population studies and pathogenesis. In: Gomez MR, ed. Tuberous Sclerosis. New York: Raven Press, 1979:207–220.
127. Green AJ, Smith M, Yates JR. Loss of heterozygosity on chromosome 16pl3.3 in hamartomas from tuberous sclerosis patients. Nat Genet 1994; 6(2):193–196.
128. Osborne JP, Fryer A, Webb D. Epidemiology of tuberous sclerosis. Ann NY Acad Sci 1991; 615:125–127.
129. Sampson JR, Scahill SJ, Stephenson JB, et al. Genetic aspects of tuberous sclerosis in the west of Scotland. J Med Genet 1989; 26:28–31.
130. Cassidy SB, Pagon RA, Pepin M, Blumhagen JD. Family studies in tuberous sclerosis. Evaluation of apparently unaffected parents. J Am Med Assoc 1983; 249: 1302–1304.
131. Fryer AE, Chalmers A, Connor JM, et al. Evidence that the gene for tuberous sclerosis is on chromosome 9. Lancet 1987; 1:659–661.
132. Connor JM, Pirrit LA, Yates JR, et al. Linkage of the tuberous sclerosis locus to a DNA polymorphism detected by v–abl. J Med Genet 1987; 24:544–546.
133. Pierson M, Leheup B. Bourneville's tuberous sclerosis. J Genet Hum 1938; 36: 181–199.
134. Haines JL, Short MP, Kwiatkowski DJ, Jewell A, Andermann E, Bejjani B, Yang CH, Gusella JF, Amos JA. Localization of one gene for tuberous sclerosis within 9q32–9q34, and further evidence for heterogeneity. Am J Hum Genet 1991; 49(4):764–772.
135. Sampson JR, Harris PC. The molecular genetics of tuberous sclerosis. Hum Mol Genet 1994; 3(Spec No):1477–1480.
136. Povey S, Burley MW, Attwood J, Benham F, Hunt D, Jeremiah SJ, Franklin D, Gillett G, Malas S, Robson EB, et al. Two loci for tuberous sclerosis: one on 9q34 and one on 16pl3. Ann Hum Genet 1994; 58(Pt 2):107–127.
137. van Slegtenhorst M, de Hoogt R, Hermans C, Nellist M, Janssen B, Verhoef S, Lindhout D, van den Ouweland A, Halley D, Young J, Burley M, Jeremiah S, Woodward K, Nahmias J, Fox M, Ekong R, Osborne J, Wolfe J, Povey S, Snell RG, Cheadle JP, Jones AC, Tachataki M, Ravine D, Kwiatkowski DJ, et al. Identification of the tuberous sclerosis gene TSC1 on chromosome 9q34. Science 1997; 277(5327):805–808.
138. Green AJ, Johnson PH, Yates JR. The tuberous sclerosis gene on chromosome 9q34 acts as a growth suppressor. Hum Mol Genet 1994; 3(10):1833–1834.
139. Young J, Povey S. The genetic basis of tuberous sclerosis. Mol Med Today 1998; 4(7):313–319.
140. Young JM, Burley MW, Jeremiah SJ, Jeganathan D, Ekong R, Osborne JP, Povey S. A mutation screen of the TSC1 gene reveals 26 protein truncating mutations and 1 splice site mutation in a panel of 79 tuberous sclerosis patients. Ann Hum Genet 1998; 62(Pt 3):203–213.
141. Kwiatkowska J, Wigowska-Sowinska J, Napierala D, Slomski R, Kwiatkowski DJ. Mosaicism in tuberous sclerosis as a potential cause of the failure of molecular diagnosis. N Eng J Med 1999; 340(9):703–707.
142. Kandt RS, Haines JL, Smith M, Northrup H, Gardner RJ, Short MP, Dumars K, Roach ES, Steingold S, Wall S, et al. Linkage of an important gene locus for tuberous sclerosis to a chromosome 16 marker for polycystic kidney disease. Nat Genet 1992; 2(1):37–41.
143. Anonymous. Identification and characterization of the tuberous sclerosis gene on chromosome 16. The European Chromosome 16 Tuberous Sclerosis Consortium. Cell 1993; 75(7):1305–1315.
144. van Bakel I, Sepp T, Ward S, Yates JR, Green AJ. Mutations in the TSC2 gene: analysis of the complete coding sequence using the protein truncation test (PTT). Hum Mol Genet 1997; 6(9):1409–1414.

145. Hodges AK, Li S, Maynard J, Parry L, Braverman R, Cheadle JP, DeClue JE, Sampson JR. Pathological mutations in TSC1 and TSC2 disrupt the interaction between hamartin and tuberin. Hum Mol Genet 2001; 10(25):2899–2905.
146. Fahsold R, Rott HD, Lorenz P. A third gene locus for tuberous sclerosis is closely linked to the phenylalanine hydroxylase gene locus. Hum Genet 1991; 88(1):85–90.
147. Platt LD, Devore GR, Horenstein J, et al. Prenatal diagnosis of tuberous sclerosis. The use of fetal echocardiography. Prenat Diagn 1987; 7:407–411.
148. von Hippel E. Über eine sehr seltene Erkrankung der Netzhaut. Albrecht von Graefes. Arch Klin Exp Ophthalmol 1904; 59:83.
149. Lindau A. Studies Über Kleinhirncysten. Bau, Pathogenese und Beziehungen zur Angiomatosis Retinae. Acta Pathol Microbiol Scand Suppl 1926; 1:1–28.
150. Augsburger JJ, Shields JA, Goldberg RE. Classification and management of hereditary retinal angiomas. Int Ophthalmol Clin 1981; 4:93–106.
151. Watzke RC, Weingeist TA, Constantine JB. Diagnosis and management of von Hippel–Lindau disease. In: Peyman GA, Apple DJ, Sanders DR, eds. Intraocular Tumors. New York: Appleton–Century–Crofts, 1977:199–217.
152. Salazar FG, Lamiell JM. Early identification of retinal angiomas in a large kindred with von Hippel–Lindau disease. Am J Ophthalmol 1980; 89:540–545.
153. Maher ER, Yates JR, Harries R, Benjamin C, Harris R, Moore AT, Ferguson-Smith MA. Clinical features and natural history of von Hippel–Lindau disease. J Med 1990; 77(283):1151–1163.
154. Maher ER, Moore AT. Von Hippel–Lindau disease. Br J Ophthalmol 1992; 76(12): 743–745.
155. Shields CL, Shields JA, Barrett J, De Potter P. Vasoproliferative tumors of the ocular fundus. Classification and clinical manifestations in 103 patients. Arch Ophthalmol 1995; 113(5):615–623.
156. Schmidt D, Neumann HP. Retinal vascular hamartoma in von Hippel–Lindau disease. Arch Ophthalmol 1995; 113(9):1163–1167.
157. Carr RE, Noble KG. Retinal angiomatosis. Ophthalmology 1980; 87:956–959.
158. Neumann HP, Eggert HR, Weigel K, et al. Hemangioblastomas of the central nervous system. A 10 year study with special reference to von Hippel-Lindau syndrome. J Neurol 1989; 70:24–30.
159. Hardwig P, Robertson DM. von Hippel–Lindau disease: a familial, often lethal, multisystem phakomatosis. Ophthalmology 1984; 91:263–270.
160. Majoor-Krakauer D, Luyten G, Niermeyer MF. von Hippel–Lindau disease. Its natural history and a protocol for diagnosis and follow-up. Am J Med Genet 1986; 25:751–752.
161. De Jong PTVM, Verkaart JF, van de Vooren MJ, et al. Twin vessels in von Hippel–Lindau disease. Am J Ophthalmol 1988; 105:165–169.
162. Lamiell JM, Salazar FS, Hsia YE. von Hippel–Lindau disease affecting 43 members of a single kindred. Medicine 1989; 68:1–29.
163. Walther MM, Reiter R, Keiser HR, Choyke PL, Venzon D, Hurley K, Gnarra JR, Reynolds JC, Glenn GM, Zbar B, Linehan WM. Clinical and genetic characterization of pheochromocytoma in von Hippel–Lindau families: comparison with sporadic pheochromocytoma gives insight into natural history of pheochromocytoma. J Urol 1999; 162(3 Pt 1):659–664.
164. Neumann HP, Berger DP, Sigmund G, Blum U, Schmidt D, Parmer RJ, Volk B, Kirste G. Pheochromocytomas, multiple endocrine neoplasia type 2, and von Hippel–Lindau disease. N Engl J Med 1993; 329(21):1531–1538.
165. Choyke PL, Glenn GM, Wagner JP, Lubensky JA, Thakore K, Zbar B, Linehan WM, Walther MM. Epididymal cystadenomas in von Hippel–Lindau disease. Urology 1997; 49(6):926–931.
166. Libutti SK, Choyke PL, Bartlett DL, Vargas H, Walther M, Lubensky I, Glenn G, Linehan WM, Alexander HR. Pancreatic neuroendocrine tumors associated with von

Hippel–Lindau disease: diagnostic and management recommendations. Surgery 1998; 124(6):1153–1159.
167. Webster AR, Richards FM, MacRonald FE, Moore AT, Maher ER. An analysis of phenotypic variation in the familial cancer syndrome von Hippel–Lindau disease: evidence for modifier effects. Am J Hum Genet 1998; 63(4):1025–1035.
168. Webster AR, Maher ER, Moore AT. Clinical characteristics of ocular angiomatosis in von Hippel–Lindau disease and correlation with germline mutation. Arch Ophthalmol 1999; 117(3):371–378.
169. Webster AR, Maher ER, Bird AC, Gregor ZJ, Moore AT. A clinical and molecular genetic analysis of solitary ocular angioma. Ophthalmology 1999; 106(3):623–629.
170. Singh AD, Nouri M, Shields CL, Shields JA, Smith AF. Retinal capillary hemangioma: a comparison of sporadic cases and cases associated with von Hippel–Lindau disease. Ophthalmology 2001; 108(10):1907–1911.
171. Singh A, Shields J, Shields C. Solitary retinal capillary hemangioma: hereditary (von Hippel–Lindau disease) or nonhereditary? Arch Ophthalmol 2001; 119(2):232–234.
172. McCabe CM, Flynn HW Jr, Shields CL, Shields JA, Regillo CD, McDonald HR, Berrocal MH, Gass JD, Mieler WF. Juxtapapillary capillary hemangiomas. Clinical features and visual acuity outcomes. Ophthalmology 2000; 107(12):2240–2248.
173. Sato Y, Waziri M, Smith W, et al. von Hippel–Lindau disease: MR imaging. Radiology 1988; 166:241–246.
174. Maher ER, Webster AR, Moore AT. Clinical features and molecular genetics of von Hippel–Lindau disease. Ophthalmic Genet 1995; 16(3):79–84.
175. Mottow-Lippa L, Tso MOM, Peyman GA, Chejfec G. von Hippel angiomatosis. A light, electron microscopic and immunoperoxidase characterization. Ophthalmology 1983; 90:848–855.
176. Richards FM, Crossey PA, Phipps ME, Foster K, Latif F, Evans G, Sampson J, Lerman MI, Zbar B, Affara NA, et al. Detailed mapping of germline deletions of the von Hippel–Lindau disease tumour suppressor gene. Hum Mol Genet 1994; 3(4): 595–598.
177. Crossey PA, Richards FM, Foster K, Green JS, Prowse A, Latif F, Lerman MI, Zbar B, Affara NA, Ferguson-Smith MA, et al. Identification of intragenic mutations in the von Hippel–Lindau disease tumour suppressor gene and correlation with disease phenotype. Hum Mol Genet 1994; 3(8):1303–1308.
178. Choyke PL, Glenn GM, Walther MM, Patronas NJ, Linehan WM, Zbar B. von Hippel–Lindau disease: genetic, clinical, and imaging features. Radiology 1995; 194(3):629–642.
179. Decker HJ, Weidt EJ, Brieger J. The von Hippel–Lindau tumor suppressor gene. A rare and intriguing disease opening new insight into basic mechanisms of carcinogenesis. Cancer Genet Cytogenet 1997; 93(1):74–83.
180. Neumann HP, Schemp W, Wienker TF. High-resolution chromosome banding and fragile site studies in von Hippel–Lindau syndrome. Cancer Genet Cytogenet 1988; 31:41–46.
181. Seizinger BR, Rouleau GA, Ozelius LJ, et al. von Hippel–Lindau disease maps to the region of chromosome 3 associated with renal cell carcinoma. Nature 1988; 332: 268–269.
182. Decker HJ, Neumann HP, Walter TA, Sandberg AA. 3p involvement in a renal cell carcinoma in von Hippel–Lindau syndrome. Region of tumor breakpoint clustering on 3p? Cancer Genet Cytogenet 1988; 33:59–65.
183. Latif F, Tory K, Gnarra J, Yao M, Duh FM, Orcutt ML, Stackhouse T, Kuzmin I, Modi W, Geil L, et al. Identification of the von Hippel–Lindau disease tumor suppressor gene. Science 1993; 260(5112):1317–1320.
184. Gnarra JR, Tory K, Weng Y, Schmidt L, Wei MH, Li H, Latif F, Liu S, Chen F, Duh FM, et al. Mutations of the VHL tumour suppressor gene in renal carcinoma. Nat Genet 1994; 7(1):85–90.

185. Tse JY, Wong JH, Lo KW, Poon WS, Huang DP, Ng HK. Molecular genetic analysis of the von Hippel–Lindau disease tumor suppressor gene in familial and sporadic cerebellar hemangioblastomas. Am J Clin Pathol 1997; 107(4):459–466.
186. Prowse AH, Webster AR, Richards FM, Richard S, Olschwang S, Resche F, Affara NA, Maher ER. Somatic inactivation of the VHL gene in von Hippel–Lindau disease tumors. Am J Hum Genet 1997; 60(4):765–771.
187. Chan CC, Vortmeyer AO, Chew EY, Green WR, Matteson DM, Shen DF, Linehan WM, Lubensky IA, Zhuang Z. VHL gene deletion and enhanced VEGF gene expression detected in the stromal cells of retinal angioma. Arch Ophthalmol 1999; 117(5): 625–630.
188. Patel RJ, Appukuttan B, Ott S, Wang X, Stout JT. DNA-based diagnosis of the von Hippel–Lindau syndrome. Am J Ophthalmol 2000; 129(2):258–260.
189. Beroud C, Joly D, Gallou C, Staroz F, Orfanelli MT, Junien C. Software and database for the analysis of mutations in the VHL gene. Nucleic Acids Res 1998; 26(1):256–258.
190. Maher ER, Webster AR, Richards FM, Green JS, Crossey PA, Payne SJ, Moore AT. Phenotypic expression in von Hippel–Lindau disease: correlations with germline VHL gene mutations. J Med Genet 1996; 33(4):328–332.
191. Zbar B, Kishida T, Chen F, Schmidt L, Maher ER, Richards FM, Crossey PA, Webster AR, Affara NA, Ferguson-Smith MA, Brauch H, Glavac D, Neumann HP, Tisherman S, Mulvihill JJ, Gross DJ, Shuin T, Whaley J, Seizinger B, Kley N, Olschwang S, Boisson C, Richard S, Lips CH, Lerman M, et al. Germline mutations in the von Hippel–Lindau disease (VHL) gene in families from North America, Europe, and Japan. Hum Mutat 1996; 8(4):348–357.
192. Allen RC, Webster AR, Sui R, Brown J, Taylor CM, Stone EM. Molecular characterization and ophthalmic investigation of a large family with type 2A Von Hippel–Lindau Disease. Arch Ophthalmol 2001; 119(11):1659–1665.
193. Chen F, Kishida T, Yao M, Hustad T, Glavac D, Dean M, Gnarra JR, Orcutt ML, Duh FM, Glenn G, et al. Germline mutations in the von Hippel–Lindau disease tumor suppressor gene: correlations with phenotype. Hum Mutat 1995; 5(1):66–75.
194. Lonser RR, Glenn GM, Walther M, Chew EY, Libutti SK, Linehan WM, Oldfield EH. von Hippel–Lindau disease. Lancet 2003; 361(9374):2059–2067.
195. Stolle C, Glenn G, Zbar B, Humphrey JS, Choyke P, Walther M, Pack S, Hurley K, Andrey C, Klausner R, Linehan WM. Improved detection of germline mutations in the von Hippel–Lindau disease tumor suppressor gene. Hum Mutat 1998; 12(6):417–423.
196. Brieger J, Weidt EJ, Gansen K, Decker HJ. Detection of a novel germline mutation in the von Hippel–Lindau tumour-suppressor gene by fluorescence–labelled base excision sequence scanning (F–BESS). Clin Genet 1999; 56(3):210–215.
197. Sgambati MT, Stolle C, Choyke PL, Walther MM, Zbar B, Linehan WM, Glenn GM. Mosaicism in von Hippel–Lindau disease: lessons from kindreds with germline mutations identified in offspring with mosaic parents. Am J Hum Genet 2000; 66(1):84–91.
198. Goldberg MF, Koenig S. Argon laser treatment of von Hippel–Lindau retinal angiomas: I. Clinical and angiographic findings. Arch Ophthalmol 1974; 92:121–125.
199. Goldberg MF. Clinicopathologic correlation of von Hippel angiomas after xenon arc and argon laser photocoagulation. In: Peyman GA, Apple DJ, Sanders DR, eds. Intraocular Tumors. New York: Appleton-Century-Crofts, 1977:219–234.
200. Nicholson DH. Induced ocular hypertension during photocoagulation of afferent artery in angiomatosis retinae. Retina 1983; 3:59–61.
201. Peyman GA, Rednam KRV, Mottow-Lippa L, Flood T. Treatment of large von Hippel tumors by eye wall resection. Ophthalmology 1983; 90:840–847.
202. Garcia-Arumi J, Sararols LH, Cavero L, Escalada F, Corcostegui BF. Therapeutic options for capillary papillary hemangiomas. Ophthalmology 2000; 107(1):48–54.
203. Raja D, Benz MS, Murray TG, Escalona-Benz EM, Markoe A. Salvage external beam radiotherapy of retinal capillary hemangiomas secondary to von Hippel–Lindau disease: visual and anatomic outcomes. Ophthalmology 2004; 111(1):150–153.

204. Aiello LP, George DJ, Cahill MT, Wong JS, Cavallerano J, Hannah AL, Kaelin WG Jr. Rapid and durable recovery of visual function in a patient with von Hippel–Lindau syndrome after systemic therapy with vascular endothelial growth factor receptor inhibitor su5416. Ophthalmology 2002, 109(9):1745–1751.
205. McKusick VA. Mendelian Inheritance in Man. Baltimore: Johns Hopkins University Press, 1983:498.
206. Shields JA. Diagnosis and Management of Intraocular Tumors. St Louis: CV Mosby, 1983:556–562, 672–682.
207. Gass JDM. Cavernous hemangioma of the retina, a neurooculo–cutaneous syndrome. Am J Ophthalmol 1971; 71:799–814.
208. Klein M, Goldberg MF, Cotlier E. Cavernous hemangioma of the retina: report of four cases. Ann Ophthalmol 1975; 7:1213–1222.
209. Lewis RA, Cohen MH, Wise GN. Cavernous hemangioma of the retina arid optic disc. Br J Ophthalmol 1975; 59:422–434.
210. Messmer E, Font RL, Laqua H, et al. Cavernous hemangioma of the retina. Immunohistochemical and ultrastructural observations. Arch Ophthalmol 1984; 102:413–418.
211. Hayman LA, Evans RA, Ferrell RE, et al. Familial cavernous angiomas: natural history and genetic study over a 5 year period. Am J Med Genet 1982; 11:147–160.
212. Goldberg RE, Pheasant TR, Shields JA. Cavernous hemangioma of the retina: a four-generation pedigree with neurocutaneous manifestations and an example of bilateral retinal involvement. Arch Ophthalmol 1979; 97:2321–2324.
213. Colvard DM, Robertson DM, Trautmann JC. Cavernous hemangioma of the retina. Arch Ophthalmol 1978; 96:2042–2044.
214. Messmer E, Laqua H, Wessing A, et al. Nine cases of cavernous hemangioma of the retina. Am J Ophthalmol 1983; 95:383–390.
215. Dobyns WB, Michels W, Groover RV, et al. Familial cavernous malformations of the central nervous system and retina. Ann Neurol 1987; 21:578–583.
216. Sarraf D, Payne AM, Kitchen ND, Sehmi KS, Downes SM, Bird AC. Familial cavernous hemangioma: an expanding ocular spectrum. Arch Ophthalmol 2000; 118(7): 969–973.
217. Couteulx SL, Brezin AP, Fontaine B, Toumier-Lasserve E, Labauge P. A novel KRIT1/CCM1 truncating mutation in a patient with cerebral and retinal cavernous angiomas. Arch Ophthalmol 2002; 120(2):217–218.
218. Gunel M, Laurans MS, Shin D, DiLuna ML, Voorhees J, Choate K, Nelson-Williams C, Lifton RP. KRIT1, a gene mutated in cerebral cavernous malformation, encodes a microtubule-associated protein. Proc Nat Acad Sci USA 2002; 99(16):10677–10682.
219. Denier C, Labauge P, Brunereau L, Cave-Riant F, Marchelli F, Arnoult M, Cecillon M, Maciazek J, Joutel A, Toumier-Lasserve E. Societe Francaise de Neurochirgurgie. Societe de Neurochirurgie de Langue Francaise. Clinical features of cerebral cavernous malformations patients with KRITl mutations. Ann Neurol 2004; 55(2):213–220.
220. Schweitzer NMJ, Vein der Pol BAE. Multiple mucosal neuroma (MMN) or multiple endocrine neoplasia (MEN) type 3 syndrome ocular manifestations. A case report. Doc Ophthalmol 1977; 44:151–159.
221. Robertson DM, Sizemore GW, Gordon H. Thickened corneal nerves as a manifestation of multiple endocrine neoplasia. Trans Am Acad Ophthalmol Otolarynol 1975; 79: 772–787.
222. Nasir MA, Yee RW, Piest KL, Reasner CA 2nd. Multiple endocrine neoplasia type III. Cornea 1991; 10(5):454–459.
223. Yanoff M, Sharaby ML. Multiple endocrine neoplasia type IIB. Arch Ophthalmol 1996; 114(2):228–229.
224. Spector B, Klintworth GK, Wells SA. Histologic study of the ocular lesions in mutliple endocrine neoplasia syndrome type II. Am J Ophthal 1981; 91:204–215.

225. Pasini B, Hofstra RM, Yin L, Bocciardi R, Santamaria G, Grootscholten PM, Ceccherini I, Patrone G, Priolo M, Buys CH, et al. The physical map of the human RET proto-oncogene. Oncogene 1995; 11(9):1737–1743.
226. Fink A, Lapidot M, Spierer A. Ocular manifestations in multiple endocrine neoplasia type 2b. Am J Ophthalmol 1998; 126(2):305–307.
227. Eng C, Mulligan LM. Mutations of the RET proto-oncogene in the multiple endocrine neoplasia type 2 syndromes, related sporadic tumours, and hirschsprung disease. Hum Mutat 1997; 9(2):97–109.
228. Feman SS, Apt L, Roth AM. The basal cell nevus syndrome. Am J Ophthalmol 1974; 78:222–228.
229. Kedem A, Even–Paz Z, Freund M. Basal cell nevus syndrome associated with malignant melanoma of the iris. Dermatologica 1970; 140:99.
230. Grand MG, Kaine J, Fulling, et al. Cerebroretinal vasculopathy. A new hereditary syndrome. Ophthalmology 1988; 95:649–659.
231. Gutmann DH, Fischbeck KH, Sergott RC. Hereditary retinal vasculopathy with cerebral white matter lesions. Am J Med Genet 1989; 34(2):217–220.
232. Ophoff RA, DeYoung J, Service SK, Joosse M, Caffo NA, Sandkuijl LA, Terwindt GM, Haan J, van den Maagdenberg AM, Jen J, Baloh RW, Barilla-LaBarca ML, Saccone NL, Atkinson JP, Ferrari MD, Freimer NB, Frants RR. Hereditary vascular retinopathy, cerebroretinal vasculopathy, and hereditary endotheliopathy with retinopathy, nephropathy, and stroke map to a single locus on chromosome 3p21.1–p21.3. Am J Hum Genet 2001; 69(2):447–453.
233. Siveke JT, Schmid H. Evidence for systemic manifestations in cerebroretinal vasculopathy. Am J Med Genet 2003; 123A(3):309.

22
Albinism

INTRODUCTION

Albinism is the general term used to describe a series of congenital and inherited diseases characterized by an abnormally low amount of melanin in normally pigmented tissues and affecting the skin, hair, and eyes (oculocutaneous albinism) or the eyes alone (ocular albinism). Several authors qualify the definition by including nystagmus, photophobia, and reduced visual acuity, using the term *albinoidism* if hypomelanosis occurs without nystagmus (1). Because of its striking appearance, the oculocutaneous form of albinism, since the dawn of history, has been known to exist in humans and in much of the animal kingdom. Only recently, however, has the complexity of the clinical, genetic, pathologic, and pathophysiologic aspects of the subject been known. At least 10 different types of oculocutaneous albinism, and at least four different types of ocular albinism are now recognizable. The number of genes involved in human albinism is even greater. In addition to the genes associated with oculocutaneous and ocular albinisms, seven genes are involved in the Hermansky–Pudlak syndrome and seven genes in the Waardenburg syndromes. This is a minimal total of 24 genes (2). However, in animals a greater number of genes are responsible for pigmentation, and a whole book has been written on the coat color of mammals (3).

An abnormality that occurs in the anatomy of the visual pathways in most cases of albinism has provided an explanation for several clinical findings of this disease that were formerly poorly understood. The clinical picture of albinism has become even more complex with the identification of several types of albinoidism (4) and the possible existence of a congenital nystagmus associated with a fundus hypopigmentation that cannot be classified into one of the existing types of albinism.

OCULOCUTANEOUS ALBINISM

Description and Clinical Findings

In oculocutaneous albinism (OCA), melanin, is absent or found in abnormally low amounts in the skin, hair and eyes. The clinical appearance is striking. The division into tyrosinase-negative and tyrosinase-positive OCA separates patients with a permanent lack of pigment from those who may accumulate some amounts of pigment during life. Although there are many differences between the different types of OCA, some general features have been noted.

At birth, a child with OCA has white skin, with no or little pigmentation. In some types of OCA, skin pigmentation may develop later in life. In others, partial skin pigmentation may assume different hues, such as the red skins of Papua New Guinea (5). In general the ability to tan indicates the presence of melanin. It may even occur rarely in those with tyrosinase-negative OCA (6). Patients with OCA tend to suffer from hyperkeratosis and skin carcinoma (both squamous cell and basal cell) much more frequently than the general population (7). They also have a higher tendency toward the dysplastic nevus syndrome and amelanotic malignant melanomas (8,9).

The hair is commonly white at birth. In some types of OCA, melanin may develop, imparting some color, such as blond, yellow, or brown.

The ocular anomalies are usually serious, as vision is always affected. The eye, with no pigment in the iris, has a pink or red reflex, characteristic of the albino appearance. The clinical examination may reveal the following features: nystagmus is practically a universal finding in those with OCA. It usually starts in the first months of life and continues therafter, although, in some cases, it may decrease. The nystagmus is usually horizontal and pendular, but seesaw and vertical nystagmus have also been described (10). Most albinos are seriously photophobic. This starts early in life and can be alleviated by reducing the amount of light that enters the eye (see "Management of Oculocutaneous Albinism").

Nystagmus that is coarse in childhood usually improves slowly and becomes less conspicuous by adolescence (11).

Visual acuity is reduced in all albinos. Commonly, there is an inverse relationship between the amount of pigmentation in the eye and the extent of decreased visual acuity and other eye problems (12). In tyrosinase-negative OCA, visual acuity is about 6/60 at aged three years (4). In a mixed group of 32 albino patients, Taylor (13) found the visual acuity range of 6/18 to 6/60 to be evenly divided. Examination of small infants with the preferential looking procedure showed the visual acuity to be better in the first years of life (14,15). At 15 weeks it was 6/15 to 6/21, which is fairly normal for this age. The acuity was much worse under higher luminance, and became worse under any luminance at aged three years (14). Relatively good visual acuities sometimes occurred, even in albinos who had no detectable fovea (15). In some albinos, mostly in those afflicted with tyrosinase-positive albinism, visual acuity may, in fact, improve with time (16). Visual acuity is significantly better under good lighting conditions (16).

Albinos do not have binocular stereoscopic vision; therefore, it is not surprising that strabismus is very common (more than 90% in one series; (13)). Usually, the angle of squint is not large and may be cosmetically acceptable. Vertical malalignment may also occur, frequently resulting in abnormal head posture (13).

High myopia, high hyperopia, and astigmatism also occur frequently in albinism.

Iris translucency is observed in every albino, even those in the heterozygote state. Its degree obviously depends on the amount of pigmentation present. The eye may be pink in appearance or the translucency may be detectable only by tests (see "Diagnosis and Tests in Oculocutaneous Albinism").

The most apparent finding in the fundus is the hypoplgmentation of the retinal pigment epithelium. This renders the choroidal blood vessels clearly visible, and gives the background a reddish appearance.

In patients with some pigmentation (tyrosinase-positive types), the color may be blond or light orange, and pigment may be seen in the choroid.

Fluorescein angiography has shown that in tyrosinase-positive OCA the abnormal pigmentation of the retinal pigment epithelium may range from scattered small transmission defects to a translucent layer without pigment (17).

The dark area of the xanthophyll pigment at the macula is not seen. Also, most patients have no foveal pit or reflex. The absence of a foveal pit has been confirmed by histologic examination (see "Pathology, Biochemistry, and Pathophysiology of Oculocutaneous Albinism"). Optic nerve hypoplasia has been noted in the majority of patients in one study (18) and appears to be much more common than previously reported. The hypoplasia can be in its typical full form or exhibit only some elements (18).

The large retinal vessels are generally normal, but an anomalous large nonci-lioretinal vessel extending from disk to fovea (18) and small vessels crossing through the foveal avascular zone or through the presumed point of fixation have been described when no fovea is present (17,18). It is not clear whether these small vessels have any influence on the visual acuity, as such vessels have also been described in normal individuals with perfect vision (19).

The Clinical and Genetic Types of Oculocutaneous Albinism

Albinism has long been recognized as an autosomal recessive disease. A genetic study of one family, in which the parents were complete albinos, but their two children were normally pigmented, was the first definite indication that at least two types of OCA exist (20). Additional genetic (21), clinical, and biochemical (22) studies have confirmed the existence of at least two nonallelic types of OCA (23). Since then, additional types have been defined and the list amended (Table 1).

Tyrosinase-Negative Oculocutaneous Albinism (OCA Type 1A)

OCA1A, tyrosinase-negative OCA (TNOCA), is the classic and most severe form of albinism. Tyrosinase activity is completely absent and no melanin pigment can be found in skin, hair, or eyes (24).

It is the classic form, in which patients have snow-white hair, white or pink nonpigmented skin, and eyes with photophobia, nystagmus, poor vision, and no detectable pigment. Visual acuity is generally somewhat worse than in tyrosinase-positive OCA.

The name TNOCA, is based on the fact that the hairbulb tyrosinase activity is negative. In 1976, King and Witkop (25) showed that a hairbulb incubated in tyrosinase may (tyrosinase-positive) or may not (tyrosinase-negative) show melanin formation. They also suggested that TNOCA is similar to the *c/c* genotype of albino mice, which have no tyrosinase activity; however, the correlation with the clinical state of the patient is not always evident. The hairbulb incubation test does not consistently yield negative results in TNOCA patients (6,26). Although the reason for this is unclear, it is assumed that tyrosinase is absent in TNOCA because of an inborn error of metabolism. It is possible that in some cases melanin may be formed, even in the absence of tyrosinase (26).

Table 1 Major Characteristics of the Different Types of Oculocutaneous Albinism

	Type	Eponym[a]	Gene	Chromosomal location	Inheritance[b]	Skin color	Hair	Iris	Hairbulb tyrosinase activity	Iris transillumination	Skin biopsy	Remarks
1	OCA1A	TNOCA	TYR	11q14-q21	AR	White or pink		Blue	None	+	Stage II and early III melanosomes with only intermediate vesicle	No tyrosinase activity
2	OCA1B	YMOCA	TYR	11q14-q21	AR	Nevi + lentigines tanning ±	White-blond	Blue-brown	None, very low or variable	+	Stage II and early III melanosomes	
3	OCA1C	MPOCA	TYR	11q14-q21	AR	Brown	Cream-platinum	Blue-pigment ring	None, low or intermediate	+	—	Similar to, except milder than OCA1B
4	OCA2(A)	TPOCA	P	15q11-q13	AR	Nevi + lentigines	White-blond	Blue-brown	Normal or high	+	Stage II and III melaosomes	
5	OCA2(B)	BOCA	P	15q11-q13	AR	Light brown	Light brown	Blue	?	+	—	Allelic to OCA2
6	OCA3	ROCA	TYRP1	9p23	AR	Bronze-red	Light brown	Brown	Normal	—	—	Found in new Guinea and Africans
7	OCA4	OCA4	MATP	5p	AR	Pale	White-yellow	Normal +	Normal	+	—	More common in Japanese patients
8	ADOCA	ADOCA	—	—	AD	White-creamy	White-blond	—	—	+	Melanosomes up to stage III	Not confirmed distinct entity

[a]former terms; see text.
[b]all are of autosomal recessive inheritance, except type of that is of autosomal dominant inheritance.

The heterozygote for TNOCA often has low tyrosinase activity (27), but the overlap with normals is great, and the reliability of the test to detect heterozygotes is inconsistent (28).

As in most other types of albinism, the optic pathways in OCA1A are misrouted, providing the opportunity for a clinical test. Schmitz et al. (29) compared the magnetic resonance imaging (MRI) of albino patients with that of controls and showed that OCA1 patients had significantly smaller chiasmatic widths, smaller optic nerves and traits, and wider angles between nerves and traits. However, these abnormalities cannot be used to distinguish between OCA1 type A and OCA1 type B (29). King et al. (30) assumed that white hair at birth indicates OCA1 phenotype and performed mutational studies. These confirmed that 85% of 120 newborns with white hair indeed carried mutations in TYR, the tyrosinase gene, in both subtype OCA1A and OCA1B. However, about 5% had OCA2 mutations (30).

OCA1A is caused by mutations in the tyrosinase gene located in chromosome 11ql4-q21 (2,11,31). The gene TYR encodes the tyrosinase polypeptide of 528 amino acids (32) or of 529 amino acids (33). In one of the first studies, a single mutation Pro81Leu was detected in 20% of patients with OCA1 (31). A multitude of various mutations, however, later were identified. By 2001, they numbered 109 (34), most being missense mutations (24). Some mutations were found in the promoter region or in splice–sites (30). The most frequent mutation was Thr373Lys missense mutation (35). Other mutations are specific to certain populations, such as the Gly47Asp mutation found in the Moroccan Jewish community, in the Canary Islands and in Puerto Rico (36). Some OCA1 patients manifest no mutation at all, possibly because the mutation has not been sought for in the promoter area or within introns (34). No tyrosinase activity can be detected in OCA1 (11,24). Tyrosinase is a catalytic enzyme that binds copper. It catalyzes the first two critical steps of melanin biosynthesis (33). The fact that complete absence of tyrosinase activity exists regardless of the type of mutation is interesting. Toyofuku et al. (24) concluded from their study that it results not from the complete loss of function, but rather from the inability of the tyrosinase to reach the target cell. Mutant tyrosinase, caused by any mutation, is retained and degraded in the endoplasmic reticulum and is not transported to the melanosomes (24). Halaban et al. (35) named the condition "an endoplasmic retention disease."

Tyrosinase–Positive Oculocutaneous Albinism (OCA Type 2)

Various names were used for this type of albinism, including tyrosinase–positive OCA (TPOCA), OCA type 2, OCA type II, OCA2. The condition is associated with mutations in the P–protein gene. One subtype of this condition is Brown OCA (BOCA) as described below. Another is a strictly ocular condition, associated with mutations of the same gene and causing autosomal recessive ocular albinism.

The TPOCA is the second most common type in whites and the most common type in blacks. Together with TNOCA, it accounts for most cases of albinism (See Epidemiology). Clinically, TPOCA may be distinguished from TNOCA by the traces of pigment that accumulate during life. However, the expression of the disease is extremely variable, ranging from patients indistinguishable from those with TNOCA to those who later in life have brown irides, blond hair, and tanned skin. The skin usually contains no generalized pigment, but has pigmented nevi and lentigines (27,37). The hairbulb incubation test shows normal or excessive, tyrosinase activity, suggesting that in this type of albinism substrate availability or transport is deficient, the tyrosinase is structurally abnormal, or the tyrosinase is blocked by an inhibitor (25). There is no evidence to prove or disprove any of these hypotheses (4). Skin biopsy specimens show dense accumulations of premelanosomes and melanosome complexes inside the melanocyte. This feature may indicate a defective ability to pass normal melanin products to keratinocytes in the skin (12). It may be possible to identify heterozygotes by iris transillumination (38). The amount of pigment a patient with TPOCA accumulates depends mainly on ethnic origin; in darker races this may be considerable (39).

Ramsay et al. (40) linked OCA2 to chromosome 15q11.2-ql2 and postulated that the P locus of mice (pink–eye dilute) on mouse chromosome 7 has the human homolog gene in chromosome 15. The P locus, the chromosomal location and the human homolog gene were all later confirmed. Rinchik et al. (41) demonstrated that deletion of both copies of the P gene is associated with OCA2, and that the human P gene encodes an integral membrane transporter protein. Lee et al. (42) determined the structure and the nucleotide sequence of the human P gene. It is quite large, contains 25 exons, spans 250– 600kb and encodes a protein of 838 amino acids that contains 12 transmembrane domains. It is an integral membrane protein of melanosomes (42). How it prevents normal melanin biosynthesis or accumulation is not yet known.

Many mutations have been reported. By 1997, 26 various mutations were known (43). Most were point missense mutations (43), but a large deletion of a whole exon was found exclusively in African communities (44). Navajo Indians also suffer from a high prevalence of OCA2: another deletion in the P gene causes the disorder (45).

Yellow Mutant Oculocutaneous Albinism (OCA Type 1B)

First described in an Amish isolate in the United States (46), yellow mutant OAC (YMOCA; Amish albinism, OCA type IB) is now known in other populations, such as American blacks, African blacks, Ceylonese (39), and British whites (1). Albinism is generally profound at birth; thereafter pigmentation develops rapidly in the skin, which has some tanning abilities, and the hair turns yellow.

The ocular signs of nystagmus, photophobia, and poor visual acuity are often as severe as in TNOCA. In many cases, however, the nystagmus improves with time and may resolve (4). Transillumination of the iris shows a cartwheel effect or a ring of pigment. Hairbulb incubation produces some pigment formation, probably of phaeomelanin. The activity of tyrosinase is absent or low.

It has been suggested that the genes of YMOCA are allelic to the genes of TNOCA and a double heterozygote yellow mutant/tyrosinase–negative albino has been described (23,47). Later, the allelic association with OCA1A was confirmed.

Skin biopsy specimens show premelanosomes in stage II and sometimes in stage III and even early state IV (2,47).

It may be difficult in some cases to distinguish, on clinical grounds, between OCA type 1B and OCA 2 (33). Finding a TYR gene mutation will confirm the diagnosis and the classification. It is likely that specific mutations of the TYR gene, limited in number, are the cause of OCA2B. This subtype probably includes the mutation that results in a temperature–sensitive tyrosinase. The enzyme is more active in cooler areas of the body thus causing selective melanogenesis (48). Mutations associated with OCAIB were reported by Sprite et al. (33). Most were missense, such as: Arg77Trp, Val275Glu, Arg299Ser, Thr325Ala, Ala355Pro and Asp448Asn. Others were small deletions or insertions (33). The mutation Val275Phe was reported to cause a very mild phenotype of OCAIB (34). Camand et al. (34) also reported that about half of the mutations were not identified. This could result from a "hidden" mutation within the gene, as in splice sites within introns, or the promoter area or in noncoding sequences (34). Another possibility would be a more complex mutational mechanism, including digenic transmission (30,34). King et al. (30) reported in 2003 that about one half of mutations involving OCAIB are also found in OCA1A. Some of the OCAIB specific mutations were Trp39Stop, Ser79Asp, Pro81Ser, Gly106Arg, Pro209Arg, Met332Thr, Gly346Stop and Arg422Trp. Some deletions and insertions also existed.

Minimal Pigment Oculocutaneous Albinism

A type of autosomal recessive OCA (49), minimal pigment OCA (MPOCA) appears to be quite rare and bears similarities to the yellow mutant type. Affected patients are born without any pigment, their hair is snow–white, and their irides are blue. During the first year of life, minimal amounts of pigment develop in the iris as a dark ring. Hairbulb tyrosinase activity is negative or very low. Skin biopsy specimens show a normal ultrastructure of the melanocyte, but variations in the pigmentation of the premelanosome.

Currently it seems certain that MPOCA is allelic to OCA1 and is caused by mutations in the TYR gene (30). It should therefore, be classified as OCAIB. If enough clinical phenotypic variance exists, it could also be classified as OCA1C.

Brown Oculocutaneous Albinism

Brown OCA (BOCA), an autosomal recessive form of OCA, has been described in 19 black Nigerian families (50). Patients have light–brown skin; light–brown hair; blue, gray, or light–brown irides; nystagmus; and hypopigmented fundi. The foveal reflex was muted in all examined. Visual activity ranged from 20/60 to 20/100. Contrary to the common TPOCA in Nigeria, these patients demonstrated no increased pigmentation with age and showed no tendency toward premalignant or malignant tumors. One patient evaluated with BOCA had normal hairbulb tyrosinase activity; however, the existence of a partial block in the distal eumelanin pathway has been suggested (51). BOCA has been reported also in South Africa. Manga et al. (52) reported the occurrence of this condition in southern Africa and identified associated mutations linked to the P-gene. The authors suggest that P-gene mutations are responsible for BOCA, and that a limited number of mutations cause this variant of OCA2. It seems therefore that BOCA is allelic to OCA2 and should probably be classified as OCA2B. It is possible that modifying genes may also play a role as such. A modifying gene has been described to change the phenotype of OCA2 (53).

Red Oculocutaneous Albinism

The red type of OCA (ROCA; OCA type III, rufous OCA), has been used to describe "the red-skinned" natives, of Papua New Guinea (5). Their skin is bronze–red and their hair is brown–red. The irides and the fundus of these people have a reddish–brown discoloration. Nystagmus and photophobia are present in a mild form, and visual acuity is only slightly reduced.

This type of OCA is much more common in African populations and has been reported in southern Africa and in African Americans (54,55). Manga et al. (55) described the differences between ROCA and BOCA. In ROCA (Rufous OCA), the skin is brick red, mahogany or bronze, the hair ginger or red–ginger; in BOCA, the skin is tan or light brown, hair is also light brown. In both cases, nystagmus is mild or absent. Boissy et al. (54). and Manga et al. (55) identified disease–bearing mutations on the TYRP gene. In fact, all identified mutations were either Serl66Stop nonsense mutation or a 1-bp deletion, 368del A. Almost all ROCA patients had one or both of these mutations. The gene TYRP1 (for tyrosinase–related protein) spans 24 kb of genomic DNA and consists of seven exons (56). It was mapped to chromosome 9p23 (57).

OCA Type 4 and MATP Gene

OCA4 is a recently identified locus associated with oculocutaneous albinism. Newton et al. surveyed 102 patients with OCA for mutations in three known genes associated with OCA. One of the 102 patients with OCA, of Turkish origin, had OCA–associated mutations in the MATP gene (58). In 2004, Rundshagen et al. (59) identified compound mutations in five out of 176 surveyed German families and Inagaki et al. (60) identified MATP mutations in 18 out of 75 (24%) of Japanese OCA patients. The disorder was named OCA type 4, since the fourth gene associated with the heterogeneic OCA disorder has been identified. All the mutations reported were either missense or frameshift mutations (60).

OCA4 is phenotypically indistinguishable from OCA1B or OCA2. The hair is white–yellow, the skin pale, visual acuity variable, and foveal and/or optic nerve dysplasia is common (59).

The gene, MATP, was cloned (58) and found to contain seven exons and spans approximately 40 kb of DNA on chromosome 5p (59). It is considered the most frequent OCA in Japan (60) and to be responsible for 5–6% of all OCA in Caucasian populations (59). The gene has 12 transmembrane regions, like the P gene, and both genes are predicted to function as transporters. In cases of mutated membrane-associated transporter protein (MATP), tyrosinase processing and intracellular trafficking to the membranes is disrupted (61).

Autosomal Dominant Oculocutaneous Albinism

Two families with an autosomal dominant transmission of OCA (ADOCA) have been described (62,63). The affected members had blond hair, hazel eyes, and typical findings of ocular albinism. The visual acuity was approximately 20/60. Brothers and sisters, as well as their sons and daughters, were similarly affected (63) The condition is rare.

The condition has not yet been confirmed as a distinct entity. It alternatively may represent a dominant allele of one of the known OCA genes or be a variant of Waardenburg syndrome.

BADS Syndrome

The BADS syndrome (Black locks, Oculocutaneous Albinism, and Deafness of the Sensorineural type) has been described in two families (39). The findings consist of patchy pigmentation of the skin, hair, and eyes, with severe sensorineural hearing loss. The preponderant nonpigmented areas have no melanocytes, which do occur normally in the pigmented areas. Nystagmus and poor vision are the rule. In one of the two original families the condition was named "the ermine phenotype" (64,65). BADS should probably be classified with the Waardenburg syndromes.

Other associations such as albinism, mental retardation and microphthalmus have been described in an Amish family (66).

OCA with generalized muscle weakness (67); or glutathione synthetase deficiency (68) may be spurious.

Pathology, Biochemistry, and Pathophysirology of Oculocutaneous Albinism

The facts that albinism has been found throughout most of the animal kingdom and that it bears amazing similarities to human albinism have been helpful to our understanding of the condition.

Melanogenesis

Human melanogenesis occurs normally in embryonal life in melanocytes, which are derived from two sources: the neural crest, which is the source for the migrating melanocytes in all parts of the human body; and the neuroectoderm, which is the derivation of the pigmented cells of the pigment epithelium (69). The melanin pathway (Fig. 1) within the melanocyte uses tyrosine to form one of two final products: common brown to black pigment (eumelanin) and the less usual yellow to red pigment (phaeomelanin). Two enzymes are active in this process: tyrosinase and dopachrome oxido–reductase.

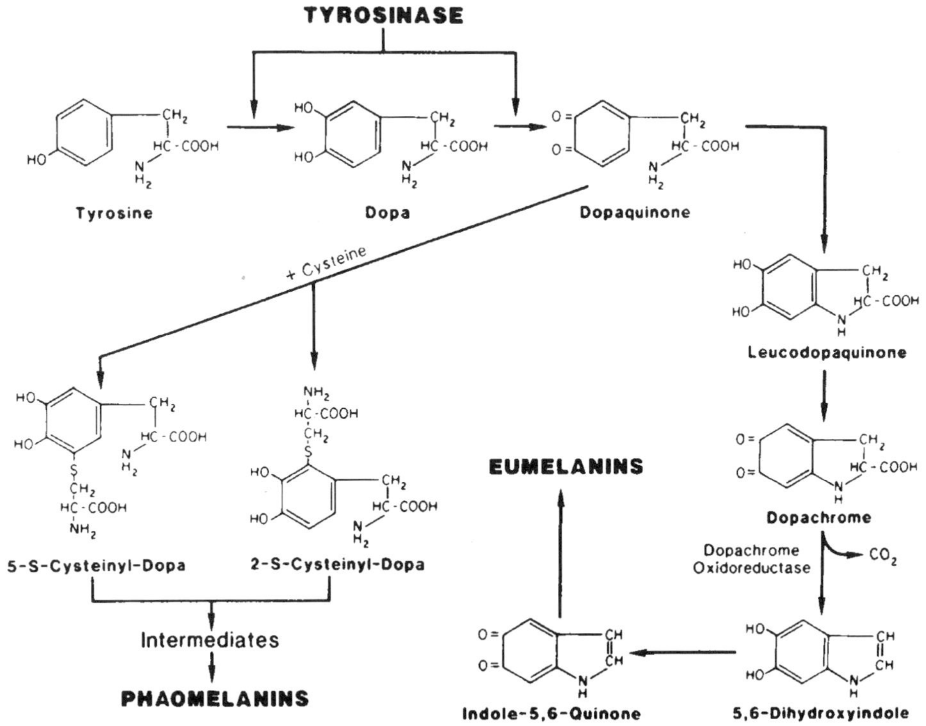

Figure 1 Simplified scheme of the melanin pathways. To produce eumelanins and phaeomelanins, two substrates are necessary (tyrosine and cysteine), and two enzymes are active (tyrosinase and DOPA–chrome oxidoreductase) (from Ref. 27).

Melanogenesis takes place within membrane–bound organelles, called melanosomes, inside the cytoplasm of the melanocyte. In the skin, melanosomes undergo four stages: in stage I, melanosomes are round and contain filaments; in stage II, deposition of pigment begins; in stage III, deposition continues, and in stage IV, a dark pigment deposit is seen. The first three stages are also called premelanosomes. Enzyme activity, which is maximum in stage I, decreases gradually until it totally disappears in stage IV. In the last stages melanin is formed through nonenzymatic polymerization (39).

Melanosomes are then transferred to the keratinocytes of the skin and hair by union and phagocytosis of dendritic extensions of melanocytes (39). This does not normally happen in ocular pigmented structures.

In the human albino, the final stage of a pigmented melanosome is rarely achieved. Usually, only melanosomes of the early stages or later stages are found, but pigmented melanosomes are not seen. The types of albinism are differentiated by the ultra–structure of the pigmented tissues.

Pathology of the Eye

The pathologic study of two human albino eyes, one with OCA2 (70), the other with OCA1 (71), showed that both lacked a foveal pit. A continuous six- to eight cell thick layer of ganglion cells traversed the site of the normal fovea, with no sign of any thinning or dipping of retinal structures (Fig. 2). Retinal pigment epithelial (RPE) cells and melanocytes in the choroid had a normal number of melanocytes, but a

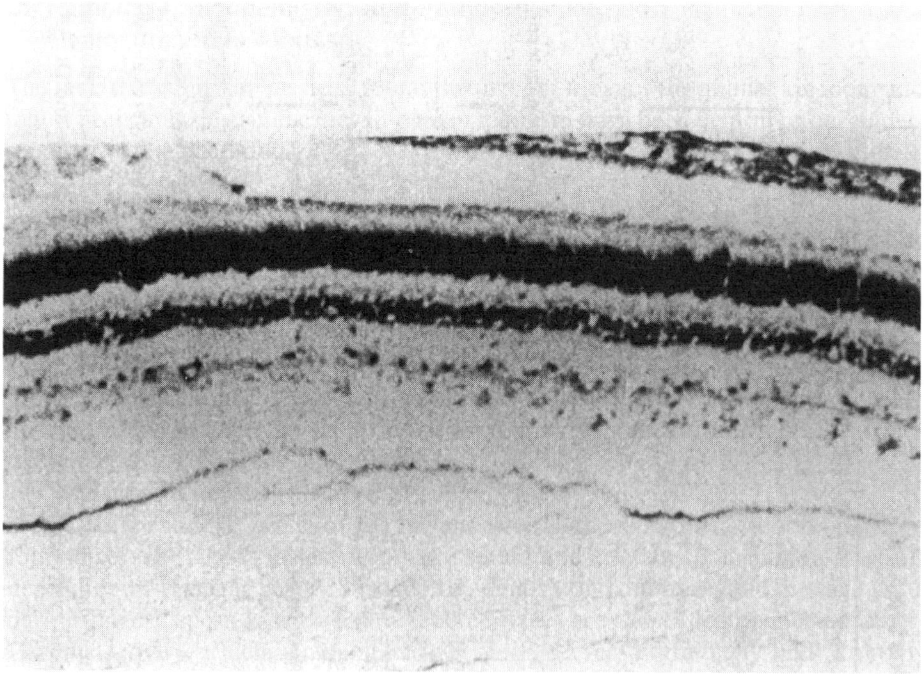

Figure 2 Histologic specimen of an eye from a patient with tyrosinase–negative oculocutaneous albinism. All retinal layers are present. In a normal eye the area represented here would include the fovea (from Ref. 71).

deficiency of melanin (70). In the OCA2 eye, stage III melanosomes with some pigmentation were found; there was a total absence of yellow macular pigment (71), A specimen from the abortion of an OCA1, 19-week-old fetus, contained a reduction in the number of ganglion cells. No rod–free area was found in the macula. The ciliary body was less developed than usual. RPE cells contained filaments without melanization, classified as stage I or II melanosomes (72). The DOPA reaction test enhanced the melanization of melanocytes in samples from normal fetuses and from tyrosinase-positive and from tyrosinase negative fetusues (73). This test has been used for skin biopsies intended for prenatal diagnosis.

Optic Pathway Anomalies

Commonly, almost half of the human retinofugal fibers (the retinal nerve fiber axons entering the optic nerve at the disk) do not decussate at the chiasm but remain in the ipsilateral side of the brain. This feature is related to phylogenetic evolution in mammals. The approximate percentage of nondecussating fibers increased from 2% to 4% in rodents, 20% in dogs and horses, 35% in cats, and 45% in primates (74). Misrouted retinofugal fibers, which decussate at the chiasm in a significantly higher percentage than normal, have been recognized as an anatomic anomaly in albino animals such as rats, mice, guinea-pigs, rabbits, cats, ferrets, and mink (75). Indirect evidence from electrophysiologic studies and the pathologic anatomy of the lateral geniculate body (LGB) indicates that this phenomenon occurs in most human albinos as well.

The abnormal retinofugal projection starts at the retina. The border between "nasal" and "temporal" ganglion cells is not at the fovea, as in the normal eye, but 20° or more into the temporal retina (74), which means some 20–25% more "nasal" fibers cross at the chiasmal decussation. Therefore, the LGB receives abnormal input of information. Not surprisingly, pathologic studies have shown anatomic anomalies in the LGB of human albinos (74,75) and in an albino monkey (76). The normal laminar pattern of the LGB had been lost. In the six–layered part, abnormal fusions between layers of the parvocellular portion and the two layers of the magnocellular portion were found. The bilaminar portion, which reflects the input from the crossed fibers, was abnormally large, and it extended from rostral to caudal tip of the nucleus. Finally, the LGB was smaller than normal and had a rotation of 30° (75). Consequently, the fibers leaving the LGB, the geniculostriate projections, are abnormal. Because cortical cells do not receive bilateral input, binocular cells are absent. Therefore, the well–known lack of binocular vision in the albino has an anatomic basis.

How does the brain cope with the abnormal input of information? Possibly, the human albino brain responds like that of the albino (Siamese) cat: one response is the Boston type, or suppression of the abnormally misrouted input. The second is the Midwestern type, in which rerouting occurs (77).

The approximately 10% of retinal nerve fibers that are not involved in vision, but terminate in the midbrain, also have an abnormal projection. Unlike the 80% crossed and 20% uncrossed retinal superior colliculus fibers in the normal individual, the albino has 95% crossed and 5% uncrossed fibers (74).

The misrouting of retinofugal fibers in the albino can be demonstrated by electrophysiologic tests (see the following section). An abnormal chiasmatic decussation was found in cases of TNOCA, TPOCA, YMOCA, BOCA, the HPS variants of

OCA (77), and in the X–linked and the autosomal recessive types of ocular albinism (78).

What causes the abnormal visual pathways of the albino? It is not the pleiotropic action of a gene, since several genes are involved, and it is inconceivable that each will also demonstrate this action on the visual pathways, as was pointed out by Witkop et al. (77). An association with lack of ocular pigment has been suggested (78), but recently Leventhal et al. (79) found similar misoriented visual pathways in normally pigmented cats that were heterozygous for albinism. The authors concluded that it is not the hypopigmentation of the retina that causes the misdirected retinal projection. In a study on the developing eyes of mice and rats, Silver and Sapiro (80) showed that the distal half of the primitive eye stalk is transiently pigmented before and during the migration of the pioneer optic axons. The growing axons try to avoid the pigmented tissue and are directed into the ventral, pigment-free zone. In albino rats, on day 15 of embryonal life, axons invaded this area because it was not pigmented and started misrouting the axons. It is possible that a lack of pigmented tissue in early embryonal life misdirects axons.

A similar misrouting of auditory pathways is also known in albinotic humans and animals. Pigment is found in the normal inner ear of all mammals (77), providing a similar process to the optic pathways.

Diagnosis and Tests in Oculocutaneous Albinism

The diagnosis of OCA is usually simple, depending on the degree of hypopigmentation and the presence of typical ocular findings. In certain types of OCA, the diagnosis is less obvious, as when pigment is present and in heterozygotes. Also, the classification of patients into subtypes of OCA may be difficult. Jay et al. (1) could not definitely diagnose and classify 36 of 201 (18%) albino patients.

The following tests are available to help in the diagnosis of patients with OCA.

Transillumination of the Iris

A hand-held light or a slit–lamp method of transillumination can be used (81). The hand-held light is directed on the sclera or lower eyelid, toward the pupil and iris. With the slit–lamp, the light should be coaxial, which enables good evaluation of the iris pigment epithelium (81). With use of the slit-lamp method, Jay et al. (38) found transillumination defects in the iris in 0.67% of the normal population; this increased to 9.72% if the room was well darkened. Thirty of 40 (75%) obligatory heterozygotes showed defects by this method. Wirtschafter et al. (82) have suggested a quantifiable method of iris translucency, in which Kodak neutral-density filters are used to match and neutralize the light emerging from the pupil.

Another sign of positive translucency is the ability to see the edge of the lens (11).

The iris translucency sign may be negative in patients with some pigmentation as in OCA2, in some cases of ocular albinism, or with increasing pigmentation.

Abnormal Fovea

An abnormal fovea is one of the hallmarks of OCA, but sometimes it may be difficult ophthalmoscopically to confirm. Using OCT, Meyer et al. (83) were unable to detect any foveal pit. A widespread thickening of fovea to 300 microns instead of the normal 150 microns was measured in the optic pit. McGuire et al. (84) also demonstrated extension of retinal neuro-sensory layers through the area in which the fovea would normally be located.

Detection of melanin pigment in the macula, as detected by ophthalmoscopy, is associated with better visual acuity (16).

Hairbulb Tyrosinase Incubation

Freshly epilated hairbulbs incubated in a concentrated L-tyrosine solution will form heavy pigment (tyrosinase-positive) or not (tyrosinase–negative) (25) or will show an intermediate response (minimal pigment type). The active melanocytes are located in the upper part of the hairbulb, just above the dermal papilla. False-negative results can be minimized by using freshly epilated hair for the test. False-positive results are obtained when melanin is formed, sometimes even in the absence of tyrosinase (26). These results may also be positive in heterozygotes. Unfortunately, the test is not foolproof, and false-negative or "false-positive" results may occur (26). The production of phaeomelanin may be assayed by incubating the hairbulb in a mixed solution of L-tyrosine and L-cysteine.

Electroretinography and Electro-oculography

Large and faster than normal ERG responses (85) and supernormal electrooculo grams (EOGs) (86) have been obtained in albino patients. It has been suggested that this phenomenon is a consequence of the large light scatter of the albino eye. Heterozygotes do not show this phenomenon. Walk et al. (87) found normal ERGs in six patients with tyrosinase-positive OCA and in three patients with autosomal dominant OCA (tyrosinase-positive), and normal or slightly higher than normal in amplitude with shorter than normal implicit times ERGs in six patients with tyrosinase–negative OCA.

In summary, an accentuated ERG, with a significantly larger than normal a wave and significantly shorter latencies of both a-wave and b-wave, are characteristic of OCA (88–90). This may be more pronounced in tyrosinase–negative OCA. The larger and faster ERGs may result from the stronger effect of the flash stimulus, owing to the translucent iris and lack of RPE absorption (89).

Visual-Evoked Potentials

Binocular stimulation yields normal responses from the striate cortex (91) in patients with OCA. However, monocular stimulation produces significantly decreased visual–evoked potential (VEP) amplitudes from the ipsilateral hemisphere, whereas those recorded from the contralateral hemisphere will be normal (Fig. 3) (91). This was first reported in 1974 and has since been confirmed in many reports. The VEP reflects the misrouting of the retinofugal fibers. In one study of 100 patients with OCA, the VEP was positive in 70% (93). Of four stimuli used in the study, flash, modulated light, pattern reversal, and pattern appearance–disappearance, the last was found to be the most sensitive and specific (28,93,94). With pattern reversal stimuli and recordings over five occipital spots (midline and two on each side), Jay and Carrol (95) sometimes recorded a P100 response with maximal amplitude over the ipsilateral scalp and, sometimes, over the contralateral scalp. By subtracting the VEP responses over the two hemispheres and stimuli of the appearing–disappearing checkerboard pattern, Van Dorp et al. (28) and Apkarian et al. (96) received a 100% recognition of the misrouted fibers in all albino subjects they examined.

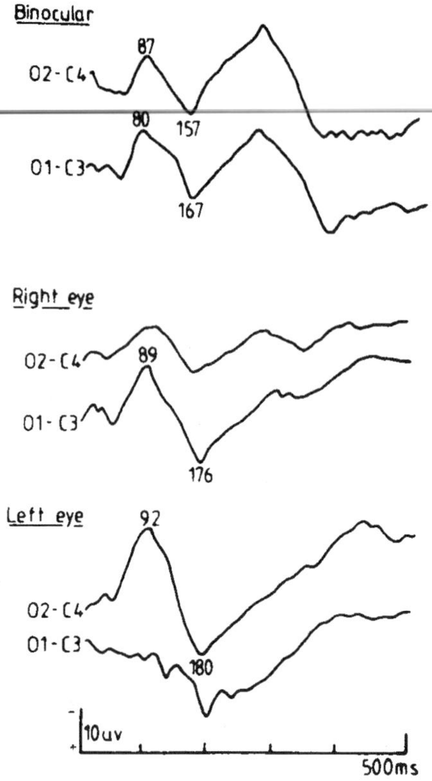

Figure 3 Visual–evoked potential from a 4.5–month–old albino baby: numbers over graphs indicate time of response in milliseconds. 02–C_a indicates the response over the right hemisphere; 0I–C_3, the response over the left hemisphere. Diffuse flash stimulation was used. Note symmetric responses on binocular stimulation and the asymmetric responses with higher amplitudes over the contralateral hemisphere following monocular stimulation (from Ref. 94).

Monocular stimulation by flash VEP resulted in a consistently shorter latency of the P_2 over the contralateral hemisphere (94).

All techniques of VEP, such as flash VEP (fVEP), pattern onset (poVEP) and pattern reversal (prVEP), showed an occipital crossed asymmetry in OCA patients, when comparing responses from each eye. A prominent negativity was recorded contralaterally and a small positive component was recorded ipsilaterally (88). Crossed asymmetry was noted more with fVEP (100%) than with poVEP (56%) or prVEP (44%) (11).

Creel et al. (90) concludes that the VEP, performed with two active electrodes (both sides of the scalp), is the most reliable concomitant for determining albinism.

Auditory Brain Stem Responses

Auditory brain stem responses (ABRs) were subnormal (about 50% of the normal amplitude) in those with Chediak–Higashi syndrome (91).

The electron microscopic examination of skin biopsy specimens may be helpful to evaluate the type of OCA, especially to distinguish it from ocular albinism.

Epidemiology and Genetics

The prevalence of all types of albinism has been reported for large populations as 1:10,000 to 1:20,000 (4,58,79). The division between tyrosinase-negative and tyrosinase positive OCA is fairly equal, with the two largest types of OCA evenly divided. Among the white population, TNOCA is somewhat more common than TPOCA, and cited figures range from 1:34,000 to 1:39,000 (4,22). The rate of heterozygotes is approximately 1:95 for each group. In the black population the ratio is different. Among Afro–Americans, the frequency of OCA2 is almost double that of OCA1 (TNOCA), with ratios of 1:15,000 and 1:28,000, respectively (4,22). Most albinism in Africa is tyrosinase-positive–OCA. However, the figures are much higher in isolates, and in certain populations. In South African blacks, the prevalence of all types of albinism was reported to be 1:3900, with a heterozygote rate of 1:32 (40,97). In the city of Harare in Zimbabwe, prevalence of OCA2 was reported as 1:2833 with a carrier frequency of 1:27 (98). In Navajo Indians, prevalence of OCA2 is in the range of 1:1500 to 1:2000 (45). Frequency of rufous OCA (OCA3, ROCA) has been estimated as 1:8500 in the black South African population (55). Frequency of OCA4, with MATP gene mutations, was found to be 24% in the Japanese population (60) and estimated to be 5–6% in the European Caucasian population (59). The heterozygote rate for Hermansky–Pudlak syndrome in Puerto Rico was reported to be 1:22 (99).

All types of OCA are transmitted by autosomal recessive genes, except the one recognized type of autosomal dominant OCA. The hereditary influence of the genes is overwhelming; there is little or no environmental contribution. Gedda et al. (100) have found an amazing similarity of findings in monozygotic twins. The different OCA types (see Table 1) are caused by different genes on different loci, except for the tyrosinase–negative types, which are allelic, including TNOCA, YMOCA, and possibly minimal pigment types. A double heterozygote for tyrosinase–negative and tyrosinase–positive OCA will have normal pigmentation, as was proved for families with albino parents of mixed types (20,21), Similarly, the genes for ocular albinism of the X-linked or autosomal recessive types are separate from those for OCA (1,101).

The cause of the large phenotypic variability of TPOCA is not entirely clear. It is probable that variable phenotypes are associated with different alleles (38). Currently, however, the effect of modifying genes cannot be ruled out.

Management of Oculocutaneous Albinism

Medical and Surgical

Taylor (13) compiled a list of attempted and failed approaches toward the treatment of OCA, including melanocytic-stimulating hormones, topically applied tyrosine, oral DOPA, *Ammi majus* plant derivatives, AMP, and prostaglandins.

Protective clothes for the skin are advised for albinos, especially those living in areas with high penetration of ultraviolet radiation, and for patients with TNOCA. Precancerous lesions and skin tumors should be watched for and removed.

Haptic contact lenses to reduce the amount of light entering the eye have failed to improve vision, even when fitted early in life (13,102,103). However, this subject needs additional investigation. Refraction should be performed and glasses prescribed for most albino patients, as high refractive errors are common. Dark–tinted glasses help to alleviate photophobia. Amber (10% transmission) aad dark amber (2% transmission) are often preferred by albino patients (104).

Strabismus surgery should be performed when the condition is cosmetically unacceptable, bearing in mind that these patients have no binocular vision. Abnormal head posture, which is not uncommon in albinos, can be eliminated by surgery, using the Kestenbaum procedure or the Faden operation (posterior fixation suture) (105).

Genetic Counseling

Given the regular Mendelian laws, the risk of an additional sibling being affected after one albino baby has been born to normal parents is 25%. The same applies to any additional children. The risk to the offspring of an albino parent married to a nonalbino person not known to be a heterozygote is based on the frequency of such heterozygotes in the population. Although the frequency varies according to the type of OCA and population considered, it is about 1:95 for the two major types of OCA in a white population. Therefore, the risk to the progeny of such an albino parent (tyrosinase-positive or tyrosinase-negative OCA) will be ($1/95 \times 1/4$) about 1:380. This may increase up to a maximum of 50% for any subsequent child to be affected if the other parent is a suspected heterozygote (e.g., has transillumination defects in the iris) or an obligatory heterozygote (e.g., one child born with albinism).

Genetic counseling should coordinate with the different types and frequencies of the gene in a particular population.

Prenatal Diagnosis

Pigment can be found in the hair follicles of a normal fetus as early as 16 weeks of gestation (106). This fact enabled Eady et al. (107) to perform amniocentesis and diagnose OCA prenatally in a 20-week-old fetus. The amniocentesis was done under real-time ultrasonic inspection, fetoscopy, and biopsy with the aid of a 20-gauge forceps from the skin of the back of the scalp. Normally, all four stages of melanosomes are found. The authors diagnosed albinism when only stage I and stage II melanosomes without pigment were noted by election microscopy (107).

This approach, using the DOPA test and electron microscopy, was widely used by Shimizu et al. (108) before week 19 of gestation. It can be used only in detecting OCA type 1 (107,110). The current approach is to perform DNA testing, once the involved mutations have been identified. DNA testing can be done as early as the 14th week of gestation. If used for the different genetic types of OCA, it can distinguish between homozygotes and heterozygotes and is more accurate (109). After the DNA has been extracted from the amniocytes, either direct mutational analysis or linkage analysis can be used (110).

Although OCA is not fatal, many parents request prenatal diagnosis, as they prefer not to have any more affected children after having had one.

OCULAR ALBINISM

At the beginning of the century, Nettleship (111) recognized ocular albinism as a separate entity from OCA and defined its X-linked mode of inheritance. Later, Falls (112) described the typical fundus changes in the female carrier of the disease, and the name Nettleship–Falls type was given to this ocular albinism.

Description and Clinical Findings

Several types of ocular albinism can be defined and all have a common definition. The eyes show hypomelanosis with nystagmus, and the hair and skin have no or little clinical manifestations. Affected eyes may demonstrate findings similar to those with OCA, but this feature varies among the different types.

The Clinical and Genetic Types

The most common type of ocular albinism is X-linked ocular albinism. Other types have been mainly described in isolates and specific families (Table 2).

X–Linked Ocular Albinism (Nettleship–Falls Type;XLOA1 OA1)

Clinical definition. Hypopigmentation of the ocular tissues, photophobia, and congenital nystagmus, with poor visual acuity (commonly, 6/60 or less) are the hallmarks of the disease. Of 29 affected patients, Johnson et al. (113) found horizontal nystagmus in 11, rotary nystagmus in three, and combined horizontal and rotary nystagmus in the rest. Refraction anomalies and strabismus (mainly exotropia) are as common (113) as they are in OCA. The iris may be blue, darkening later in life. Photophobia may be mild to severe. The fundus shows little or no pigmentation and is muted. The disease occurs in a much milder form in blacks. Pigment may be sufficient for the patient to have a brown iris and good visual acuity (114).

Detection of heterozygotes. Female carriers of the disease (heterozygotes) exhibit characteristic findings in the fundus (112,113,115). Patches of pigment alternate with patches of depigmentation, more pronounced in the periphery of the fundus (Fig. 4). Fluorescein angiography displays spotty areas of blocked fluorescence in midperiphery (116). Some female carriers may appear to be heterozygotes with nystagmus, poor vision, and pronounced fundus findings, thus confirming Lyon's hypothesis (113,117,118). Positive iris transillumination is found in some heterozygotes, although less frequently than the fundus changes (119).

Skin biopsy. By using skin biopsy specimens, O'Donnell et al. (120) found abnormal melanosomes within the epidermis and dermis of males affected by XLOA and of carrier females. These were fontana–positive and DOPA-oxidase-positive macromelanosomes detected by both light and electron microscopy. This finding was confirmed in additional studies, indicating the extensive, systemic nature of X-linked ocular albinism (121–123).

Normal melanosomes, giant pigment granules and macromelanosomes have been found in those with XLOA (Fig. 5). Surprisingly, female obligatory carriers had similar, but fewer, macromelanosomes than affected males. Studies of the retinal and iris pigment epithelium showed a similar finding in both tissues: few normal melanosomes; fewer than normal immature melanosomes; giant pigment granules; and macromelanosomes (120,124).

Giant melanosomes can be found in skin biopsy specimens of several other diseases including neurofibromatosis, Albright's syndrome, generalized lentigines, xeroderma pigmentosum, Chediak-Higashi, and dysplastic nevus syndrome (120,125).

Visual pathways. Anomalous optic projections similar to those described in OCA have also been found in ocular albinism. At least 70% of patients with XLOA or autosomal recessive ocular albinism (AROA) have misrouted retinofugal fibers (78). With proper electrophysiologic methods, it is possible to detect the abnormality in all patients with XLOA (96).

Table 2 The Clinical and Genetic Types of Ocular Albinism (OA)

	Type	Name	Inheritance	Iris transillumination	Skin biopsy	Gene	Chromosomal location	Mutations	Remarks
1	XLOA1	Ocular albinism	XL	+	Giant pigment granules; macromelanosomes	OA1	Xp22.3	Large deletions of 1–9 exons in up to 50%	Genotype/phenotype correlation poor
2	AROA-1	Autosomal recessive ocular albinism (OCA1 variant)	AR	+	Normal melanosomes	TYR	11q14-q21	Arg402Gln and another disease-bearing mutation	Variable phenotypes, mild to severe
3	AROA-2	Autosomal recessive ocular albinism (OCA2 variant)	AR	+	Normal melanosomes	P	15q11-q13		Variable phenotypes, mild to severe
4	AROA-3	Autosomal recessive ocular albinism with Waardenburg syndrome	AR digenic	+	Normal melanosomes	MITF and TYR	11q14-q21, 3p12.3-p14.1	TYR, Arg402Gln polymorphism and MITF mutation	Variable phenotypes, mild to severe
5	AIED	Åland Island Eye disease	XL	+ or −	Normal melanosomes	(? RPGR)	Xp21	—	Nyctalopia and myopia prominent
6	OASD	Ocular albinism with sensori-neural deafness	XL	+	Macromelanosomes	? OA1	Xp22.3	Possibly allelic to OA1	Causes poor vision up to blindness and deafness, later in life

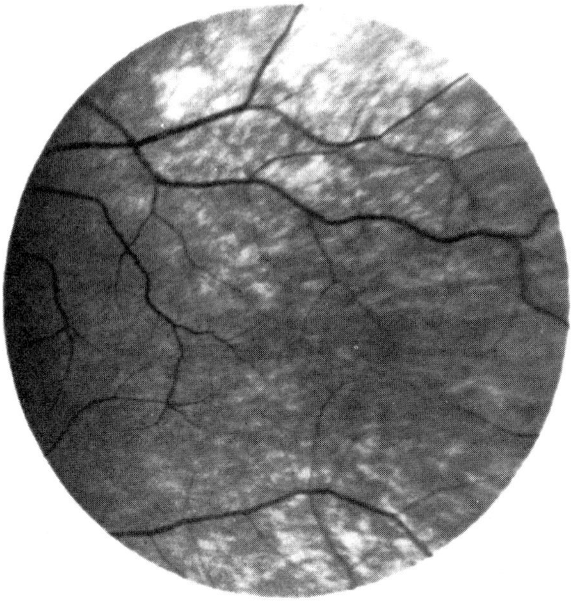

Figure 4 The fundus of a heterozygote carrier of X-linked ocular albinism: note the lines of hypopigmentation in the retinal periphery (Courtesy G. A. Fishman, MD).

Tests. Five tests can be performed to diagnose XLOA or to detect the carrier state: iris illumination, fundus examination, skin biopsy, VEP, and DNA tests. Once a skin biopsy is found positive for the typical macromelanosomes, this becomes a powerful and reliable basis for diagnosis (123). It can also be used to confirm carrier status. The most accurate test, however, is DNA testing. Hedge et al. (126) recommended a "hierarchical mutation screening protocol" that consists of two steps. First, a multiplex PCR is done to detect intragenic deletions in the OAl gene. Second, a heteroduplex analysis to scan for mutations is then performed. Table 2 lists the various genes associated with ocular albinism.

Epidemiology and genetics. In one study in England (1), 21 cases of XLOA were found among 201 albino patients, a rate of about 10%. The gene for XLOA was determined to be within a measurable distance from Xg (127,128). Later, a 700-kb deletion at the distal part of the short arm of chromosome X was found to be associated with ocular albinism only (129). In 1995, et al. (130) cloned the OAl gene. The gene spans 40 kb of genomic DNA and contains nine exons (131). Its product, the OAl protein is a melanosomal membrane glycoprotein that displays structural and functional features of G protein–coupled receptors (GPCRs) (132,133). GPCRs participate in the most common signal transduction system at the cell membrane. However, the OAl protein is intracellular, targeted to melanosomes and involved in intracellular signal transduction (132).

Diverse mutations in the OAl gene associated with ocular albinism have been reported. Large intragenic deletions were the most conspicuous, including deletion of any one of exon 1, 2, or 4, of exons 2–8, or of the whole gene (133–135). Unexpectedly a rather small study of 30 families showed that such large deletions were identified in 57% of North American families and in only 8% of European families (133). Other mutations identified were nonsense, missense, splice site, frameshift and small

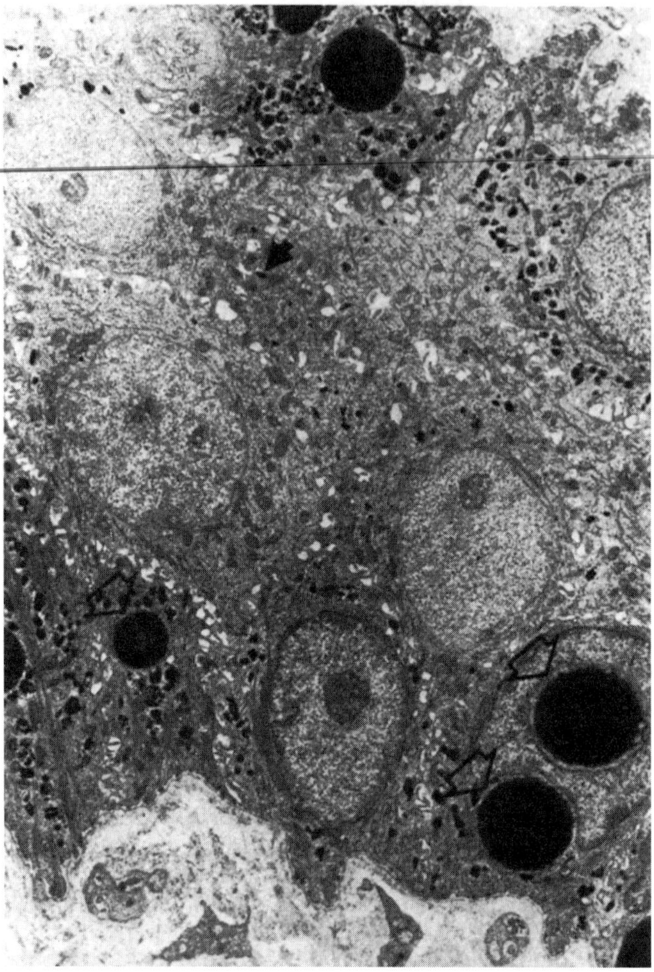

Figure 5 Electron micrograph of epidermis from a black patient with X-linked ocular albinism: Note macromelanosomes (open arrows) and normal-sized melanosomes (solid arrow). Macromelanosomes are typically found in both X-linked ocular albinism and in autosomal recessive ocular albinism, (from Ref. 114).

deletions (131,133,134). Various figures were given for detection of OAl mutations ranging from 15%, through 33% to 90% (131,134,135). No definite genotype/phenotype correlation could be established. A deletion of the whole gene including all nine exons resulted in typical ocular albinism, as in cases of point mutation (135). In a three–generation family diagnosed with congenital nystagmus an OAl deletion was identified (136). Some members showed mild signs of ocular albinism such as iris translucency and fundus hypopigmentation while other did not. All affected manifested foveal hypoplasia and nystagmus (136).

Management. The ocular problems of patients with XLOA are managed similarly to those of patients with OCA, including refraction, tinted glasses, and surgery for strabismus or head turn, when necessary. Genetic counseling is consistent with any X-linked disease, with some modifications: the risk to offspring of an affected father and a normal homozygote mother is no affected sons and all daughters as carriers, some manifesting the disease. Also, the risk to sons of a carrier mother is 50%, as is the risk for a daughter to be a carrier. Again, some carriers can have the disease.

Prenatal diagnosis is possible by prediction of the gender of the fetus and, accurately with a high success rate, by DNA testing (126).

Autosomal Recessive Ocular Albinism

Autosomal recessive ocular albinism (AROA) was defined as a separate clinical and genetic entity by O'Donnell et al. (137), in seven females and two males from five unrelated families. The affected patients had impaired vision, markedly translucent iris, congenital nystagmus with photophobia, an albinotic fundus with hypoplasia of the fovea, and (often) strabismus. The hairbulb test was positive for tyrosinase. Also, the skin biopsy specimens showed normal melanosomes without macromelanosomes, which clearly distinguished them from cases of XLAO. The VEP shows similar retinofugal fibers misrouting as XLAO, or most types of OCA (78).

Fukai et al. (138) examined 12 patients with AROA and identified mutations of the TYR gene in two of them. In each they identified one disease–bearing mutation and a polymorphism, Arg402Gln, that usually is not disease bearing (138). They concluded that this compound heterozygosity was associated with a mild form of AROA.

Some cases of AROA were found to be associated with mutations of the P gene, responsible for TPOCA (OCA2) (138).

Morell et al. (139) reported their DNA studies in patients with Waardenburg syndrome (WS II) in conjunction with ocular albinism. WSII is caused by mutations in the MITF gene (see below). It is probable that a digenic inheritance causes the WS 2 and AROA association. Affected individuals were heterozygous for a mutation of MITF and were, in addition, either heterozygous or homozygous for the Arg402Gln mutation (polymorphism) of the TYR gene. The Arg402Gln polymorphism without MITF mutation does not result in disease (139).

In summary, AROA is a heterogenous disorder associated with allelic mutations on the loci OCA1, OCA2 and WS2. Additional loci may be involved.

Forsius–Eriksson Syndrome (Forsius–Eriksson Ocular Albinism; Åland Eye Disease)

This form of ocular albinism had been described in an isolate on Åland Islands (140). The clinical characteristics include hypopigmentation of the fundus, hypoplasia of the fovea, latent or manifest nystagmus, myopia (which may increase), astigmatism, and color vision abnormalities, with a tendency to protanomaly. The hairbulb test shows a tyrosinase-positive response. The skin is normally pigmented and tans normally. However, contrary to the Nettleship–Falls type of XLOA, these patients have regular melanosomes in the skin (141) and normal optic pathways (142).

Åland eye disease is transmitted by females and affects males as an X-linked characteristic. The female carrier is clinically normal and shows no typical fundus of an XLOA carrier.

The most frequent abnormality encountered in Åland Island Eye Disease (AIED) is night blindness. The hallmark of the disorder seems to be the combination of high myopia and night blindness. The disorder is described in Chapter 15.

X–Linked Ocular Albinism with Late–Onset Sensorineural Deafness

Described in a white South African family, findings consisted of pale eyes, horizontal nystagmus, hypopigmented fundus with some pigment clumps, and hearing loss in the fifth decade of life (143). Macromelanosomes were found, similar to those with XLOA. This form of XLOA may represent the same condition described by Ziprkovski (144), and be similar to the ocular albinism and deafness described by Lewis (145) as an autosomal dominant disease.

DNA studies performed by Winship et al. (146) on the same South African family (ocular albinism, sensorineural deafness) detected tight linkage of the locus to chromosome Xp22.3. They concluded that OASD is a variant of OA1.

HERMANSKY–PUDLAK SYNDROMES (HPS)

Clinical Manifestations

In 1959, Hermansky and Pudlak (147) described a triad of findings in two unrelated patients from Czechoslovakia, consisting of albinism, hemorrhagic diathesis, and "peculiar pigmented reticular cells in the bone marrow." Except for a consistently prolonged bleeding time, hematologic tests yielded variable results. The disease was later reported in many countries, with the highest frequencies found in the Araceibo region of Puerto Rico (1:2000 affected), in an isolate in Lencois Island of Brazil (148), in some parts of Holland (149), and in a village in Valais, Switzerland (150). The British cases appeared to be milder than those described in Puerto Rico (1).

Patients with HPS have widely varying amounts of pigmentation. In general, they all have reduced visual acuity, nystagmus, translucent iris, hypopigmented fundi, and muted fovea, as in the other types of albinism (151).

In a study of 20 patients, Summers et al. (149) found nystagmus and foveal hypoplasia in all, visual acuity ranging from 6/18 to 6/120, and varying amounts of iris pigmentation.

The electroretinogram (ERG) may be normal (151) or show decreased cone and rod responses (148). The bleeding diathesis is usually mild and may not be discovered until later in life, but may also be life–threatening, especially after the ingestion of aspirin or indomethacin (151,152). The platelets from these affected persons lack the secondary phase of irreversible aggregation and normal dense bodies and are low in serotonin and nonmetabolic nucleotides (12). Hematologic testing shows a prolonged bleeding time, grossly decreased platelet aggregation in epinephrine or in collagen, and abnormally low platelet serotonin uptake (about 50% of normal) (152). Many tissues accumulate intracellular neutral lipids and ceroid (12,153). Storage of a ceroidlike material in the reticuloendothelial system may cause interstitial pulmonary fibrosis, inflammatory bowel disease, renal failure, or cardiomyopathy (149). Ultrastructurally, a lysosomal storage disease is indicated by ceroid accumulation within single membrane-bound intracellular organelles (153).

Hairbulb incubation demonstrates weak tyrosinase activity, and skin biopsy specimens reveal giant melanosomes that are single–membrane limited, with multiple microvesicles (154). The total number of melanosomes is noticeably decreased in both keratinocytes and melanocytes of the skin (153).

The disease is clearly autosomal recessive, but pseudodominance has been found because of the high frequency of the gene in isolates (99).

For the ophthalmolgist, HPS provides a diagnostic challenge, especially because of the variable phenotypic appearance and the often insignificant bleeding tendency. However, fatalities have been reported after delivery (155), minor surgical procedures, or ingestion of aspirin. An increased incidence of infections has also been noted (156).

The clinical manifestations of HPS have been the subject of several large studies performed in Puerto Rico. Izquierdo et al. (157) studied 55 Puerto–Rican patients and outlined the triad of HPS clinical findings: tyrosinase-positive oculocutaneous albinism, bleeding diathesis, and the accumulation of ceroid in tissues. Visual acuity ranged from 20/50 to 20/200. All had nystagmus. Strabismus was found in 43 of the 55 patients, and posterior embryotoxon/Axenfeld anomaly in 19 patients. Foveal aplasia was universal. Iris pigmentation ranged from minimal to normal (157). In some patients in Puerto Rico, ceroid–lipofuscin accumulation in the cells led to fatal pulmonary fibrosis; granulomatous colitis or a bleeding diathesis (158,159) can also be fatal. Ramsay (160) stressed the pleiotropic effect of the mutated HPS gene on various organelles, particularly melanosomes, platelet dense bodies and lysosomes. Skin biopsy reveals the atypical large melanosomes, progressed only to stage II of melanogenesis; reduced or absent platelet dense bodies and giant perinuclear vesicles (160). Bleeding results from the absence of platelet dense bodies.

The Clinical and Genetic Types of HPS

In the mid–1990s HPS was considered a single genetic entity without any evidence of heterogeneity (161). However, later additional loci were identified in addition to the locus that became known as HPS1 (Table 3).

HPS1 Locus and Gene

The locus has been mapped to chromosome 10q23.1–q23.3 (161). Oh et al. (162) identified the HPS1 gene by positional cloning and identified different mutations in the different affected communities. The gene consists of 20 exons and spans 30.5 kb of genomic DNA (157). The mutation identified in Puerto Rico was a 16–bp duplication within exon 15 resulting in termination at codon 586. In studies conducted in Japan and Switzerland, a point duplication at codon 441 or 324 was

Table 3 Hermansky–Pudlak (HPS) Syndrome

	Type	Gene	Chromosomal location	Clinical expression	Remarks
1	HPS-1	HPS-1	10q23.1	Severe	In all; variable OCA; variable amounts of pigmentation; bleeding diathesis; lipid storage. Abnormal melanosomes in number and shape. Macromelanosomes. Intracellular microvesicles
2	HPS-2	AP3B1	5q14.1	Severe	
3	HPS-3	HPS3	3q24	Mild	
4	HPS-4	HPS4	22q11.2-q12.2	Severe	
5	HPS-5	RU2	11p15-p13	Moderate	
6	HPS-6	RU	10q24.32	Moderate	
7	HPS-7	DTNBP1	6p22.3	Moderate	

found to result in termination at codon 451 (163). The 16–bp duplication in exon 15 of the HPS1 gene was identified in 25 of 27 Puerto Rican HPS patients (158). Gahl et al. compared their phenotype to that of 22 patients from mainland U.S. without this duplication. This mutation was associated with a broad range of pigmentation and an increased risk of restrictive lung disease in adults (158), but it did not result in any significant difference in visual acuity (159).

Oh et al. (162) defined the HPS1 protein product as a transmembrane polypeptide, apparently crucial for the normal development of intracellular organelles. It is a non–glycosylated, non–membrane protein with two distinct complexes, different in melanotic and non–melanotic cells (164).

The fact that two out of 24 Puerto Rican HPS patients did not share the typical Puerto Rican common mutation of a homozygous 16-bp duplication in exon 15 of the HPS1 gene led Hazelwood et al. (165) to the assumption that HPS is a heterogenous disorder. They examined the DNA of these patients and did not detect any mutations of the HPS1 gene (165). Additional loci were bound to exist.

The HPS2 Locus and Gene

Dell' Angelica et al. (166) identified mutations in the AP3B1 gene, a gene mapped to chromosome 5ql4.1, in two patients with typical HSC manifestations. The gene functions in protein sorting to lysosomes. The disorder results from the mutation–induced altered trafficking of the internal membrane protein (166).

HPS2 seems to be very rare.

The HPS3 Locus and Gene

Anikster et al. (167) localized and identified a new HPS susceptibility gene, while studying a small genetic isolate of HPS in central Puerto Rico. The gene HPS3 was mapped to chromosome 3q24. It consists of 17 exons and was predicted to produce a 113.7 kDa putative protein. The authors assumed that the protein functions in intracellular vesicle formation (167). Huizing et al. (168) demonstrated that the HSC1 locus is found also in other communities. They identified various mutations in five Ashkenazi Jews and in others (168). HPS3 is also expressed in a mild phenotype. Some patients had only ocular albinism as the expression of the disorder (168).

The HPS4 Locus and Gene

Suzuki et al. (169) identified an additional locus of HPS in seven patients of European origin. The locus HPS4 maps to chromosome 22ql1.2-ql2.2. Anderson et al. (170) examined the clinical characteristics of 22 non-Puerto Rican HPS patients. The phenotype of HPS4 is severe and similar to HPS1. Patients may show iris transillumination, variable hair and skin pigmentation, absent platelet dense bodies and occasionally pulmonary fibrosis and granulomatous colitis (170).

The gene HPS4 encodes a polypeptide of 708 amino acids and consists of 13 exons (169). It has been estimated that approximately half of all non–Puerto Rico HPS patients do not carry mutations of HPS1 gene (169). Anderson et al. (170) identified HPS4 mutations in seven of the 22 HPS patients they examined. HPS4 seems, therefore, one of the more important and frequent HPS genes.

The HPS5 and HPS6 Loci and Genes

Zhang et al. (171) identified and cloned two genes associated with a depigmentation disorder in mice that were known as ru and ru–2 (for ruby–eye). They identified disease–causing mutations in the human homolog of these genes, and designated them as HPS5 and HPS6.

The two genes are quite similar. HPS5 was mapped to chromosome 11pl5-pl3 and the gene was named RU2. HPS6 was mapped to chromosome 10q24.32 and named RU (171). Their protein product directly interacts in the biogenesis of lysosome–related organelles complex–2. RU2 and RU contain 1129 amino acids and 23 exons, respectively. Skin biopsy gives a similar picture in both. Melanosomes were reduced in number and abnormal in shape (171).

A 4-bp deletion with a truncated protein of RU2/HPS5 was identified in a Turkish boy and a similar mutation was identified in a Belgian woman with HPS6 disorder and a RU mutation (171).

These rare disorders seem to be milder than HPS, with less bleeding tendency and more cutaneous pigment.

The HPS7 Locus and Gene

Li et al. (172) identified the seventh locus of HPS. They demonstrated that Sdy mutant mice (with a pigmentary disorder and bleeding tendency) do not express the protein dysbindin–l. Mutations in the human ortholog, dystrobrevin–binding protein 1 (DTNBP1) are associated with HPS type 7 disorders.

The gene contains 10 exons, 352 amino acids, and maps to chromosome 6p22.3 (2). Its product is another protein component of biogenesis of lysosome–related organelles complex (BLOC–1), just as HPS5 and HPS6 are associated with BLD6–2 (172).

CHEDIAK–HIGASHI SYNDROME (CHS)

A rare autosomal recessive type of OCA, Chediak–Higashi syndrome has several similarities to HPS: (i) the variable amount of pigmentation may render the diagnosis difficult; (ii) bleeding diathesis and an increased frequency of infections have been observed; and (iii) at the cellular level, uneven distribution of pigment is more a factor than lack of pigment (173).

About 60 cases of the syndrome have been reported (174). Affected children show some skin pigmentation, which is often patchy, prompting terms like "partial" or "imperfect" OCA to be used. Their hair is light brown, and the iris is translucent and hazel or brown. A fine horizontal nystagmus is usually associated with other signs of ocular albinism, such as hypopigmentation of the fundus, muted fovea, and poor visual acuity. As in the other types of albinism, the visual–evoked response is abnormal with monocular stimulation (91).

The electroretinogram was reduced in one patient studied, with a progressive reduction in response noted on follow–up (174). In early life, these children suffer from frequent pyogenic infections, intermittent febrile episodes, and bleeding tendencies. They may undergo a lymphoma–like phase and early death (175).

The diagnosis of Chediak–Higashi syndrome can be confirmed by giant granules in the leukocytes (the Chediak anomaly). A pathologic study by Libert et al. (175) of the eyes of two patients who died from Chediak–Higashi syndrome showed that the pigment epithelium of iris, ciliary body, and retina was mostly depigmented, lacking even immature melanosomes. Some cells had large secondary lysosomes filled by melanin granules or by a lipofuscion-like material. Similar findings were seen in the skin. No melanosomes were found. As in the eye, pigment was nevertheless present inside abnormal and sometimes bizarre organelles that could be divided into three types: (i) macromelanosomes, (ii) polyphagosomes, and (iii) giant melanosomes without the normal spindle–shaped skeleton (175). Similar bizarre intracytoplasmic bodies have been found in the conjunctiva of one patient with Chediak–Higashi syndrome (174).

Chediak–Higashi syndrome is caused by mutations in a single gene with pleiotropic effect on various subcellular organelles, particularly the melanosomes, the platelet dense bodies, and the lysosomes (160). These lead to hypopigmentation, a severe immunologic deficiency that includes neutropenia and the lack of natural killer cells (NK) causing (sometimes fatal) infections in childhood, bleeding tendencies, and neurological abnormalities. Skin biopsy will detect the characteristic giant inclusion bodies and giant organelles in various cells (176). The gene is associated with normal subcellular protein traffic. The CHS mutation is responsible for protein–sorting defects (160,176). The vesicular transport to and from the lysosome is defective (177). Zhao et al. (178) studied cultured melanocytes taken from CHS patients, and concluded that these melanocytes are defective in structure and/or function and express abnormal trafficking of some cellular proteins. It may also lead to the "accelerated phase" of uncontrolled malignant lymphoproliferative disease (179).

The gene responsible for CHS, the CHS1 gene has been identified and cloned in 1996 (176,177). It is the human homolog of the mouse beige gene. CHS1 is a large gene that encodes a 429 kDa protein containing 3801 amino acids (176). Various mutations associated with CHS were identified, most of them null mutations leading to total loss of function (176,180,181). Homozygous nonsense and frameshift mutations result in premature termination and a truncated protein. Karim et al. (181) compared the genotype to the phenotype and found such correlation. All cases of early childhood onset suffer a severe disease, often fatal due to infections or bleeding, and carry a null mutation. They comprise approximately 85% of CHS. In the remaining 15%, the childhood disease is mild and a serious neurological disorder progresses in late adulthood. A third, rare, clinical group consists of infections in childhood and late mild neurological disease. The last two groups carry missense mutations (181).

Management

Systemic treatment of CHS is beyond the scope of this book.

Genetic counseling should be according to the autosomal recessive transmission of the disease. Prenatal diagnosis has been performed using a morphological approach (182). Light microscopy of hair shaft and both light and electron microscopy of polymorphonuclear cells were performed with reliable results.

DNA testing for prenatal diagnosis can be performed. However, in about half of all cases, no mutation associated with CHS can be identified; in about 20% of cases, only one mutation is identified (181). This could be due to the complexity of DNA testing of a very large gene.

ALBINOIDISM AND SUBCLINICAL ALBINISM

Albinoidism is used by some authors to describe a condition in which generalized hypopigmentation of the skin and eyes occurs without nystagmus or photophobia (4). It was reported in a few families as autosomal dominant albinoidism or punctate oculocutaneous albinoidism. There is no confirmation that these are separate clinical and genetic entities, or if they represent the heterozygote state of OCA (38). Albinism also has been used to describe the hypopigmentation occurring in a series of systemic or multi-system diseases, such as Apert syndrome, Waardenburg syndrome (see below), phenylketonuria, and Menkes' kinky-hair syndrome. The last demonstrates tyrosinase-negative hairbulb test results.

Subclinical albinism is probably far more common than albinoidism. I prefer this term to define a condition with only minor, but definite, signs of ocular hypopigmentation (if looked for), decreased visual acuity, nystagmus, and hypoplastic fovea. In a recent study of 26 patients with congentical nystagmus, but no known history of albinism, Simon et al. (183) found 12 with some characteristic of albinism, such as a detectable iris transillumination defect, choroidal depigmentation, abnormal tanning history, or abnormal macular reflex.

Subclinical albinism may represent a heterozygous state of one type of albinism or a disease entity of its own.

WAARDENBURG SYNDROME

Waardenburg syndrome (WS) is a multi–system disease that affects various tissues and structures including the eye. Pigmentary abnormalities are common and the syndrome will be discussed in this chapter.

Waardenburg syndrome is one of a large group of abnormalities stemming from an abnormal developmental pathway of the neural crest (184). It is a heterogenousdisease with several loci and several different phenotypes known. In all forms, marked interfamilial variability exists, so that a specific mutation will not predict the severity of the disorder (184).

Description and Clinical Findings

In 1951, Waardenburg (185) described a new syndrome with the following findings: lateral displacement of medial canthi and lacrimal points (dystopia canthorum); hyperplastic, broad, and high nasal root, hyperplasia of the medial portions of the eyebrows; partial or total heterochromia iridis; congenital bilateral or unilateral deafness; white forelock (poliosis); and autosomal dominant transmission.

The iris discoloration occurs as a form of hypochromia, usually light blue, that can be just a sector of the iris in one eye (Fig. 6), can involve the whole iris in one eye (heterochromia iridis), or can affect both eyes (bilateral iris hypochromia). Goldberg (186) indicated that hypochromia also involves other pigmented structures of the eye, paralleling the iris findings. Thus, a homolateral blond or albinoid fundus has been associated with a homolateral hypochromia iridis, a patchy fundus with iris bicolor, and bilateral albinoid fundus with bilateral iris hypochromia.

Some other congenital and acquired abnormalities may occur. Various anomalies of the upper limb have been described (187) along with abnormal cutaneous pigmentation, vitiligo, white skin with freckles, premature graying, and other features.

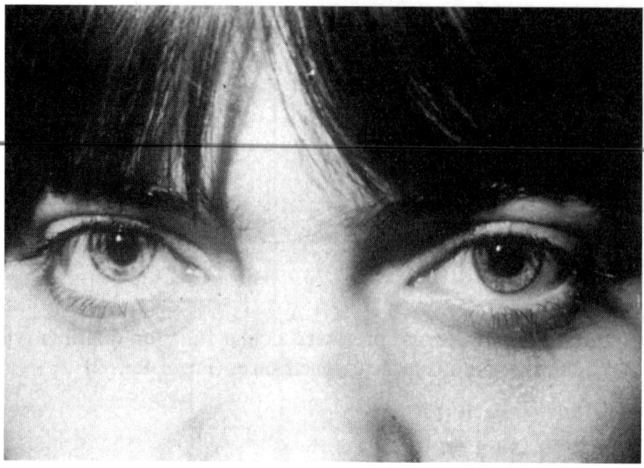

Figure 6 Hypochromia of the iris in girl with Waardenburg's syndrome: only one sector of the iris in one eye was affected. Also noted were congenital bilateral deafness and a white forelock, which is dyed.

The Clinical and Genetic Types of Waardenburg's Syndrome

The expressivity of Waardenburg's syndrome is extremely variable. No one sign described in the syndrome was found in all of the 14 cases studied by Goldberg (186) indicating that any of the signs may be missing. Nevertheless, Arias (188) suggested that at least two types of classic Waardenburg syndrome can be recognized and are separate genetic entities. In fact, at least four clinical phenotypes and at least five distinct genes are associated with Waardenburg syndromes (Table 4).

WS1 (Waardenburg Syndrome Type I)

WS1 is the classic disorder as described by Waardenburg in his original article (185). It is transmitted by an autosomal dominant gene with extremely variable expressivity, even in the same family. Pardono et al. (189) found no sign that is always present. The W index, a composite measure used in the literature to measure and confirm dystonia canthorum, confirmed the diagnosis of WS2 in 93% of such cases, but only in 60% of WS1 (189). Other measures that were used: iris pigmentation abnormalities, localized hair albinism, deafness or hearing impairment, hypopigmented skin spots, nasal root hyperplasia and inferior lacrimal dystopia (189). De Stefano et al. (190) studied 48 families of WS1 grouped by the Waardenburg consortium and determined the frequency of four abnormalities: hearing loss (partial or total)–63%, dye pigmentation anomalies–41%, white forelock–36%, and patchy skin pigmentation–35% (190).

The locus for WS1 has been found to be linked to chromosome 2q37 (191), later refined to chromosome 2q35 (2). It was suggested and confirmed to be the human homolog of the Splotch mouse. Tassabehji et al. (192) reported the association of WS1 with mutations of the PAX3 gene at this location. The gene contains eight exons and spans 100 kb of genomic DNA (193). Mutations of the PAX3 gene were found within exon 6 (in the homeobox) (194) but also within exon 2 (in the paired domain) and in exon 4 (192).

Table 4 The Waardenburg syndromes

	Name	Locus/ symbol	Tran-smis-sion	Gene	Chromoso-mal location	CLINICAL MANIFESTATIONS				Remarks
						Dystopia canthorum	Anomalous skin and eye pigmentation	Deafness	Other	
1	Waardenburg syndrome type I	WS1	AD	PAX3	2q35	Yes	Approx. 40% for each	63%	—	Modifying genes may play a role
2	Waardenburg syndrome type II A	WS2A	AD	MITF	3p12.3-p14.1	No	Mild	Often: congential and more severe	—	Digenic inheritance causes WS2+OA
3	Waardenburg syndrome type II B	WS2B	AD	?	1p13.3-p21	No	Mild	Often: congential and more severe	—	One family reported
4	Waardenburg syndrome type II C	WS2C	AD	?	8p23	No	Mild	Often: congential and more severe	—	One family reported
5	Waardenburg syndrome type III	WS3	AD	PAX3	2q35	Yes	Approx. 40% for each	63%	Musculo-skeketal limb anomalies	Allelic to WS1; also in homozygotes of WS1
6	Waardenburg syndrome type IV A	WS4A	AD	SOX10	22q13	Yes	Variable	As in WS1	Hirschprung megacolon	
7	Waardenburg syndrome type IV B	WS4B	AR	EDNRB	13q22	Yes	Variable	As in WS1	Hirschprung megacolon	

WS, Waardenburg syndrome; AD, autosomal dominant; AR, autosomal recessive; OA, ocular albinism.

Genotype/phenotype correlation seemed to be important for skin, eye and hair pigmentation. Some mutations increased the risks of involvement of these tissues up to eight times. No such correlation was found for hearing loss (190). Pandya et al. (195) stressed that the large intrafamilial phenotypic variations cannot be explained by allelic heterogeneity. They pointed out that studies of MZ twins indicate a high concordance. The authors suggested that genetic modifiers or additional genes might also play a role (195).

Homozygosity for WS1 is a rare occurrence. Zlotogora et al. (196) reported such a patient born to heterozygous parents with a mild phenotype of WS1. The child had a severe disorder that included upper-limb defects so severe that it was diagnosed as WS3. Zlotogora et al. (196) pointed out that in mice PAX3 homozygosity leads to severe neural tube defects and is probably lethal in most human cases (196).

WS2A (Waardenburg Syndrome Type IIA)

WS2, an autosomal dominant disorder, is similar to WS1 but does not manifest the lateral displacement of medial canthi and lacrimal puncti (188,197). Reynolds, however, found some differences between WS1 and WS2. Deafness was more severe in WS2 while the pigmentary and craniofacial anomalies were milder (198). The WS2 group has been subdivided according to the variable genetic background.

The gene responsible for WS2A has been mapped to chromosome 3pl2.3-pl4.1 (199). In this location microphthalmia-associated transcription factor (MITF), the human homolog of the mouse microphthalmia gene has been located (199,200). Mice carrying the microphthalmia mutation show reduced pigmentation of the eyes and coat, microphthalmia, hearing loss, and osteopetrosis (200). It has been suggested that normal (wild type) MITF converts fibroblasts into cells with characteristics of melanocytes (201). Various mutations have been described, with most being mild mutations such as missense or splice site (200). A point mutation creating a stop codon in exon 7 resulting in early termination has been reported in one North European and one Indian family (202). No clear genotype/phenotype association has been established for the different mutations. In comparison to PAX3 gene mutations, WS2 manifested differences in the absence or near absence of dystopia canthorum and of facial dysmorphism (199).

Read and Newton (184) claimed that only 15% of WS2 patients carry the MITF mutation and therefore WS2 is a heterogenous group of disorders. Additional genes may also play a role.

Digenic inheritance is the cause of a syndrome in which the clinical expression of both WS2 and ocular albinism is apparent. A mutation in exon 8 of the MITF gene and either homozygous or heterozygous missense mutation (Arg204Gln) in the TYR gene are the cause of this combined disorder (139). The family described by Bard (203) of WS with ocular albinism, hyperopia, esotropia and amblyopia likely had the same syndrome.

WS2B (Waardenburg Syndrome Type IIB)

WS2B is clinically identical to other WS2 entities. Lalwani et al. (202) reported the second WS2 locus mapped to chromosome 1pl3.3–p21 (212). No other family has been reported and the gene has not been identified.

WS2C (Waardenburg Syndrome Type IIC)

Selicomi et al. (204) have detected the third locus for WS2 (WS2C) in an Italian family. The locus was mapped to chromosome 8p23 (204). No other family has been reported and the gene has not yet been identified.

WS3 (Waardenburg Syndrome Type III; Klein–Waardenburg Syndrome)

WS3 is genetically allelic to WS1 and caused by mutations in the same gene, PAX3, mapped to chromosome 2q35. Clinically, however, it is expressed as a distinct entity. The clinical disorder includes, in addition to the WS1 usual manifestations, abnormalities of the arms. These can be sometimes severe. Mutations in the PAX3 gene may result in WS1 or in WS3 (205) or may not be associated with any Waardenburg syndrome anomalies. Zlotogora et al. (195) described a family with both parents heterozygous displaying WS1 phenotype, and their child, a homozygote to the mutated PAX3 gene, manifesting a severe WS3 phenotype. Recently, Wollnik et al. (206) reported a third family with identical findings of a homozygote child manifesting musculoskeletal anomalies of WS3. It may well be that increased loads of the abnormal mutation (by double dose as in homozygotes or in more "severe mutations") are the cause for PAX3 associated WS3. It is also possible that in some cases modifying genes play a role.

WS4 (Waardenburg Syndrome Type IV; Shah–Waardenburg Syndrome)

Waardenburg syndrome with Hirschprung disease (megacolon) has been described as an autosomal dominant disease with dystopia canthorum (197,207–209) in isolated and familial cases. The disorder is transmitted by a distinct autosomal dominant gene, SOX10 (for Sry–Boxl0) and has been mapped to chromosome 22ql3 (210,211).

WS4 with Hirschprung disease as an autosomal recessive disease has been described at least in two large families (209,212). Puffenberger et al. (212) mapped an associated recessive susceptibility gene to chromosome 13q22. The gene was identified as EDNRB for endothelin–B receptor gene (212). The iris had a bicolor patchy appearance and the intercanthal distance was normal (209).

Other Possibly Related Syndromes

Congenital sensorineural deafness, partial albinism, heterochromia iridis, and normal intercanthal distance have been described as being transmitted by the X-linked recessive mode in one family (213). Another family demonstrated a white forelock, distinct facial features, blue sclera, hypertelorism, epicanthus, strabismus, and myopia associated with skeletal and cardio-pulmonary malformations (214). The mode of transmission was autosomal or X-linked recessive.

Diagnosis

Waardenburg syndrome is diagnosed by its clinical features. No laboratory test can be used to confirm the diagnosis. Psychophysical and electrophysiologic studies of the eye yield normal results (215). Suggested linkage to the ABO blood group locus (216) has not been confirmed. The variability of the different possible findings in this syndrome, together with the multitude of organs and tissues that can be involved, necessitate awareness.

A neurocristopathy, or disease from an abnormal development of the neural crest, has been suggested to explain this multitude of findings (208,209,217). An embryonal structure not present in later life, the neural crest affects the formation of skin, bones, cartilage, viscera, and other structures built by cells from this derivation, including all melanocytes and visceral ganglia. Diseases that may be called neurocristopathies include mandibulofacial dysostosis, multiple endocrine neoplasia, neurofibromatosis, and Waardenburg syndrome, or Hirschprung's disease. Piebaldism, an autosomal dominant trait, with many similarities to Waardenburg syndrome, is also classified as a neurocristopathy (218).

DNA testing can be successfully performed for the known genes associated with WS mutations (Table 4).

Epidemiology and Genetics

Waardenburg identified 12 patients with this syndrome among 840 deaf-mutes in five Dutch institutes for the deaf. He estimated its prevalence in the general population as 1:42,000. This may be an underestimate, as in many patients the sensorineural deafness is only a minor problem or may occur late in life. Congential deafness has been reported in 25% of WS1 and in 50% of WS2 cases.

The relatively high frequency of this syndrome reflects that more than 1000 cases were reported during a period of 25 years (215). It occurs worldwide. Descriptions have included whites, blacks, Indians, and Asians (186). It is generally responsible for 2–5% of profound deafness in childhood (208), but in South Australia it is the leading cause of deafness (184).

Waardenburg syndrome is transmitted by an autosomal dominant gene (185), with an incomplete penetrance and variable expressivity.

Management

No ocular treatment is usually necessary for patients with Waardenburg syndrome. The role of the ophthalmologist is more to establish the diagnosis.

Genetic counseling should be offered, with the emphasis that autosomal dominant transmission is the rule. The incomplete penetrance and widely variable expressivity should be considered.

Prenatal diagnosis can be performed if the causative gene and mutation are known.

REFERENCES

1. Jay B, Witkop CJ, King PA. Albinism in England. Birth Defects 1982; 18:319–325.
2. Online Mendelian Inheritance in Man, OMIM (TM). McKusick–Nathans Institute for Genetic Medicine, Johns Hopkins University (Baltimore, MD) and National Center for Biotechnology Information, National Library of Medicine (Bethesda, MD), 2000. World Wide Web URL: http://www.ncbi.nlm.nih.gov/omim/.
3. Searle AG. Comparative Genetics of Coat Color in Mammals. London: Logos Press, 1968.
4. Kinnear PE, Jay B, Witkop CJ Jr. Albinism. Surv Ophthalmol, 1985; 30:75–101.
5. Hornabrook RW, McDonald WI, Carrol RL. Congenital nystagmus among the red-skins of the highlands of Papua-New Guinea. Br J Ophthalmol 1980; 64:375–380.

6. van Dorp DB, van Haeringen NJ, Glasius E. Evaluation of hairbulb incubation test and tyrosinase assay in the classification of albinism. Ophthalmol Paediatr Genet 1982; 1:189–200.
7. Bazex J, Sans B, Janeau D, et al. Oculo–cutaneous tyrosinase-positive albinism. Ann Dermatol Venereol 1982; 109:573–576.
8. Pehamberger H, Honigsmann H, Wolff K. Dysplastic nevus syndrome with multiple primary amelanotic melanomas in oculocutaneous albinism. J Am Acad Dermatol 1984; 11:731–735.
9. Lynch HT, Fusaro RM. Hereditary malignant melanoma: a unifying etiologic hypothesis. Cancer Genet Cytogenet 1986; 15:301–304.
10. Hoyt CS, Gelbart SS. Vertical nystagmus in infants with congenital ocular abnormalities. Ophthalmic Paediatr Genet 1984; 4:155–161.
11. Kriss A, Russell–Eggitt I, Harris CM, Lloyd IC, Taylor D. Aspects of albinism. Ophthalmic Paediatr & Genet 1992; 13(2):89–100.
12. Witkop CJ Jr, Hill CW, Desnick S, et al. Ophthalmologic, biochemical, platelet, and ul–trastructural defects in the various types of oculocutaneous albinism. J Invest Dermatol 1973; 60:443–456.
13. Taylor WO. Visual disabilities of oculocutaneous albinism and their alleviation. Trans Ophthalmol Soc UK 1978; 98:423–445.
14. Jacobson SG, Mohindra I, Held R, et al. Visual acuity development in tyrosinase negative oculocutaneous albinism. Doc Ophthalmol 1984; 56:337–344.
15. Mayer DL, Fulton AB, Hansen RM. Visual acuity of infants and children with retinal degenerations. Ophthalmic Paediatr Genet 1985; 5:51–56.
16. Summers CG. Vision in albinism. Trans Am Ophthalmol Soc 1996; 94:1095–1155.
17. Gregor Z. The perifoveal vasculature in albinism. Br J Ophthalmol 1978; 62:554–557.
18. Spedick MJ, Beauchamp GR. Retinal vascular and optic nerve abnormalities in albinism. J Pediatr Ophthalmol Strabismus 1986; 23:58–63.
19. Bird AC, Weale RA. On the retinal vasculature of the human fovea. Exp Eye Res 1974; 19:409–417.
20. Trevor–Roper PD. Marriage of two complete albinos with normally pigmented offspring. Br J Ophthalmol 1952; 36:107–108.
21. Nance WE, Witkop CJ, Rawls RF. Genetic and biochemical evidence for two forms of oculocutaneous albinism in man. Birth Defects 1971; 7:125–128.
22. Witkop CJ, Nance WE, Rawls RF, White JG. Autosomal recessive oculocutaneous albinism in man: evidence for genetic heterogeneity. Am J Hum Genet 1970; 22:55–74.
23. Warren ST. Allelism in human oculocutaneous albinism [letter]. Am J Hum Genet 1981; 33:479–480.
24. Toyofuku K, Wada I, Spritz RA, Hearing VJ. The molecular basis of oculocutaneous albinism type 1 (OCA1): sorting failure and degradation of mutant tyrosinases results in a lack of pigmentation. Biochem J 2001; 355(Pt 2):259–269.
25. King RA, Witkop CA. Hairbulb tyrosinase activity in oculocutaneous albinism. Nature 1976; 263:69–71.
26. Winder AF, Jay B, Kissun RD. Biochemical aspects of human albinism. Birth Defects 1976; 12:427–433.
27. King RA, Olds DP. Hairbulb tyrosinase activity in oculocutaneous albinism: suggestions for pathway control and block location. Am J Med Genet 1985; 20:49–55.
28. van Dorp DB, van Haeringen NJ, Delleman JW, Apkarian P, Westerhof W. Albinism: phenotype or genotype? Doc Ophthalmol 1983; 56:183–194.
29. Schmitz B, Schaefer T, Krick CM, Reith W, Backens M, Kasmann-Kellner B. Configuration of the optic chiasm in humans with albinism as revealed by magnetic-resonance imaging. Invest Ophthalmol Vis Sci 2003; 44(1):16–21.
30. King RA, Pietsch J, Fryer JP, Savage S, Brott MJ, Russell-Eggitt I, Summers CG, Oetting WS. Tyrosinase gene mutations in oculocutaneous albinism 1 (OCA1): definition of the phenotype. Hum Genet 2003; 113(6):502–513.

31. Giebel LB, Strunk KM, King RA, Hanifrn JM, Spritz RA. A frequent tyrosinase gene mutation in classic, tyrosinase-negative (type IA) oculocutaneous albinism. Proc Nat Acad Sci USA 1990; 87(9):3255–3258.
32. Oetting WS, King RA. Molecular basis of albinism: mutations and polymorphisms of pigmentation genes associated with albinism. Hum Mutat 1999; 13(2):99–115.
33. Spritz RA, Oh J, Fukai K, Holmes SA, Ho L, Chitayat D, France TD, Musarella MA, Orlow SJ, Schnur RE, Weleber RG, Levin AV. Novel mutations of the tyrosinase (TYR) gene in type I oculocutaneous albinism (OCA1). Hum Mutat 1997; 10(2): 171–174.
34. Camand O, Marchant D, Boutboul S, Pequignot M, Odent S, Dollfus H, Sutherland J, Levin A, Menasche M, Marsac C, Dufier JL, Heon E, Abitbol M. Mutation analysis of the tyrosinase gene in oculocutaneous albinism. Hum Mutat 2001; 17(4):352.
35. Halaban R, Svedine S, Cheng E, Smicun Y, Aron R, Hebert DN. Endoplasmic reticulum retention is a common defect associated with tyrosinase-negative albinism. Proc Nat Acad Sci USA 2000; 97(11):5889–5894.
36. Gershoni-Barach R, Rosenmann A, Droetto S, Holmes S, Tripathi RK, Spritz RA. Mutations of the tyrosinase gene in patients with oculocutaneous albinism from various ethnic groups in Israel. Am J Hum Genet 1994; 54(4):586–594.
37. O'Donnell FE Jr. Congenital ocular hypopigmentation. Int Ophthalmol Clin 1984; 24:133–142.
38. Jay B, Carruthers J, Treplin MCW, Winder AF. Human albinism. Birth Defects 1976; 12:415–426.
39. Worobec-Victor SM, Bain MAB. Oculocutaneous genetic diseases. In: Renie WA, ed. Goldberg's Genetic and Metabolic Eye Disease. Boston: Little, Brown & Co, 1986:489–541.
40. Ramsay M, Colman MA, Stevens G, Zwane E, Kromberg J, Farrall M, Jenkins T. The tyrosinase-positive oculocutaneous albinism locus maps to chromosome 15q11.2–q12. Am J Hum Genet 1992; 51(4):879–884.
41. Rinchik EM, Bultman SJ, Horsthemke B, Lee ST, Strunk KM, Spritz RA, Avidano KM, Jong MT, Nicholls RD. A gene for the mouse pink-eyed dilution locus and for human type II oculocutaneous albinism. Nature 1993; 361(6407):72–76.
42. Lee ST, Nicholls RD, Jong MT, Fukai K, Spritz RA. Organization and sequence of the human P gene and identification of a new family of transport proteins. Genomics 1995; 26(2):354–363.
43. Spritz RA, Lee ST, Fukai K, Brondum-Nielsen K, Chitayat D, Lipson MH, Musarella MA, Rosenmann A, Weleber RG. Novel mutations of the P gene in type 2 oculocutaneous albinism (OCA2). Hum Mutat 1997; 10(2):175–177.
44. Durham–Pierre D, Gardner JM, Nakatsu Y, King RA, Francke U, Ching A, Aquaron R, del Marmol V, Brilliant MH. African origin of an intragenic deletion of the human P gene in tyrosinase positive oculocutaneous albinism. Nat Genet 1994; 7(2):176–179.
45. Yi Z, Garrison N, Cohen-Barak O, Karafet TM, King RA, Erickson RP, Hammer MF, Brilliant MH. A 122.5–kilobase deletion of the P gene underlies the high prevalence of oculocutaneous albinism type 2 in the Navajo population. Am J Hum Genet 2003; 72(1):62–72.
46. Nance WE, Jackson CE, Witkop CJ Jr. Amish albinism: a distinctive autosomal recessive phenotype. Am J Hum Genet 1970; 22:579–586.
47. Hu F, Hanifin JM, Prescott GH, Tongue AC. Yellow mutant albinism: Cytochemical, ultrastructural, and genetic characterization suggesting multiple allelism. Am J Hum-Genet 1980; 32:387–395.
48. King RA, Townsend D, Oetting W, Summers CG, Olds DP, White JG, Spritz RA. Temperature–sensitive tyrosinase associated with peripheral pigmentation in oculocutaneous albinism. J Clin Invest 1991; 87(3):1046–1053.
49. King RA, Wirtschafter JD, Olds DP, Brumbaugh J. Minimal pigment: a new type of oculocutaneous albinism. Clin Genet 1986; 29:42–50.

50. King RA, Creel D, Cervenka J, et al. Albinism in Nigeria with delineation of new recessive oculocutaneous type. Clin Genet 1980; 17:259–270.
51. King RA, Lewis RA, Townsend D, et al. Brown oculocutaneous albinism. Clinical, ophthalmological, and biochemical characterization. Ophthalmology 1985; 92:1496–1505.
52. Manga P, Kromberg J, Turner A, Jenkins T, Ramsay M. In Southern Africa, brownoculocutaneous albinism (BOCA) maps to the 0CA2 locus on chromosome 15q: P-gene mutations identified. Am J Hum Genet 2001; 68(3):782–787.
53. King RA, Willaert RK, Schmidt RM, Pietsch J, Savage S, Brott MJ, Fryer JP, Summers CG, Oetting WS. MC1R mutations modify the classic phenotype of oculocutaneous albinism type 2 (OCA2). Am J Hum Genet 2003; 73(3):638–645.
54. Boissy RE, Zhao H, Oetting WS, Austin LM, Wildenberg SC, Boissy YL, Zhao Y, Sturm RA, Hearing VJ, King RA, Nordlund JJ. Mutation in and lack of expression of tyrosinase–related protein–1 (TRP–1) in melanocytes from an individual with brown oculocutaneous albinism: a new subtype of albinism classified as "0CA3." Am J Hum Genet 1996; 58(6):1145–1156.
55. Manga P, Kromberg JG, Box NF, Sturm RA, Jenkins T, Ramsay M. Rufous oculocutaneous albinism in southern African Blacks is caused by mutations in the TYRP1 gene. Am J Hum Genet 1997; 61(5):1095–1101.
56. Sturm RA, O'Sullivan BJ, Box NF, Smith AG, Smit SE, Puttick ER, Parsons PG, Dunn IS. Chromosomal structure of the human TYRP1 and TYRP2 loci and comparison of the tyrosinase-related protein gene family. Genomics 1995; 29(1):24–34.
57. Murty VV, Bouchard B, Mathew S, Vijayasaradhi S, Houghton AN. Assignment of the human TYRP (brown) locus to chromosome region 9p23 by nonradioactive in situ hybridization. Genomics 1992; 13(1):227–229.
58. Newton JM, Cohen-Barak O, Hagiwara N, Gardner JM, Davisson MT, King RA, Brilliant MH. Mutations in the human orthologue of the mouse underwhite gene (uw) underlie a new form of oculocutaneous albinism, OCA4. Am J Hum Genet 2001; 69(5):981–988.
59. Rundshagen U, Zuhlke C, Opitz S, Schwinger E, Kasmann-Kelmer B. Mutations in the MATP gene in five German patients affected by oculocutaneous albinism type 4. Hum Mutat 2004; 23(2):106–110.
60. Inagaki K, Suzuki T, Shimizu H, Ishii N, Umezawa Y, Tada J, Kikuchi N, Takata M, Takamori K, Kishibe M, Tanaka M, Miyamura Y, Ito S, Tomita Y. Oculocutaneous albinism type 4 is one of the most common types of albinism in Japan. Am J Hum Genet 2004; 74(3):466–471.
61. Costin GE, Valencia JC, Vieira WD, Lamoreux ML, Hearing VJ. Tyrosinase processing and intracellular trafficking is disrupted in mouse primary melanocytes carrying the underwhite (uw) mutation. A model for oculocutaneous albinism (OCA) type 4. J Cell Sci 2003; 116(Pt 15):3203–3212.
62. Frenk E, Calame A. Hypopigmentation oculo-cutanee familiale a transmission dominante due a un trouble de la formation des melanosomes. Schweiz Med Wochenschr 1977; 107:1964–1968.
63. King RA. Autosomal dominant oculocutaneous albinism with a mild phenotype. Am J Hum Genet 1979; 31:75A.
64. Witkop CJ. Depigmentations of the general and oral tissues and their genetic foundations. Ala J Med Sci 1979; 16(4):330–343.
65. O'Doherty NJ, Gorlin RJ. The ermine phenotype: pigmentary-hearing loss heterogeneity. Am J Med Genet 1998; 30(4):945–952.
66. Cross HE, McKusick VA, Green W. A new oculocerebral syndrome with hypopigmentation. J Pediatr 1967; 70:398–406.
67. Hamano K, Kawashima K, Joganoto M et al. Muscle involvement in a case of oculocutaneous albinism. Neuropediatrics 1986; 17:53–56.

68. Prchal JT, Crist WM, Roper M, Wellner VP. Hemolytic anemia, recurrent metabolic acidosis, and incomplete albinism associated with glutathione synthetase deficiency. Blood 1983; 62:754–757.
69. Mund ML, Rodrigues MM, Fine BS. Light and electron microscopic observations on the pigmented layers of the developing human eye. Am J Ophthaimol 1972; 73:167–182.
70. Naumann GOH, Lerche W, Schroeder W. Foveola-Aplasie bei tyrosinase-positive oculocutanen Albinismus. Klinisch–pathologishe Befunde. Graefes Arch Ophthal 1976; 200:39–50.
71. Fulton AB, Albert DM, Craft JL. Human albinism. Light and electron microscopy study. Arch Ophthalmol 1978; 96:305–310.
72. Akeo K, Shirai S, Okisaka S, Shimizu H, MiyataH, Kikuchi A, Nishikawa T, Suzumori K, Fujiwara T, Majima A. Histology of fetal eyes with oculocutaneous albinism. Arch Ophthalmol 1996; 114(5):613–616.
73. Kikuchi A, Shimizu H, Nishikawa T. Epidermal melanocytes in normal and tyrosinase-negative oculocutaneous albinism fetuses. Arch Dermatol Res 1995; 287(6):529–533.
74. Creel D. Problems of ocular miswiring in albinism, Duane's syndrome, and Marcus Gunn phenomenon. Int Ophthalmol Clin 1984; 24:165–176.
75. Guillery RW, Okoro AN, Witkop CJ Jr. Abnormal visual pathways in the brain of a human albino. Brain Res 1975; 96:373–377.
76. Gross KJ, Hickey TL. Abnormal laminar patterns in the lateral geniculate nucleus of an albino monkey. Brain Res 1980; 190:231–237.
77. Witkop CJ Jr, Jay B, Creel D, Guillery RW. Optic and otic neurologic abnormalities in oculocutaneous and ocular albinism. Birth Defects 1982; 18:299–318.
78. Creel D, O'Donnell FE Jr, Witkop CJ. Visual system anomalies in human ocular albinos. Science 1978; 201:931–933.
79. Leventhal AG, Vitek DJ, Creel DJ. Abnormal visual pathways in normally pigmented cats that are heterozygous for albinism. Science 1985; 229:1395–1397.
80. Silver J, Sapiro J. Axonal guidance during development of the optic nerve. The role of pigmented epithelia and other extrinsic factors. J Comp Neurol 1981; 202:521–538.
81. Abrams JD. Transillumination of the iris during routine slit lamp examination. Br J Ophthalmol 1964; 48:42–44.
82. Wirtschafter JD, Denslow DT, Shine IB. Quantification of iris translucency in albinism. Arch Ophthalmol 1974; 90:274–277.
83. Meyer CH, Lapolice DJ, Freedman SF. Foveal hypoplasia in oculocutaneous albinism demonstrated by optical coherence tomography. Am J Ophthalmol 2002; 133(3):409–410.
84. McGuire DE, Weinreb RN, Goldbaum MH. Foveal hypoplasia demonstrated in vivo with optical coherence tomography. Am J Ophthalmol 2003; 135(l):112–114.
85. Krill AE, Lee GB. The electroretinogram in albinos and carriers of the ocular albino-trait. Arch Ophthalmol 1963; 69:32–38.
86. Reeser F, Weinstein GW, Feiock BK, Oser RS. Electro-oculography as a test of retinal function. The normal and supernormal EOG. Am J Ophthalmol 1970; 70:505–514.
87. Walk MA, Peachey NS, Fishman GA. Electro-retinographic findings in human oculocutaneous albinism. Ophthalmology 1989; 96:1778–1785.
88. Kriss A, Russell–Eggitt I, Taylor D. Childhood albinism. Visual electrophysiological features. Ophthalmic Paediatr Genet 1990; 11(3):185–192.
89. Russell–Eggitt I, Kriss A, Taylor DS. Albinism in childhood: a flash VEP and ERG study. Br J Ophthalmol 1990; 74(3):136–140.
90. Creel DJ, Summers CG, King RA. Visual anomalies associated with albinism. Ophthalmic Paediatr Genet 1990; 11(3):193–200.
91. Creel D, Boxer LA, Fauci AS. Visual and auditory anomalies in Chediak–Higashi syndrome. Electroencephalogr Clin Neurophysiol 1983; l55:252–257.
92. Creel DJ, Witkop CJ Jr, King RA. Asymmetric visually evoked potentials in human albinos: evidence for visual system anomalies. Invest Ophthalmol 1974; 13:430–440.

93. Creel D, Spekreijse H, Reits D. Evoked potentials in albinos: efficacy of pattern stimuli in detecting misrouted optic fibers. Electroencephalogr Clin Neurophysiol 1981; 52: 595–603.
94. Harding GF, Boylan C, Clement RA. Visual evoked cortical and subcortical potentials in human albinos. Doc Ophthalmol 1986; 62:81–88.
95. Jay B, Carroll W. Albinism. Recent advances. Trans Ophthalmol Soc UK 1980; 100:467–471.
96. Apkarian P, Reits D, Spekreijse H, van Dorp D. A decisive electrophysiological test for human albinism. Electroencephalogr Clin Neurophysiol 1983; 55:513–531.
97. Kromberg JG, Jenkins T. Prevalence of albinism in the South African negro. S Afr Med J 1982; 61:383–386.
98. Kagore F, Lund PM. Oculocutaneous albinism among school children in Harare, Zimbabwe. J Med Genet 1995; 32(11):859–861.
99. Palmer DJ, Miller MT, Rao S. Hermansky–Pudlak oculocutaneous albinism. Clinical and genetic observation of six patients. Ophthalmol Paediatr Genet 1983; 3:147–156.
100. Gedda L, Berard-Magistretti S, Brenci G. Miscellaneous clinical case reports in twins. Acta Genet Med Gemellol (Roma) 1984; 33:505–508.
101. Taylor WO. Hereditary puzzles in albinism: Heterogeneity or phenotypical variation? Trans Ophthalmol Soc UK 1983; 103:318–330.
102. Burger DS, London R. Soft opaque contact lenses in binocular vision problems. J Am Optom Assoc 1993; 64(3):176–180.
103. Jurkus JM. Contact lenses for children. Optom Clin 1996; 5(2):91–104.
104. Hoeft WW, Hughes MK. A comparative study of low-vision patients: their ocular disease and preference for one specific series of light transmission filters. Am J Optom Physiol Opt 1981; 58:841–845.
105. Flander M, Young D. Atypical sensory nystagmus and its surgical management. Can J Ophthalmol 1983; 18:349–351.
106. Haynes ME, Robertson E. Can oculocutaneous albinism be diagnosed prenatally? Prenat Diagn 1981; 1:85–89.
107. Eady RA, Gunner DB, Garner A, Rodeck CH. Prenatal diagnosis of oculocutaneous albinism by electron microscopy of fetal skin. J Invest Dermatol 1983; 80:210–212.
108. Shimizu H, Ishiko A, Kikuchi A, Akiyama M, Suzumori K, Nishikawa T. Prenatal diagnosis of tyrosinase-negative oculocutaneous albinism by an electron microscopic dopa reaction test of fetal skin. Prenat Diagn 1994; 14(6):442–450.
109. Shimizu H, Niizeki H, Suzumori K, Aozaki R, Kawaguchi R, Hikiji K, Nishikawa T. Prenatal diagnosis of oculocutaneous albinism by analysis of the fetal tyrosinase gene. J Invest Dermatol 1994; 103(1):104–106.
110. Rosenmann E, Rosenmann A, Ne'eman Z, Lewin A, Bejarano-Achache I, Blumenfeld A. Prenatal diagnosis of oculocutaneous albinism type I: review and personal experience. Pediatr Dev Pathol 1999; 2(5):404–414.
111. Nettleship E. On some hereditary diseases of the eye. Trans Ophthalmol Soc UK 1909; 29:57–198.
112. Falls HP. Sex-linked ocular albinism displaying typical fundus changes in female heterozygote. Am J Ophthalmol 1951; 34:41–50.
113. Johnson GJ, Gillan JG, Pearce WG. Ocular albinism in Newfoundland. Can J Ophthalmol 1971; 6:237–248.
114. O'Donnell FE Jr, Green WR, Fleischman JA, Hambrick GW. X-linked ocular albinism in blacks. Ocular albinism cum pigmento. Arch Ophthalmol 1978; 96:1189–1192.
115. Jay B. X-linked retinal disorders and the Lyon hypothesis. Trans Ophthalmol Soc UK 1985; 104:836–844.
116. Mansour AM, Greenwald MJ, Jampol LM, Hrisomalos N. Fundal findings in a female carrier of X-linked ocular albinism. Arch Ophthalmol 1987; 105:750–751.

117. Jaeger C, Jay B. X-linked ocular albinism: a family containing a manifesting heterozygote, and an affected male married to a female with autosomal recessive ocular albinism. Hum Genet 1981; 56:299–304.
118. Rott HD, Rix R. Carrier state in X-linked ocular albinism: a proof of the validity of Lyon's hypothesis in man. Klin Monatsbl Augenheilkd 1984; 184:128–129.
119. Gillerspie FD, Covelli B. Carriers of ocular albinism with and without ocular changes. Arch Ophthalmol 1963; 70:209–213.
120. O'Donnell FE, Hambrick GW, Green WR, et al. X-linked ocular albinism. An oculocutaneous macromelanosomal disorder. Arch Ophthalmol 1976; 94:1883–1892.
121. Garner A, Jay BS. Macromelanosomes in X-linked ocular albinism. Histopathology 1980; 4:243–254.
122. Szymanski KA, Boughman JA, Nance WE, et al. Genetic studies of ocular albinism in a large Virginia kindred. Ann Ophthalmol 1984; 16:183–196.
123. Cortin P, Tremblay M, Lemagne JM. X-linked ocular albinism: relative value of skin-biopsy, iris transillumination and funduscopy in identifying affected males and carriers. Can J Ophthalmol 1981; 16:121–123.
124. Wong G, O'Donnell FE Jr, Green WR. Giant pigment granules in the retinal pigment epithelium of a fetus with X-linked ocular albinism. Ophthal Paediatr Genet 1983; 2: 47–65.
125. Hull MT, Epinette WW. Giant melanosomes in the dysplastic nevus syndrome. Electron microscopic observations. Dermatologica 1984; 168:112–116.
126. Hegde M, Lewis RA, Richards CS. Diagnostic DNA testing for X-linked ocular albinism (OA1) with a hierarchical mutation screening protocol. Genet Test 2002; 6(1):7–14.
127. Fialkow PJ, Giblett ER, Motulsky AG. Measurable linkage between ocular albinism and *Xg*. Am J Hum Genet 1967; 19:63–69.
128. Pearce WG, Johnson GJ, Sanger R. Ocular albinism and Xg [letter]. Lancet 1971; 1:1072.
129. Bassi MT, Bergen AA, Wapenaar MC, Schiaffino MV, van Schooneveld M, Yates JR, Charles SJ, Meitinger T, Ballabio A. A submicroscopic deletion in a patient with isolated X-linked ocular albinism (OA1). Hum Mol Genet 1994; 3(4):647–648.
130. Bassi MT, Schiaffino MV, Renieri A, De Nigris F, Galli L, Bruttini M, Gebbia M, Bergen AA, Lewis RA, Ballabio A. Cloning of the gene for ocular albinism type 1 from the distal short arm of the X chromosome. Nat Genet 1995; 10(1):13–19.
131. Schiaffino MV, Bassi MT, Galli L, Renieri A, Bruttini M, De Nigris F, Bergen AA, Charles SJ, Yates JR, Meindl A, et al. Analysis of the OA1 gene reveals mutations in only one-third of patients with X-linked ocular albinism. Hum Mol Genet 1995; 4(12):2319–2325.
132. Schiaffino MV, d'Addio M, Alloni A, Baschirotto C, Valetti C, Cortese K, Puri C, Bassi MT, Colla C, De Luca M, Tacchetti C, Ballabio A. Ocular albinism: evidence for a defect in an intracellular signal transduction system. Nat Genet 1999; 23(1):108–112.
133. Bassi MT, Bergen AA, Bitoun P, Charles SJ, Clementi M, Gosselin R, Hurst J, Lewis RA, Lorenz B, Meitinger T, Messiaen L, Ramesar RS, Ballabio A, Schiaffino MV. Diverse prevalence of large deletions within the OA1 gene in ocular albinism type 1 patients from Europe North America. Hum Genet 2001; 108(1):51–54.
134. Schnur RE, Gao M, Wick PA, Keller M, Benke PJ, Edwards MJ, Grix AW, Hockey A, Jung JH, Kidd KK, Kistenmacher M, Levin AV, Lewis RA, Musarella MA, Nowakowski RW, Orlow SJ, Pagon RS, Pillers DA, Punnett HH, Quinn GE, Tezcan K, Wagstaff J, Weleber RG. OA1 mutations and deletions in X-linked ocular albinism. Am J Hum Genet 1998; 62(4):800–809.
135. Tijmes NT, Bergen AB, De Jong PT. Paucity of signs in X linked ocular albinism with a 700 kb deletion spanning the OA1 gene. Br J Ophthalmol 1998; 82(4):457–458.
136. Preising M, Op de Laak JP, Lorenz B. Deletion in the OA1 gene in a family with congenital X linked nystagmus. Br J Ophthalmol 2001; 85(9):1098–1103.

137. O'Donnell FE Jr, King RA, Green RW, Witkop CJ Jr. Autosomal recessively inherited ocular albinism. Arch Ophthamol 1978; 96:1621–1625.
138. Fukai K, Holmes SA, Lucchese NJ, Siu VM, Weleber RG, Schnur RE, Spritz RA. Autosomal recessive ocular albinism associated with a functionally significant tyrosinase gene polymorphism. Nat Genet 1995; 9(1):92–95.
139. Morell R, Spritz RA, Ho L, Pierpont J, Guo W, Friedman TB, Asher JH Jr. Apparent digenic inheritance of Waardenburg syndrome type 2 (WS2) and autosomal recessive ocular albinism (AROA). Hum Mol Genet 1997; 6(5):659–664.
140. Forsius H, Eriksson AW. Ein neues Augensyndrom mit X–chromosomaler Transmission Eine Sippe mit Fundusalbinismus, Foveahypoplasie, Nystagmus, Myopie, Astigmatismus und Dyschromatopsie. Klin Monatsbl Augenheilkd 1964; 144:447–457.
141. O'Donnell FE, Green WR, McKusick VA, et al. Forsius–Eriksson syndrome: its relation to the Nettleship-Falls X-linked ocular albinism. Clin Genet 1980; 17:403–438.
142. van Dorp DB, Eriksson AW, Delleman JW, et al. Åland eye disease: no albino misrouting. Clin Genet 1985; 28:526–531.
143. Winship I, Gericke G, Beighton P. X-linked inheritance of ocular albinism with late-onset sensorineural deafness. Am J Med Genet 1984; 19:797–803.
144. Ziprkowski L, Krakowski A, Adam A, et al. Partial albinism and deaf-mutism due to a recessive sex–linked gene. Arch Dermatol 1962; 86:530–539.
145. Lewis RA. Ocular albinism and deafness. Am J Hum Genet 1978; 30:57A.
146. Winship IM, Babaya M, Ramesar RS. X-linked ocular albinism and sensorineural deafness: linkage to Xp22.3. Genomics 1993; 18(2):444–445.
147. Hermansky F, Pudlak P. Albinism associated with hemorrhagic diathesis and unusual pigmented reticular cells in the bone marrow: report of two cases with histochemical studies. Blood 1959; 14:162–169.
148. Fagadau WR, Heinemann MJ, Cotlier E. Hermansky–Pudlak syndrome: albinism with lipofuscin storage. Int Ophthalmol 1981; 4:113–122.
149. Summers CG, Knobloch WH, Witkop CJ, King RA. Hermansky–Pudlak syndrome. Ophthalmic findings. Ophthalmology 1988; 95:545–554.
150. Lattion F, Schneider DA, Prada M, et al. Syndrome d'Hermansky–Pudlak dans un village valaisan. Helv Paediatr Acta 1983; 38:495–512.
151. Kinnear PE, Tuddenham EG. Albinism with haemorrhagic diathesis: Hermansky–Pudlak syndrome. Br J Ophthalmol 1985; 69:904–908.
152. Simon JW, Adams RJ, Calhoun JH, et al. Ophthalmic manifestations of the Hermansky–Pudlak syndrome (oculocutaneous albinism and hemorrhagic diathesis). Am J Ophthalmol 1982; 93:71–77.
153. Schinella RA, Greco MA, Garay SM, Lackner H, Wolman SR, Fazzini EP. Hermansky–Pudlak syndrome: a clinicopathologic study. Hum Pathol 1985; 16:366–376.
154. Frenk E, Lattion F. The melanin pigmentary disorder in a family with Hermansky–Pudlak syndrome. J Invest Dermatol 1982; 78:141–143.
155. Reiss RE, Copel JA, Roberts NS, Hobbins JC. Hennansky–Pudlak syndrome in pregnancy: two case studies. Am J Obstet Gynecol 1985; 153:564–565.
156. Depinho RA, Kaplan KL. The Hermansky–Pudlak syndrome. Report of three cases and of pathophysiology and management considerations. Medicine 1985; 64:192–202.
157. Izquierdo NJ, Townsend W, Hussels IE. Ocular findings in the Hermansky–Pudlak syndrome. Trans Am Ophthalmol Soc 1995; 93:191–200; discussion 200–202.
158. Gahl WA, Brantly M, Kaiser-Kupfer MI, Iwata F, Hazelwood S, Shotelersuk V, Duffy LF, Kuehl EM, Troendle J, Bernardini I. Genetic defects and clinical characteristics of patients with a form of oculocutaneous albinism (Hermansky–Pudlak syndrome). N Engl J Med 1998; 338(18):1258–1264.
159. Iwata F, Reed GF, Caruso RC, Kuehl EM, Gahl WA, Kaiser–Kupfer MI. Correlation of visual acuity and ocular pigmentation with the 16–bp duplication in the HPS–1 gene of Hermansky–Pudlak syndrome, a form of albinism. Ophthalmol 2000; 107(4): 783–789.

160. Ramsay M. Protein trafficking violations. Nat Genet 1996; 14(3):242–245.
161. Fukai K, Oh J, Frenk E, Almodovar C, Spritz RA. Linkage disequilibrium mapping of the gene for Hermansky–Pudlak syndrome to chromosome 10q23.1–q23.3. Hum Mol Genet 1995; 4(9):1665–1669.
162. Oh J, Bailin T, Fukai K, Feng GH, Ho L, Mao JI, Frenk E, Tamura N, Spritz RA. Positional cloning of a gene for Hermansky–Pudlak syndrome, a disorder of cytoplasmic organelles. Nat Genet 1996; 14(3):300–306.
163. Bailin T, Oh J, Feng GH, Fukai K, Spritz RA. Organization and nucleotide sequence of the human Hermansky–Pudlak syndrome (HPS) gene. J Invest Dermatol 1997; 108(6):923–927.
164. Oh J, Liu ZX, Feng GH, Raposo G, Spritz RA. The Hermansky–Pudlak syndrome (HPS) protein is part of a high molecular weight complex involved in biogenesis of early melanosomes. Hum Mol Genet 2000; 9(3):375–385.
165. Hazelwood S, Shotelersuk V, Wildenberg SC, Chen D, Iwata F, Kaiser-Kupfer MI, White JG, King RA, Ghal WA. Evidence for locus heterogeneity in Puerto Ricans with Hermansky–Pudlak syndrome. Am J Hum Genet 1997; 61(5):1088–1094.
166. Dell'Angelica EC, Shotelersuk V, Aguilar RC, Gahl WA, Bonifacino JS. Altered trafficking of lysosomal proteins in Hermansky–Pudlak syndrome due to mutations in the beta 3A subunit of the AP-3 adaptor. Mol Cell 1999; 3(1):11–21.
167. Anikster Y, Huizing M, White J, Shevchenko YO, Fitzpatrick DL, Touchman JW, Compton JG, Bale SJ, Swank RT, Gahl WA, Toro JR. Mutation of a new gene causes a unique form of Hermansky–Pudlak syndrome in a genetic isolate of central Puerto Rico. Nat Genet 2001; 28(4):376–380.
168. Huizing M, Anikster Y, Fitzpatrick DL, Jeong AB, D'Souza M, Rausche M, Toro JR, Kaiser-Kupfer MI, White JG, Gahl WA. Hermansky–Pudlak syndrome type 3 in Ashkenazi Jews and other non-Puerto Rican patients with hypopigmentation and platelet storage-pool deficiency. Am J Hum Genet 2001; 69(5):1022–1032.
169. Suzuki T, Li W, Zhang Q, Karim A, Novak EK, Sviderskaya EV, Hill SP, Bennett DC, Levin AV, Nieuwenhuis HK, Fong CT, Castellan C, Miterski B, Swank RT, Spritz RA. Hermansky–Pudlak syndrome is caused by mutations in HPS4, the human homolog of the mouse light-ear gene. Nat Genet 2002; 30(3):321–324.
170. Anderson PD, Huizing M, Claassen DA, White J, Gahl WA. Hermansky–Pudlak syndrome type 4 (HPS-4): clinical and molecular characteristics. Hum Genet 2003; 113(l):10–17.
171. Zhang Q, Zhao B, Li W, Oiso N, Novak EK, Rusiniak ME, Gautam R, Chintala S, O'Brien EP, Zhang Y, Roe BA, Elliott RW, Eicher EM, Liang P, Kratz C, Legius E, Spritz RA, O'Sullivan TN, Copeland NG, Jenkins NA, Swank RT. Ru2 and Ru encode mouse orthologs of the genes mutated in human Hermansky–Pudlak syndrome types 5 and 6. Nat Genet 2003; 33(2):145–153.
172. Li W, Zhang Q, Oiso N, Novak EK, Gautam R, O'Brien EP, Tinsley CL, Blake DJ, Spritz RA, Copeland NG, Jenkins NA, Amato D, Roe BA, Starcevic M, Dell'Angelica EC, Elliott RW, Mishra V, Kingsmore SF, Paylor RE, Swank RT. Hermansky–Pudlak syndrome type 7 (HPS–7) results from mutant dysbindin, a member of the biogenesis of lysosome-related organelles complex 1 (BLOC–1). Nat Genet 2003; 35(1):84–89.
173. Zelickson AS, Windhorst DB, White JG, Good RA. The Chediak–Higashi syndrome: Formation of giant melanosomes and the basis of hypopigmentation. J Invest Dermatol 1967; 49:575–581.
174. Ben-Ezra D, Mengistu F, Cividalli G, et al. Chediak–Higashi syndrome ocular findings. J Pediatr Ophthalmol Strabismus 1980; 17:68–74.
175. Libert J, Dhermy P, van Hoof F, et al. Ocular findings in Chediak–Higashi disease: a light and electron microscopic study of two patients. Birth Defects 1982; 18:327–344.
176. Nagle DL, Karim MA, Woolf EA, Holmgren L, Bork P, Misumi DJ, McGrail SH, Dussault BJ Jr, Perou CM, Boissy RE, Duyk GM, Spritz RA, Moore KJ. Identification

and mutation analysis of the complete gene for Chediak–Higashi syndrome. Nat Genet 1996; 14(3):307–311.
177. Barbosa MD, Nguyen QA, Tchernev VT, Ashley JA, Detter JC, Blaydes SM, Brandt SJ, Chotai D, Hodgman C, Solan RC, Lovett M, Kingsmore SF. Identification of the homologous beige and Chediak–Higashi syndrome genes. Nature 1996; 382(6588):262–265.
178. Zhao H, Boissy YL, Abdel-Malek Z, King RA, Nordlund JJ, Boissy RE. On the analysis of the pathophysiology of Chediak–Higashi syndrome. Defects expressed by cultured melanocytes. Lab Invest 1994; 71(1):25–34.
179. Spritz RA. Multi–organellar disorders of pigmentation: tied up in traffic. Clin Genet 1999; 55(5):309–317.
180. Spritz RA. Genetic defects in Chediak–Higashi syndrome and the beige mouse. J Clin Immunol 1998; 18(2):97–105.
181. Karim MA, Suzuki K, Fukai K, Oh J, Nagle DL, Moore KJ, Barbosa E, Falik–Borenstein T, Filipovich A, Ishida Y, Kivrikko S, Klein C, Kreuz F, Levin A, Miyajima H, Regueiro J, Russo C, Uyama E, Vierimaa O, Spritz RA. Apparent genotype–phenotype correlation in childhood, adolescent, and adult Chediak–Higashi syndrome. Am J Med Genet 2002; 108(1):16–22.
182. Durandy A, Breton-Gorius J, Guy-Grand D, Dumez C, Griscelli C. Prenatal diagnosis of syndromes associating albinism and immune deficiencies (Chediak–Higashi syndrome and variant). Prenat Diagn 1993; 13(1):13–20.
183. Simon JW, Kandel GL, Krohel GB, Nelsen PT. Albinotic characteristics in congenital nystagmus. Am J Ophthalmol 1984; 97:320–327.
184. Read AP, Newton VE. Waardenburg syndrome. J Med Genet 1997; 34(8):656–665.
185. Waardenburg PJ. A new syndrome combining developmental anomalies or the eyelids, eyebrows and nose root, with pigmentary defects of the iris and head hair and with congenital deafness. Am J Hum Genet 1951; 3:195–253.
186. Goldberg MF. Waardenburg's syndrome with fundus and other anomalies. Arch Ophthalmol 1966; 76:797–810.
187. Goodman RM, Lewithal I, Solomon A, Klein D. Upper limb involvement in the Klein–Waardenburg syndrome. Am J Med Genet 1982; 11:425–433.
188. Arias S. Genetic heterogeneity of the Waardenburg syndrome. Birth Defects 1971; 7:87.
189. Pardono E, van Bever Y, van den Ende J, Havrenne PC, Iughetti P, Maestrelli SR, Costa FO, Richieri-Costa A, Frota-Pessoa O, Otto PA. Waardenburg syndrome: clinical differentiation between types I and II. Am J Med Genet 2003; 117A(3):223–235.
190. DeStefano AL, Cupples LA, Amos KS, Asher JH Jr, Baldwin CT, Blanton S, Carey ML, da Silva EO, Friedman TB, Greenberg J, Lalwani AK, Milunsky A, Nance WE, Pandya A, Ramesar RS, Read AP, Tassabejhi M, Wilcox ER, Fairer LA. Correlation between Waardenburg syndrome phenotype and genotype in a population of individuals with identified PAX3 mutations. Hum Genet 1998; 102(5):499–506.
191. Foy C, Newton V, Wellesley D, Harris R, Read AP. Assignment of the locus for Waardenburg syndrome type I to human chromosome 2q37 and possible homology to the Splotch mouse [see comment]. Am J Hum Genet 1990; 46(6):1017–1023.
192. Tassabehji M, Read AP, Newton VE, Patton M, Gruss P, Harris R, Strachan T. Mutations in the PAX3 gene causing Waardenburg syndrome type 1 and type 2. Nat Genet 1993; 3(1):26–30.
193. Macina RA, Barr FG, Galili N, Riethman HC. Genomic organization of the human PAX3 gene. DNA sequence analysis of the region disrupted in alveolar rhabdomyosarcoma. Genomics 1995; 26(1):1–8.
194. Lalwani AK, Brister JR, Fex J, Grundfast KM, Ploplis B, San Agustin TB, Wilcox ER. Further elucidation of the genomic structure of PAX3, and identification of two different point mutations within the PAX3 homeobox that cause Waardenburg syndrome type 1 in two families. Am J Hum Genet 1995; 56(1):75–83.
195. Pandya A, Xia XJ, Landa BL, Arnos KS, Israel J, Lloyd J, James AL, Diehl SR, Blanton SH, Nance WE. Phenotypic variation in Waardenburg syndrome. Mutational

heterogeneity, modifier genes or polygenic background? Hum Mol Genet 1996; 5(4): 497–502.
196. Zlotogora J, Lerer I, Bar-David S, Ergaz Z, Abeliovich D. Homozygosity for Waardenburg syndrome. Am J Hum Genet 1995; 56(5):1173–1178.
197. Arias S. Waardenburg syndrome—two distinct types [letter]. Am J Med Genet 1980; 6:99–100.
198. Reynolds JE, Meyer JM, Landa B, Stevens CA, Arnos KS, Israel J, Marazita ML, Bodurtha J, Nance WE, Diehl SR. Analysis of variability of clinical manifestations in Waardenburg syndrome. Am J Med Genet 1995; 57(4):540–547.
199. Hughes AE, Newton VE, Liu XZ, Read AP. A gene for Waardenburg syndrome type 2 maps close to the human homologue of the microphthalmia gene at chromosome 3pl2–pl4.1. Nat Genet 1994; 7(4):509–512.
200. Tassabehji M, Newton VE, Read AP. Waardenburg syndrome type 2 caused by mutations in the human microphthalmia (MITF) gene. Nat Genet 1994; 8(3):251–255.
201. Tachibana M, Takeda K, Nobukuni Y, Urabe K, Long JE, Meyers KA, Aaronson SA, Miki T. Ectopic expression of MITF, a gene for Waardenburg syndrome type 2, converts fibroblasts to cells with melanocyte characteristics. Nat Genet 1996; 14(1):50–54.
202. Lalwani AK, Attaie A, Randolph FT, Deshmukh D, Wang C, Mhatre A, Wilcox E. Point mutation in the MITF gene causing Waardenburg syndrome type II in a three–generation Indian family. Am J Med Genet 1998; 80(4):406–409.
203. Bard LA. Heterogeneity in Waardenburg's syndrome: report of a family with ocular albinism. Arch Ophthalmol 1978; 96:1193–1198.
204. Selicorni A, Guerneri S, Ratti A, Pizzuti A. Cytogenetic mapping of a novel locus for type II Waardenburg syndrome. Hum Genet 2002; 110(1):64–67.
205. Hoth CF, Milunsky A, Lipsky N, Sheffer R, Clairen SK, Baldwin CT. Mutations in the paired domain of the human PAX3 gene cause Klein–Waardenburg syndrome (WS–III) as well as Waardenburg syndrome type I (WS–I). Am J Hum Genet 1993; 52(3):455–462.
206. Wollnik B, Tukel T, Uyguner O, Ghanbari A, Kayserili H, Emiroglu M, Yuksel–Apak M. Homozygous and heterozygous inheritance of PAX3 mutations causes different types of Waardenburg syndrome. Am J Med Genet 2003; 122A(l):42–45.
207. Branski D, Dennis NR, Neale JM, Brooks LJ. Hirschsprung's disease and Waardenburg's syndrome. Pediatrics 1979; 63:803–805.
208. Omenn GS, McKusick VA. The association of Waardenburg syndrome with Hirshsprung megacolon. Am J Genet 1979; 3:217–223.
209. Liang JC, Juarez CP, Goldberg MF. Bilateral bicolored irides with Hirschsprung's disease. A neural crest syndrome. Arch Ophthalmol 1983; 101:69–73.
210. Pingault V, Bondurand N, Kuhlbrodt K, Goerich DE, Prehu MO, Puliti A, Herbarth B, Hermans-Borgmeyer I, Legius E, Matthijs G, Amiel J, Lyonnet S, Ceccherini I, Romeo G, Smith JC, Read AP, Wegner M, Goossens M. SOX10 mutations in patients with Waardenburg–Hirschsprung disease. Nat Genet 1998; 18(2):171–173.
211. Touraine RL, Attie–Bitach T, Manceau E, Korsch E, Sarda P, Pingault V, Encharazavi F, Pelet A, Auge J, Nivelon-Chevallier A, Holschneider AM, Munnes M, Doerfler W, Goossens M, Munnich A, Vekemans M, Lyonnet S. Neurological phenotype in Waardenburg syndrome type 4 correlates with novel SOX 10 truncating mutations and expression in developing brain. Am J Hum Genet 2000; 66(5):1496–1503.
212. Puffenberger EG, Hosoda K, Washington SS, Nakao K, deWit D, Yanagisawa M, Chakravart A. A missense mutation of the endothelin-B receptor gene in multigenic Hirschsprung's disease. Cell 1994; 79(7):1257–1266.
213. Ziprkowski L, Krakowski A, Adam A, et al. Partial albinism and deaf-mutism due to a recessive sex-linked gene. Arch Dermatol 1962; 86:530–539.
214. Goodman RM, Yahav Y, Frand M, et al. A New white forelock (poliosis) syndrome with multiple congenital malformations in two sibs. Clin Genet 1980; 17:437–442.

215. Delleman JW, Hageman MJ. Ophthalmological findings in 34 patients with Waardenburg's syndrome. J Pediatr Ophthalmol Strabismus 1978; 15:341–345.
216. Arias S, Mota M. Current status of the ABO-Waardenburg syndrome type I linkage. Cytogenet Cell Genet 1978; 22:291–294.
217. Le Douarin N. The Neural Crest. Cambridge: Cambridge University Press, 1982:1–259.
218. Kaplan P, De Chaderevian JP. Piebaldism–Waardenburg syndrome: histopathologic evidence for a neural crest syndrome. Am J Med Genet 1988; 31:679–688.

23
Mitochondrial DNA and Eye Disease

INTRODUCTION

The study of mitochondrial DNA (mtDNA) abnormalities has intensified in the last 10 years and revolutionized our knowledge of a previously esoteric subject. Ophthalmologists were initially among the first physicians to express interest in this genetic topic because of the intriguing facts related to the genetic transmission of Leber hereditary neuroretinopathy (LHON). Ophthalmology continues to be in the forefront of mtDNA research due to several serious eye diseases that are associated with mtDNA mutations.

Recently, Land and associates (1) described the early history of the study of mitochondrial diseases. Luft and associates (2) published in 1962 the first reported case of a woman who suffered from severe hypermetabolism of nonthyroid origin associated with mitochondrial abnormality. Using the tool of testing the enzymatic activity of skeletal muscle mitochondria, which the same group developed (3), they demonstrated high ATPase activity in the mitochondria.

The investigation of mitochondrial disease continued using clinical, morphological, biochemical, and molecular genetic methods. Mitochondrial disease was eventually found to be more common than initially expected. Several studies in the last years indicate that the incidence of mitochondrial disease is at least one in 8000 of the population (1).

The most important function of mitochondria is the respiratory chain activity. Mitochondrial enzymes play a central role in oxidative phosphorylation and, in addition, are important in fatty acid oxidation, urea synthesis, calcium and hydrogen homeostasis, free radical defence, and cellular apoptosis (1).

A common symptom of mitochondrial disease is fatigue (1), A useful test for the cellular cause of this symptom is to test the level of lactate and pyruvic acid. Characteristically, mitochondrial disease will show an increased blood lactate/pyruvate ratio, an excessive exercise-related increase in lactate levels, and a slower than usual reduction of lactate levels following rest after exercise (1).

Mitochondrial diseases may be caused by mtDNA mutations but may also result from nuclear DNA mutations.

Mitochondrial DNA is circular in form and consists of 16,569 base pairs (about 16.6 kb). It is almost fully sequenced and has none or only a few noncoding bases without introns (4). The mtDNA encodes 13 proteins of the respiratory chain (RC) complexes, 2 ribosomal RNAs, and 22 transfer RNAs (5). Of the five respiratory chain complexes, mtDNA mutations are associated with defects in some cases RC complexes I, III, IV, or V, and in combined cases, while autosomal recessive inheritance is responsible for all cases of RC complex II, most cases of complex I, IV of childhood onset, and some cases of complex IV of late onset (5).

The genetic features of mitochondrial DNA transmission are unique and considerably differ from Mendelian genetics. Thorburn and Dahl, in their review of the subject (5), listed five major differences.

First, *maternal inheritance*: mtDNA is exclusively inherited from the mitochondria of maternal cytoplasm, or almost exclusively. A human cell contains about 1000 mitochondria. Each mitochondrion contains 5–10 mtDNA copies, so that each somatic cell may contain up to 10,000 mtDNA copies (5). However, these numbers are different within germinal cells. A mature oocyte carries approximately 100,000 mtDNA copies while a spermatozoon carries only 100 copies (6). Early in the process of embryogenesis the limited number of paternal mtDNA copies are eliminated, while the number of maternal DNA copies are multiplied.

Second, *heteroplasmy*: This indicates the phenomenon of a variable ratio of mutant to wild-type ("normal") mtDNA within the cell. The percentage of mutant mtDNA may vary from 1% to 99%, according to the disease and apording to the tissue. It may be 100% (homoplasmy), as often seen in LHON. In two recent studies, the variations in heteroplasmy in different tissues were large. Kaplanova et al. found a range of heteroplasmy, in LHON from 7% in the blood to 100% in hair follicles (7).

Shanske and colleagues studied five tissues in 22 families harboring the A3243G mutation (8). Generally, the highest proportion of mutant mtDNA was found in urinary sediment, the lowest in blood, and intermediate in fibroblasts and cheek mucosa. Hair roots differed markedly one from another (8).

Third, *threshold effect*: Usually, a narrow threshold occurs and is characteristic for each specific disease. Below a certain percentage of mutant mtDNA the mitochondrial function is normal. Above it, the function is greatly impaired.

Fourth, *mitochondrial bottleneck hypothesis*: This hypothesis assumes that in the early development of the oocyte the number of mtDNA is greatly reduced or that only a few copies serve as a template for the later multiplication of these copies (5). Poulton and colleagues estimated this number as 1–5 (9).

Fifth, *selection*: The question of physiological selection of oocytes with or without certain mutations remains, by now, open (5). The possibility was brought up because in maternal inheritance the expected number of mutations is higher than the occurring number.

Pathogenic mtDNA mutations occur in at least one out of 8000 individuals (10). The risk factors and disease recurrence figures are not well known. Most of the mutations are point mutations in a single base pair, but multiple deletions of mtDNA occur in some diseases such as progressive external ophthalmoplegia (PEO) (11). The incidence of mtDNA deletion disorders does not increase with maternal age (10) and most are assumed to result from a nuclear gene defect (11).

Table 1 presents a list of named entities associated with eye abnormalities and mitochondrial DNA mutations.

Table 1 Disorders with Eye Abnormalities Associated with DNA Mutations

Acronym	Disorder	Mutations	Mutation load	Main ocular manifestations	Main systemic manifestations
LHON	Leber hereditary optic neuropathy	G11778A T14484C G 3460A +Rare mutations	Usually homoplasmy in main tissues	Optic neuropathy, Optic atrophy	Few
NARP	Neurogenic muscle weakness Ataxia Retinitis pigmentosa	T8993G T8993C	60–80% Severe: 80–90%	Retinal dystrophy Cone or cone-rod dystrophy	Mild mental retardation Muscle weakness
MILS	Maternally inherited Leigh disease	T8993G T8993C	More than 90%	RPE dystrophy Optic atrophy	Severe psychomotor delay: Seizures Fatal
MELAS	Mitochondrial encephalopathy Lactic acidosis Stroke-like episodes	A3243G (80%) A3271G(10%) G13513A G12147A	Heteroplasmy-severity association	Maculopathy Cone–rod dystrophy Hemianopsia	Seizures Recurrent strokes Deafness Ataxia Mental retardation
MIDD	Maternally inherited diabetes and deafness	A3243G (common) Several others (rare)	Heteroplasmy-severity association	Pattern maculopathy Pigmentary retinopathy	NIDDM (usually) IDDM (uncommon) Deafness Skeletal myopathy Low body weight
MERRF	Myoclonic epilepsy Ragged red fibers	A8344G (80%) T8356C G8363A	Heteroplasmy-severity association	Optic atrophy Mild pigmentary retinopathy	Myoclonus Epilepsy Ataxia
KSS	Kearns–Sayre syndrome	Single large DNA deletion (most common)		Pigmentary retinopathy Strabismus ptosis	Ataxia High CSF protein Heart conduction block
CPEO	Chronic progressive Extraocular ophthalmoplegia	Duplications Multiple deletions Rearrangements		Ptosis Strabismus Ophthalmoplegia	Mild systemic abnormalities

THE CLINICAL AND GENETIC TYPES OF MITOCHONDRIAL DNA DISEASES

Description

The eyes are often, but not always, affected in mitochondrial diseases. Several types of ocular manifestations may occur (12):

- Visual loss may be acute, as in LHON, or gradual as in NARP; the loss is bilateral but may affect each eye separately.
- Visual field loss may occur rapidly, as in optic neuropathy, or slowly, as in retinal dystrophies.
- Different ocular motility abnormalities are sometimes the hallmark of the disease.
- Bilateral ptosis may be manifested.

Systemic abnormalities associated with mtDNA mutations vary with the various diseases and with the mutation load (ratio of mutant to wild-type DNA).

Diagnosis of the specific disease can be achieved by screening for mutations of the blood DNA, muscle biopsy, blood lactate and creatine levels, and/or MRI studies.

Leber Hereditary Optic Neurorchinopathy

LHON is the most important ocular disease associated with mitochondrial mutations. It is extensively discussed in Chapter 17, which deals with inherited diseases of the optic nerve. Three main mutations associated with LHON are mutations in complex I subunits in the ATPase-6 gene (13). In mutated cells, reactive oxygen species (ROS) are formed (13), meaning that free radicals production is increased. The frequency of the various mutations is characteristic and different in specific populations. The relative frequency of the main mutations of LHON was established in Australia. Of the patients screened for LHON the G11778A mutation was detected in 6.6%, the T14484C mutation in 5.76%, and the G3460A mutation in 0.29% (14).

NARP and Maternally Inherited Leigh Syndrome

In 1990, Holt and associates (15) reported "a new mitochondrial disease", that was later termed NARP. Four members of one family suffered from several abnormalities. The clinical findings included variable developmental delay, mental retardation of mild to moderate degree, occasional seizures, ataxia, proximal neurogenic muscle weakness, and sensory neuropathy. The vision was affected by a retinal dystrophy diagnosed as retinitis pigmentosa (15). The term NARP was introduced to highlight the major signs of the syndrome: Neurogenic muscle weakness, Ataxia, Retinitis Pigmentosa (16). The mutation was identified as a point mutation at nucleotide 8993 with a T to G substitution (T8993G) that replaced a highly conserved amino acid leucine by arginine in the mitochondrial ATP 6 enzyme gene (15–17). This mutation resulting in a Leu156Arg substitution in the MTATP6 gene yields impaired oxidative phosphorylation and results in increase of intracellular free radical production (18).

A remarkable finding of the syndrome was the finding of variable heteroplasmy. The mutation load ranged in the various cells from less than 10% to close to 100%. The ratio of the mutant DNA to all mtDNA usually determines the clinical manifestation. If this "mutant load" is less than 60%, the individual is normal without any clinical manifestation. A mutant load of 60–80% is associated with

NARP, 80–90% with NARP or Leigh disease, and above 90% with Leigh disease. Exceptions may occur. In one family, five out of eight affected members had a mutant load of more than 90% but manifested NARP instead of Leigh disease. In most cases the mutation is maternally inherited but a de novo mutation has been also reported (19). A boy with Leigh disease had a mutant load of 95%. His mother and her sister had normal mtDNA.

Leigh disease is now usually called maternally inherited Leigh syndrome (MILS). The clinical course of MILS is severe, rapid, fulminating, and leads to early death in the first year of life. The child is born with hypotonia, severe psychomotor delay up to dementia, persistent lactic acidosis, seizures, and ataxia, and death occurs in the first or second year of life (20). Brain stem and respiratory abnormalities may occur (21). Chowers and associates (22) described a family with NARP and claimed that the retinal dystrophy of NARP affects primarily the cones either as cone dystrophy or as cone–rod dystrophy. They pointed out that a review of the literature points to a mainly cone abnormality in NARP rather than a classic rod–cone dystrophy as in retinitis pigmentosa (22).

In some cases NARP is associated with a T8993C mutation in place of the T8993G mutation (23). Sciacco et al. (23) stressed the variability of the phenotype in this mutation. Variable severity of the clinical manifestation of episodes of loss of consciousness, hypotonia, muscle weakness, ataxia, hypoacusia, and retinal dystrophy occurred in the same family (23). Some members had no clinical signs, in spite of carrying a high mutant load (23).

MELAS

The term MELAS is used for a syndrome that involves Mitochondrial Encephalopathy Lactic Acidosis and Stroke-like episodes. The most common mutation causing MELAS is a point mutation adenine to guanine at position 3243 (24). Eighty percent of all MELAS patients carry this A3243G mutations, 10% carry the A3271G mutation, and the rest carry other mutations (25). The point mutation is located in subunit III of cytochrome C oxidase (13). It causes enhanced ROS but no biochemical defects (13). The mutated gene is the tRNALeu (UUR) gene (26) Other mutations associated with MELAS were also reported. G > A transition at nt 13513 was associated with MELAS when the mutant load was low and with MERFF when the mutant load was high (27). One patient had LHON. G12147A mutation in the tRNA (His) gene was identified in a young man with MELAS and turned into a MELAS/MERFF phenotype later on (28). A14693G mutation may be related to existence of diabetes mellitus in patients with MELAS (29).

Patients with the common MELAS 3243 mutation vary in their phenotypic expressivity, mainly from differences in heteroplasmy (proportion of mutant mtDNA), but other genetic components may also be important (30). Neurological abnormalities are the most common manifestation. In a study of 14 patients with MELAS Morgan–Hughes et al. (30) found seizures and recurrent strokes in six, encephalopathy with deafness, ataxia, and dementia in four, progressive external ophthalmoplegia in two, and limb weakness in two (30). In a study of MELAS and related mitochondrial disorders in Korea, Chae and associates (31) found that each affected person had three or more of the following signs: recurrent stroke-like episodes, mental retardation, sensorineural hearing loss, relatives with mitochondrial disease or hyperlacticacidemia. In some cases, idiopathic cardiomyopathy, skeletal myopathy, renal disease, or diabetes mellitus were detected

(31). The brain lesions may be slowly progressive. Headache is usually the first symptom followed by hemianopsia, psychosis, and aphasia, with a later occurrence of epileptic seizures (32). Follow-up by MRI revealed the spread of the stroke-like lesion evolving over a few weeks (32).

The first report on the ocular manifestations of MELAS by Kuchle and associates was published in 1990 (33). The author described a 34-year-old patient with mitochondrial encephalomyopathy. The ocular abnormalities included homonymous hemianopsia, atypical retinitis pigmentosa, a markedly reduced ERG, myopia, and nuclear cataract (33). Eight of 14 patients with MELAS had atypical retinitis pigmentosa (24), and many of the reported patients manifested it (26). The ERG presents reduced cone and rod amplitudes but nyctalopia is not one of the symptoms (25). Possibly more common is a maculopathy manifested by macular pigmentation (25,26,34). This is usually slowly progressive and may show the typical changes of "geographic atrophy of the macula" (25).

Diabetes mellitus occasionally found in MELAS was reported to be much more common in patients who also have macular and paramacular RPE atrophy and hyperpigmentation (34).

The diagnosis of MELAS can be confirmed by identifying the A3243G mutation in the peripheral blood or in hair roots. However, the most reliable test is identification of the mutation in urinary epithelial cells (8,35).

Another method of investigation is to detect the increased lactate level in the brain using MRI. Higher levels of ventricular lactate are associated with more severe neurologic impairment (36).

A pathological study of a patient with MELAS revealed structurally abnormal, enlarged mitochondria in the iris, cornea, lens epithelium, and ciliary epithelium (26). Ragged-red fibers were seen in rectus muscles. Outer segments were degenerated in the macula and RPE dystrophy in the form of hyperpigmentation or atrophy was extensive. Optic atrophy and a PC cataract were also noted (26).

Maternally Inherited Diabetes and Deafness

The acronym MIDD stands, for maternally inherited diabetes and deafness. In its classic form, MIDD is caused by the same mitochondrial point mutation as MELAS, the A3243G mutation in the gene encoding tRNA-Leu. This gene encodes the mitochondrial transfer RNA for leucine (UUR) and contains mtDNA nucleotides from 3230 to 3304 (37). The gene is also called MTTL1. The same A3243G mutation is found in cases of MELAS, in many cases of MIDD, and sometimes in other disorders. However, the phenotype of MIDD is different from that of MELAS even in cases of exactly the same point mutation at position 3243. The reason for such a clinical difference is not known.

Guillausseau et al. reported the results of a multicenter study regarding the clinical presentation of MIDD (38). Onset is usually at a young age; the body weight is low or normal but never overweight and 73% have a family history of diabetes mellitus (DM). At onset, 87% had noninsulin dependent DM but with the years this figure dropped to 46%. Eighty-six percent showed pattern maculopathy with lines of pigmentation. Less common were skeletal myopathy (43%), neuropsychiatric abnormalities (18%), and renal disease (28%) (38). The same group of investigators demonstrated that the vast majority (83%) had type 2 DM (T2D) and only 17% had type 1 DM (T1D) (39). They suggested that the different phenotypes, MIDD1 (associated with T1D) and MIDD2 (associated with T2D), may be related to the severity of the mitochondrial disease or to additional genetic factors (39). The pathogenesis of diabetes in MIDD has not been established and it is not clear whether a difference in pathogenesis exists between MIDD and MELAS (40). MELAS uncommonly may also manifest diabetes.

It was claimed that in MIDD, the prevalence of diabetic retinopathy and of diabetic cataract is reduced (41), but this claim has not been confirmed. Holmes–Walker and colleagues (41) proposed that the reduced glucose metabolism by polyol pathway "protects" the eye from these two complications. However, in contrast, abnormal glucose tolerance increases expression of pigmentary retinopathy (41). In one study, only 6% of MIDD patients manifested diabetic retinopathy while 15% of nonmaternally inherited DM type 2 manifested it (42).

Massin and associates, in a study of 29 families with a guanine for adenine substitution at nt 3243, found that 85% of MIDD patients presented a pattern dystrophy of the macula (42). A nonuniform damage to the retina in MIDD with some areas much more affected than other areas was also shown in a study using multifocal ERG and autofluorescence of the retina (43).

A "de novo" case of MIDD from A3243G mutation has been reported in a girl whose mother and mother's brothers had normal mtDNA, thus supporting the theory mentioned above of a genetic "bottleneck" (44).

MIDD may be associated with other mtDNA mutations, when the phenotype is MIDD but the test for 3243 mutation is negative. Homoplasmic mutations, A8381G, G1888A, and T4216C were associated with different cases of MIDD (45).

Another study found that the T16189C mutation had a significant association with type 2 diabetes (46). The T14709C mutation caused MIDD that caused a similar severity of diabetes but milder RPE changes in the macular area (47). In one case, MIDD was associated with a 7 kb heteroplasmic deletion of the mitochondrial genome (48). The patient also had parotitis, maculopathy, and cataract.

Myoclonic Epilepsy and Ragged Red Fibers Syndrome

The acronym MERRF stands for myoclonic epilepsy and ragged red fibers syndrome. It is usually caused by an A8344G mutation in the gene encoding mitochondrial transfer RNA for lysine (49). The gene, also named MTTK, contains mt nucleotides 8295–8364 (37).

MERRF is one of the more common mitochondrial encephalomyopathies (49). The disease is usually severe. The more common findings are myoclonus, epilepsy, ataxia, and ragged-red fibers (determined by muscle biopsy). The less common abnormalities include hearing loss, exercise intolerance, peripheral neuropathy, optic atrophy, lactic acidosis, and dementia (49). MERRF is much less common than MELAS. Its prevalence is one-quarter that of MELAS in the United Kingdom and less than this in Finland (50). As in MELAS, higher levels of intracranial ventricular lactate are associated with more severe neurological impairment (36).

Ocular abnormalities include a mild retinal pigmentary disorder and optic neuropathy (51). Optic atrophy may occur later. The mitochondrial myopathy of extraocular muscles may be similar in MERRF, in MELAS, and in Kearns–Sayre syndrome (KSS) (52,53). Light microscopy shows granular and vesicular spots in the muscle fibers with endomysial fibrosis (52). Electron microscopy shows accumulation of abnormal enlarged mitochondria with lipid vacuoles and extensive loss of myofibrils (52). Abnormal mitochondria were also found throughout RPE cells and corneal endothelium. Ultrastructural abnormalities of the mitochondria included swelling, tubular cristae, or parallel rows of elongated cristae or "whorled" cristae (53).

The most common mutation associated with MERRF has been established as A8344G encoding mitochondrial mtRNA-Lys. It is present in 80–90% of MERRF patients (49). Most of the rest carry one of two other mutations within the tRNA-Lys gene, T8356C, or G8363A (49). Other, probably very rare, mutations associate with MERRF were reported as G8361A (49) (within the tRNA-Lys gene) and as G611A (54) (within the gene encoding transfer RNA for phenylaianine). Single reports related to A8344G mutation (within tRNA-Lys gene) associated with severe and fatal infantile cardiomyopathy (55), to G12147A mutation (within tRNA-His gene) associated with a combined MELAS/MERRF phenotype (28), and to G3255A mutation [within tRNA-Leu (UUR) gene] associated with a combined MERRF/KSS phenotype (56).

Van Goethem and associates (57) reported a patient with a homozygous autosomal recessive missense mutation in the gene encoding polymerase gamma associated with mtDNA function. This nuclear mutation is often associated with progressive external ophthalmoplegia (see later).

KSS and Chronic Progressive Extraocular Ophthalmoplegia

Mitochondrial disorders may involve the extraocular muscles and cause paresis or palsy of these muscles. Several clinical entities are known. KSS and chronic progressive extraocular ophthalmoplegia (CPEO) are the two most common disorders. In contrast to the point mutations that were described above in this chapter, this whole group of disorders is associated with larger deletions, duplications, or multiplications of the mtDNA.

KSS has an early onset in life, before the age of 15 years (26) or before the age of 20 years (58). CPEO occurs in adulthood (26).

The hallmark of the clinical manifestation of CPEO is ptosis and external ophthalmoplegia (26,59). The onset of the disorder starts with strabismus or ptosis or both and progresses slowly (59). In one study of four patients with CPEO, age of onset was seven years, 27, 38 and 44 years (59). In CPEO paresis or palsy of these muscles is often the only finding. In some cases a pigmentary retinopathy also exists (26). CPEO is considered a heterogenous group of disorders characterized by chronic, progressive, bilateral, and usually symmetric ocular motility deficits and ptosis (60). Like KSS and MELAS, CPEO is considered one of the disorders of mitochondrial encephalopathies (31). KSS has been defined as an ultimately fatal mitochondrial disorder characterized by PEO, pigmentary retinopathy, and at least one of the following: ataxia, high CSF protein content, and cardiac conduction block (58). A diffuse white matter disease can be detected in brain imaging and mental retardation or sensorineural hearing loss may occur (26).

The variability of the clinical manifestation of CPEO and KSS is considerable. In addition, different terms have been used for entities with specific clinical findings. Pearson's syndrome (PS) is the term used for an entity that includes CPEO and a severe, fatal disorder of the hematopoietic system, sideroblastic anemia (61). SANDO is the acronym for the syndrome of Sensory Ataxic Neuropathy Dysarthria and Ophthalmoparesis (62).

Respiratory complex I defects were more often associated with dilated cardiomyopathy than with hypertrophic cardiomyopathy (63).

The ocular manifestations of CPEO, KSS, and PS, in addition to the muscle defects, are various. The characteristic retinal manifestation of KSS is a pigmentary retinopathy of the salt and pepper variant, and that of CPEO is a milder defect at the RPE level (51). The pigmentary retinopathy that eventually progresses to retinitis pigmentosa involves almost all KSS patients and about half of CPEO patients. In both KSS and CPEO the muscle defect starts with strabismus or ptosis and usually progresses to total or almost total ophthalmoplegia in ten years or so. The cornea may be affected. A boy was reported who manifested corneal edema with photophobia and tearing as the presenting symptom of KSS (64). Lagophthalmus, recurrent conjunctivitis, and keratitis were also reported as part of the KSS (65). In one reported case, exposure keratitis necessitated bilateral corneal grafts (65).

KSS, CPEO, and allied disorders are caused by large deletions, duplications, or rearrangement of mitochondrial DNA (14). The three clinical conditions, KSS, CPEO, and PS, are commonly associated with single large deletions of mtDNA (58,61,66). Shanske and associates (61) described a mother with CPEO whose son suffered from PS. Both had an identical single deletion of 5355 bp in mtDNA. This family emphasizes the fact that the type of mtDNA mutation is not the only factor to establish the clinical entity. Other factors are the mutant load (degree of heteroplasmy), age of onset, and regulatory nuclear genes.

Multiple deletions of mitochondrial DNA in postmitotic tissues may also be associated with progressive external ophthalmoplegia. Von Goethem and colleagues suggested that these multiple deletions are the result of a nuclear gene defect, and reviewed four such genes with identified mutations proposed to be the cause of the mtDNA mutations (11).

Mitochondrial DNA duplications were also identified in patients with KSS, PS, and CPEO and in encephalopathy with external ophthalmoplegia (67).

Clinical KSS has been reported in a patient with a point mutation, G3249A mtDNA mutation in transfer RNA-Leu gene (68). The patient suffered from all the characteristic findings of KSS including external ophthalmoplegia, ptosis, muscle wasting, muscle weakness, difficulty in swallowing, and dystrophic features in the cornea and in the retina (68).

MANAGEMENT

Medical Treatment

No medication is available to cure any one of the mitochondrial disorders. However, several clinical trials claim some efficiency of treatment with various medications. Suzuki and associates treated MIDD patients with daily oral administration of 150 mg of CoQ10 for three years and claimed that it prevented progression of hearing loss and improved blood lactate levels after exercise (69). It had no effect on diabetes or its complications. The authors speculated that CoQ10 is effective due to its antioxidant activities. Berbel-Garcia et al. (70) found coenzyme Q10 efficient in improving lactic acidosis and serum creatine kinase levels in a MELAS patient. However, larger studies did not confirm any clinical improvement of CoQ10 administration (70). Komura and associates treated five patients with various mitochondrial encephalomyopathies by creatine supplementation for nine months to five years and claimed improvement in muscle performance (71). The authors attributed this improvement to the improved aerobic oxidative function of the mitochondria. Kubota et al. (72) treated a MELAS patient with prednisolone, glycerol, and edalavone. The authors claimed that addition of L-arginine during the acute phase of seizures improved the clinical findings and the magnetic resonance spectroscopy abnormality (72).

Experimental studies indicated that antioxidants may play a role in preventing damage of NARP or MILS (18), as increased free radical production occurs due to impaired oxidative phosphorylation (18). In another study, yeast tRNA derivatives were imported into human mitochondria taken from a patient with MERRF associated with A8344G mtDNA tRNA(Lys) mutation (73). The researchers showed that these mtRNAs are able to be expressed, can participate in mitochondrial translation and thus rescue the mitochondrial DNA mutation in cultured human cells (73).

Surgical Treatment

Surgery can be performed to ameliorate the condition of ophthalmoplegia for both strabismus and ptosis. Recession of a rectus muscle has a lower effectiveness than resection and Sorkin et al. advised to perform resections of rectus muscles only in CPEO (74). Burnstine and Putterman advised performing "upper blepharoplasty" in all cases of myopathic blepharoptosis (75). In this operation, they removed only excess skin and orbicularis fibers between eyelid margin and eyebrow in patients with ptosis without concomitant lagophthalmus and without keratopathy (75). Other methods of ptosis surgery were also advised. MIDD patients had their hearing successfully rehabilitated by a cochlear implant (76).

Genetic Counseling

Genetic counseling is based on maternal transmission of the disease. Affected or unaffected males cannot transmit the mutation. Affected females will often transmit the mutation (not always) but not necessarily transmit the disorder to their children. The transmission of the disorder and its severity depend on the mutation and the transmitted mutant load. A mutation at nt8993 may cause NARP or Leigh disease or be asymptomatic, as explained above. The T8993G mutation leads to more severe disease than the T8993C mutation (77). The clinical severity may also be predicted from the mutant load which, for 8993 mutations, is determined in fetal life, does not change during adulthood, and is similar in all tissues (77).

The authors suggested five scores for the phenotype: first, asymptomatic adult; second, an asymptomatic child who will later turn symptomatic; third, mild NARP; fourth, severe NARP; and fifth, Leigh disease. The resulting score depends on the mutant load, with less than 60% asymptomatic and more than 90% Leigh disease. In contrast, most cases of mitochondrial external ophthalmoplegias are sporadic and most of the large deletions or duplications are not transmitted. It was estimated that only one of 24 affected women will have a clinically affected child (66).

Prenatal Diagnosis

Harding and colleagues published in 1992 the first description of prenatal diagnosis for a mitochondrial DNA disease (78). Since then, reports of prenatal diagnosis using chorionic villus sampling or amniotic cell analyses were published for almost all mitochondrial disorders, including NARP and Leigh disease, MELAS, MERRF, LHON, and KSS/CPEO (5). It was found to be quite reliable for nt8993 mutations and less reliable for other mutations (77,79). The problem remains with mutant loads of 60–80% leading to NARP of different severity (79). It is even more complicated in other disorders. In prenatal diagnosis of MELAS, a similar mutant load of A3243G was found in two embryos (80). One of them developed severe MELAS while the other was initially asymptomatic and later developed mild MELAS (80).

Dahl and associates analyzed the mutant load in prenatal samples of nt8993 mutations and showed that there is no substantial tissue variation and that any sample represents the mutant load in other fetal tissue (81). This is probably the major reason for the reasonably good results obtained in prenatal diagnosis of NARP, in contrast to MELAS where the blood levels of the mutant load may be misleading (82).

Preimplantation genetic diagnosis coupled with in vitro fertilization may be the future solution for prevention of mitochondrial diseases. Embryos with very low, preferably zero, mutant load can be selected for implantation (5). Two other experimental approaches, still under investigation, are associated with micromanipulation of the ovum (5). The transfer of mother's cellular nucleus into a donor oocyte that has no disease-bearing mitochondrial mutation and transfer (dilution) of a donor cytoplasm are both potentially feasible approaches to prevention.

REFERENCES

1. Land JM, Morgan-Hughes JA, Hargreaves I, Heales IJ. Mitochondria disease: a historical biochemical and London perspective. Neurochem Res 2004; 29(3):483–491.
2. Luft R, Ikkos D, Palmieri G, et al. A case of severe hypermetabolism of non-thyroid origin with a defect in the maintanance of mitochondria respiratory control: a correlated clinical, biochemical and morphological study. J Clin Invest 1962; 41:1776–1804.
3. Ernster L, Ikkos D, Luft R. Enzymatic activities of human skeletal muscle mitochondria: a tool in clinical metabolic research. Nature 1959; 184:1851–1854.
4. Anderson S, Bankier AT, Barrell BG, et al. Sequence and organization of the human mitochondrial genome. Nature 1981; 290:457–465.
5. Thorburn DR, Dahl HH. Mitochondrial disorders: genetics counseling, prenatal diagnosis and reproductive options. Am J Med Genet 2001; 106(1):102–114.
6. Jansen RP. Germline passage of mitochondria: quantitative consideration and possible embryological sequelae. Hum Reprod 2000; 15(suppl 2):112–128.
7. Kaplanova W, Zeman J Hansikova H, et al. Segregation pattern and biochemical effect of the G3460A mt mutation in 27 members of LHON family. J Neurol Sci 2004; 223(2):149–155.
8. Shanske S, Pancrudo J, Kaufmann P, et al. Varying loads of the mitochondrial DNA A3243G mutation in different tissues: implications for diagnosis. Am J Med Genet 2004; 130A(2):134.
9. Poulton J, Macaulay V, Marchington DR. Mitochondrial genetics '98: is the bottleneck cracked? Am J Hum Genet 1998; 62:752–757.
10. Chinnery PF, Dimauro S, Shanske S, et al. Risk of developing a mitochondrial DNA deletion disorder. Lancet 2004; 364(9434):592–596.
11. Van Goethem G, Martin JJ, Van Broeckhoven C. Progressive external ophthalmoplegia characterized by multiple deletions of mitochondrial DNA: unraveling the pathogenesis of human mtDNA instability and the initiation of a genetic classification. Neuromolecular Med 2003; 3(3):129–146.
12. Mojon D. Eye diseases in mitochondrial encephalomyopathies. Ther Umsch 2001; 58(1):49–55.
13. Lenaz G, Baracca A, Carelli V, et al. Bioenergetics of mitochondrial diseases associated with mtDNA mutations. Biochim Biophys Acta 2004; 1658(1–2):89–94.

14. Marotta R, Chin J, Quigley A, et al. Diagnostic screening of mitochondrial DNA mutations in Australian adults 1990–2001. Intern Med J 2004; 34(1–2):10–19.
15. Holt IJ, Harding AE, Petty RKH, Morgan-Hughes JA. A new mitochondrial DNA heteroplasmy. Am J Hum Genet 1990; 46(3):428–433.
16. Ortiz RG, Newman NJ, Shoffner JM, et al. Variable retinal neurologic manifestations in patients harboring the mitochondrial DNA 8993 mutation. AO 1993; 111:1525–1530.
17. Tsao CY, Mendell JR, Bartholomew D. High mitochondrial DNA T8993G mutation (>90%) without typical features of Leigh's and NARP syndromes. J Child Neurol 2001; 16(7):533–5353.
18. Mattiazzi M, Vijayvergiya C, Gajewski CD, et al. The mtDNA T8993G (NARP) mutation results in an impairment of oxidative phosphorylation that can be improved by antioxidants. Hum Mol Genet 2004; 13(8):869–879.
19. White SL, Shanske S, Biros I, et al. Two cases of prenatal analysis for the pathogenetic T to G substitution at nucleotide 8993 in mitochondrial DNA. Prenat Diagn 1999; 19: 1165–1168.
20. Playan A, Solano-Palacios A, Gonzalez de LaRosa JB, et al. Leigh syndrome resulting from a de novo mitochondrial DNA mutation (T8993G). Rev Neurol 2002; 34(12): 1124–1126.
21. Hayashi N, Geraghty MT, Green WR. Ocular histopathologic study of a patient with the T8993-G point mutation in Leigh's syndrome. Ophthalmology 2000; 107:1397–1402.
22. Chowers I, Lerman-Sagie T, Elpeleg ON, Sha'ag A, Merin S. Cone and rod dysfunction in the NARP syndrome. Brit J Ophthalmol 1999; 83:190–193.
23. Sciacco M, Prelle A, D'adda E, et al. Familial mtDNA T8993C transition causing both the NARP and the MILS phenotype in the same generation (Letter). J Neurol 2003; 250:1998–1500.
24. Sue CM, Mitchell P, Crimmins DS, et al. Pigmentary retinopathy associated with the mitochondrial DNA 3242 point mutation. Neurology 1997; 49:1013–1017.
25. Latkany R, Ciulia TA, Cacchillo PF, Malkoff D. Mitochondrial maculopathy: geographic atrophy of the macula in the MELAS associated A to G 3243 mitochondrial DNA point mutation. Am J Ophthalmol 1999; 128:112–114.
26. Rumelt V, Folberg R, lonasescu V. Ocular pathology of Melas syndrome with mitochondrial DNA nucleotide 3243 point mutation. Ophthalmology 1993; 100:1757–1766.
27. Pulkes T, Eunson L, Patterson V, et al. The mt DNA G13513A transition in NDS is associated with LHON/MELAS overlap syndrome and may be a frequent cause of MELAS. Ann Neurol 2000; 47(6):841.
28. Melone MA, Tessa A, Petrini S, et al. Revelation of a new mitochondrial DNA mutation (G12147A) in a MELAS/MERRF phenotype. Arch Neurol 2004; 61(2):269–272.
29. Tzen CY, Thajeb P, Wu TY, Chen, SC. MELAS with point mutations involving tRNA-Leu (A3243G) and tRNAGlu (A14693G). Muscle Nerve 2003; 28(5):575–581.
30. Morgan-Hughes JA, Sweeney MG, Cooper JM, et al. Mitochondrial DNA (mtDNA) disease: correlation of genotype to phenotype. Biochim Biophys Acta 1995; 1271: 135–140.
31. Chae JH, Hwang H, Lim BL, et al. Clinical features of A3243G mitochondrial tRNA mutation. Brain Dev 2004; 26(7):459–462.
32. Iizuka T, Sakai F, Kan S, Suzuki N. Slowly progressive spread of the stroke-like lesions in MELAS. Neurology 2003; 61(9):1238–1244.
33. Kuchle M, Brenner PM, Englehardt A, Naumann GO. Ocular changes in MELAS syndrome. Klin Monatsbl Augenheilkd 1990; 197:258–264.
34. Latvada T, Mustonen E, Uusitalo R, Majamaa K. Pigmentary retinopathy in patients with the MELAS mutation 3243A→G in mitochondrial DNA. Graefes Arch Clin Exp Ophthalmol 2002; 240(10):795–801.
35. McDonnell MT, Schaefer AM, Blakely EL, et al. Noninvasive diagnosis of the 3243A>G mitochondrial DNA mutation using urinary epithelial cells. Eur J Hum Genet 2004; 12(9):778–781.

36. Kaufmann P, Shungu DC, Sano MC, et al. Cerebral lactic acidosis correlates with neurological impairment in MELAS. Neurology 2004; 62(8):1297–1302.
37. Online Mendelian Inheritance in Man OMIM (IM) McKusick-Nathans Institute for Genetic Medicine, Johns Hopkins University, Baltimore MD and National Center for Biotechnology Information, National Library of Medicine, Bethesda MD, 2000. URL: http://www.ncbi.nlm.nih.gov/omim/.
38. Guillausseau PJ, Massin P, Dubois-Laforgue D, et al. Maternally inherited diabetes and deafness: a multicenter study. Ann Intern Med 2001; 134(9 pt 1):777–779.
39. Guillausseau PJ, Dubois-Laforgue D, Massin P, et al. Heterogeneity of diabetes phenotype in patients with 3243 bp mutation of mitochondrial DNA. Diabetes Metab 2004; 30(2):181–186.
40. Becker R, Laube H, Lim T, Damian MS. Insulin resistance in patients with mitochondrial tRNA (Leu (UUR)) gene mutation at position 3243. Exp Clin Endocrinol Diabetes 2002; 110(6):291–297.
41. Holmes-Walker DJ, Mitchell P, Boyages SC. Does mitochondrial genome mutation in subjects with MIDD decrease seventy of diabetic retinopathy. Diabet Med 1996; 15(11):946–952.
42. Massin P, Virally-Monod V, Vialettes B, et al. Prevalence of macular pattern dystrophy in MIDD. Ophthalmology 1999; 106(9):1821–1827.
43. Bellman C, Neveu MM, Scholl HP, et al. Localized retinal electrophysiological and fundus autofluorescent imaging abnormalities in maternal inherited diabetes and deafness. Invest Ophthalmol Vis Sci 2004; 45(7):2355–2360.
44. Maassen JA, Biberoglu S, t'Hart LM, et al. A case of a de novo A3243G mutation in mitochondrial DNA in a patient with diabetes and deafness. Arch Physiol Biochem 2002; 110(3):186–188.
45. Perucca-Lostanlen D, Narbonne H, Hernandez JB, et al. Mitochondrial DNA variations in patients with MIDD syndrome. Biochem Biophys Res Commun 2000; 277(3) 771–775.
46. Poulton J, Luan J, Macaulay V, et al. Type 2 diabetes is associated with a common mitochondrial variant: evidence from a population-based case-control study. Hum Mol Genet 2002; 11(13):1581–1583.
47. Vialettes BH, Paquis-Flucklinger V, Pelissier JF, et al. Phenotypic expression of diabetes secondary to a T14709C mutation of mitochondrial DNA. Comparison with MIDD syndrome (A3243G mutation). Diabetes Care 1997; 20:1731–1737.
48. Souied EH, Sales M-J, Soubrane G, et al. Macular dystrophy, diabetes and deafness associated with a large mitochondrial DNA deletion. Am J Ophthalmol 1998; 125:100–103.
49. Rossmanith W, Raffelsberger T, Roka J, et al. The expanding mutational spectrum of MERRF substitution G8361A in the mitochondrial tRNALys gene. Ann Neurol 2003; 54(6):820–823.
50. Remes AM, Karppa M, Rusanen H, et al. Epidemiology of the mtDNA 8344 A > G mutation for the myoclonus epilepsy and ragged red fibers (MERRF) syndrome. J Neurol Neurosurg Psychiatr 2003; 74:1158–1159.
51. Isashiki Y, Nakagawa M, Ohba N, et al. Retinal manifestations in mitochondrial diseases associated with mitochondrial DNA mutation. Acta Ophthalmol Scand 1998; 76(1):6–13.
52. Takeda S, Ohama E, Ikuta F. Involvement of extraocular muscle in mitochondrial encephalomyopathy. Acta Neuropathol (Berl) 1990; 80(2):118–122.
53. Chang TS, Johns DR, Walker D, et al. Ocular clinicopathologic study of the mitochondrial encephalomyopathy overlap syndrome. Arch Ophthalmol 1993; 111:1254–1262.
54. Mancuso M, Filosto M, Mootha VK, et al. A novel mitochondrial tRNAPhe mutation causes MERRF syndrome. Neurology 2004; 62(11):2119–2121.
55. Vallance HD, Jeven G, Wallace DC, Brown MD. A case of sporadic histiocytoid cardiomyopathy caused by the A8344G (MERRF) mitochondrial DNA mutation. Pediatr Cardiol 2004; 25(5):538–540.

56. Nishigaki Y, Tadesse S, Bonilla E, et al. A novel mitochondrial tRNA (Leu(UUR)) mutation in a patient with features of MERRF and Kearns-Sayre syndrome. Neuromuscul Disord 2003; 13(4):334–340.
57. Van Goethem G, Mercelis R, Lofgren A, et al. Patient homozygous for a recessive POLG mutation presents with features of MERRF. Neurology 2003; 61(12):1811–1813.
58. Ashizawa T, Subramony SH. What is Kearns-Sayre syndrome after all? Arch Neurol 2001; 58(7):1053–1054.
59. Sommer F, Fotzsch R, Pillunat LE, Wollensak G. Chronisch progressive externe ophthalmoplegie (CPEO)-diagnostische und therapeutische probleme. Klin Monatsbl Augenheilkd 2003; 220:315–319.
60. Lee AG, Brazis PW. Chronic progressive external ophthalmoplegia. Curr Neurol Neurosci Rep 2002; 2(5):413–417.
61. Shanske S, Tank Y, Hitano M, et al. Identical mitochondrial DNA deletion in a woman with ocular myopathy and in her son with Pearson syndrome. Am J Hum Genet 2002; 71(3):679–683.
62. Okun MS, Bhatti MT. SANDO: another presentation of mitochondrial disease. Am J Ophthalmol 2004; 137(5):951–953.
63. Marin-Garcia J, Goldenthai MJ, Filiano JJ. Cardiomyopathy associated with neurologic disorders and mitochondrial phenotype. J Child Neurol 2002; 17(10):759–765.
64. Boonstra F, Claerhout I, Hoi F, et al. Corneal decompensation in a boy with Kearns-Sayne syndrome. Ophthalmic Genet 2002; 23(4):247–251.
65. Schmitz K, Lins H, Behrens-Baumann W. Bilateral spontaneous corneal perforation associated with complete external ophthalmoplegia in mitochondrial myopathy (Kearns-Sayre syndrome). Cornea 2003; 22(3):267–270.
66. Chinnery PF, DiMauro S, Shanske S, et al. Risk of developing a mitochondrial DNA deletion disorder. Lancet 2004; 364(9434):592–596.
67. Odoardi F, Rana M, Broccoiini A, et al. Pathogenic role of mtDNA duplications in mitochondrial diseases associated with mtDNA deletions. Am J Med Genet 2003; 118A(3):247–254.
68. Seneca S, Verhelst H, DeMeirleir L, et al. A new mitochondrial point mutation in the transfer RNA (Leu) gene in a patient with a clinical phenotype resembling Kearns-Sayne syndrome. Arch Neurol 2001; 58(7): 113–118.
69. Suzuki S, Hinokio Y, Ohtomo M, et al. The effects of coenzyme Q10 treatment on maternally inherited diabetes mellitus and deafness, and mitochondrial DNA 3243 (A to G) mutation. Diabetologia 1998; 41:584–588.
70. Berbel-Garcia A, Barbera-Farre JR, Etessam JP, et al. Coenzyme Q10 improves lactic acidosis, stroke-like episodes and epilepsy in a patient with MELAS. Ciin Neuropharmacol 2004; 27(4):187–191.
71. Komura K, Hobbiebrunken E, Wilichowski EK, Hanefeld FA. Effectiveness of creatine monohydrate in mitochondrial encephalomyopathies. Pediatr Neurol 2003; 28(1):53–58.
72. Kubota M, Sakakihana, Y, Mori M, et al. Beneficial effect of l-arginine for stroke-like episode in MELAS. Brain Dev 2004; 26(7):481–483.
73. Kolesnikova OA, Entelis NS, Jacquin-Becker C, et al. Nuclear DNA-encoded tRNAS targeted mitochondria can rescue a mitochondrial DNA mutation associated with the MERRF syndrome in cultured human cells. Hum Mol Genet 2004; 13(20):2519–2534.
74. Sorkin JA, Shoffner JM, Grossniklausht HE, et al. Strabismus and mitochondrial defects in chronic progressive, external ophthalmoplegia. Am J Ophthalmol 1997; 123:235–242.
75. Burnstine MA, Putterman AM. Upper blepharoplasty. A novel approach to improving myopathic blepharoptosis. Ophthalmology 1999; 106:2098–2110.
76. Rant V, Sinnathuray AR, Toner JG. Cochlear implantation in maternal inherited diabetes and deafness syndrome. J Laryngol Otol 2002; 116(5):373–375.
77. White SL, Collins VR, Wolfe R, et al. Genetic counseling and prenatal diagnosis for the mitochondrial DNA mutations at nucleotide 8993. Am Hum Genet 1999; 65(2):474–482.

78. Harding AE, Holt IJ, Sweeney MG, et al. Prenatal diagnosis of mitochondrial DNA (8993 T-G) disease. Am J Hum Genet 1992; 50:629–633.
79. Poulton J, Marchington DR. Segregation of mitochondrial DNA (mtDNA) in human oocytes and in animal models of mtDNA disease: clinical implications. Reproduction 2002; 123(6):751–756.
80. Chou YJ, Ou CY, HSU TY, et al. Prenatal diagnosis of a fetus harboring an intermediate load of the A3243G mtDNA mutation in a maternal carrier diagnosed with MELAS syndrome. Prenat Diagn 2004; 24(5):367–370.
81. Dahl HH, Thorburn DR, White SC. Towards reliable prenatal diagnosis of mtDNA mutations: studies of nt8993 mutation in oocytes, fetal tissues, children and adults. Hum Reprod 2000; 15(suppl 2):246–255.
82. Poulton J, Marchington DR. Progress in genetic counseling and prenatal diagnosis of maternally inherited mtDNA diseases. Neuromuscul Disord 2000; 10:484–487.

Index